CHEMICAL NEUROANATOMY

Chemical Neuroanatomy

Editor

P. C. Emson, Ph.D.

MRC Neurochemical Pharmacology Unit
Medical Research Council Centre
Cambridge, England

Raven Press ■ New York

Raven Press, 1140 Avenue of the Americas, New York, New York 10036

Made in the United States of America

Library of Congress Cataloging in Publication Data
Manin entry under title.

Chemical neuroanatomy.

Includes bibliographical references and index.
1. Neuroanatomy.   2. Neurochemistry.   I. Emson, P. C.
QM451.C56 1983   611′.8   83-9528
ISBN 0-89004-608-5

The material contained in this volume was submitted as previously unpublished material, except in the instances in which credit has been given to the source from which some of the illustrative material was derived.

Great care has been taken to maintain the accuracy of the information contained in the volume. However, Raven Press cannot be held responsible for errors or for any consequences arising from the use of the information contained herein.

Preface

In recent years, there has been a substantial increase in the number of techniques available for neuroanatomical studies. Some of these have represented improvements for mapping CNS pathways using methods for anterograde or retrograde labeling of neurons or their processes. However, along with these improved pathway-tracing techniques, methods have been developed to localize putative neurotransmitters (or their synthetic enzymes) to particular neurons. This type of study was pioneered by the development of catecholamine histofluorescence methods by Bengt Falck and Nils-Åke Hillarp and by the use of acetylcholinesterase staining (as a potential marker for cholinergic neurons) by Charles Shute and Peter Lewis.

Since these initial studies, the number of putative transmitter substances in the nervous system has increased dramatically with discovery of the neuronal localization of a number of neuroactive peptides including the enkephalins and substance P. In the case of the neuronally localized peptides, it is not at all clear if these compounds are neurotransmitters; however, the development of immunohistochemical techniques for peptide localization has provided neuroanatomists with a number of additional markers to characterize individual neurons and neuronal systems. A further complication that was not anticipated was that many of these neuronally localized peptides coexist in neurons known to contain better-established transmitter candidates, such as dopamine, γ-aminobutyric acid, acetylcholine, and 5-hydroxytryptamine. In nearly all of these cases, researchers have little idea of the physiological roles of the neuroactive peptides, although clues are gradually emerging.

This book attempts to superimpose what is currently known about the chemistry and distribution of putative transmitters and their receptors onto the basic organization of the mammalian nervous system. Apart from the intrinsic interest generated by this type of study, it is hoped that these efforts may encourage both the neurochemist to delve further into the organization of the mammalian brain (rather than a homogenate) and the neuroanatomist to use the antibodies and ligands developed by the neurochemist.

P. C. Emson
Cambridge, 1983

Acknowledgments

As with any task of this size, I am indebted to friends and colleagues who have read and criticized individual chapters. The secretarial assistance of Mrs. M. Wynn and Mrs. J. Ditheridge is gratefully acknowledged. Mr. G. Marshall provided help with the illustrations. Thanks are also due to Dr. D. Schneider and Ms. F. Gavin of Raven Press for their patience and tolerance during the preparation of this book.

Contents

Contributors

A. Björklund
Department of Histology
University of Lund
Biskopsgatan 5
S-223 62 Lund, Sweden

N. Brecha
Center for Ulcer Research and
*   Education*
Veterans Administration Center—
*   Wadsworth*
Los Angeles, California 90073; and
The Brain Research Institute, Jules
*   Stein Eye Institute, and Department*
*   of Medicine*
UCLA School of Medicine
Los Angeles, California 90024

B. J. Davis
Worcester Foundation for Experimental
*   Biology*
Shrewsbury, Massachusetts 01545

A. M. Graybiel
Department of Psychology and Brain
*   Science*
Massachusetts Institute of Technology
Cambridge, Massachusetts 02139

Y. Hara
Department of Neuroanatomy
Institute of Higher Nervous Activity
Osaka University Medical School
4-3-57 Nakanoshima, Kitaku
Osaka 530 Japan

S. P. Hunt
MRC Neurochemical Pharmacology
*   Unit*
Medical Research Council Centre
Hills Road
Cambridge CB2 2QH England

S. Inagaki
Department of Neuroanatomy
Institute of Higher Nervous Activity
Osaka University Medical School
4-3-57 Nakanoshima, Kitaku
Osaka 530 Japan

E. G. Jones
Department of Anatomy and
*   Neurobiology*
Washington University School of
*   Medicine*
St. Louis, Missouri 63110

Y. Kawai
Department of Neuroanatomy
Institute of Higher Nervous Activity
Osaka University Medical School
4-3-57 Nakanoshima, Kitaku
Osaka 530 Japan

O. Lindvall
Department of Neurology
University of Lund
Biskopsgatan 5
S-223 62 Lund, Sweden

J. K. McDonald
Department of Physiology
The University of Texas Health Science
*   Center*
Dallas, Texas 75235

F. Macrides
Worcester Foundation for Experimental
*   Biology*
Shrewsbury, Massachusetts 01545

R. Nieuwenhuys
Department of Anatomy and
*   Embryology*
University of Nijmegen
Geert Grooteplein N 21
6500 HB Nijmegen, The Netherlands

J. G. Parnavelas
Department of Cell Biology
The University of Texas Health Science
*   Center*
Dallas, Texas 75235

G. E. Pickard
Department of Anatomy
Columbia University
College of Physicians & Surgeons
New York, New York 10032

C. W. Ragsdale, Jr.
*Department of Psychology and Brain
  Science
Massachusetts Institute of Technology
Cambridge, Massachusetts 02139*

M. Sakanaka
*Department of Neuroanatomy
Institute of Higher Nervous Activity
Osaka University Medical School
4-3-57 Nakanoshima, Kitaku
Osaka 530 Japan*

J. A. Schulman
*MRC Neurochemical Pharmacology
  Unit
Medical Research Council Medical
  School
Hills Road
Cambridge CB2 2QH England*

M. Schultzberg
*Department of Histology
Karolinska Institute
Stockholm, Sweden*

E. Senba
*Department of Neuroanatomy
Institute of Higher Nervous Activity
Osaka University Medical School
4-3-57 Nakanoshima, Kitaku
Osaka 530 Japan*

S. Shiosaka
*Department of Neuroanatomy
Institute of Higher Nervous Activity
Osaka University Medical School
4-3-57 Nakanoshima, Kitaku
Osaka 530 Japan*

A.-J. Silverman
*Department of Anatomy
Columbia University
College of Physicians & Surgeons
New York, New York 10032*

H. W. M. Steinbusch
*Department of Pharmacology
Free University
Van der Boechorststraat 7
1081 BT Amsterdam, The Netherlands*

H. Takagi
*Department of Neuroanatomy
Institute of Higher Nervous Activity
Osaka University Medical School
4-3-57 Nakanoshima, Kitaku
Osaka 530 Japan*

K. Takatsuki
*Department of Neuroanatomy
Institute of Higher Nervous Activity
Osaka University Medical School
4-3-57 Nakanoshima, Kitaku
Osaka 530 Japan*

M. Tohyama
*Department of Neuroanatomy
Institute of Higher Nervous Activity
Osaka University Medical School
4-3-57 Nakanoshima, Kitaku
Osaka 530 Japan*

I. Walaas
*Department of Pharmacology
Yale University School of Medicine
New Haven, Connecticut 06510*

CHEMICAL NEUROANATOMY

Chemical Neuroanatomy, edited by P. C. Emson,
Raven Press, New York © 1983.

The Peripheral Nervous System

Marianne Schultzberg

Department of Histology, Karolinska Institutet, Stockholm, Sweden

The idea that acetylcholine (ACh) and norepinephrine (NE) are the transmitters in the peripheral nervous system is well established and has been reviewed in detail (56,93,140,151,241). However, pharmacological and morphological studies have provided evidence for peripheral neurotransmitters other than ACh and NE. The evidence for peripheral noncholinergic and nonadrenergic transmitters has in the past been critically evaluated by Burnstock (50) and others (57), and the idea that there might be an extensive system of peripheral neurons using a purine nucleotide as transmitter has been proposed (50,54).

Furthermore, in the last 10 years, the possibility that small biologically active peptides might function as transmitters in both the central and peripheral nervous system has received considerable attention. Some of the peptides now known to occur in peripheral neurons were originally discovered in gastrointestinal endocrine cells and were therefore first thought of as gut hormones. Conversely, other peripheral neuropeptides initially discovered in the brain have since been shown to occur also in gut endocrine cells. The identification, characterization, and localization of these substances have been greatly facilitated by the development of immunochemical methods of analysis, notably radioimmunoassay (RIA), for the measurement of small quantities of peptides in tissue extracts and immunohistochemical techniques for the localization of peptides in tissue sections. There have been a number of excellent reviews of adrenergic, cholinergic, purinergic, and 5-hydroxytryptaminergic neurons at the periphery (49,57,59,78,140,151, 224,225,341,342). This chapter therefore considers in detail the evidence for the identity and distribution of other putative peripheral transmitters, notably neuropeptides. Particular attention is given to the gastrointestinal tract, sympathetic ganglia (especially the prevertebral ganglia), and the adrenal gland, since these systems have been intensively studied and are known to have extensive peptidergic innervation.

GENERAL ORGANIZATION OF THE PERIPHERAL NERVOUS SYSTEM

Modern views on the organization of the peripheral nervous system are largely derived from Langley's classification of somatic and autonomic divisions (263). In reviewing earlier work on the peripheral nervous system, he further divided the autonomic nervous system into sympathetic and parasympathetic parts (157,263). The basic pattern of organization of sympathetic and parasympathetic divisions is well established. Preganglionic sympathetic neurons are located in the lateral horn of the spinal cord at the thoracolumbar level (T1–L3). The majority of these neurons make connections in the paravertebral ganglia of the sympathetic chain or in prevertebral ganglia. The postganglionic neurons, in turn, project to their target tissues.

Preganglionic parasympathetic nerves have either a cranial or a sacral origin. Thus, the cranial part consists of preganglionic neurons in the midbrain and hindbrain, which terminate in ganglia close to or within the target organs in the head and neck region and in the thoracic viscera, as well as in the gastrointestinal tract. The sacral part consists of preganglionic neurons in the lateral horn of the sacral spinal cord (S2–S4), which terminate in the large intestine and the urogenital tract, where the postganglionic neurons are located.

The innervation of the gastrointestinal tract can therefore be said to consist of (a) extrinsic nerves from sympathetic, mainly prevertebral, ganglia, (b) parasympathetic nerves of both cranial and sacral origin, and (c) sensory neurons terminating in the gastrointestinal tract and running in sympathetic and parasympathetic trunks. However, many aspects of gut function continue virtually unimpaired when the extrinsic nerve supply has been interrupted (26). On the basis of this evidence, Langley (263) suggested that the intrinsic gut neurons were best considered as a separate system—the enteric nervous system. Classically, ACh is regarded as the transmitter in the postganglionic parasympathetic neurons of the gut as well as other peripheral organs, whereas the postganglionic sympathetic neurons utilize NE. The identity of the transmitter(s) in sensory neurons has long remained unknown, although lately a peptide, substance P, has been suggested as a possible candidate.

Several lines of evidence have suggested that there are many other types of neurons in the gut and other parts of the peripheral nervous system in addition to the cholinergic and noradrenergic neurons. Pharmacological evidence indicates the existence of neurons that on stimulation cause atropine-resistant contractions of intestinal smooth muscle (15–17,39) and therefore presumably contain an excitatory transmitter other than ACh. There is also clear evidence for noncholinergic, nonadrenergic inhibitory neurons (29,30,52,53, 311). In the cat stomach, stimulation of the vagus in the presence of atropine caused inhibitory responses that were not blocked by adrenergic blocking agents (311). In the guinea pig tenia coli, inhibitory junction potentials were produced by stimulation of intramural nerves. Neither atropine nor guanethidine blocked these inhibitory responses (52). There are several physiological events in which the enteric inhibitory neurons have been demonstrated to play a role. Generally, these neurons are involved in inhibitory reflexes, such as the facilitation of passage of material through the alimentary canal. For instance, receptive relaxation of the stomach (1–4,22,61,347,348), the descending inhibition reflex in the intestine (26,55,139,141,198), and the reflex relaxation of the internal anal sphincter (76,156) are likely to be mediated by enteric inhibitory neurons outside of the gastrointestinal tract.

Nonadrenergic inhibitory neurons have been thought to mediate such functions as bronchodilatation (443) and relaxation of lung musculature (366) and vasodilatation in several tissues (34,51,178,218,346).

Ultrastructural studies have suggested the existence of several types of noncholinergic, nonadrenergic neurons. For instance, Baumgarten and coworkers (25) observed three different types of nerves in the gastrointestinal tract; besides cholinergic and noradrenergic nerve profiles, they found nerve terminals containing large vesicles. These fibers were named "p-type fibers" because of their similarity to the peptide-containing neurons in the hypothalamus (110). The work of Gabella (150) and Cook and Burnstock (71) revealed an even more complex picture; at least eight different types of nerve terminal profiles could be differentiated (see Fig. 1).

In addition, extracts of gut wall have been shown to possess numerous biological properties that are not attributable to ACh or NE and that could well be caused by other neuroregulatory substances. An early example is substance P, which was originally described as an active factor in extracts of equine intestine and brain that caused atropine-resistant contractions of the rabbit ileum (439).

In the last few years, numerous other examples of putative transmitters have come to light. An account of the evidence for these substances as putative transmitters as well as their histochemical distribution with correlation to functional aspects is given below. (For reviews on the general organization of the peripheral nervous system, see refs. 56,59,60,140,151,152,157,192,261,263,319,384.)

METHODOLOGY

Pharmacological and physiological studies of the nervous system have been greatly advanced by the development of histochemical techniques that made it possible to identify the cellular origin of biologically active substances that seemed likely to function as neurotransmitters. Thus, the Falck–Hillarp fluorescence technique (131,132) proved to

FIG. 1. Electron micrographs of nerve endings in the guinea pig intestine. **A:** Axon profile containing small granular vesicles in which the electron-dense material is located peripherally. ×44,500. **B:** Axon profile containing mostly small agranular vesicles and some larger granular vesicles. ×22,800. **C:** Axon profile containing small round and flattened agranular vesicles and a distinct, large granular vesicle. ×37,600. **D:** Axon profile containing round and flattened agranular vesicles and some elongated vesicles. ×17,400. **E:** Axon profile containing numerous elongate vesicles. × 27,300. **F:** Axon profile containing irregularly shaped dense-cored granular vesicles up to 95 nm in diameter. ×24,300. **G:** Axon profile containing homogeneous round dense-cored vesicles, 50 to 95 nm in diameter. ×18,600. **H:** Axon profile containing large vesicles, up to 115 nm in diameter, with granular cores of variable density. ×28,800. (From Cook and Burnstock, ref. 71, with permission.)

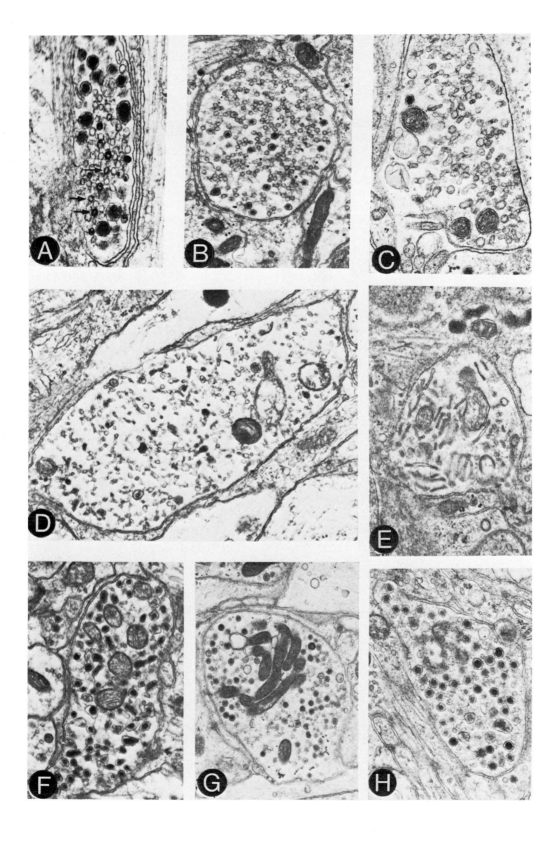

be an invaluable tool both for mapping catechol-amine-containing neurons and for functional studies of these neurons. The technique involves the use of formaldehyde, which induces conversion of catecholamines into compounds that fluoresce on illumination with ultraviolet light. Thus, the demonstration of noradrenergic nerve terminals in the enteric plexuses (224,341) (Fig. 2) led to the view that the inhibitory action of NE could be indirect, i.e., mediated by enteric neurons.

The localization of ACh has proved to be more difficult, but a histochemical method that localizes the ACh-degrading enzyme acetylcholinesterase (AChE) can be used, provided the conditions are carefully controlled. There are several reasons for interpreting the results obtained by this method with caution (395). First, AChE activity has a widespread distribution. Although there seems to be a good correlation between ACh content, choline acetyltransferase activity, and AChE content (49,167,182,281), there are several examples of the localization of AChE where there is no evi-

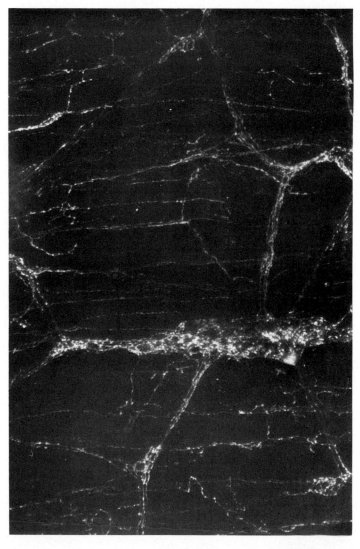

FIG. 2. Fluorescence micrograph of whole-mount preparation of longitudinal muscle and myenteric plexus from rat small intestine processed for catecholamines by the Falck–Hillarp technique. A dense network of varicose noradrenergic nerve fibers can be seen in the myenteric plexus. Fluorescent fibers also run in the interconnecting nerve strands. ×160 (Courtesy of Dr. Lars Olson, Dept. of Histology, Karolinska Institutet, Stockholm.)

dence for cholinergic nerves; for instance, AChE staining has been observed in adrenergic neurons in the rat (119,226) and in sensory neurons of rat and guinea pig (181,383). Second, there exist other cholinesterases that are unrelated to cholinergic neurons, such as butyrylcholinesterase. However, this problem can be overcome by using inhibitors for nonspecific cholinesterases. Recently, antibodies to choline acetyltransferase have been used in immunohistochemical studies, providing a more specific technique for identification of cholinergic neurons (87).

In some cases, the localization of substances in neuronal structures can be achieved by autoradiographic methods (5–7,296,310,451,452). These methods have commonly been used for the localization of 5-hydroxytryptamine (5-HT) in enteric neurons (109,162,163). The technique obviously demonstrates the capacity of a neuron to take up radiolabeled substance but does not prove that the neuron normally possesses the enzymes for its synthesis (see below). The details of the above-mentioned techniques have been extensively reviewed elsewhere (see, e.g., 59,131,132,395) and are not further discussed here.

In the last 20 years, immunochemical methods have come into wide usage and have been of special importance in localizing small peptides. Antibodies may be readily obtained by immunization of rabbits, sheep, goats, guinea pigs, or mice with peptides coupled to larger proteins, such as bovine albumin (BSA) (170). The antisera may be used in radioimmunoassay (RIA), for quantitative measurements in tissue extracts (453), and in immunohistochemistry (73,333,403). These methods offer many advantages, notably, sensitivity in detecting small amounts of the peptide; however, they are not without problems. The antigen–antibody reaction is generally highly specific, but particular care in interpretation needs to be applied, and it is seldom possible to conclude that the substance present in the tissue and reacting with the antibody actually corresponds to the antigen without careful controls.

In the case of peptides, a sequence of four to seven amino acids generally makes up the antigenic determinant. Therefore, peptides with related sequences may cross react with the same antibodies. For example, gastrin and cholecystokinin (CCK), which have a common COOH-terminal pentapeptide, both react with antibodies that are directed to the COOH terminus (102,362). It is possible to differentiate between the two peptides by using region-specific antibodies, i.e., antibodies that are raised to different parts of the molecules

(102,362). However, it is not possible to exclude the existence in the tissue of unknown molecules that may give rise to an immunoreaction. In addition, biologically active peptides are generally synthesized from larger precursors, which may be processed to several different peptides having different biological properties. Thus, caution is needed when dealing with different forms or fragments of a substance. In view of the uncertainty as to the exact nature of the substance responsible for the immunoreaction, such terms as substance P-like immunoreactivity, substance P immunoreactive, and so on, are used. Moreover, it is usually desirable to use different antisera to correlate RIA and immunohistochemistry as far as possible.

In immunohistochemistry, so-called control sera are used to check that the immunoreaction is specific for the antigen. A control serum consists of the specific antiserum, which has been preabsorbed with the antigen in order to block the specific immunoreaction. Any immunoreaction that is observed with a control serum is therefore regarded as nonspecific staining. Preabsorption of the specific antiserum with other substances, preferably in different concentrations, is a common way to investigate whether or not the antiserum cross reacts with substances other than the antigen. Desirably, decrease or inhibition of the immunoreaction is only obtained with the specific antigen.

Another problem concerns negative findings. Thus, lack of immunoreactivity may of course be due to absence of the antigen in the tissue or loss of the antigen from the tissue during the processing of the tissue; poor fixation may result in diffusion of the antigen. However, negative finding may also result from loss of immunoreactivity of the antigen, possibly caused by the fixation procedure. Finally, the levels of antigen in the tissue may be too low for detection, as is often the case for neuropeptides in axons and nerve cell bodies. This problem may be overcome by different experimental procedures. Thus, application of an inhibitor of axonal transport, such as colchicine, has been used to increase the cell body levels of amines (91,92,200,257) and can also be used to increase levels of peptides in nerve cell bodies and axons (24,207). In addition, ligation of nerves results in accumulation of axonally transported amines and peptides at the ligation site (43,90,154,303).

TRANSMITTERS

The history and properties of ACh and NE as neurotransmitters in the peripheral nervous system have been extensively reviewed in the past (see, e.g., 56,59,60,140,151,224,225,319,343). There-fore, the following section concentrates on the new-comers in this area, i.e., small biologically active peptides in particular, and briefly considers other substances such as 5-HT, dopamine, ATP, and GABA.

Substance P

Substance P was discovered in 1931 by von Euler and Gaddum as they were studying the dis-tribution of ACh (439). Their control was addition of atropine, and they found that ethanol extracts of equine intestine and brain caused contractions, which were atropine resistant, of smooth muscle from the isolated rabbit jejunum. It was not until 1970 that substance P was obtained in pure form and characterized as an undecapeptide (from bo-vine hypothalamus) (66), although its peptide na-ture had been suspected earlier (438,439). Chang et al. (67) determined the amino acid sequence of substance P and synthesized the peptide. Studer et al. (405) isolated substance P from equine intes-tine. Substance P is structurally related to a variety of peptides that have been isolated from frog skin and other tissues (122). The best known of the sub-stance P-related peptides are physalemin (120) and eledoisin (121), isolated from octopus salivary gland. Both peptides share the COOH-terminal se-quence Gly-Leu-Met-NH$_2$ which determines the biological activity of substance P. The COOH-ter-minal octapeptide is about half as active as the un-decapeptide in contracting guinea pig ileum (454). Physalemin and eledoisin have similar biological properties to substance P, e.g., vasodilatation and contraction of intestinal smooth muscle (120–122). Among another group of peptides isolated from amphibian skin, bombesin (124) has the same COOH-terminal dipeptide as substance P but shows rather different biological activities (see sec-tion on bombesin below).

The distribution of substance P was first studied by Pernow (354) who used a bioassay on guinea pig ileum or rabbit jejunum. At present, the distribu-tion of substance P is studied to a large extent by RIA and immunohistochemistry. Most substance P antibodies are directed to the COOH terminus, and cross reactivity to physalemin varies from less than 0.1% to 5%, and that to eledoisin between 0.01% and 0.03% (338). Lee et al. (277) have de-veloped an NH$_2$-terminal-directed antiserum that cross reacts less than 0.01% with physalemin and eledoisin. Cuello et al. (89) have produced a mono-clonal antibody to substance P that cross reacts less than 0.01% with eledoisin.

The initial study of the distribution of substance P showed that, in addition to the high concentra-tions in intestine and brain, the dorsal horn of the spinal cord contained large quantities, whereas only small amounts were found in the ventral horn (338). The same results have since been obtained by RIA (413), and immunohistochemical studies have shown that substance P-like material is pres-ent in numerous nerve terminals in the outer layers of the dorsal horn as well as in small-diameter cell bodies in spinal ganglia (209,210). Dorsal rhizo-tomy results in decreased concentrations of sub-stance P in the dorsal spinal cord as determined biochemically (413), and immunohistochemical studies demonstrate a marked decrease of the number of substance P-immunoreactive nerve ter-minals in the dorsal horn (209).

Both sets of findings indicate that the substance P-immunoreactive nerve terminals in the dorsal horn originate in cell bodies in the spinal ganglia. Lembeck (279) suggested that substance P may be an excitatory transmitter in primary sensory neu-rons. Both electrophysiological (250) and biochem-ical (179,412) data, in addition to the morpholog-ical data, support the view that substance P plays a role in the transmission of sensory impulses.

Vasoactive Intestinal Polypeptide

Vasoactive intestinal polypeptide (VIP) was iso-lated from porcine duodenum by Said and Mutt (376,377) and was characterized as a linear pep-tide of 28 amino acid residues (331). It is structur-ally related to secretin, glucagon, gastric inhibitory peptide (GIP), and a newly isolated peptide from porcine intestine, PHI (414,415). As the name im-plies, VIP is a potent vasodilator (376), but it also has a wide variety of other properties, e.g., relax-ation of smooth muscle in gut and respiratory tract, and stimulation of bicarbonate and water secretion from the exocrine pancreas (39,127,376). The lat-ter property is shared with secretin, which is more potent than VIP in the human (107) but less potent in the turkey (97); PHI has been shown to have similar potency to VIP in the turkey pancreas (99).

Vasoactive intestinal polypeptide has been mea-sured in tissue extracts by radioreceptor assay (33) as well as by RIA (96,153,378; see 127). Although the peptides mentioned above have biological ac-tions similar to VIP and are structurally related, they have quite different immunochemical proper-ties. In RIA, the cross reactivity of these peptides with some VIP antibodies is less than 0.005% (100). The nature of VIP in different species seems to vary slightly; chicken VIP (337) differs from porcine VIP in four amino acid residues. Studies with region-specific antibodies have shown that the human and rat intestines contain several different molecular forms of VIP, of which one corresponds to porcine VIP and the others are less basic molecules (96,98,100). At least in the rat, these different forms are found only in the muscular coat, presumably in the nerves (98,100). However, in human colon, a single form corresponding to authentic VIP is present in the muscle layers, including the myenteric plexus (96).

Vasoactive intestinal polypeptide meets many of the criteria for being a neurotransmitter (127,129,374). Thus, it has been localized in neurons (47,149; see 127,374) and shown to be present in the synaptic vesicle fraction of nerve terminals (165). Several studies have shown the release of VIP on nerve stimulation, and the effect of exogenously applied peptide mimics the response of nerve stimulation (128,129,380). It has been suggested that VIP may be the transmitter in noncholinergic, nonadrenergic inhibitory neurons in the gut (129,171; see also section on distribution below).

Enkephalins

The first isolation of an endogenous ligand for the opiate receptor (417,418; see 255) was made by Hughes and collaborators (217). They isolated from porcine brain two pentapeptides with opioid activity, i.e., analgesic activity and inhibition of electrically induced contractions of guinea pig ileum and mouse vas deferens in a naloxone-reversible fashion. The amino acid sequence of the two peptides differs only in the COOH-terminal amino acid, which is either methionine (met) or leucine (leu), hence the names met- and leu-enkephalin (216,217). It is possible to distinguish between met- and leu-enkephalin in bioassay by the oxidative destruction of met-enkephalin by cyanogen bromide (158,397) or by using region-specific antibodies in RIA (396).

Most of the enkephalin antibodies currently used in immunohistochemical studies, which may have been raised to met- or leu-enkephalin, give a positive immunoreaction with both peptides. Even when the cross reactivity is less than 1% as measured by RIA, the immunoreaction to nerve fibers with a met-enkephalin antiserum may be partially blocked by preabsorption of the antiserum with leu-enkephalin (390). Larsson et al. (265) have employed an elegant technique to overcome this problem. They examined the immunochemical properties of met- and leu-enkephalin antisera by incubating them with Sepharose beads that were previously coated with met- and leu-enkephalin, respectively. They found that their met-enkephalin

antisera contained two populations of antibodies, one specific for met-enkephalin and one that reacted with both met- and leu-enkephalin. Preabsorption of these antisera with leu-enkephalin abolished staining of leu-enkephalin-coated beads, and the antisera could therefore be used for staining met-enkephalin-containing structures. Pretreatment with cyanogen bromide or an oxidizing agent, such as acidic potassium permanganate, abolished the staining of met-enkephalin-coated beads. Therefore, a leu-enkephalin antiserum that cross reacts with met-enkephalin can be used for specific staining of leu-enkephalin provided the tissue is pretreated so that the met-enkephalin is oxidized. It was in this way possible to demonstrate separate met- and leu-enkephalin neurons both in brain and gut (265).

Met-enkephalin corresponds to NH_2-terminal pentapeptide of β-endorphin, another peptide with opioid activity, originally isolated from porcine, camel, and human pituitary in 1976 (40,287,288). Beta-endorphin in itself is the 31-amino-acid C-terminal fragment of β-lipotrophin (β-LPH), a 91-amino-acid peptide that was isolated in 1965 by Li and co-workers (285). The function of β-LPH was unknown at the time, but it now seems probable that it is the biosynthetic precursor of β-endorphin and β-melanocyte-stimulating hormone (β-MSH).

A large 31,000-dalton glycoprotein (pro-opiomelanocortin) gives rise to β-LPH and adrenocorticotrophic hormone (ACTH) (306,365). However, immunohistochemical studies with specific antibodies show that β-endorphin- and met-enkephalin-containing neurons have a quite different distribution (35), so that β-endorphin is unlikely to be a biosynthetic precursor for met-enkephalin. Recently, an increasingly impressive body of evidence for other enkephalin precursor molecules has emerged. In large part, this evidence has been obtained from peptides isolated from adrenal glands, where enkephalin-like immunoreactivity was first detected in immunohistochemical studies by Schultzberg et al. (387,391). In addition to met- and leu-enkephalin (95), large amounts of hexapeptides, heptapeptides, and larger forms of 14,000 and 21,000 daltons have since been isolated from the adrenal gland (Table 1). It is likely that opiate peptide variants also occur in the brain. Thus, an octapeptide containing leu-enkephalin with a COOH-terminal extension has been isolated from porcine hypothalamus (318). The sequence is contained within the N terminus of dynorphin, which has been isolated from pituitary and partially sequenced (168). Another leu-enkephalin-related peptide, also isolated from porcine hypothalamus (238), is α-neoendorphin, which is a pentadecapep-

TABLE 1. *Naturally occurring enkephalins (ENK) and related peptides that have been isolated and characterized*

Peptide	Source	Reference
Tyr-Gly-Gly-Phe-Met (met-ENK)	Porcine brain	217
Tyr-Gly-Gly-Phe-Met (0)-Arg	Porcine hypothalamus	215
Tyr-Gly-Gly-Phe-Met-Arg-Phe	Bovine adrenal medulla, striatum	402
Tyr-Gly-Gly-Phe-Met-Lys	Bovine adrenal medulla	282
Tyr-Gly-Gly-Phe-Met-Arg-Arg	Bovine adrenal medulla	282
Tyr-Gly-Gly-Phe-Met-Arg-Arg-Val-Gly-Arg-Pro-Glu	Bovine adrenal medulla	320
8,000-Dalton peptide with COOH-terminal met-ENK	Bovine adrenal medulla	283
14,000-Dalton peptide containing 3 met-ENK	Bovine adrenal medulla	283
34-Amino-acid peptide containing 2 met-ENK	Bovine adrenal medulla	236,244
39-Amino-acid peptide containing 1 met-ENK and 1 leu-ENK	Bovine adrenal medulla	236,244
50,000-Dalton peptide containing 6 or 7 met-ENK and 1 leu-ENK	Bovine adrenal medulla	282
Tyr-Gly-Gly-Phe-Leu (leu-ENK)	Porcine brain	217
Tyr-Gly-Gly-Phe-Leu-Arg-Arg-Ile-Arg-Pro-Lys-Leu-Lys-OH [Dynorphin (1–13)][a]	Porcine pituitary	168
Tyr-Gly-Gly-Phe-Leu-Arg-Lys-Arg-Pro-($Gly_1Tyr_2Lys_2Arg_1$) (α-neoendorphin)	Porcine hypothalamus	238
Tyr-Gly-Gly-Phe-Leu-Arg-Arg-Ile	Porcine hypothalamus	318

[a] Recent work using cloning and sequence analysis of cDNA has shown that the dynorphin/α-neoendorphin precursor contains dynorphin 1–17 (Tyr-Gly-Gly-Phe-Leu-Arg-Arg-Ile-Arg-Pro-Lys-Leu-Lys_5-Trp-Asp-Asn-Gln), rimorphin/dynorphin B (Tyr-Gly-Gly-Phe-Leu-Arg-Arg-Gln-Phe-Lys-Val-Val-Thr) as well as a α-neoendorphin (237a).

tide. From bovine adrenal medulla, two larger peptides of 34 and 39 amino acids, respectively, have been purified and sequenced (236,244). The triakontatetrapeptide contains two met-enkephalins, one at each end. The larger peptide has a met-enkephalin sequence in the middle and a leu-enkephalin sequence at the COOH terminus. More recently, a dodecapeptide which is contained within the latter peptide was isolated from bovine adrenal medulla (320). The occurrence of a large 50,000-dalton protein in bovine adrenal medulla has been demonstrated by Lewis et al. (282). Trypsinization and treatment with carboxypeptidase B provided evidence for the occurrence of six or seven met-enkephalins and one leu-enkephalin within the protein. Most likely, the large forms are biosynthetic precursors for enkephalins and enkephalin-related peptides, which are produced by the action of processing enzymes (373). Possibly a similar arrangement is true for the central nervous system. The functional significance of a precursor with a repetitive sequence is unclear, but this explains the ratio of met- and leu-enkephalin measured previously (172,186).

Somatostatin

Somatostatin was isolated and purified from bovine hypothalamus by Brazeau et al. (42). Sequence analysis revealed a tetradecapeptide with a disulfide bond between the cysteines in positions 3 and 14. Pradayrol et al. (358) isolated from porcine duodenum a peptide (somatostatin-28) that includes the somatostatin sequence in the COOH terminus. A peptide with the same sequence was recently isolated from ovine hypothalamus, in addition to a smaller peptide that comprised 25 of the amino acid residues in somatostatin-28 (41). Somatostatin occurs in large amounts in the brain and in the gastrointestinal tract, including the pancreas (21a,41,42,201,202). A significant proportion of somatostatin in the gut is present in endocrine cells (201; see 36), especially in the upper part of the tract. These cells have been identified as D cells (357); D cells in the pancreas also contain somatostatin (357). Somatostatin is known to have a number of inhibiting actions. It was originally isolated by Krulich et al. (258) as a factor inhibiting the release of growth hormone, but it is also a potent inhibitor of the release of insulin (8) and glucagon (159) from the pancreas and of gastrin and gastric acid secretion from the stomach (23,169), suggesting that it plays an important part in the regulation of these hormones.

Cholecystokinin

In 1928, a hormonal mechanism for intestinal control of gallbladder contraction was demonstrated by Ivy and Goldberg (223). They named the hormone cholecystokinin (CCK). From hog duodenum they prepared a secretin-free extract that caused contraction of the gall bladder. Fifteen years later, Harper and Raper (180) demonstrated an intestinal extract of duodenal mucosa that stimulated pancreatic enzyme secretion; they named the active principle pancreozymin. Not until 1966 was the identity of these two substances proven, when Mutt and Jorpes determined the sequence of a 33-residue peptide with both properties isolated from porcine duodenal mucosa (329). It is therefore known as cholecystokinin–pancreozymin, although the latter part of the name is now usually omitted. A 39-residue form of CCK ("CCK variant") consisting of CCK-33 and an NH_2-terminal extension has also been isolated from the same source and sequenced. Other smaller forms have also been isolated. Thus, a CCK octapeptide (CCK-8) and a closely related, slightly less acidic form have been isolated and sequenced from sheep brain (103). In addition, results from RIA measurements suggest that CCK-8 also predominates in the smooth muscle–myenteric plexus preparation of guinea pig intestine (220). Rehfeld and co-workers have suggested that the COOH-terminal tetrapeptide occurs in large amounts in the brain and gut (272,363); however, this matter is under debate, as others have failed to identify this molecular form.

The COOH-terminal pentapeptide of CCK is shared with gastrin—another classical gut hormone. Gastrin was isolated from porcine antrum by Gregory and Tracy (174,175). Including the tetrapeptide, there are at least five different forms of gastrin (270,271,361,363,365), most of which probably mainly occur in endocrine cells in the gut. It has also been reported that gastrin-like immunoreactivity occurs in the vagus nerve of dogs and cats (429). Dockray et al. (104) showed in a study of a large number of dogs and cats that G-17 occurred in the vagus nerve of relatively few animals, whereas CCK-8 appeared to be the main representative of this group of peptides. By ligation and nerve section, it was possible to establish that in the cat, CCK-8 was produced in cell bodies of nodose ganglion and transported toward the gut in afferent fibers (104). The functional significance of this remains to be shown.

Neurotensin

Carraway and Leeman first discovered neurotensin as a factor in hypothalamic extracts that caused vasodilatation and increased vascular permeability followed by cyanosis (63). It has been isolated and sequenced from bovine hypothalamus and small intestine (63–65). The biologically active region of neurotensin is localized in the COOH

terminus (45). A peptide extracted from frog skin, xenopsin (see 45), has a similar COOH-terminal sequence and has been shown to have similar biological actions. Immunochemical measurements of neurotensin show that about 10 times more activity is found in the gastrointestinal tract than in the brain. A large proportion of the neurotensin in the gut is localized in endocrine cells (48,136,184, 407), which are most numerous in the ileal mucosa. Ultrastructural studies suggest that neurotensin occurs in a distinct cell type (48). Neurotensin has a number of actions in the alimentary canal, such as inhibiting gastric acid secretion (21) and increasing plasma levels of glucagon and glucose (46,65,332). However, it has also been shown to induce contraction of intestinal smooth muscle (63).

Bombesin

Many of the small biologically active peptides that occur in the mammalian nervous and endocrine systems have counterparts that are found in high concentrations in amphibian skin. Erspamer and his co-workers have isolated and characterized numerous amphibian skin peptides (124,126). Among these are the ceruleins, which are closely related to mammalian cholecystokinins, and physalemin, related to substance P. In addition, it is now clear that the bombesin family of peptides from amphibian skin also has mammalian counterparts. The amphibian peptide bombesin is a molecule of 14 amino acid residues (19); its biological activity seems to reside in the COOH-terminal octapeptide, which is also common to several other amphibian peptides, e.g., litorin, ranatensin, and alytesin (19,20,44,315). Recently, McDonald et al. (313) isolated from porcine nonantral stomach a peptide of 27 amino acid residues that shows an identical sequence in nine of the 10 COOH-terminal amino acids. The mammalian bombesin-like peptide also has similar biological properties to the amphibian molecule. In extracts of guinea pig stomach and intestines, bombesin-like immunoreactivity seems to occur in two molecular forms, one that might represent the heptacosapeptide isolated from pig (313) and one smaller form (220). The two COOH-terminal amino acids of bombesin (14 and 27) are identical with the COOH-terminal dipeptide of substance P. Many antibodies to substance P and bombesin are directed to the COOH terminus of these peptides and may show cross reactivity.

Bombesin has a wide range of biological actions. It causes an increase in blood pressure; stimulates smooth muscle contraction; stimulates secretion of gastric acid, gastrin, and CCK; stimulates pancreatic secretion; and lowers body temperature (31,32,46,62,123,316).

Other Peptides

In addition to the peptides already discussed, there may be other as yet undiscovered peptides occurring in the peripheral nervous system. Furthermore, there are some peptides occurring in the endocrine cells of gut and pancreas, such as insulin, glucagon, bradykinin, and secretin, which have been demonstrated by immunohistochemistry to occur in the brain (74,181,295,330,411) and which may well occur in peripheral nerves too, but in very small amounts, since they have not been detected so far. There is, however, suggestive evidence for a few additional peptides in the peripheral nervous system. Angiotensin II-like immunoreactivity occurs in both central and peripheral neurons (148,155). One of the most recent peptides to be found in peripheral neurons appears to be a form of pancreatic polypeptide (PP). Kimmel and co-workers (242,243) isolated and sequenced avian pancreatic polypeptide (APP) from chicken pancreas. Human (HPP) and bovine (BPP) homologs have also been isolated (288), as well as the ovine (OPP), porcine (PPP), and canine (CPP) peptides. There are only minor differences in the sequence of the mammalian peptides, but the avian peptide differs in more than half ot the 36 amino acid residues.

Although APP does not cross react in a RIA using an antibody raised to HPP or BPP, antibodies to APP give a positive immunoreaction with neuronal and endocrine structures in mammalian species (see below). The identity of the peptide that is recognized by the APP antibodies has recently been clarified and it is now believed to be neuropeptide Y (413a).

Luteinizing hormone-releasing hormone (LHRH)-like immunoreactivity has until recently only been found in central neurons but has recently also been shown by immunohistochemistry to occur in sympathetic ganglia in the frog (228,229). The occurrence of another central neuropeptide, thyrotropin-releasing hormone (TRH), in tissue extracts of different parts of the gastrointestinal tract has been shown in RIA (280,328).

Other Putative Transmitters

Apart from neuropeptides, other types of substances have been localized in peripheral neurons. Thus, ATP or a related nucleotide has been proposed as a transmitter in the noncholinergic, non-adrenergic inhibitory neurons (50). The morphological evidence is based on the uptake of radiolabeled ATP or adenosine, which is converted to labeled ATP and was localized in nerves (50). A fluorescence histochemical method using quinacrine was developed by Olson and co-workers (14,349). Quinacrine has been shown to bind ATP (222). However, the relationship between quinacrine-binding structures and ATP is still not fully elucidated. Stimulation of the vagus nerve results in a release of adenosine and inosine, which are interpreted as the breakdown products of ATP. Both ATP and ADP cause a rapid hyperpolarization of smooth muscle that is unaffected by tetrodotoxin, suggesting a direct effect on the muscle cells (50,54).

Serotonin is known to be a transmitter in central neurons, and there is also considerable evidence for transmitter function in the gut (57,108,161,162; see also 78). Autoradiographic and immunohistochemical data show uptake of radiolabeled 5-HT into enteric neurons (109,160,163,368) and the occurrence of tryptophan hydroxylase in submucous and myenteric neurons (161). Serotonin has an excitatory action on gastrointestinal smooth muscle (449,450), and it is believed that 5-HT gives rise to slow excitatory postsynaptic potentials (449). However, it is difficult positively to identify 5-HT-containing neurons in the normal gut. Recently, the development of antibodies to 5-HT (401; and Steinbusch and Nieuwenhuys, *this volume*) has made possible a more direct localization of 5-HT in neurons.

GABA is also known to be a transmitter in the central nervous system. Recent autoradiographic studies have shown the uptake of radiolabeled GABA into gut neurons (231). The significance of this finding is still unclear but is compatible with a population of GABA-containing peripheral neurons.

Intrinsic amine-handling neurons are characterized by their content of aromatic amino acid decarboxylase and monoamine oxidase and their ability to take up and retain catecholamines and indoleamines (137,142). It seems, however, as though these neurons do not in fact synthesize catecholamines, since tyrosine hydroxylase (TH) and dopamine β-hydroxylase (DBH) cannot be detected in extrinsically denervated intestine (146). Enteric noradrenergic cell bodies have been described to occur almost exclusively in guinea pig colon (138). Some cell bodies reacting with DBH antiserum were, however, observed in guinea pig stomach and rat esophagus and colon (388). It is, however, possible that the DBH antiserum cross reacts with an unknown molecule not related to noradrenergic neurons. Grzanna and Coyle (176) showed DBH-like immunoreactivity in almost all of the ganglion cells in the rat submandibular ganglion, which does not contain NE. The relationships among the amine-handling neurons, the DBH-immunoreactive neurons, and the tryptophan hydroxylase-containing neurons are still uncertain, but it is possible that the latter neurons may belong to the same population as the amine-handling neurons. The development of antibodies to 5-HT (401; and Steinbusch and Nieuwenhuys, *this volume*) and NE and epinephrine (434) may help to resolve this question.

Dopamine is another neurotransmitter in the central nervous system. Hirst and Silinsky (199) have suggested that it is the transmitter in inhibitory interneurons in the gut, but it has not been demonstrated in enteric neurons so far. However, it is believed that dopamine is the transmitter in the well-known small intensively fluorescent cells (SIF cells) (118) in the carotid body and sympathetic ganglia (see 86,118).

DISTRIBUTION

Gastrointestinal Tract

In the following section, the distribution of putative neurotransmitters in the gut neurons is discussed. An attempt is made to relate the distribution to the biological actions of the substances in order to provide a basis for understanding possible physiological roles. It is now known that many active peptides of the gut have a dual localization, in neurons and endocrine cells. Thus, the biological actions of exogenously administered peptides may reflect either the responses of target organs normally receiving a blood-borne stimulus or a response normally evoked by locally released peptides from nerve terminals. Obviously, therefore, considerable caution needs to be applied in interpreting the significance of the biological actions of exogenously administered peptides. The organization and distribution of the enteric nerves and the nervous control of gastrointestinal functions have been reviewed in detail previously (22,56, 60,140,145,150–152,192,224,254,261,319,341, 384).

Substance P

The gastrointestinal tract is densely innervated by substance P-immunoreactive neurons as shown by immunohistochemistry (75,134,232,233,276,

309,339,352,386,388,408). Several lines of evidence indicate that the majority of substance P-immunoreactive fibers in the gut are of intrinsic origin. Thus, substance P-containing nerve cell bodies in the gut were demonstrated (a) by *in vivo* localization in untreated and colchicine- or vinblastine-treated animals (145,388); studies on tissue sections and whole mount preparations gave a similar answer (145,388); (b) by *in vitro* studies of organotypic tissue cultures (386); mouse small intestine was cultured for 3 weeks in which time the extrinsic nerves degenerated; and (c) by *in oculo* studies of intestinal tissue (389). Different regions of intestine from fetal and adult rats were transplanted to the anterior chamber of the rat eye and subjected to immunohistochemical staining. In the latter experimental model, ingrowth of fibers from the host iris is possible but can be prevented by denervation of the iris at the time of implantation. However, a small number of substance P-immunoreactive fibers in the gut may be of extrinsic origin, since ligation of the mesenteric nerves results in an accumulation of immunoreactive material on the central side, suggesting that substance P is being transported towards the gut.

Denervation of the guinea pig ileum indicates that the extrinsic nerves are related mainly to small arteries in the submucosa (75). The number of substance P-immunoreactive neurons in the enteric plexuses of the rat and guinea pig is generally 2% to 5% of the total number of cell bodies in the submucous plexus and about 10% to 15% of those in the myenteric plexus, as determined from immunohistochemical examination of colchicine- or vinblastine-treated animals (388; see also 145). Immunohistochemical studies reveal a fairly even distribution of substance P-immunoreactive fibers along the digestive tract of rat and guinea pig. Substance P-immunoreactive fibers occur in all layers of the gastrointestinal wall (Fig. 3A). Different types of lesion experiments on the guinea pig small intestine showed that there are a number of well-defined projections of neurons containing substance P-like immunoreactivity (81). However, the stomach seems to be somewhat less well innervated than the intestines; the estimation of substance P by bioassay and RIA shows a similar differentiated distribution (339,354).

Franco et al. (134) have shown that substance P is released on electrical stimulation from enteric nerves. The distribution of substance P-containing nerve fibers in the gut provides a basis for understanding the physiological significance of the biological actions of substance P. Although substance P is also present in endocrine cells, the largest

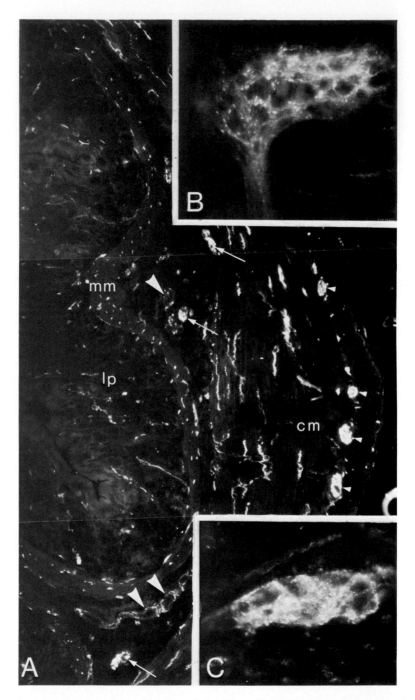

FIG. 3. Immunofluorescence micrographs of sections of the guinea pig rectum (**A**) and proximal colon (**C**) and rat colon (**B**) after incubation with substance P antiserum. **A**: Numerous substance P-immunoreactive nerve fibers can be seen in the inner circular smooth muscle layer (cm), the submucous *(small arrows)* and myenteric *(small arrowheads)* plexus, and the lamina muscularis mucosae (mm). Substance P-immunoreactive fibers surround some blood vessels *(large arrowheads)* in the submucosa, and some fibers can be seen in the lamina propria (lp) between the glands. × 160. **B, C**: A network of substance P-immunoreactive fibers surrounding ganglion cells in the myenteric (**B**) and submucous (**C**) plexus. ×350 and ×420, respectively. (Figure 3A is from Schultzberg et al., ref. 388, with permission.)

amounts of substance P are found in nervous structures (135). This supports the view that its biological actions are exerted by neuronally released substance P. However, it cannot be excluded that part of the actions are caused by substance P released from endocrine cells.

Substance P is known to cause atropine-resistant contractions of intestinal smooth muscle (354,439,455), and since a very dense innervation is observed in the smooth muscle layers, particularly the circular layer (see Fig. 3A), a direct action of substance P on smooth muscle is likely. This is further supported by pharmacological experiments in which tetrodotoxin inhibition of neuronal transmission had no effect on substance P-induced contractions (58,135,183,317,354,372, 439,455).

However, there is evidence that substance P also affects cholinergic transmission (28,112,183), and electrophysiological studies have shown that substance P depolarizes myenteric neurons (173,239,240) by a direct action (444; see also 317). There is also a dense innervation by substance P-containing fibers in the enteric plexuses (see Fig. 3B,C), suggesting that it may have excitatory actions on myenteric neurons. Furthermore, substance P is known as a potent vasodilator (439), and many fibers can be seen to be close to blood vessels in the gastrointestinal wall (see Fig. 3A). Substance P-immunoreactive nerve fibers are also abundant in the mucosa, often occurring in the superficial parts, as is the case especially in the rat small intestine (388).

Low concentrations of substance P have been observed in extracts of gut from mice inoculated with *Trypanosoma cruzi* virus (Chaga's disease). The lesions in the myenteric plexus characteristic of this condition simultaneously caused a decrease in the number of dense-cored vesicles and a decreased concentration of substance P (11). Smaller amounts of substance P have also been observed in segments of gut from patients with Hirschsprung's disease, in which the distal colon is aganglionic (113,410). The significance of the lowered levels of substance P in these diseases is, however, still unknown, but it is conceivable that it reflects the fact that substance P fibers in the gut are mainly of intrinsic origin.

Vasoactive Intestinal Polypeptide

Immunohistochemical studies of the distribution of VIP in the gastrointestinal tract indicate that VIP is one of the most abundant neuropeptides in the gut (12,79,111,147,232,233,264,269,276,378, 386,388,431). The concentrations of immunoreactive VIP in gut are also higher than those of other neuropeptides. The distribution of VIP in the gut seems to be related entirely to nervous structures. Like substance P, the occurrence of VIP in neuronal cell bodies has been demonstrated by different techniques *in vivo* (145,388) (Fig. 4), *in vitro* (386), and *in oculo* (389). These experiments strongly suggest that the major part of the VIP-immunoreactive fibers in the gut represent processes of such intrinsic VIP neurons. The VIP-immunoreactive cells predominate in the submucous plexus (see Fig. 4), with about 20% to 25% of the total in the guinea pig intestine and as much as around 50% in the rat intestine. The myenteric plexus contains about 5% of VIP-immunoreactive neurons in both species. These values were obtained by examining sections of gut from animals treated with colchicine or vinblastine (388; see also 145).

Some of the VIP-containing neurons may project out of the gut. Thus, ligation of the mesenteric nerves results in accumulation of VIP-immunoreactive material on the gut side (93a). The regional distribution of VIP-immunoreactive neurons seems to be approximately uniform throughout the gut as estimated from immunohistochemical studies of, e.g., the rat and guinea pig (388). In the pig, the concentration of VIP immunoreactivity in the muscle layers including the myenteric plexus is also very much the same throughout the gut, whereas in the mucosa, about 20 to 50 times more VIP-like material was found in the colon than in the stomach (98). The distribution of VIP-immunoreactive fibers in the different layers of the gastrointestinal wall provides a morphological framework for the biological actions of VIP in the gut.

Vasoactive intestinal polypeptide was discovered because of its strong vasodilator action and its relaxation of smooth muscle (376). The VIP-immunoreactive fibers are numerous in the smooth muscle layers in all parts of the gut, and it is conceivable that VIP has a direct action on the smooth muscle cells (39,423). Vasoactive intestinal polypeptide is proposed as the neurotransmitter in enteric inhibitory neurons (129,171). Thus, it is released by stimulation of the vagus nerve or by mechanical stimulation of the stomach, actions that excite the enteric inhibitory neurons in gastric reflex relaxation (129,380). Vasoactive intestinal polypeptide is also released by stimulation of the pelvic nerve or by stimulation of the rectal mucosa and for this reason may be involved in the colonic vasodilatation accompanying the defecation reflex (129). Lesions of nerves in the myenteric plexus in whole-mount preparations of guinea pig ileum

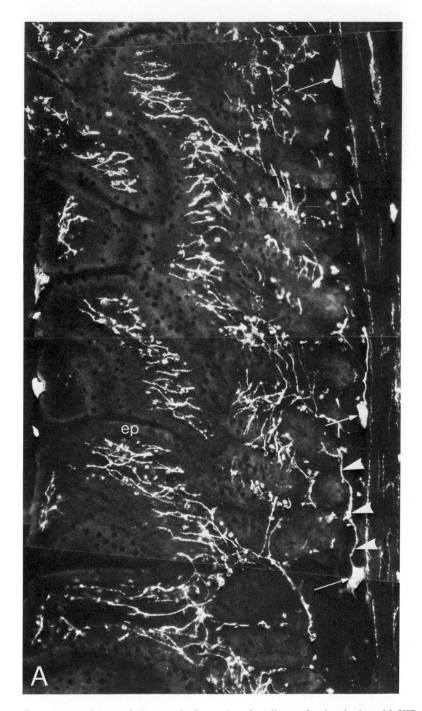

FIG. 4. Immunofluorescence micrograph (montage) of a section of rat ileum after incubation with VIP antiserum. A dense network of VIP-immunoreactive nerve terminals is observed in the mucosa extending up into the villi and possibly following small blood vessels. The fibers often run closely to the epithelium (ep). The VIP-immunoreactive cell bodies occur in the submucous plexus *(arrows)*. Note the process of one of the cells *(arrowheads)*. ×160. (From Schultzberg et al., ref. 388, with permission.)

(144) have shown that VIP neurons in this plexus project in an anal direction, which is the arrangement for enteric inhibitory neurons mediating the descending inhibition in peristalsis (141,198). Moreover, VIP-immunoreactive neurons in the myenteric plexus of the guinea pig cecum were shown to project to the tenia coli in a similar fashion as the enteric inhibitory neurons (147).

Another feature of the VIP innervation of the gut is the particular density of fibers observed in the smooth muscle in sphincter regions, suggesting a functional role for the peptide (12). In fact, VIP has been shown to decrease the lower esophageal sphincter pressure (360), and this action is specifically inhibited by infusion of VIP antiserum (171). On the other hand, VIP has also been demonstrated to decrease the flow through the cat pyloric sphincter, suggesting that it increases tone in this tissue (111). Recent findings have shown that VIP also may excite intestinal muscle, possibly through stimulating cholinergic neurons (227,237), and Williams and North (447) have shown that VIP excites neurons in the myenteric plexus.

Nerve terminals with VIP-like immunoreactivity are often seen close to blood vessels (Fig. 5A), which is compatible with the potent vasodilatory action of the peptide (376). Release of VIP has, in fact, been shown to occur on activation of enteric neurons mediating intestinal hyperemia (114,129). Particularly dense networks of fibers are found in the lamina propria of the mucous layer (see Fig. 4). Possible targets of these fibers are small blood vessels or capillaries. However, VIP fibers often run close to the epithelium, the functional implication of which is supported by the finding that VIP stimulates production of intestinal juices (359,393). As is well known, it has been suggested that VIP is involved in the watery diarrhea syndrome, and the effects caused by VIP resemble the signs in this disease (37,321,322,375).

Enkephalins

Immunohistochemical localization of enkephalin-containing neurons in the gastrointestinal tract (13,115,232,233,276,292,356,386,388) demonstrates that although the enkephalin-immunoreactive fibers are numerous, they are somewhat more restricted than those of substance P and VIP. Thus, enkephalin-immunoreactive fibers mainly run in the smooth muscle layers and in the myenteric plexus (see Fig. 5B). The fibers are relatively sparse in the submucous plexus and in the mucosa.

In the external muscle layers, the fibers are particularly numerous in the circular layer in the small intestine, possibly as part of the deep muscular plexus (see Fig. 5B). The regional distribution of enkephalin-immunoreactive fibers in the rat and guinea pig (388) is on the whole even. The longitudinal muscle layer in the guinea pig stomach is particularly densely innervated as compared to the other parts.

Radioimmunological measurements (292), in agreement with immunohistochemical studies (292,388), show that the guinea pig gastrointestinal tract contains more enkephalin-immunoreactive material than that of the rat. Most enkephalin-immunoreactive material was measured in the guinea pig duodenum (292). Also, the enkephalin-containing fibers probably represent processes of intrinsic gut neurons, as indicated by *in vivo* studies (145,388), *in vitro* studies (386), and *in oculo* studies (389). Furthermore, synthesis of enkephalin has been demonstrated in preparations of the myenteric plexus attached to the longitudinal muscle of guinea pig ileum (399). Inhibition of synthesis by cycloheximide results in loss of enkephalins from the intestinal tissue (313). In addition, release of enkephalin has been shown from the myenteric plexus of guinea pig ileum (392).

Enkephalin-immunoreactive nerve cells constitute about 5% to 15% of the total number of cells in the myenteric plexus, as estimated from immunohistochemical studies on colchicine- or vinblastine-treated tissue from rat and guinea pig (388; see also 145). No positive cells have so far been observed in the submucous plexus of these species. However, large numbers of enkephalin-immunoreactive cells were observed in the submucous plexus of dog intestine (C. Vaillant, *personal communication*).

Both met- and leu-enkephalin-like immunoreactivity have been observed in nerve fibers and cells and have been measured in large amounts in the gastrointestinal tract of rat and guinea pig (216,292). Whether or not the two peptides occur in the same neurons has been difficult to determine, since most enkephalin antibodies in use today react with both peptides in sufficient degree to give a positive immunoreaction in immunohistochemical studies. Thus, for example, a met-enkephalin antiserum (K 329C) cross reacts with leu-enkephalin to the extent of less than 1% in RIA, but addition of 0.2 mM of leu-enkephalin to this antiserum results in a visible decrease in the immunofluorescence observed in sections of tissue stained with this antiserum (390). However, Larsson et al.

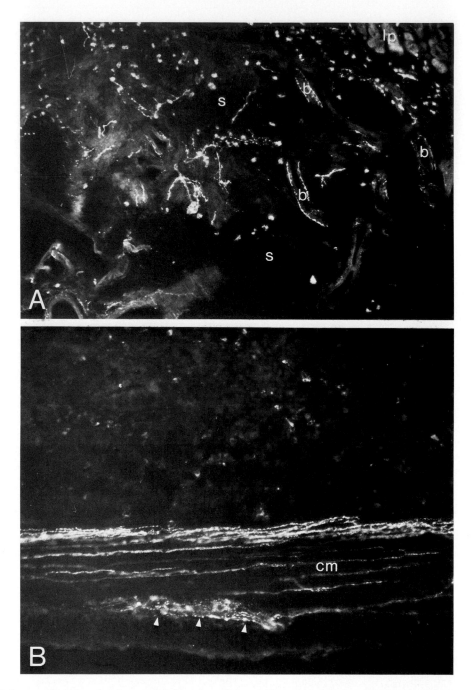

FIG. 5. Immunofluorescence micrographs of sections of the cardia region of the rat stomach (**A**) and of the guinea pig ileum (**B**) after incubation with VIP and enkephalin antisera, respectively. **A**: Numerous VIP-immunoreactive fibers are seen around and close to blood vessels (b) in the submucosa (s) of the cardia. lp, lamina propria. ×180. **B**: Numerous enkephalin-immunoreactive nerve fibers are observed in the circular smooth muscle layer (cm), particularly in the innermost part, possibly in the so-called deep muscular plexus. A dense innervation is also seen in the myenteric plexus (*arrowheads* in **B**). ×160. (Figure 5A is from Schultzberg et al., ref. 388, with permission.)

(265) have described a technique by which it was possible to localize met- and leu-enkephalin in separate neurons (see above). Whether or not there are only separate met- and leu-enkephalin neurons or, in addition, neurons containing both peptides has still to be determined. Beta-endorphin antiserum also demonstrates weakly fluorescent fibers in the gut, but the cross reactivity of the antiserum with met-enkephalin may be sufficient to give a possible immunoreaction with nerves containing high amounts of enkephalin (388).

Enkephalin inhibits contractions of gastrointestinal smooth muscle caused by electrical stimulation (217,433). The effect is reversed by naloxone (432,440) and is therefore mediated by opiate receptors. In the guinea pig ileum, the type of receptor responsible for the inhibitory action of morphine is the so-called μ-receptor (293). Enkephalin has been shown to inhibit the release of ACh from the myenteric plexus (440) where, as mentioned above, the innervation by enkephalin-immunoreactive nerve terminals is dense. Electrophysiological studies show that leu- and met-enkephalin inhibit firing from myenteric neurons (345) and that both peptides cause hyperpolarization of such neurons (379). The action of enkephalins on intestinal contractions may therefore be caused by inhibition of firing through hyperpolarization with an increase in conductance of cholinergic myenteric neurons (344; see also 101,185,256). Enkephalin may also have a direct effect on smooth muscle (446).

Somatostatin

Immunohistochemical studies of the distribution of somatostatin in the gastrointestinal tract (82,83,201,206,276,386,388) show that somatostatin-immunoreactive nerve fibers are more sparse than those of the previously mentioned peptides and that they are mostly restricted to the enteric plexuses (82,83,388; see Fig. 7 below). Often the fibers closely surround a few of the neurons in one ganglionic plexus, whereas other cells are surrounded by a looser network (82). Small numbers of somatostatin-immunoreactive fibers can be seen in the muscle layers. The mucosa and submucosa are generally sparsely innervated except around the basal crypt of the glands in the intestinal mucosa (Fig. 6A). The origin of the fibers in the gut is probably intrinsic, as shown by *in vivo* (145,388), *in vitro* (386), and *in oculo* (389) experiments. However, findings from ligation of the mesenteric nerves point to the possibility that some somatosta-

tin-containing fibers also originate in prevertebral sympathetic ganglia (see below).

The somatostatin-immunoreactive nerve cells in the gut, as estimated from colchicine- or vinblastine-treated animals, are most numerous in the submucous plexus (see Fig. 6C), where the number reaches 20% of the total in the rat and guinea pig ileum and guinea pig colon. In the myenteric plexus only about 2% to 3% of the total number of cells contain somatostatin, except in the rat colon where they reach 14% (388; see also 145). When interpreting the biological actions of somatostatin, it must be taken into consideration that a large proportion of somatostatin in the gut is present in endocrine cells (201; see 36). Thus, somatostatin released into the bloodstream may well contribute to its physiological actions. However, in the following, the actions of somatostatin are discussed in relation to the morphological distribution of immunoreactive nerves.

Somatostatin inhibits firing of myenteric neurons, possibly through hyperpolarization (445). It also inhibits the release of ACh from myenteric neurons (70,143,177). The preferential distribution of somatostatin-immunoreactive nerve terminals in the enteric plexuses may serve as the source of the somatostatin exerting these effects. Costa et al. (82) have shown by lesions in whole-mount preparations of myenteric plexus adhering to longitudinal muscle that somatostatin neurons project anally within the plexus (Fig. 7). They suggest that the somatostatin neurons may be interneurons in the descending inhibitory reflex (77,80,141, 198,400).

Cholecystokinin

The distribution of CCK-immunoreactive neurons in the gastrointestinal tract has been studied by Larsson and Rehfeld (272) and Schultzberg et al. (388). The nerve fibers are comparatively sparse, being most numerous in the circular smooth muscle layer and in the myenteric plexus. The main origin of CCK-immunoreactive fibers in the gut is probably in intrinsic neurons. Estimation of the number of CCK-immunoreactive cells by immunohistochemical studies of vinblastine-treated colon from guinea pig shows that these neurons are most numerous in the submucous plexus (see Fig. 6B) where they reach about 12% of the total number of cells *(unpublished observations)*. However, some of the CCK-immunoreactive fibers may also represent vagal fibers, since the vagus nerve con-

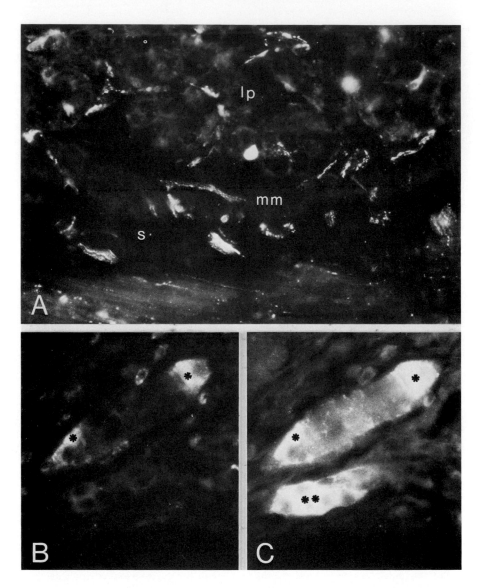

FIG. 6. Immunofluorescence micrographs of sections of the rat ileum (**A**) and the guinea pig proximal colon (**B,C**) after incubation with somatostatin (**A,C**) and CCK (**B**) antisera, respectively. A: Many somatostatin-immunoreactive fibers are observed around the crypts in the basal parts of the lamina propria (lp). Some fibers can also be seen in the lamina muscularis mucosae (mm) and in the submucosa (s). **B,C:** Micrographs of the same section of guinea pig proximal colon showing groups of submucous ganglion cells. The guinea pig was treated with vinblastine. After photography of the CCK-like immunoreactivity (**B**) and removal of the CCK antiserum according to Tramu et al. (421), the section was reincubated with somatostatin antiserum (**C**). The CCK-immunoreactive cells (**B**) in the submucous plexus also show somatostatin-like immunoreactivity *(single asterisks)*. Note that some cell bodies are somatostatin *(double asterisks* in **C**) but not CCK immunoreactive. ×460. (From Schultzberg et al., ref. 388, with permission.)

tains CCK-like material (303,429). It may be noted that in the guinea pig proximal colon, many of the CCK-immunoreactive nerve cells also contain somatostatin-immunoreactive material (388; see Fig. 6B,C). The functional implications of this finding are still unknown. It is possible that the two peptides have a common precursor, but immunochemical studies have so far not given positive results in this direction (J. F. Rehfeld, *unpublished observations*).

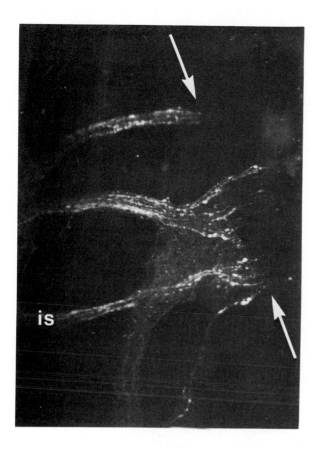

FIG. 7. Immunofluorescence micrograph of whole-mount preparation of the guinea pig small intestine after incubation with somatostatin antiserum. An accumulation of somatostatin-immunoreactive material is observed on the oral side after crushing *(line between arrows)* the nerves in the myenteric plexus and incubation *in vitro*. is, internodal strand. ×210. (From Costa et al., ref. 82, with permission.)

Cholecystokinin and structurally related peptides have direct effects on smooth muscle in the gastrointestinal tract, e.g., on gallbladder and on antral circular muscle in the dog (324,325). However, in the guinea pig ileum, there is evidence that CCK contracts longitudinal muscle by release of ACh and perhaps also substance P from the myenteric plexus (221,437). The histochemical localization of CCK in the gut reveals that many fibers surround nerve cells in the myenteric plexus (388), which may suggest that these fibers are a source of the CCK exerting these actions. The major part of CCK in the gut is, however, localized in endocrine cells, and it is therefore possible that CCK released from these cells participates in these actions.

Neurotensin

Immunohistochemical studies of the distribution of neurotensin in the gastrointestinal tract (388) show that only very few fibers occur in the rat, whereas no fibers could be detected in the guinea pig. The fibers are mainly localized in the circular muscle layer and in the myenteric plexus. No nerve cells containing neurotensin have so far been observed.

Although neurotensin-containing nerve fibers are scarce, neurotensin-containing endocrine cells are abundant (48,136,184,407), and it is therefore possible that some of the effects of exogenously administered neurotensin represent actions normally mediated by hormonal pathways. Neurotensin causes contraction of the guinea pig ileum (63,246,371,394) and tenia coli (69,246,248). Tetrodotoxin was shown to block the effect on guinea pig ileum, indicating that it is nerve mediated (246). Kitabgi and Freychet (247) have also shown that the contractile action of neurotensin in isolated longitudinal muscle from guinea pig ileum is mediated by the release of ACh. However, part of the neurotensin-induced contractions is insensitive to atropine, which suggests that neurotensin acts via ACh and another excitatory factor. Desensitization of the isolated muscle preparation to substance P results in inhibition of the atropine-resistant part of the neurotensin-induced contractions (323).

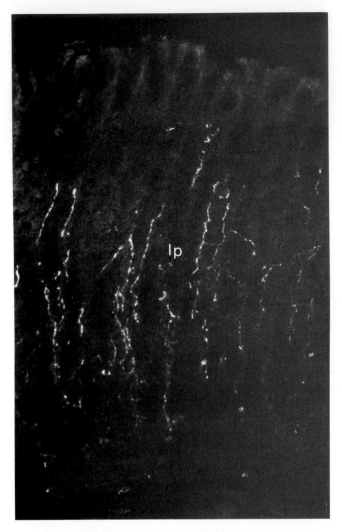

FIG. 8. Immunofluorescence micrograph of section of the corpus region of the rat stomach after incubation with bombesin antiserum. Numerous bombesin-immunoreactive nerve fibers are observed in the lamina propria (lp) between the glands. ×180. (Courtesy of Dr. Camille Vaillant, Department of Physiology, Liverpool University, Liverpool.)

Bombesin

Immunohistochemical studies of rat gastrointestinal tract (38,106) show that bombesin-like immunoreactivity is exclusively located in neuronal structures. Dense innervation was observed in the stomach and colon, whereas the small intestine was more sparsely innervated. In the stomach, abundant nerve fibers were seen in the mucosa (Fig. 8), especially in the acid-secreting region. Many fibers were also found in the myenteric plexus, whereas the muscular layers were more sparsely innervated.

Measurements of bombesin-like material in the guinea pig gastrointestinal tract show that the major part is localized in the muscular layers including the myenteric plexus, whereas only trace amounts occur in the mucosa (220). The bombesin-immunoreactive material extracted from the guinea pig ileum longitudinal muscle was shown to consist of two molecular forms.

Bombesin is shown to have a number of actions, one of which is stimulation of contractions of intestinal muscle (44,62,125). Bombesin has also a potent gastrin-releasing effect, which might account for atropine-resistant vagal release of gastrin (105,416). Furthermore, bombesin releases GIP and PP, but since few bombesin-immunoreactive fibers are observed in areas containing GIP or PP cells, it is not likely to be a direct physiological action.

Other Peptides

In addition to the above-mentioned peptides, there are a few others that have been demonstrated in the gastrointestinal tract. The details of their distribution are, however, not fully known. Angiotensin II has been detected in nerve fibers in the rat gut by immunohistochemical techniques (148,155). Pancreatic polypeptide-like material has recently been observed with antibodies to the COOH-terminal hexapeptide in nerve fibers in rat, dog, man, cat, and mouse intestine (C. Vaillant, *unpublished observations*) and with antibodies to APP in rat, cat, and dog intestine (294). Thyrotropin-releasing hormone-like immunoreactivity has been measured in rat gastrointestinal tract in amounts of about 2 ng/g of tissue (280,324).

Other Putative Transmitters

As mentioned earlier, ATP or a related purine has been proposed as the transmitter in enteric inhibitory neurons (50,54). These neurons are interneurons in the gut that cause hyperpolarization and relaxation of intestinal muscle. The neurons project anally and mediate descending inhibitory reflexes throughout the gastrointestinal tract (139,141,198,230). Burnstock has shown that ATP produces relaxation of intestinal muscle in a way that mimics nerve stimulation of enteric inhibitory neurons; for instance, it causes rapid hyperpolarization of smooth muscle via an increase in K^+ conductivity. Release of ATP (54) and the amplitude of inhibitory junction potentials (212) are Ca^{2+} dependent.

The existence of 5-HT-containing neurons in the gastrointestinal tract has been studied with a number of techniques. Studies on intestinal tissue cultures visualized neurons with bright yellow fluorescence (108), which was identified by microspectrofluorophotometry as caused by 5-HT. *In vivo*, the histofluorescence technique has to be preceded by loading the neurons with the precursor amino acid tryptophan and by inhibition of monoamine oxidase (108). Uptake and conversion of tritiated tryptophan to [^{3}H]-5-HT indicates synthesis of 5-HT in the gut (108,109,160,162,368). This was shown also in preparations that lack the mucosa containing the 5-HT-containing enterochromaffin cells (108,368). Immunohistochemical studies using antibodies to tryptophan hydroxylase—the enzyme converting tryptophan to 5-HT—visualize neurons in both of the enteric plexuses (161). Serotonin is released on electrical stimulation in a nerve-mediated fashion (see 78). Stimulation of enteric noncholinergic interneurons results in slow excitatory postsynaptic potentials (EPSP) which are associated with increased membrane resistance. The EPSPs are mimicked both by substance P and 5-HT (173,239). The action of 5-HT is blocked by methysergide (439,450) or densitization ot 5-HT (340), which also inhibits the EPSPs. Intrinsic amine-handling neurons are localized by uptake of catecholamines followed by histofluorescence techniques (80,138). The neurons occur both in the submucous and myenteric plexus. Nerve fibers run within the plexuses as well as in the deep muscular plexus and the mucosa.

Sympathetic Ganglia

Main attention is given to prevertebral sympathetic ganglia, i.e., the inferior mesenteric ganglion and the celiac–superior mesenteric ganglion complex. These ganglia are the most thoroughly studied with regard to the occurrence of peptides and are also of interest since they provide the gastrointestinal wall with noradrenergic inhibitory nerves. Comparisons with ganglia in the sympathetic chain are also made. General organization and properties of sympathetic neurons have been reviewed previously (225,259,260).

Substance P

Fine networks of substance P-containing nerve fibers have been found in the prevertebral ganglia of rat, cat, and guinea pig (205). The fibers are mainly thin and varicose (Fig. 9A), probably representing nerve terminals. Smooth nerve fibers have also been observed; treatment with colchicine results in accumulation of substance P-immunoreactive material in nerve fiber bundles that probably represent axons running through the ganglia, since no positive ganglion cells have been observed.

It has been suggested that peripheral branches of substance P-containing primary sensory neurons (209,210) terminate in the prevertebral ganglia as well as run through them on their way to the gastrointestinal tract. Retrograde tracing experiments with horseradish peroxidase have provided direct evidence for a connection between dorsal root ganglia and prevertebral ganglia (116). Ligation of the

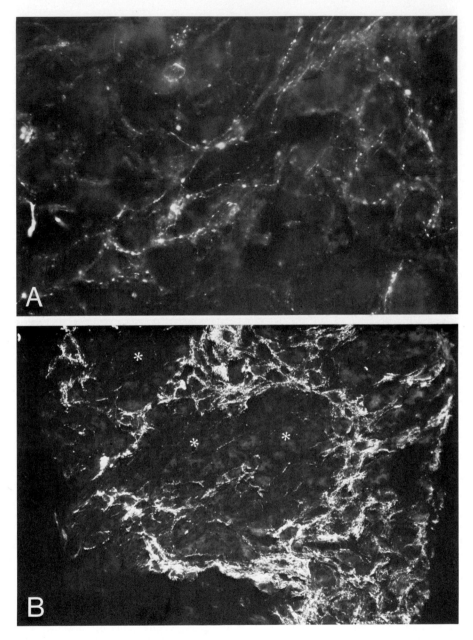

FIG. 9. Immunofluorescence micrographs of sections of the guinea pig inferior mesenteric (**A**) and celiac–superior mesenteric (**B**) ganglion after incubation with substance P and VIP antisera, respectively. **A:** Numerous varicose substance P-immunoreactive fibers are observed surrounding the ganglion cells. ×350. A dense network of VIP-immunoreactive nerve terminals is observed in **B**. The fibers are varicose and often run two or more together. Note that in some regions, only few VIP-immunoreactive fibers occur (*asterisks* in **B**). ×140.

mesenteric nerves connecting the prevertebral ganglia with the gut causes an accumulation of substance P-immunoreactive material on the ganglion side (93a). Further, Konishi et al. (250) have shown that the amounts of immunoreactive substance P in the inferior mesenteric ganglion decreased markedly after section of the lumbar splanchnic and intermesenteric nerves. Substance P is released by high K^+ concentration from prevertebral ganglia of the guinea pig, and the principal ganglion cells respond to substance P with an atropine-resistant depolarization (250). In other sympathetic ganglia, such as the stellate and superior cervical ganglia, only a sparse, more patchy network of substance P-containing fibers has been observed.

Vasoactive Intestinal Polypeptide

Extensive networks of VIP-containing nerve terminals have been observed in the rat and guinea pig prevertebral ganglia (204). The fibers are varicose and seem to run two or more together (see Fig. 9B). The network of fibers is unevenly distributed over the ganglia, some regions are densely innervated with fibers surrounding the ganglion cells, whereas others are almost devoid of fibers. In addition, there are VIP-containing cells that appear to be located in the more sparsely innervated areas of the ganglia. These cells may give rise to parts of the network of VIP-containing fibers. However, in addition, there are probably projections from VIP-immunoreactive neurons in the gastrointestinal wall to the ganglia. Electrophysiological (88,234,315,409) and anatomical (259,260,262) evidence for such projections has been described earlier. However, it is also possible that some of the VIP-containing fibers in the ganglia represent peripheral branches of VIP-immunoreactive neurons in spinal ganglia (303). Like substance P fibers, the VIP-immunoreactive fibers in the superior cervical ganglion are more sparse than in the prevertebral ganglia.

Enkephalins

Immunohistochemical studies of the prevertebral ganglia have also revealed a dense innervation by enkephalin-immunoreactive fibers in rat and guinea pig (387,390) and in man (129,190,353). The fibers are varicose and surround the ganglion cells in a dense network. Both met- and leu-enkephalin have been demonstrated to be present in the ganglia (95). Ultrastructural studies of human sympathetic ganglia showed that enkephalin-like material occurred in large dense-core vesicles and some small clear vesicles in nerve fibers (187). Some enkephalin-immunoreactive SIF cells can be seen in untreated ganglia (Fig. 10A), and colchicine treatment increases the number. These cells may give rise to some of the enkephalin-containing fibers, but fibers may also originate in the central nervous system, since enkephalin-immunoreactive fibers have been observed in the vagus nerve and in ventral spinal roots (303). Both met- and leu-enkephalin have been shown to inhibit cholinergic transmission in the prevertebral ganglia of guinea pig (251). In the superior cervical ganglion, comparatively few enkephalin-immunoreactive fibers can be seen (Fig. 11A). However, some of the principal ganglion cells in the rat ganglion have been shown to contain enkephalin-like material. The number of cells seen increased after colchicine treatment; by study of consecutive sections, evidence has been obtained that some cells contained both enkephalin and norepinephrine (390; see Fig. 11B,C).

Somatostatin

Somatostatin differs from the three previously mentioned neuropeptides in that there is a relatively sparse population of somatostatin-immunoreactive fibers in the prevertebral ganglia. In contrast, there are a large number of principal ganglion cells that contain somatostatin-like immunoreactivity. About two-thirds of the noradrenergic ganglion cells are somatostatin immunoreactive (203; see Fig. 12A,B). As the noradrenergic ganglion cells project to the gut, it is tempting to assume that at least some of these fibers also contain somatostatin. Moreover, in this context, it is interesting to note that both substances inhibit release of ACh from enteric neurons (70,140,143,177,274,275). Indirect evidence for this view is provided by ligation of the mesenteric nerves, which results in accumulation of somatostatin-immunoreactive material on the ganglion side (J. M. Lundberg and T. Hökfelt, *unpublished observations*). However, it has not yet been possible to demonstrate the coexistence of somatostatin and NE in nerve terminals in the gut. Although denervation of the gut (guinea pig ileum) did not result in a change in the network of somatostatin fibers in the gut (82), it may well be that the contribution from the prevertebral ganglia is too small relative to the intrinsic somatostatin neurons for immunohistochemical detection. The superior cervical gan-

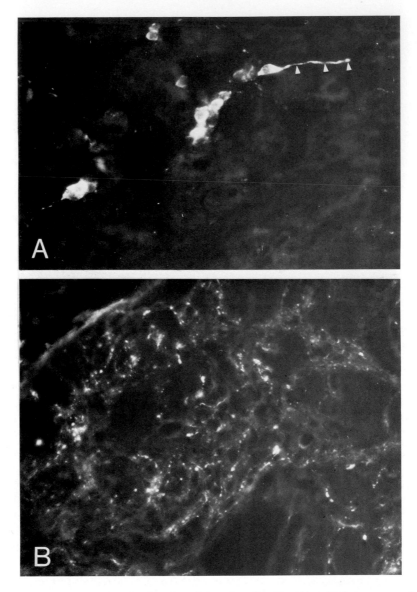

FIG. 10. Immunofluorescence micrographs of sections of the guinea pig celiac (**A**) and inferior mesenteric (**B**) ganglion after incubation with enkephalin and bombesin antisera, respectively. **A:** Enkephalin-immunoreactive SIF cells. Note the process from one of these SIF cells (*arrowheads* in **A**). ×300. **B:** Many fine varicose bombesin-immunoreactive nerve fibers are observed around the ganglion cells. ×350. (**A** is from M. Schultzberg et al., ref. 390, with permission.)

glion contains only a small number of somatostatin-immunoreactive cells.

Cholecystokinin

A dense network of CCK-immunoreactive fibers has been demonstrated in the celiac–superior mesenteric ganglion complex (272). A similarly dense network has been observed also in the inferior mes-

enteric ganglion *(unpublished observations)*. The fibers most probably originate in the gastrointestinal wall, since ligation of the mesenteric nerves caused an accumulation of CCK-like material on the gastrointestinal side (93a). The possibility exists, however, that at least some CCK-immunoreactive fibers originate in spinal ganglia (303). The superior cervical ganglion receives only a sparse innervation of CCK-immunoreactive fibers.

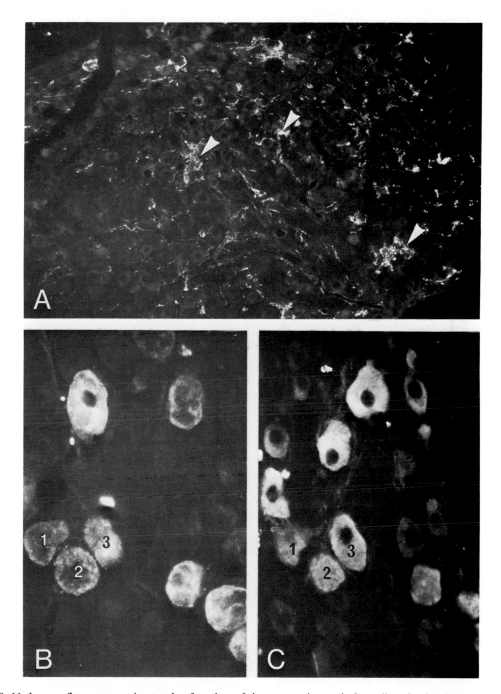

FIG. 11. Immunofluorescence micrographs of sections of the rat superior cervical ganglion after incubation with en-kephalin (**A,B**) and tyrosine hydroxylase (TH) (**C**) antisera. **B,C:** Consecutive sections of a superior cervical ganglion from a rat treated with colchicine. ×300. **A:** Enkephalin-immunoreactive varicose nerve terminals, often occurring in patches (*arrowheads* in **A**). ×140. **B:** The occurrence of enkephalin-immunoreactive principal ganglion cells after treatment with colchicine. Note that the enkephalin-immunoreactive cells (numbered 1–3) are TH positive (**C**). (From M. Schultzberg et al., ref. 390, with permission.)

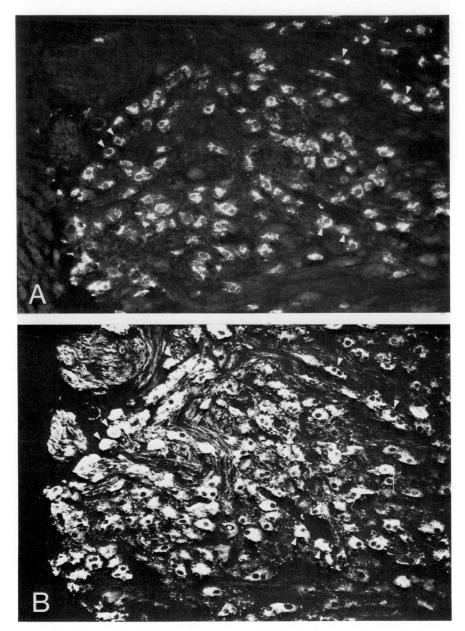

FIG. 12. Immunofluorescence micrographs of consecutive sections of guinea pig celiac ganglion after incubation with somatostatin **(A)** and DBH **(B)** antisera, respectively. A large proportion of the principal ganglion cells are somatostatin immunoreactive **(A)**. Note that many of the ganglion cells are present in both sections and contain both somatostatin- **(A)** and DBH-like **(B)** immunoreactivity *(arrowheads)*. ×140.

Neurotensin

No neurotensin-containing nerve fibers have so far been observed in the rat or guinea pig prevertebral ganglia, but a sparse innervation has been seen in these ganglia in the cat (302).

Bombesin

Recent studies have shown a dense network of bombesin-immunoreactive nerve fibers in the prevertebral ganglia of both rat and guinea pig (385) (see Fig. 10B). The fibers are varicose and appear to run in groups of two or more in a similar way to the VIP-immunoreactive fibers. No positive cell bodies have been detected so far, even after colchicine treatment. The innervation of the superior cervical ganglion is sparse.

Other Peptides

Recent immunohistochemical studies using antibodies to avian PP have shown the occurrence of immunoreactive material in numerous cell bodies in the superior cervical, stellate, and celiac ganglia of the rat and cat (301). In the frog, LHRH-like immunoreactivity has been demonstrated in nerve fibers in paravertebral ganglia (228,229). Denervation experiments coupled with HRP tracing suggested that the LHRH immunoreactive fibers represent preganglionic fibers (228). It was suggested that LHRH may coexist with ACh in these neurons.

Other Putative Transmitters

Recent immunohistochemical studies with antibodies to 5-HT have shown the occurrence of 5-HT-containing SIF cells in the rat superior cervical ganglion (435). The immunoreactive cells occurred in clusters mostly located at the cranial or caudal poles of the ganglion and appear to represent a population separate from those containing NE. In addition, dopamine has been demonstrated to occur in SIF cells in sympathetic ganglia (see 86,118). The superior cervical ganglion, and possibly also other sympathetic ganglia, therefore contain three types of SIF cells, histochemically characterized as containing norepinephrine (117; see 86,118), dopamine, and 5-HT (435), respectively.

Adrenal Glands

The presence of enkephalin-like material in adrenal medullary cells was originally suggested on the basis of immunohistochemical studies (387,391). This suggestion has now been amply confirmed by the isolation from bovine adrenals of met- and leu-enkephalin as well as several new opiate peptides (see above). From the immunohistochemical studies, it is evident that there are species differences in the abundance of enkephalin-like material. Thus, in the guinea pig, a large proportion of the chromaffin cells show enkephalin-like immunoreactivity. The fluorescence intensity of the positive cells varies from very weak to very bright (Fig. 13A,B), suggesting the presence of different amounts of the immunoreactive material. In the cat, the proportion of enkephalin-immunoreactive cells was larger than in the guinea pig, but a more uniform fluorescence intensity was observed. The relative abundance of enkephalin-containing cells indicates that both NE- and epinephrine-containing cells also contain the peptide(s), since in the cat the NE-containing cells constitute 20% to 50% of the medullary cells (193,194).

Examination of the human adrenal gland shows that a large number of the cells in the medulla contain enkephalin-like material (300). Most of the cells also contained DBH and PNMT, indicating coexistence with both NE and epinephrine. In the rat adrenal gland, only a few enkephalin-immunoreactive cells were observed in untreated animals (391). These cells were DBH positive but PNMT negative, i.e., contained NE but not epinephrine. However, transection of the greater splanchnic nerve results in a marked increase in the number of enkephalin-immunoreactive cells visualized, so that cells that were positive for both PNMT and enkephalin were now seen (391). Moreover, treatment with reserpine increases synthesis of enkephalins by adrenal chromaffin cells (448). Together, these observations suggest that enkephalin production might in some way be related to catecholamine turnover.

There are now several studies that demonstrate that enkephalin-like material is associated with the chromaffin granules. Viveros et al. (436) have shown that enkephalins and related low-molecular-weight opiates comigrate with catecholamines in density gradients of dog adrenal medullary tissue. In addition, ultrastructural studies of the rat adrenal gland show an association of enkephalin-like material with storage granules in the medullary cells (188). The functional implications of the occurrence of enkephalins in chromaffin cells are still unknown. A hormonal role cannot be excluded, although it is well known that enkephalins are rapidly degraded by hydrolytic enzymes in the blood. Nevertheless, it has recently been shown that intact met-enkephalin circulates in human plasma (68). One possibility is also that the higher-molecular-weight forms containing the enkephalin sequence are secreted into the bloodstream as hormones and that the smaller pentapeptides act locally on the chromaffin cells themselves or on the incoming nerves.

Release of enkephalin and catecholamines on stimulation of the adrenal gland *in vivo* and *in vitro* during perfusion has been shown recently (404,436). Enkephalin-like immunoreactivity has also been observed in varicose nerve terminals in the adrenal gland (387,391) (see Fig. 13A). A few

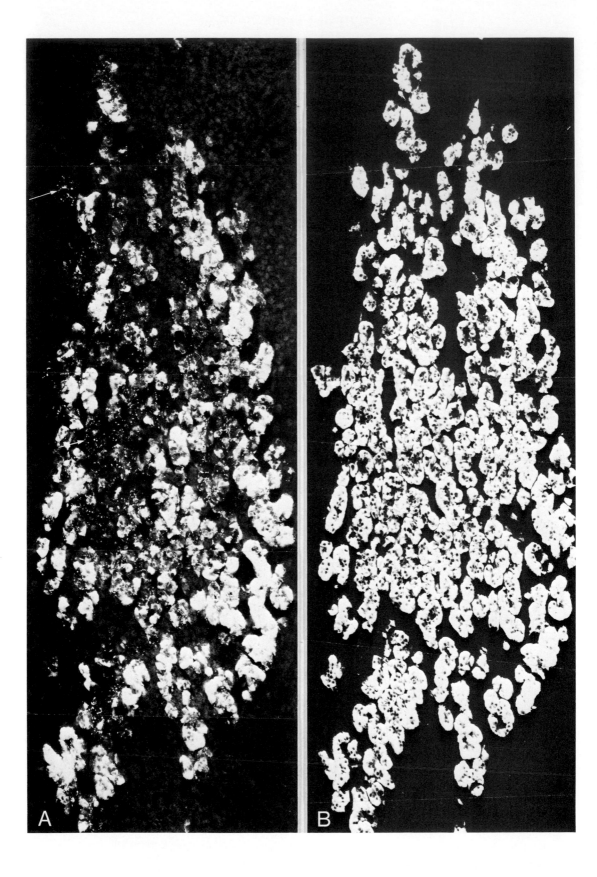

fibers were seen in the adrenal cortex radiating towards the medulla, and many fibers occurred in the medulla. Transection of the greater splanchnic nerve results in a marked decrease in the number of fibers. The adrenal glands are innervated by preganglionic cholinergic neurons in the lateral horn of the spinal cord in the segments between T3 and L3 (84,85,245,312,370,420,456; see 86). Enkephalin-like material has been observed in ventral spinal roots (303), and possibly the enkephalin-immunoreactive fibers are a separate population of preganglionic neurons other than the cholinergic neurons. Alternatively, enkephalin-like material could coexist with ACh in some or all of the preganglionic cholinergic neurons.

In man, somatostatin-like immunoreactivity was observed in many of the adrenal medullary cells, both in normal glands and in pheochromocytoma (300). A few scattered somatostatin-immunoreactive cells have also been observed in the guinea pig adrenal *(unpublished observations).* In the cat, a large number of cells in the adrenal medulla contain neurotensin-like immunoreactivity (302). The significance of these findings has yet to be clarified. Furthermore, PP-like material has been observed in a number of adrenal medullary cells in the rat and cat (301).

Other Peripheral Organs

Urogenital Tract

The organs of the urogenital tract are innervated by sympathetic and parasympathetic nerves. The former mainly originate in the prevertebral ganglia and in ganglia located close to the organ. The parasympathetic postganglionic neurons are located close to or within the target organ. As in the gastrointestinal tract, there is evidence for types of nerves other than the cholinergic and noradrenergic in the urogenital tract. Thus, pharmacological studies of the urinary bladder have shown the presence of noncholinergic excitatory nerves; indeed, these appear to be the major portion of excitatory nerves in this organ (18,50,54,94). Noncholinergic, nonadrenergic excitatory responses have also been obtained from stimulation of nerves to the seminal vesicle (335,336). An inhibitory innervation of the dog retractor penis has been demonstrated, the stimulation of which has again been shown to be resistant to cholinergic and adrenergic inhibitors (297). More recently, immunohistochemical studies have shown the presence of peptidergic neurons in the urogenital tract. The most abundant peptides are substance P and VIP, whereas enkephalin- and somatostatin-immunoreactive neurons are more sparse. Presumably, release of the peptides accounts for the effects mentioned above.

Substance P.

Substance P-immunoreactive nerves have been observed in the guinea pig (211) and cat (9) urogenital tract. Only sparse substance P-immunoreactive fibers were observed in the guinea pig kidney, and no fibers were seen in the rat or cat (9). The fibers mostly run alongside blood vessels but also close to smooth muscle fibers in the renal pelvis. Numerous substance P-immunoreactive fibers occur in the ureter, especially in the epithelium and underlying connective tissue (see Fig. 14A; 9,211). The smooth muscle layers are also densely innervated, and fibers were also seen close to blood vessels (9,211). The trigonum was the most densely innervated part of the urinary bladder. The distribution of fibers was similar to that in the ureter. Small ganglia in the wall of the bladder contain some substance P-immunoreactive fibers but no positive nerve cells, suggesting an extrinsic origin of the substance P-containing fibers. The distribution of fibers in the wall of the urethra is similar to that in the ureter and bladder, but the innervation is more sparse. Substance P also occurs in nerve fibers in both the male and female genital tract (9). The vagina is particularly densely innervated. The fibers occur in the connective tissue close to the epithelium in relation to blood vessels and the smooth muscle bundles. The uterus, oviduct, ovaries, and the male genital organs, except the prostate gland, are sparsely innervated by substance P-immunoreactive fibers.

Vasoactive intestinal polypeptide.

This peptide has been demonstrated in abundant nerve fibers in the urogenital tract of the cat (10,266) and also in the pig, guinea pig, rat, and

---

FIG. 13. Immunofluorescence micrographs of consecutive sections of the guinea pig adrenal gland after incubation with enkephalin (**A**) and DBH (**B**) antisera, respectively. A large proportion of the adrenal medullary cells contain enkephalin-like immunoreactivity (**A**). Many of the cells are both enkephalin (**A**) and DBH (**B**) immunoreactive. Note also the occurrence of varicose enkephalin-immunoreactive nerve fibers in the adrenal medulla (*arrows* in **A**). ×110. (From M. Schultzberg et al., ref. 391, with permission.)

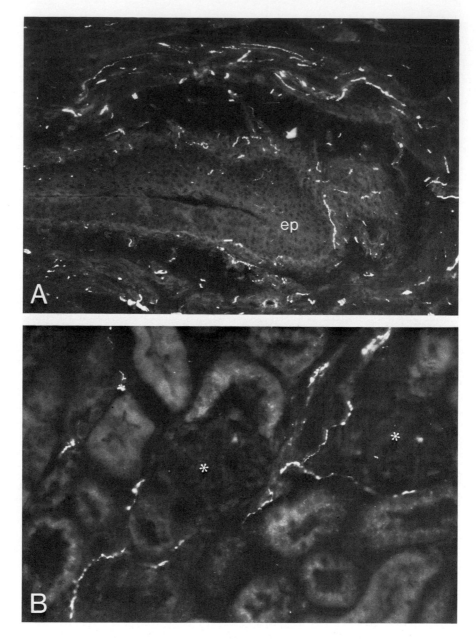

FIG. 14. Immunofluorescence micrographs of sections of the guinea pig ureter (**A**) and kidney (**B**) after incubation with substance P and VIP antisera, respectively. **A**: Numerous substance P-immunoreactive fibers in the wall of the ureter and under the epithelium, sometimes extending into the epithelium (ep). ×140. **B**: The renal cortex including renal corpuscles (*asterisks* in **B**). Note the occurrence of VIP-immunoreactive nerve fibers between the renal tubules. ×350.

mouse (10,211,267). In addition, the human female genital tract has been shown to receive a sparse innervation by VIP-immunoreactive fibers (305). A few VIP-immunoreactive fibers were observed in the guinea pig kidney, mainly following blood vessels in the cortex (see Fig. 14B). Some fibers also occurred in the renal pelvis in relation to smooth muscle cells (211). No fibers have been observed in the kidney of cat, rat, pig, or mouse (10,266,267). The VIP-immunoreactive fibers are abundant in the ureter, and in the cat, concentrations of about 200 pmoles/g of immunoreactive VIP have been reported in extracts of ureter, whereas the urinary bladder contains about 10 times less (267). The VIP-immunoreactive fibers in the ureter were observed in the smooth muscle, around blood vessels, and in the connective tissue under the epithelium.

A similar distribution pattern was seen in the urinary bladder and the urethra, although smaller numbers of fibers were present there. However, the smooth muscle of the trigonum (see Fig. 15A,B) and around the openings of the ureters into the bladder are densely innervated by VIP-immunoreactive fibers. Many nerve cell bodies in small ganglia in the wall of the bladder and some in the urethral wall showed VIP-like immunoreactivity (10). Both male and female genital tracts also contain large amounts of VIP (266,267). In the male, a particularly dense innervation was observed in the epididymis, the seminal vesicles, vas deferens, and the prostate (10,266). In the female, the vagina and uterus are most densely innervated (267). The VIP-immunoreactive fibers occur in the smooth muscle, around blood vessels, and subepithelially in these organs, and in the uterus many fibers were also seen in the endometrium. The VIP-like immunoreactivity as measured in human female genital tract (305) was about 30 times lower than that in the cat (267). A large proportion of the VIP-immunoreactive fibers in the cat female genital tract appear to originate in the paracervical ganglion, since removal of this ganglion results in a large decrease of VIP fibers in all of these organs except the ovaries (10).

The physiological significance of the VIP-containing nerves in the urogenital tract is still unknown, but the localization of such nerves close to blood vessels suggests that it acts on the blood flow, since VIP is known to be a potent vasodilator (376). Rather high concentrations of VIP (300 ng/ml) have been shown to cause contraction of the detrusor muscle in the guinea pig urinary bladder, but the response, although dose dependent, is only about 10% of the nerve-induced response (235). Therefore, it may be that this response is of minor importance and that VIP has another function in the bladder.

Other peptides.

Enkephalin- and somatostatin-immunoreactive nerves have also been found in the urogenital tract (211,430; and *unpublished observations*). Somatostatin-immunoreactive nerve fibers occur in the smooth muscle layers of ureter and urinary bladder. Some nerve cells in ganglia in the wall of the urinary bladder were somatostatin immunoreactive, and a dense network of enkephalin-immunoreactive fibers was observed in these ganglia. A dense plexus of nerve fibers reacting with antibodies to APP has been observed in the rat and cat vas deferens (301).

Respiratory Tract

The respiratory tract is innervated by sympathetic and parasympathetic nerves. Bronchodilatation is caused by sympathetic stimulation, whereas parasympathetic stimulation causes bronchoconstriction and stimulation of bronchial glands. However, there is pharmacological evidence for noncholinergic, nonadrenergic inhibitory nerves in the vagus, supplying lung musculature (366). Stimulation of the vagus nerve in the presence of atropine gives bronchodilator responses (443). Moreover, nerve profiles of another type than cholinergic and adrenergic, i.e., containing large opaque vesicles (LOV), have been identified in chicken, mouse, and human lung (72,219,366).

There is thus suggestive evidence for the existence of putative transmitters other than ACh and NE. One of the neuropeptides, VIP, has been shown to occur in nerve fibers in the respiratory tract of several mammals (379). The VIP-immunoreactive fibers are observed in smooth muscle in the tracheobronchial wall and around small blood vessels and seromucous glands in the mucosa of the nose, epipharynx, mesopharynx, larynx, and tracheobronchial wall (422,427). Some nerve cells in the tracheobronchial wall also showed VIP-like immunoreactivity. The VIP-immunoreactive fibers in the nasal mucosa seem to originate in the pterygopalatine ganglion, since removal of this ganglion results in an almost complete loss of VIP fibers (425).

Vasoactive intestinal polypeptide is known to cause a potent relaxation of lung musculature (376), and recent studies of cat nasal mucosa show

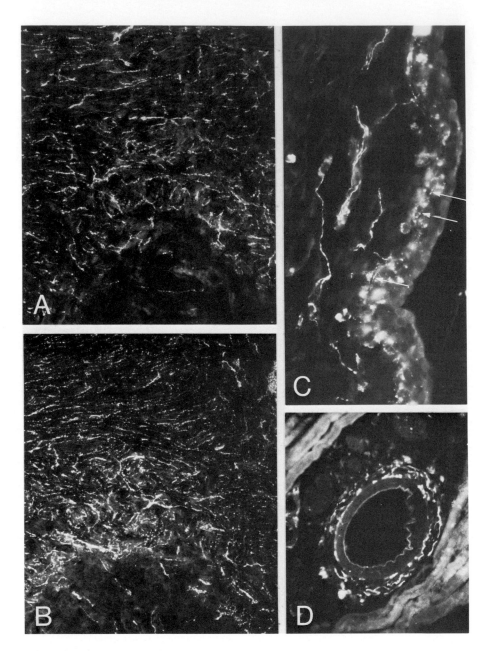

FIG. 15. Immunofluorescence micrographs of sections of the guinea pig urinary bladder (**A,B**) and the rat trachea (**C**) and tongue (**D**) after incubation with VIP (**A**), DBH (**B**), and substance P (**C,D**) antisera, respectively. **A:** Numerous VIP-immunoreactive fibers are observed in the smooth muscle in the trigonum region of the urinary bladder. ×140. **B:** The dense noradrenergic innervation of the same area in a semiconsecutive section. ×140. **C:** Many substance P-immunoreactive fibers can be seen in the connective tissue under the lining epithelium of the trachea. Note also some positive fibers in the epithelium (*arrows* in **C**). ×350. **D:** An artery in the tongue of the rat surrounded by numerous substance P-immunoreactive fibers. ×140.

that close intraarterial infusion of VIP causes increased blood flow, a decrease in systemic arterial blood pressure, and dilatation of both resistance and capacitance blood vessels (308). The responses were atropine resistant. Furthermore, stimulation of the vidian nerve results in an atropine-resistant increase of VIP concentration in nasal venous plasma accompanied by dilatation of nasal resistance vessels (426).

Immunohistochemical studies with antiserum to APP showed the occurrence of immunoreactive nerve fibers in the cat nasal mucosa (301), and local infusion of APP reduced the vasodilatatory response to parasympathetic nerve stimulation (299).

Some substance P-immunoreactive fibers innervate the respiratory tract and were mainly observed in the epithelium and close to blood vessels *(unpublished observations)* (see Fig. 15C,D).

Pancreas

The exocrine secretion of the pancreas has long been thought to be regulated mainly by hormones. Thus, secretin, which was discovered in 1902 by Bayliss and Starling (27), stimulates secretion of bicarbonate and water from the pancreas of mammals, whereas CCK causes enzyme secretion.

In dogs and cats, vagal stimulation produces an enzyme-rich pancreatic juice. Moreover, there is now increasing evidence that in the dog there are vagovagal reflexes controlling pancreatic enzyme secretion after feeding (398). In the pig, vagal nerve stimulation evokes the release not just of enzymes but also of a watery bicarbonate-rich juice. In the presence of atropine, the secretion of enzymes is inhibited, whereas the increased flow of water and bicarbonate persists (191). More recently, it has been suggested that VIP is the mediator of this atropine-resistant response (130). This suggestion is based on several lines of evidence. Immunohistochemical studies have shown that VIP-immunoreactive nerve fibers are abundant in the exocrine parenchyma close to the acini and in the wall of blood vessels (268,406). The endocrine islets contain only a few fibers. Perfusion of the porcine pancreas *in vitro* with VIP gives a marked increase in water and bicarbonate secretion, mimicking the response to vagal nerve stimulation (289). Vagal stimulation also causes an increase of the VIP concentration in the venous outflow from porcine pancreas (130) that is accompanied by the secretory response of the exocrine

pancreas. Atropine and adrenergic blocking agents do not block the increased VIP output. Pancreatic blood flow was also increased by vagal stimulation, and it was suggested that VIP also mediates this response since it is known to have potent vasodilatatory activity (376,419). Vasoactive intestinal polypeptide has also been shown to have a potent action on the secretion of water and bicarbonate from the turkey pancreas (97). Unlike the cases in the pig and man (107,253), VIP is more potent than secretin in inducing this response in the turkey (97) but not in endocrine cells. It is possible that it has a neurotransmitter role in controlling pancreatic fluid secretion (130).

Vasoactive intestinal polypeptide has, in addition, been shown to stimulate the release of insulin and glucagon (382) in a glucose-dependent manner from the porcine pancreas (289). The origin of the VIP acting on the endocrine pancreas is not likely to be hormonal, since the basal as well as postprandial concentration of VIP is much lower than the minimum concentration needed for increasing insulin and glucagon secretion (381). It was suggested that the origin of VIP eliciting this response is neuronal, since at least in the pig, VIP is released from the pancreas by vagal stimulation in the presence of atropine (130), and such stimulation also causes an increase in the release of insulin and glucagon (213,214). The stimulatory action of gastrins and CCKs on the protein secretion from the endocrine pancreas is well known (290,291). No effect on the release of insulin or glucagon is obtained with these hormones except in very high doses (290,291). However, it has been shown that the COOH-terminal tetrapeptide of gastrin and CCK is highly potent in releasing insulin and glucagon from the perfused porcine pancreas (364). It was suggested that tetrapeptide-immunoreactive nerves in the pancreas constitute the origin of the tetrapeptide acting on the endocrine islets in the pancreas (363,364).

Sweat Glands

Sweat glands are innervated by sympathetic cholinergic nerves originating in paravertebral sympathetic ganglia. Sympathetic stimulation causes sweat secretion accompanied by vasodilatation. However, pharmacological experiments have shown that part of the vasodilatatory response is atropine resistant (133). Recently, VIP-immunoreactive nerves have been shown to occur in sweat glands of the cat, where they surround the acini and blood vessels (304). Ligation of the sciatic nerve carrying nerves innervating the sweat glands of the hind paw resulted in accumulation of VIP-like material mainly on the cell body side (164,304), and lumbosacral sympathectomy caused disappearance of VIP-immunoreactive fibers in the sweat glands (304). The origin of these fibers is therefore likely to be neurons in the lower

sympathetic chain ganglia that contain VIP-like immunoreactivity.

Most of the VIP-immunoreactive neurons also exhibited a strong or medium staining for AChE (see Fig. 16A,B), suggesting that VIP is present in cholinergic sympathetic neurons. The pattern of VIP-immunoreactive fibers in the sweat glands and at the ligation of the sciatic nerve closely resembles

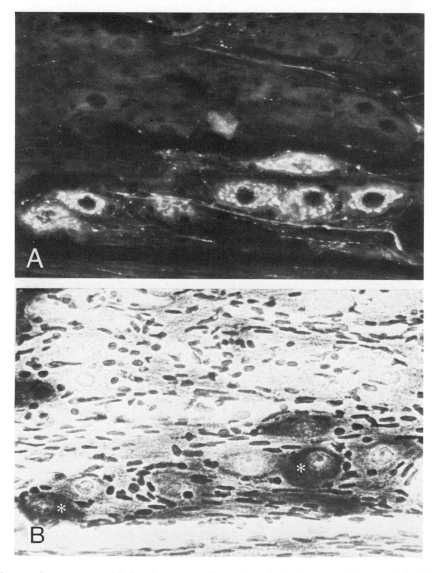

FIG. 16. Immunofluorescence and light micrographs of a section of the L7 sympathetic ganglion of the cat after incubation with antiserum to VIP (**A**), followed by AChE staining (**B**). The section was first processed for immunohistochemistry and, after photography, for AChE staining. A group of VIP-immunoreactive cell bodies is seen in **A**. Some of these are strongly AChE positive *(asterisks)*, whereas some VIP-immunoreactive cells have only a medium or low AChE activity. ×400. (From J. M. Lundberg et al., ref. 304, with permission.)

that of the AChE-positive fibers. Secretion is assumed to be mediated directly by ACh released from nerves (93). However, sweat secretion is accompanied by increased blood flow (133), which cannot be blocked by atropine. Since VIP is known to be a potent vasodilator (376), the possibility exists that VIP is the mediator of the atropine-resistant increase in blood flow accompanying sweat secretion, either directly by relaxing the vascular smooth muscle or indirectly via activation of the kallikrein–bradykinin system (195–197).

Salivary Glands

In addition to sweat glands and pancreas, VIP has been found in nerves serving exocrine glands, e.g., the submandibular salivary gland, glands in the nasal mucosa, the tongue, and tracheobronchial wall (47,422,424,427). It has been shown that stimulation of the cat chordalingual nerve, which results in a marked salivary secretion from the submandibular gland, was accompanied by an increase in plasma VIP levels in the venous effluent from the gland (298). Close intraarterial infusion of VIP antiserum reduced both vasodilatation and secretion. Infusion of VIP itself caused an atropine-resistant vasodilatation but not salivary secretion, whereas ACh infusion resulted in both salivary secretion and vasodilatation. Acetylcholine was, however, less potent than VIP in causing vasodilatation. When ACh and VIP were infused together, a marked potentiation of both secretion and vasodilatation was observed. These findings support the view that ACh and VIP could be acting together in promoting salivary secretion, and they provide a possible functional significance for the coexistence of ACh and VIP in these sympathetic neurons (298).

More recently, Lundberg at al. (299) showed that APP, in contrast to VIP, caused a marked reduction of the local blood flow in the cat submandibular gland. The APP reduced both the vasodilatory response to parasympathetic nerve stimulation and to stimulation by VIP, whereas the ACh-induced response was not affected. The APP also reduced the salivary secretion from the gland. The effects were atropine resistant. In immunohistochemical studies, an antiserum to APP demonstrated nerve fibers around blood vessels in rat submaxillary gland and cat submandibular gland (301). These observations suggest that the inhibitory actions of PP-like peptide(s) may be of physiological significance in salivary gland function (301).

SUMMARY

There is now compelling evidence for the existence of noncholinergic, nonadrenergic neurons in the peripheral nervous system. In addition to neurons that probably contain and release 5-HT and purines, there is an increasing body of data to suggest the occurrence of many small biologically active peptides in peripheral neurons. Studies on the physiology of the peripheral peptidergic nervous system are at a relatively early stage. Even so, the following conclusions now appear justified.

Substance P-, VIP-, enkephalin-, somatostatin-, CCK-, neurotensin-, bombesin-, and PP-like peptides occur in peripheral nerves that have characteristic patterns of distribution; the gastrointestinal tract is particularly rich in peptide immunoreactive neurons. In addition, there may well be other peptides, still not discovered, that occur in neurons.

Biochemical studies have shown that many of the peptides occur in more than one molecular form, exemplified by the gastrin–CCK family of peptides in the gut and the enkephalin-related peptides isolated from the adrenal medulla.

The peptides have a wide range of biological actions; the actions on the gastrointestinal tract have received particular attention. However, since some of the peptides occur in both endocrine and nerve cells in the gut, the physiological effects of these peptides may be exerted via endocrine, neurocrine, or possibly paracrine pathways.

An increasing number of peptides are now recognized to occur in neurons that contain classical transmitters (208). Although it is generally conceived that the neuropeptides occur in synaptic vesicles, it remains to be elucidated whether they occur in separate vesicles or concomitant with ACh or NE.

ACKNOWLEDGMENTS

Much of the original work described here was supported by grants from Karolinska Institutet and the Swedish Medical Research Council (04X-2887; 04X-04495) and was performed in collaboration with Dr. J. M. Lundberg in Professor T. Hökfelt's laboratory (Department of Histology, Karolinska Institutet), to whom I am grateful for generous support and advice. The author thanks Ms. W. Hiort for expert photographic assistance and Ms. E. McElroy for excellent help in typing this manuscript. Dr. G. J. Dockray and Professor R. A. Gregory are gratefully acknowledged for invaluable discussions and the development of ideas. The author thanks Dr. R. D. Cook, Professor G.

Burnstock, Dr. J. B. Furness, Dr. Lars Olson, and Dr. C. Vaillant for generously providing micrographs for this chapter. The author was in receipt of a fellowship from the Royal Society European Scientific Exchange Programme, when this chapter was written (1981).

REFERENCES

1. Abrahamsson, H. (1973): Vagal relaxation of the stomach induced from the gastric antrum. *Acta Physiol. Scand.,* 89:406–414.

2. Abrahamsson, H., and Jansson, G. (1969): Elicitation of reflex vagal relaxation of the stomach from pharynx and esophagus in the cat. *Acta Physiol. Scand.,* 77:172–178.

3. Abrahamsson, H., and Jansson, G. (1973): Reflex vagal inhibition of esophageal motility. *Acta Physiol. Scand.,* 89:600–602.

4. Abrahamsson, H., and Jansson, G. (1973): Vago-vagal gastro–gastric relaxation in the cat. *Acta Physiol. Scand.,* 88:209–295.

5. Aghajanian, G. K., and Bloom, F. E. (1966): Electron-microscopic autoradiography of rat hypothalamus after intraventricular H^3-norepinephrine. *Science,* 153:308–310.

6. Aghajanian, G. K., and Bloom, F. E. (1967): Localization of tritiated serotonin in rat brain by electron-microscopic autoradiography. *J. Pharmacol. Exp. Ther.,* 156:23–30

7. Aghajanian, G. K., Bloom, F. E., Lovell, R. A., Sheard, M. H., and Freeman, D. X. (1966): The uptake of 5-hydroxytryptamine ^3H from the cerebral ventricles: Autoradiographic localization. *Biochem. Pharmacol.,* 15:1401–1403.

8. Alberti, K. G. M. M., Christensen, S. E., Iversen, J., Seyerhansen, K., Christensen, N. J., Hansen, A. A. P., Lundbaek, K., and Örskov, H. (1973): Inhibition of insulin secretion by somatostatin. *Lancet,* 1:1299–1301.

9. Alm, P., Alumets, J., Brodin, E., Håkanson, R., Nilsson, G., Sjöberg, N.-O., and Sundler, F. (1978): Peptidergic (substance P) nerves in the genitourinary tract. *Neuroscience,* 3:419–425.

10. Alm, P., Aluments, J., Håkanson, R., and Sundler, F. (1977): Peptidergic (vasoactive intestinal peptide) nerves in the genitourinary tract. *Neuroscience,* 2:751–754.

11. Almeida, H. O., Tafuri, W. L., Cunha-Melo, J. R., Freire-Maia, L., Raso, P., and Brenzer, Z. (1977): Studies on the vesicular component of the Auerbachs plexus and the substance P content of the mouse colon in the acute phase of the experimental *Trypanosoma cruzi* infection. *Virchows Arch. Pathol. Anat. Histol.,* 376:353–360.

12. Alumets. J., Fahrenkrug, J., Håkanson, R., Schaffalitzky de Muckadell, O., Sundler, F., and Uddman, R. (1979): A rich VIP nerve supply is characteristic of sphincters. *Nature,* 280:155–156.

13. Alumets, J., Håkanson, R., Sundler, F., and Chang, K. J. (1978): Leu-enkephalin-like material in nerves and enterochromaffin cells in the gut. *Histochemistry,* 56:187–196.

14. Ålund, M., and Olson, L. (1979): Depolarization-induced decreases in fluorescence intensity of gastrointestinal quinacrine-binding nerve. *Brain Res.,* 166:121–137.

15. Ambache, N. (1951): Unmasking, after cholinergic paralysis by botulinum toxin of a reversed action of nicotine on the mammalian intestine, revealing the probable presence of local inhibitory ganglion cells in the enteric plexus. *Br. J. Pharmacol.,* 6:51–67.

16. Ambache, N., and Freeman, M. A. (1968): Atropine-resistant longitudinal muscle spasms due to excitation of non-cholinergic neurones in Auerbach's plexus. *J. Physiol. (Lond.),* 199:705–728.

17. Ambache, N., Verney, J., and Zar, M. A. (1970): Evidence for the release of two atropine-resistant spasmogens from Auerbach's plexus. *J. Physiol. (Lond).,* 207:761–782.

18. Ambache, N., and Zar, M. A. (1970): Non-cholinergic transmission by postganglionic motor neurones in the mammalian bladder. *J. Physiol. (Lond.),* 210:761–783.

19. Anastasi, A., Erspamer, V., and Bucci, M. (1971): Isolation and structure of bombesin and alytesin, two analogous active peptides from the skin of the European amphibians, *Bombina* and *Alytes. Experientia,* 27:166–167.

20. Anastasi, A., Erspamer, V., and Endean, R. (1975): Amino acid composition and sequence of litorin, a bombesin-like nonapeptide from the skin of the Australian leptodactylid frog *Litoria rea. Experientia,* 31:510–511.

21. Andersson, S., Chang, E., Folkers, K., and Rosell, S. (1976): Inhibition of gastric acid secretion in dogs by neurotensin. *Life Sci.,* 19:367–371.

21a. Arimura, A., Sato, H., Dupont, A., Nishi, N., and Schally, A. V. (1975): Somatostatin: Abundance of immunoreactive hormone in rat stomach and pancreas. *Science,* 189:1007–1009.

22. Barclay, A. E. (1936): *The Digestive Tract: A Radiological Study of Its Anatomy, Physiology and Pathology,* 2nd ed. Cambridge University Press, Cambridge.

23. Barros D'Sa, A. A. J., Bloom, S. R., and Baron, J. H. (1975): Direct inhibition of gastric acid by growth-hormone release-inhibiting hormones in dogs. *Lancet,* 1:886–887.

24. Barry, J., Dubois, M. P., and Poulain, P. (1973): LRF producing cells of the mammalian hypothalamus. A fluorescent antibody study. *Z. Zellforsch. Mikrosk. Anat.,* 146:351–366.

25. Baumgarten, H. G., Holstein, A. F., and Owman, C. (1970): Auerbach's plexus of mammals and man: Electron microscopic identification of three different types of neuronal processes in myenteric ganglia of the large intestine from rhesus monkeys, guinea-pigs and man. *Z. Zellforsch.,* 106:376–397.

26. Bayliss, W. M., and Starling, E. H. (1899): The movement and innervation of the small intestine. *J. Physiol. (Lond.),* 24:99–143.

27. Bayliss, W. M., and Starling, E. H. (1902): The mechanism of pancreatic secretion. *J. Physiol. (Lond.),* 28:325–353.

28. Béléslin, D., and Varagić, V. (1960): The effect of substance P on the responses of the isolated guinea-pig ileum to acetylcholine, nicotine, histamine and 5-hydroxytryptamine. *Arch. Int. Pharmacodyn.*, 126:321–327.

29. Bennett, M. R., and Burnstock, G. (1968): Electrophysiology of the innervation of the intestinal smooth muscle. In: *Handbook of Physiology, Section 6: Alimentary Canal. IV: Motility,* edited by C. F. Code, pp. 1709–1732. American Physiological Society, Washington.

30. Bennett, M. R., Burnstock, G., and Holman, M. E. (1966): Transmission from perivascular inhibitory nerves to the smooth muscle of the guinea-pig taenia coli. *J. Physiol. (Lond.),* 182:527–540.

31. Bertaccini, G., Erspamer, V., Melchiorri, P., and Sopranzi, N. (1974): Gastrin release by bombesin in the dog. *Br. J. Pharmacol.,* 52:219–225.

32. Bertaccini, G., Impicciatore, M., Molina, E., and Zappia, L. (1974): Action of bombesin on human gastrointestinal motility. *Rend. Gastroenterol.,* 6:45–51.

33. Besson, J., Laburthe, M., Bataille, D., Dupont, C., and Rosselin, G. (1978): Vasoactive intestinal peptide (VIP): Tissue distribution in the rat as measured by radioimmunoassay and by radioreceptorassay. *Acta Endocrinol. (Kbh.),* 87:799–810.

34. Biber, B., Lundgren, O., and Svanvik, J. (1971): Studies on the intestinal vasodilatation observed after mechanical stimulation of the mucosa of the gut. *Acta Physiol. Scand.,* 82:177–190.

35. Bloom, F. E., Battenberg, E., Rossier, J., Ling, N., and Guillemin, R. (1978): Neurons containing β-endorphin in rat brain exist separately from those containing enkephalin: Immunocytochemical studies. *Proc. Natl. Acad. Sci. U.S.A.,* 75:1591–1595.

36. Bloom, S. R. (1978): *Gut Hormones.* Churchill Livingstone, Edinburgh.

37. Bloom, S. R., and Gardner, J. D. (1978): The VIP controversy. *Dig. Dis.,* 23:370–376.

38. Bloom, S. R., Ghatei, M. A., Wharton, J. W., Polak, J. M., and Brown, M. R. (1979): Distribution of bombesin in human alimentary tract. *Gastroenterology,* 76:1103.

39. Bodanszky, M., Klausner, Y. S., and Said, S. I. (1976): Biological activities of synthetic peptides corresponding to fragments of and to the entire sequence of the vasoactive intestinal peptide. *Proc. Natl. Acad. Sci. U.S.A.,* 70:382–384.

40. Bradbury, A. F., Smyth, D. G., and Snell, C. R. (1976): Lipotropin C-fragment—an endogenous peptide with potent analgesic activity. In: *Opiates and Endogenous Opioid Peptides,* edited by H. W. Kosterlitz, pp. 9–17. Elsevier/North Holland Biomedical Press, Amsterdam.

41. Brazeau, P., Ling, N., Esch, F., Böhlen, P., Benoit, P., and Guillemin, R. (1981): High biological activity of the synthetic replicates of somatostatin-28 and somatostatin-25. *Regul. Peptides,* 1:255–264.

42. Brazeau, P., Vale, W., Burgus, R., Ling, N., Butcher, M., Rivier, J., and Guillemin, R. (1973): Hypothalamic polypeptide that inhibits the secretion of immunoreactive pituitary growth hormone. *Science,* 179:77–79.

43. Brimijoin, S., Lundberg, J. M., Brodin, E., Hökfelt, T., and Nilsson, G. (1980): Axonal transport of substance P in the vagus and sciatic nerves of the guinea pig. *Brain Res.,* 191:443–457.

44. Broccardo, M., Falconieri Erspamer, G., Melchiorri, P., Negri, L., and De Castiglione, R. (1975): Relative potency of bombesin-like peptides. *Br. J. Pharmacol.,* 55:221–227.

45. Brown, M., Rivier, J., Kobayashi, R., and Vale, W. (1978): Neurotensin-like and bombesin-like peptides: CNS distribution and actions. In: *Gut Hormones,* edited by S. R. Bloom, pp. 550–558. Churchill Livingstone, Edinburgh.

46. Brown, M. R., and Vale, W. W. (1976): Effects of neurotensin and substance P on glucoregulation. *Endocrinology,* 98:819–822.

47. Bryant, M. G., Polak, M. M., Modlin, L., Bloom, S. R., Albuquerque, R. H., and Pears, A. G. E. (1976): Possible dual role for vasoactive intestinal peptide as gastrointestinal hormone and neurotransmitter substance. *Lancet,* 1:991–993.

48. Buchan, A. M. J., Polak, J. M., Sullivan, S., Bloom, S. R., Brown, M., and Pearse, A. G. E. (1978): Neurotensin in the gut. In: *Gut Hormones,* edited by S. R. Bloom, pp. 544–549. Churchill Livingstone, Edinburgh.

49. Buckley, G., Consolo, S., and Sjöqvist, F. (1967): Cholinacetylase in innervated and denervated sympathetic ganglia and ganglion cells of the cat. *Acta Physiol. Scand.,* 71:348–356.

50. Burnstock, G. (1972): The purinergic nervous system. *Pharmacol. Rev.,* 24:509–581.

51. Burnstock, G. (1979): Cholinergic and purinergic regulation of blood vessels. In: *Handbook of Physiology, Section 2: Circulation, Vol. IV: Vascular Smooth Muscle,* edited by D. Bohr, A. Somlyo, and H. Sparks. Williams & Wilkins, Baltimore *(in press).*

52. Burnstock, G., Campbell, G., Bennett, M., and Holman, M. E. (1963): The effects of drugs on the transmission of inhibition from autonomic nerves to the smooth muscle of the guinea-pig taenia coli. *Biochem. Pharmacol.,* 12(Suppl.), 467:134.

53. Burnstock, G., Campbell, G., Bennett, M., and Holman, M. E. (1964): Innervation of the guinea-pig taenia coli: Are there intrinsic inhibitory nerves which are distinct from sympathetic nerves? *Int. J. Neuropharmacol.,* 3:163–166.

54. Burnstock, G., Cocks, T., Kasakov, L., and Wong, H. (1978): Direct evidence for ATP release from nonadrenergic, noncholinergic ("purinergic") nerves in the guinea-pig taenia coli and bladder. *Eur. J. Pharmacol.,* 49:145–149.

55. Burnstock, G., and Costa, M. (1973): Inhibitory innervation of the gut. *Gastroenterology,* 64:141–144.

56. Burnstock, G., and Costa, M. (1975). *Adrenergic Neurons, Their Organization, Function and Development in the Peripheral Nervous System.* John Wiley & Sons, New York.

57. Burnstock, G., Hökfelt, T., Gershon, M. D., Iversen, L. L., Kosterlitz, H. W., and Szurszewski, J. H. (1979): Nonadrenergic, noncholinergic autonomic neurotransmission mechanisms. *Neurosi. Res. Prog. Bull.,* 17:379–519.

58. Bury, R. W., and Mashford, M. L. (1977): A phar-macological investigation of synthetic substance P on the isolated guinea-pig ileum. *Clin. Exp. Pharmacol. Physiol.*, 4:453–461.
59. Campbell, G. (1970): Autonomic nervous system to effector tissues. In: *Smooth Muscle,* edited by E. Bülbring, A. F. Brading, A. W. Jones, and T. Tomita, pp. 451–485. Williams & Wilkins, Baltimore.
60. Campbell, G., and Burnstock, G. (1968): The comparative physiology of gastrointestinal motility. In: *Handbook of Physiology, Section 6: Alimentary Canal, Motility, Vol. IX,* edited by C. F. Code, pp. 2213–2266. American Physiological Society, Washington.
61. Cannon, W. B., and Lieb, C. W. (1911): The receptive relaxation of the stomach. *Am. J. Physiol.*, 29:441–454.
62. Caprilli, R., Melchiorri, P., Improta, G., Vernia, P., and Frieri, G. (1975): Effects of bombesin and bombesin-like peptides on gastrointestinal myoelectric activity. *Gastroenterology,* 68:1228–1235.
63. Carraway, R., and Leeman, S. E. (1973): The isolation of a new hypotensive peptide, neurotensin, from bovine hypothalami. *J. Biol. Chem.,* 248:6854–6861.
64. Carraway, R., and Leeman, S. E. (1974): The amino acid sequence, chemical synthesis, and radioimmunoassay of neurotensin. *Fed. Proc.,* 23:548.
65. Carraway, R., and Leeman, S. E. (1975): The amino acid sequence of a hypothalamic peptide, neurotensin. *J. Biol. Chem.,* 250:1907–1911.
66. Chang, M. M., and Leeman, S. E. (1970): Isolation of a sialogogic peptide from bovine hypothalamic tissue and its characterization as substance P. *J. Biol. Chem.,* 245:4784–4790.
67. Chang, M. M., Leeman, S. E., and Niall, H. D. (1971): Amino-acid sequence of substance P. *Nature [New Biol.],* 232:86–87.
68. Clement-Jones, V., Lowry, P. J., Rees, L. H., and Besser, G. M. (1980): Met-enkephalin circulates in human plasma. *Nature,* 283:295–297.
69. Cooks, T., and Burnstock, G. (1979): Effects of neuronal polypeptides on intestinal smooth muscle: A comparison with non-adrenergic, non-cholinergic nerve stimulation and ATP. *Eur. J. Pharmacol.,* 54:251–259.
70. Cohen, M. L., Rosing, E., Wiley, K. S., and Slater, I. H. (1978): Somatostatin inhibits adrenergic and cholinergic neurotransmission in smooth muscle. *Life Sci.,* 23:1659–1664.
71. Cook, R. D., and Burnstock, G. (1976): The ultrastructure of Auerbach's plexus in the guinea pig. I. Neuronal elements. *J. Neurocytol.,* 5:171–194.
72. Cook, R. D., and King, A. S. (1970): Observations on the ultrastructure of the smooth muscle and its innervation in the avian lung. *J. Anat.,* 106:273–283.
73. Coons, A. H. (1958): Fluorescent antibody methods. In: *General Cytochemical Methods,* edited by J. F. Danielli, pp. 399–422. Academic Press, New York.
74. Corrêa, F. M. A., Innis, R. B., Uhl, G. R., and Snyder, S. H. (1979): Bradykinin-like immunoreactive neuronal systems localized histochemically in rat brain. *Proc. Natl. Acad. Sci. U.S.A.,* 76:1489–1493.
75. Costa, M., Cuello, A. C., Furness, J. B., and Franco, R. (1980): Distribution of enteric neurons showing immunoreactivity for substance P in the guinea-pig ileum. *Neuroscience,* 5:323–331.
76. Costa, M., and Furness, J. B. (1973): The innervation of the internal anal sphincter in the guinea-pig. *Gastroenterology,* 5:37–38.
77. Costa, M., and Furness, J. B. (1976): The peristaltic reflex: An analysis of the nerve pathways and their pharmacology. *Naunyn Schmiedebergs Arch. Pharmacol.,* 294:47–60.
78. Costa, M., and Furness, J. B. (1979): On the possibility that an idoleamine is a neurotransmitter in the gastrointestinal tract. *Biochem. Pharmacol.,* 28:565–571.
79. Costa, M., Furness, J. B., Buffa, R., and Said, S. I. (1980): Distribution of enteric nerve cell bodies and axons showing immunoreactivity for vasoactive intestinal polypeptide in the guinea-pig ileum. *Neuroscience,* 5:587–596.
80. Costa, M., Furness, J. B., and Gabella, G. (1971): Catecholamine containing nerve cells in the mammalian myenteric plexus. *Histochemie,* 25:103–106.
81. Costa, M., Furness, J. B., Lewellyn-Smith, I. J., and Cuello, A. C. (1981): Projections of substance P-containing neurons within the guinea-pig small intestine. *Neuroscience,* 6:411–424.
82. Costa, M., Furness, J. B., Llewellyn-Smith, I. J., Davies, B., and Oliver, J. (1980): An immunohistochemical study of the projections of somatostatin-containing neurons in the guinea-pig intestine. *Neuroscience,* 5:841–852.
83. Costa, M., Patel, Y., Furness, J. B., and Arimura, A. (1977): Evidence that some intrinsic neurons of the intestine contain somatostatin. *Neuroscience Lett.,* 6:215–222.
84. Coupland, R. E. (1965): *The Natural History of the Chromaffin Cell,* pp. 1–279. Longmans, London.
85. Coupland, R. E. (1972): The chromaffin system: In: *Catecholamines,* edited by H. Blaschko and E. Muscholl, pp. 16–45. Springer, Berlin.
86. Coupland, R. E., and Fujita, T. (1976): *Chromaffin, Enterochromaffin and Related Cells.* Elsevier, Amsterdam.
87. Cozzari, C., and Hartman, B. K. (1980): Preparation of antibodies specific to choline acetyltransferase from bovine caudate nucleus and immunohistochemical localization of the enzyme. *Proc. Natl. Acad. Sci. U.S.A.,* 77:7453–7457.
88. Crowcroft, P. J., Holman, M. E., and Szurszewski, J. H. (1971): Excitatory input from the distal colon to the inferior mesenteric ganglion in the guinea-pig. *J. Physiol. (Lond.),* 219:443–461.
89. Cuello, A. C., Galfree, G., and Milstein, C. (1979): Detection of substance P in the central nervous system by a monoclonal antibody. *Proc. Natl. Acad. Sci. U.S.A.,* 76:3532–3536.
90. Dahlström, A. (1965): Observations on the accu-

mulation of noradrenaline in the proximal and distal parts of peripheral adrenergic nerves after compression. *J. Anat.*, 99:677–689.

91. Dahlström, A. (1968): Effect of colchicine on transport of amine storage granules in sympathetic nerves of rat. *Eur. J. Pharmacol.*, 5:111–112.

92. Dahlström, A. (1971): Effects of vinblastine and colchicine on monoamine containing neurons of the rat, with special regard to the axoplasmic transport of amine granules. *Acta Neuropathol. [Suppl.] (Berl.)*, 5:226–237.

93. Dale, H. H., and Feldberg, W. (1934): The chemical transmission of secretory impulses to the sweat glands of the cat. *J. Physiol. (Lond.)*, 82:121–128.

93a. Dalsgaard, C.-J., Hökfelt, T., Schultzberg, M., Lundberg, J. M., Terenius, L., Dockray, G. J., Cuello, C., and Goldstein, M. (1983): Origin of peptide-containing fibres in the inferior mesenteric ganglion of the guinea pig: Immunohistochemical studies with antisera to substance P, enkephalin, vasoactive intestinal polypeptide, cholecystokinin/gastrin and bombesin. *Neuroscience (in press)*.

94. Dean, D. M., and Downie, J. W. (1978): Interaction of prostaglandins and adenosine 5-triphosphate in non-cholinergic neurotransmission in rabbit detrusor. *Prostaglandins*, 16:245–251.

95. DiGiulio, A. M., Yang, H.-Y. T., Lutold, B., Fratta, W., Hong, J., and Costa, E. (1978): Characterization of enkephalin-like material extracted from sympathetic ganglia. *Neuropharmacology*, 17:989–992.

96. Dimaline, R., and Dockray, G. J. (1978): Multiple immunoreactive forms of vasoactive intestinal peptide in human colonic mucosa. *Gastroenterology*, 75:387–392.

97. Dimaline, R., and Dockray, G. J. (1979): Potent stimulation of the avian exocrine pancreas by porcine and chicken vasoactive intestinal peptides. *J. Physiol. (Lond.)*, 294:153–163.

98. Dimaline, R., and Dockray, G. J. (1979): Molecular variants of vasoactive intestinal polypeptide in dog, rat and hog. *Life Sci.*, 25:1893–1900.

99. Dimaline, R., and Dockray, G. J. (1980): Actions of a new peptide from porcine intestine (PHI) on pancreatic secretion in the rat and turkey. *Life Sci.*, 27:1947–1951.

100. Dimaline, R., Vaillant, C., and Dockray, G. J. (1980): The use of region-specific antibodies in the characterization and localization of vasoactive intestinal polypeptide-like substances in the rat gastrointestinal tract. *Regul. Peptides*, 1:1–16.

101. Dingledine, R., and Goldstein, A. (1976): Effect of synaptic transmission blockade on morphine action in the guinea-pig myenteric plexus. *J. Pharmacol. Exp. Ther.*, 196:97–106.

102. Dockray, G. J. (1979): Immunochemistry of gastrin and cholecystokinin: Development and application of region specific antisera. In: *Gastrins and the Vagus*, edited by J. F. Rehfeld and E. Amdrup, pp. 73–83. Academic Press, New York.

103. Dockray, G. J., Gregory, R. A., Hutchinson, J. B., Harris, I. J., and Runswick, M. J. (1978): Isolation, structure and biological activity of two cholecysto-kinin octapeptides from sheep brain. *Nature*, 274:711–713.

104. Dockray, G. J., Gregory, R. A., Tracy, H. J., and Zhu, W.-Y. (1981): Transport of cholecystokinin-octapeptide-like immunoreactivity toward the gut in afferent vagal fibres in cat and dog. *J. Physiol. (Lond.)*, 314:501–511.

105. Dockray, G. J., and Tracy, H. J. (1980): Atropine does not abolish cephalic vagal stimulation of gastrin release in dogs. *J. Physiol. (Lond.)*, 306:473–480.

106. Dockray, G. J., Vaillant, C., and Walsh, J. H. (1979): The neuronal origin of bombesin-like immunoreactivity in the rat gastrointestinal tract. *Neuroscience*, 4:1561–1568.

107. Domschke, S., Domschke, W., Rösch, W., Konturek, S. J., Sprügel, W., Mitznegg, P., Wünsch, E., and Demling, L. (1966): Vasoactive intestinal peptide: A secretin-like partial agonist for pancreatic secretion in man. *Gastroenterology*, 73:478–480.

108. Dreyfus, C. F., Bornstein, M. B., and Gershon, M. D. (1977): Synthesis of serotonin by neurons of the myenteric plexus *in situ* and in organotypic tissue culture. *Brain Res.*, 128:125–139.

109. Dreyfus, C. F., Sherman, D. L., and Gershon, M. D. (1977): Uptake of serotonin by intrinsic neurons of the myenteric plexus grown in organotypic tissue culture. *Brain Res.*, 128:109–123.

110. Du Vigneaud, V. (1956): Hormones of the posterior pituitary glands: Oxytocin and vasopressin. In: *Harvey Lectures, 1954–1955*, pp. 1–26. Academic Press, New York.

111. Edin, R., Lundberg, J. M., Ahlman, H., Kewenter, J., Dahlström, A., Fahrenkrug, J., and Hökfelt, T. (1979): On the VIP-ergic innervation of the feline pylorus. *Acta Physiol. Scand.*, 107:185–187.

112. Edin, R., Lundberg, J. M., Lidberg, P., Dahlström, A., and Ahlman, H. (1980): Atropine sensitive contractile motor effects of substance P on the feline pylorus and stomach. *Acta Physiol. Scand.*, 119:207–209.

113. Ehrenpreis, T., and Pernow, B. (1952): On the occurrence of substance P in Hirschprung's disease. *Acta Physiol. Scand.*, 27:380–388.

114. Eklund, S., Jodal, M., Lundgren, O., and Sjöqvist, A. (1979): Effects of vasoactive intestinal polypeptide on blood flow, motility and fluid transport in the gastrointestinal tract of the cat. *Acta Physiol. Scand.*, 105:461–468.

115. Elde, R., Hökfelt, T., Johansson, O., and Terenius, L. (1976): Immunohistochemical studies using antibodies to leucine-enkephalin. Initial observations on the nervous system of the rat. *Neuroscience*, 1:349–351.

116. Elfvin, L.-G., and Dalsgaard, C. J. (1977): Retrograde axonal transport of horseradish peroxidase in afferent fibers of the inferior mesenteric ganglion of the guinea-pig. Identification of the cells of origin in dorsal root ganglia. *Brain Res.*, 126:149–153.

117. Elfvin, L.-G., Hökfelt, T., and Goldstein, M. (1975): Fluorescence microscopical, immunohistochemical and ultrastructural studies on sympathetic ganglia of the guinea pig with special reference to

the SIF cells and their catecholamine content. *J. Ultrastruct. Res.*, 51:377–396.

118. Eränkö, O. (1976): *SIF Cells, Structure and Function of the Small Intensely Fluorescent Sympathetic Cells (Fogarty International Center Proceedings No. 30).* United States Government Printing Office, Washington, D.C.

119. Eränkö, O., and Härkönen, A. (1964): Noradrenaline and acetylcholinesterase in sympathetic ganglion cells of the rat. *Acta Physiol. Scand.*, 61:299–300.

120. Erspamer, V., Anastasi, A., Bertaccini, G., and Cei, J. M. (1964): Structure and pharmacological actions of physalaemin, the main active polypeptide of the skin of *Physalaemus fuscumaculatus. Experientia,* 20:489–490.

121. Erspamer, V., and Falconieri Erspamer, G. (1962): Pharmacological actions of eledoisin on extravascular smooth muscle. *Br. J. Pharmacol.,* 19:337–354.

122. Erspamer, V., Falconieri Erspamer, G., and Linari, G. (1977): Occurrence of tachykinins (physalemin- or substance P-like peptides) in the amphibian skin and their actions on smooth muscle preparations. In: *Substance P, Nobel Symposium 37,* edited by U.S. von Euler and B. Pernow, pp. 67–74. Raven Press, New York.

123. Erspamer, V., Improta, G., Melchiorri, P., and Sopranzi, N. (1974): Evidence of cholecystokinin release by bombesin in the dog. *Br. J. Pharmacol.,* 52:227–232.

124. Erspamer, V., and Melchiorri, P. (1973): Active polypeptides of the amphibian skin and their synthetic analogues. *Pure Appl. Chem.,* 35:463–494.

125. Erspamer, V., and Melchiorri, P. (1975): Actions of bombesin on secretions and motility of the gastrointestinal tract. In: *Gastrointestinal Hormones,* edited by J. C. Thompson, pp. 575–589. University of Texas Press, Austin.

126. Erspamer, V., Melchiorri, P., Falconieri Erspamer, C., and Negri, L. (1978): Polypeptides of the amphibian skin, active on the gut and their mammalian counterparts. In: *Gastrointestinal Hormones and Pathology of the Digestive System,* edited by M. Grossman, V. Speranza, N. Basso, and E. Lezoche, pp. 51–64. Plenum Press, New York.

127. Fahrenkrug, J. (1979): Vasoactive intestinal polypeptide: Measurement, distribution and putative neurotransmitter function. *Digestion,* 19:149–169.

128. Fahrenkrug, J., Galbo, H., Holst, J. J., Schaffalitzky de Muckadell, O. B. (1978): Influence of the autonomic nervous system on the release of vasoactive intestinal polypeptide from the porcine gastrointestinal tract. *J. Physiol. (Lond.),* 230:405–422.

129. Fahrenkrug, J., Haglund, U., Jodal, M., Lundgren, O., Olbe, L., and Schaffalitzky De Muckadell, O. B. (1978): Nervous release of vasoactive intestinal polypeptide in the gastrointestinal tract of cats: Possible physiological implications. *J. Physiol. (Lond.),* 284:291–305.

130. Fahrenkrug, J., Schaffalitzky de Muckadell, O. B., Holst, J. J., and Lindkaer Jensen, S. (1979): Role of VIP in the vagally mediated pancreatic secretion of fluid and bicarbonate. *Am. J. Physiol.,* 237:E535–E541.

131. Falck, B. (1962): Observations on the possibilities of the cellular localization of monoamines by a fluorescence method. *Acta Physiol. Scand. [Suppl.],* 197:1–25.

132. Falck, B., Hillarp, N.-A., Thieme, G., and Torp, A. (1962): Fluorescence of catecholamines and related compounds with formaldehyde. *J. Histochem. Cytochem.,* 10:348–354.

133. Fox, R. H., and Hilton, S. M. (1958): Bradykinin formation in human skin as a factor in heat vasodilatation. *J. Physiol. (Lond.),* 142:219–232.

134. Franco, R., Costa, M., and Furness, J. B. (1979): Evidence for the release of endogenous substance P from intestinal nerves. *Naunyn Schmiedebergs Arch. Pharmacol.,* 306:185–201.

135. Franco, R., Costa, M., and Furness, J. B. (1979): Evidence that axons containing substance P in the guinea-pig ileum are of intrinsic origin. *Naunyn Schmiedebergs Arch. Pharmacol.,* 307:57–63.

136. Frigerio, B., Ravazola, M., Ito, S., Buffa, R., Capella, C., Solcia, E., and Orci, L. (1977): Histochemical and ultrastructural identification of neurotensin cells in the dog ileum. *Histochemistry,* 54:123–131.

137. Furness, J. B., and Costa, M. (1971): Monoamine oxidase histochemistry of enteric neurons in the guinea-pig. *Histochemie,* 28:324–336.

138. Furness, J. B., and Costa, M. (1971): Storage-uptake and synthesis of catecholamines in the intrinsic adrenergic nerones in the proximal colon of the guinea-pig. *Z. Zellforsch. Mikrosk. Anat.,* 120:364–385.

139. Furness, J. B., and Costa, M. (1973): The nervous release and the action of substances which affect intestinal muscle through neither adrenoceptors nor cholinoceptors. *Phil. Trans. R. Soc. [Biol.],* 265:123–133.

140. Furness, J. B., and Costa, M. (1974): The adrenergic innervation of the gastrointestinal tract. *Ergeb. Physiol.,* 69:1–52.

141. Furness, J. B., and Costa, M. (1977): The participation of enteric inhibitory nerves in accommodation of the intestine to distension. *Clin. Exp. Pharmacol. Physiol.,* 4:37–41.

142. Furness, J. B., and Costa, M. (1978): Distribution of intrinsic nerve cell bodies and axons which take up aromatic amines and their precursors in the small intestine of the guinea-pig. *Cell Tissue Res.,* 188:527–543.

143. Furness, J. B., and Costa, M. (1979): Actions of somatostatin on excitatory and inhibitory nerves in the intestine. *Eur. J. Pharmacol.,* 56:69–74.

144. Furness, J. B., and Costa, M. (1979): Projections of intestinal neurons showing immunoreactivity for vasoactive intestinal polypeptide are consistent with these neurons being the enteric inhibitory neurons. *Neurosci. Lett.,* 15:199–204.

145. Furness, J. B., and Costa, M. (1980): Types of nerves in the enteric nervous system. *Neuroscience,* 5:1–20.

146. Furness, J. B., Costa, M., and Freeman, C. G. (1979): Absence of tyrosine hydroxylase activity

and dopamine β-hydroxylase immunoreactivity in intrinsic nerves of the guinea-pig ileum. *Neuroscience*, 4:305–310.

147. Furness, J. B., Costa, M., and Walsh, J. H. (1981): Evidence for and significance of the projection of VIP neurons from the myenteric plexus to the taenia coli in the guinea-pig. *Gastroenterology*, 80:1557–1561.

148. Fuxe, K., Ganten, D., Hökfelt, T., and Bolme, P. (1976): Immunohistochemical evidence for the existence of angiotensin II-containing nerve terminals in the brain and spinal cord of the rat. *Neurosci. Lett.*, 2:229–234.

149. Fuxe, K., Hökfelt, T., Said, S. I., and Mutt, V. (1977): Vasoactive intestinal polypeptide and the nervous system: Immunohistochemical evidence for localization in central and peripheral neurons, particularly intracortical neurons of the cerebral cortex. *Neurosci. Lett.*, 5:241–246.

150. Gabella, G. (1972): Fine structure of the myenteric plexus in the guinea pig. *J. Anat.*, 111:69–97.

151. Gabella, G. (1976): *Structure of the Autonomic Nervous System*. Chapman and Hall, London.

152. Gabella, G. (1979): Innervation of the gastrointestinal tract. *Int. Rev. Cytol.*, 59:129–193.

153. Gaginella, T. S., Mekhjian, H. S., and O'Dorisio, T. M. (1978): Vasoactive intestinal peptide: Quantification by radioimmunoassay in isolated cells, mucosa, and muscle of the hamster intestine. *Gastroenterology*, 74:718–721.

154. Gamse, R., Lembeck, F., and Cuello, A. C. (1979): Substance P in the vagus nerve: Immunochemical and immunohistochemical evidence for axoplasmic transport. *Naunyn Schmiedebergs Arch. Pharmacol.*, 306:37–44.

155. Ganten, D., Fuxe, K., Phillips, M. I., Mann, J. F. E., and Ganten, U. (1978): The brain isorenin–angiotensin system: Biochemistry, localization, and possible role in drinking and blood pressure regulation. In: *Frontiers in Neuroendocrinology, Vol. 5*, edited by W. F. Ganong and L. Martini, pp. 61–69. Raven Press, New York.

156. Garrett, J. R., and Howard E. R. (1972): Effects of rectal distension on the internal anal sphincter of cats. *J. Physiol. (Lond.)*, 222:90P–91P.

157. Gaskell, W. H. (1916): *The Involuntary Nervous System*. Longmans Green, London.

158. Gentleman, S., Ross, M., Lowney, L. I., Cox, B. M., and Goldstein, A. (1976): Pituitary endorphins. In: *Opiates and Endogenous Opioid Peptides*, edited by H. W. Kosterlitz, pp. 27–34. North-Holland, Amsterdam.

159. Gerich, J. E., Lorenzi, M., Schneider, V., Kwan, C. W., Karam, J. H., Guillemin, R., and Forsham, P. H. (1974): Inhibition of pancreatic glucagon response to arginine by somatostatin in normal man and in insulin-dependent diabetics. *Diabetes*, 23:876–880.

160. Gershon, M. D., and Altman, R. F. (1971): An analysis of the uptake of 5-hydroxytryptamine by the myenteric plexus of the small intestine of the guinea pig. *J. Pharmacol. Exp. Ther.*, 179:29–41.

161. Gershon, M. D., Dreyfus, C. F., Pickel, V. M., Joh, T. H., and Reis, D. J. (1977): Serotonergic neurons in the peripheral nervous system: Identification in gut by immunohistochemical localization of tryptophan hydroxylase. *Proc. Natl. Acad. Sci. U.S.A.*, 74:3086–3089.

162. Gershon, M. D., Robinson, R. G., and Ross, L. L. (1976): Serotonin accumulation in the guinea pig's myenteric plexus: Ion dependence, structure activity relationship, and the effect of drugs. *J. Pharmacol. Exp. Ther.*, 198:548–561.

163. Gershon, M. D., and Ross, L. L. (1976): Location of sites of 5-hydroxytryptamine storage and metabolism by radioautography. *J. Physiol. (Lond.)*, 186:477–492.

164. Giachetti, A., and Said, S. I. (1979): Axonal transport of vasoactive intestinal peptide in sciatic nerve. *Nature*, 281:574–575.

165. Giachetti, A., Said, S., Reynolds, R. C., and Koniges, F. C. (1977): Vasoactive intestinal polypeptide in brain: Localization in and release from isolated nerve terminals. *Proc. Natl. Acad. Sci. U.S.A.*, 74:3424–3428.

166. Giacobini, E. (1959): The distribution and localization of cholinesterase in nerve cells. *Acta Physiol. Scand. [Suppl.]*, 156:1–45.

167. Giacobini, E., Palmborg, B., and Sjöqvist, F. (1967): Cholinesterase activity in innervated and denervated sympathetic ganglion cells of the cat. *Acta Physiol. Scand.*, 69:355–361.

168. Goldstein, A., Tachibana, S., Lowney, L. I., Hunkapiller, M., and Hood, L. (1979): Dynorphin-(1–13), an extraordinarily potent opioid peptide. *Proc. Natl. Acad. Sci. U.S.A.*, 76:6666–6670.

169. Gomez-Pan, A., Reed, J. D., Albinus, H., Shaw, B., Hull, R., Besser, G. M., Coy, D. H., Kastin, A. J., and Schally, A. V. (1975): Direct inhibition of gastric acid and pepsin secretion by growth-hormone release-inhibiting hormone in cats. *Lancet*, 1:888–890.

170. Goodfriend, T. L., Levine, L., and Fasman, G. D. (1964): Antibodies to bradykinin and angiotensin: A use of carbodiimides in immunology. *Science*, 144:1344–1346.

171. Goyal, R. K., and Rattan, S. (1980): VIP as a possible neurotransmitter of noncholinergic nonadrenergic inhibitory neurones. *Nature*, 288:378–380.

172. Gros, C., Pradelles, P., Rouget, C., Bepoldin, O., and Dray, F. (1978): Radioimmunoassay of methionine- and leucine-enkephalins on regions of rat brain and comparison with endorphins estimated by a radioreceptor assay. *J. Neurochem.*, 31:29–39.

173. Grafe, P., Mayer, C. J., and Wood, J. H. (1979): Evidence that substance P does not mediate slow synaptic excitation within the myenteric plexus. *Nature*, 279:720–721.

174. Gregory, R. A., and Tracy, H. J. (1964): The constitution and properties of two gastrins extracted from hog antral mucosa. *Gut*, 5:103–114.

175. Gregory, R. A., and Tracy, H. J. (1972): Isolation of two "big gastrins" from Zollinger–Ellison tumour tissue. *Lancet*, 2:797–799.

176. Grzanna, R., and Coyle, J. T. (1978): Dopamine β-hydroxylase in rat submandibular ganglion cells which lack norepinephrine. *Brain Res.*, 115:206–214.

177. Guillemin, R. (1976): Somatostatin inhibits the release of acetylcholine induced electrically in the myenteric plexus. *Endocrinology*, 99:1653–1654.

178. Haddy, F. J., and Scott, J. B. (1968): Metabolically linked vasoactive chemicals in local regulation of blood flow. *Physiol. Rev.*, 48:688–707.

179. Harmar, A., Schofield, J. G., and Keen, P. (1980): Cycloheximide-sensitive synthesis of substance P by isolated dorsal root ganglia. *Nature*, 284:267–269.

180. Harper, A. A., and Raper, H. S. (1943): Pancreozymin, a stimulant of the secretion of pancreatic enzymes in extracts of the small intestine. *J. Physiol. (Lond.)*, 102:115–125.

181. Havrankova, J., Schmechel, D., Roth, J., and Brownstein, M. (1978): Identification of insulin in rat brain. *Proc. Natl. Acad. Sci. U.S.A.*, 75:5737–5741.

182. Hebb, C. O. (1957): Biochemical evidence for the neural function of acetylcholine. *Physiol. Rev.*, 37:196–220.

183. Hedqvist, P., and Von Euler, U. S. (1975): Influence of substance P on the response of guinea pig ileum to transmural nerve stimulation. *Acta Phsyiol. Scand.*, 95:341–343.

184. Helmstaedter, V., Taugner, C., Feurle, G. E., and Forssman, W. G. (1977): Localization of neurotensin-immunoreactive cells in the small intestine of man and various mammals. *Histochemistry*, 53:35–41.

185. Henderson, G., Hughes, J., and Kosterlitz, H. W. (1975): The effects of morphine on the release of noradrenaline from the cat isolated nictitating membrane and the guinea-pig ileum myenteric-longitudinal muscle preparation. *Br. J. Pharmacol.*, 53:505–512.

186. Henderson, J., Hughes, J., and Kosterlitz, H. W. (1978): *In vitro* release of Leu- and Met-enkephalin from the corpus striatum. *Nature*, 271:677–679.

187. Hervonen, A., Pelto-Huikko, M., Helen, P., and Alho, H. (1980): Electron-microscopic localization of enkephalin-like immunoreactivity in axon terminals of human sympathetic ganglia. *Histochemistry*, 70:1–6.

188. Hervonen, A., Pelto-Huikko, M., and Linnoila, I. (1980): Ultrastructural localization of enkephalin-like immunoreactivity in the rat adrenal medulla. *Am. J. Anat.*, 157:445–448.

189. Hervonen, A., Pickel, V. M., Joh, T. H., Reis, D. J., Linnoila, I., Kanerva, L., and Miller, R. J. (1980): Immunocytochemical demonstration of the catecholamine-synthesizing enzymes and neuropeptides in the catecholamine-storing cells of human fetal sympathetic nervous system. In: *Histochemistry and Cell Biology of Autonomic Neurons, SIF Cells, and Paraneurons*, edited by O. Eränkö, S. Soinila, and H. Paivärinta, pp. 373–378. Raven Press, New York.

190. Hervonen, A., Pickel, V. M., Joh, T. H., Reis, D. J., Linnoila, I., and Miller, R. J. (1981): Immunohistochemical localization of the catecholamine-synthesizing enzymes, substance P, and enkephalin in the human fetal sympathetic ganglion. *Cell Tissue Res.*, 214:33–42.

191. Hickson, J. C. D. (1970): The secretion of pancreatic juice in response to stimulation of the vagus nerves in the pig. *J. Physiol. (Lond.)*, 206:275–297.

192. Hillarp, N.-Å. (1960): Peripheral autonomic mechanisms. In: *Handbook of Physiology, Section I: Neurophysiology, Vol. II*, edited by J. Field, pp. 979–1005. Williams & Wilkins, Baltimore.

193. Hillarp, N.-Å., and Hökfelt, B. (1953): Evidence of adrenaline and noradrenaline in separate adrenal medullary cells. *Acta Physiol. Scand.*, 30:55–68.

194. Hillarp, N.-Å., and Hökfelt, B. (1954): Cytological demonstration of noradrenaline in the suprarenal medulla under conditions of varied secretory activity. *Endocrinology*, 55:255–260.

195. Hilton, S. M., and Lewis, G. P. (1955): The cause of vasodilatation accompanying activity in the submandibular salivary gland. *J. Physiol. (Lond.)*, 128:235–248.

196. Hilton, S. M., and Lewis, G. P. (1955): The mechanism of the functional hyperaemia in the submandibular salivary gland. *J. Physiol. (Lond.)*, 129:253–271.

197. Hilton, S. M., and Lewis, G. P. (1956): The relationship between glandular activity, bradykinin formation and functional vasodilatation in the submandibular salivary gland. *J. Physiol. (Lond.)*, 134:471–483.

198. Hirst, G. D. S., and McKirdy, H. C. (1974): A nervous mechanism for descending inhibition in guinea-pig small intestine. *J. Physiol. (Lond.)*, 238:129–143.

199. Hirst, G. D. S., and Silinsky, E. M. (1975): Some effects of 5-hydroxytryptamine, dopamine and noradrenaline on neurones in the submucous plexus of guinea-pig small intestine. *J. Physiol. (Lond.)*, 251:231–235.

200. Hökfelt, T., and Dahlström, A. (1971): Effects of two mitosis inhibitors (colchicine and vinblastine) on the distribution and axonal transport of noradrenergic storage particles, studied by fluorescence and electron microscopy. *Z. Zellforsch. Mikrosk. Anat.*, 119:460–482.

201. Hökfelt, T., Efendic, S., Hellerström, C., Johansson, O., Luft, R., and Arimura, A. (1975): Cellular localization of somatostatin in endocrine-like cells and neurons of the rat with special reference to the A cells of the pancreatic islets and to the hypothalamus. *Acta Endocrinol. [Suppl.] (Kbh.)*, 200:5–41.

202. Hökfelt, T., Elde, R., Johansson, O., Luft, R., Nilsson, G., and Arimura, A. (1976): Immunohistochemical evidence for separate populations of somatostatin-containing and substance P-containing primary afferent neurons in the rat. *Neuroscience*, 1:131–136.

203. Hökfelt, T., Elfvin, L.-G., Elde, R., Schultzberg, M., Goldstein, M., and Luft, R. (1977): Occurrence of somatostatin-like immunoreactivity in some peripheral sympathetic noradrenergic neurons. *Proc. Natl. Acad. Sci. U.S.A.*, 74:3587–3591.

204. Hökfelt, T., Elfvin, L.-G., Schultzberg, M., Fuxe, K., Said, S. I., Mutt, V., and Goldstein, M. (1977): Immunohistochemical evidence of vasoactive intestinal polypeptide-containing neurons and nerve fibers in sympathetic ganglia. *Neuroscience*, 2:885–896.

205. Hökfelt, T., Elfvin, L.-G., Schultzberg, M., Goldstein, M., and Nilsson, G. (1977): On the occurrence of substance P-containing fibers in sympathetic ganglia: Immunohistochemical evidence. *Brain Res.*, 132:29–41.

206. Hökfelt, T., Johansson, O., Efendić, S., Luft, R., and Arimura, A. (1975): Are there somatostatin-containing nerves in the rat gut? Immunohistochemical evidence for a new type of peripheral nerves. *Experientia*, 31:852–854.

207. Hökfelt, T., Johansson, O., Kellerth, J.-O., Ljungdahl, Å., Nilsson, G., Nygårds, A., and Pernow, B. (1977): Immunohistochemical distribution of substance P. In: *Substance P, Nobel Symposium 37*, edited by U. S. von Euler and B. Pernow, pp. 117–145. Raven Press, New York.

208. Hökfelt, T., Johansson, O., Ljungdahl, Å., Lundberg, J. M., and Schultzberg, M. (1980): Peptidergic neurons. *Nature*, 284:515–521.

209. Hökfelt, T., Kellerth, J.-O., Nilsson, G., and Pernow, B. (1975): Experimental immunohistochemical studies on the localization and distribution of substance P in cat primary sensory neurons. *Brain Res.*, 100:235–252.

210. Hökfelt, T., Kellerth, J.-O., Nilsson, G., and Pernow, B. (1975): Substance P: Localization in the central nervous system and in some primary sensory neurons. *Science*, 190:889–890.

211. Hökfelt, T., Schultzberg, M., Elde, R., Nilsson, G., Terenius, L., Said, S., and Goldstein, M. (1978): Peptide neurons in peripheral tissues including the urinary tract: Immunohistochemical studies. *Acta Pharmacol. Toxicol. (Kbh.)*, 43:79–89.

212. Holman, M. E., and Weinrich, J. P. (1975): Effects of calcium and magnesium of inhibitory junctional transmission in smooth-muscle of guinea-pig small intestine. *Pfluegers Arch.*, 30:109–119.

213. Holst, J. J., Fahrenkrug, J., Schaffalitzky de Muckadell, O. B., Lindkaer Jensen, S., and Nielsen, O. V. (1977): Vagal control of glucagon release in pigs. *Diabetologia*, 13:402.

214. Holst, J. J., Schaffalitzky de Muckadell, O. B., and Fahrenkrug, J. (1979): Nervous control of pancreatic exocrine secretion in pigs. *Acta Physiol. Scand.*, 105:33–51.

215. Huang, W.-Y., Chang, R. C. C., Kastin, A., Coy, D. H., and Schally, A. V. (1979): Isolation and structure of pro-methionin-enkephalin: Potential enkephalin precursor from porcine hypothalamus. *Proc. Natl. Acad. Sci. U.S.A.*, 76:6177–6180.

216. Hughes, J., Kosterlitz, H. W., and Smith, T. W. (1977): The distribution of methionine-enkephalin and leucine-enkephalin in the brain and peripheral tissues. *Br. J. Pharmacol.*, 61:639–647.

217. Hughes, J., Smith, T. W., Kosterlitz, H. W., Fothergill, L. A., Morgan, B. A., and Morris, H. R. (1975): Identification of two related pentapeptides from the brain with potent opiate agonist activity. *Nature*, 258:577–579.

218. Hultén, L. (1969): Reflex control of colonic motility and blood flow. *Acta Physiol. Scand. [Suppl.]*, 335:77–93.

219. Hung, K.-S., Hertwic, M. S., Hardy, J. D., and Loosli, C. G. (1972): Innervation of pulmonary alveoli of the mouse lung: An electron microscopic study. *Am. J. Aat.*, 135:477–496.

220. Hutchison, J. B., Dimaline, R., and Dockray, G. J. (1981): Neuropeptides in the gut: Quantification and characterization of cholecystokinin octapeptide-, bombesin-, and vasoactive intestinal polypeptide-like immunoreactivities in the myenteric plexus of the guinea-pig small intestine. *Peptides*, 2:23–30.

221. Hutchison, J. B., and Dockray, G. J. (1981): Evidence that the action of cholecystokinin octapeptide on the guinea pig ileum longitudinal muscle is mediated in part by substance P release from the myenteric plexus. *Eur. J. Pharmacol.*, 69:87–93.

222. Irvin, J. L., and Irvin, E. M. (1954): The interaction of quinacrine with adenine nucleotides. *J. Biol. Chem.*, 210:45–56.

223. Ivy, A. C., and Oldberg, E. (1928): A hormone mechanism for gall bladder contraction and evacuation. *J. Physiol.*, 86:599–613.

224. Jacobowitz, D. (1965): Histochemical studies of the autonomic innervation of the gut. *J. Pharmacol. Exp. Ther.*, 149:358–364.

225. Jacobowitz, D. (1970): Catecholamine fluorescence studies of adrenergic neurons and chromaffin cells in sympathetic ganglia. *Fed. Proc.*, 29:1929–1944.

226. Jacobowitz, D., and Koelle, G. B. (1965): Histochemical correlations of acetylcholinesterase and catecholamines in postganglionic autonomic nerves of the cat, rabbit and guinea pig. *J. Pharmacol. Exp. Ther.*, 148:225–237.

227. Jaffer, S. S., Farrar, J. T., Yau, W. M., and Makhlouf, G. M. (1974): Mode of action and interplay of vasoactive intestinal peptide (VIP), secretin and octapeptide of cholecystokinin (OCTA-CCK) on duodenal and ileal muscle *in vitro*. *Gastroenterology*, 66:A62–71.

228. Jan, L. Y., Jan, Y. N., and Brownfield, M. S. (1980): Peptidergic transmitters in synaptic boutons of sympathetic ganglia. *Nature*, 288:380–382.

229. Jan, Y. N., Jan, L. Y., and Kuffler, S. W. (1979): A peptide as a possible transmitter in sympathetic ganglia of the frog. *Proc. Natl. Acad. Sci. U.S.A.*, 76:1501–1505.

230. Jansson, G. (1969): Extrinsic nervous control of gastric motility. An experimental study in the cat. *Acta Physiol. Scand. [Suppl.]*, 326:1–42.

231. Jessen, K. R., Mirsky, R., Dennison, M. E., and Burnstock, G. (1979): GABA may be a neurotransmitter in the vertebrate peripheral nervous system. *Nature*, 281:71–74.

232. Jessen, K. R., Polak, J. M., Van Noorden, S., Bloom, S. R., and Burnstock, G. (1980): Peptide-containing neurones connect the two ganglionated plexuses of the enteric nervous system. *Nature*, 283:391–393.

233. Jessen, K. R., Saffrey, M. J., Van Noorden, S., Bloom, S. R., Polak, J. M., and Burnstock, G. (1980): Immunohistochemical studies of the enteric nervous system in tissue culture and *in situ*: Localization of vasoactive intestinal polypeptide (VIP), substance P, and enkephalin immunoreactive nerves in the guinea-pig gut. *Neuroscience*, 5:1717–1735.

234. Job, C., and Lundberg, A. (1952): Reflex excitation of cells in the inferior mesenteric ganglion on stim-

ulation of the hypogastric nerve. *Acta Physiol. Scand.,* 26:366–382.

235. Johns, A. (1979): The effect of vasoactive intestinal polypeptide on the urinary bladder and taenia coli of the guinea-pig. *Can. J. Physiol. Pharmacol.,* 57:106–108.

236. Jones, B. N., Stern, A. S., Lewis, R. V., Kimura, S., Stein, S., Udenfriend, S., and Shively, J. E. (1980): Structure of two adrenal polypeptides containing multiple enkephalin sequences. *Arch. Biochem. Biophys.,* 204:392–395.

237. Kachelhoffer, J., Mendel, C., Dauchel, J., Hohmatter, D., and Grenier, J. F. (1976): The effects of VIP on intestinal motility. Study on *ex vivo* perfused isolated canine jejunal loops. *Am. J. Dig. Dis.,* 21:957–962.

237a. Kakidani, H., Furutani, Y., Takahashi, H., Noda, M., Morimoto, Y., Hirose, T., Asai, M., Inayama, S., Nakanishi, S., and Numa, S. (1982): Cloning and sequence analysis of cDNA for porcine β-neoendorphin/dynorphin precursor. *Nature,* 298:245–249.

238. Kangawa, K., Matsuo, H., and Igarashi, M. (1979): α-Neo-endorphin: A "big" leu-enkephalin with potent opiate activity from porcine hypothalami. *Biochem. Biophys. Res. Commun.,* 86:153–160.

239. Katayama, Y., and North, R. A. (1978): Does substance P mediate slow excitation within the myenteric plexus? *Nature,* 274:387–388.

240. Katayama, Y., North, R. A., and Williams, J. T. (1979): The action of substance P on neurons of the myenteric plexus of the guinea-pig small intestine. *Proc. R. Soc. Lond. [Biol.],* 206:191–208.

241. Katz, B. (1966): The production of endplate potentials in muscles paralysed by tetrodotoxin. *J. Physiol. (Lond.),* 185:5–6P.

242. Kimmel, J. R., Hayden, L. J., and Pollock, H. G. (1975): Isolation and characterization of a new pancreatic polypeptide hormone. *J. Biol. Chem.,* 250:9369–9376.

243. Kimmel, J. R., Pollock, H. G., and Hazelwood, R. L. (1968): Isolation and characterization of chicken insulin. *Endocrinology,* 83:1323–1330.

244. Kimura, S., Lewis, R. V., Stern, A. S., Rossier, J., Stein, S., and Udenfriend, S. (1980): Probable precursors of (leu)enkephalin and (met)enkephalin in adrenal medulla: Peptides of 3–5 kilodaltons. *Proc. Natl. Acad. Sci. U.S.A.,* 77:1681–1685.

245. Kiss, T. (1951): Experimentell-morphologische Analyse der Nebenniereninnervation. *Acta Anat.,* 13:81–89.

246. Kitabgi, P., and Freychet, P. (1978): Effects of neurotensin on isolated intestinal smooth muscles. *Eur. J. Pharmacol.,* 50:349–357.

247. Kitabgi, P., and Freychet, P. (1979): Neurotensin contracts the guinea-pig longitudinal ileal muscle by inducing acetylcholine release. *Eur. J. Pharmacol.,* 56:403–406.

248. Kitabgi, P., Hamson, G., and Worcel, N. (1979): Electrophysiological study of the action of neurotensin on the smooth muscle of the guinea-pig taenia coli. *Eur. J. Pharmacol.,* 56:87–93.

249. Konishi, S., and Otsuka, M. (1974): Excitatory action of hypothalamic substance P on spinal motoneurones of newborn rats. *Nature,* 252:734–735.

250. Konishi, S., Tsunoo, A., and Otsuka, M. (1979): Substance P and noncholinergic excitatory synaptic transmission in guinea pig sympathetic ganglia. *Proc. Jpn. Acad.,* 55:B525–530.

251. Konishi, S., Tsunoo, A., and Otsuka, M. (1979): Enkephalins presynaptically inhibit cholinergic transmission in sympathetic ganglia. *Nature,* 282:515–516.

252. Konturek, S. J., Domschke, S., Domschke, W., Wünsch, E., and Demling, L. (1977): Comparison of pancreatic responses to portal and systemic secretin and VIP in cats. *Am. J. Physiol.,* 232:E156–E158.

253. Konturek, S. J., Thor, P., Dembinski, A., and Kroi, R. (1975): Comparison of secretin and vasoactive intestinal peptide on pancreatic secretion in dogs. *Gastroenterology,* 68:1527–1535.

254. Kosterlitz, H. W. (1968): Intrinsic and extrinsic nervous control of motility of the stomach and the intestines. In: *Handbook of Physiology, Section 6: The Alimentary Canal, Vol. 4,* edited by C. F. Code, pp. 2147–2171. Williams & Wilkins, Baltimore.

255. Kosterlitz, H. W., and Paterson, S. J. (1980): Characterization of opioid receptors in nervous tissue. *Proc. R. Soc. Lond. [Biol.],* 210:113–122.

256. Kosterlitz, H. W., and Waterfield, A. A. (1975): *In vitro* models in the study of structure activity relationships of narcotic analgesics. *Annu. Rev. Pharmacol.,* 15:29–47.

257. Kreutzberg, G. (1969): Neuronal dynamics and axonal flow. IV. Blockage of intra-axonal enzyme transport. *Proc. Natl. Acad. Sci. U.S.A.,* 62:722–728.

258. Krulich, L., Dhariwal, A. P. S., and McCann, S. M. (1968): Stimulatory and inhibitory effects of purified hypothalamic extracts on growth hormone release from rat pituitary *in vitro. Endocrinology,* 83:783–790.

259. Kuntz, A. (1938): The structural organization of the coeliac ganglia. *J. Comp. Neurol.,* 69:1–12.

260. Kuntz, A. (1940): The structural organization of the inferior mesenteric ganglia. *J. Comp. Neurol.,* 72:371–382.

261. Kuntz, A. (1946): *The Autonomic Nervous System.* Bailliere, Tindall & Cox, London.

262. Kuntz, A., and Saccomanno, G. J. (1944): Reflex inhibition of intestinal motility mediated through decentralized prevertebral ganglia. *J. Physiol.,* 7:163–170.

263. Langley, J. H. (1921): *The Autonomic Nervous System, Part I.* W. Heffer and Sons, Cambridge.

264. Larsson, L.-I. (1977): Ultrastructural localization of a new neuronal peptide (VIP). *Histochemistry,* 54:170–176.

265. Larsson, L.-I., Childers, S., and Snyder, S. H. (1979): Met- and leu-enkephalin immunoreactivity in separate neurones. *Nature,* 282:407–410.

266. Larsson, L.-I., Fahrenkrug, J., and Schaffalitzky de Muckadell, O. (1977): Occurrence of nerves containing vasoactive intestinal polypeptide immunoreactivity in the male genital tract. *Life Sci.,* 21:503–508.

267. Larsson, L.-I., Fahrenkrug, J., and Schaffalitzky de Muckadell, O. B. (1977): Vasoactive intestinal polypeptide occurs in nerves of the female genitourinary tract. *Science,* 197:1374–1375.

268. Larsson, L.-I., Fahrenkrug, J., and Schaffalitzky de Muckadell, O. B. (1978): Innervation of the pancreas by vasoactive intestinal polypeptide (VIP) immunoreactive nerves. *Life Sci.,* 22:773–780.

269. Larsson, L.-I., Fahrenkrug, J., Schaffalitzky de Muckadell, O., Sundler, F., Håkanson, R., and Rehfeld, J. F. (1976): Localization of vasoactive intestinal polypeptide (VIP) to central and peripheral neurons. *Proc. Natl. Acad. Sci. U.S.A.,* 73:3197–3200.

270. Larsson, L.-I., and Rehfeld, J. F. (1977): Evidence for a common evolutionary origin of gastrin and cholecystokinin. *Nature,* 269:335–338.

271. Larsson, L.-I., and Rehfeld, J. F. (1977): Characterization of antral gastrin cells with region-specific antibodies. *J. Histochem. Cytochem.,* 25:1317–1321.

272. Larsson, L.-I., and Rehfeld, J. F. (1979): Localization and molecular heterogeneity of cholecystokinin in the central and peripheral nervous system. *Brain Res.,* 165:201–218.

273. Larsson, L.-I., and Rehfeld, J. F. (1979): A peptide resembling COOH-terminal tetrapeptide amide of gastrin from a new gastrointestinal endocrine cell type. *Nature,* 277:575–578.

274. Lawson, H. (1934): Role of inferior mesenteric ganglia in diphasic response of colon to sympathetic stimuli. *Am. J. Physiol.,* 109:257–273.

275. Lawson, H., and Holt, J. P. (1937): Control of large intestine by decentralized inferior mesenteric ganglion. *Am. J. Physiol.,* 118:780–785.

276. Leander, S., Håkanson, R., and Sundler, F. (1981): Nerves containing substance P, vasoactive intestinal polypeptide, enkephalin, or somatostatin in the guinea-pig taenia coli: Distribution, ultrastructure and possible functions. *Cell Tissue Res.,* 215:21–39.

277. Lee, C. M., Emson, P. C., and Iversen, L. L. (1980): The development and application of a novel N-terminal directed substance P antiserum. *Life Sci.,* 27:535–543.

278. Leeman, S. E., Mroz, E. A., and Carraway, R. (1977): Substance P and neurotensin. In: *Peptides in Neurobiology,* edited by H. Gainer, pp. 99–144. Plenum Press, New York.

279. Lembeck, F. (1953): Zur Frage der zentralen Übertragung afferenter Impulse. III. Mitteilung. Das Vorkommen und die Bedeutung der Substanz P in den dorsalen Wurzeln des Rückenmarks. *Naunyn Schmiedebergs Arch. Pharmakol.,* 219:197–213.

280. Leppäluoto, J., Koivusalo, F., and Kraama, R. (1978): Thyrotropin-releasing factor: Distribution in neural and gastrointestinal tissues. *Acta Physiol. Scand.,* 104:175–179.

281. Lewis, P. R., Shute, C. C. D., and Silver, A. (1967): Confirmation from choline acetylase analyses of a massive cholinergic innervation to the rat hippocampus. *J. Physiol. (Lond.),* 191:215–224.

282. Lewis, R. V., Stern, A. S., Kimura, S., Rossier, J., Stein, S., and Udenfriend, S. (1980): An about 50,000-dalton protein in adrenal medulla: A common precursor of (met)- and (leu)-enkephalin. *Science,* 208:1459–1461.

283. Lewis, R. V., Stern, A. S. Kimura, S., Stein, S., and Udenfriend, S. (1980): Enkephalin biosynthetic pathway: Proteins of 8000 and 1400 daltons in bovine adrenal medulla. *Proc. Natl. Acad. Sci. U.S.A.,* 77:5018–5020.

284. Lewis, R. V. Stern, A. S., Rossier, J., Stein, S., and Udenfriend, S. (1979): Putative enkephalin precursors in bovine adrenal medulla. *Biochem. Biophys. Res. Commun.,* 89:822–829.

285. Li, C. H. (1964): Lipotropin, a new active peptide from pituitary glands. *Nature,* 201:924.

286. Li, C. H., and Chung, D. (1976): Isolation and structure of an untriakontapeptide with opiate activity from camel pituitary glands. *Proc. Natl. Acad. Sci. U.S.A.,* 73:145–148.

287. Li, C. H., Chung, D., and Doneen, B. A. (1976): Isolation, characterization and opiate activity of beta-endorphin from human pituitary glands. *Biochem. Biophys. Res. Commun.,* 72:1542–1547.

288. Lin, T.-M., and Chance, R. E. (1974): Bovine pancreatic polypeptide (BPP) and avian pancreatic polypeptide (APP). *Gastroenterology,* 67:737–738.

289. Lindkaer Jensen, S., Fahrenkrug, J., Holst, J. J., Vagn Nielsen, O., and Schaffalitzky de Muckadell, O. B. (1978): Secretory effects of vasoactive intestinal polypeptide (VIP) on the isolated, perfused porcine pancreas. *Am J. Physiol.,* 235:E387–E391.

290. Lindkaer Jensen, S., Rehfeld, J. F., Holst, J. J., Fahrenkrug, J., Nielsen, O. V., and Schaffalitzky de Muckadell, O. B. (1980): Secretory effects of gastrins on isolated, perfused porcine pancrease. *Am J. Physiol.,* 238:E186–E192.

291. Lindkaer Jensen, S., Rehfeld, J. F., Holst, J. J., Nielsen, O. V., Fahrenkrug, J., and Schaffalitzky de Muckadell, O. B. (1981): Secretory effects of cholecystokinins on isolated, perfused porcine pancreas. *Acta Physiol. Scand.,* 111:225–233.

292. Linnoila, R. I., Di Augustine, R. P., Miller, R. J., Chang, K. J., and Cuatrecasas, P. (1978): An immunohistochemical and radioimmunological study of the distribution of (met^5)- and (leu^5)-enkephalin in the gastrointestinal tract. *Neuroscience,* 3:1187–1196.

293. Lord, J. A. H., Waterfield, A. A., Hughes, J., and Kosterlitz, H. W. (1977): Endogenous opioid peptides: Multiple agonists and receptors. *Nature,* 67:494–499.

294. Lorén, I., Alumets, J., Håkanson, R., and Sundler, F.(1979): Immunoreactive pancreatic polypeptide (PP) occurs in the central and peripheral nervous system: Preliminary immunocytochemical observations. *Cell Tissue Res.,* 200:179–186.

295. Lorén, I., Alumets, J., Håkanson, R., Sundler, F., and Thorell, J. (1979): Gut-type glucagon immunoreactivity in nerves of the rat brain. *Histochemistry,* 61:335–341.

296. Lubinska, L. (1959): Region of transition between preserved and regenerating parts of myelinated nerve fibres. *J. Comp. Neurol.,* 113:315–335.

297. Luduena, F. P., and Grigar, E. O. (1966): Pharmacological study of autonomic innervation of dog retractor penis. *Am. J. Physiol.,* 210:435–445.

298. Lundberg, J. M., Änggård, A., Fahrenkrug, J.,

Hökfelt, T., and Mutt, V. (1980): Vasoactive intestinal polypeptide in cholinergic neurons of exocrine glands: Functional significance of co-existing transmitters for vasodilation and secretion. *Proc. Natl. Acad. Sci. U.S.A.,* 77:1651–1655.

299. Lundberg, J. M., Änggård, A., Hökfelt, T., and Kimmel, J. (1980): Avian pancreatic polypeptide (APP) inhibits atropine resistant vasodilation in cat submandibular salivary gland and nasal mucosa: Possible interaction with VIP. *Acta Physiol. Scand.,* 110:199–201.

300. Lundberg, J. M., Hamberger, B., Schultzberg, M., Hökfelt, T., Granberg, P.-O., Efendic, S., Terenius. L., Goldstein, M., and Luft, R. (1979): Enkephalin- and somatostatin-like immunoreactivities in human adrenal medulla and pheochromocytoma. *Proc. Natl. Acad. Sci. U.S.A.,* 76:4079–4083.

301. Lundberg, J. M., Hökfelt, T., Änggård, A., Kimmel, J., Goldstein, M., and Markey, K. (1980): Co-existence of an avian pancreatic polypeptide (APP) immunoreactive substance and catecholamines in some peripheral and central neurons. *Acta Physiol. Scand.,* 110:107–109.

302. Lundberg, J. M., Hökfelt, T., Änggård, A., Uvnäs-Wallensten, K., Brimijoin, S., Brodin, E., and Fahrenkrug, J. (1980): Peripheral peptide neurons: Distribution, axonal transport, and some aspects on possible function. In: *Neural Peptides and Neuronal Communication,* edited by E. Costa and M. M. Trabucchi, pp. 25–36. Raven Press, New York.

303. Lundberg, J., Hökfelt, T., Nilsson, G., Terenius, L., Rehfeld, J., Elde, R. P., and Said, S. (1978): Peptide neurons in the vagus, splanchnic and sciatic nerves. *Acta Physiol. Scand.,* 104:499–501.

304. Lundberg, J. M., Hökfelt, T., Schultzberg, M., Uvnäs-Wallensten, K., Köhler, L., and Said, S. (1979): Occurrence of VIP-like immunoreactivity in cholinergic neurons of the cat: Evidence from combined immunohistochemistry and acetylcholine esterase staining. *Neuroscience,* 4:1539–1559.

305. Lynch, E. M., Wharton, J., Bryant, M. G., Bloom, S. R., Polak, J. M., and Elder, M. G. (1980): The differential distribution of vasoactive intestinal polypeptide in the normal human female genital tract. *Histochemistry,* 67:169–177.

306. Mains, R. E., Eipper, B. A., and Ling, N. (1977): Common precursor to corticotropins and endorphins. *Proc. Natl. Acad. Sci. U.S.A.,* 74:3014–3018.

307. Mall, F. P. (1896): On the reversal of the intestine. *Johns Hopkins Med. J.,* 1:37–75.

308. Malm, L., Sundler, F., and Uddman, R. (1981): Effects of vasoactive intestinal polypeptide on resistance and capacitance vessels in the nasal mucosa. *Acta Otolaryngol.,* 90:304–308.

309. Malmfors, G., Leander, S., Brodin, E., Håkanson, R., Holmin, T., and Sundler, F. (1981): Peptide-containing neurons intrinsic to the gut wall. *Cell Tissue Res.,* 214:225–238.

310. Marks, B. H., Samorajski, T., and Webster, E. J. (1962): Radioautographic localization of norepinephrine-H^3 in the tissues of mice. *J. Pharmacol. Exp. Ther.,* 138:376–381.

311. Martinson, J., and Muren, A. (1963): Excitatory and inhibitory effects of vagus stimulation on gastric motility in the cat. *Acta Physiol. Scand.,* 57:309–316.

312. Maycock, W. D. A., and Heslop, T. S. (1939): An experimental investigation of the nerve supply of the adrenal medulla of the cat. *J. Anat.,* 73:551–558.

313. McDonald, T. J., Jörnvall, H., Nilsson, G., Vagne, M., Ghatei, M., Bloom, S. R., and Mutt, V. (1979): Characterization of a gastrin releasing peptide from porcine nonantral gastric tissue. *Biochem. Biophys. Res. Commun.,* 90:227–233.

314. McKnight, A. T., Sosa, R. P., Hughes, J., and Kosterlitz, H. W. (1978): Biosynthesis and release of enkephalins. In: *Developments in Neuroscience, Vol. 4: Characteristics and Function of Opioids,* edited by J. M. Van Ree and L. Terenius, pp. 259–269. North-Holland, Amsterdam.

315. McLennan, H., and Pascoe, J. H. (1954): The origin of certain nonmedullated nerve fibres which form synapses in the inferior mesenteric ganglion of the rabbit. *J. Physiol. (Lond.),* 124:145–156.

316. Melchiorri, P. (1978): Bombesin and bombesin-like peptides of amphibian skin. In: *Gut Hormones,* edited by S. R. Bloom, pp. 534–540. Churchill Livingstone, Edinburgh.

317. Milenov, K., Oehme, P., Bienert, M., and Bergmann, J. (1978): Effect of substance P on mechanical and myoelectrical activities of stomach and small intestine in conscious dog. *Arch. Int. Pharmacodyn.,* 233:251–260.

318. Minamino, N., Kangawa, K., Fukuda, A., and Matsuo, H. (1980): A new opioid octapeptide related to dynorphin from porcine hypothalamus. *Biochem. Biophys. Res. Commun.,* 95:1475–1481.

319. Mitchell, G. A. A. (1953): *Anatomy of the Autonomic Nervous System.* Livingstone, Edinburgh.

320. Mizuno, K., Minamino, N., Kangawa, K., and Matsuo, H. (1980): A new endogenous opioid peptide from bovine adrenal medulla: Isolation and amino acid sequence of a dodecapeptide (BAM-12P). *Biochem. Biophys. Res. Commun.,* 95:1482–1488.

321. Modlin, I. M., Bloom, S. R., Barnes, A., and Welbourn, R. B. (1978): Cure of intractable watery diarrhoea by excision of a VIPoma. *Br. J. Surg.,* 65:234–236.

322. Modlin, I. M., Bloom, S. R., and Mitchell, S. J. (1978): Experimental evidence for vasoactive intestinal peptide as the cause of the watery diarrhoea syndrome. *Gastroenterology,* 75:1051–1054.

323. Monier, S., and Kitabgi, P. (1980): Substance P-induced autodesensitization inhibits atropine-resistant neurotensin-stimulated contractions in guinea-pig ileum. *Eur. J. Pharmacol.,* 65:461–462.

324. Morgan, K. G., Schmalz, P., Go, V. L. W., and Szurszewski, J. H. (1978): Effects of pentagastrin G_{17}, and G_{34} on the electrical and mechanical activities of canine antral smooth muscle. *Gastroenterology,* 75:405–412.

325. Morgan, K. G., Schmalz, P. F., Go, V. L. M., and Szurszewski, J. H. (1978): Electrical and mechanical effects of molecular variants of CCK on antral smooth muscle. *Am. J. Physiol.,* 235:E324–E329.

326. Morgan, K. G., Schmalz, P. F., and Szurszewski, J.

H. (1978): The inhibitory effects of vasoactive intestinal polypeptide on the mechanical and electrical activity of canine antral smooth muscle. *J. Physiol. (Lond.),* 282:437–450.

327. Morita, K., North, R. A., and Katayama, Y. (1980): Evidence that substance P is a neurotransmitter in the myenteric plexus. *Nature,* 287:151–152.

328. Morley, J. E., Garvin, T. J., Pekary, E., and Hershman, J. M. (1977): Thyrotropin-releasing hormone in the gastrointestinal tract. *Biochem. Biophys. Res. Commun.,* 79:314–318.

329. Mutt, V., and Jorpes, J. E. (1966): Cholecystokinin and pancreozymin, one single hormone? *Acta Physiol. Scand.,* 66:196–202.

330. Mutt, V., Carlquist, M., and Tatemoto, K. (1979): Secretin-like bioactivity in extracts of porcine brain. *Life Sci.,* 25:1703–1708.

331. Mutt, V., and Said, S. I. (1974): Structure of the porcine vasoactive intestinal octacosapeptide: The amino acid sequence. Use of kallikrein in its determination. *Eur. J. Biochem.,* 42:581–589.

332. Nagai, K., and Frohman, L. A. (1976): Hyperglycaemia and hyperglucagonemia following neurotensin administration. *Life Sci.,* 19:273–280.

333. Nairn, R. C. (1969): *Fluorescent Protein Tracing.* Livingstone, Edinburgh.

334. Nakajima, T., Tanimra, T., and Pisano, J. J. (1970): Isolation and structure of a new vasoactive polypeptide. *Fed. Proc.,* 29:282.

335. Nakanishi, H., and Takeda, H. (1972): The possibility that adenosine triphosphate is an excitatory transmitter in guinea-pig seminal vesicle. *Jpn. J. Pharmacol.,* 22:269–270.

336. Nakanishi, H., and Takeda, H. (1973): The possible role of adenosine triphosphate in chemical transmission between the hypogastric nerve terminal and seminal vesicle in the guinea-pig. *Jpn. J. Pharmacol.,* 23:479–490.

337. Nilsson, A. (1974): Structure of the vasoactive intestinal octacosapeptide from chicken intestine. Amino acid sequence. *FEBS Lett.,* 60:322–326.

338. Nilsson, G., and Brodin, E. (1977): Tissue distribution of substance P-like immunoreactivity in dog, cat, rat and mouse. In: *Substance P. Nobel Symposium 37,* edited by U. S. von Euler and B. Pernow, pp. 49–54. Raven Press, New York.

339. Nilsson, G., Larsson, L.-I., Håkanson, R., Brodin, E., Sundler, F., and Pernow B. (1975): Localization of substance P-like immunoreactivity in mouse gut. *Histochemistry,* 43:97–99.

340. Nishi, S., and North, R. A. (1973): Presynaptic action of noradrenaline in the myenteric plexus. *J. Physiol. (Lond.),* 231:29P–30P.

341. Norberg, K.-A. (1964): Adrenergic innervation of the intestinal wall studied by fluorescence microscopy. *Int. J. Neuropharmacol.,* 3:379–382.

342. Norberg, K.-A. (1967): Transmitter histochemistry of the sympathetic adrenergic nervous system. *Brain Res.,* 5:125–170.

343. Norberg, K.-A., and Hamberger, B. (1964): The sympathetic adrenergic neuron. Some characteristics revealed by histochemical studies on the intraneuronal distribution of the transmitter. *Acta Physiol. Scand. [Suppl.],* 238:1–42.

344. North, R. A., Katayama, Y., and Williams, J. T. (1979): On the mechanism and site of action of enkephalin on single myenteric neurons. *Brain Res.,* 165:67–77.

345. North, R. A., and Williams, J. T. (1976): Enkephalin inhibits firing of myenteric neurones. *Nature,* 264:460–461.

346. Öberg, B. (1976): Overall cardiovascular regulation. *Annu. Rev. Physiol.,* 38:537–370.

347. Ohga, A., Nakazato, Y., and Saito, K. (1969): An analysis of the vago–vagal reflex relaxation of the stomach. *J. Jpn. Soc. Physiol.,* 31:92–93.

348. Ohga, A., Nakazato, Y., and Saito, K. (1970): Considerations of the efferent nervous mechanism of the vago–vagal reflex relaxation of the stomach in the dog. *Jpn. J. Pharmacol.,* 20:116–130.

349. Olson, L., Ålund, M., and Norberg, K. (1976): Fluorescence-microscopical demonstration of a population of gastrointestinal nerve fibres with a selective affinity for quinacrine. *Cell Tissue Res.,* 171:407–423.

350. Orci, L., Baetens, O., Rufener, C., Brown, M., Vale, W., and Guillemin, R. (1976): Evidence for immunoreactive neurotensin in dog intestinal mucosa. *Life Sci.,* 19:559–562.

351. Pearcy, J. F., and Liere, E. J. Van (1926): Studies on the visceral nervous system. XVII. Reflexes from the colon. 1. Reflexes to the stomach. *Am. J. Physiol.,* 78:64–73.

352. Pearse, A. G. E., and Polak, J. M. (1975): Immunocytochemical localization of substance P in mammalian intestine. *Histochemistry,* 41:373–395.

353. Pelto-Huikko, M., Hervonen, A., Helen, P., Linnoila, I., Pickel, V. M., and Miller, R. J. (1980): Localization of (Met⁵)- and (Leu⁵)-enkephalin in nerve terminals and SIF cells in adult human sympathetic ganglia. In: *Histochemistry and Cell Biology of Autonomic Neurons, SIF Cells, and Paraneurons,* edited by O. Eränkö, S. Soinila, and H. Paivärinta, pp. 379–383. Raven Press, New York.

354. Pernow, B. (1953): Studies on substance P. Purification, occurrence, and biological actions. *Acta Physiol. Scand. [Suppl.],* 29;1–90.

355. Petrusz, P., Sar, M., Ordronneau, P., and Dimeo, P. (1976): Specificity in immunocytochemical staining. *J. Histochem. Cytochem.,* 24:1110–1115.

356. Polak, J. M., Bloom, S. R., Sullivan, S. N., Facer, P., and Pearse, A. G. E. (1977): Enkephalin-like immunoreactivity in the human gastrointestinal tract. *Lancet,* 1:972–974.

357. Polak, J. M., Pearse, A. G. E., Grimelius, L., Bloom, S. R., and Arimura, A. (1975): Growth-hormone release-inhibiting hormone in gastrointestinal and pancreatic D cells. *Lancet,* 1:1220–1222.

358. Pradayrol, L., Chayville, J., and Mutt, V. (1978): Pig duodenal somatostatin: Extraction and purification. *Metabolism,* 27(Suppl. 1):1197–1200.

359. Racusen, L. C., and Binder, H. J. (1977): Alteration of large intestinal electrolyte transport by vasoactive intestinal polypeptide in the rat. *Gastroenterology,* 73:790–796.

360. Rattan, S., Said, S. I., and Goyal, R. K. (1977): Effect of vasoactive intestinal polypeptide (VIP) on the lower oesophageal sphincter pressure (LESP). *Proc. Soc. Exp. Biol. Med.,* 155:40–43.

361. Rehfeld, J. F. (1972): Three components of gastrin in human serum. *Biochem. Biophys. Acta,* 285:364–372.
362. Rehfeld, J. F. (1978): Immunochemical studies on cholecystokinin. II. Distribution and molecular heterogeneity in the central nervous system and the small intestine of man and hog. *J. Biol. Chem.,* 253:4022–4030.
363. Rehfeld, J. F., and Larsson, L.-I. (1979): The predominating molecular form of gastrin and cholecystokinin in the gut is a small peptide corresponding to their COOH-terminal tetrapeptide amide. *Acta Physiol. Scand.,* 105:117–119.
364. Rehfeld, J. F., Larsson, L.-I., Goltermann, N. R., Schwartz, T. W., Holst, J. J., Lindkaer Jensen, S., and Morley, J. S. (1980): Neural regulation of pancreatic hormone secretion by the C-terminal tetrapeptide of CCK. *Nature,* 284:33–38.
365. Rehfeld, J. F., and Stadil, F. (1973): Gel filtration studies on immunoreactive gastrin in serum from Zollinger–Ellison patients. *Gut,* 14:369–374.
366. Richardson, J., and Béland, J. (1976): Nonadrenergic inhibitory nervous system in human airways. *J. Appl. Physiol.,* 41:764–771.
367. Roberts, J. L., and Herbert, E. (1977): Characterization of a common precursor to corticotrophin and β-lipotropin: Identification of β-lipotropin peptides and their arrangement relative to corticotrophin in the precursor synthesized in a cell-free system. *Proc. Natl. Acad. Sci. U.S.A.,* 74:5300–5304.
368. Robinson, R., and Gershon, M. D. (1971): Synthesis and uptake of 5-hydroxytryptamine by the myenteric plexus of the small intestine of the guinea pig. *J. Pharmacol. Exp. Ther.,* 179:29–41.
369. Robinson, P. M., McLean, J. R., and Burnstock, G. (1971): Ultrastructural identification of nonadrenergic inhibitory nerve fibres. *J. Pharmacol. Exp. Ther.,* 179:149–160.
370. Robinson, R., and Monro, A. F. (1958): Adrenal activity in subjects with complete transverse lesions of the spinal cord. *Nature,* 182:805.
371. Rökaeus, A., Burcher, E., Chang, D., Folkers, K., and Yagima, H. (1977): Actions of neurotensin and (Gln⁴)-neurotensin on isolated tissues. *Acta Pharmacol. Toxicol. (Kbh.),* 41:141–147.
372. Rosell, S., Björkroth, U., Chang, D., Yamaguchi, I., Wan, Y.-P., Rackur, G., Fisher, G., and Folkers. K. (1977): Effects of substance P and analogs on isolated guinea-pig ileum. In: *Substance P. Nobel Symposium 37,* edited by U. S. von Euler and B. Pernow, pp. 83–88. Raven Press, New York.
373. Rossier, J., Trifaro, J. M., Lewis, R. Y., Lee, R. W. H., Stern, A., Kimura, S., Stein, S., and Udenfriend, S. (1980): Studies with (³⁵S) methionine indicate that the 22,000-dalton (met)enkephalin-containing protein in chromaffin cells is a precursor of (met)enkephalin. *Proc. Natl. Acad. Sci. U.S.A.,*77:6889–6891.
374. Said, S. I. (ed.) (1982): *Advances in Peptide Hormone Research, Vol. 1: Vasoactive intestinal polypeptide.* Raven Press, New York.
375. Said, S. I., and Faloona, G. R. (1975): Elevated plasma tissue levels of VIP in the watery diarrhoea syndrome due to pancreatic, bronchogenic and other tumours. *N. Engl. J. Med.,* 293:155–160.

376. Said, S. I., and Mutt, V. (1970): Polypeptide with broad biological activity. Isolation from small intestine. *Science,* 169:1217–1218.
377. Said, S. I., and Mutt, V. (1972): Isolation from porcine intestine of a vasoactive octocosapeptide related to secretin and glucagon. *Eur. J. Biochem.,* 28:199–204.
378. Said, S. I., and Rosenberg, R. N. (1976): Vasoactive intestinal polypeptide: Abundant immunoreactivity in neural cell lines and normal tissue. *Science,* 192:907–908.
379. Sakai, K. K., Hymson, D. L., and Shapiro, R. (1978): The mode of action of enkephalins in the guinea-pig ileum. *Neurosci. Lett.,* 10:317–322.
380. Schaffalitzky de Muckadell, O. B., Fahrenkrug, J., and Holst, J. J. (1977): Release of vasoactive intestinal polypeptide (VIP) by electric stimulation of the vagal nerves. *Gastroenterology,* 72:373–375.
381. Schaffalitzky de Muckadell, O. B., Fahrenkrug, J., Holst, J. J., and Lauritsen, K. B. (1977): Release of vasoactive intestinal polypeptide (VIP) by intraduodenal stimuli. *Scand. J. Gastroenterol.,* 12:793–799.
382. Schebalin, M., Said, S. I., and Makhlouf, G. M. (1977): Stimulation of insulin and glucagon secretion by synthetic vasoactive intestinal peptide. *Am. J. Physiol.,* 232:E197–E200.
383. Schlaepfer, W. W. (1968): Acetylcholinesterase activity of motor and sensory nerve fibres in the spinal nerve roots of the rat. *Z. Zellforsch. Mikrosk. Anat.,* 88:441–456.
384. Schofield, G. C. (1968): Anatomy of muscular and neural tissues in the alimentary canal. In: *Handbook of Physiology, Section 6: Alimentary Canal, Vol. 4: Motility,* edited by C. F. Code, pp. 1579–1627. Williams & Wilkins, Baltimore.
385. Schultzberg, M. (1980): Immunohistochemical evidence for bombesin-like immunoreactivity in nerve fibres in sympathetic ganglia. *Regul. Peptides,* 1:S101.
386. Schultzberg, M., Dreyfus, C. F., Gershon, M. D., Hökfelt, T., Elde, R., Nilsson, G., Said, S., and Goldstein, M. (1978): VIP, enkephalin, substance P-, and somatostatin-like immunoreactivity in neurons intrinsic to the intestine: Immunohistochemical evidence from organotypic tissue cultures. *Brain Res.,* 155:239–248.
387. Schultzberg, M., Hökfelt, T., Lundberg, J. M., Terenius, L., Elfvin, L.-G., and Elde, R. (1978): Enkephalin-like immunoreactivity in nerve terminals in sympathetic ganglia and adrenal medulla and in adrenal medullary gland cells. *Acta Physiol. Scand.,* 103:475–477.
388. Schultzberg, M., Hökfelt, T., Nilsson, G., Terenius, L., Rehfeld, J. F., Brown, M., Elde, R., Goldstein, M., and Said, S. I. (1980): Distribution of peptide- and catecholamine-containing neurons in the gastrointestinal tract of rat and guinea-pig: Immunohistochemical studies with antisera to substance P, vasoactive intestinal polypeptide, enkephalins, somatostatin, gastrin/cholecystokinin, neurotensin and dopamine β-hydroxylase. *Neuroscience,* 5:689–744.
389. Schultzberg, M., Hökfelt, T., Olson, L., Ålund, M., Nilsson, G., Terenius, L., Elde, R., Goldstein, M.,

and Said, S. (1980): Substance P, VIP, enkephalin, and somatostatin immunoreactive neurons in intestinal tissue transplanted to the anterior eye chamber. *J. Autonom. Nerv. Syst.,* 1:291–303.

390. Schultzberg, M., Hökfelt, T., Terenius, L., Elfvin, L.-G., Lundberg, J. M., Brandt, J., Elde, R. P., and Goldstein, M. (1979): Enkephalin immunoreactive nerve fibers and cell bodies in sympathetic ganglia of the guinea-pig and rat. *Neuroscience,* 4:249–270.

391. Schultzberg, M., Lundberg, J. M., Hökfelt, T., Terenius, L., Brandt, J., Elde, R. P., and Goldstein, M. (1978): Enkephalin-like immunoreactivity in gland cells and nerve terminals of the adrenal medulla. *Neuroscience,* 3:1169–1186.

392. Schultz, R., Wüster, M., Simantov, R., Snyder, S. H., and Herz, A. (1977): Electrically stimulated release of opiate-like material from the myenteric plexus of the guinea-pig ileum. *Eur. J. Pharmacol.,* 41:347–348.

393. Schwartz, C. J., Kimberg, D. V., and Scherrin, H. E. (1974): Vasoactive intestinal peptide stimulation of adenylate cyclase and active electrolyte secretion in intestinal mucosa. *J. Clin. Invest.,* 54:536–544.

394. Segawa, T., Hosokawa, M., Kitagawa, K., and Yajima, H. (1977): Contractile activity of synthetic neurotensin and related polypeptides on guinea-pig ileum. *J. Pharm. Pharmacol.,* 29:57–58.

395. Silver, A. (1974): *The Biology of Cholinesterases.* North-Holland, Amsterdam.

396. Simantov, R., and Snyder, S. H. (1976): Brain-pituitary opiate mechanisms: Pituitary opiate receptor binding, radioimmunoassays for methionine enkephalin and leucine enkephalin, and ^{3}H-enkephalin interactions with the opiate receptor. In: *Opiates and Endogenous Opioid Peptides,* edited by H. W. Kosterlitz, pp. 41–48. North-Holland, Amsterdam.

397. Smith, T. W., Hughes, J., Kosterlitz, H. W., and Sosa, R. P. (1976): Enkephalins: Isolation, distribution and function. In: *Opiates and Endogenous Opioid Peptides,* edited by H. W. Kosterlitz, pp. 57–62. Elsevier/North Holland, Amsterdam.

398. Solomon, T. E., and Grossman, M. I. (1979): Response of transplanted pancreas to intestinal stimulants in dogs: Effects of atropine and comparison to intact pancreas. *Am. J. Physiol.,* 236:E186–E190.

399. Sosa, R. P., McKnight, A. T. Hughes, J., and Kosterlitz, H. W. (1977): Incorporation of labelled aminoacids into the enkephalins, *FEBS Lett.,* 84:195–198.

400. Stadaas, J. O., Schrumpf, E., and Hanssen, K. F. (1978): Somatostatin inhibits motility in response to distention. *Scand. J. Gastroenterol.,* 13:145–158.

401. Steinbusch, H. W. M., Verhofstad, A. A. J., and Joosten, H. W. J. (1978): Localization of serotonin in the central nervous system by immunohistochemistry: Description of a specific and sensitive technique and some applications. *Neuroscience,* 3:811–819.

402. Stern, A. S., Lewis, R. V., Kimura, S., Rossier, J., Gerber, L. D., Brink, L., Stein, S., and Udenfriend, S. (1979): Isolation of the opioid heptapeptide met-enkephalin (Arg^6, Phe^7) from bovine adrenal medullary granules and striatum. *Proc. Natl. Acad. Sci. U.S.A.,* 76:6680–6683.

403. Sternberger, L. A. (1974): *Immunocytochemistry.* Prentice Hall, Englewood Cliffs, New Jersey.

404. Stine, S. M., Yang, H.-Y. T., and Costa, E. (1980): Release of enkephalin-like immunoreactive material from isolated bovine chromaffin cells. *Neuropharmacology,* 19:683–685.

405. Studer, R. O., Trazeciak, H., and Lergier, W. (1973): Isolierung und Aminosäuresequenz von Substanz P aus Pferdedarm. *Helv. Chim. Acta,* 56:860–866.

406. Sundler, F., Alumets, J., Håkanson, R., Fahrenkrug, J., and Schaffalitzky de Muckadell, O. (1978): Peptidergic (VIP) nerves in the pancreas. *Histochemistry,* 55:173–176.

407. Sundler, F., Håkanson, R., Hammer, R. A., Alumets, J., Carraway, R., Leeman, S. E., and Zimmerman, E. A. (1977): Immunohistochemical localization of neurotensin in endocrine cells of the gut. *Cell Tissue Res.,* 178:313–321.

408. Sundler, F., Håkanson, R., Larsson, L.-I., Brodin, E., and Nilsson, G. (1977): Substance P in the gut: An immunochemical and immunohistochemical study of its distribution and development. In: *Substance P. Nobel Symposium 37,* edited by U. S. Von Euler and B. Pernow, pp. 59–65. Raven Press, New York.

409. Szurszewski, J. H., and Weems, W. A. (1976): Control of gastrointestinal motility by prevertebral ganglia. In: *Physiology of Smooth Muscle,* edited by E. Bülbring and M. F. Shuba, pp. 313–379. Raven Press, New York.

410. Tafuri, W. L., Maria, T. A., Pitella, J. E. H., and Bogliolo, L. (1974): An electron microscope study of the Auerbach's plexus and determination of substance P of the colon in Hirschsprung's disease. *Virchows Arch. Pathol. Anat. Physiol.,* A362:41–50.

411. Tager, H., Hohenboken, N., Markese, J., and Dinerstein, R. J. (1980): Identification and localization of glucagon-related peptides in rat brain. *Proc. Natl. Acad. Sci. U.S.A.,* 77:6229–6233.

412. Takahashi, T., Konishi, S., Powell, D., Leeman, S. E., and Otsuka, M. (1974): Identification of the motoneuron-depolarizing peptide in bovine dorsal root as hypothalamic substance P. *Brain Res.,* 73:59–69.

413. Takahashi, T., and Otsuka, M. (1975): Regional distribution of substance P in the spinal cord and nerve roots of the cat and the effect of dorsal root section. *Brain Res.,* 87:1–11.

413a. Tatemoto, K., Carlquist, M., and Mutt, U. (1982): Neuropeptide Y—A novel brain peptide with structural similarities to peptide YY and pancreatic polypeptide. *Nature,* 296:659–660.

414. Tatemoto, K., and Mutt, V. (1978): Chemical determination of polypeptide hormones. *Proc. Natl. Acad. Sci. U.S.A.,* 75:4115–4119.

415. Tatemoto, K., and Mutt, V. (1980): Isolation of two novel candidate hormones using a chemical method for finding naturally occurring polypeptides. *Nature,* 285:417–418.

416. Taylor, I. L., Walsh, J. H., Carter, D., Wood, J., and Grossman, M. I. (1979): Effects of atropine and bethanechol on bombesin-stimulated release of

pancreatic polypeptide and gastrin in dog. *Gastroenterology*, 77:714–718.

417. Terenius, L., and Wahlström, A. (1974): Inhibitor(s)of narcotic receptor binding in brain extracts and cerebrospinal fluid. *Acta Pharmacol. Toxicol. [Suppl.]* 1:55.

418. Terenius, L., and Wahlström, A. (1975): Search for an endogenous ligand for the opiate receptor. *Acta Physiol. Scand.*, 94:78–81.

419. Thulin, L., and Olsson, P. (1973): Effects of intestinal peptide mixture G2 and vasoactive intestinal peptide VIP on splanchnic circulation in the dog. *Acta Chir. Scand.*, 139:691–697.

420. Tournade, A., Chabrol, M., and Wagner, P. E. (1925): Le système nerveux adrénaline-sécréteur. *C. R. Soc. Biol. (Paris)*, 93:933.

421. Tramu, G., Pillez, A., and Leonardelli, J. (1978): An efficient method of antibody elution for the successive or simultaneous location of two antigens by immunocytochemistry. *J. Histochem. Cytochem.*, 26:322–324.

422. Uddman, R., Alumets, J., Densert, O., Håkanson, R., and Sundler, F. (1978): Occurrence and distribution of VIP nerves in the nasal mucosa and tracheobronchial wall. *Acta Otolaryngol.*, 86:443–448.

423. Uddman, R., Alumets, J., Edvinsson, L., Håkanson, R., and Sundler, F. (1978): Peptidergic (VIP) innervation of the esophagus. *Gastroenterology*, 75:5–8.

424. Uddman, R., Fahrenkrug, J., Malm, J., Alumets, J., Håkanson, R., and Sundler, F. (1980): Neuronal VIP in salivary glands: Distribution and release. *Acta Physiol. Scand.*, 110:31–38.

425. Uddman, R., Malm, L., and Sundler, F. (1980): The origin of vasoactive intestinal polypeptide (VIP) nerves in the feline nasal mucosa. *Acta Otolaryngol.*, 89:152–156.

426. Uddman, R., Malm, L., and Fahrenkrug, J. (1981): VIP increases in nasal blood during stimulation of the vidian nerve. *Acta Otolaryngol.*, 91:135–138.

427. Uddman, R., and Sundler, F. (1979): Vasoactive intestinal polypeptide nerves in human upper respiratory tract. *ORL J. Otorhinolaryngol. Rolat. Spec.*, 41:221–226.

428. Uvnäs-Wallensten, K., Efendic, S., and Luft, R. (1978): Occurrence of somatostatin-like immunoreactivity in the vagal nerves. *Acta Physiol. Scand.*, 102:248–250.

429. Uvnäs-Wallensten, K., Rehfeld, J. F., and Uvnäs, B. (1977): Heptadecapeptide gastrin in the vagal nerve. *Proc. Natl. Acad. Sci. U.S.A.*, 74:5707–5710.

430. Vaalasti, A., Linnoila, I., and Hervonen, A. (1980): Immunohistochemical demonstration of VIP, (met^5)- and (leu^5)-enkephalin immunoreactive nerve fibres in the human prostate and seminal vesicles. *Histochemistry*, 66:89–98.

431. Vaillant, C., Dimaline, R., and Dockray, G. J. (1980): The distribution and cellular origin of vasoactive intestinal polypeptide in the avian gastrointestinal tract and pancreas. *Cell Tissue Res.*, 211:511–523.

432. Van Nueten, J., Van Ree, J. M., and Vanhoutte, P. M. (1977): Inhibition by met-enkephalin of peristaltic activity in the guinea-pig ileum, and its reversal by naloxone. *Eur. J. Pharmacol.*, 41:341–342.

433. Vaught, J. L., and Takemori, A. E. (1978): Characterization of leucine and methionine enkephalin and their interaction with morphine on the guinea-pig ileal longitudinal muscle. *Res. Commun. Chem. Pathol. Pharmacol.*, 21:391–407.

434. Verhofstad, A. A. J., Steinbusch, H. W. M., Penke, B., Varga, J., and Joosten, H. W. J. (1980): Use of antibodies to norepinephrine and epinephrine in immunohistochemistry. In: *Histochemistry and Cell Biology of Autonomic Neurones, SIF Cells, and Paraneurones*, edited by O. Eränkö, S. Soinila, and H. Paivärinta, pp. 185–193. Raven Press, New York.

435. Verhofstad, A. A. J., Steinbusch, H. W. M., Penke, B., Varga, J., and Joosten, H. W. J. (1981): Serotonin-immunoreactive cells in the superior cervical ganglion of the rat. Evidence for the existence of separate serotonin- and catecholamine-containing small ganglionic cells. *Brain Res.*, 212:39–49.

436. Viveros, O. H., Diliberto, E. J., Hazum, E., and Chang, K.-J. (1979): Opiate-like materials in the adrenal medulla: Evidence for storage and secretion with catecholamines. *Mol. Pharmacol.*, 16:1101–1108.

437. Vizi, E. S., Bertaccini, G., Impicciatore, M., and Knoll, J. (1973): Evidence that acetylcholine released by gastrin and related polypeptides contributes to their effect on gastrointestinal motility. *Gastroenterology*, 64:268–277.

438. von Euler, U. S. (1963): Substance P in subcellular particles in peripheral nerves. *Ann. N.Y. Acad. Sci.*, 104:449–461.

439. von Euler, U. S., and Gaddum, J. H. (1931): An unidentified depressor substance in certain extracts. *J. Physiol. (Lond.)*, 72:74–87.

440. Waterfield, A. A., Smokcum, R. W. J., Hughes, J., Kosterlitz, H. W., and Henderson, G. (1977): *In vitro* pharmacology of the opioid peptides, enkephalins and endorphins. *Eur. J. Pharmacol.*, 43:107–116.

441. Watson, S. J., Akil, H., Richard, C. W. III, and Barchas, J. D. (1978): Evidence for two separate opiate peptide neuronal systems. *Nature*, 275:226–228.

442. Wharton, J., Polak, J. M., Bryant, M. G., Van Noorden, S., Bloom, S. R., and Pearse, A. G. E. (1979): Vasoactive intestinal polypeptide (VIP)-like immunoreactivity in salivary glands. *Life Sci.*, 25:273–280.

443. Widdicombe, J. G. (1963): Regulation of tracheobronchial smooth muscle. *Physiol. Rev.*, 43:1–37.

444. Williams, J. T., and North, R. A. (1978): Effect of substance P on intestinal smooth muscle cells. *Fed. Proc.*, 37:1422.

445. Williams, J. T., and North, R. A. (1978): Inhibition of firing of myenteric neurons by somatostatin. *Brain. Res.*, 155:165–168.

446. Williams, J. T., and North, R. A. (1979): Effects of endorphins on single myenteric neurons. *Brain Res.*, 165:57–75.

447. Williams, J. T., and North, R. A. (1979): Vasoactive intestinal polypeptide excites neurones of the myenteric plexus. *Brain Res.*, 175:174–177.

448. Wilson, S. P., Chang, K.-J., and Viveros, H. (1980): Synthesis of enkephalins by adrenal medullary chromaffin cells: Reserpine increases incorporation of radiolabelled amino acids. *Proc. Natl. Acad. Sci. U.S.A.,* 77:4364–4368.

449. Wood, J. D., and Mayer, C. J. (1978): Slow synaptic excitation mediated by serotonin in Auerbach's plexus. *Nature,* 276:836–837.

450. Wood, J. D., and Mayer, C. J. (1978): Functional significance of slow EPSP in myenteric ganglion cells. In: *Neurosci. Abstr.,* 4:586.

451. Wolfe, D. E., and Potter, L. T. (1963): Localization of norepinephrine in the atrial myocardium. *Anat. Rec.,* 145:301.

452. Wolfe, D. E., Potter, L. T., Richardson, K. C., and Axelrod, J. (1963): Localising tritiated norepineph-rine in sympathetic axons by electron microscopic autoradiography. *Science,* 138:440–444.

453. Yalow, R. S. (1978): Radioimmunoassay: A probe for the fine structure of biologic systems. *Science,* 200:1236–1245.

454. Yanaihara, N., Yanaihara, C., Hirohashi, M., Sato, H., Iizuka, Y., Hashimoto, T., and Sakagami, M. (1977): Substance P analogs: Synthesis, and biological and immunological properties. In: *Substance P. Nobel Symposium 37,* edited by U. S. von Euler and B. Pernow, pp. 27–33. Raven Press, New York.

455. Yau, W. M. (1978): Effect of substance P on intestinal muscle. *Gastroenterology,* 74:228–231.

456. Young, J. Z. (1939): Partial degeneration of the nerve supply of the adrenal. A study in autonomic innervation. *J. Anat.,* 73:540–550.

Chemical Neuroanatomy, edited by P. C. Emson,
Raven Press, New York © 1983.

Cytochemistry of the Spinal Cord

S. P. Hunt

MRC Neurochemical Pharmacology Unit, Medical Research Council Centre, Cambridge, England

The current interest in histochemistry has stemmed largely from the success in isolating and raising antibodies to a large number of small peptides and other putative neurotransmitter substances. Once antibodies became available, immunocytochemical techniques were used to localize the antigens in nervous tissue from a variety of animals and man (28,39). Such has been the success of this approach that there has been an avalanche of immunocytochemical data which, to a large extent, has complemented previous morphological observations (28).

In some areas such as the dorsal horn of the spinal cord, the intricate structure had proved particularly difficult to analyze with traditional neuroanatomical methods. The seminal discovery of substance P (58,60,95) within dorsal root sensory fibers and the subsequent localization of a wide variety of peptides within intrinsic neurons of the dorsal horn have radically changed this situation, and an unexpectedly high degree of organization is emerging.

A large part of the interest in the spinal cord has, of course, been in mechanisms of pain transmission (1) and the analgesia that can be caused by enkephalin and other peptides and amines when perfused over the spinal cord or injected at various levels of the brainstem (144–146). However, although many of the neuropeptides are found in sensory areas of the spinal cord, they are also found to varying extents in the ventral horn and around the central canal and may interact with other well-established neurotransmitter substances in these areas.

This chapter attempts to synthesize histochemical and neuroanatomical data on the spinal cord. It is not an inclusive treatise on spinal cord anatomy, a large part of which has been recently reviewed (23,143).

GENERAL ORGANIZATION OF THE SPINAL CORD

The gray matter of the spinal cord has been divided into 10 layers following the system introduced by Rexed (122) (Fig. 1). The marginal layer has been designated layer I, and the substantia gelatinosa, layer II, which was further divided into inner (II_i) and outer layers (II_o). Spinothalamic and other ascending pathways arise from neurons in layers I through VI, excluding, for the most part, layer II (143). Motor neurons are found within ventral horn layers VII through IX, and the gray matter surrounding the central canal is designated layer X. Sensory fibers from the dorsal root terminate throughout the spinal cord but predominantly within the dorsal horn and especially in layers I and II (see Figs. 3, 5).

THE ORGANIZATION OF PRIMARY SENSORY NEURONS

Cell Bodies

Sensory neurons within the dorsal root ganglia have been divided into two classes on the basis of perikaryal size (2,87–89) (Fig. 2). Large neurons are thought to give rise to large-diameter myelinated axons and are generally nonnociceptive, whereas smaller neurons give rise to finely myelinated small-diameter ($A\delta$) or unmyelinated (C) fibers which may have either nociceptive or nonnociceptive receptive field properties (16,92,98). There is, however, little direct evidence for the relationship between perikaryal size and axon diameter, and, indeed, only within the mouse and rat have cell size measurements been fitted to two distinct cell populations on the basis of perikaral size (87–89). Yoshida and Matsuda (148) injected the

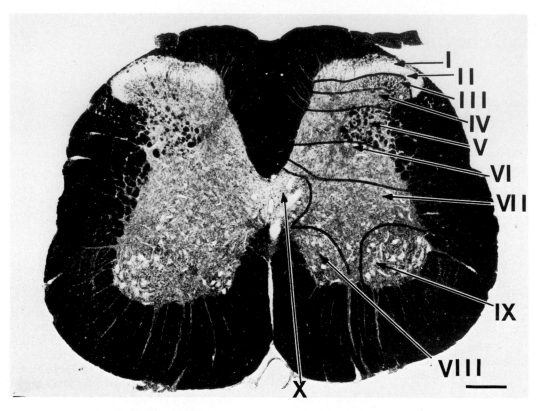

FIG. 1. Coronal section of the rat lumbar cord (L4) showing the lamina designations of Rexed (122). This is an unstained preparation, and dark areas indicate areas of myelination. The substantia gelatinosa, layer II, is conspicuous by the absence of myelinated fibers. Scale bar, 400 μm.

enzyme horseradish peroxidase (HRP) into single dorsal root ganglion cells of the mouse *in vitro* and measured conduction velocities. Small cell bodies had axons with slow conduction velocities, reflecting unmyelinated axons, and large perikarya had myelinated axons and fast conduction velocities.

In a detailed study of this problem, Lawson (87,88) has found that the small-cell compartment could be selectively manipulated by the neurotoxic drug capsaicin. Neonatal administration of the drug subcutaneously (80–90 mg/kg) resulted in a loss of 90% to 95% of unmyelinated fibers and 30% of the smaller diameter myelinated fibers (that is, the C and Aδ fiber groups) (74–76,105,106). Within the dorsal root ganglion, a major loss of neurons occurred from the small-cell compartment, and the larger neurons were left virtually undamaged (S. N. Lawson, *personal communication*). This clearly suggests that C and Aδ fibers originate from small perikarya with diameters ranging from 15 to 25 μm in the mouse.

Termination of Axons

At the light microscopic level, using Golgi methods, Cajal (22) and later the Scheibels (131,132) suggested that thicker (i.e., larger myelinated) fibers within the dorsal root pass medially before plunging ventrally through gelatinosa, arching back, and terminating within the substantia gelatinosa and deeper layers. A finer plexus of primary afferent fibers entered the superficial layers directly from the dorsal root and terminated in the marginal layer and the substantia gelatinosa. Ranson (118–120) later suggested that the finer fiber component was made up of primary afferent Aδ and C fibers and that the thick- and fine-fiber systems could be selectively lesioned by virtue of the distinct medial passage of large-diameter axons, a point exploited in the recent tracing studies of Light and Perl (see below). Ranson also concluded that the substantia gelatinosa received an exclusively unmyelinated fiber input, whereas Aδ fibers terminated primarily within layer I. This second division of the fine-fiber system received support from later Golgi studies (23,143).

The results of degeneration studies were broadly in agreement with the Golgi work (84). At the light microscopic level in the cat and rat, termination of primary afferents within the substantia gelatinosa was initially felt to be minimal (114,115,140). However, by using short survival times (24–48 hr), Heimer and Wall (57) were able to demonstrate dense terminal degeneration within the deeper half of the substantia gelatinosa and to a lesser extent in layer I in both the rat and the cat. In the monkey, the situation appears to be slightly different. At the electron microscopic level, large fibers or at least the axon terminals of large myelinated fibers degenerate before those of fine myelinated fibers, and the C fibers are the last fiber component to degenerate (117).

From the analysis of these relative rates of degeneration, it was concluded (117) that Aδ fibers terminated mainly within layer I and C fibers in layer II which was in good agreement with Ran-son's earlier studies of silver-stained tissue. The result was, however, not in agreement with that of Gobel and Binck (52). Following peripheral trigeminal nerve injury in the cat, fine axon and terminal changes occurred first and were confined to layer I. Later changes thought to be related to Aδ fibers were restricted to layer II. However, in a later study, Arvidsson and Gobel (5) produced data to suggest that in fact the situation in the cat may not be so different from that in other animals (see below).

The introduction of anterograde HRP tracing methods has greatly helped to establish unequivocally the mode of termination of both fiber groups and individual sensory axons with an identified receptive field.

Light and Perl (90,91), using a selective lesioning procedure, confirmed the original suspicion that large fibers terminate exclusively below layer II, whereas fine fibers terminate within layers I and II, occasionally with collaterals to layer V. Large fibers have been, in many cases, intracellularly filled with HRP, and their receptive fields analyzed

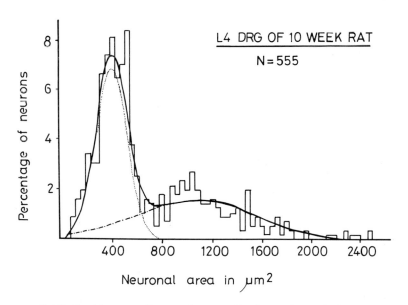

FIG. 2. A frequency distribution histogram of neuronal cross-sectional areas from a single rat L4 dorsal root ganglion. The measurements were made on all neurons with nucleoli in one 1.5-μm epon section every 100 μm throughout the ganglion. The data are displayed as a histogram, superimposed on which are the normal distributions of the small- and large-cell populations calculated from the best-fit parameters provided by the Maximum Likelihood Program by G. S. Ross, Rothamsted, Harpenden, Herts. Also superimposed is the summed calculated frequency distribution of these two populations. The χ^2 test between this (expected) and the data (observed) shows there is no significant difference at the 5% level. Similar histograms from mouse L3 and rat T13 and L4 ganglia can always be fitted by two normal distributions, which represent two separate morphological neuronal types, the large light and small dark cell populations, which are probably equivalent to types A and B described by Andres in 1961(2). (From Lawson, ref. 87, with permission.)

(19,20). The organization of the afferent axonal arborization within layers III and IV of the spinal cord (of the cat in most cases) is generally distinct and related to each type of cutaneous afferent unit. Brown comments (19) that this specificity "extends to the branching pattern of the collaterals, the arrangement of the terminal arborization, the laminar distribution of the synaptic boutons and the bouton arrangement of the terminal axons."

Light and Perl (92) have extended this type of analysis to small myelinated $A\delta$ fibers. They found that high-threshold mechanoreceptors had terminals within layer I and collaterals in layer V, with the occasional "spray" in the midline over the central canal. In contrast, low-threshold "D-hair" $A\delta$ fibers terminated extensively within lamina III. To date, no C fibers have been individually filled. However, there is indirect evidence that C fibers terminate throughout layers I and II. Arvidsson and Gobel (5) noted that the smallest-diameter trigeminal ganglion cell bodies were filled by HRP application to the inferior alveolar nerve but not following tooth pulp injections of the enzyme. Within the brainstem, terminal labeling within the spinal trigeminal nucleus was largely restricted to layer I after tooth pulp injections but extended into layer II in alveolar nerve experiments. This suggests that the smallest perikarya, which presumably have unmyelinated axons, project onto layers I and II.

The situation has been investigated in the rat cord by observing the anterograde movement of HRP after direct injection into the dorsal root ganglion at L5 and L6 (Fig. 3). As has been previously demonstrated (56,149), after application of HRP to the cut sciatic nerve of the rat, the rate of transport of HRP in small-diameter fibers is faster than that in large-diameter fibers. Moreover, direct injection into the ganglion resulted in a Golgi-like labeling of dorsal root afferents which could also be visualized at the electron microscopic level (69). At 3 to 5 days survival, we found labeling throughout layers I and II, with a particularly high concentration of labeled fibers within layer I outer (I_o) and the inner portion of layer II (II_i) (Fig. 3A). At 7 days (Fig. 3B) and longer survival periods, labeling in these axons was diminished, and coarse fibrous labeling was seen in layers I, II_o, and III as well as in deeper layers of the cord.

These tracing experiments were repeated in animals that had received a neonatal dose of the neurotoxic drug capsaicin (Fig. 3C,D). Capsaicin has been shown to destroy primarily unmyelinated primary afferents (Fig. 4) without affecting the central nervous system (74–76,104–106,130). Increasing doses of the drug result in the destruction of increasing numbers of small myelinated fibers (J. I. Nagy, L. L. Iversen, S. P. Hunt, and D. W. Chapman, *in preparation*). In animals in which C fibers had been preferentially lost, very little labeling was seen within layer II_i (Fig. 3C,D), although some termination within layers I and II_o also seemed probable from immunohistochemical data (see below). Layer II_i, therefore, receives only C-fiber input without an $A\delta$ component, a result in agreement with physiological reports in the monkey (14,15).

In the rat, some 70% of the recorded population of peripheral nerve C fibers were polymodal nociceptors, and 12% mechanorecptors (98), although these proportions show considerable interspecies variation (16). In the cat and monkey, neurons within layer II_i respond primarily to nonnoxious C-fiber stimulation, which may imply that the principal input to this region of the rat substantia gelatinosa is also nonnociceptive.

The pattern of termination of dorsal root fibers was also studied after injections of [^{3}H]proline into the dorsal root ganglion with survival periods of 6 to 24 hr (Fig. 5). In normal animals, labeling was

---

FIG. 3. The anterograde movement of the enzyme horseradish peroxidase (HRP) following injection into dorsal root ganglia L4 and L5 in the rat, visualized in parasagittal sections. **A:** Three days after injection of enzyme, three tiers of anterograde labeling are seen within the superficial spinal cord. Intense bursts of label are seen in layer I *(arrowhead)*, and bands of label within layers II_o and II_i. Many labeled fibers are seen within Lissauer's tract (Lt). **B:** Seven days after injection of enzyme, labeling within layer II has largely disappeared, but intense labeling of fibers within layer III is now seen. Some enzyme is also found in layer I. This is thought to reflect the slower labeling of large-diameter fiber systems. **C:** Three days after HRP injection into the lumbar ganglion of an adult animal treated 2 days after birth with the drug capsaicin (50 mg/kg). Intense labeling is seen within layer II_o, with some in I. The deeper layer of labeling within layer II_i is not apparent. **D:** Five days after HRP injection into L4/L51 of a capsaicin-treated animal. Extensive labeling of coarse fibers within layers I and II_o is seen. The implication of these studies is that the destruction of unmyelinated (C) fibers following capsaicin treatment results in a loss of primary afferent input primarily to layers I and II_i but that there may be increased input to layer II_o by the remaining small-caliber primary afferents, perhaps because of sprouting. Tetramethyl benzidene substrate. Scale bar, 90 μm. (From S. P. Hunt and J. I. Nagy, *unpublished observations.*)

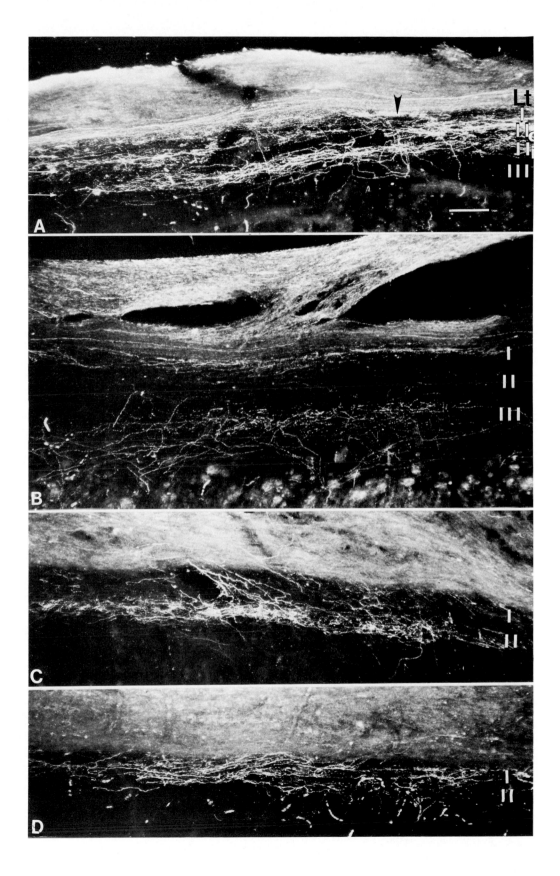

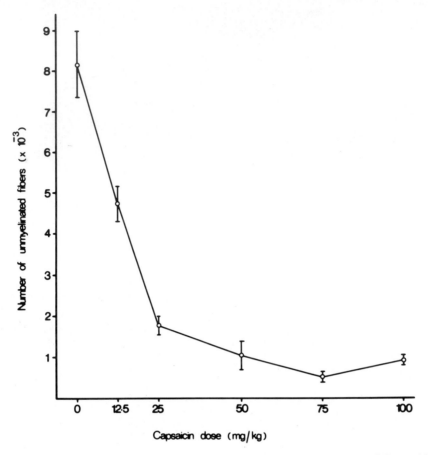

FIG. 4. The effects of various doses of capsaicin given 2 days after birth on the unmyelinated fibers within the third lumbar dorsal root (L3) of the adult rat: 90% of unmyelinated fibers are lost following injection of 25 to 50 mg of the drug. (From Nagy et al., ref 105a, with permission.)

seen throughout the dorsal horn but with concentrations of silver grains within layers I and II (Fig. 5). These concentrations disappeared after high-dose neonatal capsaicin injections, but silver grains were still seen over all dorsal horn layers.

These observations on the rat, which revealed discrete layers of heavy primary afferent termination within gelatinosa, are similar to studies in the cat (84) and monkey (121) in which the heaviest zone of primary afferent terminal labeling was seen also within layers I and II.

In summary, a large number of studies tend to suggest that C fibers terminate throughout layers I and II, whereas Aδ fibers terminate only within layers I and II$_o$. Larger-diameter myelinated fibers terminate deep to layer II.

FIG. 5. Labeling of the superficial layers of the lumbar dorsal horn by a variety of histochemical procedures. Parasagittal sections. **A:** The distribution of substance P-like immunoreactivity predominantly within layers I and II$_o$ with positive fibers running in Lissauer's tract (Lt). **B:** The total pattern of primary afferent termination is seen in this autoradiograph made 6 hr after an injection of 40 μCi of [^{3}H]proline into lumbar ganglia L4 and L5. Parts **A** and **B** were chosen to correspond as closely as possible. It is immediately apparent that there is an intense band of primary afferent termination within layer II$_i$ which is not seen with SP histochemistry (**A**). **C:** Photomicrograph taken rostral to **B.** Labeling within layer II is diminished, but there is still extensive labeling within layers I and III–IV. **D:** Retrogradely labeled cells in layer I and III following injection of HRP into the white matter of the cervical spinal cord. Projection cells are rarely found within the substantia gelatinosa (cf. 45). Tetramethyl benzidene reaction. Scale bar, 100μm. (S. P. Hunt and J. I. Nagy, *unpublished observations.*)

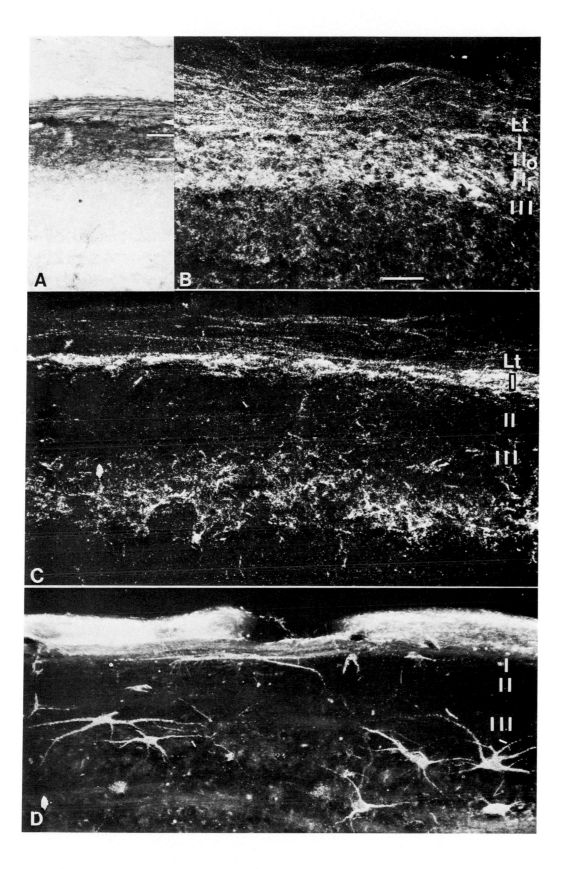

Histochemistry of Dorsal Root Afferents

A number of peptides and the enzyme fluoride-resistant acid phosphatase (FRAP) have been found within discrete populations of small dorsal root ganglion cells of the rat and mouse. Hökfelt et al. originally demonstrated that the peptides substance P (SP) (Fig. 6) and somatostatin (SOM) were present in discrete, nonoverlapping populations of small-diameter ganglion cells and terminated in slightly different regions of the superficial dorsal horn in rat (58).

We have found that the enzyme FRAP, which is only demonstrable in the rodent dorsal root ganglion (82), is found in approximately twice as many small sensory perikarya as SP and SOM but does not coexist with either of these peptides (Fig. 7) (104). Some FRAP-positive primary afferent terminals are found within layer II of the spinal cord (Fig. 8), overlapping with the distribution of SOM-positive terminals but incompletely with the more superficially distributed SP. After neonatal capsaicin treatment sufficient to destroy mainly the unmyelinated fibers of the dorsal root, SP and SOM concentrations within the dorsal root are reduced by about 90%, but less so in the dorsal horn (50% and 20%, respectively) (105). The distribution and depletion of SP could be detected histochemically, as could the complete loss of FRAP from the dorsal horn (76,105). These results suggested that there are at least three discrete populations of C fibers containing either SP, SOM, or FRAP (Fig. 9). These terminate differentially within layers I and II of the dorsal horn, SP within layers I and II_o, SOM in II_i, and the largest group, containing FRAP, within layer II_i.

Comparison with the data from the anterograde tracing experiments described above suggests that the loss of input from layer II_i corresponds primarily to the loss of FRAP-positive C fibers, whereas the loss of C fibers from layer I is confirmed by the loss of SP from this layer and from layer II_o. The distribution of SP-positive afferents is not restricted to layers I and II. Many fibers run through the superficial layers to terminate within deeper layers. These fibers disappear after capsaicin treatment, may "contact" intrinsic SP-containing neurons (see Fig. 18E), and may reflect a population of fine fibers terminating in deep layers of the dorsal horn that has been described by other workers (Fig. 9) (67,105).

Peptide- and FRAP-containing C-fiber systems are further distinguished by their response to damage of the peripheral nerve (10,72,79). Following crush or ligation and section of the sciatic nerve, there is a fall in the content of FRAP within the zone of primary afferent termination within the dorsal horn (27,36,82). This recovers after prolonged survival periods of up to 6 months. Substance P content, however, only falls following section but not crush of the peripheral nerve (Fig. 5) (10), and recovery of substance P content has not yet been reported. In human material obtained 25 months following amputation of one leg, a loss of substance P was observable throughout the corresponding side of the lumbar and sacral (L4–S2) dorsal horn (Fig. 10) (72). The lack of recovery suggests primary afferent degeneration (3), and there was some evidence for an increase in the amounts of enkephalin immunoreactivity on the lesioned side (72) of the cord. Evidence has also been presented to show a loss of SP in patients with diminished pain sensitivity (111) and that peripheral structures are innervated by primary afferent SP (29,30,37).

A number of other peptides have been described within certain primary afferent neurons. These include a cholecystokinin-like peptide (CCK) (76,99), which has a similar distribution to primary afferent substance P within the dorsal horn; vasoactive intestinal polypeptide-like immunoreactivity (VIP) (97), which is confined largely to layer I of the spinal cord; and angiotensin II-like immunoreactivity (24,43). Levels of SP, CCK, and VIP-like immunoreactivity all decline following neonatal capsaicin treatment (76).

FIG. 6. The peripheral (**A,B**) and central (**C**) patterns of termination of substance P-containing dorsal root ganglion cells (**D**). Sternberger's immunoperoxidase technique (138) with interference contrast optics. **A:** Substance P-containing primary afferents ramify around a fungiform taste bud (t) in the rat tongue. Scale bar, 160 μm. (From Nagy et al., ref. 103, with permission.) **B:** A bundle of SP-containing fibers *(arrowhead)* ramify within the skin of a rat, coming into close contact with hair shafts (h) and passing dorsally as free nerve endings within the most superficial regions of the dermis. Scale bar, 18 μm. (S. P. Hunt, *unpublished observation*). **C:** The pattern of SP-containing primary afferent termination within the superficial dorsal horn of the rhesus monkey. Scale bar, 600 μm. (S. P. Hunt, *unpublished observation*). **D:** Substance P-containing small-diameter dorsal root ganglion cell *(arrowhead)*. Section taken from cervical dorsal root ganglion of rhesus monkey. Scale bar, 25 μm. (M. Ninkovic, *unpublished observation*.)

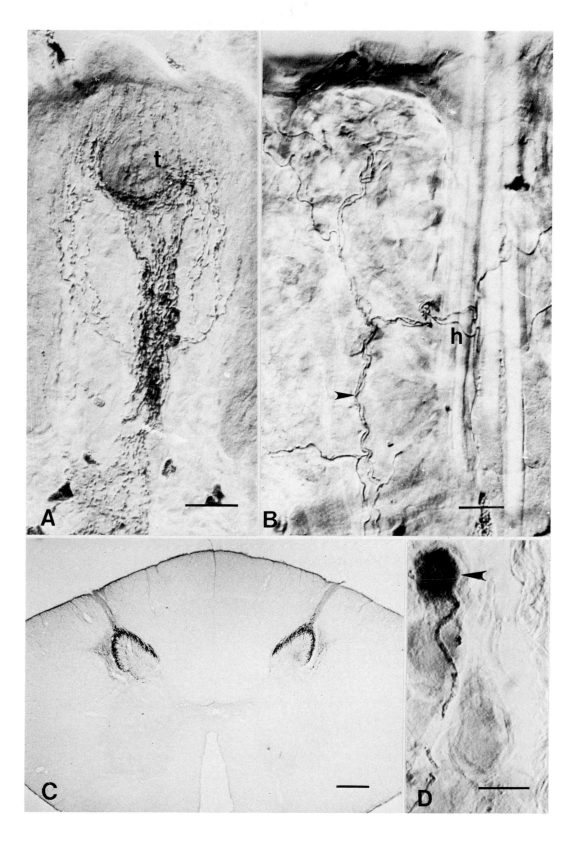

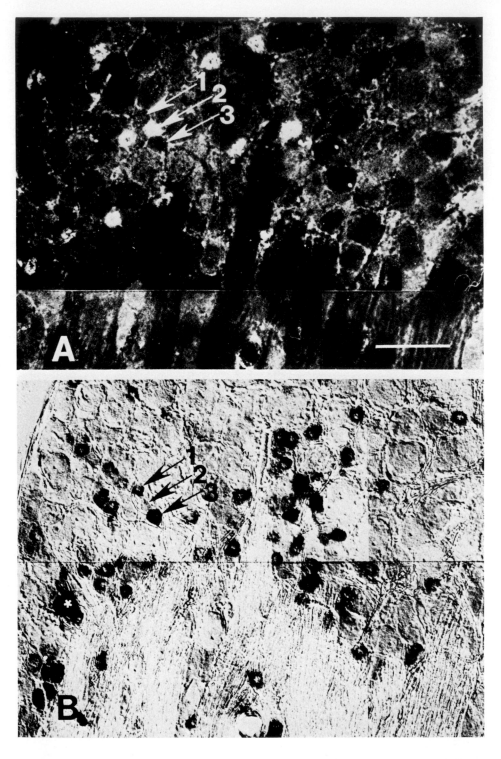

FIG. 7. Sequential labeling of a section of the rat lumbar dorsal root ganglion with (**A**) antisera to somatostatin using indirect immunofluorescence and (**B**) the Gomori reaction for acid phosphatase. Separate populations of small neurons were revealed. Substance P-containing cell bodies form a third population of neurons. Scale bar, 100 μm. (From Nagy and Hunt, ref. 104, with permission.)

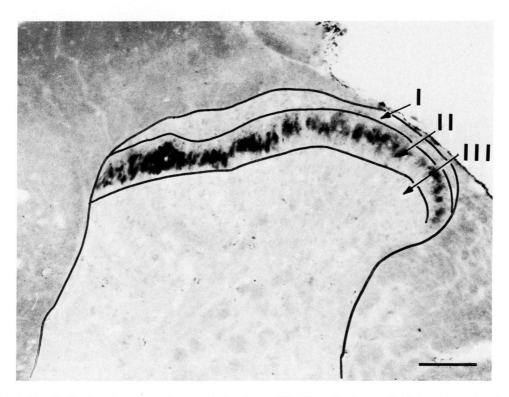

FIG. 8. The distribution of fluoride-resistant acid phosphatase (FRAP) within the superficial dorsal horn. Activity is largely confined to the intermediate portions of layer II and is derived from a population of dorsal root ganglion cells. The FRAP disappears following capsaicin treatment or rhizotomy. Scale bar, 180 μm.

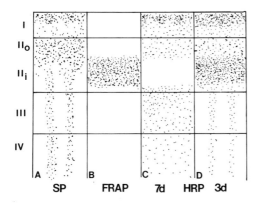

FIG. 9. Summary of the relationships between various primary afferent histochemical markers within the dorsal horn of the spinal cord. **A:** SP immunoreactivity. **B:** FRAP histochemistry. **C:** Anterograde labeling of myelinated fibers 7 days after HRP injections of the dorsal root ganglion. **D:** Anterograde labeling of unmyelinated fibers 3 days after HRP injection into the dorsal root ganglion.

Electron Microscopy of the Dorsal Horn

In their thorough study of synaptology in the monkey superficial dorsal horn, Ralston and Ralston (116,117) document the type and number of synapses within each layer and the ways in which these numbers change between layers. They list three broad classes of synaptic profile: round and clear, pleomorphic, and a mixture of both clear round and large granular vesicles (LGVs). In their study of normal and experimental material, they came to a number of important conclusions. One subclass of the "round clear" synaptic type formed axonal dilatations that make multiple synaptic contacts, usually in glomerular formations (C type). These almost totally (75%) disappear after dorsal root section or are labeled after [³H]leucine injections into the dorsal root ganglion (80%). They form 10% of the synaptic population of layer II but only 3% to 5% of layer I and are thought to be of primary afferent origin.

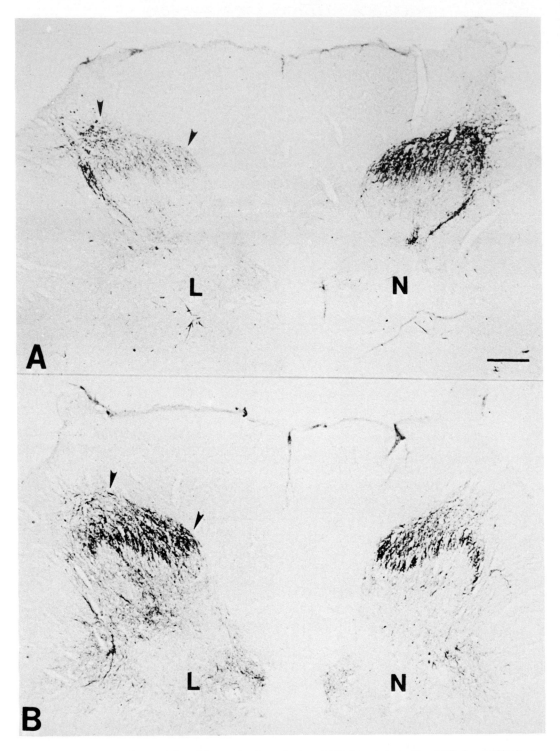

FIG. 10. Immunoperoxidase staining of human lumbar spinal cord **(A)** for substance P and **(B)** for methionine-enkephalin-like immunoreactivity 25 months after limb amputation. Substance P immunoreactivity is lost from side of lesion (L), particularly in the medial two-thirds of the dorsal horn *(arrowheads)*. There was some indication of increased levels of enkephalin **(A)** on the side of the lesion compared with the normal side (N). Scale bar, 1.2 mm. (From Hunt et al., ref. 72, with permission.)

Pleomorphic synaptic terminals never degenerated, whereas about 15% of the LGVs disappeared from layers I and II_o. The LGVs formed up to 15% of the total synaptic population in layers I and II_o. The C-type glomerular synapse would appear to correspond to a similar axon terminal population described earlier in the rat and cat. Synaptic glomeruli are rare in layer I and become more common toward the layer I/II_o border. Coimbra et al. (26), using FRAP histochemistry at the EM level, were able to localize the enzyme almost exclusively to C-type axonal endings, particularly within the intermediate portions of layer II. These degenerate following dorsal root section (26) or intrathecal capsaicin treatment (110). This observation, therefore, also suggests that the 70% of C-type terminations that contain FRAP and degenerate following dorsal root section represent one type of primary afferent ending. In some cases, FRAP-positive "C" terminals were presynaptic to other vesicle-containing profiles, often with round vesicles and LGVs, or postsynaptic to pleomorphic vesicle-containing dendritic profiles (26).

The nature of primary afferent termination within layer I of the spinal cord has been reinvestigated at the electron microscopic level following filling of sensory fibers with HRP (53,55). Two types thought to be either C or $A\delta$ fibers were filled and studied. Both types entered into glomerular arrangements, and were both pre- and postsynaptic to other elements of the neuropil. The discrepancy between this study (55), demonstrating fairly extensive axoaxonic interactions within the dorsal horn, and other studies in the rat and monkey in which such interactions are relatively rare (66,116,117,150) is difficult to explain but may reflect species differences.

The termination of peptide-containing afferents has been more difficult to analyze. Initial observations on substance P-containing terminals within the dorsal horn and, in fact, later work on other peptide-containing systems within the spinal cord suggested a common morphology for "peptidergic" terminals (9,25,66,112) (Fig. 11), including large numbers of round synaptic vesicles and LGVs and the making of asymmetric or symmetric synaptic contacts. The distribution and type of contact made by substance P-containing afferents have, however, proved particularly difficult to analyze, as there are both intrinsic and descending sources of the peptide (46,62,67). However, Barber et al. (9) demonstrated that substance P was found associated with LGVs and made axodendritic and occasionally axosomatic contacts. Little evidence was presented to show a glomerular localization for substance P. This would support the observations that peptides and FRAP are in separate dorsal root ganglion cells which terminate in the dorsal horn with minimal overlap and which have terminals that have different ultrastructures and synaptic relationships.

BIOCHEMICALLY SPECIFIC POPULATIONS OF SPINAL CORD NEURONS

Dorsal Horn

Cell Types

Within the dorsal horn of the spinal cord, a number of morphologically discrete populations of interneurons have been described on the basis of their peptide or glutamic acid decarboxylase (GAD) content (Figs. 12, 13) (GAD is regarded as a specific marker for GABAergic neurons). Correlation of histochemically defined cell types with those described from Golgi preparations has been particularly difficult because of the poor dendritic labeling of cells in histochemical studies and the failure of workers to agree on an acceptable classification of gelatinosa neurons. Most published studies would support the presence of at least two distinct cell types (15,22,23,131) as named by Gobel (50,51): the stalked cell and the islet cell (the limitrophe and central neurons of Cajal) (22) (Fig. 14). The perikaryon of the stalked cell lies on the I/II_o border with spiny dendrites which pass diagonally into more ventral laminae. The axon ramifies within layer I. Islet cells are found throughout layer II and have long rostrocaudally directed dendrites with restricted spread in the mediolateral plane and an axon that ramifies within the vicinity of the neuron's dendritic tree.

Both cell types have been described and characterized following intracellular injections of HRP with, in some cases, electron microscopic analysis (54). Two points of particular importance emerged. The receptive field properties of neurons could not be predicted on the basis of their morphology (although islet cells within II_i tended to be nonnociceptive), and islet cell dendrites are packed with synaptic vesicles and presynaptic to other dendrites and in some cases to axon terminals thought to be of primary afferent origin.

Peptide-Containing Neurons

In an immuohistochemical study of the rat spinal cord using local injections of colchicine to

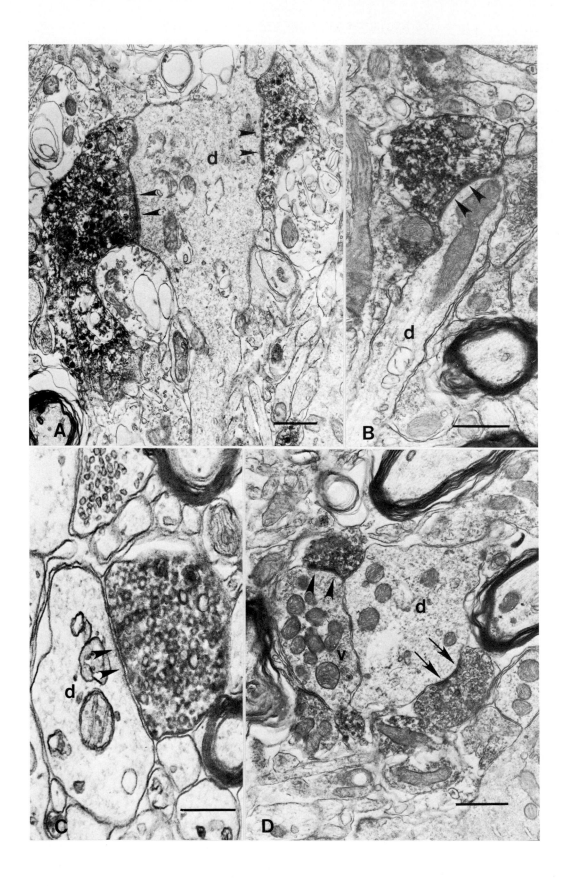

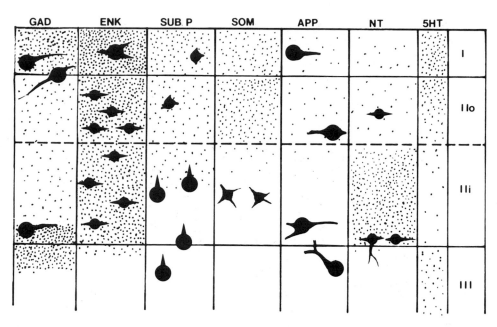

FIG. 12. A summary of the various immunoreactive cell types found within the dorsal horn of the rat spinal cord. *Stippling* is terminal immunoreactivity. GAD, glutamic acid decarboxylase; ENK, enkephalin; SUB P, substance P; SOM, somatostatin; APP, avian pancreatic polypeptide; NT, neurotensin-like immunoreactivity. The serotonin (5HT) immunoreactivity shown is derived from cell bodies in the raphe nuclei. (From Hunt et al., ref. 67, with permission.)

build up perikaryal levels of peptides, it was suggested that certain islet cells within layer II may contain enkephalin (ENK) (67) but that the only cell type that looked at all like a stalked cell was that containing GAD (67,123). This would suggest an inhibitory link between layers II and I. In the cat (49), however, a similar study suggested that most enkephalin-containing neurons were found within layer I, although, as in the rat, enkephalin immunoreactivity is found densely throughout layers I and II (38,42,59,63,66,128,133,135). Although able to confirm the presence of enkephalin-positive perikarya within layer I in the rat, reexamination of the cat normal spinal cord or following colchicine treatment revealed a number of enkephalin-positive neurons within layer II which would seem to be of the islet and, less commonly, stalked cell types (Fig. 14) (69,70).

In the rhesus monkey and human spinal cord, enkephalin-positive perikarya can be seen without resorting to colchicine pretreatment (Fig. 15) (72,85). Positive neurons are found throughout layers I through III but were clustered in layer III. In some cases, an axon could be seen to pass dorsally into the mass of enkephalin-positive fibers. Aronin et al. (4) report that many of these enkephalin-positive neurons have vesicle-containing dendrites, which would support the general thesis that

←

FIG. 11. Immunocytochemical localization of cholecystokinin (CCK)-like (**A**), glutamic acid decarboxylase (GAD)-like (**B,D**), and methionine-enkephalin (ENK)-like (**C**) immunoreactivity within the superficial dorsal horn of the rat using Sternberger's immunoperoxidase technique (138). **A:** CCK-like immunoreactivity localized in axon terminals making synaptic contacts *(arrowheads)* with a dendritic profile (d) in layer I of the lumbar dorsal horn. Scale bar, 0.5 μm. **B:** GAD-like immunoreactivity within an axon terminal making synaptic contact *(arrowheads)* with a dendrite (d) in layer II of the rat dorsal horn. Scale bar, 1 μm. **C:** An enkephalin-containing profile makes synaptic contact *(arrowheads)* with a dendritic element (d) in layer II. Scale bar, 0.25 μm. (From Hunt et al., ref. 66, with permission.) **D:** GAD-containing profile making a synaptic contact *(arrowheads)* with a vesicle-containing profile (v) which may be an axon terminal. A second labeled profile makes synaptic contact *(arrow)* with a dendrite (d). Layer III. Scale bar, 0.5 μm.

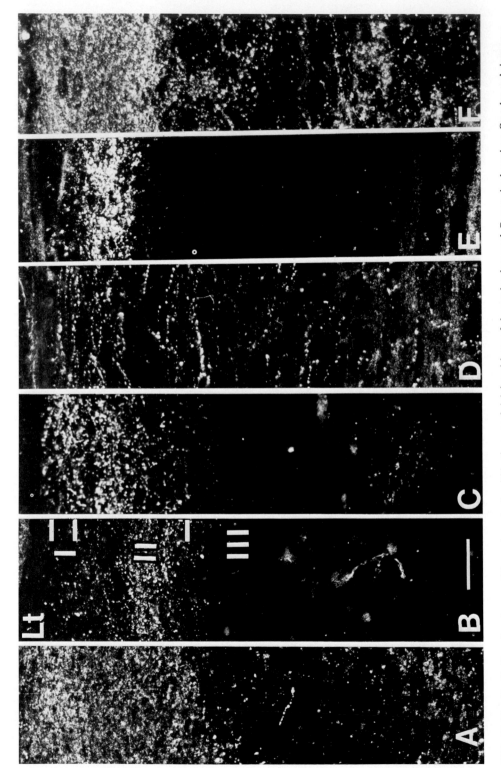

FIG. 13. The distribution of various peptides and serotonin within the superficial dorsal horn of the rat lumbar cord. Parasagittal sections; Sternberger's immunoperoxidase technique using dark-field illumination (138). **A:** Methionine-enkephalin. **B:** Neurotensin. **C:** Avian pancreatic polypeptide. **D:** Serotonin. **E:** Somatostatin. **F:** Substance P-like immunoreactivity. Scale bar, 100 μm.

a population of islet cells contain enkephalins and have dendrites that are presynaptic to other elements of the neuropil.

However, a difficulty arises if it is accepted that islet cells are at least in part the enkephalinergic neurons of the substantia gelatinosa. Within gelatinosa, opiate receptors are found both on intrinsic elements and on primary afferent fibers (6, 86,107,108). This has led to the suggestion that the direct inhibitory action of enkephalin on primary afferents was responsible for the analgesia caused by opiates (77,78,102,145). However, investigation of the relationship between enkephalinergic terminals and primary afferents at the electron microscopic level in the rat (31,66), cat (48), and monkey (4) has failed to find evidence for more than the occasional axoaxonic interaction. Although methodological difficulties may in part be responsible for this negative finding, the results as they stand are not completely compatible with the suggestion that islet cells are the enkephalinergic interneuron, as these cells do seem to have direct interactions with primary afferents within glomeruli. Perhaps the most parsimonious explanation is that there are several biochemical subclasses of islet cells and stalked cells and that not all subclasses of islet cells are in synaptic relationship with primary afferents.

A second histochemically distinct type of cell is that containing neurotensin-like immunoreactivity (NT) (44,67,134,141) (Fig. 12). These lie along the II/III border zone, with axon terminals forming a dense band within layer II_i and grouped less densely in layer I (Fig. 13). Electron microscopy suggests that most NT-positive terminals form asymmetric contacts with dendritic profiles and that axoaxonic interactions are rarely seen (108). The distribution of neurotensin receptors mapped with [^{3}H]neurotensin matches the distribution of immunoreactive axon terminals within layers I and II, and, unlike opiate and histamine receptors, these are unaffected by dorsal root section (41,107,108) (Figs. 15, 16).

The distribution of intrinsic substance P immunoreactivity has been studied after rhizotomy and hemisection (67). The remaining immunoreactivity has a distribution similar to but obviously less dense than the normal substance P (SP) pattern (in I and II). The deposits of immunoreactive material are, however, punctate rather than fibrous. After colchicine injections, cell bodies are found throughout layers I through V but particularly in II_i. The situation was entirely similar for intrinsic somatostatin-containing interneurons (21,34,67) which

account for up to 80% of the measurable somatostatin within the dorsal horn. Substance P-containing interneurons have in many cases bipolar dendritic trees and are invested with a plexus of primary afferent substance P-containing fibers (see Fig. 18E) (67,105). These fibers disappear following dorsal root section or neonatal capsaicin treatment (105).

Avian pancreatic polypeptide-like immunoreactivity (APP) has also been found within intrinsic interneuronal systems within the dorsal horn (65,96). This is of particular interest as it has been shown to coexist with norepinephrine or epinephrine in certain medullary cell groups (A1–A3) and within the locus ceruleus (A6) (65,96). The APP is present in large neurons scattered throughout the dorsal horn (65), with concentrations of terminal immunoreactivity in layers I and II_o. High concentrations of APP also occur in relation to the sacral parasympathetic system (65). In the sacral cord, enkephalin coexists with APP (65). It has also been shown that enkephalin immunoreactivity is found within parasympathetic motor neurons, but whether these are the neurons that also contain APP has not been directly demonstrated (47).

A number of peptide-containing interneurons were found within deeper layers of the dorsal horn and around the central canal. The majority of these cells were multipolar and could be labeled with antisera to SOM, ENK, SP, CCK, or APP (34,65,67,95).

GABA and Glycine

The distribution of [^{3}H]GABA-accumulating synapses and perikarya has been studied after *in vivo* subarachnoid perfusions of the tritiated amino acid (123). Cell bodies were seen principally within layer II_o and on the II/III border. Similar results were seen with GAD immunohistochemistry (Figs. 11, 12) (7,67). In all studies, it was suggested that the labeled gelatinosa cells were "stalked" cells. The GAD structures were seen to be concentrated within the superficial dorsal horn and concentrated into two zones within layer I and within layer III (8,101). At the electron microscopic level, some [^{3}H]GABA-accumulating profiles were thought to be dendritic, whereas the majority were axon terminals making axodendritic and occasionally axosomatic synaptic contacts. By using immunohistochemistry at the electron microscopic level 24 to 48 hr following dorsal root section, some GAD positive axon terminals were found to synapse on degenerating primary afferent axon terminals within

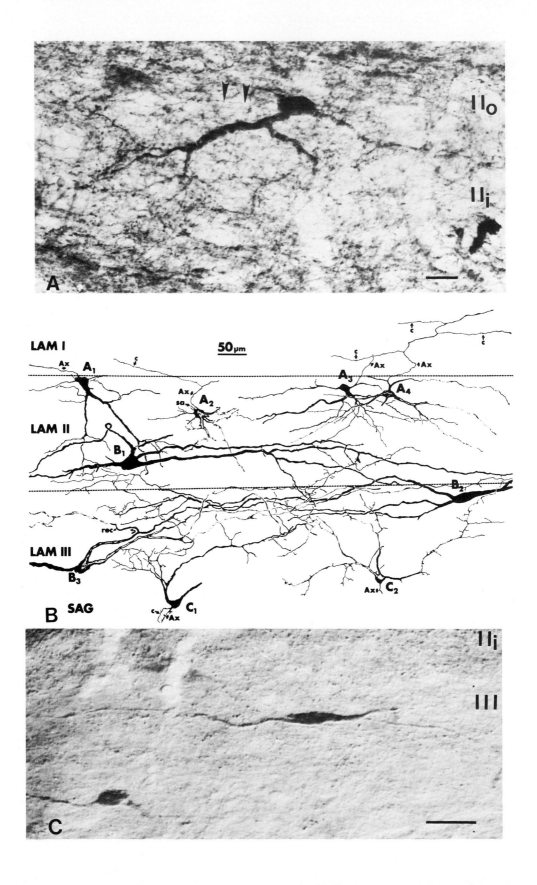

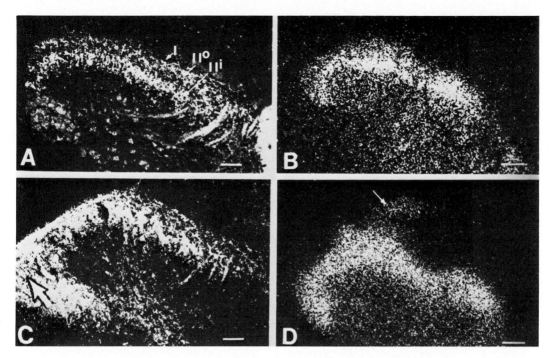

FIG. 15. Correspondence between the distribution of neuropeptides and their receptors in the superficial layers of the rat dorsal horn. Neurotensin-like (**A**) and Met-enkephalin-like (**C**) immunoreactivity were localized by immunoperoxidase staining. The autoradiographic distributions of [³H] neurotensin and opiate ([³H]etorphine) binding sites are shown in **B** and **D**, respectively. **D**. *Arrow* shows the presence of opiate receptors on incoming dorsal root fibers. **C**: *Arrow* indicates presence of Met-enkephalin-like immunoreactivity within the dorsal white matter—an area that does not show a corresponding density of opiate receptors. Receptors were localized using the technique of Young and Kuhar (147). Scale bar, 100 μm. (From Ninkovic et al., ref. 108, with permission.)

layer III (8). This may well be the morphological basis for primary afferent depolarization which is thought to be mediated by GABA (8).

Within layers III through V [³H]glycine was accumulated by neurons and terminals (123).

Glutamate and Aspartate

L-Glutamate is the only putative amino acid transmitter for which dorsal root levels exceed those of the ventral root; this has led to speculation that this amino acid may be a neurotransmitter of primary afferent neurons (32). [³H]-D-Aspartate injected into the dorsal horn is taken up by small (1) cells in layer II (127), and it has been suggested that there is some retrograde transport of the amino acid (139) to the perikarya of large cervical dorsal root ganglion cells (M. Cuenod, *personal communication*).

In a recent series of experiments (Fig. 17) (S. P. Hunt and D. van de Kooy, *in preparation*), when slices of spinal cord were incubated in micromolar

FIG. 14. The two most characteristic cell types of the substantia gelatinosa, the stalked cell (**A** and **B**) and the islet cell (**B** and **C**), can in some cases be shown to contain enkephalin-like immunoreactivity. **A:** Stalked cell stained for ENK with Sternberger's immunoperoxidase technique. The cell body lies in layer II$_o$, and a fine axon can be seen *(arrowheads)*. Cat lumbar spinal cord. Scale bar, 15 μm. **B:** Composite drawing of Golgi cell types. (From Beal and Cooper, ref. 13, with permission.) Stalked cells are represented by cell types A$_1$–A$_4$, and islet cells by neurons B$_1$–B$_3$. Monkey spinal cord. **C:** Islet cell labeled with enkephalin antisera using immunoperoxidase technique. Monkey spinal cord. Scale bar, 25 μm. **A** and **C** from immersion-fixed material (S. P. Hunt, *unpublished observations*).

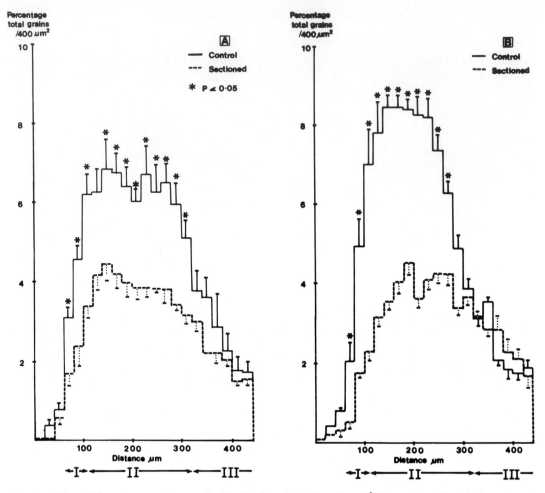

FIG. 16. Effect of dorsal root section on the distribution of specific opiate ([³H]etorphine, **A**) and histamine H_1 ([³H]mepyramine, **B**) binding sites in the cervical dorsal horn of the monkey. I represents the marginal layer; II, the substantia gelatinosa; and III, the nucleus proprius. Transparent grids were used to count silver grains within an area of 400 μm^2. Nonspecific binding levels for opiate and H_1 receptors were defined using 1 μM levorphanol and 2 μM promethazine, respectively; they were subtracted from each density measurement to show the distribution of specific binding sites. Each series of grain counts was repeated 10 times in each animal on several different tissue sections, and each point represents data from four animals ($N = 4$), each having received unilateral dorsal root sections 8 days prior to death. Sectioned and control sides were compared, and results are expressed as percentage frequencies of total grains; values on histograms are means ± SEM. Nonspecific binding levels represented 1.30 ± 0.10% of total grains for [³H]etorphine binding and 1.60 ± 0.16% for [³H]mepyramine binding sites. Results were analyzed using a two-tailed t-test and a significance level of $p < 0.05$. Both opiate and histamine H_1 receptor densities were significantly reduced by dorsal root section in all four animals by 43.5 ± 4.50% and 52.3 ± 4.89%, respectively (mean ± SEM). These reductions in receptor density represent specifically only those areas showing a significant loss. (From Ninkovic et al., ref. 107, with permission.)

FIG. 17. A: Uptake of [³H]-D-aspartate into a vibratome slice of unfixed rat lumbar (L6) spinal cord. In this dark-field autoradiograph, heavy uptake into layers I and II can be seen. There is also some uptake by elements lying along the ventral margin of the spinal cord *(arrow)*. These 300-μm tissue slices were incubated in Ringer solution with [³H]-D-aspartate (2 μM) for 25 min, rinsed, and fixed in 2.5% gluteraldehyde before embedding in paraffin wax, sectioning, and treatment with routine autoradiographic procedures. Exposure time, 24 days. Dark-field (**B**) and bright-field (**C**) photomicrographs of labeled dorsal root ganglion cells following (**B**) intrathecal perfusion with [³H]-D-aspartate (200 μCi in 40 μl artificial CSF) and a survival time of 18 hr or (**C**) direct injection of [³H]-D-aspartate (30 $\mu Ci/0.2$ μl) into the spinal cord and a survival time of 18 hr. Scale bar, 50 μm (**B,C**) and 200 μm (**A**). (S. P. Hunt and D. Van de Kooy, *unpublished observations*.)

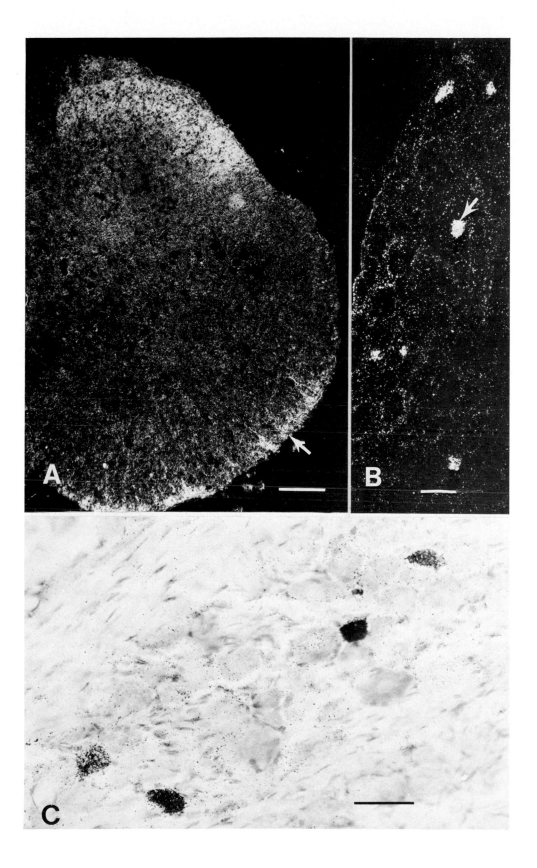

[^{3}H]-D-aspartate, there was intense uptake into layers I and II. Intrathecal or local injection of [^{3}H]-D-aspartate into the lumbar spinal cord resulted in the retrograde labeling of small dorsal root ganglia only (diameter 20 μm) and never the larger neurons. In lumbar sensory ganglia L4 and L5, the total number of labeled cells was small with rarely more than 10 labeled cells in each 20-μm section. Dorsal root section, however, had no effect on the pattern or intensity of [^{3}H]-D-aspartate uptake by the spinal cord slices. This suggests that there may be a small subpopulation of glutamate- or aspartate-releasing primary afferent neurons and a larger pool of gelatinosa neurons also capable of taking up and perhaps releasing these amino acids.

Acetylcholine

By using an antibody to choline acetyltransferase, high levels of immunoreactivity have been found within the substantia gelatinosa of the cat (81). In the rat, this layer also contained high levels of acetylcholinesterase. Perikarya have, however, rarely been seen with either marker. With the putative nicotinic receptor ligand [^{125}I]-α-bungarotoxin, concentrations of receptor were found within layers I and III (71) and on certain large dorsal root ganglion cells (113). There was a small reduction in labeling density after dorsal root sections, which implies a presynaptic toxin-binding component (M. Ninkovic, *unpublished observation*). Acetylcholinesterase levels do not change following rhizotomy *(unpublished observations)*.

Ventral Horn

Peptide-Containing Neurons

The number of peptide-containing neurons within the ventral horn appears to be limited. Following cervical section, levels of enkephalin within the lumbar ventral cord (67) are unchanged. Immunoreactive axons appear to end in relation to small neurons rather than the adjacent larger motor (cf. 35) neurons (Fig. 18). Peptides are also found in association with certain "specializations" of the neuropil within the cord such as the lateral sympathetic motor column, parasympathetic sacral neurons, and Onuf's nucleus in the lower lumbar cord. Markers including APP, CCK, SP, and ENK are found at these sites, but it is not known to what extent these are descending or intrinsic systems (46,67,69,96).

GABA and Glycine

The distribution of GABA or GAD-containing neurons has been studied both by uptake of [^{3}H]GABA either in slices or after *in vivo* injections and by immunohistochemical methods. GABA is taken up into small cells located preferentially within the medial and dorsal parts of the spinal cord but in nerve terminals throughout the gray matter (61,94). Iversen and Bloom (73) calculated from electron microscopic observations that some 25% of all spinal cord synaptosomes were labeled with [^{3}H]GABA but that there was also some glial uptake.

With immunohistochemistry following colchicine injections in the rat, GAD and perikarya were found in cells of the ventral horn (7) with small to medium-sized perikarya. The distribution of terminals appeared similar to that seen in [^{3}H]GABA uptake experiments.

Uptake of [^{3}H]glycine by spinal cord slices was seen into nerve endings, unmyelinated axons, and glial cell bodies (61,93,100). No perikaryal labeling was seen. Direct injections of [^{3}H] glycine into the spinal cord, however, revealed the presence of labeled cell bodies mainly in the ventral horn. At the electron microscopic level, Matus and Dennison (100) report that all labeled axon terminals contained flattened synaptic vesicles. Most labeled terminals make axosomatic and axodendritic synaptic contacts and comprise about 25% of the total synaptic population. Certain of these "glycinergic" neurons are believed to be Renshaw cells mediating recurrent inhibition of motor neurons, and others may be interneurons mediating direct or reciprocal inhibition of motor neurons.

Acetylcholine

Motor neurons of the ventral horn contain and release acetylcholine. This is seen in the high content of both acetylcholinesterase and choline acetyltransferase (81). Recurrent collaterals of these neurons are thought to activate Renshaw cells at a nicotinic cholinergic synapse. With the putative nicotinic receptor ligand μ-bungarotoxin, extensive labeling of medium-sized cells was seen within the ventral and medial ventral horn (71). These may well be the Renshaw cells.

DESCENDING PATHWAYS

With retrograde and anterograde tracing methods, a large number of brain areas from the me-

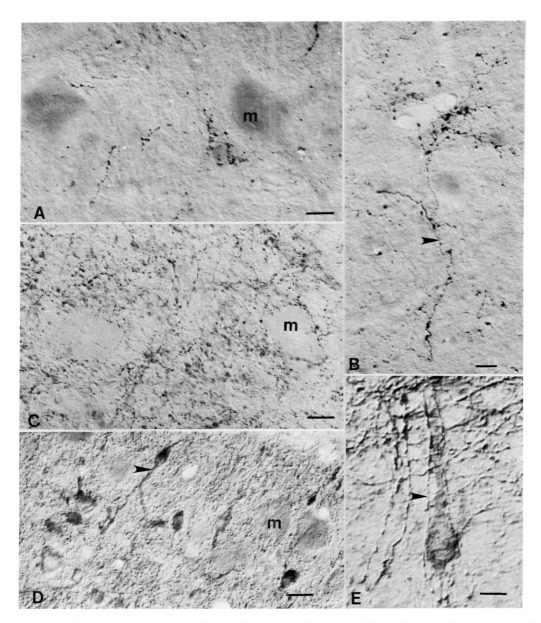

FIG. 18. A,B,C,E: Patterns of innervation by peptide-containing fibers. **A,B:** Enkephalin-positive fibers *(arrowhead)* innervate small perikarya but not the larger adjacent motor neurons (m) within the ventral horn of the rat. **C:** Substance P-positive fibers are found closely associated with most cell bodies found within the ventral horn. **E:** In the dorsal horn, substance P-containing fibers *(arrowhead)* "innervate" substance P-positive interneurons. **D:** GAD-positive interneurons *(arrowhead)* found in the ventral horn between motor neurons (m). All immunoperoxidase preparations photographed with interference contrast optics. Scale bar, 10 μm. (Figure 18E is from Hunt et al., ref. 67, with permission.)

dulla, the hypothalamus, and the cortex have been found to project onto the spinal cord (11,40,83). A number of peptide and other putative neurotransmitter substances have been found within certain of these neurons: occasionally several of these substances are found within the same neuron (62,64,68,80,129).

The Monoamines

Serotonin- (18,136,137), norepinephrine- (33, 109,142), epinephrine- (124), and dopamine (17)-containing neurons have been shown to project onto the spinal cord, although in some cases the exact details of area of termination are unknown.

Dopamine

Dopamine-containing neurons within the hypothalamic A11 group were labeled following cord injections of retrograde tracers (17,19). The area of dopaminergic termination within the spinal cord was shown by histofluorescent techniques following neonatal depletion of norepinephrine-containing systems and found to terminate throughout the dorsal and ventral horn (G. Skageberg and A. Björklund, *personal communication*).

Norepinephrine and Epinephrine

These projection systems arise from the medullary A1 through A3 cell groups and from the A5 and A6 cell groups (109,124,142). The A5 norepinephrine (NE) neurons project primarily to the lateral sympathetic motor column, whereas the remaining cell groups send projections to the dorsal horn (A1–A3) and ventral horn (A6) terminating apparently in association with motor neurons. Within the medulla, certain NE and epinephrine (E)-containing cells also contain an APP-like immunoreactive substance (65). Preliminary observations suggest that these neurons do not project to the spinal cord but send axons rostrally (D. van de Kooy and S. P. Hunt, *unpublished observations*).

Serotonin

Serotonin-containing cell bodies have been described in cell groups lying principally in the hindbrain from the caudal medulla to the hypothalamus (136,137). The medullary and pontine raphe nuclei are the principal source of spinal pathways, but not all neurons with descending axons contain serotonin, the proportions varying according to the nucleus and the species under investigation

(18,64,68). The dorsal horn receives input via the dorsolateral funiculus from the nucleus raphe magnus (NRM) (11,40), whereas the more caudally situated n. raphe obscurus (NRO) and pallidus (NRP) innervate the intermediate and ventral horns, ending in close association with motor neurons. Stimulation of these ventral horn inputs has a depressant action on certain spinal cord reflexes (40).

Serotonin-containing fibers terminate throughout the dorsal horn, but less strongly within layer II$_i$ (Fig. 19) (137). In an electron microscopic study of [^{3}H]serotonin uptake in the spinal trigeminal nucleus of the cat, Ruda and Gobel (125,126) conclude that there are up to seven distinct types of serotonin-accumulating axon terminals and that axoaxonic interactions are extremely rare. They suggest (126) that there may be three circuits by which serotonergic afferents may inhibit or reduce the output of layer I projection neurons. These are the direct inhibition of the layer I projection neuron by serotonergic terminals in layer I; inhibition of excitatory interneurons such as the stalked cell (although this neuron may in fact be inhibitory); and excitation of an inhibitory interneuron.

Histamine

The existence of a histamine-containing descending pathway has recently been suggested by the immunohistochemical localization of a histamine-like immunoreactivity within cell bodies in the pons and medulla (H. W. M. Steinbusch, *personal communication*) and the presence of H$_1$ histamine receptors, localized with [^{3}H]mepyramine, within both the dorsal and ventral horns of the spinal cord, in many cases over motor neurons (107). Section of the dorsal root results in a 40% drop in receptor binding within the substantia gelatinosa after 7 days, a result that parallels the loss of opiate receptors under similar conditions (Fig. 20). Also H$_1$ receptors were found over small dorsal root ganglion cells, which by serial sectioning techniques were also found to have opiate receptors on their perikarya (107).

Peptide-Containing Systems and Coexistence

The peptides SP and TRH have been found to coexist with serotonin in certain raphe neurons (Fig. 19) (46,80). Johansson et al. (80) have estimated that in the rat, out of all immunoreactive neurons in the medulla, twice as many 5-HT (56%) as TRH (23%) and SP (21%) cells were found, although within individual nuclei, these pro-

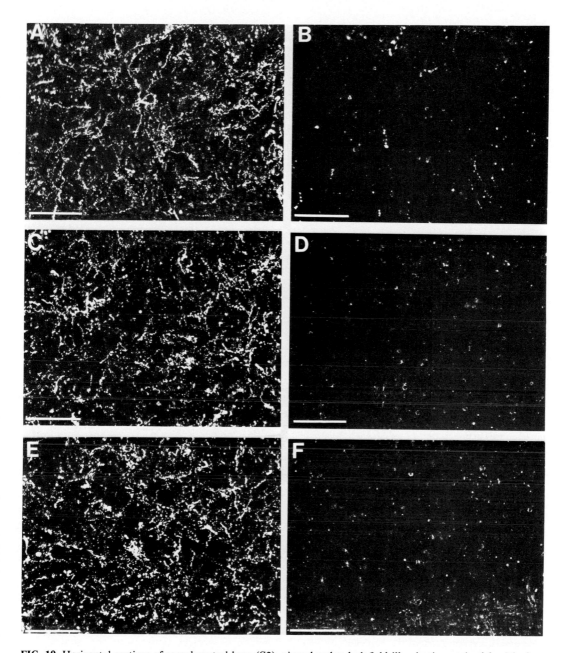

FIG. 19. Horizontal sections of sacral ventral horn (S2), viewed under dark-field illumination, stained for 5-hydroxytryptamine (**A,B**), thyrotropin-releasing hormone (**C,D**), and substance P (**E,F**). **A,C,E** are from a control animal, whereas **B,D,F** are from an animal pretreated with 200 µg 5,7-dihydroxytryptamine (free base) i.c.v. 3 weeks previously. This neurotoxin selectively destroys serotonergic axons originating from the hindbrain raphe nuclei and terminating within the spinal cord. This treatment also results in the loss of peptides that coexist with serotonin. (From Gilbert et al., ref. 46, with permission.)

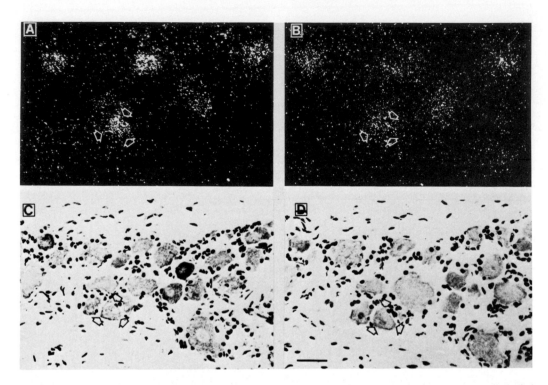

FIG. 20. Histamine H_1 (**A**) and opiate (**B**) receptors in serial 5-μm sections of the C4 dorsal root ganglion of the rhesus monkey. **A:** Dark-field autoradiograph of [^{3}H]mepyramine binding sites. **C:** Light-field photomicrograph of the same section stained with methylene blue. **B:** Dark-field autoradiograph of [^{3}H]etorphine binding sites. **D:** Light-field photomicrograph of the same sections stained with methylene blue. Silver grains are tightly associated with specific cell bodies, following both radioligands. *Arrows* indicate a cell body that is easily distinguishable on both serial sections and is apparently labeled by both opiate and H_1 receptors. Several other examples of dual labeling can be seen in this pair of serial sections. Scale bar, 40 μm. (From Ninkovic et al., ref. 107, with permission.)

portions varied. Some neurons contained both 5-HT and SP, others 5-HT, SP, and TRH, and other populations contained 5-HT alone. Within the ventral horn of the spinal cord, overlapping distributions of 5-HT, TRH, and SP were seen, particularly in association with motor neurons. Evidence that these peptide-containing fibers coexist within serotinergic neurons comes from the application of the neurotoxin 5,7-DHT which selectively destroys serotinergic systems. There is a concomitant loss of both SP and TRH throughout the ventral horn (Fig. 19). A severe depletion is also found within the lateral sympathetic motor column (46).

In the cat (12,68) and rat (42,64), a large number of raphe neurons contain both enkephalin and serotonin and project onto the spinal cord: other nonserotinergic enkephalin-containing pathways have also been described using a double-labeling technique, and it was found that the proportion of

single- and double-labeled neurons varied among nuclei. Within NRM of 78 neurons analyzed, 63% contained both ENK and 5-HT, 9% 5-HT only, and 28% ENK alone: that is, there were more neurons containing ENK than 5-HT. Within NRP, which contained many more labeled neurons, of 99 positive neurons, 38% were double labeled, 45% contained 5-HT alone, and 17% ENK only.

The TRH-containing neurons of the brainstem appear to project entirely to the ventral horn (46,80), whereas the exact mode of termination of SP descending axons is obscured by the large amounts of primary afferent and intrinsic SP. By radioimmunoassay, approximately 25% of SP in the dorsal horn is accounted for by descending systems (46).

There is preliminary evidence to suggest that a number of hypothalamic peptide-containing pathways project to the spinal cord, notably those containing oxytocin, vasopressin, somatostatin, and perhaps other peptides (129).

CONCLUSION

One of the most striking conclusions that can be drawn from this brief review of spinal cord cytochemistry is that the peptides that have been localized are almost entirely within unmyelinated primary afferents and interneuronal systems. Large-diameter myelinated afferents and spinal cord projection neurons are invariably unstained.

The second important general conclusion is that a neuronal system that may appear homogeneous by one anatomical criterion may well be divisible with other cytochemical techniques. Thus, the unmyelinated fibers of the dorsal root are divisible into at least three cytochemical groupings with apparently different areas of termination within the spinal cord. Similarly, gelatinosa neurons that appear to be distinct subtypes from Golgi studies can in fact be divided into a number of subgroups by virtue of their histochemical characteristics. Thus, certain islet cells may contain enkephalin or neurotensin, and certain stalked cell populations may contain enkephalin and/or GABA. These subtle biochemical distinctions are also seen in descending pathways that terminate within the spinal cord. Serotonin-containing cells of the raphe contain varying amounts of peptides such as SP, ENK, and TRH. These biochemically distinct subgroups may also terminate in distinct areas of the spinal cord; TRH, for example, is only found within the ventral horn and not the dorsal horn, and SP is found within serotonergic axons that terminate in all areas of the spinal cord.

The function(s) of these various peptides within the spinal cord and their interactions pre- and post-synaptically are at present poorly understood but, in time, will no doubt expand present concepts of neurotransmission or neuromodulation.

ACKNOWLEDGMENTS

Many of the experiments described in the text were carried out with the excellent technical assistance of Annette Bond and David Chapman. I would also like to thank Dr. L. L. Iversen for his support and encouragement and my collaborators, Mary Ninkovic and J. Nagy, in many of the studies

Expert secretarial assistance was given by Mary Wynn and Jan Ditheridge.

REFERENCES

1. Akil, H., Mayer, D. J., and Liebeskind, J. C. (1976): Reduction of stimulation-produced analgesia by the narcotic antagonist, naloxone. *Science,* 191:961–962.
2. Andres, K. H. (1961): Untersuchungen über den Feinbau von spinal ganglien. *Z. Zellforsch. Mikrosk. Anat.,* 55:1–48.
3. Aldskogius, H., and Arvidsson, J. (1978): Nerve cell degeneration and death in the trigeminal ganglion of the adult rat following peripheral nerve transection. *J. Neurocytol.,* 7:229–250.
4. Aronin, N., DiFiglia, M., Liotta, A. S., and Martin, J. B. (1981): Ultrastructural localization and biochemical features of immunoreactive Leu-enkephalin in monkey dorsal horn. *J. Neurosci.* 1:561–577.
5. Arvidsson, J., and Gobel, S. (1981): An HRP study of the central projections of primary trigeminal neurons which innervate tooth pulps in the cat. *Brain Res.,* 219:1–16.
6. Atweh, S. F., and Kuhar, M. J. (1977): Autoradiographic localization of opiate receptors in rat brain. I. Spinal cord and lower medulla. *Brain Res.,* 124:53–67.
7. Barber, R. P., Vaughn, J. E., and Roberts, E. (1982): The cytoarchitecture of GABAergic neurons in rat spinal cord. *Brain Res.,* 238:305–328.
8. Barber, R. P., Vaughn, J. E., Saito, K., McLaughlin, B., and Roberts, E. (1978): GABAergic terminals are presynaptic to primary afferent terminals in the substantia gelatinosa of the rat spinal cord. *Brain Res.,* 141:35–55.
9. Barber, R. P., Vaughn, J. E., Slemmon, J. R., Salvaterra, P. M., Roberts, E., and Leeman, S. E. (1979): The origin, distribution and synaptic relationships of substance P axons in rat spinal cord. *J. Comp. Neurol.,* 184:3311–3352.
10. Barbut, D., Polak, J. M., and Wall, P. D. (1981): Substance P in spinal cord dorsal horn decreases following peripheral nerve injury. *Brain Res.,* 205:289–298.
11. Basbaum, A. I., Clanton, C. H., and Fields, H. L. (1978): Three bulbospinal pathways from the rostral medulla of the cat: An autoradiographic study of pain-modulating systems. *J. Comp. Neurol.,* 178:209–224.
12. Basbaum, A. I., Glazer, E. J., Steinbusch, H., and Verhofstad, A. (1980): Serotonin and enkephalin coexist in neurons involved in opiate and stimulation produced analgesia. *Neurosci. Abstr.,* 6:540.
13. Beal, J. A., and Cooper, M. H. (1978): The neurons in the gelatinosal complex (lamina II and III) of the monkey *(Macaca mulatta).* A Golgi study. *J. Comp. Neurol.,* 179:89–122.
14. Bennett, G. J., Abdelmoumene, M., Hayashi, J., and Dubner, R. (1980): Physiology and morphology of substantia gelatinosa neurons intracellularly stained with horseradish peroxidase. *J. Comp. Neurol.,* 194:781–808.
15. Bennett, G. J., Hayashi, H., Abdelmoumene, M., and Dubner, R. (1979): Physiological properties of stalked cells of the substantia gelatinosa intracel-

lularly stained with horseradish peroxidase. *Brain Res.,*164:285–289.

16. Bessou, P., and Perl, E. R. (1979): Response of cutaneous sensory units with unmyelinated fibres to noxious stimuli. *J. Neurophysiol.,* 32:1025–1043.

17. Björklund, A., and Skageberg, G. (1979): Evidence for a major spinal cord projection from the diencephalic A11 dopamine cell group in the rat using transmitter-specific fluorescent retrograde tracing. *Brain Res.,* 177:170–175.

18. Bowker, R. M., Westlund, K. N., and Coulter, J. D. (1981): Origins of serotonergic projections to the spinal cord in rat: An immunocytochemical retrograde transport study. *Bruin Res.,* 226:187–199.

19. Brown, A. G. (1981): The primary afferent input: Some basic principles. In: *Spinal Cord Sensation,* edited by A. G. Brown and M. Rethelyi, pp. 23–32. Socttish Academic Press, Edinburgh.

20. Brown, A. G. (1981): *Organization in the Spinal Cord.* Springer Verlag, Berlin, Heidelberg, New York.

21. Burnweit, C., and Forssmann, W. G. (1979): Somatostatinergic nerves in the cervical spinal cord of the monkey. *Cell Tissue Res.,* 200:83–90.

22. Cajal Ramon, Y. S. (1909): *Histolgie du Systeme Nerveus de l'Homme et des Vertebres, Vol. I* (1952 reprint). Instituto Ramon y Cajal, Madrid.

23. Cervero, F., and Iggo, A. (1980): The substantia gelatinosa of the spinal cord: A critical review. *Brain,* 103:717–772.

24. Changaris, D. G., Keil, L. C., and Severs, W. B. (1978): Angiotensin II immunohistochemistry of the rat brain. *Neuroendocrinology,* 25:257–274.

25. Chan-Palay, V., and Palay, S. L. (1977): Ultrastructural identification of substance P cells and their processes in rat sensory ganglia and their terminals in the spinal cord by immunocytochemistry. *Proc. Natl. Acad. Sci. U.S.A.,* 74:4050–4054.

26. Coimbra, A., Sodre-Borges, B. P., and Magalhaes, M. M. (1974): The substantia gelatinosa Rolandi of the rat. Fine structure, cytochemistry (acid phosphatase) and changes after dorsal root section. *J. Neurocytol.,* 3:199–217.

27. Csillik, B., and Knyihar, E. (1978): Biodynamic plasticity in the Rolando substance. *Prog. Neurobiol.,* 10:203–230.

28. Cuello, A. C. (1978): Immunocytochemical studies of the distribution of neurotransmitters and related substances in CNS. In: *Handbook of Psychopharmacology,* Vol. 9, edited by L. L. Iversen, S. D. Iversen, and S. H. Snyder, pp. 69–124. Plenum Press, New York.

29. Cuello, A. C., del Fiacco, M., and Paxinos, G. (1978): The central and peripheral ends of the substance P-containing sensory neurons in the rat trigeminal system. *Brain Res.,* 152:499–509.

30. Cuello, A. C., Polak, J. M., and Pearse, A. G. E. (1976): Substance P: A naturally occurring transmitter in human spinal cord. *Lancet,* 2:1054–1056.

31. Cuello, A. C., Priestley, J. V., and Milstein, C. (1982): Immunocytochemistry with internally labelled monoclonal antibodies. *Proc. Natl. Acad. Sci. U.S.A.,* 79:665–669.

32. Curtis, D. R., and Johnston, G. A. R. (1974): Amino acid transmitters in the mammalian central nervous system. *Ergeb. Physiol.,* 69:97–188.

33. Dahlström, A., and Fuxe, K. (1964): Evidence for the existence of monoamine neurons in the central nervous system. I. Demonstration of monoamines in the cell bodies of brain stem neurons. *Acta Physiol. Scand. [Suppl.],* 232:1–55.

34. Dalsgaard, C. J., Hökfelt, T., Johansson, O., and Elde, R. (1981): Somatostatin immunoreactive cell bodies in the dorsal horn and the parasympathetic intermediolateral nucleus of the rat spinal cord. *Neurosci. Lett.,* 27:335–340.

35. Davies, J., and Dray, A. (1976): Effects of enkephalin and morphine on Renshaw cells in feline spinal cord. *Nature,* 262:603–604.

36. Devor, M., and Claman, D. (1980): Mapping and plasticity of acid phosphatase afferents in the rat dorsal horn. *Brain Res.,* 190:17–28.

37. Edvinsson, L., and Uddman, R. (1982): Immunohistochemical localization and dilatory effect of substance P on human cerebral vessels. *Brain Res.,* 232:466–471.

38. Elde, R., Hökfelt, T., Johansson, O., and Terenius, L. (1976): Immunohistochemical studies using antibodies to leucine-enkephalin: Initial observations on the nervous system of the rat. *Neuroscience,* 1:349–351.

39. Emson, P. C. (1979): Peptides as neurotransmitter candidates in the mammalian CNS. *Prog. Neurobiol.,* 13:61–116.

40. Fields, H. L., and Basbaum, A. I. (1978): Brain stem control of spinal pain-transmission neurons. *Annu. Rev. Physiol.,* 40:217–248.

41. Fields, H. L., Emson, P. C., Leigh, B. K., Gilbert, R. F. T., and Iversen, L. L. (1980): Multiple opiate receptor sites on primary afferent fibres. *Nature,* 284:351–353.

42. Finley, J. C. W., Maderdrut, J. L., and Petrusz, P. (1981): The immunocytochemical localization of enkephalin in the central nervous system of the rat. *J. Comp. Neurol.,* 198:541–566.

43. Fuxe, K., Ganten, D., Hökfelt, T., and Bolme, P. (1976): Immunohistochemical evidence for the existence of angiotensin-II containing nerve terminals in the brain and spinal cord in the rat. *Neurosci. Lett.,* 2:229–234.

44. Gibson, S. J., Polak, J. M., Bloom, S. R., and Wall, P. D. (1981): The distribution of nine peptides in rat spinal cord with special emphasis on the substantia gelatinosa and on the area around the central canal (lamina X) *J. Comp. Neurol.,* 201:65–80.

45. Giesler, G. J., Menetrey, D., and Basbaum, A. I. (1978): Differential origins of spinothalamic tract projections to medial and lateral thalamus in the rat. *J. Comp. Neurol.,* 184:107–126.

46. Gilbert, R. F. T., Emson, P. C., Hunt, S. P., Bennett, G. W., Marsden, C. A., Sandberg, B. E. B., Steinbusch, H. W. M., and Verhofstad, A. A. J. (1982): The effects of monoamine neurotoxins on peptides in the rat spinal cord. *Neuroscience,* 7:69–87.

47. Glazer, E. J., and Basbaum, A. I. (1980): Leucine enkephalin: Localization in and axoplasmic transport by sacral parasympathetic preganglionic neurons. *Science,* 208:1479–1480.
48. Glazer, E. J., and Basbaum, A. I. (1981): Serial analysis of leu-enkephalin synaptic relationships in cat dorsal horn. *Pain [Suppl.],* 1:158.
49. Glazer, E. J., and Basbaum, A. I. (1981): Immunohistochemical localization of leucine-enkephalin in the spinal cord of the cat: Enkephalin containing marginal neurons and pain modulation. *J. Comp. Neurol.,* 196:358–376.
50. Gobel, S. (1978): Golgi studies of the neurons in layer I of the dorsal horn of the medulla (trigeminal nucleus caudalis). *J. Comp. Neurol.,* 180:375–394.
51. Gobel, S. (1978): Golgi studies of the neurons in layer II of the dorsal horn of the medulla (trigeminal nucleus caudalis). *J. Comp. Neurol.,* 180:395–414.
52. Gobel, S., and Binck, J. M. (1977): Degenerative changes in primary trigeminal axons and in neurons in nucleus caudalis following tooth pulp extirpations in the cat. *Brain Res.,* 132:347–354.
53. Gobel, S., and Falls, W. M. (1979): Anatomical observations of horseradish peroxidase-filled terminal primary axonal arborisations in layer II of the substantia gelatinosa of Rolando. *Brain Res.,* 175:335–340.
54. Gobel, S., Falls, W. M., Bennett, G. J., Abdelmoumene, M., Hayashi, H., and Humphrey, E. (1980): An E.M. Analysis of the synaptic connections of horseradish peroxidase-filled stalked cells and islet cells in the substantia gelatinosa of adult cat spinal cord. *J. Comp. Neurol.,* 194:761–780.
55. Gobel, S., Falls, W. M., and Humphrey, E. (1981): Morphological and synaptic connections of ultrafine primary axons in lamina I of the spinal dorsal horn: Candidates for the terminal axonal arbors of primary neurons with unmyelinated (C) axons. *J. Neurosci.,* 1:1163–1179.
56. Grant, G., Arvidsson, J., Robertson, B., and Igge, J. (1979): Transganglionic transport of horseradish peroxidase in primary sensory neurons. *Neurosci. Lett.,* 12:23–28.
57. Heimer, L., and Wall, P. D. (1968): The dorsal root distribution to the substantia gelatinosa of the rat with a note on the distribution in the cat. *Exp. Brain Res.,* 6:89–99.
58. Hökfelt, T., Elde, R., Johansson, O., Luft, R., Nilsson, G., and Arimura, A. (1976): Immunohistochemical evidence for separate populations of somatostatin-containing and substance P-containing primary afferent neurons in the rat. *Neuroscience,* 1:131–136.
59. Hökfelt, T., Elde, R., Johansson, D., Terenius, L., and Stein, L. (1977): Distribution of enkephalin-like immunoreactivity in the rat central nervous system. I. Cell bodies. *Neurosci. Lett.,* 5:25–31.
60. Hökfelt, T., Kellerth, J. O., Nilsson, G., and Pernon, B. (1975): Experimental immunohistochemical studies on the localization and distribution of substance P in cat primary sensory neurons. *Brain Res.,* 100:235–252.
61. Hökfelt, T., and Ljungdahl, A. (1975): Uptake mechanisms as a basis for the histochemical identification and tracing of transmitter-specific neuron populations. In: *The Use of Axonal Transport for Studies of Neuronal Connectivity,* edited by W. M. Cowan and M. Cuénod, pp. 249–306. Elsevier, Amsterdam.
62. Hökfelt, T., Ljungdahl, A., Steinbusch, H., Verhofstad, A., Nilsson, G., Brodin, E., Pernow, B., and Goldstein, M. (1978): Immunohistochemical evidence of substance P-like immunoreactivity in some 5-hydroxytryptamine containing neurons in the rat central nervous system. *Neuroscience,* 3:517–538.
63. Hökfelt, T., Ljungdahl, A., Terenius, L., Elde, R., and Nilsson, G. (1977): Immunohistochemical analysis of peptide pathways possibly related to pain and analgesia: Enkephalin and substance P. *Proc. Natl. Acad. Sci. U.S.A.,* 74:3081–3085.
64. Hökfelt, T., Terenius, L., Kuypers, H. G. J. M., and Dann, O. (1979): Evidence for enkephalin immunoreactive neurons in the medulla oblongata projecting to the spinal cord. *Neurosci. Lett.,* 14:55–60.
65. Hunt, S. P., Emson, P. C., Gilbert, R., Goldstein, M., and Kimmell, J. R. (1981): Presence of avian pancreatic polypeptide-like immunoreactivity in catecholamine and methionine-enkephalin containing neurons within the central nervous system. *Neurosci. Lett.,* 21:125–130.
66. Hunt, S. P., Kelly, J. S., and Emson, P. C. (1980): The electron microscopic localization of methionine-enkephalin within the superficial layers (I and II) of the spinal cord. *Neuroscience,* 5:1871–1890.
67. Hunt, S. P., Kelly, J. S., Emson, P. C., Kimmell, J. R., Miller, R., and Wu, J.-Y. (1981): An immunohistochemical study of neuronal populations containing neuropeptides or GABA within the superficial layers of the rat dorsal horn. *Neuroscience,* 6:1883–1898.
68. Hunt, S. P., and Lovick, T. A. (1982): The distribution of 5-IIT, Met enkephalin and β-lipotropin like immunoreactivity in neuronal perikarya in the cat brain stem. *Neurosci., Lett.,* 30:139–145.
69. Hunt, S. P., Nagy, J. I., and Ninkovic, M. (1982): Peptides and the organisation of the dorsal horn. In: *Brain Stem Control of Spinal Mechanisms,* edited by A. Bjorklund and B. Sjolund, pp. 159–178. Elsevier/North Holland, Amsterdam.
70. Hunt, S. P., Ninkovic, M., Gleave, J. R. W., Iversen, S. D., and Iversen, L. L. (1982): *Interrelationships Between Enkephalin and Opiate Receptors in the Spinal Cord. Eleventh Pfizer International Symposium: Neuropeptides: Basic and Clinical Aspects,* edited by G. Fink and L. J. Whalley, pp. 13–23. Churchill Livingstone, Edinburgh
71. Hunt, S. P., and Schmidt, J. (1978): Some observations on the binding patterns of α-bungarotoxin in the central nervous system of the rat. *Brain Res.,* 157:213–232.
72. Hunt, S. P., Rossor, M. N., Emson, P. C., and Clement-Jones, V. (1982): Substance P and enkephalins in spinal cord after limb amputation. *Lancet,* 1:1023.

73. Iversen, L. L., and Bloom, F. E. (1972):Studies of the uptake of [³H]GABA and [³H]glycine in slices and homogenates of rat brain and spinal cord by electron microscopic autoradiography. *Brain Res.,* 41:131–143.

74. Jancso, G., and Kiraly, E. (1980): The distribution of chemosensitive primary sensory afferents in the central nervous system of the rat. *J. Comp. Neurol.,* 190:781–792.

75. Jancso, G., Kiraly, E., and Jancso-Gabor, A. (1977): Pharmacologically induced selective degeneration of chemosensitive primary sensory neurons. *Nature,* 270:741–743.

76. Jancso, G., Hökfelt, T., Lundberg, J., Kiraly, E., Halasz, N., Nilsson, G., Terenius, L., Rehfeld, J., Steinbusch, H., Verhofstad, A., Elde, R., Said, S., and Brown, M. (1981): Immunohistochemical studies on the effect of capsaicin on spinal and medullary peptide and monoamine neurons using antisera to substance P, gastrin/CCK, somatostatin, VIP, enkephalin, neurotensin and 5-hydroxytryptamine. *J. Neurocytol,* 10:963–980.

77. Jessell, T., and Iversen, L. L. (1977): Opiate analgesics inhibit substance P release from rat trigeminal nucleus. *Nature,* 268:549–551.

78. Jessell, T. M., Mudge, A. W., Leeman, S. E., and Yaksh, T. L. (1979): Release of substance P and somatostatin *in vivo,* from primary afferent terminals in mammalian spinal cord. *Neurosci. Abstr.,* 5:2078.

79. Jessell, T., Tsumoo, A., Kanazawa, I., and Otsuka, M. (1979): Substance P depletion in the dorsal horn of rat spinal cord after section of peripheral processes of primary sensory neurones. *Brain Res.,* 168:247–259.

80. Johansson, O., Hökfelt, T., Pernow, B., Jeffcoate, S. L., White, N., Steinbusch, H. W. M., Verhofstad, A. A. J., Emson, P. C., and Spindel, E. (1981): Immunohistochemical support for three putative transmitters in one neuron: Coexistence of 5-hydroxytryptamine, substance P- and thyrotropin releasing hormone-like immunoreactivity in medullary neurons projecting to the spinal cord. *Neuroscience.,* 6:1857–1882.

81. Kimura, H., McGeer, P. L., Peng, J. H., and McGeer, E. G. (1981): The central cholinergic system studied by choline acetyltransferase immunohistochemistry in the cat. *J. Comp. Neurol.,* 200:151–201.

82. Knyihar-Csillik, E., and Csillik, B. (1981): FRAP: Histochemistry of the primary nociceptive neuron. *Prog. Histochem. Cytochem.,* 14:1.

83. Kuypers, H. G. J. M., and Maisky, V. A. (1975): Retrograde axonal transport of horseradish peroxidase from spinal cord to brain stem groups in the cat. *Neurosci. Lett.,* 1:9–14.

84. LaMotte, C. (1977): Distribution of the tract of Lissauer and the dorsal root fibers in the primate spinal cord. *J. Comp. Neurol.,* 172:529–561.

85. LaMotte, C. C., and Lanerolle, N. C. (1981): Human spinal cord neurons: Innervation by both substance P and enkephalin. *Neuroscience,* 6:713–723.

86. LaMotte, C., Pert, C. M., and Snyder, S. H. (1976): Opiate receptor binding in primate spinal cord: Distribution and changes after dorsal root section. *Brain Res.,* 112:407–412.

87. Lawson, S. N. (1979): The postnatal development of large light and small dark neurons in mouse dorsal root ganglia: A statistical analysis of cell numbers and size. *J. Neurocytol.,* 8:275–294.

88. Lawson, S. N., and Nickels, S. M. (1980): The use of morphometric techniques to analyse the effect of neonatal capsaicin treatment on rat dorsal root ganglia and dorsal roots. *J. Physiol. (Lond.),* 303:12P.

89. Lieberman, A. R. (1976): Sensory ganglia. In: *The Peripheral Nerve,* edited by D. N. Landon, pp. 188–278. Chapman and Hall, London.

90. Light, A. R., and Perl, E. R. (1977): Differential termination of large diameter and small diameter primary afferent fibres in the spinal dorsal grey matter as indicated by labelling with horseradish peroxidase. *Neurosci. Lett.,* 6:59–63.

91. Light, A. R., and Perl, E. R. (1979): Re-examination of the dorsal root projection to the dorsal horn including observations on the differential termination of coarse and fine fibers. *J. Comp. Neurol.,* 186:117–132.

92. Light, A. R., and Perl, E. R. (1979): Spinal termination of functionally identified primary afferent neurons with slowly conducting myelinated fibers. *J. Comp. Neurol.,* 186:133–150.

93. Ljungdahl, A., and Hökfelt, T. (1973): Accumulation of ³H-glycine in interneurons of the cat spinal cord. *Histochemie,* 33:277–280.

94. Ljungdahl, A., and Hökfelt, T. (1973): Autoradiographic uptake patterns of [³H]GABA and [³H]glycine in central nervous tissue with special reference to the cat spinal cord. *Brain Res.,* 62:587–595.

95. Ljungdahl, A., Hökfelt, T., and Nilsson, G. (1978): Distribution of substance P-like immunoreactivity in the central nervous system of the rat. I. Cell bodies and nerve terminals. *Neuroscience,* 3:861–944.

96. Lundberg, J. M., Hökfelt, T., Angaard, A., Kimmel, J., Goldstein, M., and Markey, K. (1980): Coexistence of an avian pancreatic polypeptide (APP) immunoreactive substance and catecholamines in some peripheral and central neurons. *Acta Physiol. Scand.,* 110:107–109.

97. Loren, I., Emson, P. C., Fahrenkrug, J., Bjorklund, A., Alumets, J., Hakanson, R., and Sundler, F. (1979): Distribution of vasoactive intestinal polypeptide in the rat and mouse brain. *Neuroscience,* 5:1953–1976.

98. Lynn, B., and Carpenter, S. E. (1981): Primary afferent units from the hairy skin of the rat hind limb. *Brain Res.,* 238:13–28.

99. Marley, P. D., Nagy, J. I., Emson, P. C., and Rehfeld, J. F. (1982): Cholecystokinin in the rat spinal cord: Distribution and lack of effect of neonatal capsaicin treatment and rhizotomy. *Brain Res.,* 238:494–498.

100. Matus, A. I., and Dennison, M. E. (1971): Autoradiographic localisation of tritiated glycine at "flat-vesicle" synapses in spinal cord. *Brain Res.,* 32:195–197.

101. McLaughlin, B. J., Barker, R., Saito, K., Roberts,

E., and Wu, J.-Y. (1975): Immunocytochemical localization of glutamate decarboxylase in the rat spinal cord. *J. Comp. Neurol.,* 164:305–322.

102. Mudge, A. W., Leeman, S. E., and Fischbach, G. D. (1979): Enkephalin inhibits release of substance P from sensory neurons in culture and decreases action potential duration. *Proc. Natl. Acad. Sci. U.S.A.,* 76:526–530.

103. Nagy, J. I., Goedert, M., Hunt, S. P., and Bond, A. (1982): The nature of the substance P-containing nerve fibers in taste papillae of the rat tongue. *Neuroscience 7:3137–3152.*

104. Nagy, J. I., and Hunt, S. P. (1981): Fluoride-resistant acid phosphatase-containing neurones in dorsal root ganglia are separate from those containing substance P or somatostatin. *Neuroscience,* 7:88–97.

105. Nagy, J. I., Hunt, S. P., Iversen, L. L., and Emson, P. C. (1981): Biochemical and anatomical observations on the degeneration of peptide-containing primary afferent neurons after neonatal capsaicin. *Neuroscience,* 6:1923–1934.

105a. Nagy, J. I., Iversen, L. L., Goedert, M., Chapman, D., and Hunt, S. P. (1982): Dose dependent effects of capsaicin on primary sensory neurons in the neoratal rat. *J. Neurosci. (in press).*

106. Nagy, J. I., Vincent, S. R., Staines, W. A., Fibiger, H. C., Reisine, T. D., and Yamamura, H. I. (1980): Neurotoxic action of capsaicin on spinal substance P neurones. *Brain Res.,* 186:435–444.

107. Ninkovic, M., Hunt, S. P., and Gleave, J. (1982): Localization of opiate and histamine H$_1$-receptors in primate sensory ganglia and spinal cord. *Brain Res.,* 241:197–206.

108. Ninkovic, M., Hunt, S. P., and Kelly, J. S. (1981): Effect of dorsal rhizotomy on the autoradiographic distribution of opiate and neurotensin receptors and neurotensin-like immunoreactivity within the rat spinal cord. *Brain Res.,* 230:11–119.

109. Nygren, L.-G., and Olson, L. (1977): A new major projection from locus coeruleus: The main source of noradrenergic nerve terminals in the ventral and dorsal columns of the spinal cord. *Brain Res.,* 132:85–93.

110. Palermo, N. N., Brown, K. H., and Smith, D. L. (1981): Selective neurotoxic action of capsaicin on glomerular C-type terminals in rat substantia gelatinosa. *Brain Res.,* 208:506–510.

111. Pearson, J., Brandeis, L., and Cuello, A. C. (1982): Depletion of substance P-containing axons in substantia gelatinosa of patients with diminished pain sensitivity. *Nature,* 295:61–63.

112. Pickel, V. M., Reis, D. J., and Leeman, S. E. (1977): Ultrastructural localization of substance P in neurons of rat spinal cord. *Brain Res.,* 122:533–540.

113. Polz-Tejera, G., Hunt, S. P., and Schmidt, J. (1980): Nicotinic receptors in sensory ganglia. *Brain Res.,* 195:223–230.

114. Ralston, H. J. III (1965): The organization of the substantia gelatinosa Rolandi in the cat lumbar sacral spinal cord. *Z. Zellforsch.,* 67:1–23.

115. Ralston, H. J. III (1968): Dorsal root projections to dorsal horn neurons in the cat spinal cord. *J. Comp. Neurol.,* 132:303–330.

116. Ralston, J. H. III (1979): The fine structure of laminae I, II and III of the macaque spinal cord. *J. Comp. Neurol.,* 184:619–642.

117. Ralston, H. J. III, and Ralston, D. D. (1979): The distribution of dorsal root axons in laminae I,II and III of the macaque spinal cord: A quantitative electron microscope study. *J. Comp. Neurol.,* 184:643–684.

118. Ranson, S. W. (1913): The course within the spinal cord of the non-medullated fibres of the dorsal roots: A study of Lissauer's tract in the cat. *J. Comp. Neurol.,* 23:259–281.

119. Ranson, S. W. (1914): An experimental study of Lissauer's tract and the dorsal roots. *J. Comp. Neurol.,* 24:531–545.

120. Ranson, S. W. (1914): The tract of Lissauer and the substantia gelatinosa Rolandi. *Ann. J. Anat.,* 16:97–126.

121. Rethelyi, M., Trevino, D. L., and Perl, E. R. (1979): Distribution of primary afferent fibers within the sacro coccygeal dorsal horn: An autoradiographic study. *J. Comp. Neurol.,* 185:603–622.

122. Rexed, B. (1952): The cytoarchitectonic organization of the spinal cord in the cat. *J. Comp. Neurol.,* 96:415–496.

123. Ribeiro-da-Silva, A., and Coimbra, A. (1980): Neuronal uptake of [^{3}H]GABA and [^{3}H]glycine in laminae I–III (substantia gelatinosa Rolandi) of the rat spinal cord. An autoradiographic study. *Brain Res.,* 188:499–464.

124. Ross, C. A., Armstrong, D. M., Ruggeiro, D. A., Pickel, V. M., Joh, T. H., and Reis, D. J. (1981): Adrenaline neurons in the rostral ventrolateral medulla innervate thoracic spinal cord: A combined immunocytochemical and retrograde transport demonstration. *Neurosci. Lett.,* 25:251–256.

125. Ruda, M. A., Allen, B., and Gobel, S. (1981): Ultrastructural analysis of serotinergic medial brainstem afferents to the superficial dorsal horn. *Brain Res.,* 205:175–180.

126. Ruda, M. A., and Gobel, S. (1980): Ultrastructural characterization of axonal endings in the substantia gelatinosa which take up [^{3}H]serotonin. *Brain Res.,* 184:57–83.

127. Rustioni, A., and Cuénod, M. (1982): Selective retrograde transport of D-aspartate in spinal interneurons and cortical neurons of rats. *Brain Res.,* 236:143–155.

128. Sar, M., Stumpf, W. E., Miller, R. J., Chang, K.-J., and Cuatrecasas, P. (1978): Immunohistochemical localization of enkephalin in rat brain and spinal cord. *J. Comp. Neurol.,* 182:17–38.

129. Sawchenko, P. E., and Swanson, L. W. (1982): Immunohistochemical identification of neurons in the paraventricular nucleus of the hypothalamus that project to the medulla or to the spinal cord in the rat. *J. Comp. Neurol.,* 205:260–272.

130. Scadding, J. W. (1980): The permanent anatomical effect of neonatal capsaicin on somatosensory nerves. *J. Anat.,* 131:473–484.

131. Scheibel, M. E., and Scheibel, A. B. (1968): Terminal axonal patterns in the cat spinal cord. II. The dorsal horn. *Brain Res.,* 9:32–58.

132. Scheibel, M. E., and Scheibel, A. B. (1969): Ter-

minal patterns in cat spinal cord. III. Primary afferent collaterals. *Brain Res.,* 13:417–443.

133. Seybold, V., and Elde, R. (1980): Immunohistochemical studies of peptidergic neurons in the dorsal horn of the spinal cord. *J. Histochem. Cytochem.,* 28:367–370.

134. Seybold, V. S., and Elde, R. P. (1982): Neurotensin immunoreactivity in the superficial laminae of the dorsal horn of the rat. I. Light microscopic studies of cell bodies and proximal dendrites. *J. Comp. Neurol.,* 205:89–100.

135. Simantov, R., Kuhar, M. J., Uhl, G. R., and Snyder, S. H. (1977): Opioid peptide enkephalin: Immunohistochemical mapping in rat central nervous system. *Proc. Natl. Acad Sci. U.S.A.,* 74:2167–2171.

136. Steinbusch, H. W. M. (1981): Distribution of serotonin-immunoreactivity in the central nervous system of the rat: Cell bodies and terminals. *Neuroscience,* 6:557–618.

137. Steinbusch, H. W. M., Verhofstad, A. J., and Joosten, H. W. J. (1978): Localization of serotonin in the central nervous system by immunohistochemistry: Description of a specific and sensitive technique and some applications. *Neuroscience,* 3:811–819.

138. Sternberger, L. A. (1979): *Immunocytochemistry,* 2nd ed. John Wiley & Sons, New York.

139. Streit, P. (1980): Selective retrograde labeling indicating the transmitter of neuronal pathways. *J. Comp. Neurol.,* 191:429–463.

140. Szentagothai, J. (1964): Neuronal and synaptic arrangement in the substantia gelatinosa Rolandi. *J. Comp. Neurol.,* 122:219–239.

141. Uhl, G. R., Goodman, R. R., and Snyder, S. H. (1979): Neurotensin-containing cell bodies fibres and nerve terminals in the brain stem of the rat: Immunohistochemical mapping. *Brain Res.,* 167:77–92.

142. Westlund, K. N., Bowker, R. M., Ziegler, M. G., and Coulter, J. D. (1981): Origins of spinal noradrenergic pathways demonstrated by retrograde transport of antibody to dopamine-β-hydroxylase. *Neurosci. Lett.,* 25:239–242.

143. Willis, W. D., and Coggeshall, R. E. (1978): *Sensory Mechanisms of the Spinal Cord.* Plenum Press, New York.

144. Yaksh, T. L. (1980): Direct evidence that spinal serotonin and noradrenaline terminals mediate the spinal antinociceptive effects of morphine in the periaqueductal gray. *Brain Res.,* 160:180–185.

145. Yaksh, T. L., Jessell, T. M., Gamse, R., Mudge, A. W., and Leeman, S. E. (1980): Intrathecal morphine inhibits substance P release from mammalian spinal cord *in vivo. Nature,* 286:155–157.

146. Yaksh, T. L., and Rudy, T. A. (1978): Narcotic analgetics: CNS sites and mechanisms of action as revealed by intracerebral injection techniques. *Pain,* 4:299–359.

147. Young, W. S., and Kuhar, M. J. (1979): A new method for receptor autoradiography: [^{3}H]Opioid receptor labelling in mounted tissue sections. *Brain Res.,* 179:255–270.

148. Yoshida, S., and Matsuda, Y. (1979): Studies on sensory neurons of the mouse with intracellular-recording and horseradish peroxidase-injection techniques. *J. Neurophysiol.,* 42:1134–1144.

149. Zenker, W., Mysicka, A., and Neuhuber, W. (1980): Dynamics of the transganglionic movement of horseradish peroxidase in primary sensory neurons. *Cell Tissue Res.,* 207:479–489.

150. Zhu, C. G., Sandri, C., and Akert, K. (1981): Morphological identification of axo–axonic and dendro–dendritic synapses in the rat substantia gelatinosa. *Brain Res.,* 230:25–40.

Chemical Neuroanatomy, edited by P. C. Emson,
Raven Press, New York © 1983.

Retinal Neurotransmitters: Histochemical and Biochemical Studies

Nicholas Brecha

*Center for Ulcer Research and Education, Veterans Administration Center—Wadsworth, Los Angeles,
California 90073 and the Brain Research Institute, Jules Stein Eye Institute, and Department of
Medicine, UCLA School of Medicine, Los Angeles, California 90024*

The retina is a specialized structure of the nervous system which transduces light into biologically meaningful signals, processes these signals, and subsequently transmits this visual information to the central nervous system. Simple as well as complex retinal processing, including the detection of brightness, contrast, movement, and color, are accomplished by the interaction of retinal neurons at both electrical and chemical synaptic junctions. Evidence to date indicates that the preponderance of synaptic interactions between retinal neurons are mediated by chemical substances, and therefore a detailed understanding of the histochemical, biochemical, and anatomical organization of the retina is critical for an evaluation of its functional organization.

In this chapter, I intend to review the literature through early 1981 pertaining to the histochemical and biochemical organization of the retina. In order to provide a context for the presentation of these studies, a brief synopsis of each of the different retinal cell types is given. Detailed reviews of the structural and functional organization of the retina have been presented elsewhere (22,45,52,60,61,140,245,261,299).

MORPHOLOGICAL ORGANIZATION OF THE RETINA

The vertebrate retina is an extracranial derivative of neuroectoderm which arises from an outpouching of the diencephalon during early embryogenesis. Morphologically, the retina is characterized by a distinct laminar organization of its cells and processes. Proceeding from the distal surface adjacent to the pigment epithelium toward the proximal or vitreal surface, these layers are designated as the photoreceptor layer (PRL), outer nuclear layer (ONL), outer plexiform layer (OPL), inner nuclear layer (INL), inner plexiform layer (IPL), ganglion cell layer (GCL), and optic axon layer (OAL) (Fig. 1).

Six main neuronal cell types—photoreceptor, bipolar, horizontal, amacrine, interplexiform, and ganglion—are found within the retina (23,45). In addition, glia, of which the majority are a specialized radial glia known as Müller cells, also are found within the retina. Retinal neurons are distinguished from one another by several features including the location, size, and shape of their cell bodies as well as the morphology and arborization pattern of their processes (45). In the past, these morphological differences have served as the sole criteria by which retinal neurons and their subtypes were distinguished. However, the recent identification of histochemically unique cell populations has provided an additional basis on which to characterize these cells. In addition, these histochemical studies have provided the basis for a better understanding of the functional organization of the retina (82).

The major morphological features of each of the six retinal neuronal cell types are described below (Fig. 1).

Photoreceptor cells, which include rods and cones, lie immediately adjacent to the pigment epithelium within the ONL and give rise to processes whose terminals are located in the OPL. Bipolar and horizontal cell processes form synaptic contacts with photoreceptor terminals.

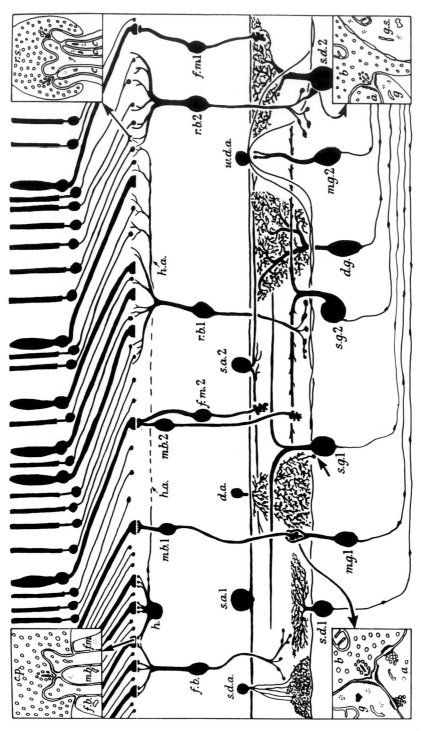

FIG. 1. Schematic representation of the primate retina illustrating its basic organizational features. Photoreceptor cells (c.p., cones; r.s., rods) make synaptic contact with bipolar cells (f.b., flat bipolar cell; m.b.1 and m.b.2, midget bipolar cells; f.b.2 and f.m.1, flat midget bipolar cells; r.b.1 and r.b.2, rod bipolar cells) and horizontal cells (c.h., type A horizontal cell; r.h., type B horizontal cell; r.h.a., type A horizontal cell axon; r.h.a., type B horizontal cell axon) in the outer plexiform layer. Bipolar cells in turn make synaptic contact with amacrine cells (s.d.a., stratified diffuse amacrine cell; s.a.1 and s.a.2, unistratified amacrine cells; d.a., narrow-field diffuse amacrine cell; w.d.a., wide-field diffuse amacrine cell) and ganglion cells (s.d.1 and s.d.2, stratified diffuse ganglion cells; m.g.1 and m.g.2, midget ganglion cells; s.g.1 and s.g.2, stratified ganglion cells; d.g., diffuse ganglion cell) in the inner plexiform layer. Interplexiform, displaced amacrine, and displaced ganglion cells are not shown. A detailed description of this figure may be found in Boycott and Dowling (22). (From Boycott and Dowling, ref. 22, with permission.)

Horizontal cells, of which there are several distinct subtypes, lie within the distal portion of the INL and give rise to processes that are confined exclusively to the OPL. These processes ramify over relatively large areas within the OPL and make synaptic contacts with other horizontal cells as well as with photoreceptor and bipolar cell processes.

Bipolar cells, whose somata are located within the middle portion of the INL, have processes that arborize in both the OPL and IPL. In the OPL, bipolar cell processes have relatively small fields and contact photoreceptor terminals and horizontal cell processes. Within the IPL, bipolar cell processes generally have small fields, often ramify within selected laminae of the IPL, and are in synaptic contact with both amacrine cell processes and ganglion cell dendrites.

Amacrine cells, of which there are a large number of morphological subtypes, are located primarily within the proximal INL. In addition, displaced amacrine cells are present within the IPL and GCL. Amacrine cells give rise to processes that are confined to the IPL and have fields of variable sizes that often arborize within selected laminae of the IPL. These processes are in synaptic contact with bipolar, interplexiform, and ganglion cell dendrites as well as with other amacrine cell processes.

Interplexiform cells also are located in the proximal INL, usually at the junction of the INL and IPL. Interplexiform cells are characterized by processes that arborize in both the OPL and IPL (23). However, unlike bipolar cells, these cells provide for centrifugal information flow from the IPL to the OPL (122). In general, interplexiform cell processes in the OPL form presynaptic contacts with horizontal and bipolar cells. In the IPL, the majority of interplexiform cell processes make postsynaptic contacts with amacrine cell processes (62,151).

Ganglion cells are located within the GCL, and displaced ganglion cells are located within the proximal INL and IPL. Ganglion cells, like amacrine cells, consist of many distinct morphological subtypes. These cells have dendritic fields of variable sizes that often arborize within selected laminae of the IPL. As mentioned above, ganglion cells are in synaptic contact with both bipolar and amacrine cell processes. Ganglion cells give rise to the optic nerve and are the only retinal neurons that conduct visual information to central visual structures.

Retinal neurons interconnect in various ways to form a number of neuronal pathways that undergo complex and as yet poorly understood interactions in the processing of visual stimuli (see reviews cited

above). The essential organizational feature of the retina, as suggested by light and electron microscopy as well as electrophysiology, is one of parallel neuronal pathways consisting of photoreceptor, bipolar, and ganglion cells. The information processing in these pathways is modified by lateral interconnections of horizontal cells in the OPL and amacrine cells in the IPL. Interplexiform cells, which ramify in both plexiform layers, provide a pathway for a centrifugal information flow from the IPL to the OPL.

HISTOCHEMICAL AND BIOCHEMICAL ORGANIZATION OF THE RETINA

Morphological studies in combination with both histochemistry and biochemistry have provided powerful experimental tools for identifying the location of putative neurotransmitter systems in several areas of the nervous system including the retina. A neurotransmitter is defined here as a substance that is synthesized, stored, and released by neurons and interacts with a specific membrane receptor site on an adjacent neuron (42,231,328). Most of the substances considered in this review meet several of the commonly accepted criteria for a neurotransmitter and might reasonably be considered as retinal neurotransmitter substances.

The following sections summarize much of the existing biochemical and histochemical evidence supporting a neurotransmitter role for acetylcholine; several amino acids, including γ-aminobutyric acid (GABA), glycine, aspartate, glutamate, and taurine; dopamine; indoleamines (serotonin and melatonin); and a variety of different neuropeptides in the vertebrate retina. Several other reviews of retinal neurotransmitters have also been published (20,113,212,299,315).

Acetylcholine

Biochemistry

Acetylcholine (ACh) is reported to be present in all vertebrate retinas studied to date [see Graham (113) for review; 3,212,270]. Specific high-affinity uptake systems for choline (2,14,198,199,213,215) as well as the synthesis of ACh from choline (3,14,127,163,165,197,198,215) have been observed in the retina. In addition, the release of ACh by either K^+ or light stimulation in a Ca^{2+}-dependent manner (14,197,200,213,214,217) has been noted.

The synthetic enzyme choline acetyltransferase (ChAT) and the degradative enzyme acetylcholinesterase (AChE) are both present in the retina (see Graham, ref. 113, for review; 2,69,203,212,213, 265,270,271). Microdissection of the retinal layers (178,265,266) as well as chemical lesion studies using intraocular injections of either monosodium glutamate[1] (179,265) or kainic acid[2] (18,281) demonstrate that these enzymes are concentrated in proximal retinal regions.

The specific high-affinity binding of α-bungaro-toxin (α-BuTX), a nicotinic cholinergic ligand, and quinuclidinyl benzilate (QNB), a muscarinic cho-linergic ligand, to retinal homogenates has been described (131,205,207,300,320,321,323,334,338, 339). These binding studies provide good evidence for cholinergic synaptic systems in the retina.

Histochemistry

Identification of retinal cholinergic systems ini-tially relied on the localization of AChE. More re-cently, cholinergic systems have been identified by using high-affinity uptake of choline as well as α-BuTX and QNB localization techniques.

Selected amacrine cells of chick and rabbit re-tinas accumulate choline (14,198). These cells are located within the proximal INL and GCL, and their processes are distributed within two discrete bands within the IPL (14,198) (Fig. 2). Further-more, a double-label study using choline uptake and retrograde labeling of ganglion cells by axonal transport in rabbit retina has conclusively demon-strated that the choline-accumulating cells located in the GCL are displaced amacrine cells (120). These histochemical studies have thus established the existence of a distinct population of choline-ac-cumulating amacrine and displaced amacrine cells.

Since the 1950s, AChE has been used as an in-dicator of cholinergic systems within the retina (19,285). This enzyme has been most often re-ported in amacrine and displaced amacrine cells [see Graham (113) for comparisons; 19,104,222, 224,225,285]. In some vertebrate retinas, AChE is also associated with horizontal cell bodies (251,290) and horizontal and bipolar cell processes (19,58,69,104,119). Ultrastructural studies de-scribe the presence of AChE at photoreceptor syn-

INL

IPL

GCL

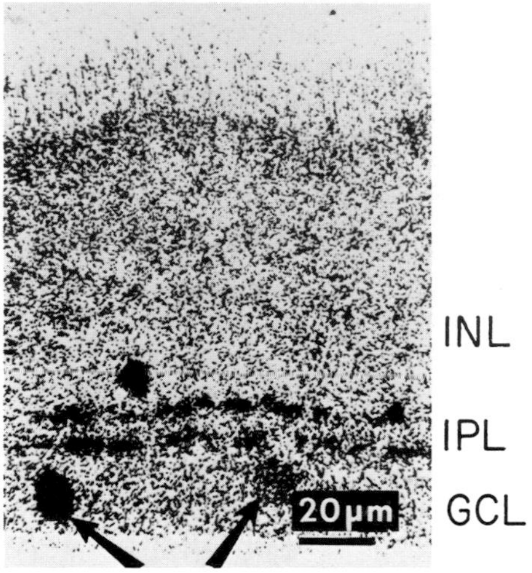

FIG. 2. Choline-accumulating amacrine and displaced amacrine cells *(arrows)* in the rabbit retina. Choline-accmulating processes are located in two bands of the IPL. (From Masland and Mills, ref. 198, with permission.)

aptic complexes in teleost and amphibian retinas (58,69,70).

In the IPL of chick, mouse, and goldfish, pro-cesses of bipolar, amacrine, and ganglion cells are postsynaptic to synapses labeled with α-BuTX (55,247,320,342). However, the presynaptic cells differ. In chick, both bipolar and amacrine pro-cesses are presynaptic elements (320); whereas, in mouse and goldfish retinas, only amacrine cells are presynaptic elements in synapses labeled with α-BuTX (247,342). In the OPL, electrophysiological evidence for a nicotinic mechanism is weak. Al-though small bipolar cell processes appear labeled with α-BuTX in goldfish and pigeon retina (283,334), it has been suggested that in goldfish the α-BuTX binding sites on bipolar cell bodies and dendrites in the OPL represent patches of acetyl-choline receptors that were synthesized in the cell body and are diffusing throughout the plasma membrane. Thus, the presence of these binding sites, in the absence of specialized junctions, may not be indicative of nicotinic cholinergic function (342).

A single light microscopic study has localized QNB to selected laminae of chick IPL (300), pro-viding evidence that muscarinic cholinergic sys-tems are localized to the IPL.

In conclusion, biochemical studies have provided evidence indicating that ACh, AChE, and ChAT are present in the retina, primarily within its prox-

---

[1]Monosodium glutamate at concentrations used in these lesion studies destroys most if not all retinal cells except photoreceptor and Müller cells (226).

[2]Kainic acid at concentrations used in these lesion studies destroys most if not all retinal cells in the INL while not affecting cells located in the ONL and GCL (18,281).

imal regions. The presence of choline uptake systems, the synthesis of choline from ACh, and the release of ACh from the retina have been described. Finally, binding studies suggest the presence of cholinergic synaptic receptors in the retina. Histochemical studies describe amacrine cells that accumulate choline and stain for AChE, correlating with the localization of α-BuTX and QNB binding patterns in the IPL. Additional histochemical evidence for cholinergic systems in the IPL is the recent localization of ChAT to the chick IPL (D. M. K. Lam, *personal communication*). The existence of a cholinergic photoreceptor–bipolar cell system in selected retinas including the goldfish is implied by the localization of α-BuTX to bipolar cell processes, matching AChE staining patterns, and the observation that some cone photoreceptors in the turtle retina contain ACh. Therefore, both biochemical and histochemical studies provide convincing evidence for cholinergic amacrine cell systems in the mammalian and nonmammalian retina.

Amino Acids

Gamma-Aminobutyric Acid

Biochemistry.

Gamma-aminobutyric acid (GABA) is present in the retina [see Graham (113) for review; 53,146, 157,81,227,228,238,239,271,291,293,318] and is reported to be most concentrated in the proximal INL, IPL, and GCL (15,112,114,145,147,158,206, 316). In some nonmammalian species, a high GABA content has been reported in distal retinal regions (112). A specific high-affinity uptake system for GABA has been demonstrated in the retina (18,111,158,168,218,219,252,256,281, 282,291,296,311,317). In addition, several studies have described a K^+, light, and/or electrically stimulated release of GABA from the retina (10,11,126,127,148,167,168,176,190,212,240, 252,256,294,319), although other studies have not (144,148,212,214,217,240,252,256,294,319). The reasons for these contradictory observations are not fully understood and may result from species variation or from differing experimental protocols. Resolution of these differences is important and requires further study.

The rate-limiting synthetic enzyme L-glutamate decarboxylase (GAD) and the degradative enzyme α-aminobutyric acid transaminase (GABA-T) also have been localized within the retina [see Graham (113) for review; 126,157,164,165,271]. The highest levels of GAD and GABA-T activity are found in the proximal retina (53,112,114,158). This observation is supported by lesion studies that have demonstrated that GAD activity is reduced following intravitreal treatments with either monosodium glutamate or kainic acid (179,180,281).

Specific, low- and high-affinity GABA binding sites have been demonstrated in retinal homogenates of goldfish, chicken, rat, pig, sheep, and cow (98,253,256–258,335). The binding characteristics in the retina of both GABA and its agonist muscimol are similar if not identical to those reported for the central nervous system. Thus, these binding studies have provided evidence for the presence of GABAergic synaptic systems in the retina and that these synaptic systems are similar to those in the brain.

Histochemistry.

The identification of GABAergic systems in the retina is based primarily on the localization of neurons that accumulate GABA and to a lesser degree on the localization of either GAD immunoreactivity or GABA and muscimol binding sites.

Gamma-aminobutyric acid is accumulated by seemingly specific populations of retinal cells in both mammalian and nonmammalian retinas (24, 35,77,78,86,114,126,127,165,192–194,209,248, 296,317) (Fig. 3; also see Fig. 7A) as well as by Müller cells in some mammalian retinas (35, 83,193,194,216). In general, horizontal, amacrine, and displaced amacrine cell populations accumulate GABA in nonmammalian retinas. In most mammalian retinas, only amacrine and displaced amacrine cells are reported to be GABA accumulating. However, the accumulation of GABA by a population of ganglion cells rather than displaced amacrine cells has not been thoroughly explored. A stratified distribution of GABA over the IPL is a commonly reported feature for all of these retinas. In the cat retina, in addition to several populations of GABA-accumulating amacrine cells (248), a population of GABA-accumulating interplexiform cells has recently been described (209).

The best studied GABA-accumulating cells are the teleost cone horizontal (H1) and amacrine (Ab pyriform) cells (162,167,190) (Fig. 3). The H1 cone horizontal cells lie within the most distal lamina of the INL and give rise to processes that contact cone photoreceptors (298). All H1 horizontal cells appear to accumulate GABA. Furthermore, GABA uptake by these cells is enhanced by slowly flashing light, and they release GABA in dark conditions (167,190). GABA-accumulating Ab amacrine cells, of which there are at least two subpopulations on the basis of soma size, ramify in the

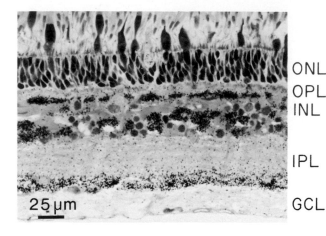

ONL

OPL

INL

IPL

GCL

FIG. 3. GABA-accumulating retinal cells in the goldfish retina. The H1 horizontal cells and Ab pyriform amacrine cells with somata of various diameters are labeled. In addition, a dense accumulation of label is present in the proximal portion of the IPL. (Photomicrograph courtesy of Dr. S. Yazulla.)

proximal one-third of the IPL (sublamina b). An ultrastructural study demonstrated that these amacrine cells are synaptically linked to depolarizing bipolar cells (190). The uptake of GABA by Ab pyriform amacrine cells is reportedly greatest when they are exposed to darkness or to blue or green lights; red light apparently suppresses uptake (190). Studies of GABAergic systems in the teleost retina therefore have demonstrated at least two GABA-accumulating retinal cell populations that are sensitive to light conditions.

Glutamate decarboxylase-containing horizontal and amacrine cell populations have been studied in several vertebrate retinas (9,24,25,123,124,169, 312,331; *unpublished observations*). In the goldfish retina, GAD immunoreactivity is localized to H1 horizontal cells, Ab pyriform amacrine cells, and the proximal one-third of the IPL (169). This staining pattern closely matches the GABA uptake pattern (190) and correlates well with biochemical studies describing GAD activity in isolated horizontal cells (164) (Fig. 4). Light microscopic studies of other mammalian and nonmammalian retinas note that amacrine and presumed displaced amacrine cells contain GAD immunoreactivity. In the retinas of frogs and squirrel monkeys, GAD immunoreactivity is distributed in a homogenous manner across all laminae of the IPL (Fig. 5) (25; and *unpublished observations*). In contrast, GAD immunoreactivity in the pigeon, rat, and rabbit IPL is distributed in at least four distinct bands (9,24,312; and *unpublished observations*) (Fig. 6). The distribution of GAD immunoreactive staining in these retinas generally matches GABA uptake patterns, but the lack of detailed light and electron microscopic studies makes exact comparisons difficult.

Ultrastructural immunohistochemical analysis of rat and rabbit retinas demonstrate that GAD-containing amacrine cell processes form the majority of their synaptic contacts with other amacrine cell processes (24,312,331). In addition, they form synaptic contacts with bipolar and ganglion cell

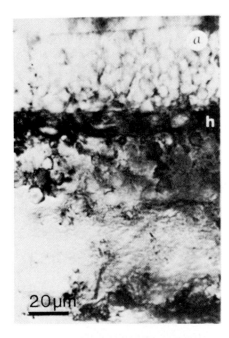

FIG. 4. Glutamate decarboxylase immunoreactive staining of horizontal cells in the goldfish retina. Note the correspondence between the GABA uptake pattern (Fig. 3) and the GAD staining pattern for these cells. h, horizontal cell body. (From Lam et al., ref. 169, with permission.)

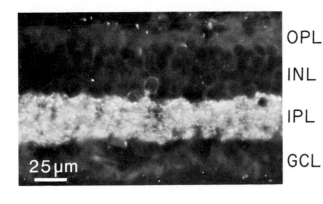

FIG. 5. Glutamate decarboxylase immunoreactive staining pattern in the squirrel monkey retina. The GAD staining is distributed in a homogeneous manner across the IPL. The GAD antiserum used for this study was generously supplied by Dr. W. Oertel.

processes (24,312,331). The existence of GABA-ergic synaptic contacts with ganglion, bipolar, and amacrine cell processes is in contrast to the more limited synaptic arrangements found for catechol-amine-containing and indoleamine-accumulating neurons (see below). The apparent diversity of GABAergic synaptic systems may simply reflect a large number of GABAergic cell populations found in the retina as suggested by both GABA uptake and GAD immunohistochemical studies. Each of

these GABAergic subtypes may contact a particular cell type within the IPL.

The degradative enzymes GABA-T and succinic semialdehyde dehydrogenase have been localized to most retinal layers (99,133,204). The seemingly ubiquitous distribution of these enzymes in the retina does not allow for a detailed correlation between their distribution and cell types with which they may be associated.

Muscimol is associated with specific GABA-ac-

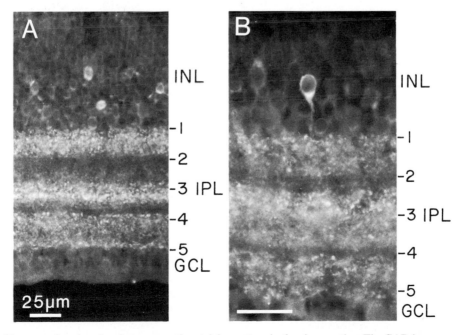

FIG. 6. Glutamate decarboxylase immunoreactive staining pattern in the pigeon retina. The GAD immunoreactivity is located in (1) somata of various diameters which are scattered throughout the proximal INL and (2) processes that are distributed in a stratified manner in the IPL. **A:** Low-power photomicrograph. **B:** High-power photomicrograph illustrating a well-labeled soma and its primary process. The GAD antiserum used for this study was generously supplied by Dr. W. Oertel.

cumulating cells and GABA membrane binding sites in the goldfish and chick retina (335,336). Incubation of chicken retina in muscimol results in the uptake of this substance into both amacrine and horizontal cell populations (Fig. 7B) in a pattern similar to that observed for GABA (Fig. 7A). But the details of these two uptake patterns differ, especially within the IPL. Muscimol and GABA uptake occurs in a diffuse manner across the IPL; however, muscimol uptake is more concentrated to laminae 2 and 4 of the IPL, whereas GABA uptake is more concentrated to lamina 5 of the IPL. In

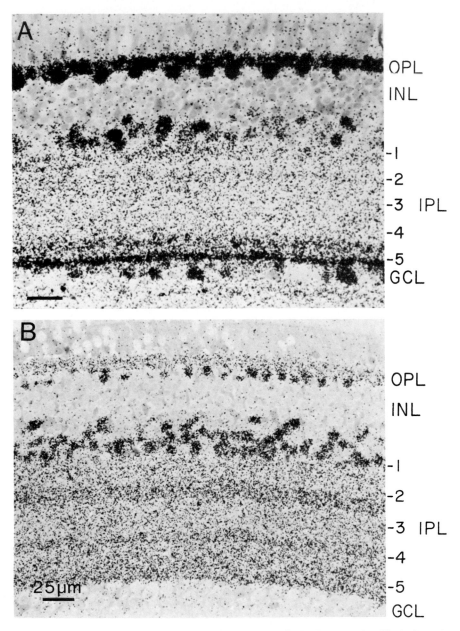

FIG. 7. GABA and muscimol uptake patterns in the chicken retina. **A:** GABA is accumulated by horizontal, amacrine, and displaced amacrine cells. There is light labeling of the entire IPL with particularly dense labeling of lamina 5. **B:** Muscimol is accumulated by horizontal and amacrine cells. There is labeling of the entire IPL in addition to somewhat more densely concentrated labeling of laminae 2 and 4. (From Yazulla and Brecha, ref. 335, with permission.)

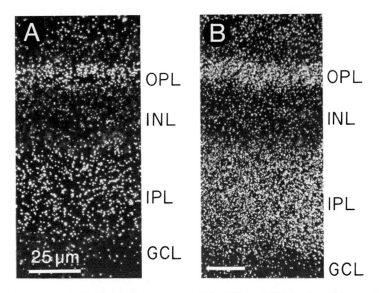

FIG. 8. GABA (**A**) and muscimol (**B**) labeling patterns of the OPL and IPL in the chicken retina. These retinal sections were processed by a dry autoradiographic procedure. Note the lack of staining of somata and the homogeneous distribution of label over the plexiform layers. (From Yazulla and Brecha, ref. 336, with permission.)

striking contrast are the labeling patterns observed with dry autoradiographic techniques that demonstrate GABA and muscimol binding sites. The GABA and muscimol binding sites are distributed in a homogeneous manner over the IPL and OPL (Fig. 8) and are not concentrated to those laminae that show a dense accumulation of GABA uptake (335,336).

Moreover, an ultrastructural analysis of the muscimol labeling pattern in the IPL, involving a statistical analysis of the correlation of the distance between silver grains (representative of a muscimol binding site) and the nearest synaptic specialization, demonstrates that muscimol binding is associated with amacrine cell synaptic complexes (336) (Fig. 9). These labeled synaptic complexes are dis-

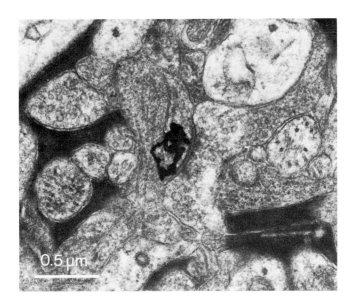

FIG. 9. Electron microscopic autoradiograph of an amacrine cell synapse and associated muscimol labeling in the chicken IPL. (From Yazulla and Brecha, ref. 336, with permission.)

tributed most densely in laminae 2 and 4 of the IPL, closely matching the muscimol uptake pattern within the IPL (Fig. 10).

These studies indicate that synaptic binding sites may not necessarily be revealed by uptake studies, and as demonstrated for the chicken IPL, GABA-sensitive muscimol binding sites are more concentrated in laminae, 2 and 4 of the IPL than in lamina 5 of the IPL (336). A similar conclusion regarding differences in the localization of GABA uptake and synaptic binding sites for GABA has been reported in the goldfish IPL (335a).

In conclusion, biochemical studies have revealed the presence of GABA, GAD, and GABA-T within the retina. A high-affinity uptake system for GABA and high-affinity GABA binding sites are also present in the retina. Histochemical studies both suggest the presence of GABAergic amacrine and horizontal cells within the retina and demonstrate the presence of GABAergic synaptic sites in the IPL. Most studies have identified GABAergic retinal neurons at the light microscopic level; however, with the exception of the goldfish and cat, more detailed morphological studies are lacking. Such studies would be of value in determining how many classes of GABA-accumulating retinal cells there are in any single species as well as clarifying the differences that exist in GAD immunohistochemical and GABA and muscimol staining patterns.

The teleost retina also contains a well-documented GABAergic horizontal cell system. Evidence for this system includes the presence of GAD in isolated and intact horizontal cells and the accumulation of GABA by these cells. GABAergic horizontal cell systems are also likely to be present in other vertebrate retinas. Biochemical and histochemical studies thus suggest that GABAergic systems are present in selected amacrine cell populations and, in some species, in interplexiform and horizontal cell populations.

Benzodiazepines.

Biochemistry. Studies of GABAergic systems in the central nervous system have demonstrated a functional relationship between GABA and benzodiazepine binding sites (304). Specific high-affinity binding sites for benzodiazepine are present in both mammalian and nonmammalian retinal homogenates (21,129,130,232,242,259,286; and *unpublished observations*). Muscimol and GABA will increase the apparent affinity of, but not the number of, binding sites in retinal homogenates (130,242) in a manner similar to that reported for the rat brain (304). However, studies of bovine retina report either no change or a reduction in benzodiazepine binding in the presence of GABA or muscimol (232,259). Reasons for this discrepancy are not known.

Intravitreal treatment with monosodium glutamate or kainic acid results in a 90% reduction in benzodiazepine binding in the rat retina (286). These data and the recent histological localization of benzodiazepine binding sites suggest that these sites are located on neuronal processes within the IPL (340; and *unpublished observations*).

Histochemistry. Benzodiazepine binding sites are localized in the IPL of the pigeon and rat retina (340; and *unpublished observations*) (Fig. 11). This localization pattern is abolished by pretreatment of the retina by benzodiazepine drugs, suggesting that these binding sites are specific for benzodiazepines. In addition, the number of silver grains, which represent benzodiazepine binding sites, over the IPL is markedly increased by the addition of 100 μM GABA or muscimol to the incubation mixture (Fig. 11B). This enhancement of benzodiazepine binding probably results from the increase in the apparent affinity for the benzodiazepine ligand and not from an increase in the number of benzodiazepine binding sites (130).

In conclusion, retinal benzodiazepine binding

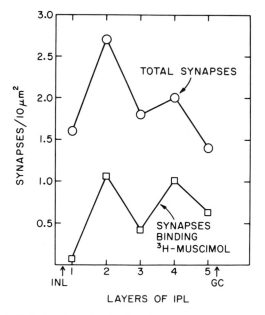

FIG. 10. Laminar distribution of the density of amacrine cell synapses (○) and amacrine cell synapses associated with muscimol (□) in the IPL. (From Yazulla and Brecha, ref. 336, with permission.)

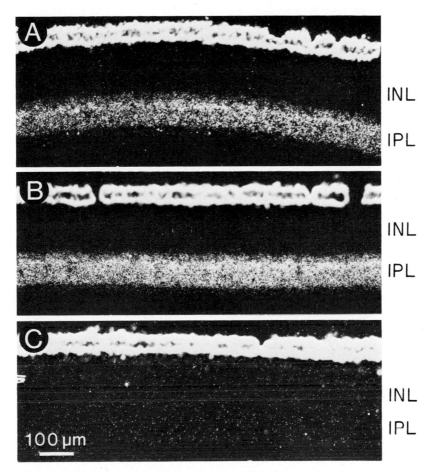

FIG. 11. Benzodiazepine (flunitrazepam) binding patterns in the IPL of the pigeon retina. **A:** Retinal section incubated in 3.3×10^{-9} M [³H]-flunitrazepam. **B:** Experimental section incubated in 3.3×10^{-9} M [³H]-flunitrazepam and 100 μM muscimol, illustrating an enhancement of benzodiazepine binding in the presence of muscimol. **C:** Control section incubated in 3.3×10^{-9} M [³H]-flunitrazepam and 1×10^{-6} M clonazepam demonstrating the inhibition of flunitrazepam binding. These three sections were adjacent to one another and processed together with a dry autoradiographic procedure.

sites are similar in nature to benzodiazepine binding sites described in the brain. Furthermore, benzodiazepine binding sites are associated with GABA binding sites in the retina.

Glycine

Biochemistry.

Glycine is present in the retina and found at the greatest concentrations within the INL and IPL [see Voaden (314) for review; 15,145–147,181, 206,228,238,291,316,333]. Specific low- and high-affinity uptake systems for glycine have been described (34,168,218,276,317). In addition, most studies report that glycine is released in a stimulus-specific manner from the retina (54,94,95,127, 144,152,166,171,176,217,218,240,274,313).

Histochemistry.

Glycine is accumulated by amacrine and displaced amacrine cells (34,35,78,79,86,95,127, 150,152,190,191,193,248,317). A population of glycine-accumulating interplexiform cells is also reported to be present in goldfish (189). Finally, the uptake and concentration of this amino acid by frog photoreceptor terminals have been described (195). No other studies have suggested glycine to be a photoreceptor transmitter, and further studies are needed to confirm and clarify this potentially important observation.

In conclusion, biochemical studies have described the presence of glycine in proximal retinal regions, a specific high-affinity uptake system for glycine, as well as the light-modulated release of glycine. However, to date, no studies have evaluated the retina for glycine binding sites. Histochemical studies suggest that only amacrine cells accumulate glycine. A detailed electron microscopic study of glycine-accumulating amacrine cells and the localization of their synaptic sites are needed. Overall, these biochemical and histochemical studies are indicative of glycinergic systems within the proximal retina.

Glutamate and Aspartate

Biochemistry.

Both glutamate and aspartate are present in the retina (56,114,178,181,228,238,239,291,293). Microdissection studies demonstrate that the highest concentrations of these two amino acids are found within the IPL and GCL, although moderate levels are also present in distal retinal regions (15,145,147,206,316,333). Specific low- and high-affinity uptake systems for both glutamate and aspartate are present in rat and rabbit retinas (218,220,307,329). Aspartate uptake systems are inhibited by glutamate, and, likewise, glutamate uptake systems are inhibited by aspartate, suggesting a common transport system for both of these amino acids (307,329). There is no effect of light stimulation on the release of glutamate from the retina (54,144,214,217,240), but low-frequency flashing light stimulation does result in a decrease in the release of aspartate from the retina (212,214,217). Finally, some evidence for glutamate receptor sites has been presented (18). Glutamate shows a higher affinity for these binding sites than does either aspartate or dihydrokainate, suggesting that these sites are specific for glutamate.

Histochemistry.

The majority of histochemical studies report that glutamate and aspartate are accumulated only by Müller cells (35,78,83,86,147,329). One report, however, describes the accumulation of glutamate by rod photoreceptors in cat, monkey, and human retinas (35).

In goldfish retina, low concentrations of kainic acid selectivity destroy horizontal, cone bipolar, and the majority of amacrine cells (337). These authors (337) argue that if low concentrations of kainic acid destroy only those retinal cells with glutamate receptors, the destruction of these retinal cell types could suggest that "glutamatergic" systems are present in both distal and proximal retinal regions (337).

In conclusion, biochemical studies imply the existence of glutamate and aspartate retinal neuronal systems. Histochemical studies, however, do not provide strong support for such a suggestion. Indeed, a reexamination of glutamate and aspartate uptake patterns in the vertebrate retina is important and necessary in view of these biochemical data.

Taurine

Biochemistry.

Taurine is present in the retina (145,181, 182,228,229,292) at concentrations that are several times greater than that of any other amino acid (147,206,238,239). Most studies report that taurine is concentrated in retinal regions (145,147,206,228,237,295,297,316,333) distal to photoreceptor cells (53,121,229,275,277). Specific low- and high-affinity uptake systems for taurine are present in many retinas (80,149,159,160, 218,219,237,267,274,275,292,295,297), and these uptake systems are associated only with photoreceptor cells (275,276). In addition, a K^+- or light-stimulated release of taurine from the retina has been reported (54,144,149,174,176,214,217,240, 241,268,274). The presence of cysteine sulfinate (CSA) decarboxylase in the retina also has been described (102,188,201). Specific low- and high-affinity taurine binding sites are also present in the chicken retina (175). Further studies are needed to determine the precise location of these binding sites in the retina.

Histochemistry.

Taurine is accumulated by the pigment epithelium as well as by retinal neurons and Müller cells (80,149,159,160,246,316). In all retinas examined to date, taurine is accumulated by photoreceptor cells; in some retinas, by seemingly specific amacrine cell populations (80,149,159,160,237,246, 316).

In conclusion, biochemical studies provide convincing evidence that taurine is concentrated within photoreceptor cells. Furthermore, these cells are likely to be the only retinal neurons having a high-affinity uptake system for taurine. Some evidence has also been provided for CSA decarboxylase activity and taurine synaptic sites in the retina. Histochemical studies demonstrating uptake of taurine by photoreceptor cells correlate well with biochemical studies. Uptake studies also suggest the presence of taurine-accumulating amacrine cell populations in some species. However, evidence supporting a neurotransmitter role for taurine in the retina is still incomplete. Indeed, much of the biochemical and histochemical data can just as well be interpreted to suggest that taurine is absolutely critical for the normal maintenance of the retina and that it is not a retinal transmitter substance.

Other Amino Acids

Several studies have provided summary tables giving the relative concentrations of the different amino acids found in the retina. A number of amino acids including glutamine and β-alanine are present in concentrations similar to those of GABA and glycine (53,56,145,180,206,238,239,293,316, 333). However, the current consensus is that these two above-mentioned amino acids are not neuroactive substances in the retina (12,36).

General histochemical surveys of the uptake patterns of several amino acids in the rabbit retina have been presented (35,78,86). Amino acids that are not likely to be neuroactive substances in the retina are distributed in a diffuse manner over the entire INL, IPL, and GCL. This labeling pattern is likely caused by the nonspecific uptake systems possessed by these retinal cells.

Catecholamines: Dopamine, Norepinephrine, Epinephrine

Biochemistry

Dopamine is the predominant catecholamine found in the retina [see Graham (113) for review; 103,134,135,280]. Very low or nondetectable levels of norepinephrine have been reported for most retinas (68,115,116,134,135,223,280), and moderate levels of epinephrine have been reported in frog and toad retina (67,68). Specific high-affinity uptake systems for dopamine (89,272,306) as well as the release of dopamine by either light or K^+ stimulation in a Ca^{2+}-dependent manner have been described (13,66,127,272,306). In the rabbit retina, dopamine release is modulated by the neuropeptide α-melanocyte-stimulating hormone but not by GABA, glutamate, or glycine (13).

The monoaminergic enzymes monoamine oxidase and DOPA decarboxylase are distributed in most retinal layers [see Graham (113) for review; 4,5,8,103,208,280,287,288,302]. Tyrosine hydroxylase, the rate-limiting enzyme necessary for the synthesis of dopamine, is present in the retinas of all species studied to date (134,135,165,280). Moreover, the synthesis of dopamine from either tyrosine or L-DOPA has been reported (127, 134,135,165,272).

Specific high-affinity dopamine binding sites have been described in the retina of every species studied to date (184,186,253–255,279,325,326). Dopamine binding sites have been identified using spiroperidol but not with domperidone. These studies suggest that the retina contains a homogeneous subclass of dopamine receptors (143) that are linked to an adenylate cyclase system (see below) [but see also Makman et al. (186)].

A dopamine-sensitive adenylate cyclase system has been demonstrated within the IPL and OPL (32,33,40,41,51,103,172,183,185,230,253, 254,278–280,306,324–327). This system is stimulated by low concentrations of dopamine and dopamine agonists but is unaffected by a variety of other substances including serotonin, GABA, glycine, aspartate, glutamate, morphine, substance P, somatostatin, and D-ala-2-D-leu-5-enkephalin (280,326,327). These data suggest that retinal dopamine receptors are most likely linked to an adenylate cyclase and can thus be classified as D_1 dopamine receptors (143) [but see Makman et al. (186)].

Histochemistry

The localization of retinal catecholamines is based on extensive histofluorescence studies. Most studies have employed the Falck–Hillarp histofluorescence techniques (82). More recently, catecholaminergic retinal neurons have been identified and characterized using high-affinity uptake, immunohistochemistry, and electron microscopic techniques.

Dopamine and L-DOPA are accumulated by amacrine cells and their processes (86,127,153–155). In goldfish retina, dopamine is accumulated by interplexiform cells and is most heavily concentrated within somata of the proximal INL as well as within presynaptic terminals located in the OPL (190,272). The uptake of dopamine and L-DOPA into specific retinal cell populations matches in detail both the Falck–Hillarp histofluorescence and tyrosine hydroxylase immunohistochemical staining patterns found within the retina.

Histofluorescence studies have demonstrated distinct catecholamine-containing amacrine and/or interplexiform cell populations in the retina [see Ehinger (82) for review; 1,63,64,70,72–76, 81, 84, 85, 87, 88, 101, 102, 116, 118, 119, 142, 170, 187, 221,223,310] (Figs. 12, 13). In the teleost retina, catecholamine-containing cells are estimated to

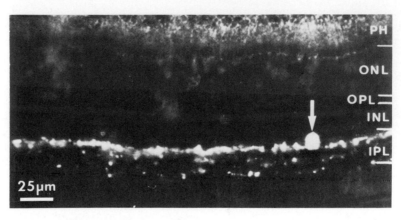

FIG. 12. Catecholamine-containing amacrine cell in the rabbit retina as demonstrated with the Falck–Hillarp technique. A fluorescent cell body in the INL is indicated *(arrow),* and fluorescent processes are distributed in three laminae of the IPL. (From Ehinger and Florén ref. 88, with permission.)

represent 5% to 10% of the total number of cells within the INL (82). In addition, the cebus monkey retina contains a catecholamine-containing cell population that is located in the middle portion of the INL (85). Pharmacological and microspectrofluorometric studies suggest that dopamine is the predominant retinal catecholamine (84,87,116, 118,119,187,221); however, these studies have not proved convincingly that dopamine is the only retinal catecholamine. In view of this uncertainty, it is still best to refer to these as catecholamine-containing cells.

Catecholamine-containing amacrine cells are located typically in the proximal INL as well as within the GCL. They give rise to varicose processes that are distributed in selected laminae of the IPL (Fig. 12). In most cases, these processes are concentrated in lamina 1 of the IPL; in addition, these processes are present within laminae 3

and 5 of the IPL. In several vertebrates, catecholamine-containing cells are thought to represent amacrine cell populations based on their appearance and size, and the location of their somata and processes (76,82,84).

Catecholamine-containing interplexiform cells are present in certain species including the teleost and New World monkey (70,85,87,170) (Fig. 13). These cells are located in the proximal INL and give rise to a dense plexus of varicose processes in the IPL, INL, and OPL. In the IPL, these processes are distributed in a laminar fashion similar to that reported for other types of catecholamine-containing amacrine cells. In the distal INL, these processes arborize around horizontal cells and form a dense plexus within the proximal OPL. These histofluorescence studies have firmly established the existence of a catecholamine-containing interplexiform cell population in some species.

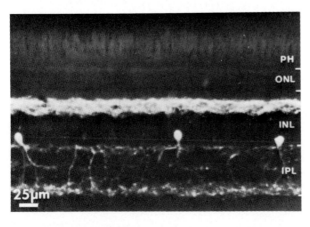

FIG. 13. Catecholamine-containing interplexiform cells in the perch retina as demonstrated with the Falck–Hillarp technique. These cells are located in the proximal INL and give rise to processes that ramify in both plexiform layers (OPL and IPL). PH, photoreceptor layer. (From Ehinger, ref. 82, with permission.)

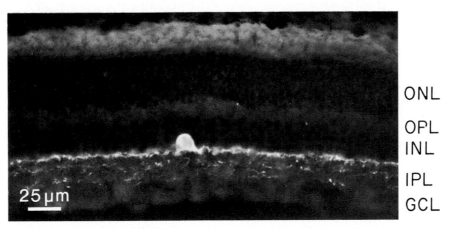

ONL
OPL
INL
IPL
GCL

FIG. 14. Tyrosine hydroxylase immunoreactive amacrine cell in the rabbit retina. Note the virtually identical appearance of this cell and the fluorescence cell and its processes illustrated in Fig. 12. Tyrosine hydroxylase antiserum used for this study was generously supplied by Drs. A. W. Tank and N. Weiner.

Recently, tyrosine hydroxylase-like (TH) immunoreactive cells have been observed in goldfish, pigeon, rat, rabbit, and monkey retinas (123,124; and *unpublished observations*) (Figs. 14, 15). In general, TH immunoreactivity is present in distinct amacrine and/or interplexiform cell populations which are identical in appearance to catechol-amine-containing retinal cells based on the Falck–Hillarp technique (Figs. 12, 14).

Finally, monoamine oxidase is found in both distal and proximal retinal regions in several mammalian and nonmammalian species (99,208). However, the lack of morphological specificity in monoamine oxidase staining does not allow for an

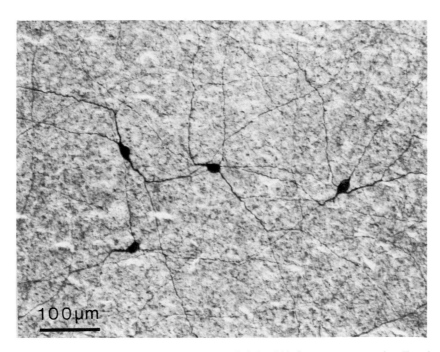

FIG. 15. Tyrosine hydroxylase immunoreactive amacrine cells in a rabbit flat-mount preparation. Tyrosine-containing cells typically give rise to two or three primary processes. Tyrosine hydroxylase antiserum used for this study was generously supplied by Drs. A. W. Tank and N. Weiner.

adequate evaluation of which cell populations contain this enzyme.

Catecholamine-containing retinal cell populations will preferentially accumulate monoamines and monoamine-related neurotoxins, including 5,6-dihydroxytryptamine (64,88,90,91,96,101). This neurotoxin, which causes distinct ultrastructural changes in monoaminergic neurons, has been used to selectively label monoamine-related retinal cell populations (i.e., catecholamine-containing and indoleamine-accumulating neurons) so that their synaptic relationships can be observed.

Catecholamine-containing amacrine cells in the mudpuppy and rabbit retina appear to form conventional pre- and postsynaptic contacts with other amacrine cell processes (1,64) as determined by a special pharmacological-histochemical procedure using 5,6-dihydroxytryptamine (64). With similar histochemical procedures, catecholamine-containing interplexiform cells in the goldfish and cebus monkey retina have been observed to form synaptic contacts with amacrine cell somata and processes. In the OPL, these cells form presynaptic contacts with bipolar and selected horizontal cell somata and processes (62,63,65). Interplexiform cells do not contact photoreceptor cells (62,63,65). These studies suggest that catecholaminergic retinal systems form synaptic contacts only with amacrine cells in the IPL. This general observation does not appear to be dependent on which retinal cell type (i.e., amacrine cell or interplexiform cell) contains the catecholamine. Moreover, this synaptic arrangement suggests that catecholamine cells interact only with other amacrine cells. In contrast, GAD-containing amacrine cells form synaptic contacts with all cell types in the IPL, and indoleamine-accumulating amacrine cells form synaptic contacts only with bipolar cell processes in the IPL (see below).

Ultrastructural studies of conventionally prepared retinal tissue have noted the existence of different-sized dense-cored vesicles located in amacrine cell somata and processes (187,243). The early suggestion that catecholamine cells contain large dense-cored vesicles (187,243) must be reevaluated in light of (a) the poor correlation between the distribution of catecholamine-containing processes and large dense-cored vesicle-containing profiles (62–65,82); (b) the localization using monoamine neurotoxins of small rather than large dense-cored vesicles within catecholamine-containing processes (1,62–65); and (c) the recent identification of neuropeptide-like-containing amacrine cells which also may contain large dense-cored vesicles.

In conclusion, biochemical evidence indicates that dopamine is the principal catecholamine in the retina; however, epinephrine and norepinephrine are also likely to be present in the retina of some species. Indeed, a reevaluation of the catecholamine content in the retina of various vertebrates using modern analytical techniques would be of great interest. Furthermore, although tyrosine hydroxylase activity has been demonstrated in several retinas, only one study in the chicken retina has evaluated the presence of dopamine-β-hydroxylase activity in the retina. Certainly, the presence of this catecholamine enzyme would suggest that norepinephrine and/or epinephrine metabolic systems are present in the retina. Biochemical studies have presented convincing evidence that dopamine is taken up and released from retina and that most dopamine binding sites can be classified tentatively as D_1 receptors which are linked to a dopamine-sensitive adenylate cyclase system. Histochemical studies also suggest the presence of distinct catecholamine-containing retinal cell populations. These amacrine and/or interplexiform cell populations have been identified using high-affinity uptake, histofluorescence, and immunohistochemical techniques. Electron microscopic studies have confirmed these observations and have described the association of catecholamine-containing profiles with only amacrine cells in the IPL. In the OPL, catecholamine-containing interplexiform cells contact both bipolar and horizontal cells. Overall, the presence of catecholamine retinal cell populations that are likely to contain dopamine has been established.

Indoleamines: Serotonin and Melatonin

Serotonin

Biochemistry.

A low concentration of serotonin has been detected in the retina of several vertebrates (8,92,103,116,233,288,301). Specific high-affinity uptake systems for serotonin are present in chick, rabbit, and bovine retina (89,233,303,305,308, 309), suggesting that specific uptake systems for serotonin or a closely related indoleamine are present in the retina. In addition, serotonin is released from bovine retinal homogenates and synaptosomes by K^+ stimulation in a Ca^{2+}-dependent manner (233,234,308,309).

As mentioned above, the monoaminergic enzymes monoamine oxidase (4,5,287,301,302) and 5-hydroxytryptophan decarboxylase (DOPA decarboxylase) (4,5,8,103,280,287,288) are present in ocular tissue including the retina. Tryptophan hydroxylase, the rate-limiting enzyme for the synthesis of serotonin, is found in the bovine retina but not in the mouse or rabbit retina (103,233, 287,288). These studies suggest that the necessary metabolic enzymes for serotonin synthesis are present in some vertebrate retinas.

Histochemistry.

The identification of serotonin-containing retinal cell populations has been attempted using the Falck–Hillarp histofluorescence and high-affinity uptake procedures. To date, the high-affinity uptake of indoleamines has been the most widely used technique for identifying indoleamine-containing cells.

Histofluorescence studies, which have primarily used the Falck–Hillarp technique, have failed to demonstrate indoleamine fluorescence in any adult retina. This negative observation has been reported repeatedly (103) despite the recent employment of modifications of the Falck–Hillarp technique designed to increase indoleamine levels in the retina (102,103).

In contrast, the embryonic chick retina does contain a transiently appearing population of amacrine cells that show indoleamine fluorescence following Falck–Hillarp processing (118) [but see Florén (101)]. These cells are located in the proximal INL and give rise to processes that arborize in the IPL. Moreover, intraperitoneal injections of *para*-chlorophenylalanine, an indoleamine-depleting agent, selectively eliminate their fluorescence while only slightly affecting the fluorescence of catecholamine-containing cells. These observations suggest the existence of a serotonin-containing amacrine cell population in the embryonic chicken retina.

Indoleamine-accumulating amacrine cell populations are present in most retinas [see Ehinger and Florén (92) for review; 1,63–65,88–91,93,101, 102,234] (Fig. 16). Indoleamine-accumulating amacrine cells are located in the proximal INL, give rise to processes in the IPL, and are morphologically distinct from catecholamine-containing cells (Figs. 12,14,16). Furthermore, they outnumber catecholamine-containing cells by severalfold (65,88,89,92).

With 5,6-dihydroxytryptamine used as an ultrastructural marker, indoleamine-accumulating amacrine cells in the rabbit and cebus monkey retina appear to form the majority if not all of their synaptic contacts with bipolar cell terminals (64,65,93). This synaptic arrangement suggests that indoleamine-accumulating cells have different synaptic functions within the IPL than either the catecholaminergic and GABAergic systems.

At best, evidence for serotonin as a retinal neurotransmitter is incomplete. Serotonin is undoubtedly present in some retinas, such as the chicken, but not others. Furthermore, serotonin uptake systems and the release of preloaded serotonin have been described in the retina. To date, no data have been presented describing the effects of light on the release of preloaded or endogenous serotonin within the retina. The monoaminergic enzymes 5-hydroxytryptophan decarboxylase and monoamine oxidase are present in most retinas; however, the rate-limiting enzyme tryptophan hydroxylase has been identified only in the bovine retina. An extensive survey of the occurrence of tryptophan hydroxylase in several different vertebrate retinas is needed. The presence of this enzyme would suggest the existence of an indoleaminergic system in the retina. Finally, no studies have reported the presence of specific serotonin binding sites in retinal homogenates. Histochemical studies have only demonstrated a transiently appearing serotonin-

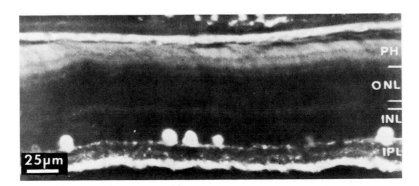

FIG. 16. Indoleamine-accumulating neurons in the rabbit retina 4 hr after an intravitreal injection of 50 μg of 5,7-dihydroxytryptamine. Note the prominent labeling within the proximal IPL. (From Ehinger and Florén, ref. 88, with permission.)

fluorescing amacrine cell population in the embryonic chick retina. In contrast, histochemical uptake
studies have reported the presence of indoleamine-
accumulating amacrine cells within the retinas of
most vertebrates, and ultrastructural studies suggest that these cells contact only bipolar cells. The
available data thus suggest that in some retinas, including the chicken and cow, serotonin should be
considered a serious retinal transmitter candidate,
but in other species, including the rabbit, indoleamines may not be retinal transmitter substances.

Melatonin

Melatonin is present in the retinas of several different vertebrate species (6,106,117,235,236). In
the trout retina, melatonin-like (MEL) immunoreactivity is greatest during the light phase of a 12-
hr light/dark cycle (106). In contrast, in both
chick and rat retinas, MEL immunoreactivity is
severalfold greater at the midpoint of the dark
phase of a 12-hr light/dark cycle (117,236). Furthermore, in the chick retina, levels of MEL immunoreactivity fluctuate in a rhythmic manner
during constant darkness and are rapidly reduced
by brief light stimulation during dark conditions.
These data suggest that MEL levels exhibit a circadian rhythm that can be entrained by light
(117).

N-Acetyltransferase (NAT) and hydroxyindole-
O-methyltransferase (HIOMT) are the enzymes
that synthesize melatonin from serotonin. The activity of these two enzymes is present in ocular tissue including the retina (5,7,17,38,46,50,103,
210,211,244,249,289,322). Activity of NAT and
HIOMT is usually reported to be greater within
the retina than in other ocular tissues (48,
49,117,250). Moreover, both NAT and HIOMT
activities from ocular and retinal tissue appear to
be associated with a circadian rhythm (17,117,
210). Finally, synthesis of melatonin from serotonin has been reported for both trout and rat retina
(47,107).

Histochemistry.

N-Acetylindolealkylamine-like (melatonin and/
or N-acetylserotonin) immunoreactivity is apparently localized to every cell in the ONL of the rat
retina (37–39). These cells stain with more intensity during dark conditions than in light conditions
(39); this observation is consistent with radioimmunoassay studies (117,236) that describe a
greater MEL content during this period. These histochemical studies suggest that MEL is present in
all cells located in the ONL, but whether all or
some proportion of these cells synthesize melatonin

or N-acetylserotonin, or both, has yet to be
determined.

In conclusion, biochemical studies have provided
some evidence for the existence of a melatonin system within the retina. These studies have described
the presence of endogenous melatonin, the existence of the melatonin metabolic enzymes NAT
and HIOMT, and the synthesis of melatonin from
its precursor, serotonin. Indeed, further biochemical studies aimed at determining the location in the
retina of MEL immunoreactivity, the release of
MEL immunoreactivity, as well as the existence
and characterization of melatonin receptor sites
would be of great interest. Histochemical studies,
although of preliminary nature, suggest that those
cells that are involved with melatonin are located
within distal retinal regions. Additional studies
clarifying the exact location of melatonin in the
retina are needed.

Neuropeptides

The exact biological function(s) of neuropeptides remains an enigma, although there is increasing evidence that they play a neurotransmitter
and/or "neuromodulator" role in the nervous system (42,43,125,136).

Within the last 4 years, several reports have appeared describing neuropeptide-like immunoreactivity in different vertebrate retinas as determined
by either radioimmunoassay or immunohistochemical techniques. To date, the presence of enkephalin-like (ENK), β-endorphin-like, cholecystokinin-
like (CCK), glucagon-like (GLU), neurotensin-
like (NT), somatostatin-like (SRIF), substance P-
like (SP), vasoactive intestinal polypeptide-like
(VIP), and thyrotropin-releasing hormone-like
(TRH) immunoreactivity has been described in
retinal tissue. The following sections review much
of the evidence reporting the presence of these neuropeptides in the retina.

Substance P

Biochemistry.

Bioassay studies first noted substance P-like biological activity in bovine and dog retina about 25
years ago (71,330). More recently, SP immunoreactivity has been described by the use of radioimmunoassays in several mammalian and nonmammalian retinas (Table 1) (100,139,260).

Substance P biological activity and immunoreactivity have also been reported in pigeon, rat,
and bovine optic nerve extracts, suggesting the
existence of SP-containing ganglion cells (71,

TABLE 1. *Immunoreactive substance P in the retina and optic nerve*

Species	Concentration	Reference
Frog *(Rana catesbeiana)*	218 ± 26.2 pg/mg wet wt	100
Chick (2 days old)	25 ± 1.4 pg/mg wet wt	100
Pigeon	3 ± 1 pmoles/g wet wt	260
Pigeon optic nerve	35 ± 13 pmoles/g wet wt	260
Pigeon *(Columba livia)*	45.8 ± 7 fmoles/mg protein	unpublished data
Rat (Osborne–Mendel)	65 ± 10.6 pg/mg wet wt	100
Rat	89 ± 19.4 ng/g wet wt	139
Rat optic nerve	87 ± 18.6 ng/g wet wt	139
Guinea pig	69 ± 13.6 pg/mg wet wt	100
Rabbit	38 ± 7.2 pg/mg wet wt	100
Cow	32 ± 3.0 pg/mg wet wt	100
Monkey *(Macaca mulatta)*	7 ± 1.2 pg/mg wet wt	100

139,260,330). These data must be evaluated carefully, because optic nerve fractions may be contaminated by SP-, ENK-, and/or VIP-containing nerves which are present near the optic nerve and within the ciliary ganglion (99a).

Histochemistry.

Specific SP immunoreactivity is present in the amacrine, interplexiform, and perhaps ganglion cells in a wide variety of vertebrates (26,31, 123,124,141) (Tables 2 and 3).

TABLE 2. *Localization of neuropeptide immunoreactivity in the retina of various vertebrates*

Species	Neuropeptide						
	SP	ENK	SS	NT	VIP	GLU	CCK
Fish							
Goldfish *(Carassius auratus)*	+	+	+	+		+	+
File perch *(Damanichthys vacca)*	+	+		+			
Cohoe salmon	+	+					
Sturgeon poacher	+						
Plainfin midshipman *(Porichthys pacifica)*	+						
Surfsmelt *(Hypomesus pretisus)*	+						
Rockfish *(Sevastes caurinus)*	+	+					
Channel catfish		+					
Carp	+	+	+			+	
Amphibians							
Xenopus laevis	+						
Toad *(Bufo marinus)*	+		+				
Frog *(Rana pipiens)*	+	+	+	+			+
Tiger salamander *(Ambysoma tigrinum)*	+	+					
Mudpuppy *(Necturus maculosus)*	+	+	+	+	+	+	+
Reptiles							
Turtle *(Chrysemys scripta)*	+	+				+	
Lizard *(Anolis carolinensis)*	+	+					
Lizard *(Uta stansburiana)*	+						
Lizard *(Gecko gecko)*	+	+					
Birds							
Pigeon *(Columba livia)*	+	+	+	+	+	+	
Chicken *(Gallus domesticus)*	+	+	+	+	+	+	
Mammals							
Rat	+				+		
Rabbit	+		+		+		
Cat	+		+		+		
New World monkey *(Saimira sciureus)*	+		+		+		
Old World monkey *(Macaca nemestrima)*	+		+		+		
Old World monkey *(Macaca facicularis)*	+		+		+		

TABLE 3. *Distribution of substance P-like immunoreactivity in the retina*

	GCL	IPL	INL	OPL	Cell types
Fish					
Goldfish *(Carassius auratus)*	+	3	+		1
Pile perch *(Damanichthys vacca)*		1,5	+		1[a]
Cohoe salmon		1,5	+		1[a]
Sturgeon poacher		1	+		1
Plainfin midshipman *(Porichthys pacifica)*		1,5	+		1[a]
Surfsmelt *(Hypomesus pretiosus)*		5	+		1
Rockfish *(Sebastes caurinus)*		1,2,4,5	+		1[a]
Carp		3	+		1
Amphibians					
Xenopus laevis	+	1,2,4,5	+		2[a]
Toad *(Bufo marinus)*	+	1,2,3,4,5	+		3
Frog *(Rana pipiens)*		3,5	+		1[a]
Tiger Salamander *(Ambystoma tigrinum)*		3,5	+		1[a]
Mudpuppy *(Necturus maculosus)*		1,5			
Reptiles					
Turtle *(Chrysemys scripta)*		M[b]	+		1[a]
Lizard *(Anolis carolinensis)*		3	+		1
Lizard *(Uta stansburiana)*	+	3	+		1
Lizard *(Gecko gecko)*		1,3,5	+		1
Birds					
Pigeon *(Columba livia)*		3	+		1
Chicken *(Gallus domesticus)*		3	+		1
Mammals					
Rat		M[b]	+		1[a]
Rabbit	+	1,3,5	+	+	4
Cat	+	3			1
New World monkey *(Saimira sciureus)*	+	1,3,5	+		2[a]
Old World monkey *(Macaca nemestrima)*	+	1,3,5	+	+	5
Old World monkey *(Macaca facicularis)*	+	3	+	+	1[a]

[a]Possibly more cell types.
[b]M, multistratified.

A population of unistratified SP-containing amacrine cells is present in the goldfish and carp retina (31). In the goldfish retina, these cells typically give rise to a single process which ramifies within lamina 3 of the IPL (Fig. 17). These cells are usually located at the border of the INL and IPL and measure about 9 μm in diameter. The SP-containing amacrine cells in the goldfish retina are distributed throughout the entire retina. In both the goldfish and carp retina, these immunoreactive cells resemble unistratified cell types observed in Golgi impregnation studies (45).

In the pigeon retina, SP immunoreactivity is observed within a population of unistratified amacrine cells that are distributed throughout the retina (141). These cells are located at the border of the INL and IPL, measure about 7 μm in diameter, and are characterized by a single process that descends to and ramifies in lamina 3 of the IPL (Fig. 18). The appearance of these immunoreactive cells is strikingly similar to cell types depicted by Cajal (45) and Boycott and Dowling (22) in their studies of bird retina.

In the rabbit retina, SP immunoreactivity is present in somata located in the INL and GCL and processes in the IPL (29a) (Figs. 19 and 20). Substance P immunoreactive processes are distributed within laminae 1, 3, and 5 of the IPL, although they are most dense in lamina 5. At least three distinct populations of retinal cells contain SP. There are two amacrine cell populations: one is located at the border of the INL and IPL and gives rise to a single, stout process which descends to and ramifies within lamina 5 of the IPL (Figs. 19 and 20), whereas a second amacrine cell type gives rise to several processes that ramify in laminae 1 and 3 before terminating within lamina 5 of the IPL. Finally, SP-containing cells whose somata are located in the GCL give rise to several processes that ramify within lamina 5 of the IPL (Fig. 20). To date, an axon-like process has not been observed to be associated with these cells; however, the pres-

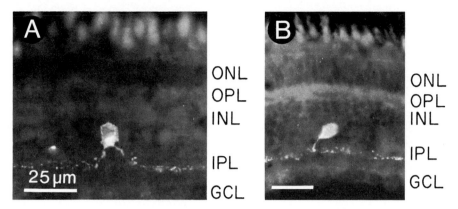

FIG. 17. Unistratified SP immunoreactive amacrine cells in the goldfish retina. These cells give rise to one or two processes which descend to and ramify in lamina 3 of the IPL. (From Brecha et al., ref. 31, with permission.)

ence of immunoreactive processes in the GCL suggests the possible existence of SP-containing ganglion cells within the rabbit retina. Further studies are needed to resolve this issue.

In the Old and New World monkey retina, SP is also present within somata in the INL, IPL, and GCL, as well as processes in the IPL (26,123,124) (Fig. 21). The SP processes are distributed within laminae 1, 3, and 5 of the IPL. These processes are most dense in lamina 3 of the Old World monkey retina and lamina 5 of the New World monkey retina. There are at least four distinct SP-containing retinal cell populations in the Old World monkey retina (26). Substance P-containing amacrine cells whose somata are located at the border of the INL and IPL give rise to a single stout process which descends to and ramifies in lamina 3 of the IPL (Fig. 21A). A SP-containing cell population that is located within the IPL gives rise to processes that ramify within lamina 3 of the IPL (Fig. 21B). These cells do not appear to give rise to an axon, nor are they labeled by retrograde transport of horseradish peroxidase (HRP) following HRP injections into central visual nuclei (A. Hendrickson, *personal communication*). These data suggest that these cells are displaced amacrine cells rather than displaced ganglion cells. Finally, two other types of immunoreactive cells are located within the GCL;

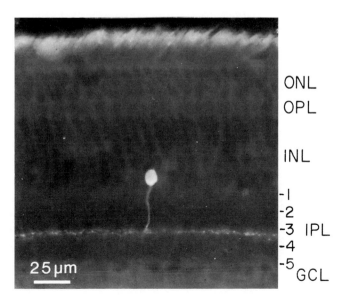

FIG. 18. Unistratified SP-containing amacrine cell in the pigeon retina. The SP-containing amacrine cells in the pigeon retina are located in the proximal INL and give rise to a single process which ramifies in lamina 3 of the IPL. (From Karten and Brecha, ref. 141, with permission.)

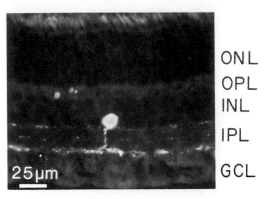

ONL
OPL
INL

IPL

GCL

FIG. 19. Unistratified SP immunoreactive amacrine cell in the rabbit retina. This type of SP-containing amacrine cell gives rise to a single stout process which ramifies in lamina 5 of the IPL. Note the laminar distribution of SP-containing processes in laminae 1,3, and 5 of the IPL.

one of these SP-containing cell populations gives rise to a single process which ascends to and ramifies in lamina 3 of the IPL (Fig. 21C). This type of cell is virtually identical in appearance to the SP-containing amacrine cell located in the INL (Fig. 21A). A second cell type gives rise to several processes which ramify within lamina 5 of the IPL. Whether these latter two cell populations are displaced amacrine cells or ganglion cells has yet to be established.

In both the rabbit and Old World monkey retina, a few immunoreactive processes are observed in the distal INL and the OPL. Although the somata giving rise to these processes have not been identified, their presence implies the existence of SP-containing interplexiform cells.

In view of earlier reports of SP biological activity and immunoreactivity in optic nerve extracts and the presence of SP-containing cell populations in the GCL of the rabbit and monkey retina, the existence of SP-containing ganglion cells in these retinas should also be considered. Double-label experiments using retrograde transport techniques in combination with immunohistochemistry could provide a final identification and classification of the immunoreactive neurons in the GCL.

Physiology.

The effects of exogenous applied substance P in the amphibian and teleost retina have been described in two recent abstracts (57,109). An electrophysiological study using the mudpuppy eyecup preparaton and iontophoretic techniques showed that synthetic substance P increased spontaneous activity and excited all ganglion cells sampled. This excitatory effect was rapid, with an onset similar to that of glutamate, but longer lasting (57). A second study, using the carp eyecup preparation in which synthetic substance P was applied by a nebulizer system, reported that substance P excited most on- and off-center ganglion cells (109). The localization of SP immunoreactivity to amacrine cells in mudpuppy and carp retinas and the excitatory action of this substance on ganglion cell discharge are consistent with the idea that substance P plays a functional role in the retina.

Enkephalin

Biochemistry.

Enkephalin-like immunoreactivity is present in frog, toad, and chicken retinal extracts (97,128,

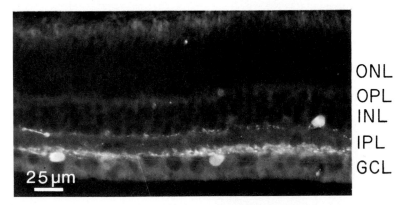

ONL
OPL
INL
IPL
GCL

FIG. 20. Substance P immunoreactive amacrine and perhaps displaced amacrine cell or ganglion cell in the rabbit retina. The SP-containing cells in the GCL typically give rise to processes that ramify only in lamina 5 of the IPL.

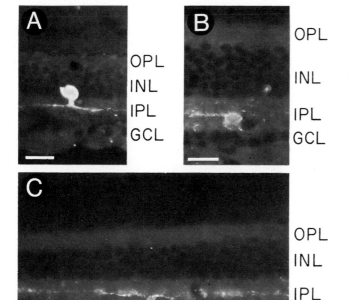

FIG. 21. Substance P immunoreactive amacrine and perhaps displaced amacrine or ganglion cells in the Macaca retina. **A:** An SP-containing unistratified amacrine cell which ramifies in lamina 3 of the IPL. **B:** An SP-containing displaced amacrine cell which is located within lamina 3 of the IPL and ramifies in this lamina. **C:** An SP-containing displaced amacrine cell or perhaps a ganglion cell within the GCL. This cell type is similar in appearance to SP-containing unistratified amacrine cells.

132,137) (Table 4). In addition, both high-pressure liquid chromatography (HPLC) and gel filtration chromatographic studies suggest the existence of authentic met⁵-enkephalin in the 11-day embryonic chick retina (132). A moderate concentration of β-endorphin-like immunoreactivity is present in frog retina as well (137).

The existence of stereospecific, displaceable binding of several different opiate ligands to retinal homogenates has been reported (128,202; and *unpublished observations*). Naloxone, met⁵ enkephalin, or etorphine binding to rat retinal homogenates is saturable, inhibited by naloxone or met⁵-enkephalin, and is characterized as a high-affinity system (128). In addition, opiate binding sites in the rat retina respond to Na⁺ concentrations in a manner similar to that reported for rat brain (128). The retinal opiate-binding system is similar to that re-

TABLE 4. *Immunoreactive enkephalin and β-endorphin in the retina*

Species	Concentrations	References
Enkephalin		
Frog *(Rana pipiens)* [met⁵-ENK]	50 pg/retina	137
Frog *(Rana pipiens)* [leu⁵-ENK]	35 pg/retina	137
Frog	4.6 ng/retina	97
Toad *(Bufo marinus)*	6 ng/mg protein	128
Chick (5 days old)	7.8 ng/retina	97
Embryonic chick (11 days old) [met⁵-ENK]	608 ± 108 pg/mg protein	132
Embryonic chick (11 days old) [leu⁵-ENK]	8.4 ± 33 pg/mg protein	132
Rat	<0.005 ng/retina	97
Cow	<0.1 ng/retina	97
Monkey	<0.01 ng/retina	97
β-Endorphin		
Frog *(Rana pipiens)*	30 ng/retina	137

TABLE 5. *Distribution of enkephalin-like immunoreactivity in the retina*

Species	GCL	IPL	INL	OPL	Cell types
Fish					
Goldfish *(Carassius auratus)*		1,5	+		1
Pile perch *(Damanichthys vacca)*		1	+		1
Cohoe salmon		M[b]	+		1[a]
Channel catfish		3	+		1
Carp		1,5	+		1
Amphibians					
Frog *(Rana pipiens)*		3,4,5	+		1[a]
Tiger salamander *(Ambystoma tigrinum)*		5	+		1[a]
Mudpuppy *(Necturus maculosus)*	+	1,2,3,4,5	+		2
Reptiles					
Turtle *(Chrysemys scripta)*		1,4,5	+		1
Lizard *(Anolis carolinensis)*		1,3,5	+		1[a]
Lizard *(Gecko gecko)*		3	+		1
Birds					
Pigeon *(Columba livia)*		1,3,4,5	+		1
Chicken *(Gallus domesticus)*		1,3,4,5	+		1

[a]Possibly more cell types.
[b]M, multistratified.

ported in the brain and could be mediated by ENK-containing amacrine cells like those described in nonmammalian retinas (see below). However, the apparent lack of ENK immunoreactivity in the mammalian retina as determined by both radioimmunoassay (128) and immunohistochemistry (Tables 2 and 4) suggests that another, as yet unidentified, opiate-like substance may be present in mammalian retina.

Histochemistry.

Specific ENK immunoreactive amacrine cells are present in both central and peripheral retinal regions of several nonmammalian retinas (28) Tables 2 and 5). Because there is cross reactivity of the enkephalin antisera used in these studies with leu[5]-enkephalin, met[5]-enkephalin, as well as dynorphin (110,269), it is not possible to determine whether the observed immunoreactive staining is

FIG. 22. Enkephalin-containing amacrine cells located in the yellow field of the pigeon retina. These cells give rise to multistratified processes that ramify in laminae 1, 3, 4, and 5 of the IPL. Enkephalin antiserum used for this study was generously supplied by Dr. K.-J. Chang.

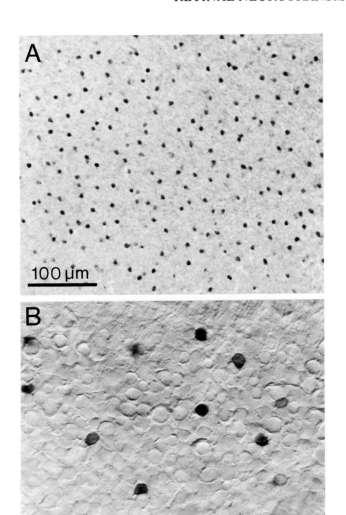

FIG. 23. Enkephalin immunoreactive somata in a flat-mount preparation of the retina. **A:** Low-power photomicrograph. **B:** High-power photomicrograph. Enkephalin antiserum used for this study was generously supplied by Dr. K.-J. Chang.

specific to the pentapeptides leu[5]-enkephalin and met[5]-enkephalin or to some other enkephalin-like peptide.

Enkephalin immunoreactivity is present in what appears to be a distinct class of multistratified amacrine cells in both the pigeon and chicken retina (28) (Fig. 22). These multistratified amacrine cells are characterized by a single process which descends to the border of the IPL before arborizing into several secondary processes. These processes ramify in lamina 1 and give rise to processes that descend to and ramify within laminae 3, 4, and 5 of the IPL. The ENK immunoreactive somata usually are located within the second and third tiers of cells of the proximal INL, are ovoid in shape, and measure about 7.5 µm in diameter. In the pigeon

retina, ENK-containing amacrine cells are distributed within all retinal regions (Fig. 23). The density of ENK immunoreactive cells is greater in central regions of the retina than in peripheral retinal regions (Fig. 24), and this density appears to be proportional to the overall cell density within the INL and GCL (16,105).

As mentioned above, radioimmunoassay studies have described ENK immunoreactivity in retinal extracts from 11-day-old embryonic chicken (132), and these observations have been confirmed in a recent immunohistochemical study (29). In embryonic chicken retina, very faint ENK immunoreactivity is first detected at day 13 within centrally located somata in the proximal INL. At day 18 or 19, ENK-containing immunoreactive cells have a

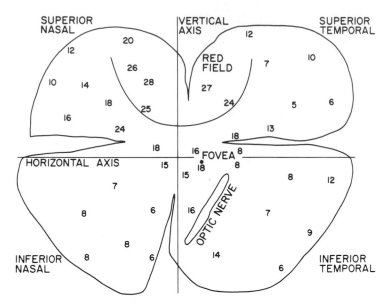

FIG. 24. Line drawing of a flat-mounted pigeon retina demonstrating the number of enkephalin (ENK)-containing amacrine cells in 100 μm $\times$ 100 μm fields. This figure demonstrates that there is a greater density of ENK-containing amacrine cells in central than in peripheral retinal regions.

heavily staining somata but weakly staining primary and secondary processes (Fig. 25). However, within 6 to 12 hr after hatching, ENK-containing cells are identical in both their morphological appearance as well as their staining characteristics to ENK-containing cells observed in the adult retina (Fig. 26). These observations suggest that the presence of "adult" levels of ENK immunoreactivity in the retina is correlated with hatching, light stimulation or both. (Fig. 27). Regardless of what event triggers the increase in ENK immunoreactivity, the rapid increase of ENK immunoreactive staining implies a dramatic increase in the biosynthesis of enkephalin. This increase could be mediated by a specific enkephalinase that cleaves leu[5]- and/or met[5]-enkephalin from a larger enkephalin peptide. If this sequence of events were true, perhaps the ENK immunoreactivity observed before hatching is due to some cross reactivity between the antiserum and a larger enkephalin-like peptide.

Physiology.

The evidence for a functional role of enkephalin in the teleost retina has been presented in a recent abstract (59). When applied by an atomizer system to an eyecup preparation, D-ala[2]-met[5]-Enkephalinamide enhanced spontaneous activity and the light-evoked response of on-center ganglion cells. In contrast, this peptide also inhibited spontaneous activity and the light-evoked response of off-center ganglion cells. These effects were reversible and prevented by pretreatment of the retina with naloxone. Similar but irreversible effects on ganglion cell activity were observed following morphine application. The physiological actions of this enkephalin analog in the retina are consistent with histochemical observations demonstrating multistratified ENK-containing amacrine cells in the goldfish and carp retina *(unpublished observations).*

Earlier studies demonstrated that GABA was accumulated by selected Ab pyriform amacrine cells of the teleost retina in dark conditions (190) and released from these cells by K^+ stimulation in a Ca^{2+}-dependent manner (166). Recently, C. A. Chin and D. M. K. Lam *(personal communication)* have demonstrated that met[5]-enkephalin and morphine suppress this K^+-stimulated, Ca^{2+}-dependent release of preloaded GABA in a dose-related manner. Moreover, naloxone blocks the suppressive action of met[5]-enkephalin. These data suggest that enkephalins have a general effect in the teleost retina; they may excite ganglion cells by disinhibition via an inhibitory GABAergic amacrine cell.

Somatostatin

Biochemistry.

Somatostatin-like biological activity and immunoreactivity are present in the retina of all species

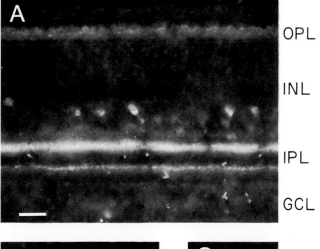

OPL

INL

IPL

GCL

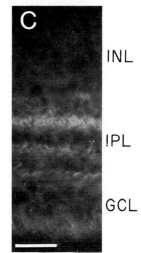

INL

IPL

GCL

20 μm

FIG. 25. Enkephalin immunoreactive staining within the central portion of the chick retina about 36 hr before hatching (stage 44). Note the poor staining of amacrine cells and their processes (**A,B**) and the high nonspecific staining within the IPL (**C**). **A:** Low-power photomicrograph. **B:** High-power photomicrograph. **C:** Control section incubated in enkephalin antiserum absorbed with 10 μM leu⁵-enkephalin. Enkephalin antiserum used for this study was generously supplied by Dr. K.-J. Chang.

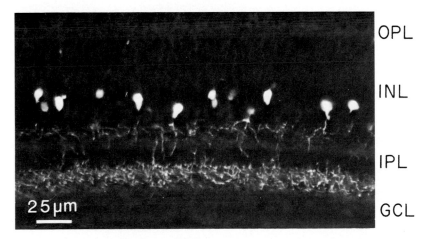

OPL

INL

IPL

GCL

25 μm

FIG. 26. Enkephalin (ENK) immunoreactive staining within the central portion of the 3-day-old chick retina. Note the dense staining of multistratified amacrine cells which are identical in appearance to ENK-containing amacrine cells observed in the adult retina. Enkephalin antiserum used for this study was generously supplied by Dr. K.-J. Chang.

EMBRYONIC RETINA   YOUNG RETINA

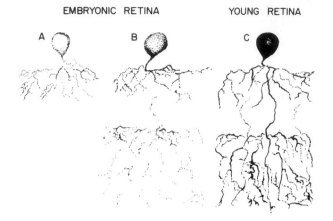

FIG. 27. Schematic representation of the appearance of immunoreactive enkephalin (ENK) in the embryonic and young chick retina. The ENK immunoreactivity is first present within amacrine cell somata and later within amacrine cell processes.

studied to date (30,100,108,161,262–264,284,332) (Table 6). Both rat and human retinal extracts inhibit the release of growth hormone from rat anterior pituitary cells in a manner that is similar to that reported for SRIF from hypothalamic extracts (262,264). Radioimmunoassay studies demonstrate that synthetic somatostatin and retinal extracts have similar displacement curves, suggesting the presence of authentic somatostatin in these extracts (262,264,332). Finally, gel chromatographic studies demonstrate that SRIF immunoreactivity from the goldfish retina elutes in two peaks, one corresponding to synthetic somatostatin (332). Other chromatogaphic studies of rat and human retinal extracts demonstrate that immunoreactive

SRIF first purified by immunoaffinity chromatography elutes as a single peak corresponding to synthetic somatostatin (262,264). These bioassay, radioimmunoassay, and gel chromatography experiments all suggest the presence of authentic somatostatin in the vertebrate retina.

The location in the retina of SRIF immunoreactivity has been suggested by several indirect biochemical techniques. First, no differences in SRIF immunoreactivity are observed between retinal extracts from Osborne–Mendal albino rats and PETH rats which undergo hereditary degeneration of their photoreceptor cells (262). Second, no change in retinal SRIF is observed in retinal extracts 1 year after transection of the optic nerves

TABLE 6. *Immunoreactive somatostatin in the retina and optic nerve*

Species	Concentration	References
Goldfish	4.0 ± 1.8 pmoles/mg protein	332
Frog *(Rana catesbeiana)*	46 ± 2.8 pg/mg wet wt	100
Frog *(Rana pipiens)*	2.9 ± 0.1 pmoles/mg protein	332
Frog *(Rana pipiens)* optic nerve	11.6 ± 2.3 pmoles/mg protein	332
Frog *(Rana esculenta)*	390 ± 110 pg/mg protein	108
Chick (2 days old)	102 ± 7.3 pg/mg wet wt	100
Pigeon *(Columba livia)*	527 ± 76 fmoles/mg protein	30
Rat (Wistar)	13.24 ± 2.88 ng/g tissue	284
Rat (Charles River)	0.621 ± 0.44 pg/mg protein	262
Rat (Osborne–Mendel)	0.960 ± 0.09 pg/mg protein	262
Rat (PETH)	1.46 ± 0.16 pg/mg protein	262
Rat (Osborne–Mendel)	52 ± 4.7 pg/mg wet wt	100
Rat	1.34 ± 0.07 ng/retina	161
Guinea pig	21 ± 1.9 pg/mg wet wt	100
Rabbit	7 ± 0.6 pg/mg wet wt	100
Cow	49 ± 8.2 pg/mg wet wt	100
Cow	11.4 pmoles/mg protein	332
Monkey *(Macaca mulatta)*	28 ± 3.5 pg/mg wet wt	100
Human	492–1,480 pg/mg protein	264

(262). These studies suggest that retinal SRIF is not present in either photoreceptor or ganglion cells. Additionally, a loss of SRIF immunoreactivity does occur in frog and rat retinas following the intraocular injection of either monosodium glutamate or kainic acid (100,161). These lesion experiments support the hypothesis that immunoreactive SRIF in the retina is contained in bipolar, horizontal, interplexiform, and/or amacrine cell populations.

Histochemistry.

Somatostatin-containing cells are present within amacrine and displaced amacrine cells of goldfish, frog, pigeon, and rat retina (30,332) (Table 2). A single study reports that SRIF-containing somata are found throughout the INL and GCL and that SRIF-containing processes are found in both the OPL and IPL (156). This pattern of immunoreactivity implies the existence of SRIF-containing bipolar, horizontal, interplexiform, amacrine, and ganglion cell populations. The large number of SRIF immunoreactive cells reported in this study (156) is in marked contrast to other immunohistochemical (332,340) and radioimmunoassay (100,161,262) studies. The reasons for this disparity are not known.

In the goldfish retina, specific SRIF immunoreactivity is localized in three types of amacrine cells and one other cell type whose somata are located within the GCL (332). Immunoreactive amacrine cells give rise to either large unbranched processes or fine varicose processes which ramify in lamina 1 of the IPL. In addition, some amacrine cells give rise to a fine process which descends to and ramifies in lamina 5 of the IPL (332). The somata located in the GCL give rise to processes that arborize in lamina 5 of the IPL. These cells are likely to be displaced amacrine cells in view of the lack of staining in the GAL and optic nerve.

Pigeon and chicken retinas also contain a distinct population of SRIF-containing amacrine cells (27,30) (Fig. 28). These cells give rise to a single process which descends to lamina 1 of the IPL before ramifying into several secondary processes. Some of these secondary processes then descend to and ramify within laminae 3 and 4 of the IPL. The somata of these SRIF immunoreactive cells measure about 7 μm in diameter and are located in the proximal INL in all retinal regions.

Neurotensin

Biochemistry.

Neurotensin-like immunoreactivity is present in pigeon retinal extracts (30) (Table 7).

Histochemistry.

Specific NT immunoreactivity is localized in distinct populations of amacrine cells in several vertebrate retinas (Table 2). These immunoreactive cells, like other peptide-containing retinal cells, are distributed in both central and peripheral regions.

In the pigeon retina, NT immunoreactivity is localized to a distinct population of multistratified amacrine cells (27,30) (Fig. 29) which measure about 7.0 μm in diameter. The NT-containing amacrine cells are distributed in all retinal regions, and their relative density across the retina appears to match the density of cells in the INL and GCL. These cells give rise to a single process which descends to lamina 1 of the IPL before branching into several secondary processes which give rise to processes that descend to and ramify in lamina 3 and 4 of the IPL.

Preabsorption and double-label studies (30) suggest that although they are similar in appearance, NT-, SS-, and ENK-containing amacrine cells are likely to constitute separate amacrine cell (30) populations (Figs. 22 and 28–30).

Vasoactive Intestinal Polypeptide

Biochemistry.

Vasoactive intestinal polypeptide-like immunoreactivity is present in retinal extracts from the rat and pigeon (Table 7).

A recent abstract reports that low concentrations of synthetic vasoactive intestinal polypeptide will stimulate adenylate cyclase activity in the bovine and rabbit retina in a manner similar to that described in rat brain (173). The presence of a vasoactive intestinal polypeptide-sensitive adenylate cyclase system also has been observed in teleost retina (J. E. Dowling, *personal communication*). Both of these studies suggest a functional linkage between vasoactive intestinal polypeptide and adenylate cyclase systems in the retina. Whether or not these systems are also related to the dopamine-sensitive adenylate cyclase system is not known.

Histochemistry.

Immunohistochemical studies describe the occurrence of specific VIP immunoreactivity in amacrine cells of the retina (177; and *unpublished observations*) (Table 2). The VIP-containing amacrine cells, like other peptide-containing amacrine cells, are distributed in both central and peripheral retinal regions.

In the pigeon retina, VIP immunoreactivity is present within medium-sized somata that are located at the border of the INL and IPL and in processes that are present within laminae 1, 3, and 5

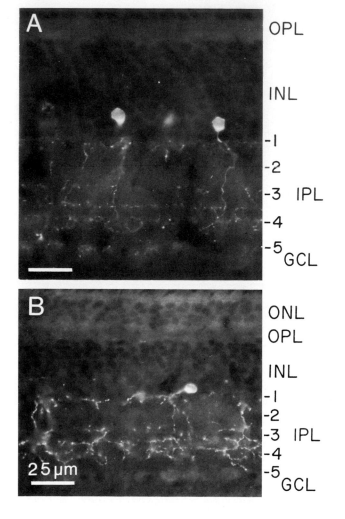

FIG. 28. Somatostatin immunoreactive staining in the pigeon retina. These cells give rise to multistratified processes which ramify in laminae 1, 3 and 4 of the IPL. **A:** Central retina. **B:** Peripheral retina. Somatostatin antisera used for this study was generously supplied by Drs. W. Vale and T. Yamada.

TABLE 7. *Immunoreactive neurotensin, vasoactive intestinal polypeptide, and cholecystokinin in the retina*

Species	Neuropeptide concentrations[a]		
	Neurotensin	Vasoactive intestinal polypeptide	Cholecystokinin
Pigeon *(Columba livia)*	15.4 ± fmoles/mg protein (30)	0.49 ± 0.004 pmoles/mg protein (*unpublished data*)	—
Rat	—	1.100 ± 0.46 pmoles/mg protein (*unpublished data*)	0.2 ng/retina (97)
Frog	—	—	1.7 ng/retina (97)
Chick (15 days old)	—	—	0.04 ng/retina (97)
Cow	—	—	3.4 ng/retina (97)
Monkey	—	—	0.6 ng/retina (97)

[a]Reference number in parentheses.

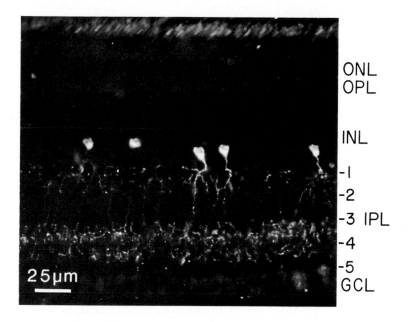

FIG. 29. Neurotensin immunoreactive staining in the pigeon retina. These cells give rise to multistratified processes which ramify in laminae 1, 3, and 4 of the IPL. Neurotensin antisera used in this study was generously supplied by Dr. M. Brown and Mr. J. Koeing.

of the IPL. The greatest density of VIP-containing processes is in lamina 5. The VIP-containing amacrine cells typically give rise to a single process which descends and ramifies in two bands at the border of laminae 2 and 3 and within lamina 5 of the IPL (Fig. 30). An occasional immunoreactive soma has been observed to give rise to processes that ramify in lamina 1 of the IPL. Whether or not these cells also give rise to processes that ramify in more proximal regions of the IPL remains to be investigated. The pigeon retina may thus contain uni-, bi-, and/or tristratified VIP immunoreactive amacrine cells.

In the rat retina, VIP immunoreactivity is observed within a population of bistratified amacrine cells that ramify in the most proximal and distal portions of the IPL (177). Amacrine cells containing VIP also are observed in rabbit and monkey retina. These cells are located in the proximal INL and give rise to multistratified processes which ramify throughout the IPL *(unpublished observations).*

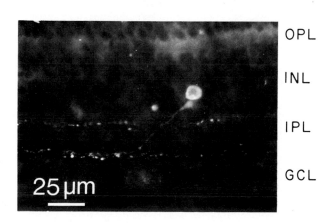

FIG. 30. Vasoactive intestinal polypeptide immunoreactive staining in the pigeon retina. The VIP-containing cells, of which there are at least two subtypes, give rise to processes that may ramify in laminae 1, 3, and/or 5 of the IPL. Vasoactive intestinal polypeptide antiserum used in this study was generously supplied by Dr. J. Walsh.

Glucagon

Histochemistry.

Specific glucagon-like immunoreactivity is localized to amacrine cells in several vertebrates. In the pigeon retina, medium-sized GLU immunoreactive somata are located at the border of the INL and IPL (Fig. 31). Glucagon immunoreactivity is observed in processes that ramify in lamina 1 of the IPL and in a narrow band at the border of laminae 2 and 3 of the IPL. On occasion, in peripheral retinal regions, GLU-containing processes are distributed in a narrow band at the border of laminae 4 and 5 of the IPL. These observations suggest the possible existence of uni-, bi-, and/or tristratified GLU-containing amacrine cells. In pigeon and turtle retinas, a dense accumulation of coarse GLU-containing processes is also observed at the ora serrata (Figs. 31B and 32). The functional role of this plexus of GLU-containing processes is not known.

Cholecystokinin

Biochemistry.

Cholecytokinin-like immunoreactivity is present in both mammalian and nonmammalian retinal extracts (97) (Table 7).

Histochemistry.

Cholecystokinin immunoreactive amacrine cells have been identified in both frog and mudpuppy retina. The CCK-containing amacrine cells, like other neuropeptide-containing amacrine cells, are distributed in both central and peripheral retinal regions. In frog retina, specific CCK immunoreactivity is present in amacrine cells which give rise to a single primary process which, in turn, branches to form a very dense plexus of fine processes within the distal two-thirds of the IPL (Fig. 33).

Thyrotropin-Releasing Hormone

Biochemistry.

Thyrotropin-releasing hormone-like immunoreactivity is present in both mammalian and nonmammalian retinas (100,108,138,196,273,341) (Table 8). The existence of low to moderate levels of TRH immunoreactivity in extracts of the rat retina as compared to hypothalamic extracts has been reported by two separate groups (196,273) but not by a third (100). The evidence that authentic thyrotropin-releasing hormone is present in rat retinal extracts includes the degradation of TRH immunoreactivity by the peptidase pyroglutamate aminopeptidase. Additionally, TRH immunoreactivity coelutes with synthetic thyrotropin-releasing hormone on gel filtration chromatography (196,273).

Thyrotropin-releasing hormone immunoreactivity fluctuates with lighting conditions; levels are highest during light periods and lowest during dark periods (273). Whether or not this light-versus-dark difference is related to circadian rhythms

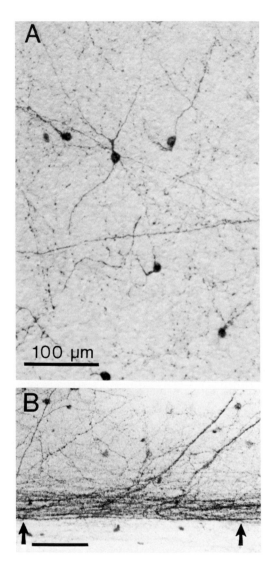

FIG. 31. Glucagon-containing amacrine cells in the pigeon retina from a flat-mount preparation. **A:** Central retina. **B:** Peripheral retina. Note the dense plexus of processes at the peripheral margin of the retina. *(arrows).* Glucagon antiserum for this study was generously supplied by Dr. N. Track.

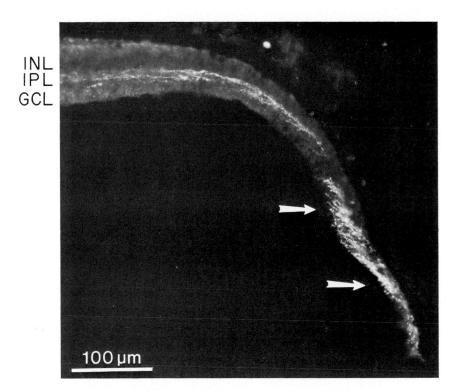

FIG. 32. Glucagon immunoreactive processes in the pigeon retina. A dense accumulation of processes is present at the margin of the retina in the ora serrata *(arrows).* Glucagon antiserum for this study was generously supplied by Dr. N. Track.

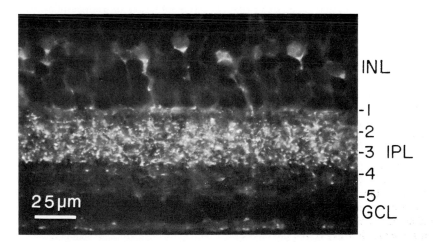

FIG. 33. Cholecystokinin-containing amacrine cells in the frog retina. These cells give rise to processes that ramify predominantly within laminae 2 and 3 of the IPL. Cholecystokinin antiserum used for this study was generously supplied by Dr. G. Rosenquist.

TABLE 8. *Immunoreactive thyrotropin-releasing hormone in the retina*

Species	Concentration	Reference
Eel *(Anguilla rostrata)*	64 ± 17.6 pg/mg wet wt	100
Frog *(Rana catesbeiana)*	95 ± 12.5 pg/mg wet wt	100
Frog *(Rana pipiens)*	3.3 ± 0.4 μg/g protein	138
Frog *(Rana esculenta)*	69 ± 19 pg/mg	108
Chick (2 days old)	<0.1 pg/mg wet wt	100
Rat (Osborne–Mendel), dark adapted	75 pg/mg protein	273
Rat (Osborne–Mendel), light adapted	300 pg/mg protein	273
Rat (Charles River)	75–200 pg/retina	196
Rat	800 pg/retina	341
Rat (Osborne–Mendel)	<0.1 pg/mg wet wt	100
Guinea pig	<0.3 pg/mg wet wt	100
Rabbit	<0.3 pg/mg wet wt	100
Cow	<0.1 pg/mg wet wt	100
Monkey *(Macaca mulatta)*	<0.1 pg/mg wet wt	100

must await a more rigorous analysis. A recent developmental study in the rat has shown that TRH immunoreactivity is not detectable before the eyes open, low at eye opening (day 8), and very high 30 days after eye opening. At somewhat later time periods, TRH immunoreactivity declines to more intermediate levels characteristic of the adult retina (196). Interestingly, the appearance of TRH immunoreactivity in the developing rat retina is prevented by maintaining the rat pups in the dark. These data support the notion that retinal levels of this TRH immunoreactive substance are dependent on light stimulation (196).

Specific TRH binding sites have been described in sheep retinal homogenates (44). This study demonstrated that retinal and pituitary TRH binding sites have similar binding characteristics and pharmacological properties, implying the existence of TRH receptors within the retina.

The TRH immunoreactivity in frog retina is dramatically reduced following intraocular injections of kainic acid (100), suggesting that this peptide may be associated with horizontal, bipolar, amacrine, and/or interplexiform cells. However, to date, no immunohistochemical localization of TRH in the retina has been reported.

In conclusion, a wide variety of neuropeptides have been described in the retina, and these substances are localized to distinct retinal cell populations. Additional biochemical studies are needed to clarify the role of neuropeptides in the retina. They should comprise biosynthetic studies, a determination of the exact identity of the immunoreactive substances, and release studies. In addition, a characterization and localization of neuropeptide binding sites would be important. Several additional histochemical studies are also needed and should include detailed quantitative analyses of neuropeptide cell populations as well as an ultrastructural analysis of neuropeptide-containing cells. The determination of the coexistence of neuropeptides with a "conventional" neurotransmitter substance in the same cell type also would be of great interest. Overall, biochemical and histochemical studies provide convincing evidence for the existence of neuropeptide-containing amacrine cell populations within the vertebrate retina.

SUMMARY

Although a variety of neurotransmitter candidates have been implicated in retinal function, few have been definitively assigned to any one retinal cell population or retinal microcircuit. To date, the best characterized cell type is the teleost GABAergic cone horizontal cell. In addition, there is excellent evidence for the existence of a dopaminergic interplexiform cell population in the teleost and cebus monkey retina. A number of other putative transmitter substances are present in amacrine cells, including acetylcholine, GABA, glycine, dopamine, and perhaps an indoleamine. A wide variety of neuropeptide-like substances, including cholecystokinin, enkephalin, glucagon, neurotensin, somatostatin, substance P, and vasoactive intestinal polypeptide also are localized to distinct populations of amacrine cells. These studies demonstrate the histochemical variety of amacrine cell types but also emphasize the failure to correlate known and suspected neurotransmitter substances to most other retinal cell types. These data suggest that many, if not most, retinal neurotransmitter substances are as yet unidentified. Indeed, this lack of correlation suggests that major efforts are now needed to identify additional neuroactive substances belonging to the retina.

ACKNOWLEDGMENTS

I would like to express my deepest appreciation to Susan Badyna for her assistance in preparing this chapter and Marianne Cilluffo for preparing much of the unpublished material presented in this chapter. I also thank J. P. Card, G. Engbretson, and S. Yazulla for their timely and helpful criticisms without which this chapter would not have been completed. Finally, I thank K. Keyser, N. Bogan, and D. Marshak for their reading and helpful comments. This work was supported by NEI Grants EY 02146 to H. J. Karten and EY 04067 to the author, and NIAMDD 17328 to J. Walsh.

REFERENCES

1. Adolph, A., Dowling, J. E., and Ehinger, B. (1980): Monoaminergic neurons of the mudpuppy retina. *Cell Tissue Res., 210:269–282.*
2. Atterwill, C. K., and Neal, M. J. (1978): Subcellular distribution of [3-H]-choline, choline acetyltransferase, acetylcholinesterase and butrylcholinesterase activities in rabbit retina. *Exp. Eye Res.,* 27:659–672.
3. Bader, C. R., Baughman, R. W., and Moore, J. L. (1978): Different time course of development for high-affinity choline uptake and choline acetyltransferase in the chick retina. *Proc. Natl. Acad. Sci. U.S.A.,* 75:2525–2529.
4. Baker, P. C. (1966): Monoamine oxidase in the eye, brain, and whole embryo of developing *Xenopus laevis. Dev. Biol.,* 14:267–277.
5. Baker, P. C., Hoff, K. M., and Clise, R. L. (1971): The effects of light and dark backgrounds upon indoleamine enzymes in developing *Xenopus laevis. Comp. Gen. Pharmacol.,* 2:397–401.
6. Baker, P. C., and Hoff, K. M. (1971): Melatonin localization in the eyes of larval *Xenopus. Comp. Biochem. Physiol.,* 39A:879–881.
7. Baker, P. C., Quay, W. B., and Axelrod, J. (1965): Development of hydroxyindole-*O*-methyltransferase activity in the eye and brain of the amphibian *Xenopus laevis. Life Sci.,* 4:1981–1987.
8. Baker, P. C., and Quay, W. B. (1969): 5-Hydroxytryptamine metabolism in early embryogenesis and the development of brain and retinal tissues. *Brain Res.,* 12:273–295.
9. Barber, R., and Saito, K. (1976): Light microscopic visualization of GAD and GABA-T in immunocytochemical preparations of rodent CNS. In: *GABA in Nervous System Function,* edited by E. Roberts, T. N. Chase, and T. B. Tower, pp. 113–132. Raven Press, New York.
10. Bauer, B. (1978): Photic release of radioactivity from rabbit retina preloaded with [3H] GABA. *Acta Ophthalmol. (Kbh.),* 56:270–283.
11. Bauer, B., and Ehinger, B. (1977): Light evoked release of radioactivity from rabbit retinas preloaded with [3-H]-GABA. *Experientia,* 33:470–471.
12. Bauer, B., and Ehinger, B. (1977): Stimulated release of [³H] β-alanine from rabbit retina. *Brain Res.,* 120:447–457.
13. Bauer, B., Ehinger, B., and Aberg, L. (1980): [3H]-Dopamine release from the rabbit retina. *Albrecht von Graefes Arch. Klin. Ophthalmol.,* 215:71–78.
14. Baughman, R. W., and Bader, C. R. (1977): Biochemical characterization and cellular localization of the cholinergic system in the chicken retina. *Brain Res.,* 138:469–486.
15. Berger, S. J., McDaniel, M. L., Carter, J. G., and Lowry, O. H. (1977): Distribution of four potential transmitter amino acids in monkey retina. *J. Neurochem.,* 28:159–163.
16. Binggeli, R. L., and Paule, W. J. (1969): The pigeon retina: Quantitative aspects of the optic nerve and ganglion cell layer. *J. Comp. Neurol.,* 137:1–18.
17. Binkley, S., Hryshchyshyn, M., and Reilly, K. (1979): *N*-Acetyltransferase activity responds to environmental lighting in the eye as well as in the pineal gland. *Nature,* 281:479–481.
18. Biziere, K., and Coyle, J. T. (1979): Localization of receptors for kainic acid on neurons in the inner nuclear layer of retina. *Neuropharmacology,* 18:409–413.
19. Boell, E. J., Greenfield, P., and Shen, S. C. (1955): Development of cholinesterase in the optic lobe of the frog *(Rana pipiens). J. Exp. Zool.,* 129:415–452.
20. Bonting, S. L. (1976): *Transmitters in the Visual Process.* Pergamon Press, Oxford, New York.
21. Borbe, H. O., Muller, W. E., and Wollert, U. (1980): The identification of benzodiazepine receptors with brain-like specificity in bovine retina. *Brain Res.,* 182:466–469.
22. Boycott, B. B., and Dowling, J. E. (1969): Organization of the primate retina: Light microscopy. *Phil. Trans. R. Soc. Lond. [Biol.],* 255:109–184.
23. Boycott, B. B., Dowling, J. E., Fisher, S. L., Kolb, H., and Laties, A. M. (1975): Interplexiform cells of the mammalian retina and their comparisons with catecholamine-containing retinal cells. *Proc. R. Soc. Lond. [Biol.],* 191:353–368.
24. Brandon, C., Lam, D. M. K., and Wu, J.-Y. (1979): The γ-aminobutyric acid system in rabbit retina: Localization by immunocytochemistry and autoradiography. *Proc. Natl. Acad. Sci. U.S.A.,* 76:3557–3561.
25. Brandon, C., Lam, D. M. K., Su, Y. Y. T., and Wu, J. -Y. (1980): Immunocytochemical localization of GABA neurons in the rabbit and frog retina. *Brain Res. Bull.,* 5:21–29.
26. Brecha, N., Hendrickson, A., Florén, I., and Karten, H. J. (1982): Localization of substance P-like immunoreactivity within the monkey retina. *Invest. Opthalmol. Vis. Sci.,* 23:147–153.
27. Brecha, N., and Karten, H. J. (1980): Localization of enkephalin, substance P, neurotensin and somatostatin immunoreactivity within amacrine cells of the retina. *Anat. Rec.,* 196:225.

28. Brecha, N., Karten, H. J., and Laverack, C. (1979): Enkephalin-containing amacrine cells in the avian retina: Immunohistochemical localization. *Proc. Natl. Acad. Sci. U.S.A.*, 76:3010–3014.

29. Brecha, N., Karten, H. J., and Davis, B. (1980): Localization of neuropeptides, including vasoactive intestinal polypeptide and glucagon within the adult and developing retina. *Soc. Neurosci. Abstr.*, 6:346.

29a. Brecha, N. C., Karten, H. J., and Famiglietti, E. V., Jr. (1983): Localization of substance P-like immunoreactivity within the rabbit retina (*in preparation*).

30. Brecha, N., Karten, H. J., and Schenker, C. (1981): The localization of neurotensin-like and somatostatin-like immunoreactivity within amacrine cells of the retina. *Neuroscience*, 6:1329–1340.

31. Brecha, N., Sharma, S. C., and Karten, H. J. (1981): Localization of substance P-like immunoreactivity in the adult and developing goldfish retina. *Neuroscience*, 6:2737–2746.

32. Brown, J. H., and Makman, M. H. (1972): Stimulation by dopamine of adenylate cyclase in retinal homogenates and of adenosine 3′,5′-cyclic monophosphate formation in intact retina. *Proc. Natl. Acad. Sci. U.S.A.*, 69:539–543.

33. Brown, J. H., and Makman, M. H. (1973): Influence of neuroleptic drugs and apomorphine on dopamine sensitive adenylate cyclase of retina. *J. Neurochem.*, 21:477–479.

34. Brunn, A., and Ehinger, B. (1972): Uptake of the putative neurotransmitter, glycine, into the rabbit retina. *Invest. Ophthalmol.*, 11:191–198.

35. Brunn, A., and Ehinger, B. (1974): Uptake of certain possible neurotransmitters into retinal neurons of some mammals. *Exp. Eye Res.*, 19:435–447.

36. Brunn, A., Ehinger, B., and Forsberg, A. (1974): *In vitro* uptake of β-alanine into rabbit retinal neurons. *Exp. Brain Res.*, 19:239–247.

37. Bubenik, G. A., Brown, G. M., and Grota, L. J. (1976): Differential localization of *N*-acetylated indolealdylamines in CNS and the harderian gland using immunohistology. *Brain Res.*, 118:417–427.

38. Bubenik, G. A., Brown, G. M., Uhlir, I., and Grota, L. J. (1974): Immunohistological localization of *N*-acetylindolealkylamines in pineal gland, retina and cerebellum. *Brain Res.*, 81:233–242.

39. Bubenik, G. A., Purtill, R. A., Brown, G. M., and Groto, L. J. (1978): Melatonin in the retina and the harderian gland. Ontogeny, diurnal variations and metatonin treatment. *Exp. Eye Res.*, 27:323–333.

40. Bucher, M. B., and Schorderet, M. (1974): Apomorphine-induced accumulation of cyclic AMP in isolated retina of the rabbit. *Biochem. Pharmacol.*, 23:3079–3082.

41. Bucher, M. B., and Schorderet, M. (1975): Dopamine- and apormorphine-sensitive adenylate cyclase in homogenates of rabbit retina. *Naunyn Schmiedebergs Arch. Pharmacol.*, 288:103–107.

42. Burnstock, G. (1976): Do some nerve cells release more than one transmitter? *Neuroscience*, 1:239–248.

43. Burnstock, G., Hokfelt, T., Gershon, M. D., Iversen, L. L., Kosterlitz, H. W., and Szurszewski, J. H. (1979): Non-adrenergic, non-cholinergic autonomic neurotransmission mechanisms. *Neurosci. Res. Prog. Bull.*, 17:379–519.

44. Burt, D. R. (1979): Thyrotropin releasing hormone: Apparent receptor binding in retina. *Exp. Eye Res.*, 29:353–365.

45. Cajal, S. R. (1893): La retine des vertebres. *La Cellule*, 9:17–257.

46. Cardinali, D. P., Larin, F., and Wurtman, R. J. (1972): Action spectra for effects of light on hydroxyindole-*O*-methyl transferase in rat pineal retina and harderian gland. *Endocrinology*, 91:877–886.

47. Cardinali, D. P., and Rosner, J. M. (1971): Metabolism of serotonin by the rat retina *in vitro*, J. *Neurochem.*, 18:1769–1770.

48. Cardinali, D. P., and Rosner, J. M. (1971): Retinal localization of the hydroxyindole-*O*-methyl transferase (HIOMT) in the rat. *Endocrinology*, 89:301–303.

49. Cardinali, D. P., and Rosner, J. M. (1972): Ocular distribution of hydroxyindole-*O*-methyltransferase (HIOMT) in the duck *(Anas platyrhinchas). Gen. Comp. Endocrinol.*, 18:407–409.

50. Cardinali, D. P., and Wurtman, R. J. (1972): Hydroxyindole-*O*-methyl transferase in rat pineal, retina and harderian gland. *Endocrinology*, 91:247–252.

51. Clement-Cormier, Y., and Redburn, D. A. (1977): Dopamine-sensitive adenylate cyclase in retina: Subcellular distribution. *Biochem. Pharmacol.*, 27:2281–2282.

52. Cohen, A. I. (1963): Vertebrate retinal cells and their organization. *Biol. Rev.*, 38:427–459.

53. Cohen, A. I., McDaniel, M., and Orr, H. (1973): Absolute levels of some free amino acids in normal and biologically fractionated retinas. *Invest. Ophthalmol.*, 12:686–693.

54. Coull, B. M., and Cutler, K. W. P. (1978): Light evoked release of endogenous glycine into the perfused vitreous of the intact rat eye. *Invest. Ophthalmol.*, 17:682–684.

55. Daniels, M. P., and Vogel, Z. (1980): Localization of α-bungarotoxin binding sites in synapses of the developing chick retina. *Brain Res.*, 201:45–56.

56. Davis, J. M., Himwich, W. A., and Agrawal, H. C. (1969): Some amino acids in the developing visual system. *Dev. Psychobiol.*, 2:34–39.

57. Dick, E., Miller, R., and Behbehani, M. M. (1980): Opiods and substance P influence ganglion cells in amphibian retina. *Invest. Opthalmol. Vis. Sci.*, 19 (Suppl.):132.

58. Dickson, D. H., Flumerfelt, B. A., Hollenbert, M. J., and Gwyn, D. G. (1971): Ultrastructural localization of cholinesterase activity in the outer plexiform layer of the newt retina. *Brain Res.*, 35:229–303.

59. Djamgoz, M. B. A., and Stell, W. K. (1980): Physiological evidence for opioid pathways in goldfish retina. *Soc. Neurosci. Abstr.*, 6:613.

60. Dowling, J. E. (1968): Synaptic organization of

the frog retina: An electron microscopic analysis comparing the retinas of frogs and primates. *Proc. R. Soc. Lond.* [*Biol.*], 170:205–228.

61. Dowling, J. E., and Boycott, B. B. (1966): Organization of the primate retina: Electron microscopy. *Proc. R. Soc. Lond.* [*Biol.*], 116:80–111.

62. Dowling, J. E., and Ehinger, B. (1975): Synaptic organization of the amine-containing interplexiform cells of the goldfish and cebus monkey retinas. *Science*, 188:270–273.

63. Dowling, J. E., and Ehinger, B. (1978): The interplexiform cell system. I. Synapses of the dopaminergic neurons of the goldfish retina. *Proc. R. Soc. Lond.* [*Biol.*], 201:7–26.

64. Dowling, J. E., and Ehinger, B. (1978): Synaptic organization of the dopaminergic neurons in the rabbit retina. *J. Comp. Neurol.*, 180:203–220.

65. Dowling, J. E., Ehinger, B., and Floren, I. (1980): Fluorescence and electron microscopial observations on the amine-accumulating neurons of the cebus monkey retina. *J. Comp. Neurol.*, 192:665–685.

66. Dowling, J. E., and Watling, K. J. (1981): Dopaminergic mechanisms in the teleost retina. II. Factors affecting the accumulation of cyclic AMP in pieces of intact carp retina. *J. Neurochem.*, 36:469–579.

67. Drujan, B. D., and Diaz Borges, J. M. (1968): Adrenaline depletion induced by light in the dark-adapted retina. *Experientia*, 24:676–677.

68. Drujan, B. D., Diaz Borges, J. M., and Alvarez, N. (1965): Relationship between the contents of adrenaline, noradrenaline and dopamine in the retina and its adaptational state. *Life Sci.*, 4:473–477.

69. Drujan, B. D., Diaz Borges, J. M., and Brzin, M. (1979): Histochemical and cytochemical localization of acetylcholinesterase in retina and optic tectum of teleost fish. *Can. J. Biochem.*, 57:43–48.

70. Drujan, B. D., Negishi, K., and Laufer, M. (1980): Studies on putative neurotransmitters in the distal retina. *Neurochemistry* 1:143–150.

71. Duner, H., von Euler, U. S., and Pernow, B. (1954): Catecholamines and substance P in the mammalian eye. *Acta Physiol. Scand.*, 31:113–118.

72. Ehinger, B. (1966): Adrenergic nerves to the eye and to related structures in man and in the cynomolgus monkey *(Macaca irus)*. *Invest. Ophthalmol.*, 5:42–52.

73. Ehinger, B. (1966): Adrenergic neurons in the retina. *Life Sci.*, 5:129–131.

74. Ehinger, B. (1966): Distribution of adrenergic nerves in the eye and some related structures in the cat. *Acta Physiol. Scand.*, 66:123–128.

75. Ehinger, B. (1966): Adrenergic retinal neurons. *Z. Zellforsch.*, 71:146–152.

76. Ehinger, B. (1967): Adrenergic nerves in the avian eye and ciliary ganglion. *Z. Zellforsch.*, 82:577–588.

77. Ehinger, B. (1970): Autoradiographic identification of rabbit retinal neurons that take up GABA. *Experientia*, 26:1063–1064.

78. Ehinger, B. (1972): Cellular localization of the uptake of some amino acids into the rabbit retina. *Brain Res.*, 46:297–311.

79. Ehinger, B. (1972): Uptake of tritiated glycine into neurons of the human retina. *Experientia*, 28:1042–1043.

80. Ehinger, B. (1973): Glial uptake of taurine in the rabbit retina. *Brain Res.*, 60:512–516.

81. Ehinger, B. (1973): Ocular adrenergic neurons of the flying fox *Pteropus giganteus* Brunn. (Megachiroptera). *Z. Zellforsch.*, 139:171–178.

82. Ehinger, B. (1976): Biogenic monoamines as transmitters in the retina. In: *Transmitters in the Visual Process*, edited by S. L. Bonting, pp. 145–163. Pergamon Press, Oxford.

83. Ehinger, B. (1977): Glial and neuronal uptake of GABA, glutamic acid, glutamine and glutathione in the rabbit retina. *Exp. Eye Res.*, 25:221–234.

84. Ehinger, B., and Falck, B. (1969): Morphological and pharmacohistochemical characteristics of adrenergic retinal neurons of some mammals. *Albrecht Von Graefes Arch. Klin. Ophthalmol.*, 178:295–305.

85. Ehinger, B., and Falck, B. (1969): Adrenergic retinal neurons of some New World monkeys. *Z. Zellforsch.*, 100:364–375.

86. Ehinger, B., and Falck, B. (1971): Autoradiography of some suspected neurotransmitter substances: GABA, glycine, glutamic acid, aspartic acid, histamine, dopamine and L-DOPA. *Brain Res.*, 33:157–172.

87. Ehinger, B., Falck, B., and Laties, A. M. (1969): Adrenergic neuron in teleost retina. *Z. Zellforsch.*, 97:285–297.

88. Ehinger, B., and Floren, I. (1976): Indoleamine-accumulating neurons in the retina of rabbit, cat and goldfish. *Cell Tissue Res.*, 175:37–48.

89. Ehinger, B., and Floren, I. (1978): Quantitation of the uptake of indoleamines and dopamine in the rabbit retina. *Exp. Eye Res.*, 26:1–11.

90. Ehinger, B., and Floren, I. (1978): Chemical removal of indoleamine accumulating terminals in rabbit and goldfish retina. *Exp. Eye Res.*, 26:321–328.

91. Ehinger, B., and Florén, I. (1979): Absence of indoleamine accumulating neurons in the retina of humans and cynomolgus monkeys. *Albrecht von Graefes Arch. Ophthalmol.*, 209:145–153.

92. Ehinger, B., and Florén, I. (1980): Retinal indoleamine accumulating neurons. *Neurochemistry*, 1:209–229.

93. Ehinger, B., and Holmgren, I. (1979): Electron microscopy of the indoleamine-accumulating neurons in the retina of the rabbit. *Cell Tissue Res.*, 197:175–194.

94. Ehinger, B., and Lindberg, B. (1974): Light-evoked release of glycine from the retina. *Nature*, 251:727–728.

95. Ehinger, B., and Lindberg-Bauer, B. (1976): Light evoked release of glycine from cat and rabbit retina. *Brain Res.*, 113:535–549.

96. Ehinger, B., and Nordenfelt, L. (1977): Destruction of retinal dopamine-containing neurons in rabbit and goldfish. *Exp. Eye Res.*, 24:179–187.

97. Eiden, L. E., Beinfeld, M. C., and Eskay, R. L. (1980): RIA and HPLC evidence for the presence

of methionine enkephalin and cholecystokinin in the neuron retina of several vertebrate species. *Soc. Neurosci. Abstr.*, 6:680.

98. Enna, S. J., and Snyder, S. H. (1976): Gamma-aminobutyric acid (GABA) receptor binding in mammalian retina. *Brain Res.*, 115:174–179.

99. Eranko, O., Niemi, M., and Merenmies, E. (1961): Histochemical observations on esterases and oxidative enzymes of the retina. In: *The Structure of the Eye*, edited by G. K. Smelser, pp. 159–171. Academic Press, New York.

99a. Erichsen, J. T., Karten, H. J., Eldred, W. D., and Brecha, N. C. (1982): Localization of substance P-like and enkephalin-like immunoreactivity within preganglionic terminals of the avian ciliary ganglion: Light and electron microscopy. *J. Neurosci.*, 2:994–1003.

100. Eskay, R. L., Long, R. T., and Iuvone, P. M. (1980): Evidence that TRH, somatostatin and substance P are present in neurosecretory elements of the vertebrate retina. *Brain Res.*, 196:554–559.

101. Florén, I. (1979): Indoleamine accumulating neurons in the retina of chicken and pigeon. *Acta Ophthamol. (Kbh.)*, 57:198–210.

102. Florén, I. (1979): Arguments against 5-hydroxytryptamine as neurotransmitter in the rabbit retina. *J. Neural Transm.*, 46:1–15.

103. Florén, I., and Hansson, H. C. (1980): Investigations into whether 5-hydroxytryptamine is a neurotransmitter in the retina of rabbit and chicken. *Invest. Ophthalmol. Vis. Sci.*, 19:117–125.

104. Francis, C. N. (1953): Cholinesterase in the retina. *J. Physiol. (Lond.)*, 120:435–439.

105. Galifret, Y. (1968): Les diverses aires fonctionnelles de la retine du pigeon. *Z. Zellforsch. Mikrosk. Anat.*, 86:535–545.

106. Gern, W. A., Owens, D. W., and Ralph, C. L. (1978): The synthesis of melatonin by the trout retina. *J. Exp. Zool.*, 206:263–270.

107. Gern, W. A., and Ralph, C. L. (1979): Melatonin synthesis of the retina. *Science*, 204:183–184.

108. Giraud, P., Gillioz, P., Conte-Devolx, B., and Oliver, C. (1979): Distribution de thyroliberine (TRH), γ-melanocyte-stimulating hormone (γ-MSH) et somatostatine dans les tissues de la grenouille verte *(Rana esculenta)*. *C. R. Acad. Sci. [D] (Paris)*, 288:127–129.

109. Glickman, R. D., Adolph, A. R., and Dowling, J. E. (1980): Does substance P have a physiological role in the carp retina? *Invest. Ophthalmol. Vis. Sci.*, 19 (Suppl.):281.

110. Goldstein, A., Tachibana, S., Lowney, L., Munkapillar, M., and Hood, L. (1979): Dynorphin-(1–13), an extraordinarily potent opioid peptide. *Proc. Natl. Acad. Sci. U.S.A.*, 76:6666–6670.

111. Goodchild, M., and Neal, M. J. (1973): The uptake of [³H]-aminobutyric acid by the retina. *Br. J. Pharmacol.*, 47:529–542.

112. Graham, L. T., Jr., (1972): Intraretinal distribution of GABA content and GAD activity. *Brain Res.*, 36:476–479.

113. Graham, L. T., Jr., (1974): Comparative aspects of neurotransmitters in the retina. In: *The Eye*, Vol. 6, edited by H. Davson and L. T. Graham, Jr., pp. 283–342. Academic Press, New York.

114. Graham, L. T., Jr., C. F. Baxter, and R. N. Lolley, (1970): *In vivo* influence of light and darkness on the GABA system in the retina of the frog *(Rana pipiens)*. *Brain Res.*, 20:379–388.

115. Haggendal, J., and Malmfors, T. (1963): Evidence of dopamine-containing neurons in the retina of rabbits. *Acta Physiol. Scand.*, 59:295–296.

116. Haggendal, J., and Malmfors, T. (1965): Identification and cellular localization of the catecholamines in the retina and the choroid of the rabbit, *Acta Physiol. Scand.*, 64:58–66.

117. Hamm, H. E., and Menaker, M. (1980): Retinal rhythms in chicks: Circadian variation in melatonin and serotonin *N*-acetyltransferase activity. *Proc. Natl. Acad. Sci. U.S.A.*, 77:4998–5002.

118. Hauschild, D. C., and Laties, A. M. (1973): An indoleamine-containing cell in chick retina. *Invest. Ophthalmol.*, 12:537–540.

119. Hayashi, T. (1980): Histochemical localization of dopamine and acetylcholinesterase activity in the carp retina. *Acta Histochem. Cytochem.*, 13:330–342.

120. Hayden, S. A., Mills, J. W., and Masland, R. M. (1980): Acetylcholine synthesis by displaced amacrine cells. *Science*, 210:435–437.

121. Hayes, K. C., Carney, R. E., and Schmidt, S. Y. (1975): Retinal degeneration associated with taurine deficiency in the cat. *Science*, 188:949–951.

122. Hedden, W. L., and Dowling, J. E. (1978): The interplexiform cell system II. Effects of dopamine on goldfish retinal neurons. *Proc. R. Soc. Lond. [Biol.]*, 201:27–55.

123. Hendrickson, A., Floren, I., and Brecha, N. C. (1981): Neurotransmitter localization in the *Macaca* monkey retina. *Anat. Rec.*, 199:109A.

124. Hendrickson, A., Florén, I., Patterson, B., Brecha, N. C., and Hunt, S. P. (1981): Neurotransmitter localization in the *Macaca* monkey retina. *Invest. Ophthalmol. Vis. Sci.*, 20 (Suppl.):237.

125. Hökfelt, T., Johansson, O., Ljungdahl, A., Lundberg, J. M., and Schultzberg, M. (1980): Peptidergic neurons. *Nature*, 284:515–521.

126. Hollyfield, J. G., Rayborn, M. E., Sarthy, P. V., and Lam, D. M. K. (1979): The emergence, localization and maturation of neurotransmitter systems during development of the retina in *Xenopus laevis* I. γ-Aminobutyric acid. *J. Comp. Neurol.*, 188:587–598.

127. Hollyfield, J. G., Rayborn, M. E., Sarthy, P. V., and Lam, D. M. K. (1980): Retinal development: Time and order of appearance of specific neuronal properties. *Neurochemistry*, 1:93–101.

128. Howells, R. D., Groth, J., Hiller, J. M., and Simon, E. J. (1980): Opiate binding sites in the retina: Properties and distribution. *J. Pharmacol. Exp. Ther.*, 215:60–64.

129. Howells, R. D., Hiller, J. M., and Simon, E. J. (1979): Benzodiazepine binding sites are present in retina. *Life Sci.*, 25:2131–2136.

130. Howells, R. D., and Simon, E. J. (1980): Benzodiazepine binding in chicken retina and its interaction with γ-aminobutyric acid. *Eur. J. Pharmacol.*, 67:133–137.

131. Hruska, R. E., White, R., Azari, J., and Yamamura, H. I. (1978): Muscarinic cholinergic recep-

tors in mammalian retina. *Brain Res.*, 148:493–498.

132. Humbert, J., Pradelles, P., Gros, C., and Dray, F. (1979): Enkephalin-like products in embryonic chicken retina. *Neurosci. Lett.*, 12:259–263.

133. Hyde, J. C., and Robinson, N. (1974): Localization of sites of GABA catebolism in the rat retina. *Nature*, 248:432–433.

134. Iuvone, P. M., Galli, C. L., Garrison-Gund, C. K., and Neff, N. H. (1978): Light stimulates tyrosine hydroxylase activity and dopamine synthesis in retinal amacrine cells. *Science*, 202:901–902.

135. Iuvone, P. M., Galli, C. L., and Neff, N. H. (1978): Retinal tyrosine hydroxylase: Comparison of short-term and long-term stimulation by light. *Mol. Pharmacol.*, 14:1212–1219.

136. Iversen, L. L., Nicoll, R. A., and Vale, W. W. (1978): Neurobiology of peptides. *Neurosci. Res. Prog. Bull.*, 16:211–370.

137. Jackson, I. M. D., Bolaffi, J. L., and Guillemin, R. (1980): Presence of immunoreactive β-endorphin and enkephalin-like material in the retina and other tissues of the frog, *Rana pipiens. Gen. Comp. Endocrinol.*, 42:505–508.

138. Jackson, I. M., and Reichlin, S. (1977): Thyrotropin-releasing hormone: Abundance in the skin of the frog, *Rana pipiens. Science*, 198:414–415.

139. Kanazawa, I., and Jessell, T. (1976): Post mortem changes and regional distribution of substance P in the rat and mouse nervous system. *Brain Res.*, 117:362–367.

140. Kaneko, A. (1979): Physiology of the retina. *Annu. Rev. Neurosci.*, 2:169–191.

141. Karten, H. J., and Brecha, N. (1980): Localisation of substance P immunoreactivity in amacrine cells of the retina. *Nature*, 283:87–88.

142. Kato, S., Nakamura, T., and Negishi, K. (1980): Postnatal development of dopaminergic cells in the rat retina. *J. Comp. Neurol.*, 191:227–236.

143. Kebabian, J. W., and Calne, D. B. (1979): Multiple receptors for dopamine. *Nature*, 277:93–96.

144. Kennedy, A. J., and Neal, M. J. (1978): The effect of light and potassium depolarization on the release of endogenous amino acids from the isolated rat retina. *Exp. Eye Res.*, 26:71–75.

145. Kennedy, A. J., Neal, M. J., and Lolley, R. N. (1977): The distribution of amino acids within the rat retina. *J. Neurochem.*, 29:157–159.

146. Kennedy, A. J., and Voaden, M. J. (1974): Free amino acids in the photoreceptor cell of the frog retina. *J. Neurochem.*, 23:1093–1095.

147. Kennedy, A. J., and Voaden, M. J. (1974): Distribution of free amino acids in the frog retina. *Biochem. Soc. Trans.*, 2:1256–1258.

148. Kennedy, A. J., and Voaden, M. J. (1974): Factors affecting the spontaneous release of (^{3}H)-aminobutyric acid from the frog retina *in vitro. J. Neurochem.*, 22:63–71.

149. Kennedy, A. J., and Voaden, M. J. (1976): Studies on the uptake and release of radioactive taurine by the frog retina. *J. Neurochem.*, 27:131–137.

150. Kennedy, A. J., Voaden, M. J., and Marshall, J. (1974): Glutamate metabolism in the frog retina. *Nature*, 252:50–52.

151. Kolb, H., and West, R. W. (1977): Synaptic con-

nections of the interplexiform cell in the retina of the cat. *J. Neurocytol.*, 6:155–170.

152. Kong, Y.-C., Fung, S.-C., and Lam, D. M. K. (1980): Postnatal development of glycinergic neurons in the rabbit retina. *J. Comp. Neurol.*, 193:1127–1135.

153. Kramer, S. G. (1971): Dopamine: A retinal neurotransmitter-retinal uptake, storage and light-stimulated release of [^{3}H]-dopamine *in vivo. Invest. Ophthalmol.*, 10:438-452.

154. Kramer, S. G. (1976): Dopamine in retinal neurotransmission: In: *Transmitters in the Visual Process*, edited by S. L. Bonting, pp. 165–198. Pergamon Press, Oxford.

155. Kramer, S. G., Potts, A. M., and Mangnall, Y. (1971): Dopamine: A retinal neurotransmitter II. Autoradiographic localization of ^{3}H-dopamine in the retina. *Invest. Ophthalmol.*, 10:617–624.

156. Krisch, B., and Leonhardt, H. (1979): Demonstration of a somatostatin-like activity in retinal cells of the rat. *Cell Tissue Res.*, 204:127–140.

157. Kuriyama, K., and Kimura, H. (1976): Distribution and possible functional roles of GABA in the retina, lower auditory pathway and hypothalamus. In: *GABA in Nervous System Function*, edited by E. Roberts, T. N. Chase, and D. B. Tower, pp. 203–216. Raven Press, New York.

158. Kuriyama, K., Sisken, B., Haber, B., and Roberts, E. (1968): The γ-aminobutyric acid system in rabbit retina. *Brain Res.*, 9:165–168.

159. Lake, N., Marshall, J., and Voaden, M. J. (1977): The entry of taurine into the neural retina and pigment epithelium of the frog. *Brain Res.*, 128:497–503.

160. Lake, N., Marshall, J., and Voaden, M. J. (1978): High affinity uptake sites for taurine in the retina. *Exp. Eye Res.*, 27:713–718.

161. Lake, N., and Patel, Y. C. (1980): Neurotoxic agents reduce retinal somatostatin. *Brain Res.*, 181:234–236.

162. Lam, D. M. K. (1972): The biosynthesis and content of gamma-aminobutyric acid in the goldfish retina. *J. Cell Biol.*, 54:225–231.

163. Lam, D. M. K. (1972): Biosynthesis of acetylcholine in turtle photoreceptors. *Proc. Natl. Acad. Sci. U.S.A.*, 69:1987–1991.

164. Lam, D. M. K. (1975): Biosynthesis of γ-aminobutyric acid by isolated axons cone horizontal cells in the goldfish retina. *Nature*, 254:345–347.

165. Lam, D. M. K. (1975): Synaptic chemistry of identified cells in the vertebrate retina. In: *Cold Spring Harbor Symp. Quant. Biol.*, 40:571–579.

166. Lam, D. M. K., Marc, R. E., Sarthy, P. V., Chin, C. A., Su, Y. Y. T., Brandon, C., and Wu, J.-Y. (1980): Retinal organization: Neurotransmitters as physiological probes. *Neurochemistry*, 1:183–190.

167. Lam, D. M. K., and Steinman, L. (1971): The uptake of γ-aminobutyric acid in the goldfish retina. *Proc. Natl. Acad. Sci. U.S.A.*, 68:2777–2781.

168. Lam, D. M. K., Su, Y. Y. T., Chin, C. A., Brandon, C., Wu, J.-Y., Marc, R. E., and Lasater, E. M. (1980): GABA-ergic horizontal cells in the teleost retina. *Brain Res. Bull.*, 5:137–140.

169. Lam, D. M. K., Su, Y. Y. T., Swain, L., Marc, R.

E., Brandon, C., and Wu, J.-Y. (1979): Immuno-cytochemical localization of L-glutamic acid de-carboxylase in the goldfish retina. *Nature,* 278:565–567.

170. Laties, A. M., and Jacobowitz, D. (1966): A com-parative study of the autonomic innervation of the eye in the monkey, cat and rabbit. *Anat. Rec.,* 156:383–396.

171. Lindberg-Bauer, B. (1975): Light evoked release of glycine from rabbit retina. *Acta Ophthalmol. (Kbh.),* 125:30–31.

172. Lolley, R. N., Schmidt, S. Y., and Farber, D. B. (1974): Alterations in cyclic AMP metabolism as-sociated with photoreceptor cell degeneration in the C3H mouse. *J. Neurochem.,* 22:701–707.

173. Longshore, M. A., and Makman, M. H. (1980): Presence of vasoactive intestinal peptide (VIP) sensitive adenylate cyclase in retina and compari-son with activity in brain. *Soc. Neurosci. Abstr.,* 6:622.

174. Lopez-Colome, A. M., Erlij, D., and Pasantes-Mo-rales, H. (1976): Different effects on light and po-tassium stimulated release of taurine from retina. *Brain Res.,* 113:527–534.

175. Lopez-Colome, A. M., and Pasantes-Morales, H. (1980): Taurine interactions with chick retinal membranes. *J. Neurochem.,* 34:1047–1052.

176. Lopez-Colome, A. M., Salceda, R., and Pasantes-Morales, H. (1978): Potassium-stimulated release of GABA, glycine and taurine from the chick ret-ina. *Neurochem. Res.,* 3:431–441.

177. Lorén, I., Tornqvist, K., and Alumets, J. (1980): VIP (vasoactive intestinal polypeptide)-immuno-reactive neurons in the retina of the rat. *Cell Tis-sue Res.,* 210:167–170.

178. Lowry, O. H., Roberts, N. R., and Lewis, C. (1956): The quantitative histochemistry of the ret-ina. *J. Biol. Chem.,* 220:879–892.

179. Lund Karlsen, R., and Fonnum, F. (1976): The toxic effect of sodium glutamate on rat retina: Changes in putative transmitters and their corre-sponding enzymes. *J. Neurochem.,* 27:1437–1441.

180. Macione, S. (1972): Localization of GABA sys-tem in rat retina. *J. Neurochem.,* 19:1397–1400.

181. Macaione, S., Ruggeri, P., Dulca, F., and Tucci, G. (1974): Free amino acids in developing rat ret-ina. *J. Neurochem.,* 22:887–891.

182. Macaione, S., Tucci, G., DeLuca, G., and Digior-gio, R. M. (1976): Subcellular distribution of taur-ine and cysteine sulphinate decarboxylase activity in ox retina. *J. Neurochem.,* 27:1411–1415.

183. Magistretti, P., and Schorderet, M. (1978): Dif-ferential effects of benzamides and thioanthenes on dopamine-elicited accumulation of cyclic AMP in isolated rabbit retina. *Naunyn Schmiedbergs Arch. Pharmacol.,* 303:189–191.

184. Magistretti, P. J., and Schorderet, M. (1979): Do-pamine receptors in bovine retina: Characteriza-tion of the ^{3}H-spiroperdol binding and its use for screening dopamine receptor affinity of drugs. *Life Sci.,* 25:1675–1686.

185. Makman, M. H., Brown, J. H., and Mishira, R. K. (1975): Cyclic AMP in retina and caudate nu-cleus: Influence of dopamine and other agents. *Adv. Cyclic Nucleotide Res.,* 5:661–679.

186. Makman, M. H., Drorkin, B., Horowitz, S. G., and Thal, L. J. (1980): Properties of dopamine ag-onist and antagonist binding sites in mammalian retina. *Brain Res.,* 194:403–418.

187. Malmfors, T. (1963): Evidence of adrenergic neu-rons with synaptic terminals in the retina of rats demonstrate with fluorescence and electron mi-croscopy. *Acta Physiol. Scand.,* 58:99–100.

188. Mandel, P., Pasantes-Morales, H., and Urban, P. F. (1976): Taurine: A putative transmitter in ret-ina. In: *Transmitters in the Visual Process,* edited by S. L. Bonting, pp. 89–105. Pergamon Press, Oxford.

189. Marc, R. E., Lam, D. M. K., and Stell, W. L. (1979): Glycinergic pathways in the goldfish ret-ina. *Invest. Ophthalmol. Vis. Sci. [Suppl.],* 18:34.

190. Marc, R. E., Stell, W. K., Bok, D., and Lam, D. M. K. (1978): GABA-ergic pathways in the gold-fish retina. *J. Comp. Neurol.,* 182:221–246.

191. Marshall, J., and Voaden, M. J. (1974): A study of [^{3}H]glycine accumulation by the isolated pi-geon retina utilizing scintillation radioautography. *Biochem. Soc. Trans.,* 2:268–270.

192. Marshall, J., and Voaden, M. J. (1974): An auto-radiographic study of the cells accumulating [^{3}H]-aminobutyric acid in the isolated retinae of pigeon and chicken. *Invest. Ophthalmol.,* 13:602–607.

193. Marshall, J., and Voaden, M. J. (1974): An inves-tigation of the cells incorporating [^{3}H]-GABA and [^{3}H]-glycine in the isolated retina of the rat. *Exp. Eye Res.,* 18:367–370.

194. Marshall, J., and Voaden, M. J. (1975): Autora-diographic identification of the cells accumulating ^{3}H-γ-aminobutyric acid in mammalian retinae: A species comparison. *Vision Res.,* 15:459–461.

195. Marshall, J., and Voaden, M. J. (1976): Further observations on the uptake of [^{3}H]-glycine by iso-lated retina of frog. *Exp. Eye Res.,* 22:189–191.

196. Martino, E., Seo, H., Lernmark, A., and Refetoff, S. (1980): Ontogenetic patterns of thyrotropin-re-leasing hormone-like material in rat hypothala-mus, pancreas, and retina: Selective effect of light deprivation. *Proc. Natl. Acad. Sci. U.S.A.,* 77:4345–4348.

197. Masland, R. H., and Livingstone, C. J. (1976): Ef-fect of stimulation with light on the synthesis and release of acetylcholine by an isolated mammalian retina. *J. Neurophysiol.,* 39:1210–1219.

198. Masland, R. H., and Mills, J. W. (1979): Auto-radiographic identification of acetylcholine in the rabbit retina. *J. Cell Biol.,* 83:159–178.

199. Masland, R. H., and Mills, J. W. (1980): Choline accumulation by photoreceptor cells of the rabbit retina. *Proc. Natl. Acad. Sci. U.S.A.,* 77:1671–1675.

200. Massey, S. C., and Neal, M. J. (1979): The light evoked release of acetylcholine from the rabbit ret-ina *in vivo* and its inhibition by γ-aminobutyric acid. *J. Neurochem.,* 32:1327–1329.

201. Mathur, R. L., Klethi, J., Ledig, M., and Mandel, P. (1976): Cysteine sulfinate carboxylase in the visual pathway of adult chicken. *Life Sci.,* 18:75–80.

202. Medzihradsky, F. (1976): Stereospecific binding of etorphine in isolated neural cells and in retina,

determined by a sensitive microassay. *Brain Res.,* 108:212–219.

203. Mindel, J. S., and Mittag, T. W. (1976): Choline acetyltransferase in ocular tissues of rabbits, cats, cattle and man. *Invest. Ophthalmol.,* 15:808–814.

204. Moore, C. L., and Gruberg, E. R. (1974): The distribution of succinic semialdehyde dehydrogenase in the brain and retina of the tiger salamander *(Ambystoma tigrinum). Brain Res.,* 67:467–478.

205. Moreno-Yanes, J. A., and Mahler, H. R. (1979): Subcellular distribution [³H]-quinuclidinyl benzylate binding activity in vertebrate retina and its relationship to other cholinergic markers. *J. Neurochem.,* 33:505–516.

206. Morjaria, B., and Voaden, M. J. (1979): The formation of glutamate, aspartate and GABA in the rat retina: Glucose and glutamate as precursors. *J. Neurochem.,* 33:541–551.

207. Muller, W. E. (1977): Cholinergic receptor binding in bovine retina. *Neurosci. Lett.,* 5:345–349.

208. Mustakallio, A. (1967): Monoamine oxidase activity in the various structures of the mammalian eye. *Acta Ophthalmol. [Suppl.] (Kbh.),* 93:1–62.

209. Nakamura, Y., McGuire, B. A., and Sterling, P. (1980): Interplexiform cell in cat retina: Identification by uptake of γ-[³H] aminobutyric acid and serial reconstruction. *Proc. Natl. Acad. Sci. U.S.A.,* 77:658–661.

210. Nagle, C. A., Cardinali, D. P., and Rosner, J. M. (1972): Light regulation of rat retinal hydroxyindole-*O*-methyl transferase (HIOMT) activity. *Endocrinology,* 91:423–426.

211. Nagle, C. A., Cardinali, D. P., and Rosner, J. M. (1973): Retinal and pineal hydroxyl-*O*-methyl transferase in the rat: Changes following cervical sympathectomy, pinealectomy or blinding. *Endocrinology,* 92:1560–1564.

212. Neal, M. J. (1976): Minireview: Amino acid transmitter substances in the vertebrate retina. *Gen. Pharmacol.,* 7:321–332.

213. Neal, M. J. (1976): Acetylcholine as a retinal transmitter substance. In: *Transmitters in the Visual Process,* edited by S. L. Bonting, pp. 127–143. Pergamon Press, Oxford.

214. Neal, M. J., Collins, G. G., and Massey, S. C. (1979): Inhibition of aspartate release from the retina of the anaesthetised rabbit by stimulation with light flashes. *Neurosci. Lett.,* 14:214–245.

215. Neal, M. J., and Gilroy, J. (1975): High affinity choline transport in the retina. *Brain Res.,* 93:548–551.

216. Neal, M. J., and Iversen, L. L. (1972): Autoradiographic localisation of ³H-GABA in rat retina. *Nature,* 235:217–218.

217. Neal, M. J., and Massey, S. C. (1980): The release of acetylcholine and amino acids from the rabbit retina *in vivo. Neurochemistry,* 1:191–208.

218. Neal, M. J., Peacock, D. G., and White, R. D. (1973): Kinetic analysis of amino acid uptake by the rat retina *in vitro. Br. J. Pharmacol.,* 47:656–657.

219. Neal, M. J., and Starr, M. S. (1973): Effect of inhibitors of gamma-aminobutyrate aminotransferase on accumulation of [³H]-gamma-aminobu-

tyric acid by retina. *Br. J. Pharmacol.,* 47:543–555.

220. Neal, M. J., and White, R. D. (1978): Discrimination between descriptive models of L-glutamate uptake by the retina using non-linear regression analysis. *J. Physiol. (Lond.),* 277:387–394.

221. Negishi, K., Hayashi, T., Nakamura, T., and Drujan, B. D. (1979): Histochemical studies on catecholaminergic cells in the carp retina. *Neurochem. Res.,* 4:473–482.

222. Nichols, C. W., Hewitt, J., and Laties, A. M. (1972): Localization of acetylcholinesterase in the teleost retina. *J. Histochem. Cytochem.,* 20:130–136.

223. Nichols, C. W., Jacobowitz, D., and Hottenstein, M. (1967): The influence of light and dark on the catecholamine content of the retina and choroid. *Invest. Ophthalmol.,* 6:642–646.

224. Nichols, C. W., and Koelle, G. B. (1967): Acetylcholinesterase: Method for demonstration in amacrine cells of rabbit retina. *Science,* 155:477–478.

225. Nichols, C. W., and Koelle, G. B. (1968): Comparison of the localization of acetylcholinesterase and non-specific cholinesterase activities in mammalian and avian retinas. *J. Comp. Neurol.,* 133:1–16.

226. Olney, J. W. (1969): Glutamate-induced retinal degeneration in neonatal mice. Electron microscopy of acutely evolving lesion. *J. Neuropathol. Exp. Neurol.,* 28:455–474.

227. Oraedu, A. C. I., Voaden, M. J., and Marshall, J. (1980): Photochemical damage in the albino rat retina: Morphological changes and endogenous amino acids. *J. Neurochem.,* 35:1361–1369.

228. Orr, H. T., Cohen, A. I., and Carter, J. A. (1976): The levels of free taurine, glutamate, glycine and γ-amino-butyric acid during the postnatal development of the normal and dystrophic retina of the mouse. *Exp. Eye Res.,* 23:377–384.

229. Orr, H. T., Cohen, A. I., and Lowry, O. H. (1976): The distribution of taurine in the vertebrate retina. *J. Neurochem.,* 26:609–611.

230. Orr, T. H., Lowry, A., Cohen, I., and Ferrendelli, J. A. (1976): Distribution of 3',5'-cyclic AMP and 3',5'-cyclic GMP in rabbit retina *in vivo:* Selective effects of light and dark adaption and ischemia. *Proc. Natl. Acad. Sci. U.S.A.,* 73:4442–4445.

231. Orrego, F. (1979): Criteria for the identification of central neurotransmitters, and their application to studies with some nerve tissue preparations *in vitro. Neuroscience,* 4:1037–1057.

232. Osborne, N. N. (1980): Benzodiazepine binding to bovine retina. *Neurosci. Lett.,* 16:167–170.

233. Osborne, N. N. (1980): *In vitro* experiments on the metabolism, uptake and release of 5-hydroxytryptamine in bovine retina. *Brain Res.,* 184:283–297.

234. Osborne, N. N., and Richardson, G. (1980): Specificity of serotonin uptake by bovine retina: Comparison with tryptamine. *Exp. Eye Res.,* 31:31–39.

235. Pang, S. F., Brown, G. M., Grota, L. J., Chambers, J. W., and Rodman, R. L. (1977): Determination of *N*-acetylserotonin and melatonin activi-

ties in the pineal gland, retina, harderian gland, brain and serum of rats and chickens. *Neuroendocrinology*, 23:1–13.

236. Pang, S. F., Yu, H. S., Suen, H. C., and Brown, G. M. (1980): Melatonin in the retina of rats: A diurnal rhythm. *J. Endocrinol.*, 87:89–93.

237. Pasantes-Morales, H., Bonaventure, N., Wioland, N., and Mandel, P. (1973): Effect of intravitreal injections of taurine and GABA on chicken electroretinogram. *Int. J. Neurosci.*, 5:235–241.

238. Pasantes-Morales, H., Klethi, J., Ledig, M., and Mandel, P. (1972): Free amino acids of chicken and rat retina. *Brain Res.*, 41:494–497.

239. Pasantes-Morales, H., Klethi, J., Ledig, M., and Mandel, P. (1973): Influence of light and dark on the free amino acid pattern of the developing chick retina. *Brain Res.*, 57:59–65.

240. Pasantes-Morales, H., Klethi, J., Urban, P. F., and Mandel, P. (1974): The effect of electrical stimulation, light and amino acids on the efflux of [^{35}S]taurine from the retina of domestic fowl. *Exp. Brain Res.*, 19:131–141.

241. Pasantes-Morales, H., Urban, P. F., Klethi, J., and Mandel, P. (1973C): Light stimulated release of [^{35}S]taurine from chicken retina. *Brain Res.*, 51:375–378.

242. Paul, S., Zatz, M., and Skolnick, P. (1980): Demonstration of "brain-specific" benzodiazepine receptors in rat retina. *Brain Res.*, 187:243–246.

243. Pellegrino de Iraldi, A., and Etehevevry, G. J. (1967): Granulated vesicles in retinal synapses and neurons. *Z. Zellforsch.*, 81:283–296.

244. Pevet, P., Balemans, M. G. M., Bary, F. A. M., and Noorde-Graat, E. M. (1978): The pineal gland of the male (*Talpa europaea*, L.). Activity of hydroxyindole-*O*-methyl transferase (HIOMT) in the formation of melatonin/5-methoxytryptophol in the eyes and the pineal gland. *Ann. Biol. Anim. Biochem. Biophys.*, 18:259–264.

245. Polyak, S. (1941): *The Retina*. University of Chicago Press, Chicago.

246. Pourcho, R. G. (1977): Distribution of [^{35}S]taurine in mouse retina after intravitreal and intravascular injection. *Exp. Eye Res.*, 25:119–127.

247. Pourcho, R. G. (1979): Localization of cholinergic synapses in mammalian retina with peroxidase-conjugated α-bungarotoxin. *Vision Res.*, 19:287–292.

248. Pourcho, R. G. (1980): Uptake of [^{3}H]glycine and [^{3}H]GABA by amacrine cells in the cat retina. *Brain Res.*, 198:333–346.

249. Quay, W. B. (1965): Retinal and pineal hydroxyindole-*O*-methyl transferase activity in vertebrates. *Life Sci.*, 4:983–991.

250. Quay, W. B., Smart, L. T., and Hafeez, M. A. (1969): Substrate specificity and tissue localization of acetylserotonin methyltransferase in eyes of trout (*Salmo gairdneri*). *Comp. Biochem. Physiol.*, 28:947–953.

251. Reale, E., Luciano, L., and Spitznas, M. (1971): The fine structural localization of acetylcholinesterase activity in the retina and optic nerve of rabbits. *J. Histochem. Cytochem.*, 19:85–96.

252. Redburn, D. A. (1977): (14C) GABA uptake and release from rabbit retina synaptosomes. *Exp. Eye Res.*, 25:265–275.

253. Redburn, D. A., Clement-Cormier, Y., and Lam, D. M. K. (1980): GABA and dopamine receptor binding in retinal synaptosomal fractions. *Neurochemistry*, 1:167–181.

254. Redburn, D. A., Clement-Cormier, Y., and Lam, D. M. K. (1980): Dopamine receptors in the goldfish retina: ^{3}H-Spiroperidol and ^{3}H-domperidone binding; and dopamine-stimulated adenylate cyclase activity. *Life Sci.*, 27:23–31.

255. Redburn, D. A., and Kyles, C. B. (1980): Localization and characterization of dopamine receptors within two synaptosome fractions of rabbit and bovine retina. *Exp. Eye Res.*, 30:699–708.

256. Redburn, D. A., Kyles, C. B., and Ferkany, J. (1979): Subcellular distribution of GABA receptors in bovine retina. *Exp. Eye Res.*, 28:525–532.

257. Redburn, D. A., and Mitchell, C. K. (1980): GABA receptor binding in bovine retina. *Brain Res. Bull.*, 5:189–193.

258. Redburn, D. A., and Mitchell, C. K. (1981): GABA receptor binding in bovine retina: Effects of triton X-100 and perchloric acid. *Life Sci.*, 28:541–549.

259. Regan, J. W., Roeske, W. R., and Yamamura, H. I. (1980): ^{3}H-Flunitrazepam binding to bovine retina and the effect of GABA thereon. *Neuropharmacology*, 19:413–415.

260. Reubi, J. C., and Jessell, T. M. (1978): Distribution of substance P in the pigeon brain. *J. Neurochem.*, 31:359–361.

261. Rodieck, R. W. (1973): *The Vertebrate Retina*, W. H. Freeman, San Francisco.

262. Rorstad, O. P., Brownstein, M. J., and Martin, J. B. (1979): Immunoreactive and biologically active somatostatin-like material in rat retina. *Proc. Natl. Acad. Sci. U.S.A.*, 76:3019–3023.

263. Rorstad, O. P., Hoyte, K. M., and Martin, J. B. (1978): Demonstration of immunoreactive and bioassayable somatostatin-like activity in retinal-uveal tissue of the rat and human retina. *Clin. Res.*, 26:846A.

264. Rorstad, O. P., Senterman, M. K., Hoyte, K. M., and Martin, J. B. (1980): Immunoreactive and biologically active somatostatin-like material in the human retina. *Brain Res.*, 199:488–492.

265. Ross, C. D., Cohen, A. I., and McDougal, D. B. (1975): Choline acetyltransferase and acetylcholinesterase in normal and biologically fractionated mouse retinas. *Invest. Ophthalmol.*, 14:756–761.

266. Ross, C. D., and McDougal, D. B. (1976): The distribution of choline acetyltransferase activity in vertebrate retina. *J. Neurochem.*, 26:521–526.

267. Salceda, R. (1980): High-affinity taurine uptake in developing retina. *Neurochem. Res.*, 5:561–572.

268. Salceda, R., Lopez-Colome, A. M., and Pasantes-Morales, H. (1977): Light-stimulated release of (^{35}S)taurine from frog retinal rod outer segments. *Brain Res.*, 135:186–191.

269. Sar, M., Stumpf, W. E., Miller, R. J., Chang, K.-J., and Cuatrecasas, P. (1978): Immunohisto-

chemical localization of enkephalin in rat brain and spinal cord. *J. Comp. Neurol.*, 182:17–38.

270. Sarthy, P. V., and Lam, D. M. K. (1979): Endogenous levels of neurotransmitter candidates in photoreceptor cells of the turtle retina. *J. Neurochem.*, 32:455–461.

271. Sarthy, P. V., and Lam, D. M. K. (1979): Isolated cells from a mammalian retina. *Brain Res.*, 176:208–212.

272. Sarthy, P. V., and Lam, D. M. K. (1979): The uptake and release of [^{3}H]-dopamine in the goldfish retina. *J. Neurochem.*, 32:1269–1277.

273. Schaeffer, J. M., Brownstein, M. J., and Axelrod, J. (1977): Thyrotropin-releasing hormone-like material in the rat retina: Changes due to environmental lighting. *Proc. Natl. Acad. Sci. U.S.A.*, 74:3579–3581.

274. Schmidt, S. Y. (1978): Taurine fluxes in isolated cat and rat retinas: Effects of illumination. *Exp. Eye Res.*, 26:529–535.

275. Schmidt, S. Y. (1980): High-affinity uptake of [^{3}H]taurine in isolated cat retinas: Effects of NA$^+$ and K$^+$. *Exp. Eye Res.*, 31:373–379.

276. Schmidt, S. Y., and Berson, E. L. (1978): Taurine uptake in isolated retinas of normal rats and rats with hereditary retinal degradation. *Exp. Eye Res.*, 27:191–198.

277. Schmidt, S. Y., Berson, E. L., and Hayes, K. C. (1976): Retinal degeneration in cats fed casein: I. Taurine deficiency. *Invest. Ophthalmol.*, 15:47–52.

278. Schorderet, M. (1977): Pharmacological characterization of the dopamine mediated accumulation of cyclic AMP in intact retina of the rabbit. *Life Sci.*, 20:1741–1748.

279. Schorderet, M., and Magistretti, P. J. (1980). The isolated retina of mammals: A useful preparation for enzymatic (adenylyl cyclase) and/or binding studies of dopamine receptors. *Neurochemistry*, 1:337–353.

280. Schwarcz, R., and Coyle, J. T. (1976): Adenylate cyclase activity in chick retina. *Gen. Pharmacol.*, 7:349–354.

281. Schwarcz, R., and Coyle, J. T. (1977): Neurotoxic effects after kainic acid intraocular injection. *Invest. Ophthalmol.*, 16:141–148.

282. Schwarcz, R., Scholz, D., and Coyle, J. T. (1978): Structure-activity relations for the neurotoxicity of kainic acid derivatives and glutamate analogues. *Neuropharmacology*, 17:145–151.

283. Schwartz, I. R., and Bok, D. (1979): Electron microscopic localization of [^{125}I] α-bungarotoxin binding sites in the outer plexiform layer of the goldfish retina. *J. Neurocytol.*, 8:53–66.

284. Shapiro, B., Kronheim, S., and Pimstone, B. (1979): The presence of immunoreactive somatostatin in rat retina. *Horm. Metab. Res.*, 11:79–80.

285. Shen, S. L., Greenfield, P., and Boell, E. J. (1956): Localization of acetylcholinesterase in chick retina during histogenesis. *J. Comp. Neurol.*, 106:433–461.

286. Skolnick, P., Paul, S., Zatz, M., and Eskay, R. (1980): Brain-specific benzodiazepine receptors are localized in the inner plexiform layer of rat retina. *Eur. J. Pharmacol.*, 66:133–136.

287. Smith, M. D. (1973): 5-Hydroxytryptamine decarboxylase (5-HTPD) and monoamine oxidase (MAO) in the maturing mouse eye. *Comp. Gen. Pharmacol.*, 4:175–178.

288. Smith, M. D., and Baker, P. C. (1974): The maturation of indoleamine metabolism in the lateral eye of the mouse. *Comp. Biochem. Physiol.*, 49A:281–286.

289. Smith, M. D., and Baker, P. C. (1974): The maturation of melatonin synthesis in the lateral eyes of the mouse. *Comp. Gen. Pharmacol.*, 5:275–277.

290. Spira, A. W. (1976): The localization of cholinesterase in the retina of the fetal and newborn guinea pig. *J. Comp. Neurol.*, 169:393–408.

291. Starr, M. S. (1973): Effect of dark adaptation on the GABA system in retina. *Brain Res.*, 59:331–338.

292. Starr, M. S. (1973): Effects of changes in the ionic composition of the incubation medium on the accumulation and metabolism of [^{3}H]γ-aminobutyric acid and [^{14}C]taurine in isolated rat retina. *Biochem. Pharmacol.*, 22:1693:1700.

293. Starr, M. S. (1975): A comparative study of the utilization of glucose, acetate, glutamine and GABA as precursors of amino acids by retinae of the rat, frog, rabbit and pigeon. *Biochem. Pharmacol.*, 24:1193–1197.

294. Starr, M. S. (1975): The effect of light stimulation on the synthesis and release of GABA in rat and frog retinae. *Brain Res.*, 100:343–353.

295. Starr, M. S. (1978): Uptake of taurine by retina in different species. *Brain Res.*, 151:604–608.

296. Starr, M. S., and Voaden, M. J. (1972): The uptake of ^{14}C-aminobutyric acid by the isolated retina of the rat. *Vision Res.*, 12:549–559.

297. Starr, M. S., and Voaden, M. J. (1972): The uptake, metabolism and release of ^{14}C-taurine by rat retina *in vitro. Vision Res.*, 12:1261–1269.

298. Stell, W. K. (1967): The structure and relationships of horizontal cells and photoreceptor–bipolar synaptic complexes in goldfish retina. *Am. J. Anat.*, 121:401–424.

299. Stell, W. K. (1972): The morphological organization of the veretebrate retina. In: *Handbook of Sensory Physiology,* edited by M. G. F. Fuortes, pp. 111–213. Springer-Verlag, Berlin.

300. Sugiyama, H., Daniels, M. P., and Nirenberg, M. (1977): Muscarinic acetylcholine receptors of the developing retina. *Proc. Natl. Acad. Sci. U.S.A.*, 74:5524–5528.

301. Suzuki, O., Noguchi, E., Miyake, S., and Yagi, K. (1977): Occurrence of 5-hydroxytryptamine in chick retina. *Experientia*, 33:927–928.

302. Suzuki, O., Noguchi, E., and Yagi, K. (1977): Monoamine oxidase in developing chick retina. *Brain Res.* 135:305–313.

303. Suzuki, O., Noguchi, E., and Yagi, K. (1978): Uptake of 5-hydroxytryptamine by chick retina. *J. Neurochem.*, 30:295–296.

304. Tallman, J. F., Thomas, J. W., and Gallager, P. W. (1978): GABAergic modulation of benzodiazepine site sensitivity. *Nature*, 274:383–385.

305. Thomas, T. N., Buckholtz, N. S., and Zemp, J. W. (1979): 6-Methoxy-1,2,3,4-tetrahydro-β-carboline effects on retinal serotonin. *Life Sci.,* 25:1435–1442.

306. Thomas, T. N., Clement-Cormier, Y. C., and Redburn, D. A. (1978): Dopamine uptake and dopamine-sensitive adenylate cyclase activity of retinal synaptosomal fractions. *Brain Res.,* 155:391–396.

307. Thomas, T. N., and Redburn, D. A. (1978): Uptake of [14C]aspartic acid and [14C]glutamic acid by retinal synaptosomal fractions. *J. Neurochem.,* 31:63–68.

308. Thomas, T. N., and Redburn, D. A. (1979): 5-Hydroxytryptamine. A neurotransmitter of bovine retina. *Exp. Eye Res.,* 28:55–61.

309. Thomas, T. N., and Redburn, D. A. (1980): Serotonin uptake and release by subcellular fractions of bovine retina. *Vision Res.,* 20:1–8.

310. Tork, I., and Stone, J. (1979): Morphology of catecholamine-containing amacrine cells in the cat's retina, as seen in retinal whole mounts. *Brain Res.,* 169:261–273.

311. Tunnicliff, G., Firneisz, G., Ngo, T. T., and Martin, R. O. (1975): Developmental changes in the kinetics of γ-aminobutyric acid transport by chick retina. *J. Neurochem.,* 25:649–652.

312. Vaughn, J. E., Famiglietti, E. V., Jr., Barber, R. P., Saito, K., Roberts, E., and Ribak, C. E. (1981): GABAergic amacrine cells in rat retina: Immunocytochemical identification and synaptic connectivity. *J. Comp. Neurol.,* 197:113–127.

313. Voaden, M. J. (1974): Light and the spontaneous efflux of radioactive glycine from the frog retina. *Exp. Eye Res.,* 18:467–475.

314. Voaden, M. J. (1976): γ-Aminobutyric acid and glycine as retinal neurotransmitters. In: *Transmitters in the Visual Process,* edited by S. E. Bonting, pp. 107–125. Pergamon Press, Oxford.

315. Voaden, M. J. (1979): The chemical specificity of neurons in the retina. *Prog. Brain Res.,* 51:389–402.

316. Voaden, M. J., Lake, N., Marshall, J., and Morjaria, B. (1977): Studies on the distribution of taurine and other neuroactive amino acids in the retina. *Exp. Eye Res.,* 25:249–257.

317. Voaden, M. J., Marshall, J., and Murani, N. (1974): The uptake of 3H-γ-aminobutyric acid and 3H-glycine by the isolated retina of the frog. *Brain Res.,* 67:115–132.

318. Voaden, M. J., Morjaria, B., and Oraedu, A. C. I. (1980): The localization and metabolism of glutamate, aspartate and GABA in the rat retina. *Neurochemistry,* 1:151–165.

319. Voaden, M. J., and Starr, M. S. (1972): The efflux of radioactive GABA from rat retina *in vitro. Vision Res.,* 12:559–566.

320. Vogel, Z., Maloney, G. J., Ling, A., and Daniels, M. P. (1977): Identification of synaptic acetylcholine receptor sites in retina with peroxidase-labeled α-bungarotoxin. *Proc. Natl. Acad. Sci. U.S.A.,* 74:3268–3272.

321. Vogel, Z., and Nirenberg, M. (1976): Localization of acetylcholine receptors during synaptogenesis in retina. *Proc. Natl. Acad. Sci. U.S.A.,* 73:1806–1810.

322. Wainwright, S. D. (1979): Development of hydroxyindole-*O*-methyltransferase activity in the retina of the chick embryo and young chick. *J. Neurochem.,* 32:1099–1101.

323. Wang, G.-K., and Schmidt, J. (1976): Receptors for α-bungarotoxin in the developing visual system of the chick. *Brain Res.,* 114:524–529.

324. Wassenaar, J. S., and Korf, J. (1976): Characterization of catecholamine receptors in rat retina. In: *Transmitters in the Visual Process,* edited by S. L. Bonting, pp. 199–218. Pergamon Press, Oxford.

325. Watling, K. J., Dowling, J. E., and Iversen, L. L. (1979): Dopamine receptors in the retina may all be linked to adenylate cyclase. *Nature,* 281:578–580.

326. Watling, K. J., Dowling, J. E., and Iversen, L. L. (1980): Dopaminergic mechanisms in the carp retina: Effects of dopamine, K^+ and light on cyclic AMP synthesis. *Neurochemistry,* 1:519–537.

327. Watling, K. J., and Dowling, J. E. (1981): Dopaminergic mechanisms in the teleost retina I. Dopamine-sensitive adenylate cyclase in homogenates of carp retina; Effects of agonists, antagonists and ergots. *J. Neurochem.,* 36:559–568.

328. Werman, R. (1966): Criteria for identification of a central nervous system transmitter. *Comp. Biochem. Physiol.,* 18:745–766.

329. White, R. D., and Neal, M. J. (1976): The uptake of L-glutamate by the retina. *Brain Res.,* 111:79–93.

330. Winder, A. F., and Patsalos, P. N. (1974): Substance P and retinal neurotransmission. *Biochem. Soc. Trans.,* 4:1260–1261.

331. Wood, J. G., McLaughlin, B. J., and Vaughn, J. E. (1976): Immunocytochemical localization of GAD in electron microscopic preparations of rodent CNS. In: *GABA in Nervous System Function,* edited by E. Roberts, T. N. Chase, and D. B. Tower, pp. 133–148. Raven Press, New York.

332. Yamada, T., Marshak, D., Basinger, S., Walsh, J., Morley, J., and Stell, W. (1980): Somatostatin-like immunoreactivity in the retina. *Proc. Natl. Acad. Sci. U.S.A.,* 77:1691–1695.

333. Yates, R. A., and Keen, P. (1976): The distribution of free amino acids in subdivisions of rat and frog retina obtained by a new technique. *Brain Res.,* 107:117–126.

334. Yazulla, S. (1979): Synaptic layers of the retina: a comparative analysis with [125I]-α-bungarotoxin. In: *Neural Mechanisms of Behavior in the Pigeon,* edited by A. M. Granda and J. H. Maxwell, pp. 353–369. Plenum Press, New York.

335. Yazulla, S., and Brecha, N. (1980): Binding and uptake of the GABA analogue, 3H-muscimol, in the retinas of goldfish and chicken. *Invest. Ophthalmol. Vis. Sci.,* 19:1415–1426.

335a. Yazulla, S. (1981): GABAergic synapses in the goldfish retina: An autoradiographic study of 3H-muscimol and 3H-GABA binding. *J. Comp. Neurol.,* 200:83–93.

336. Yazulla, S., and Brecha, N. (1981): Localized binding of [³H]muscimol to synapses in chicken retina. *Proc. Natl. Acad. Sci. U.S.A.,* 78:643–647.

337. Yazulla, S., and Kleinschmidt, J. (1980): The effects of intraocular injection of kainic acid on the synaptic organization of the goldfish retina. *Brain Res.,* 182:287–301.

338. Yazulla, S., and Schmidt, J. (1976): Radioautographic localization of ¹²⁵H-α-bungarotoxin binding sites in the retinas of goldfish and turtle. *Vision Res.,* 16:878–880.

339. Yazulla, S., and Schmidt, J. (1977): Two types of receptors for α-bungarotoxin in the synaptic layers of the pigeon retina. *Brain Res.,* 138:45–57.

340. Young, W. S., and Kuhar, M. J. (1979): Autoradiographic localization of benzodiazepine receptors in the brains of humans and animals. *Nature,* 280:393–395.

341. Youngblood, W. W., Humm, J., and Kizer, J. S. (1979): TRH-like immunoreactivity in rat pancreas and eye, bovine and sheep pineals, and human placenta: Non-identity with synthetic Pyrogly-His-Pro-NH₂ (TRH). *Brain Res.,* 163:101–110.

342. Zucker, C., and Yazulla, S. (1981): Localization of synaptic and non-synaptic nicotinic-acetylcholine receptors in the goldfish retina. *J. Comp. Neurol.,* 204:188–195.

Chemical Neuroanatomy, edited by P. C. Emson,
Raven Press, New York © 1983.

The Raphe Nuclei of the Rat Brainstem: A Cytoarchitectonic and Immunohistochemical Study

*H. W. M. Steinbusch and R. Nieuwenhuys

*Department of Anatomy and Embryology, University of Nijmegen,
6500 HB Nijmegen, The Netherlands*

Since the monoamine serotonin (5-hydroxytryptamine, 5-HT) was found biochemically in the brain by Twarog and Page (310) and by Bogdansky et al. (39), and its intraneuronal localization was first demonstrated histochemically by Falck (84), Falck et al. (85), and Falck and Owman (86,87), numerous studies on the organization of the central serotoninergic neuron populations have been performed. With the aid of the formaldehyde-induced fluorescence (FIF) technique and/or immunocytochemistry, serotonin-containing neurons have been demonstrated in a variety of invertebrate species [e.g., the cockroach, *Periplaneta americana* (223); the flatworm, planaria *Dugesia tigrina, Phagocata oregonensis,* and *Procotyla fluviatilis* (333)] and vertebrate species [e.g., the lamprey, *Lampetra fluviatilis* (20,285,290); the lizard, *Lacerta siccula* and *Lacerta muralis* (188); the rat (100,284); cat (237,337); man (215)].

Unfortunately, the FIF method has a low sensitivity toward serotonin. Moreover, β-carboline, the yellow fluorescent product formed, is highly sensitive to irradiation, resulting in a rapid fading of the fluorescence (263). Another complication is the poor quality of the sections as a result of the freeze-drying of the tissue.

The basic mapping of the central monoaminergic system of the rat has been carried out with the FIF technique by Dahlström and Fuxe (69). During recent years, several modifications of the FIF technique have been introduced, such as the use of glyoxylic acid (29,33,97,171,178,186, 214,309,329), the employment of hypertonic formaldehyde perfusion (14), the application of magnesium ions (179,180), the combination of formaldehyde and glutaraldehyde (98,99), and recently the aluminum–formaldehyde (ALFA) method (7, 181). Although these methodological modifications of the FIF technique markedly increase the sensitivity for catecholamines, they do not seem to represent any clear advantage with regard to the visualization of serotonin. However, during the last few years, several other methods have been found to be highly useful for neuroanatomical studies on central serotoninergic neurons. These techniques include (a) autoradiographic demonstration of [^{3}H]serotonin uptake after injection into the brain ventricles (54,56,59–61,73,148,162,164,268), (b) immunocytochemistry using antibodies to the enzymes tryptophan hydroxylase (TrH) and DOPA decarboxylase (DDC) as markers for serotonin (124,140,235) (see Fig. 1), (c) the selective destruction of indolamine-containing neurons by pharmacological manipulations, e.g., with 5,6-dihydroxytryptamine (144,206), 5,7-dihydroxytryptamine (21,71,142,199,252), or *p*-chloroamphetamine (3,190,292), or the use of selective serotonin uptake inhibitors (166), or (d) biochemical determination of serotonin and/or the rate-limiting enzyme of the synthesis for serotonin (tryptophan hydroxylase) in small amounts of tissue (77,150,187,195,217,251,269,295,303,308,335).

In this chapter, the present knowledge of the organization of serotoninergic neurons in the brain of the rat is summarized with emphasis on our own investigations. These investigations are based on an immunocytochemical technique that helps to directly localize serotonin.

The localization of the serotonin immunoreactive cell bodies in the rhombencephalon and mesencephalon of the rat has already been the subject of two previous papers. The first of these (286) was

---

Present address: Department of Pharmacology, Free
University, 1081 BT Amsterdam, The Netherlands.

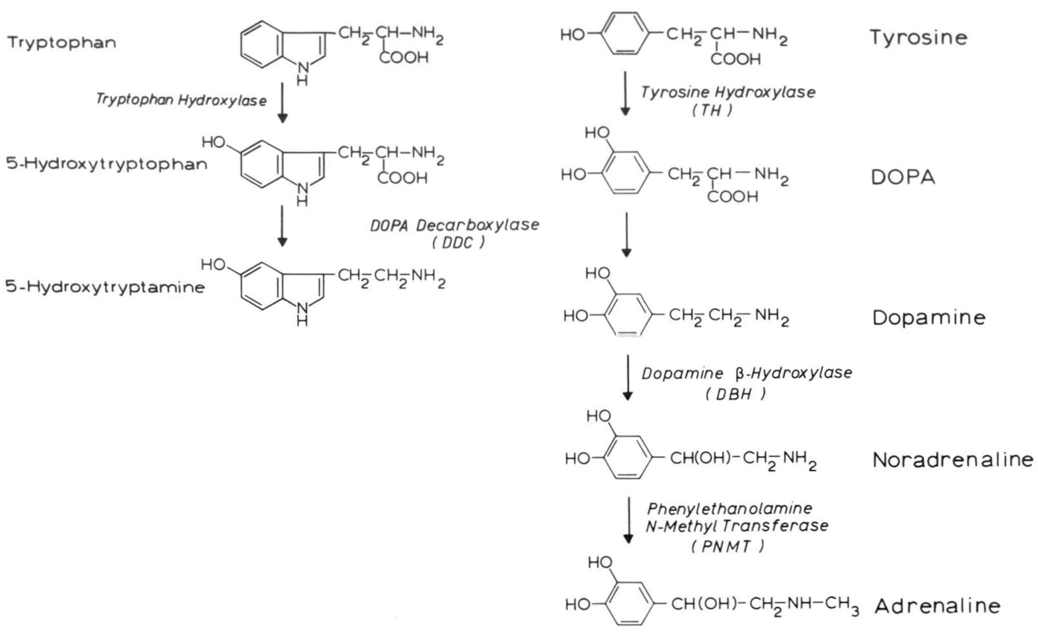

FIG. 1. Biosynthetic pathways of serotonin (**left**) and dopamine, norepinephrine, and epinephrine (**right**). Note that the enzyme DOPA decarboxylase (DDC, aromatic L-amino acid decarboxylase) is involved in both pathways.

mainly devoted to the serotoninergic innervation of the hypothalamo–hypophyseal system. In the second (284), a comprehensive mapping of serotoninergic cell bodies and terminal fibers throughout the central nervous system (CNS) of the rat was presented. These two studies were based upon 10-μm-thick cryostat sections, which were stained using the immunofluorescence technique.

In the present work, the following two experimental modifications have been applied. In preceding experiments, we pretreated the animals only with intraventricular injections of colchicine. However, it appeared to be favorable to visualize serotonin immunoreactive neurons in vibratome sections obtained from animals that were pharmacologically treated with either nialamide or L-tryptophan. In the mapping paper, we used schematic drawings in which we indicated with symbols the density of serotonin-positive neurons within a certain area. In the present study, vibratome sections in which serotonin-containing neurons were visualized were counterstained with cresyl violet. This procedure enabled us to delineate in our sections the seven raphe nuclei as cytoarchitectonic entities and, hence, to determine exactly which serotonin-positive cells were localized within and which were located beyond the boundaries of these nuclei. The relationships between serotonin im-

munoreactive neurons and other transmitter-specified elements, cell bodies as well as fibers, are discussed in some detail and summarized here in five tables. A preliminary report of this work was presented at the Fourth European Neuroscience Meeting (Brighton, England, September, 1980).

METHODOLOGY

Preparation of the Antiserum

The preparation of the immunogen for serotonin has been described previously (284,289). The serotonin antigen was modified to yield a higher molar ratio between serotonin and its carrier protein (bovine serum albumin), as has been described by Steinbusch and Nieuwenhuys (286) and Steinbusch et al. (291). The antibody to tyrosine hydroxylase was a generous gift of Dr. M. Goldstein.

Preparation of Tissues

The animals were pharmacologically pretreated according to five different procedures:

1. Intraventricular injection of colchicine (Sigma, St. Louis) (60 μg/20 μl 0.9% sodium chloride) into the lateral ventricles 24 hr prior to sacrifice.

2. Intraperitoneal injection with nialamide (Sigma) (150 mg/kg body wt) 2 hr before death.
3. Intraperitoneal injection with nialamide and, subsequently, 60 min before perfusion, an intraperitoneal injection with L-tryptophan (100 mg/kg body wt).
4. Intraperitoneal injection with reserpine (10 mg/kg body wt) 4 hr prior to perfusion.
5. Intracerebral injection of 5,7-dihydroxytryptamine creatinine sulfate (Sigma) (10 μg) with a survival time of 20 to 25 days.

Adult male albino rats (160–180 g) were anesthetized with sodium pentobarbital (Nembutal®; 60 mg/kg body wt, intraperitoneal). Because it is known that the serotonin concentration in the CNS of the rat shows a circadian rhythm (42,143,241), we sacrificed all animals at the same time of day.

In order to visualize serotonin immunoreactive cell bodies and dendrites, the peroxidase–antiperoxidase (PAP) technique of Sternberger et al. (293) as applied by Grzanna et al. (116) was used. Animals were perfused through the left ventricle of the heart with 40 ml ice cold Ca^{2+}-free Tyrode's solution. This solution was saturated with a mixture of 95% O_2/5% CO_2 starting 1 hr before perfusion. This preperfusion was followed by pressure perfusion with 400 ml ice-cold 4% (wt/vol) paraformaldehyde dissolved in 0.1 M sodium phosphate buffer, pH 7.3. Brains were promptly removed and cut into 5 to 8-mm slabs in either transverse, sagittal, or horizontal directions. The tissue pieces were postfixed for 90 min at 4°C in the same fixative and washed for at least 4 hr in 5% sucrose dissolved in 0.1 M sodium phosphate buffer at 4°C. It should be noted that after this fixation procedure, at least 50% of the tritiated serotonin was retained in the tissue (262). This percentage is considerably higher than the 3% serotonin that was retained after the FIF procedure.

Immunocytochemical Procedures: Immunofluorescence and Immunohistochemistry

The immunofluorescence procedure has been described in detail elsewhere (284).

In the immunohistochemical procedure, tissue pieces were mounted onto chucks of a vibratome stage with a cyanoacrylate adhesive. After a drying period of 5 min, the tissue slices were kept in ice cold, 0.1 M sodium phosphate buffer, pH 7.3, until they were sectioned. Serial sections of 50 or 100 μm thickness were cut at a vibration rate of 8 to 9 scale units and a feeding speed of 2 to 4 scale units

and collected in counting tubes filled with the same buffer (128).

The sections were first incubated overnight in the refrigerator with a rabbit antiserotonin serum (286,291) (76 mg/ml) or preimmune serum, diluted 1 : 1,500 with phosphate-buffered saline (PBS) that contained 0.2% (vol/vol) Triton X-100. All subsequent steps were carried out at room temperature. Sections were washed for 10 min with PBS containing 0.2% Triton X-100 followed by a wash for 10 min in PBS with 0.1% Triton X-100 and finally for an additional 10-min wash in PBS alone. Then they were incubated with goat antirabbit antiserum (1 mg/ml) diluted 1 : 30 with PBS for 2 hr (goat antirabbit IgG, Fc-specific; Nordic, Tilburg, The Netherlands). Following two 10-min washes in PBS, the rabbit PAP complex (DAKO, Denmark) was applied in a dilution of 1 : 90 in PBS. After 1 hr of incubation, the sections were washed two times for 10 min with PBS. Then they were put in a solution containing 3,3-diaminobenzidine HCl (Sigma, 0.75 mg/ml) and $CaCl_2$ (120/μM) in 50 mM Tris HCl, pH 7.7; after 10 min, H_2O_2 was added to yield a final concentration of 0.003%, and the reaction was carried out for an additional 15 min. Sections were briefly rinsed in PBS and floated on glass slides coated with chrome alum gelatine. They were then air-dried overnight. Sections were postfixed with 2% glutaraldehyde in PBS. For permanent storage, sections were dehydrated and coverslipped with DePeX® (Gurr).

To study the cytoarchitecture of the brain, some animals were fixed with 4% paraformaldehyde. Brains were dissected, dehydrated, and embedded in paraffin. Transverse and sagittal sections of 15 μm thickness were cut on a rotary microtome and stained with cresyl violet or according to the technique of Klüver and Barrera.

The boundaries of the seven raphe nuclei were determined principally in cresyl-violet-stained 50-μm-thick vibratome sections. Serotonin immunoreactive neurons were visualized in 50-μm-thick vibratome sections. The size of the cell bodies within the confines of the raphe nuclei was studied in Nissl- and Klüver–Barrera-stained paraffin material as well as in vibratome sections processed for immunohistochemistry. Their diameters were determined from drawings at a magnification of 800 using a Zeiss drawing prism by averaging the lengths measured in two directions perpendicular to each other. The arithmetic averages of the data obtained have been used for classification of the cell types.

The length of the processes of the serotonin-immunoreactive cells was determined in 100-μm-thick vibratome sections with the aid of a semi-automatic system for measuring cellular tree structures in three dimensions, as described by Overdijk et al. (221) and by Uylings (315).

RESULTS

In this section the cytoarchitecture of the raphe nuclei and of the serotoninergic neurons present in the brainstem of the rat are described. The description of the serotonin immunoreactive perikarya and their dendrites present in each of the seven raphe nuclei are based on vibratome sections immunohistochemically stained with an antibody against serotonin. Nomenclature and definitions of the raphe nuclei are based on the atlases of König and Klippel (156), Meesen and Olszewski (194), Wünscher et al. (340), and the descriptions of Braak (41), Felten and Cummings (89), and Taber et al. (300). The localization of the cell bodies is indicated in 21 representative sections through the brainstem (Figs. 2–12). The dimensions of the serotoninergic cell bodies appeared to be significantly larger than the sizes of the cells observed in the Nissl-stained paraffin sections. The measurements of the dendritic patterns of these neurons, which were obtained with a semiautomatic measuring system, have to be regarded as preliminary. For a detailed description of serotonin immunoreactive fibers and terminals refer to a previous paper (284).

Although serotoninergic neurons are confined to the rhombencephalon and the tegmentum of the midbrain, serotonin-positive fibers and terminals appeared to be present in practically all parts of the CNS. In the diencephalon, the following types of nonneuronal cells showed a specific serotonin immunoreactivity: pinealocytes, pinealocyte-like elements in the epithalamic lamina intercalaris (Fig. 13A–D), tanycytes and other glial elements in the infundibular region, and mast cells in the median eminence. In the rhombencephalon, superficially situated glial cells were demonstrated at the basal surface of the brainstem (Figs. 14C,D; 15; and 16B).

The Raphe Nuclei

Nucleus Raphe Obscurus

Cytoarchitecture.
The nucleus raphe obscurus is a small nucleus situated in the caudal part of the rhombencephalon. It extends from level P 7000 to P 5250 in our atlas (Figs. 3B and 4A,B). The nucleus is situated dorsal to the nucleus raphe pallidus and ventral to the fasciculus longitudinalis medialis. It extends rostral to the caudal pole of the nucleus raphe magnus and caudal to the level of the decussatio pyramidis. The nucleus is confined to a narrow median and paramedian zone. At its caudal side, it is laterally bordered by the nucleus reticularis paramedianus. Rostrally, the nucleus raphe obscurus is flanked by the inferior olive complex. In most places, the boundaries of the nucleus are distinct. The cellular density is small, especially in its dorsal region.

The nucleus raphe obscurus contains two types of neurons, which may be designated as small and large (respectively <18 μm and 28–36 μm). The small elements have a spherical shape and a diameter of 17 ± 2 μm. The large neurons are bipolar or tripolar. Their length and diameter measure 29 ± 3 μm and 26 ± 2 μm, respectively. Both cell types are present equally and distributed evenly within the nucleus.

Serotonin immunoreactive perikarya and dendrites.
Perikarya. Serotonin-positive cell bodies can be found throughout the nucleus raphe obscurus, with highest concentrations in the intermediate part of its rostrocaudal extension. The serotoninergic neurons here form two parallel vertical laminae adjacent to the midline (Figs. 15 and 17B).

Two types of cell bodies were identified: medium-sized and large (respectively, 18–27 μm and 28–36 μm). The medium-sized elements are round with an elongated shape. Their length and diameter measure 27 ± 5 μm and 18 ± 3 μm, respectively. The large neurons are multipolar with length and diameter of 32 ± 4 μm and 23 ± 3 μm, respectively. The medium-sized cells were predominantly found in the dorsal parts of the nucleus, the large cell type more ventrally.

Comparison of the results obtained from the normal and the immunohistochemical material rendered it likely that the two serotonin-positive cell types both belong to the medium-sized cells observed in the Nissl material.

Dendrites. Both types of serotonin-immunoreactive neurons in the nucleus raphe obscurus have three to four dendrites, which are mainly oriented in a dorsolateral direction (Figs. 15 and 17B). Their average length is between 40 and 100 μm.

Nucleus Raphe Pallidus

Cytoarchitecture.
The nucleus raphe pallidus is one of the two caudal components of the raphe nuclear group. It extends from level P 7000 to P 5250 in our atlas

(Figs. 3B and 4A,B). The nucleus is situated ventral to the nucleus raphe obscurus. Its ventral border touches the basal surface of the brain. The nucleus has approximately the same longitudinal extent as the nucleus raphe obscurus. These nuclei are separated from each other by transversely running fibers. The nucleus raphe pallidus is a mass of relatively densely packed cells situated in the median region adjoining the dorsomedial edges of the pyramidal tracts. The caudal part of the nucleus is laterally well delineated by the nucleus reticularis paramedianus. The medial and rostral parts of the nucleus raphe pallidus are flanked by the nucleus reticularis gigantocellularis, medullae oblongatae. In this area, the borders of the nucleus are ill-defined.

The nucleus raphe pallidus contains two cell types: small and very large (respectively, <18 μm and >36 μm). The medium-sized elements are round or oval with a diameter of 17 ± 3 μm. The large neurons are fusiform or elongated; their length and diameter measure 37 ± 6 μm and 27 ± 6 μm, respectively. The highest proportion of cells belongs to the medium-sized cell type. These cells are present predominantly in the ventral part of the nucleus raphe pallidus. The large cells were evenly distributed over the nucleus.

Serotonin immunoreactive perikarya and dendrites.

Perikarya. Serotoninergic cell bodies were found throughout the nucleus raphe pallidus, with highest concentrations in the ventrocaudal, ventrointermediate, and the entire rostral part (Figs. 14A,B; 15; 17A; and 18A, C).

Two cell types were observed: medium and large. The medium-sized cells have an oval shape with length and diameter of 24 ± 5 μm and 16 ± 4 μm, respectively. The large neurons are multipolar, with length and diameter of 36 ± 5 μm and 30 ± 5 μm, respectively. The medium-sized perikarya are predominantly found ventrally, where almost no large cells were detected. In the dorsal part of the nucleus, both cell types were present in about equal numbers.

Comparison of the cell bodies in the normal, Nissl material, and in the immunohistochemical material reveals that there is a good correspondence between the two cell types described.

Dendrites. The two types of serotoninergic cells are different with regard to both the number and the preferential direction of their dendrites. The medium-sized cells have two or three main dendrites, whereas the large neurons have four or five dendrites. The direction of their dendrites varies with their position within the nucleus. The direc-

tion of the dendrites arising from cells situated medially is hard to determine because of the high density of these elements. The processes of the cells situated in the dorsal part of the nucleus raphe pallidus were directed dorsally or ventrolaterally (Figs. 15; 17A; and 18A).

Nucleus Raphe Magnus

Cytoarchitecture.

The nucleus raphe magnus is a large cell group situated in the rostral part of the medulla oblongata. It extends from level P 5000 to level P 3900 in our atlas (Fig. 5A,B). It is localized dorsal to the lemniscus medialis and ventral to the fasciculus longitudinalis medialis. The nucleus extends rostrally to the level of the caudal pole of the nucleus corporis trapezoidii and caudally to the caudal pole of the nucleus nervi facialis and the nucleus raphe obscurus. The caudal part of the nucleus grades into the rostral pole of the nucleus raphe pallidus. Caudally, the nucleus raphe magnus expands laterally to the nucleus nervi facialis. Rostrally, the nucleus narrows to a thin median sheet bordered on either side by the lemniscus medialis. The delimitations of the ventral, lateral, and dorsorostral borders of the nucleus are arbitrary.

The nucleus raphe magnus can be distinguished from the surrounding reticular formation by having a greater cell density. The nucleus contains two types of neurons: medium-sized and large. The medium-sized cells are multipolar, with an oval shape. Their length and diameter are 21 ± 4 μm and 18 ± 3 μm, respectively. The large cells are fusiform with length and diameter of 35 ± 5 μm and 23 ± 5 μm, respectively. Both cell types were found equally and were distributed uniformly within the nucleus raphe magnus.

Serotonin immunoreactive perikarya and dendrites.

Perikarya. Serotonin-positive cell bodies are not equally distributed over the nucleus (Figs. 16A and 18A,C). The neurons are mainly localized in its ventrocaudal part. In the dorsal part of the nucleus raphe magnus, only a small number of serotoninergic cells appear to be present. The cells are oriented perpendicular to the midline.

One type of cell body could be demonstrated: polygonal with a dimension of 34 ± 5 μm. This cell type resembles the large neurons observed in the Nissl-stained material.

Dendrites. The serotoninergic cell bodies of the nucleus raphe magnus have four to eight dendrites with only a few branches. The average length of these dendrites is between 150 and 450 μm. They

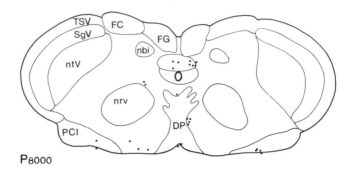

P8000

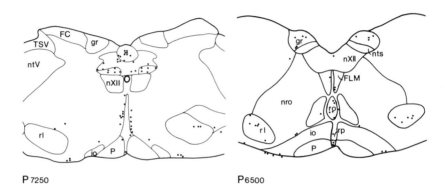

P 7250   P 6500

FIGS. 2–12. *(above and following pages)* Atlas of serotonin immunoreactive neurons in the brainstem and pons of the rat. Every cell at a certain level in a 50-μm-thick vibratome section has been plotted. Note that the majority of the serotoninergic perikarya are not strictly confined to the raphe nuclei. Abbreviations used in the figures: atv, area tegmentalis ventralis Tsai; CC, crus cerebri; ct, nucleus corporis trapezoidei; CT, corpus trapezoidei; DP, decussatio pyramidis; DT, decussationes tegmenti; FC, fasciculus cuneatus; FG, fasciculus gracilis; FL, fasciculus longitudinalis; FLDG, fasciculus longitudinalis dorsalis, pars tegmentalis; FLM, fasciculus longitudinalis medialis; FOR, formatio reticularis; gr, nucleus gracilis; io, nucleus olivaris inferior; iom, nucleus accessorius olivaris medialis; ip, nucleus interpeduncularis; LC, locus ceruleus; LM, lemniscus medialis; lo, nucleus linearis oralis; nbi, nucleus basilaris internus Cajal; ncs, nucleus centralis superior; ncu, nucleus cuneiformis; nE, nucleus Edinger–Westphal; np, nucleus parabrachialis ventralis; nrp, nucleus reticularis paramedianus; nrv, nucleus reticularis medullae oblongatae, pars ventralis; ntd, nucleus tegmenti dorsalis; ntdl, nucleus tegmenti dorsalis lateralis; ntm, nucleus tractus mesencephali; nts, nucleus tractus solitarius; ntV, nucleus tractus spinalis nervi trigemini; nIII, nucleus motorius nervi oculomotorii; nIV, nucleus nervi trochlearis; nV, nucleus motorius nervi trigemini; nVI, nucleus nervi abducentis; nVII, nucleus nervi facialis; nXII, nucleus nervi hypoglossi; os, nucleus olivaris superior; P, tractus corticospinalis; PCI, pedunculus cerebellaris inferior; PCM, pedunculus cerebellaris medius; PCMA, pedunculus corporis mamillaris; PCS, pedunculus cerebellaris superior; ph, nucleus prepositus hypoglossi; po, nucleus pontis; r, nucleus ruber; rgi, nucleus reticularis gigantocellularis; rl, nucleus reticularis lateralis; rm, nucleus raphe magnus; ro, nucleus raphe obscurus; rp, nucleus raphe pallidus; rpc, nucleus reticularis parvocellularis; rpo, nucleus raphe pontis; rpoc, nucleus reticularis pontis caudalis; rpoo, nucleus reticularis pontis oralis; rtp, nucleus reticularis tegmenti pontis; sg, nucleus suprageniculatis facialis; SGC, substantia grisea centralis lateralis; SGCv, substantia grisea centralis ventralis; SGv, substantia grisea ventralis; SN, substantia nigra; tmV, nucleus tractus mesencaphali nervi trigemini; TRS, tractus rubrospinalis; TSV, tractus spinalis nervi trigemini; TTS, tractus tectospinalis; vm, nucleus vestibularis medialis; vt, nucleus tegmenti ventralis; VII, nervus facialis.

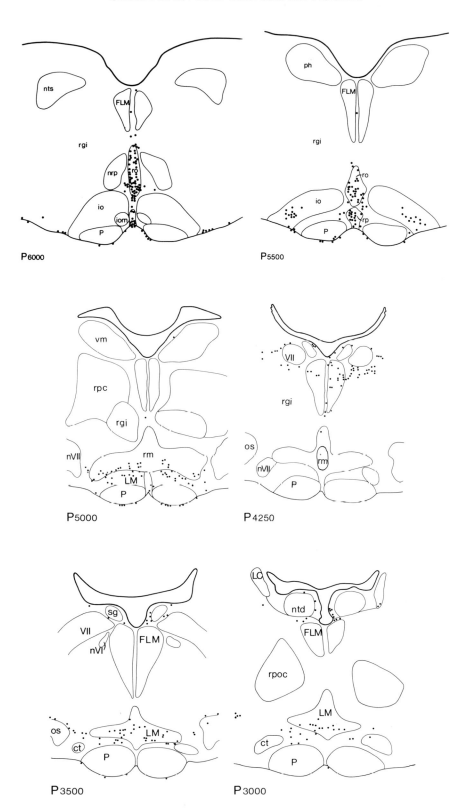

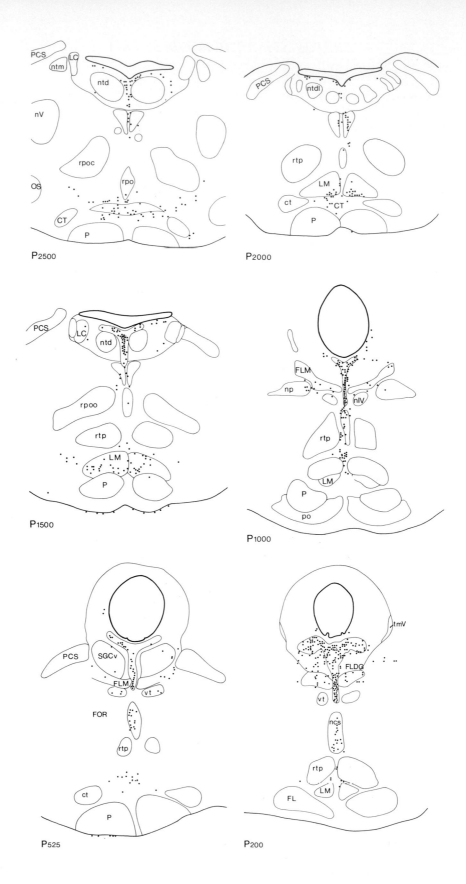

P₂₅₀₀

P₂₀₀₀

P₁₅₀₀

P₁₀₀₀

P₅₂₅

P₂₀₀

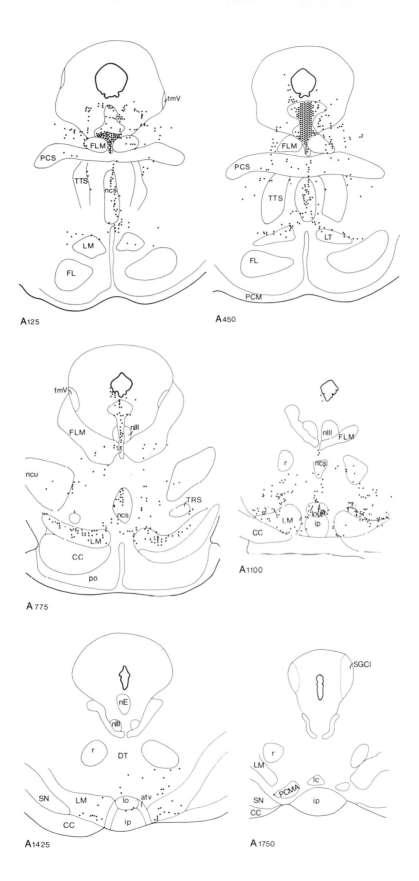

A125

A450

A775

A1100

A1425

A1750

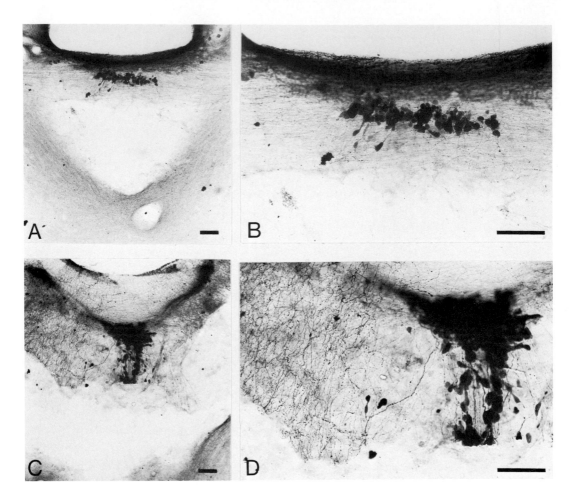

FIG. 13. Photomicrographs of a horizontal (**A,B**) and transverse (**C,D**) sections through the epithalamic lamina intercalaris after incubation with serotonin antiserum. A large number of serotonin-positive pinealocyte-like elements are observed. **D:** In addition, a strong serotoninergic innervation of the ventricular walls is shown. (*Bars,* 75 μm)

are predominantly oriented perpendicular to the midline. The processes of the cells that are located adjacent to the midline pass this area and then arch back to extend dorsally or ventrally. The dendrites, which are directed laterally, extend into the reticular formation over a distance of 350 to 700 μm.

Nucleus Raphe Pontis

Cytoarchitecture.

The nucleus raphe pontis is a vertically oriented and elongated cell mass which, as its name implies, is situated in the pons. It can be observed from level P 2600 to level P 1500 in our atlas (Figs. 7A,B and 8A). The nucleus is situated dorsal to the lemniscus medialis and ventral to the fasciculus longitudinalis medialis. Rostrally, it extends to the level of the nucleus reticularis pontis oralis and the locus ceruleus. Caudally, the cells of the nucleus raphe pontis are situated immediately dorsal to the lemniscus medialis at the level of the rostral pole of the nucleus reticularis pontis caudalis. From caudal to rostral, the nucleus shifts gradually from a ventral to a more dorsal position.

The dorsal and ventral borders are distinct; however, the lateral aspects are not sharp.

Three types of cell bodies were demonstrated: small, medium-sized, and large. The small cells are ellipsoid. Their length and diameter measure 15 ± 3 μm and 13 ± 3 μm, respectively. The medium-sized cells have a multipolar appearance, with a di-

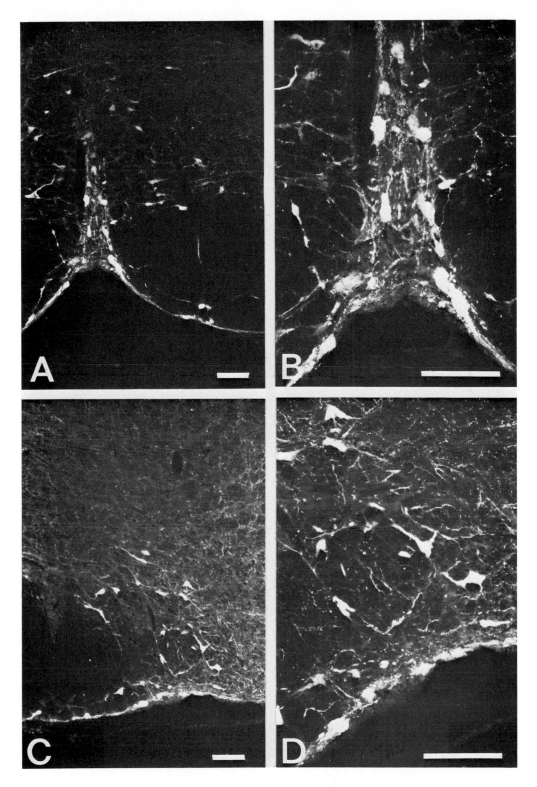

FIG. 14. Photomicrographs of transverse sections through (**A**, **B**) the nucleus raphe pallidus and (**C**, **D**) the nucleus reticularis gigantocellularis after incubation with antiserum to serotonin. Note in **B** and **D** the superficially situated glia cells. (*Bars*, 75 μm)

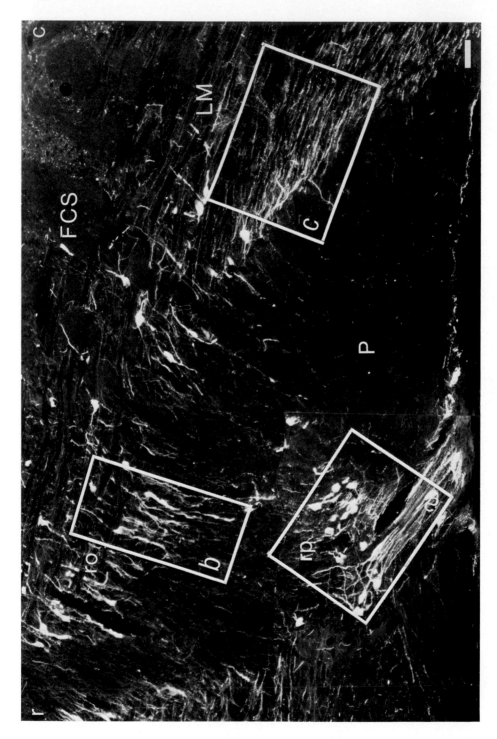

FIG. 15. Photomicrograph of a midsagittal section through the caudal brainstem after incubation with serotonin antiserum. Serotonin immunoreactive neurons are demonstrated in the nucleus raphe pallidus (rp) and the nucleus raphe obscurus (ro). Some serotonin-positive cells are shown in the reticular formation dorsal to the tractus corticospinalis (P) and ventral to the fibrae corticospinalis (FCS). Some serotoninergic fibers are seen in the area dorsocaudal to the pyramidal tract (P). Ventral to this same tract, a few superficially situated serotoninergic glia cells are visible (LM, lemriscus medialis). (*Bar*, 75μm)

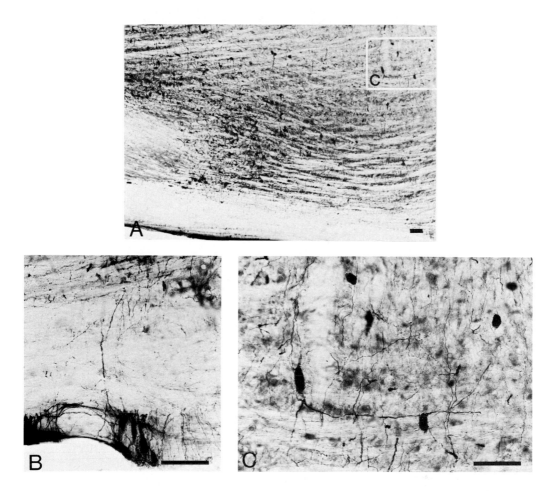

FIG. 16. Photomicrographs of a sagittal section through (**A,C**) the nucleus raphe magnus after incubation with serotonin antiserum. **B:** Superficially situated serotonin immunoreactive glia cells are demonstrated ventral to the pyramidal tract. (*Bars,* 75 μm)

mension of 21 ± 4 μm. The large neurons are bi- or sometimes multipolar, with length and diameter of 27 ± 4 μm and 22 ± 4 μm, respectively. The small, medium-sized, and large cell types were equally present and distributed evenly over the nucleus raphe pontis.

Serotonin immunoreactive perikarya and dendrites.

Perikarya. The serotonin-positive neurons are scattered throughout the nucleus with their highest concentration caudally. However, it should be mentioned that the total number of serotoninergic neurons is relatively small. Moreover, no immunoreactive cells were found in the median plane.

Three cell types were observed: medium-sized; large, fusiform; and large, multipolar. The me-dium-sized perikarya have an oval or bipolar shape with a diameter of 22 ± 3 μm. The large, fusiform cells are oriented perpendicular to the midline. Their length and diameter measure 29 ± 4 μm and 23 ± 3 μm, respectively. The large, multipolar cells are situated with their long axis parallel to the median plane. Their length and diameter are 29 ± 4 μm and 24 ± 3 μm, respectively. The large, fusiform cells are equally dispersed over the nucleus raphe pontis. The large, multipolar cells are mainly found caudally in the vicinity of the midline, whereas the medium-sized cells were observed in the ventrorostral part of the nucleus, close to the median plane.

The three serotoninergic cell types correspond to the medium-sized and large cell types in normal histological material.

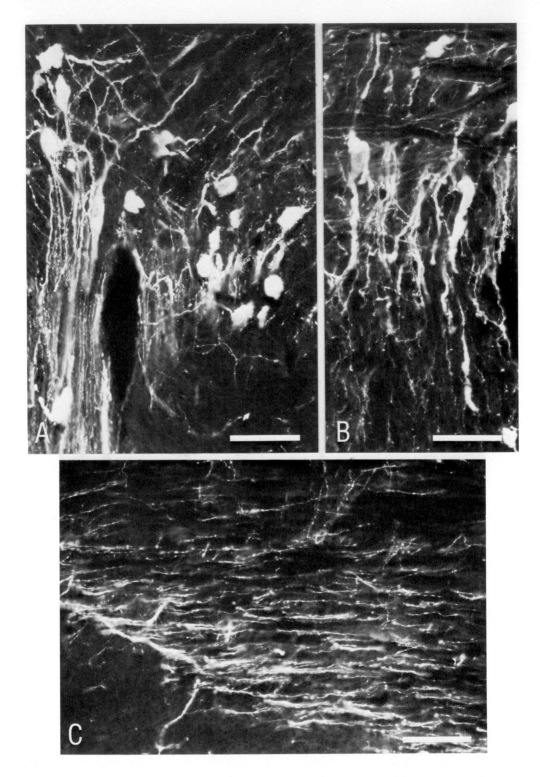

FIG. 17. Photomicrographs of a midsagittal section after incubation with serotonin antiserum showing (**A**) the nucleus raphe pallidus, (**B**) the nucleus raphe obscurus, and (**C**) descending serotoninergic fibers just dorsocaudal to the tractus corticospinalis. These fibers show only a sparse number of varicosities. (*Bars,* 75 μm)

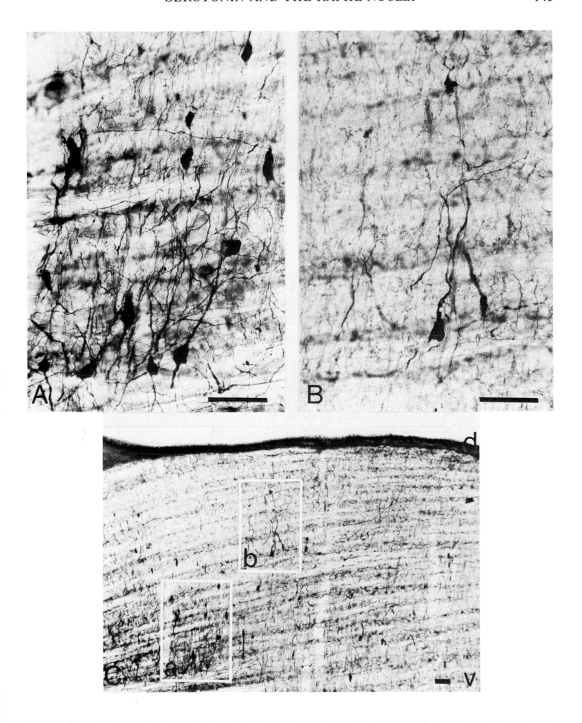

FIG. 18. Photomicrographs of a sagittal section through the nucleus raphe pontis (**A,C**) and the caudal part of the nucleus raphe dorsalis (**B,C**) after incubation with serotonin antiserum. Note the dense serotoninergic innervation of the substantia grisea (d, dorsal; v, ventral). (*Bars,* 75 μm)

Dendrites. With regard to their dendrites, the medium-sized neurons show two characteristics. At their medial side, there is one long, unbranched process, which can be followed over a distance of 77 ± 9 μm. Laterally, these neurons have small, highly branched processes. The long process reaches the midline and continues dorsally. We found that the processes arising from neurons situated rostrolaterally are much longer (115 ± 20 μm) than those of the elements situated in the remainder of the nucleus.

The dendrites of the large, fusiform cells do not show any special direction. They can be followed over a distance of 40 to 80 μm.

The dendrites of the large, multipolar cells resemble those of the medium-sized cells with only one difference: the long, medially oriented process, during its course to the midline, gives rise to many ventrally oriented ramifications.

Nucleus Raphe Dorsalis

Cytoarchitecture.

The nucleus raphe dorsalis is the largest raphe nucleus. It is located in the rostral part of the tegmentum pontis and in the caudal part of the tegmentum mesencephali. It extends from level P 2000 to level A 1400 in our atlas (Figs. 7A,B; 8A,B; 9A,B; and 10A,B). The nucleus is situated dorsal to the fasciculus longitudinalis medialis and ventral to the rostral part of the fourth ventricle and the aquaductus cerebri. It is rostrally bordered to the nucleus Edinger–Westphal. Caudally, the nucleus extends to the level of the rostral pole of the nucleus tegmentalis dorsalis of Gudden. The dorsal part of the nucleus fans out laterally, forming at the level of the nucleus nervi trochlearis a ventromedial group, a dorsomedian group, and two bilateral wings of cells. The most rostral part of the nucleus is a cluster of cells situated close to the median plane. In most places, its boundaries are distinct. At some places, however, this cell mass fuses with other groups of cells, thus making its delineation arbitrary. This happens to be the case at the border zone between the ventral part of the nucleus and the brachium conjunctivum and at the dorsal borders of its bilateral wings. In the latter region, the cell mass under discussion grades into the substantia grisea centralis.

Four areas with particularly high cell density were defined in the nucleus raphe dorsalis: one in the caudal, rhombencephalic part (pars caudalis) and three in the rostral, mesencephalic part. The latter are designated as dorsomedian, ventromedial, and lateral. The dorsomedian part of the nucleus can be seen as the spherical cluster that has the highest cell density within the nucleus.

Three types of neurons were observed: small, medium, and large. The small cells are spherical and have a diameter of 14 ± 3 μm. The median cells are of a fusiform shape; they are generally oriented in a rostrocaudal direction. Their length and diameter are 24 ± 6 μm and 20 ± 3 μm, respectively. The large cells are multipolar, with a diameter of 35 ± 4 μm. The small cells appeared to be particularly numerous in the lateral parts of the nucleus. The medium-sized cells were equally distributed. They frequently occurred in pairs. A special orientation of the medium-sized cells was observed in the narrow area between the two medial longitudinal fascicles. In this region, they were mostly lying dorsoventrally. The large cells were only found in the bilateral wings of the nucleus raphe dorsalis.

Serotonin immunoreactive perikarya and dendrites.

Perikarya. Serotonin-positive cell bodies are not equally distributed over the nucleus. Most of these neurons were demonstrated in its dorsomedian and ventromedial, mesencephalic part. Moreover, a substantial number of serotoninergic cell bodies were observed in the caudal, rhombencephalic part and in the bilateral wings, situated in the mesencephalic part. Only a few serotonin-containing perikarya were located in the remaining areas of the nucleus raphe dorsalis (Figs. 19 and 20A,B).

Four cell types were observed: small, medium, large, and very large. The small cells are round, oval, or sometimes bipolar with a diameter of 10 ± 3 μm.

The medium-sized perikarya have a fusiform or bipolar shape with length and diameter of 24 ± 4 μm and 18 ± 4 μm, respectively. The large neurons have a fusiform appearance with length and diameter of 31 ± 2 μm and 18 ± 2 μm, respectively. The very large cells are multipolar with a diameter of 39 ± 5 μm. The small cells were found in the ventromedial part and in the most rostral area of the caudal, rhombencephalic part of the nucleus. We observed about five times as many small cell bodies as medium-sized somata in the ventromedial region. Only a few small neurons were localized rostrally in the caudal, rhombencephalic part, close to the ventricular surface.

The medium-sized perikarya were found uniformly distributed over the nucleus, with highest concentration in the caudal, rhombencephalic and the dorsomedian, mesencephalic part of the nucleus. The cell bodies in the caudal area are mostly

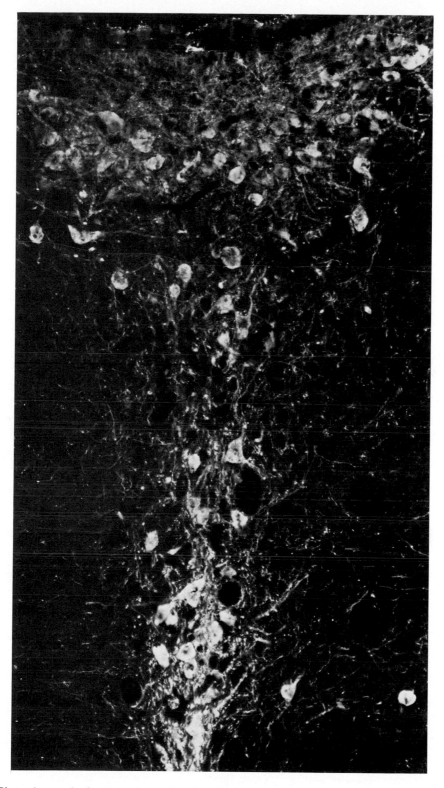

FIG. 19. Photomicrograph of a transverse section through the nucleus raphe dorslis (level P 1500, Fig. 8A) after incubation with serotonin antiserum. Note the presence of a serotonin-positive plexus in the rostral part of the fourth ventricle and the fusing of the serotoninergic cells in the ventromedial part of this nucleus. (×360)

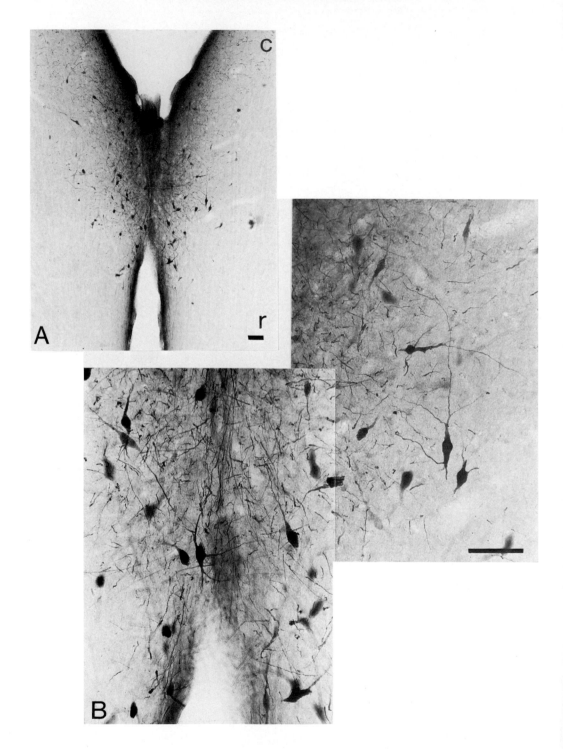

FIG. 20. Photomicrographs of a horizontal section through the dorsal part of the nucleus raphe dorsalis. **B:** A serotoninergic supraependymal plexus is present in the aquaductus cerebri. Note in **B** the dendritic pattern of the serotonin-positive neurons (c, caudal; r, rostral). (*Bars*, 75 μm)

oriented in a dorsoventral direction, whereas the perikarya in the dorsomedian part are generally oriented rostrocaudally.

The large neurons were located in the ventromedial and lateral parts of the nucleus. In the ventromedial part of the nucleus, the serotoninergic neurons are confined to the midline and are only few in number. A small percentage of large neurons were found in the dorsalmost part of the lateral region of the nucleus raphe dorsalis. Here, they are in close proximity to the very large cell elements.

The very large cells were only localized in the lateral, mesencephalic part of the nucleus, where they form the major cell type.

With regard to size and shape of the cell bodies, our results are in general agreement with other studies on the nucleus raphe dorsalis (69,132,300). From our results, it appears that the serotonin-immunoreactive neurons correspond to the medium-sized fusiform and the large multipolar neurons observed in the normal material.

Dendrites. For the sake of clarity, the dendritic patterns of the cells occurring in the four areas with high cell density are discussed separately. The dendrites belonging to the small serotoninergic neurons show different characteristics depending on their position either in the caudal part or the ventromedial part of the nucleus raphe dorsalis. The small cells situated in the most rostral area of the caudal part of the nucleus give rise to long processes that can be followed over a length of 400 to 500 μm and terminate as a part of the supraependymal plexus. Another feature of these processes is that from them, single branches originate, which issue close to the perikaryon. The dendrites belonging to the small cells situated in the ventromedial part of this nucleus could not be investigated because of the great number of serotonin-immunoreactive perikarya and the serotoninergic innervation of this region.

The dendritic patterns of the medium-sized serotonin-positive neurons differ between their two main locations. The dendrites in the caudal, rhombencephalic part show different characteristics depending on the position of their perikarya in this region. The cells situated in the midline have only very short, rather thick dendrites, which, in general, are oriented dorsoventrally. These dendrites can be followed over a length between 15 and 40 μm. The medium-sized cells situated laterally in this area have in general two or three processes. A short, rather coarse one is directed ventromedially with a length of 20 ± 10 μm. The other process(es) extend(s) dorsolateralward and can be fol-

lowed parallel to the surface of the fourth ventricle over a distance of between 150 and 250 μm. Both the short ventromedial and the long dorsolateral dendrites are generally unbranched. There have never been observed any processes entering the nucleus tegmentalis dorsalis of Gudden. The dendrites of the medium-sized cells in the dorsomedian mesencephalic part show different patterns related to the position of their perikarya. Because of the great number of serotonin-immunoreactive neurons in the medial area, it was not possible to trace their individual dendrites. However, the direction and length of the dendrites belonging to the laterally situated neurons could be determined. These cells are generally provided with two dendrites, a longer one and a shorter one. The longer dendrite shows no special orientation and can be followed over a distance of 60 μm. The shorter dendrite, with a length of 15 μm, is directed dorsally, but none of these processes has been observed actually to reach the surface (Fig. 20A,B).

The dendrites belonging to the large cell type, situated either in the ventromedial or the lateral mesencephalic part of the nucleus raphe dorsalis, show different characteristics. The dendrites of the larger cells in the ventromedial part of the nucleus could not be determined because of the dense cell packing in that area. The large, fusiform neurons situated in the caudal region of the lateral parts spread their axons dorsocaudally, reaching the ventricular surface and continuing caudally as a part of the supraependymal plexus.

The very large multipolar serotonin-immunoreactive cells situated in the lateral, mesencephalic parts of the nucleus raphe dorsalis generally show at their caudal side one process, which rapidly ramifies into two branches. These two branches can be followed over a short distance of between 20 and 40 μm. At their rostral side, the serotoninergic cells show very long dorsally directed processes, which sometimes can be followed over a length of 100 to 250 μm, and much shorter ventral processes with a length of 80 to 100 μm. However, the former processes do not reach the dorsal surface.

Nucleus Centralis Superior

Cytoarchitecture.

The nucleus centralis superior is a distinct nucleus situated in the caudal part of the tegmentum mesencephali. It extends from level P 1000 to level A 1200 in our atlas (Figs. 8B; 9A,B; 10A,B; and 11A,B). The caudal part of the nucleus is situated ventral to the nucleus ventralis tegmenti. Its intermediate and rostral parts are located ventral to the pedunculus cerebellaris superior. The caudal part of the nucleus is situated dorsal to the nucleus reticularis tegmenti pontis. The intermediate part lies dorsally to the lemniscus triangularis, and the rostral part dorsal to the lemniscus medialis.

The caudalmost neurons of the nucleus form a narrow band of cells in the median plane between the nuclei reticularis tegmenti pontis. More rostrally, the nucleus shifts to a position dorsal to the nucleus reticularis tegmenti pontis, but it is still confined to the median plane. The neurons of its intermediate part are diffusely arranged; however, they do not reach the borders of the tractus tectospinalis. Its most rostral part is difficult to delineate. The nucleus centralis superior contains three cell types, small ellipsoid, medium-sized ellipsoid, and medium-sized fusiform, with the following dimensions for length and diameter, respectively: 13 ± 3 μm, 12 ± 2 μm; 18 ± 4 μm, 13 ± 4 μm; and 19 ± 4 μm, 16 ± 4 μm. The cells of all of these types are evenly distributed over the nucleus.

Serotonin immunoreactive perikarya and dendrites.

Perikarya. Serotoninergic cell bodies are not evenly distributed over the nucleus. Most of the immunoreactive cells were found in the intermediate part, between the tectospinal tracts. In addition, some cell bodies were found in the ventrocaudal part. Two cell types could be observed: small and medium. The small cells are ellipsoid with length and diameter of 15 ± 3 μm and 12 ± 2 μm, respectively. The medium-sized cells are fusiform with length and diameter of 21 ± 4 μm and 17 ± 3 μm, respectively. The small cell type is mostly found in the medial part of the nucleus, whereas the medium-sized cells are more often observed in the lateral areas.

Comparison of the results obtained from the normal and the immunohistochemical material revealed that the two serotoninergic cell types correspond to the small ellipsoid and medium-sized fusiform perikarya observed in the Nissl material.

Dendrites. The dendrites of the serotoninergic perikarya are in general oriented in a rostrocaudal direction. The dendrites of the small ellipsoid cells are coarse and short, 10 to 20 μm. The processes of the medium-sized cells can be followed over a much longer distance, 150 to 250 μm.

Nucleus Linearis Oralis

Cytoarchitecture.

The nucleus linearis oralis is the most rostral raphe nucleus. This rather small, distinct cell mass extends from level A 1100 to level A 1750 in our atlas (Figs. 11B and 12A,B). The nucleus is situated dorsal to the nucleus interpeduncularis. Rostrally, the nucleus extends to the level of the pedunculus corporis mamillaris. The most caudal cells of the nucleus linearis oralis were found at the level of the rostral pole of the rubrospinal tracts.

Two types of cell bodies were demonstrated: small and medium. The small cells are ellipsoid with length and diameter of 15 ± 2 μm and 12 ± 2 μm, respectively. The medium-sized cells also have an ellipsoid appearance. Their length and diameter measure 18 ± 4 μm and 13 ± 3 μm, respectively, the latter being the most frequent. The cells of the two types are evenly distributed within the nucleus.

Serotonin immunoreactive perikarya and dendrites.

Perikarya. The serotoninergic cell bodies are unevenly distributed over the nucleus linearis oralis. The highest proportion of these elements was found caudally; some were observed in its intermediate part, but no serotonin-containing cells were demonstrated rostrally (Fig. 21A,C).

One one type of serotonin-positive cell body was found: small, piriform cells measuring 16 ± 3 μm and 12 ± 3 μm in length and diameter, respectively.

This latter cell type resembles the small ellipsoidal neurons demonstrated in the Nissl material.

Dendrites. The dendrites of the cell bodies situated in the dorsal part of the nucleus are oriented in a caudorostral direction. They are short and thick, their length being 15 to 25 μm. The dendrites of the neurons located ventrally in the nucleus are exclusively directed ventrally; they extend into the dorsal half of the nucleus interpeduncularis (Fig. 21A,C).

Serotoninergic Cell Bodies Beyond the Raphe Nuclei

Besides the serotoninergic neurons situated within the confines of the raphe nuclei, we were able with our current procedure to visualize serotonin-immunoreactive cells in several other rhombencephalic and mesencephalic areas. The shape and size of these serotonin immunoreactive perikarya have not been determined; however, it has been observed that the dimensions of the serotoninergic neurons visualized in the proximity of the various raphe nuclei do not differ substantially from the serotonin-positive cells within the boundaries of the raphe nuclei themselves (see, for

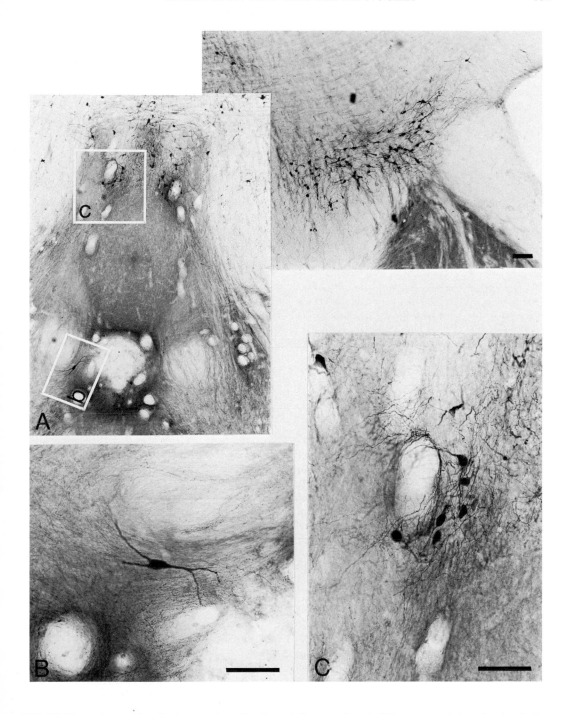

FIG. 21. Photomicrographs of a horizontal section through the ventral part of the mesencephalon after incubation with serotonin antiserum. Note in **A** the serotonin immunoreactive cells in the area of the lemniscus medialis. These cells were designated by Dahlström and Fuxe (69) as the B9 cell group. **B:** Serotonin-positive neuron ventral in the area tegmentalis ventralis of Tsai. **C:** Perikarya in the nucleus linearis oralis. (*Bars*, 75 μm)

example, Figs. 14C,D; 15; 16A–C; 18A–C; and 21A, which show the cells within and beyond the boundaries of the raphe nuclei). Our findings, which have been divided into two categories, sparse and substantial, are now briefly discussed.

In the medulla oblongata, we demonstrated a few cells in the nucleus commissuralis, in the area dorsomedially to the nucleus reticularis medullae oblongatae, pars ventralis, in the region adjacent to the decussatio pyramidis, in the nucleus intercalatus, in the nucleus reticularis lateralis, in the rostral part of the nucleus gracilis, and in the nucleus reticularis paramedianus. More rostrally, at level P 6000, we observed some cells in the midline between both fasciculi longitudinale mediale. Around level P 5500, we observed a substantial number of serotonin-positive cells ventrolaterally to the inferior olive complex (Fig. 14C,D). In the rostral part of the medulla oblongata, we found a large number of neurons in the dorsal part of the lemniscus medialis and in the zone between the nucleus raphe magnus and the nucleus nervi facialis. Moreover, dorsally, at level P 4250, we saw a substantial number of serotoninergic neurons ventral and lateral to the nervus facialis (Fig. 16C), a few cells between the nucleus vestibularis medialis and the floor of the fourth ventricle, and in the dorsal part of the fasciculi longitudinalis medialis.

In the pons, we observed a small number of serotoninergic neurons in the area surrounding the nucleus suprageniculatis facialis and, at that same level, P 3500, within and ventral to the lemniscus medialis and more laterally in the region dorsal to the nucleus olivaris superior. More rostrally, at level P 2500, we localized a substantial number of serotonin-positive cells dorsal and lateral to the nucleus tegmentalis dorsalis of Gudden and some cells between the fasciculi longitudinale mediale. A large number of serotonin-immunoreactive cells were demonstrated in the area of the lemniscus medialis and a few cells in a zone between the nucleus reticularis pontis caudalis and the nucleus corporis trapezoidii.

In the rostral part of the pons, at level P 1500, we demonstrated a few cells in the ventral part of the locus ceruleus and in the subceruleus area, in the region under the floor of the fourth ventricle, between the nucleus raphe dorsalis and the locus ceruleus, and, finally, in the region of the lemniscus medialis or immediately adjacent to it.

In the mesencephalon, we found caudally, at level P 1000, some serotoninergic neurons in the substantia griseum centralis (Fig. 20A), in the fasciculus longitudinalis medialis, and in the rostral part of the nucleus parabrachialis ventralis. In addition, some serotonin-positive neurons were observed between the rostral pole of the nucleus raphe pontis and the nucleus reticularis tegmenti pontis and in a region ventral to the nucleus raphe pontis. Rostrally, at level P 525, we localized serotonin-positive cells in an area dorsal to the tractus corticospinalis and medial to the nucleus corporis trapezoidii. In the medial and especially in the rostral part of the mesencephalon, we observed that most of the serotonin-positive neurons are not confined to the three mesencephalic raphe nuclei, although the nucleus raphe dorsalis contains the highest accumulation of serotoninergic perikarya in comparison with the other six raphe nuclei. Cell bodies were demonstrated at level A 775, in the lemniscus medialis, and in the region bordered by the fasciculus longitudinalis medialis, the nucleus cuneiformis, the lemniscus medialis, and the nucleus centralis superior (Fig. 20A). Some scattered cells were visualized within the borders of the nucleus cuneiformis. More rostrally, at level A 1100, we observed the highest concentration of extrarapheal serotoninergic neurons in the region dorsal to the lemniscus medialis and ventral to the nucleus ruber, especially in the lateral parts. A few cells were situated within the nucleus ruber.

The most rostral area in which we demonstrated serotonin-immunoreactive neurons in the untreated rat is situated between the pedunculi corporis mamillaris and the lemniscus medialis, where a few cells were found (Fig. 22B).

Interestingly, there exists from caudal to rostral a steady shift of the serotoninergic neurons from a dorsal to a ventral position. With our current procedure, we were also able to visualize serotonin-immunoreactive cells in the habenular region (Fig. 13A–D). These cells, found in the area of the subcommissural organ, are of pinealocyte rather than neuronal nature. However, some of these cells are provided with processes and differ in this respect from the cells of the pineal gland proper. Finally,

FIG. 22. Photomicrographs of transverse cryostat sections through the brainstem of a rat at postnatal day 1 after incubation with serotonin antiserum. **A:** Note that the nucleus raphe dorsalis and the nucleus centralis superior have not completed their migration. **B:** Note the lack of a sertoninergic supraependymal plexus in the aquaductus cerebri (AC). **C:** Note that the serotonin-positive neurons will migrate not medially but ventrolaterally, forming in the adult rat the B9 cell group (ip, nucleus interpeduncularis). (*Bars,* 75 μm)

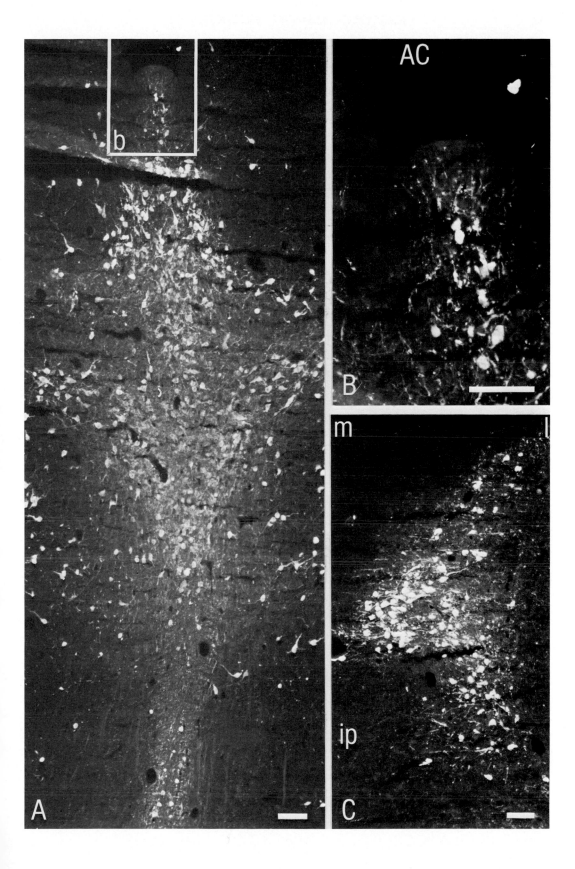

it should be noted that no serotonin-positive cells have been observed in the area of the hypothalamus or in any other diencephalic or telencephalic regions in rats that were either untreated or pretreated with either nialamide or L-tryptophan. However, in rats pretreated with a combination of both drugs, we were able to visualize a number of serotonin immunoreactive neurons in the substantia nigra (Fig. 23A,B) and ventrally in the nucleus dorsomedialis hypothalami (Fig. 24A,B).

Extraencephalic Serotoninergic Cells

Three extraencephalic regions reveal the presence of serotoninergic cells. Two of these areas contain neurons that are either situated supraependymally or superficially. One sphere is composed of superficially located serotonin immunoreactive glia cells.

Supraependymal Serotoninergic Neurons

Within the ventricles, we have observed on the roof of the rhombencephalon, on the basal surface of the fourth ventricle, and in the aqueductus cerebri some serotonin-positive neurons. The highest concentration of these neurons is found in the rostral part of the bottom of the fourth ventricle. Caudally, these neurons are only observed at the lateral ventricular walls. All of these cells are medium-sized with a fusiform–bipolar appearance. We have not observed a special orientation. Their length and diameter measure 25 ± 6 and 18 ± 3 μm, respectively. These elements were observed to have two processes, which could be followed over only a very short distance. No evidence has been found that these processes enter the ependyma.

Superficially Located Serotoninergic Neurons

The second group of extraencephalic serotonin-containing cells, consisting of only a sparse number of cells (ca. 20), is located in the region bordered dorsally by the area tegmentalis of Tsai and the nucleus mamillaris posterior. The cells are situated adjacent to the basal brain surface. All of these cells are large and tri- or multipolar. The processes of these elements usually show the following pattern. One process runs caudally, another is oriented rostrally, and a third one extends into the border zone between the nucleus interpeduncularis and the area tegmentalis ventralis of Tsai (Fig. 21A,B).

Superficially Located Serotoninergic Glial Cells

The third group of extraencephalic cells was observed adjacent to the rhombencephalic part of the tractus corticospinalis and ventral to the caudal part of the inferior olive complex (Figs. 14C,D; 15; and 16B). Two types of cells are found: (a) cells that are fusiform, oriented mediolaterally, with a length of 24 ± 5 μm and a diameter of 18 ± 3 μm and (b) cells that are small and round with a diameter of 17 ± 3 μm. The fusiform cell type is demonstrated ventral to the medial part of the tractus corticospinalis. These give rise to short processes, some of which enter the tractus corticospinalis. Other processes are directed laterally, and one particularly long process passes rostrally. The round cell type is localized ventrally to the lateral aspects of that same tract. These cells are in possession of a thick, short process, which is oriented medially, and thinner long processes, which run laterally.

DISCUSSION

Specificity of the Immunoreaction

The validity of immunocytochemical methods depends mainly on the specificity of the antibody used. The specificity of the serotonin antiserum employed in our procedure was tested as follows:

1. Liquid-phase absorption of the antiserum with increasing concentrations of serotonin (5-HT), 5-methoxytryptamine (5-MT), tryptamine (TRY), dopamine (DA), norepinephrine (NE), epinephrine (EP), octopamine (OCT), and histamine (HIST). This test demonstrated a cross reactivity to DA and 5-MT of less than 2%; the other agents showed negligible binding (Table 1).

2. Liquid-phase absorption experiments using the conjugates BSA–5-HT; BSA–DA; BSA–NE, and BSA–EP revealed that the antiserum could only be blocked with the BSA–serotonin conjugate.

3. Intraventricular and intraraphe injections with 5,7-dihydroxytryptamine (10 μg/μl) resulted in an almost complete elimination of 5-HT immunoreactive fibers. This finding has been biochemically confirmed by McRae-Degueurce and Pujol (193).

4. Administration of the serotonin neurotoxin para-chloroamphetamine (PCA; 2×10 mg/kg i.p.) 4 hr prior to sacrifice (154) resulted in a

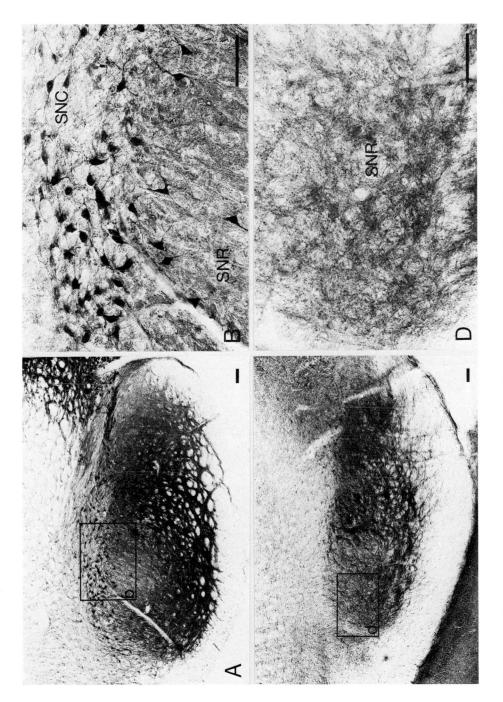

FIG. 23. Photomicrographs of transverse immunoperoxidase-stained vibratome sections through the substantia nigra after incubation with serotonin antiserum from (**A,B**) a rat pretreated with nialamide and L-tryptophan and (**C,D**) a rat pretreated with nialamide. **A,B:** Note the appearance of serotonin immunoreactive cell bodies in the substantia nigra, pars compacta. Note the presence of a dense serotoninergic innervation of the substantia nigra, pars reticulata. (*Bars*, 75 μm)

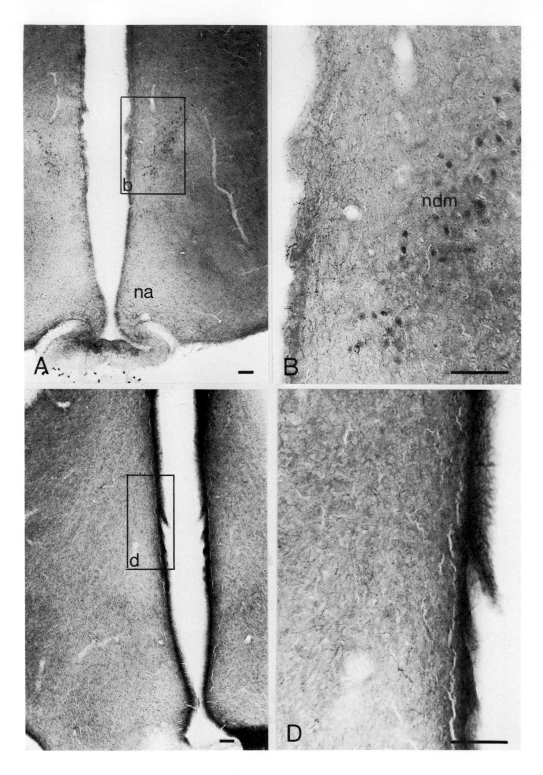

FIG. 24. Photomicrographs of transverse vibratome-stained sections through the hypothalamus after incubation with serotonin antiserum from (**A,B**) a rat pretreated with nialamide and L-trypotophan and (**C,D**) a rat pretreated with L-tryptophan. Note in **A** and **B** the appearance of serotonin immunoreactive cell bodies in the ventral part of the nucleus dorsomedalis hypothalami (ndm). Note in **B** the serotoninergic supraependymal plexus in the third ventricle (na, nucleus arcuatus). (*Bars,* 75 μm)

TABLE 1. *Results of blocking experiments*[a]

	Concentration (μM)													
	1	2	4	8	16	32	64	128	256	512	1,024	2,048	4,096	8,192
5-HT	+++	++	+	+	+	−	−	−	−	−	−	−	−	−
5-MT	+++	+++	+++	+++	+++	++	++	+	+	+	−	−	−	−
DA	+++	+++	+++	+++	+++	+++	+++	+++	+++	++	+	+	+	+
NE	+++	+++	+++	+++	+++	+++	+++	+++	+++	+++	+++	+++	+++	+++
OCT	+++	+++	+++	+++	+++	+++	+++	+++	+++	+++	+++	+++	+++	+++
EP	+++	+++	+++	+++	+++	+++	+++	+++	+++	+++	+++	+++	+++	+++
SYN	+++	+++	+++	+++	+++	+++	+++	+++	+++	+++	+++	+++	+++	+++
HIST	+++	+++	+++	+++	+++	+++	+++	+++	+++	+++	++	++	++	++

[a]Fluorescence intensity in comparable cryostat sections of the rat medulla oblongata stained with samples of an antiserum to serotonin immunogen purified from BSA antibodies. These samples were incubated with different concentrations of substances as indicated. +++, normal fluorescence; ++, some inhibition; +, strong inhibition; −, no fluorescence. 5-HT, serotonin; 5-MT, 5-methoxytryptamine; DA, dopamine; NE, norepinephrine; OCT, octapamine; EP, epinephrine; SYN, synephrine; HIST, histamine.

considerable decrease of 5-HT immunoreactivity.

5. Electrolytic lesions of either the nucleus raphe dorsalis or the nucleus centralis superior resulted in a complete disappearance of the 5-HT immunoreactivity.

6. Intraperitoneal injection with reserpine (10 mg/kg body wt) 4 hr before sacrifice resulted in a total disappearance of the serotoninergic fibers, although the blocking effect on the serotonin-positive perikarya was not complete.

7. No staining was observed in areas containing a large amount of possible cross-reacting compounds such as NE in the locus ceruleus or DA in the substantia nigra.

With regard to the specificity of our serum, the following two additional notes are relevant:

1. Close correlation with the findings of Pickel et al. (235) using an antibody to tryptophan hydroxylase (TrH, E.C. 1.14.16.4), the rate-limiting enzyme in the synthesis of serotonin from tryptophan, revealed a good correspondence. However, TrH-positive staining was often associated with heavily myelinated tracts, i.e., the tractus corticospinalis, lemniscus medialis, and the fasciculus longitudinalis medialis.

2. Since our fixation procedure resembles that of the FIF technique, the possibility of cross reactivity of the serotonin antibody toward β-carbolines has been suggested by Buckholtz (47), Deitrich (72), and Komulainen et al. (155).

We consider the cross reactivity mentioned above unlikely for the following two reasons. (a) β-Carbolines are not water-stable products. The FIF technqiue is carried out in a completely dry environment after the perfusion, but this is not so in the immunocytochemical technique. Thus, it may be expected that any β-carbolines formed will be washed out of the tissue during our procedure. (b) High concentrations of β-carbolines have been demonstrated in the nucleus arcuatus of the rat using ultraviolet laser fluorimetry and organic extraction (272). However, in our material, this area reveals only a sparse to low immunoreactivity.

In later sections of the present chapter, some data from the literature obtained with antibodies against small neuropeptides are discussed. It should be emphasized that these data should be judged with caution, because adequate control experiments have sometimes been neglected. It is also worthy of note that in immunocytochemical studies with antisera to small peptides, cross reactivity with analogues, fragments, or sequences of larger peptide should be excluded. The insufficient availability of these compounds makes liquid- or solid-phase absorption tests difficult to perform.

Ontogenesis of Serotoninergic Neurons

Neuroblasts are generally produced in the proliferative zone near the ventricular surface, from where they migrate radially to their final position where their maturation occurs. Of all transmitter-specified neuron populations investigated so far, the serotonin group is the first to appear. Using the FIF technique, Olson and Seiger (220) found that indoleamine-containing neuronal cell bodies can be observed in the rat at day 13 of gestation and in man during the seventh week of gestation (219).

The immature serotoninergic elements constitute two superficially situated columns, which are localized bilaterally at some distance from the median plane, in the stretch of the brainstem situated between the pontine and mesencephalic flexures.

From this finding, it may be surmised that the synthesis of serotonin begins after the completion of a ventrally directed radial migration of the prospective serotoninergic elements. At this stage, serotonin cannot be designated as a neurotransmitter, because the development of synaptic contacts has yet to be started. This raises the question of what specific role serotonin might play during ontogenesis other than that concerned with chemical neurotransmission. One hypothesis is that serotonin acts as a "differentiation signal" during early neurogenesis for those cells that will eventually receive a 5-HT innervation. Regulation of the timing of the target cell differentiation by a presumptive neurotransmitter substance implies a high degree of specificity in the interaction of cells in the neural tube, which is maintained during later developmental processes such as synaptogenesis (160,161). Thus, according to this hypothesis, serotonin and other neuroactive principles participate in the building of their own circuitry in the developing brain.

On the 14th day of gestation, the existence of three groups of indoleaminergic neurons was demonstrated in the rat by Cadilhac and Pons (53) using the FIF technique. The rostral and most prominent group is situated at the ventral surface between the mesencephalic and pontine flexures. The cells in this group showed a strong yellow fluorescence, indicating a high amount of indoleamines. In addition, they observed that these cells are not evenly scattered in this region but are rather arranged in two or three layers. Some rostrally directed axons were seen. The second group was localized in the rhombencephalon just behind the pontine flexure. It occupied the entire ventral part of the pons. The third group was found more caudally at the level of the cervical flexure. Only a few cells in this group give rise to descending axons. The serotoninergic axons grow out later and usually reach their area of termination shortly after birth (177,220). From birth on, the development of the serotoninergic neurons is accelerated, and they reach their mature state in the rat brain at about the 6th postnatal week (6). Moreover, the study of Hedner and Lundborg (121) showed that the rate-limiting step in the development is the availability of tryptophan hydroxylase.

The study in the rat by Levitt and Moore (169), who also used the FIF technique, started at day 18 of gestation and was primarily focused on the time of fusion of the initially bilaterally located prospective raphe cell groups. The development of these groups can be seen as a two-step procedure: first, a bilateral, ventrally oriented migration of the neuroblasts from the proliferative zone towards a region adjacent to the midline and, second, a medial migration, bringing about the fusion of the bilateral groups of neuronal elements.

Using immunocytochemistry in combination with antibodies to serotonin, we were able to confirm the findings of the authors mentioned above. Preliminary results were achieved in Chinese hamster *(Cricetulus griseus)* embryos at 14 days of gestation (Fig. 25A–D) and in rats on the first postnatal day (Fig. 22A–C). According to the work of Gribnau and Geijsberts (115), who described a system of staging of mammalian embryos, the Chinese hamster embryos studied are comparable to rat embryos aged 14.5 days of gestation. Our preparations showed that at that stage, the serotonin immunoreactive cell groups are not yet fused (Fig. 25A,B,D). We observed that some of the neuroblasts pass the midline (Fig. 25B,D). Observations in the young rats revealed that most of the serotonin-positive neurons indeed migrate in the direction of the raphe nuclei (Fig. 22A). However, from a comparison of our material from neonatal rats with that of adults, it can be inferred that in the ventrorostral part of the mesencephalon, migration is not directed medially but rather occurs in the opposite direction (Fig. 22C). These laterally migrating serotoninergic cells will probably constitute the B9 cell group in the adult rat, which is equivalent to the serotonin-positive cells in and around the mesencephalic part of the lemniscus medialis.

In adult rats, all of the seven raphe nuclei fuse except for the rhombencephalic part of the nucleus raphe dorsalis. Our observations warrant the tentative conclusion that the serotonin-positive neurons situated in the reticular formation are neurons that during ontogenesis did not complete their migration toward the raphe region.

Serotoninergic Cells in the Adult Rat

In general, our results regarding the distribution of serotonin immunoreactive perikarya are in conformity with earlier FIF observations in the rat by Dahlström and Fuxe (69), in the cat by Lackner (159), Pin et al. (237), Poitras and Parent (238), and Wiklund et al. (337), in the squirrel monkey *(Saimiri sciureus)* by Hubbard and Di Carlo (132), in the pigmy primate *(Cebullae pigmae)* by Jacobowitz and MacLean (135), and in the human fetus brain by Nobin and Björklund (213). However, we observed in our material that only a minority of the neurons in the nucleus raphe obscurus, the nucleus raphe magnus, the nucleus raphe pontis, the nucleus centralis superior, and the nucleus linearis oralis are serotonin immunoreactive.

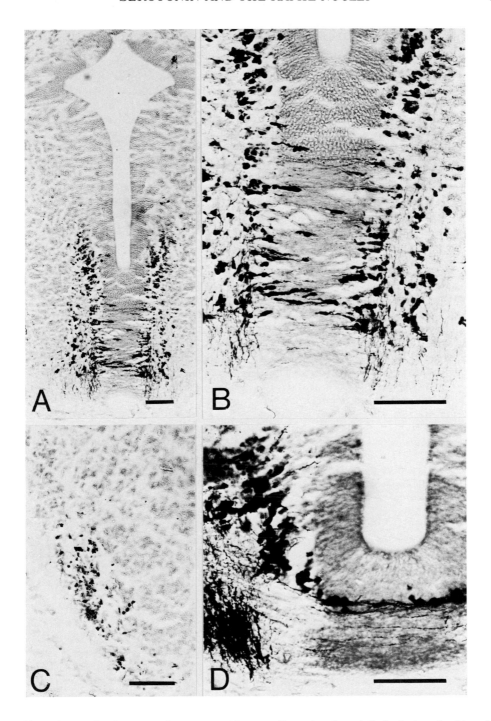

FIG. 25. Photomicrographs of transverse immunoperoxidase–paraffin sections through the brainstem of a chinese hamster embryo at 14 days of gestation, after incubation with serotonin antiserum, at the level between the pontine and mesencephalic flexures (**A, B**) in the median plane, (**C**) ventrolaterally, and (**D**) just caudal to the pontine flexure. Note in **B** and **D** that at this stage the serotoninergic cell groups are not yet fused. *(Bars, 75 μm)*

A much higher number of serotonin-positive elements were seen in the nucleus raphe pallidus and the nucleus raphe dorsalis. Moreover, it should be mentioned that most of the serotonin immunoreactive neurons are not situated within the seven raphe nuclei. It was for this reason that Dahlström and Fuxe (69) introduced a new classification of the indoleamine-containing cells in the rat brain stem, i.e., nine groups designated B_1 through B_9.

Nevertheless, we have not attempted to determine precisely the ratio between serotoninergic and nonserotoninergic neurons in the different raphe nuclei. Wiklund et al. (337), who used the FIF method in combination with Nissl stain, determined this ratio for the raphe nuclei of the cat as follows: nucleus raphe obscurus, 35%; nucleus raphe pallidus, 50%; nucleus raphe magnus, 15%; nucleus raphe pontis, 10%; nucleus raphe dorsalis, 70%; nucleus centralis superior, 35%; and nucleus linearis oralis, 25%. The percentage of serotonin-positive cells in the nucleus raphe dorsalis corresponds with that observed by Descarries et al. (74) in their autoradiographic study.

To date, the most comprehensive mapping of indoleaminergic neurons has been carried out by Wiklund et al. (337) using the FIF technique in the brainstem of the cat. Two major differences between their results and ours should be mentioned. The first is that we were unable to confirm their observations regarding the presence of serotoninergic neurons in the lateral part of the reticular formation. This could be a species difference between rat and cat. The second is that we observed a much larger number of serotonin-positive neurons within the area of the lemniscus medialis in the mesencephalon than they did.

In addition to these two major differences, the following two minor controversial points should be mentioned. (a) We observed serotoninergic cells at the basal surface of the rhombencephalon in the area ventral to the tractus corticospinalis (Figs. 14C,D; 15; and 16B). These cells have not been described before. It was not possible to relate them to normal material, since they are hard to demonstrate in 15-μm-thick Nissl sections. Conceivably, these neurons drifted during the early development of the pyramidal tract. Since the maturation of serotoninergic neurons starts ventrally, as has been

described above, these cells may have been precluded from migrating dorsomedially. (b) Indoleamine-containing cells in the area of the subcommissural organ of the rat have been described previously by Björklund et al. (31), Møllgard and Wiklund (200), and Wiklund (336), who all used the FIF method. The latter authors described, in addition, yellow fluorescent cells within the stria medullaris and in the nucleus habenularis medialis. Although we have used the same pharmacological pretreatments the authors mentioned, we could confirm the presence of serotonin-containing cells only in the area of the subcommissural organ (Fig. 13A–D).

Finally, several authors who used autoradiography (22,61,149,225) reported the uptake of [^{3}H]serotonin in perikarya in several hypothalamic nuclei including the nucleus ventromedialis hypothalami, the nucleus dorsomedialis hypothalami, and the nucleus paraventricularis hypothalami.

With regard to our own observations, even after pretreatment with nialamide or L-tryptophan to enhance the concentration of endogenous serotonin, we remained unable to confirm with immunofluorescence serotonin-positive perikarya in the hypothalamus (Figs. 23C,D and 24C,D). However, using the same pharmacological treatment in combination with the use of vibratome sections (which were immunohistochemically stained for serotonin), we were able to visualize serotoninergic cells in the ventral part of the nucleus dorsomedialis hypothalamus (Fig. 24A,B), and in the substantia nigra, pars compacta, and the area tegmentalis ventralis of Tsai (Fig. 23A,B). No staining was observed in other dopaminergic, noradrenergic, or adrenergic neuron populations.

The immunoreactive cells in the nucleus dorsomedialis hypothalami indeed contain serotonin, although their content *in vivo* is very small. The same cells are definitely not dopaminergic, as previously suggested by one of us (284). This appeared from the fact that these cells in immunofluorescence did not react with an antibody to tyrosine hydroxylase. Applying this antibody, we were able to demonstrate dopaminergic cells in neighboring areas such as the nucleus arcuatus and the zona incerta but none in the nucleus dorsomedialis hypothalami itself (Fig. 26). Although these cells were not dem-

---

FIG. 26. Photomicrograph of transverse cryostat-stained sections through the hypothalamus after incubation with an antibody to tyrosine hydroxylase. Dopaminergic neurons can be visualized in the nucleus arcuatus (na) and in the zona incerta (zi). A very dense innervation with catecholaminergic fibers has been found in the median eminence (ME). A large number of serotoninergic fibers pass through the medial forebrain bundle (MFB). No dopaminergic neurons are visualized in the nucleus dorsomedialis hypothalami (ndm) (nvm, nucleus ventromedialis hypothalami; F, fornix; IIIv, third ventricle). (*Bar,* 75 μm)

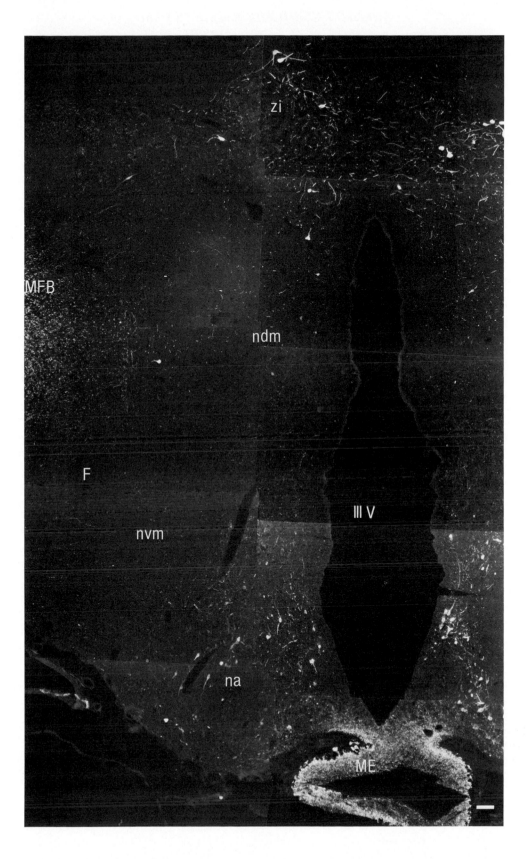

onstrated by Pickel et al. (235) using immunohistochemistry in combination with an antibody to tryptophan hydroxylase, they must contain the enzyme system to convert the applied L-tryptophan to serotonin. The neurons under discussion do not contain indoleamine other than serotonin.

The biochemical studies of Green et al. (114) and the microspectrofluorometric work of Björklund et al. (26–29) indicated that other indoleamines, namely, 5-methoxytryptamine or tryptamine, are present in the rat central nervous system. The latter author stated that these non-5-HT indoleamines are situated in brain areas other than those in which the 5-HT and catecholamine neuron populations are located, including the hypothalamus. However, Jonsson et al. (141), using a microspectrofluorimetric analysis, and Bosin et al. (40), Nakasimhachari et al. (207), and Prozialeck et al. (240), using several sensitive gas chromatographic–mass spectrophotometric methods, were unable to detect any 5-methoxytryptamine in the hypothalamus of the rat.

With regard to the serotonin immunoreactive cells in the substantia nigra, pars compacta, and the area tegmentalis ventralis of Tsai, there are several possible explanations.

It is possible that since the substantia nigra and the area tegmentalis ventralis of Tsai receive a medium-dense serotoninergic innervation, the released serotonin could be taken up by dopaminergic cells, since the monamine oxidase has been inhibited by nialamide. Subsequently, the serotonin taken up would be recognized by immunocytochemistry. However, in all other dopaminergic as well as noradrenergic neuron populations that receive an equal or even higher serotoninergic innervation, we have not demonstrated a serotonin-positive staining of their perikarya.

Another possibility is that L-tryptophan is taken up by serotoninergic neurons in which L-tryptophan is converted to 5-hydroxytryptophan. This intermediate product could be released from the neuron and subsequently be taken up by dopaminergic cells. These cells contain the same enzyme, ADDC, to convert 5-hydroxytryptophan further to serotonin (Fig. 1). However, we have to raise the same objections, viz., that in that case we should have to find a serotonin-positive staining in all catecholaminergic cells.

A further explanation could be that the addition of L-tryptophan increases the activity of the enzyme ADDC, which in its turn will result in a build-up of dopamine. Because of the low amount of cross reactivity of the serotonin antibody toward dopamine, we would then have seen dopaminergic rather than serotoninergic structures. However, as has been explained elsewhere (291), with the applied fixation procedure we are not able to fix catecholamines.

The last and, in our opinion, most likely explanation of the phenomena observed is that the immunoreactive cells in the substantia nigra, pars compacta, and in the area tegmentalis ventralis of Tsai contain minute amounts of serotonin, which normally cannot be detected. Evidence for this last explanation has been obtained from three additional experiments. No serotonin immunoreactive cell bodies were observed after pretreatment with the specific 5-HT depletor 5,7-dihydroxytryptamine. Second, in the substantia nigra, immunocytochemical staining of adjacent sections with an antibody to tyrosine hydroxylase revealed a striking similarity between serotonin and catecholamine immunohistochemistry (Figs. 23A,B and 27). Third, electrolytic lesions in the area immediately rostral to the nucleus raphe dorsalis and the nucleus centralis superior resulted in an almost complete disappearance of serotoninergic fibers in forebrain areas. However, some fibers still remained in the hypothalamus. Thus, those fibers must have an intrahypothalamic source, as previously mentioned by Van de Kar and Lorens (317).

Finally, three additional observations should be mentioned in this context. (a) Serotonin-positive cells have been observed in the reptilian homolog area of the substantia nigra in untreated animals *(Varanus exanthimaticus)* (J. G. Wolters, *personal communication*). (b) Serotonin immunoreactivity in cells of the area of the substantia nigra is much stronger at fetal stages than in adult material. (c) It has been suggested by Burnstock (49,50) that sympathetic neurons can synthesize and release two different monoamines.

Thus, it might be well possible that we have shown for the first time the presence of two endogenous monoamines within the same neurons of the CNS. Moreover, it is our impression that these cells produce much higher concentrations of serotonin during development than in the adult state and that during maturation these cells receive a changing phenotypic expression, so that they primarily produce dopamine instead of serotonin. (An alternate explanation is equally plausible: the tyrosine hydroxylase in the DA neurons, which is known to differ in properties from that in NE neurons, may have some ability to hydroxylate tryptophan under conditions in which this amino acid is present in high concentrations.)

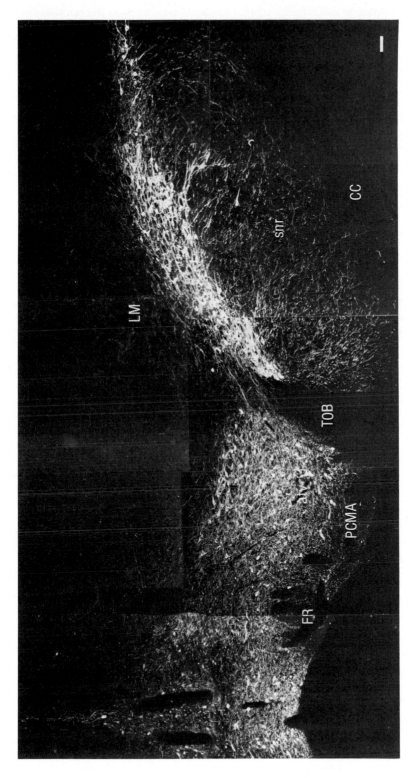

FIG. 27. Photomicrograph of a transverse cryostat-stained section through the substantia nigra after incubation with an antibody to tyrosine hydroxylase. A large number of dopaminergic cells are found in the substantia nigra, pars compacta and in the area tegmentalis ventralis of Tsai (atv) (CC, crus cerebri; FR, fasciculus retroflexus; LM, lemniscus medialis; PCMA, pedunculus cerebellaris mamillaris anterior; snr, substantia nigra, pars reticulata; TOB, tractus opticus basalis). (*Bar*, 75 μm)

Comparison of the Various Raphe Nuclei

Cytoarchitecture

The raphe nuclei are all situated in the median and paramedian zone of the brainstem. Comparison of these nuclei revealed that they differ not only in cell density but also in the types of cells they contain. On the basis of dimensions, four cell types can be distinguished: small, medium, large, and very large. Each of these four cell types can be further divided according to shape.

The small cells appear to be present in two forms: (a) spherical or ellipsoidal in the nucleus raphe obscurus, the nucleus raphe pallidus, the nucleus raphe pontis, the nucleus raphe dorsalis, the nucleus centralis superior, and the nucleus linearis oralis and (b) round or oval in the nucleus raphe pallidus.

The medium-sized cells were present in three forms: (a) multipolar in the nucleus raphe magnus and the nucleus raphe pontis, (b) fusiform in the nucleus raphe dorsalis and the nucleus centralis superior, and (c) ellipsoidal in the nucleus centralis superior.

The large cells can be divided into three types: (a) bi- or tripolar in the nucleus raphe obscurus, (b) fusiform in the nucleus raphe magnus, and (c) multipolar in the nucleus raphe dorsalis.

Finally, very large cells, which appeared as fusiform or elongated neurons, were demonstrated only in the nucleus raphe dorsalis.

Our cytoarchitectural analysis of the raphe nuclei of the rat is in general agreement with studies in the rabbit (89), cat (300), and man (41). Moreover, the raphe nuclei in the rat show, with regard to their localization, a striking resemblance to those of other species. Because of a different classification of neurons, our results differ somewhat from those of Felten and Cummings (89). The present study confirms the neuronal heterogeneity among the various raphe nuclei and shows that each of these nuclei represents a cytoarchitectonic entity.

Serotoninergic Neurons

Since the initial description of indoleamine-containing neurons in the brainstem of the rat (69,70), numerous histofluorescence studies in several species appeared. The study of Wiklund et al. (337) showed that the various raphe nuclei differ not only in total number of serotoninergic cells but also in the presence of various cell types. Four categories of cells were found on the basis of dimensions: small, medium, large, and very large. Each of these categories can be further divided according to shape.

Small serotoninergic cells, which were only present in the three mesencephalic raphe nuclei, occur in three forms: spherical, ellipsoidal, and piriform. The small spherical cells were observed in the nucleus raphe dorsalis. The small ellipsoidal cells were found in the nucleus centralis superior, and the small piriform cells were demonstrated in the nucleus linearis oralis.

Medium-sized serotoninergic cells, present in all of the raphe nuclei except for the nucleus raphe magnus, occur in two forms: (a) spherical and ellipsoidal and (b) fusiform or bipolar. The former was observed in the four rhombencephalic raphe nuclei, i.e., nucleus raphe obscurus, the nucleus raphe pallidus, nucleus raphe magnus, and the nucleus raphe pontis. The latter form was found in two of the mesencephalic raphe nuclei, i.e., the nucleus raphe dorsalis and the nucleus centralis superior.

Large serotoninergic cells were found in two forms: fusiform and multipolar. The large fusiform

TABLE 2. *Transmitter-specified perikarya within the raphe nuclei*

	Nucleus raphe obscurus	Nucleus raphe pallidus	Nucleus raphe magnus	Nucleus raphe pontis	Nucleus raphe dorsalis	Nucleus centralis superior	Nucleus linearis oralis
Serotonin (284)	+	+	+	+	+	+	+
Dopamine (127,205,216,337)					+	+	+
Norepinephrine (117,118)					+		
GABA/GAD (23,24,208)					+		
CCK (318)					+		+
leu-ENK (111,204,311)		+	+		+		
met-ENK (123,311)		+	+		+		
Substance P (63,174)	+	+	+		+		
VIP (182,273,321)					+		

cell type was demonstrated in the nucleus raphe magnus, the nucleus raphe pontis, and the nucleus raphe dorsalis. The large multipolar neurons have been found in the nucleus raphe pallidus and in the nucleus raphe pontis.

Very large serotoninergic cells, finally, were present in the nucleus raphe dorsalis only in a multipolar appearance (Fig. 20B).

These observations reveal that the seven raphe nuclei differ considerably from each other with regard to both their cytoarchitecture and the typology of their constituent serotoninergic cells. However, some similarities were observed among the four rhombencephalic raphe nuclei and the three mesencephalic raphe nuclei.

In summary, it may be stated that the raphe nuclei have two features in common: (a) their position in the midsagittal plane of the brainstem and (b) the presence of considerable numbers of serotoninergic neurons within their borders.

However, the considerable differences among these nuclei with regard to cytoarchitecture, dendritic patterns, and afferent and efferent connections render it highly unlikely that these nuclei together constitute a single functional entity.

Transmitter-Specified Cells in the Raphe Nuclei

Catecholamine-Containing Cells

It has been observed that the three mesencephalic raphe nuclei (i.e., the nucleus raphe dorsalis, the nucleus centralis superior, and the nucleus linearis oralis) contain, in addition to serotoninergic neurons, catecholaminergic elements (Table 2). In the nucleus raphe dorsalis, dopaminergic as well as noradrenergic cells have been found. Hökfelt et al. (127) described the presence of small TH-positive cell bodies in the area immediately ventral to the aqueductus cerebri. Ochi and Shimizu (216), using formaldehyde-induced fluorescence histochemistry, demonstrated the presence of medium-sized catecholaminergic neurons. Microspectrofluorometry identified the catecholamine as dopamine. These dopaminergic perikarya were situated in the midline of the ventromedial part. Nagatsu et al. (205), treating sections of unperfused tissue with antibodies to tyrosine hydroxylase or dopamine-β-hydroxylase (DBH), demonstrated dopaminergic cell bodies in the nucleus raphe dorsalis in the part just above and medial to the FLM. The cells were small to medium-sized. Grzanna and Molliver (117,118), using a homologous antibody to DBH,

demonstrated that norepinephrine immunoreactive cells are present in the lateral parts of the NRD. Yet, when we used a primarily catecholamine-directed antibody that visualizes the noradrenergic neurons of the locus ceruleus as well as the dopaminergic neural perikarya in the substantia nigra, no immunohistochemical staining was observed in the ventromedial part of the nucleus raphe dorsalis. We were able to confirm the presence of noradrenergic cells situated in the lateral part of that nucleus (287) (Fig. 28A–C). Using the antibody to TH, we were able to demonstrate the presence of dopaminergic cell bodies in the ventromedial part of the nucleus raphe dorsalis. The inability of our procedure to label these cells is probably a matter of sensitivity.

In the nucleus centralis superior, dopaminergic neurons were described by Hökfelt et al. (127), Nagatsu et al. (205), and Ochi and Shimizu (216) in the rat and recently by Wiklund et al. (337) in the cat.

In the nucleus linearis oralis, dopaminergic cell bodies have been found in the rat by Hökfelt et al. (127) and in the cat by Wiklund et al. (337). We have not been able to confirm their observations in this nucleus with our catecholamine antibody.

Intermingling of serotoninergic and catecholaminergic neurons beyond the raphe nuclei.

Two areas have been found in which serotoninergic and catecholaminergic cell bodies coincide: (a) Some serotonin-immunoreactive perikarya have been found in the locus ceruleus. This region, which is often denoted as the A6 group, contains large numbers of noradrenergic neurons (118). Similar observations have been made previously by Sladek and Walker (275), who used the FIF technique in the primate *(Macaca arctoides)* and by Léger et al. (163), who used a combined fluorescence histochemical and autoradiographic approach in the cat. However, as has already been mentioned by Sladek and Walker (275), one could argue that the small number of serotoninergic neurons situated in the locus ceruleus–subceruleus might not exert a significant influence on the noradrenergic ceruleal neurons. (b) In the region between the nucleus interpeduncularis and the lemniscus medialis, which forms part of the area tegmentalis of Tsai, serotonin immunoreactive cells have been observed. This same region is known to contain large numbers of dopaminergic neurons and is designated by Dahlström and Fuxe (69) as the A10 group.

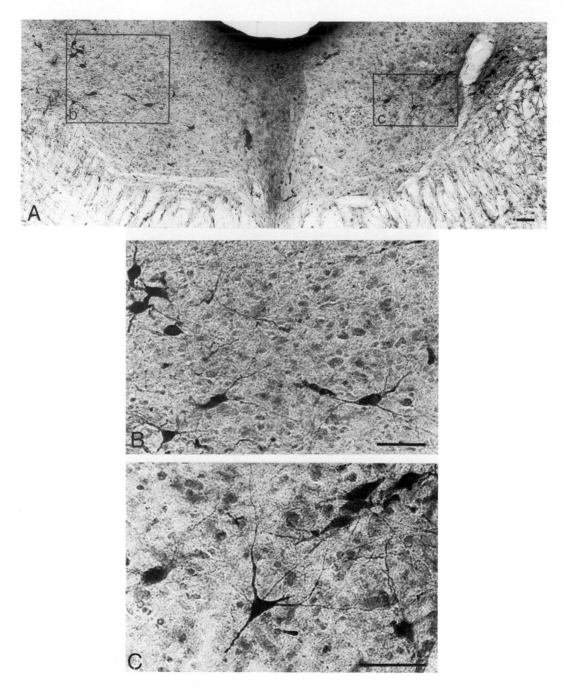

FIG. 28. Photomicrographs of a transverse, 100-μm-thick vibratome section (level P 600) through the nucleus raphe dorsalis incubated with an antibody to norepinephrine. The noradrenergic cell bodies are situated in the lateral parts of the nucleus raphe dorsalis and near the lateral corner of the periaquaductal central gray. (*Bars,* 75 μm)

Amino-Acid-Containing Cells

Six amino acids have been proposed to act as neurotransmitter candidates: GABA, glycine, glutamate, aspartate, proline, and taurine. Of these six compounds, only GABA has been demonstrated in one of the raphe nuclei (see Table 2). GABA-positive cells have been described in the nucleus raphe dorsalis by Belin et al. (23,24) and Gamrami et al. (107), using autoradiography to localize [^{3}H]GABA, by Nanopoulos et al. (208), using immunohistochemistry in combination with antibodies to glutamate decarboxylase (GAD), an enzyme involved in the synthesis of glutamate, and by Pfister et al. (234), using a modified ninhydrin reaction. Interestingly, the area containing GABA-accumulating neurons and those containing GAD-positive perikarya did not show any overlap. The former were localized caudally, whereas the GAD immunoreactive and the ninhydrin-positive cells appeared to be present in the dorsomedian and ventromedial mesencephalic part of the nucleus raphe dorsalis.

Finally, preliminary observations by J. F. Pujol and H. W. M. Steinbusch *(unpublished observations)* suggest the coexistence of GAD and serotonin in neurons of the nucleus raphe dorsalis.

Peptide-Containing Cells

From the results of Wiklund et al. (337), it is obvious that the raphe nuclei are not exclusively serotoninergic. Peptidergic neurons have been found within the confines of the nucleus raphe obscurus, the nucleus raphe pallidus, the nucleus raphe magnus, the nucleus raphe dorsalis, and in the nucleus linearis oralis. No peptide-containing cell bodies have been demonstrated within the borders of the nucleus raphe pontis and the nucleus centralis superior (Table 2).

Within the confines of the nucleus raphe obscurus, only substance P-like immunoreactive neurons have been described by Ljungdahl et al. (174). No special localization has been mentioned. In the nu-

cleus raphe pallidus and the nucleus raphe magnus, met-ENK-like immunoreactive neurons (123,311) as well as substance P-positive perikarya (62, 174) have been observed. Both cell types were randomly distributed over the two nuclei. Within the borders of the nucleus raphe dorsalis of the rat, the presence of neurons containing one of the following four neuropeptides have been observed. Enkephalin-like-containing cell bodies in the dorsal region of the bilateral wings of the nucleus have been described by Glazer et al. (111), Hökfelt et al. (123,129,131), Moss et al. (204), and Uhl et al. (311). Vasoactive intestinal polypeptide (VIP)-like-containing neurons have been localized by Lorén et al. (182) and Sims et al. (273) in the caudal and the dorsomedian parts of the nucleus raphe dorsalis. Concerning the exact number of VIP neurons in the central gray, no data are available. However, the authors stated that the VIP-containing cells in the central gray of the midbrain show a distribution similar to that of the enkephalin-positive neurons. Substance P-like immunoreactive neurons have been localized to the rostral part of the nucleus raphe dorsalis by Ljungdahl et al. (174).

Cholecystokinin octapeptide (CCK)-like immunoreactive neurons have been found by Vanderhaeghen et al. (318) in the caudal, rhombencephalic part and in the bilateral wings of the nucleus raphe dorsalis. The study of Van Der Kooy et al. (321) revealed that CCK-like immunoreactive cell bodies were situated both rostral and caudal to the serotonin-positive perikarya in the nucleus raphe dorsalis. Finally, in the nucleus linearis oralis, some CCK-containing neurons were described by Vanderhaeghen et al. (318).

Presence of Neuropeptides in Serotoninergic Neurons

In several raphe nuclei, cells containing serotonin as well as a peptide have been found (Table 3). Hökfelt et al. (130) and Chan-Palay et al. (64), although using different procedures, oberved in the

TABLE 3. *Cell bodies in raphe nuclei containing two neurotransmitters*

	Nucleus raphe obscurus	Nucleus raphe pallidus	Nucleus raphe magnus	Nucleus raphe pontis	Nucleus raphe dorsalis	Nucleus centralis superior	Nucleus linearis oralis
Serotonin + substance P (64,130)	+	+	+				
Serotonin + leu-ENK (111)			+		+		

nucleus raphe obscurus, the nucleus raphe pallidus, and the nucleus raphe magnus, numerous cell bodies containing substance P as well as serotonin. The ratio of coexistent : noncoexistent neurons has not been determined. Chan-Palay (62) postulated a concept of dynamic interrelationships between 5-HT and substance P in a single neuron. A neuron with both substances in coexistence may have fluctuating levels of one or both substances depending on parameters of time cycle and physiological demands for one or another mediator during specific types or phases of activity. Hökfelt et al. (130) pointed out that the two different compounds may either be present in different synaptic vesicles or may coexist within the same vesicles. The recent work of Pelletier et al. (233) suggested that the majority of the vesicles in the serotoninergic neurons situated in the caudal, rhombencephalic raphe area contain serotonin as well as substance P. However, no evidence has been reported as yet for a simultaneous release of both neurotransmitter candidates.

Another coexistence has been described recently by Glazer et al. (111), who demonstrated the presence of leu-ENK and serotonin in cells of the nucleus raphe magnus and in the nucleus raphe dorsalis.

Efferent Connections of the Raphe Nuclei

The efferents of the raphe nuclei can be divided into transmitter-specified and non-transmitter-specified classes.

Transmitter-Specified Connections

Of all the transmitter-defined neurons within the various raphe nuclei, relatively little is known about the efferents. Apart from serotoninergic fibers, efferents containing other neurotransmitters have been observed to originate from the raphe nuclei, e.g., substance P, thyrotropin-releasing hormone, and methionine-enkephalin. All of these fibers appeared to originate from the medullary raphe nuclear group and to descend to lower levels. They project to the dorsal and ventral horns of the spinal cord. The study of Gilbert et al. (110), who combined biochemical and immunocytochemical results, revealed that substance P and TRH are present in the same nerve terminals as serotonin in the different regions of the spinal cord. Moreover, with chemical detection techniques, it was observed that these three compounds are released simultaneously after electrical stimulation. This finding suggests that the three transmitters mentioned above are present within the same terminal.

The projections of the enkephalin-immunoreactive cells are unknown. It may, however, be mentioned that the met-ENK-positive fibers in the spinal cord do not disappear totally after a total transection of the cord (131). Moreover, Hökfelt et al. (123) found met-ENK cell bodies in the dorsal horn of the spinal cord. They considered these enkephalin-containing neurons to be local interneurons.

The areas that receive a high to very high innervation (4+) of serotonin immunoreactive fibers have been previously described by Steinbusch (284). A survey of literature focused on the correlation of these 4+ density areas with the presence of known transmitter-containing neurons in the same areas is summarized in Table 4. Some examples are shown in the diencephalon: the medial forebrain bundle (Fig. 29) and the nucleus ventralis corporis geniculati lateralis (Fig. 30). This survey revealed that serotoninergic neuron populations may influence specified transmitter-containing target neurons by direct axosomatic or axodendritic innervation. However, the data assembled in this survey have to be taken with caution and may lead to erroneous interpretations. As an example, we would like to discuss the relationships among transmitters in the nucleus suprachiasmaticus. The ventrolateral part of that nucleus receives a high to very high innervation of serotonin immunoreactive fibers. According to the work of Sofroniew (277) and L. Gross, F. van Lecuwen, H. W. M. Steinbusch (personal communication), vasopressin-positive neurons are present in the dorsomedial part of the nucleus suprachiasmaticus (Fig. 31A,B). Possibly the dendrites of the vasopressinergic cells enter the ventrolateral part of the nucleus suprachiasmaticus. But it cannot be excluded that the serotoninergic fibers do not make any synaptic contacts with the "vasopressinergic" neurons. In addition to vasopressin immunoreactive neurons, the nucleus suprachiasmaticus has also been shown to contain VIP-positive perikarya (182,273) and peptide-β-containing cell bodies (183). However, the latter authors did not describe any special distribution of these two transmitter-specified cell types within the nucleus suprachiasmaticus. Because we are not at present able to relate the various areas receiving a high or very high serotoninergic innervation specifically to one of the seven raphe nuclei, we must take all of the serotonin-positive neurons in the raphe nuclei together. The results are discussed from caudal to rostral.

The serotoninergic raphe nuclei have large efferent connections or output mechanisms to several catecholaminergic centers, viz., to the rostral part of the dopaminergic substantia nigra, pars com-

TABLE 4. Existence of transmitter-containing cell bodies in nuclei of the brain of the rat with a high to very high serotoninergic innervation[a]

	DA	NE	EP	AChE	leu-ENK	met-ENK	Peptide-β	Somato-statin	VIP	Vaso-pressin
Telecephalon										
Ventromedial part of nucleus caudatus								+		
Ventrolateral parts of nucleus accumbens								+		
Dorsolateral part of the nucleus interstitialis commissural anterioris										
Nucleus amygdaloideus basalis									+	
Nucleus amygdaloideus medialis posterior									+	
Nucleus amygdaloideus posterior									+	
Diencephalon										
Nucleus suprachiasmaticus							+		+	+
Nucleus periventricularis thalami										
Nuelcus medialis thalami, pars medialis										
Nucleus subthalamicus										
Nucleus ventromedialis hypothalami	+									
Ventral part of the nucleus mamillaris medialis				+						
Medial part of the nucleus corporis geniculati lateralis										
Mesencephalon										
Rostral part of the nucleus tractus opticus, pars medialis										
Rostral part of the substantia nigra, pars compacta	+					+				
Substantia nigra, pars lateralis						+				
Rhombencephalon										
Locus ceruleus		+								
Dorsolateral part of the nucleus reticularis pontis oralis										
Nucleus matorius nervi trigemini										
Nucleus nervi facialis			+							
Nucleus tractus spinalis nervi trigemini					+	+				
Caudal part of the nucleus tractus solitarii					+	+				
Spinal cord										
Cervical: cornu dorsale; lamina II and II, medial part of lamina VIII, which includes the nucleus commissuralis, and the nucleus ventromedialis of lamina IX						+				
Thoracic: cornu dorsale in lamina II and III, nucleus intermedio-lateralis of lamina VII						+				
Lumbar: cornu dorsale of lamina II and II, medial part of lamina VIII						+				

[a]Data from refs. 51,94,103,104,126,162,164,182,183,224,235,258,273,275,287.

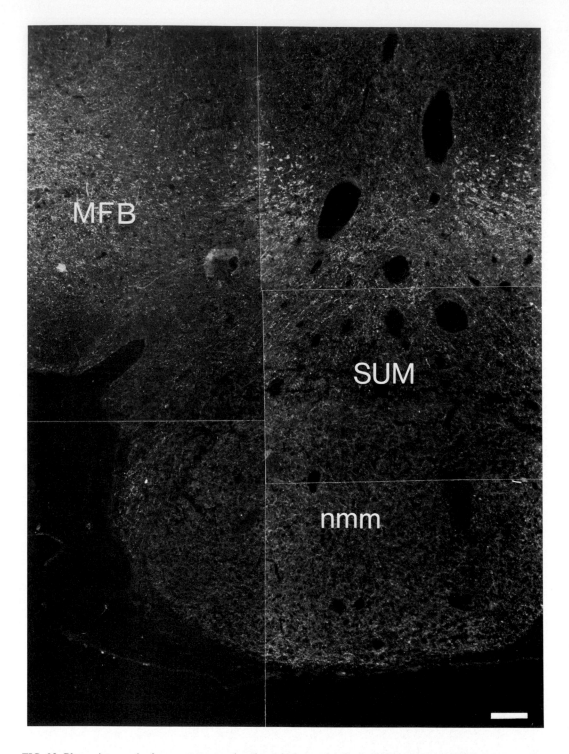

FIG. 29. Photomicrograph of a transverse section through the caudal diencephalon at level A 2600 after incubation with serotonin antiserum. A strong serotoninergic innervation is present within the medial forebrain bundle (MFB), whereas only a few fibers are seen within the nucleus mamillaris medialis (nmm). Note medial to the MFB and dorsal to the decussatio supramamillaris (SUM) fibers belonging to the ventral ascending serotoninergic bundle. (*Bar,* 75 μm)

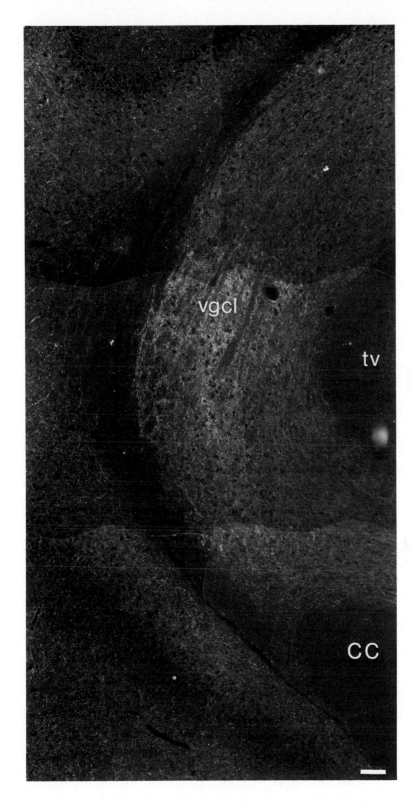

FIG. 30. Photomicrograph of a transverse section through the diencephalon at level A 2800 after incubation with serotonin antiserum. A strong serotoninergic plexus is present in the nucleus ventralis corporis geniculati lateralis (vgcl), and a few fibers are observed in the nucleus ventralis thalami (tv). The crus cerebri (CC) lacks any fibers. (*Bar*, 75 μm)

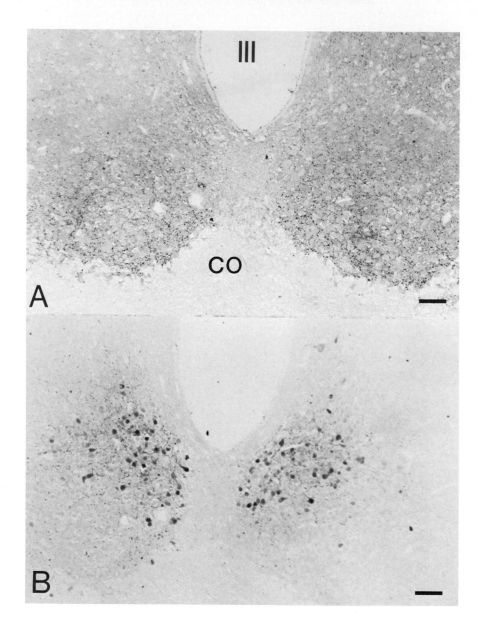

FIG. 31. Serial transverse semithin sections of the rat suprachiasmatic nucleus immunohistochemically stained with (**A**) antiserotonin and (**B**) antivasopressin serum. Note that whereas the serotonin immunoreactive perikarya are situated dorsomedially, the vasopressinergic fibers are located in the ventral part of the nucleus suprachiasmaticus (III, third ventricle; CO, chiasma opticum). (*Bars, 75 µm*) (Photomicrographs are kindly supplied by L. Gross and F. van Leeuwen.)

pacta (Fig. 23C,D), and to some hypothalamic nuclei as the nucleus ventromedialis hypothalami (104), to the noradrenergic locus ceruleus (104,163,235,275,284) and to the adrenergic cells present in the caudal part of the nucleus tractus solitarii (126). A strong serotoninergic innervation of two cholinergic centers was demonstrated, i.e.,

to the medial part of the nucleus corporis geniculati lateralis (Fig. 30), as histochemically reported by Parent (224), and to the striatum, as reported pharmacologically by Garattini et al. (108) and Samanin et al. (256) or histochemically by Parent et al. (226) (Fig. 32A,B).

In addition, we have observed 3+ to 4+ sero-

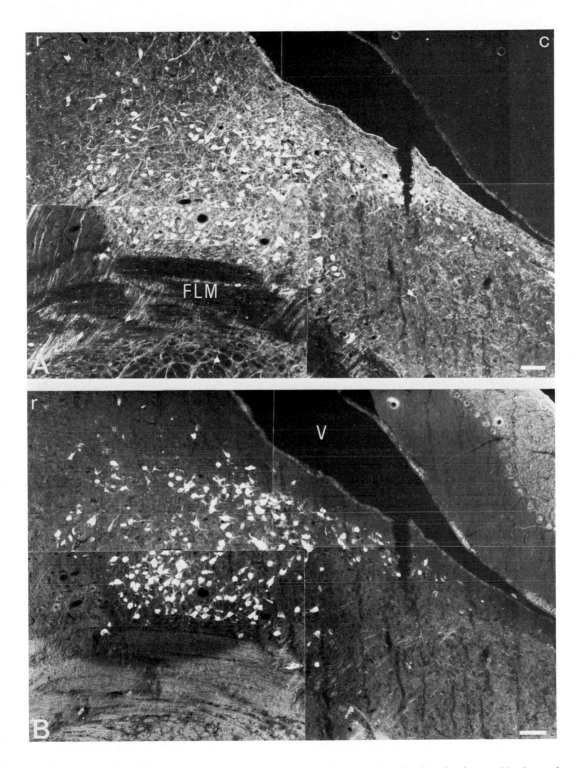

FIG. 32. Photomicrographs of the same sagittal section through the nucleus raphe dorsalis after combined use of immunofluorescent staining for serotonin and injection of propidium iodide in the caudatoputamen. **A:** Numerous serotonin-positive perikarya are seen. **B:** The same section photographed with a filter combination specific for propidium iodide, showing the cells that have efferents to the caudatoputamen complex (FLM, fasciculus longitudinalis medialis; V, ventricle). (*Bars,* 75 μm)

toninergic innervation of six peptide-specified neuron populations, i.e., leu-ENK, met-ENK, peptide-β, somatostatin, VIP, and vasopressin. Two of these, leu-ENK and met-ENK, have been visualized in the brainstem; the other four are localized in the diencephalon and the telencephalon. Taking into consideration that the nucleus raphe dorsalis, the nucleus centralis superior, and the nucleus linearis oralis have substantial ascending projections to the forebrain (69), we can state that these three mesencephalic raphe nuclei project to peptide-β-positive cells in the nucleus suprachiasmaticus (183), to somatostatinergic cells in the ventromedial part of the nucleus caudatus and the ventrolateral part of the nucleus accumbens (76,94), to VIP-containing cells in the amygdala complex (182,273), to the vasopressin immunoreactive neurons (52,281), to the LHRH-containing cells (139) through an innervation of the nucleus suprachiasmaticus, and, finally, to the CCK-positive neurons by means of an innervation of the substantia nigra, the nucleus mamillaris medialis, the tractus periventricularis thalami, the amygdala complex, the nucleus accumbens, and the nucleus caudatus (318).

In the caudal rhombencephalon and in the spinal cord, several areas containing neurons the transmitters of which are known appear to receive a dense to very dense serotoninergic innervation. Because it is known that the rhombencephalic raphe nuclei project mainly caudally (69), the dense serotoninergic terminal plexus in the following areas presumably have their parent cell bodies in these nuclei: (a) leu-ENK- as well as met-ENK-containing neurons situated in the nucleus tractus spinalis nervi trigemini and the caudal part of the nucleus tractus solitarii, (b) numerous met-ENK- and substance P-immunoreactive cell bodies as observed by Hökfelt et al. (123,129) in laminae I to IV of the cornu dorsale of the spinal cord at all levels. However, these findings are not confirmed by Sar et al. (258).

It is now possible to trace efferent connections and to determine their transmitter by a combination of immunofluorescence with retrograde transport of fluorescent tracers as has recently been described by our laboratory (287,288,323) (Fig. 32A,B). Other approaches include the use of retrograde transport of tritiated transmitters as has been mentioned by Streit et al. (294), the combination of retrograde fluorescent tracers with the FIF method (32), the anterograde transport of [^{3}H]-5-HTP (119), or immunofluorescence (131).

Finally, we would like to reemphasize that we have only discussed the areas with a high to very high serotoninergic innervation. If we assume that serotonin-related transmission or modulation can take place in all regions where we have observed serotonin-immunoreactive terminals or varicosities, it would follow that the serotoninergic elements in the raphe nuclei together have efferent connections with almost all grisea in the brain of the rat.

Transmitter-Nonspecified Efferent Connections

The ascending as well as descending projections from the raphe nuclei have been thoroughly studied with anterograde degeneration techniques (43,44,65,301), autoradiography (15,36,37,65, 201), histofluorescence combined with chemical lesions, i.e., dihydroxytryptamines (5,9,105,313), retrograde transport of HRP (146,175,189,230,271), and, finally, with the retrograde transport of fluorescent tracers (25,32,319,322). These studies have revealed the presence of ascending as well as descending axons, distributing fibers to numerous grisea, as summarized in Fig. 33.

The widespread distribution of the mesencephalic raphe projections suggest highly collateralized axon systems. For instance, single neurons in the nucleus raphe dorsalis are in a position to exert control over both ends of the massive nigrostriatal and striatonigral pathways (210). Using double labeling with fluorescent tracers, neurons were demonstrated that send collaterals to the caudate–putamen as well as to the substantia nigra (320,322). Moreover, using a triple-labeling technique, De Olmos and Heimer (218) demonstrated cells in the nucleus raphe dorsalis that project to the medial thalamus, the olfactory cortex, as well as to the septum. However, these authors showed that whereas the number of double-labeled cells in various combinations was relatively large, triple-labeled cells occur more rarely. In addition, they observed that dorsal raphe neurons have mostly ipsilateral projections and to a much smaller extent contralateral projections.

Five major efferent fiber systems from the raphe nuclei have been described: (a) the dorsal ascending or mesostriatal pathway, (b) the medial ascending pathway, (c) the ventral ascending or mesolimbic system, (d) a descending projection from the nucleus raphe dorsalis to the locus ceruleus, and (e) the descending bulbospinal pathway. In addition, three smaller pathways should be mentioned: (f) the cerebellar pathway, (g) the descending propriobulbar pathway, and (h) a pathway ascending from some caudal raphe nuclei to the dorsal part of the mesencephalon.

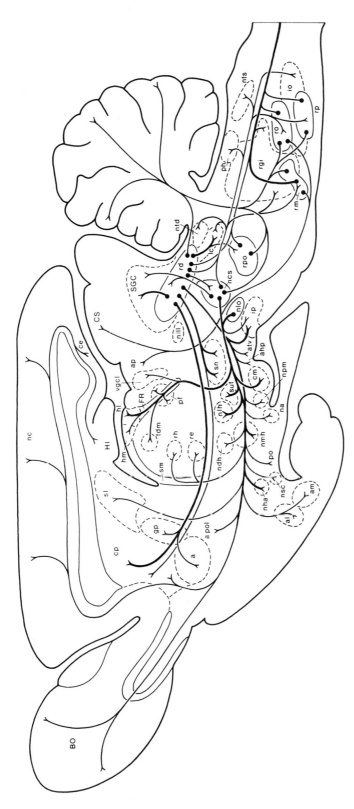

FIG. 33. Ascending and descending projections from the raphe nuclei. List of abbreviations: a, nucleus accumbens; ahp, area hypothalami posterior; al, nucleus amygdaloideus lateralis; am, nucleus amygdaloideus medialis; ap, area pretectalis; apol. area preopticus lateralis; BO, bulbus olfactorius; ce, cortex entorhinalis; cm, nucleus centromedianus thalami; cp, nucleus caudatus putamen; CS, colliculus superios; FR, fasciculus retroflexus; gp, globus pallidus; HI, hippocampus; hl, nucleus habenulae lateralis; hm, nucleus habenulae medialis; io, nucleus olivaris inferior; ip, nucleus interpeduncularis; na, nucleus arcuatus; nc, neocortex; ncs, nucleus centralis superior; ndh, nucleus dorsalis hypothalami; nf, nucleus fastiguus; nha, nucleus hypothalami anterior; nlh, nucleus lateralis hypothalami; nlo, nucleus linearis oralis; nmh, nucleus medialis hypothalami; npd, nucleus parabrachialis dorsalis; npm, nucleus premamillaris; npv, nucleus paraventricularis hypothaami; nsc, nucleus suprachiasmaticus; ntd, nucleus tegmentalis dorsalis; nts, nucleus tractus solitarius; nIII, nucleus motorius nervi oculomotorii; pf, nucleus parafascicularis; PF, cortex prefrontalis; ph, nucleus prepositus hypoglossi; po, nucleus pontis; pv, nucleus periventricularis thalami; rd, nucleus raphe dorsalis; re, nucleus reuniens; rgi, nucleus reticularis gigantocellularis; rh, nucleus rhomboideus; rm, nucleus raphe magnus; ro, nucleus raphe obscurus; rp, nucleus raphe pallidus; rpo, nucleus reticularis pontis oralis; SGC, substantia grisea centralis; sl, nucleus lateralis septi; sm, striae medialis; sn, substantia nigra; sut, nucleus subthalamicus; tdm, nucleus dorsomedialis thalami; vgcl, nucleus ventralis corporis geniculati lateralis; vm, nucleus vestibularis medialis.

The dorsal ascending pathway arises from the medial and rostral parts of the nucleus raphe dorsalis. Its fibers do not enter the medial forebrain bundle but are situated dorsolaterally to that bundle. The main area of termination of this pathway is the caudatoputamen complex, although some fibers reach the nucleus accumbens and the globus pallidus. No fibers enter the substantia nigra (75, 137,147,196,250,259,287,288,298,299,319,322).

The medial ascending pathway originates from the nucleus raphe dorsalis and projects mainly to the substantia nigra (37,80,92,222,228). However, the parent neurons of this projection have been found to send collaterals to the caudatoputamen complex (320).

The ventral ascending pathway arises from the three mesencephalic raphe nuclei. Its fibers are directed ventrolaterally (Fig. 29) and then curve rostrally to course through the ventral tegmentum, after which the medial forebrain bundle in the lateral hypothalamus is entered (65). In the mesencephalon, the bundle distributes many fibers to the nucleus interpeduncularis and some to the area tegmentalis ventralis. The major input to the nucleus interpeduncularis comes from the nucleus raphe dorsalis; some fibers originate, however, from the nucleus centralis superior. The input to the area tegmentalis ventralis arises mainly from the nucleus centralis superior (38). Before entering the medial forebrain bundle (MFB), some fibers originating from the nucleus raphe dorsalis innervate the posterior hypothalamic area. Rostrally, fibers leave the MFB to enter the fasciculus retroflexus and to distribute to the nucleus parafascicularis, the nucleus dorsomedialis thalami, the nucleus medialis habenulae, and the corpus geniculatum laterale (36,65). The major component of this fiber contingent terminates in the nucleus lateralis habenulae (227). Further rostrally, fibers leave the MFB to enter the corpus mamillare, the nucleus subthalamicus (65), the nucleus preopticus (229), the nucleus lateralis hypothalami, the nucleus arcuatus, the nucleus medialis hypothalami, the nucleus hypothalamicus anterior (317), the nucleus suprachiasmaticus (8), the septum, the bulbus olfactorius (10) by way of the striae medullares, the nucleus reuniens, and the nucleus rhomboideus (147,282) and the amygdala complex by means of the striae terminalis (137,227,326).

A minor input to the head of the nucleus caudatus has been observed by Sato et al. (259). Finally, some fibers were demonstrated that travel via the cingulum bundle (65), reaching the prefrontal, frontal, neo-, entorhinal, and hippocampal cortex (11–13,65,109,137,147,175,230,231,267, 282,304,307). The study of Pasquier et al. (229), who combined lesion experiments with quantitative spectrofluorometry for serotonin in the cat, demonstrated that the projection from the nucleus centralis superior to the preoptic area and the amygdala is stronger than the one arising from nucleus raphe dorsalis.

A major descending projection has been described from the nucleus raphe dorsalis to the locus ceruleus (58,202,222,255). Some of these fibers continue to the nucleus tegmentalis dorsalis (Gudden) and to the nucleus raphe pontis (254).

The descending bulbospinal pathway mainly arises from the nucleus raphe magnus. During its course, the bundle receives fibers from the nucleus raphe dorsalis, the nucleus raphe pontis, the nucleus raphe obscurus, and the nucleus raphe pallidus (19,32,57,151,158,165,189,192,306,327). This pathway runs principally in the dorsolateral funiculus to innervate the substantia gelatinosa, i.e., laminae I, II, V, and VI (18,19,93), whereas fibers from the nucleus raphe pallidus and the nucleus raphe obscurus descend in the lateral and ventral funiculi to terminate in the ventral horn (189). Bobillier et al. (37) suggested that the medullary raphe nuclei should be considered collectively as an extension of the limbic system, modulating sensory input and both somatic and autonomic output by way of raphe–spinal projections.

The fibers of the cerebellar pathway emerge from the nucleus raphe dorsalis, the nucleus centralis superior, the nucleus raphe pontis, the nucleus raphe magnus, the nucleus raphe obscurus, and the nucleus raphe pallidus and pass via the pedunculus cerebellaris medius to the cerebellum, where they distribute to the cortex (271). Some fibers originating from the caudal part of the nucleus raphe dorsalis innervate the flocculus (146).

The descending propriobulbar pathway consists of fibers passing from the nucleus raphe dorsalis and the nucleus centralis superior to the nucleus raphe magnus, the nucleus paragigantocellularis, the nucleus prepositus hypoglossi, the nucleus parvocellularis, the nucleus tractus solitarii, the nucleus raphe obscurus, the nucleus raphe pallidus, and the oliva inferior.

A pathway ascending from some caudal raphe nuclei to the mesencephalon arises from the nucleus raphe obscurus and the nucleus raphe magnus and terminates in the colliculum superior and in the pretectal area.

If we compare the results obtained by non-transmitter-specifying techniques (axon degeneration, autoradiography) with the one revealing the serotoninergic raphe efferents, one remarkable discrepancy appears, and that is that the fasciculus retroflexus and the striae medullaris, which do contain labeling following tritiated amino acid injections in the mesencephalic raphe nuclei, do not contain any serotoninergic fibers.

The areas that are in conformity with each other regarding the efferent non-transmitter-specified projections and the serotonin immunoreactivity are, from caudal to rostral, the nucleus tractus solitarii, the locus ceruleus, the nucleus raphe dorsalis, the substantia nigra, the nucleus subthalamicus, the nucleus corpus geniculatum laterale, the nucleus suprachiasmaticus, the nucleus amygdaloideus posterior, the nucleus accumbens, and the caudate–putamen complex. Areas that receive a very high serotonin innervation but where no connection with the raphe system has been demonstrated, using the classic neuroanatomical techniques, are the following: the nucleus nervi fascialis, the nucleus motorius nervi trigemini, the nucleus reticularis pontis oralis, the nucleus tractus opticus, pars medialis, the nucleus mamillaris medialis, the nucleus ventromedialis hypothalami, the nucleus periventricularis thalami, the nucleus amygdaloideus medialis posterior, the nucleus amygdaloideus basalis, and the nucleus interstitialis commissurae anterioris. All other areas in the CNS receive to a greater or lesser extent (3+ to 1+) serotoninergic innervation. These findings imply that the raphe nuclei have projections that are more extensive than was once thought.

In addition to the areas that receive a serotoninergic innervation from 4+ to 1+, there were only a small number of regions that show no serotonin immunoreactivity. These areas consist of coarse, well-myelinated fiber tracts, viz., cranial nerves, pedunculus cerebellaris inferior and medius, tractus corticospinalis (Figs. 14A,C; 15; and 16B), tractus olivocerebellaris, lemniscus lateralis, fasciculus mamillotegmentalis, commissura posterior and anterior, tractus opticus, fornix (Fig. 24C), chiasma opticum, corpus callosum, ansa lenticularis, and the capsula interna and externa.

The Dendritic Pattern of Serotoninergic Raphe Cells

Although immunofluorescence and autoradiography have already contributed to a comprehensive knowledge of the distribution of serotoninergic perikarya and their fibers and terminals, little is known about their dendrites. This is an important deficit, because it is the size, shape, and orientation of the dendrites of a neuron that determine the territory from which it can receive its input. For this reason, it would be extremely informative to analyze the dendritic pattern of serotoninergic neurons. The latter has been recently attempted by Felten and Harrigan (90), combining results achieved with the FIF and Golgi techniques. However, their study did not reveal whether the dendritic trees of serotoninergic neurons differ from those of nonserotoninergic neurons in the raphe nuclei. To study specifically the dendritic arborization of serotoninergic neurons in the seven raphe nuclei, we applied an immunohistochemical technique to visualize these neurons in 100-μm-thick vibratome sections of adult rats. This approach explicitly demonstrates serotonin immunoreactive neurons in their entirety, thus yielding a transmitter-specific Golgi-like image.

The serotoninergic neurons within the raphe nuclei can be considered to belong to the category of leptodendritic cells (242,243). The leptodendritic neurons are characterized by the presence of only a few, although relatively long, dendrites arising from a fusiform perikaryon.

The results obtained with our immunohistochemical technique revealed that the various raphe nuclei differ with respect to the appearance and orientation of their serotoninergic dendrites; i.e., each nucleus displays a typical and characteristic dendritic pattern. Possible relationships with other transmitter-specified systems have been found in the nucleus raphe magnus and in the lateral parts of the nucleus raphe dorsalis, where the dendrites of the serotonin immunoreactive cells radiate in areas with a large number of enkephalin-like (123,258,311) and substance P-like-containing neurons (129,174).

The function of the dendritic serotonin is at present unclear. It was observed by Joh et al. (140), using immunohistochemistry in combination with antibodies to tryptophan hydroxylase, that at the light microscopic level the dendrites of raphe neurons were TrH positive and that at the electron microscopic level the enzyme within the dendrite was primarily associated with subcellular organelles having the characteristics of microtubules. Ultrastructurally, Pickel et al. (235), using the immunohistochemical visualization of TH, DBH, and TrH, showed that these three monoaminergic enzymes are distributed in an almost identical way. These findings suggest that the enzyme TrH may be transported from sites of synthesis in the cell body to the dendrite. However, the presence of serotonin and its synthetizing enzyme in the dendrites does not necessarily imply a release of the transmitter in these areas. It is known that neurons in the substantia nigra interact by means of dendrodendritic junctions and that dopamine is involved in this transmission (30), but corresponding contacts among dendrites of serotoninergic elements have not been described so far.

Scheibel and Scheibel (261) reported in an electron microscopic study the close association of raphe neurons with blood vessels. However, as already pointed out above, especially in the caudal raphe nuclei, only a small percentage of the total neurons contain serotonin. Cummings and Felten (67) reported the attachment of serotoninergic dendrites to blood capillaries or to tanycytes. Their light microscopic study was, however, based on Golgi and histofluorescence material and thus cannot give evidence for actual release from or uptake into serotoninergic dendrites. No synaptic contacts have been described for these dendrovascular relationships. This could point to a chemoreceptor function of these transmitter-specified dendrites.

Finally, the observation that dendrites may form bundles deserves some comments. The existence of dendritic bundles was established by Scheibel and Scheibel (260) in a study of the lumbosacral spinal cord of the cat and the monkey. Later, corresponding structures were described in the reticular formation by Scheibel and Scheibel (261). Dendritic bundles are groupings of dendrites that course along very closely together, i.e., from 1 μm apart to direct membrane opposition. However, no direct ultrastructural evidence has been obtained that within these bundles dendrodendritic contacts are present. Although Roney et al. (248) stated that they are a general feature in the mammalian brain, nevertheless, we have found no evidence of dendritic bundles other than the monoaminergic ones mentioned above. No amino acid- or peptide-positive dendrite bundling has been demonstrated.

Afferent Connections to the Raphe Nuclei

The studies focused on the afferents to the raphe have been divided into transmitter-specified and non-transmitter-specified cases. A summary of these afferent systems is presented for the four rhombencephalic raphe nuclei in Fig. 34 and for the three mesencephalic raphe nuclei in Fig. 35.

Transmitter-Specified Connections

For our description of the transmitter-specified afferents to the raphe nuclei, we have only used results based on immunocytochemistry. It is noteworthy that the presence of amines, amino acids, and peptides in the raphe areas has been detected with biochemical techniques. However, because of the punch technique, it is not possible to relate the biochemical measurements thus obtained precisely to the defined raphe nuclei. Despite this shortcoming, the method gives us additional information about the presence of various neuroactive compounds. A close correlation has been observed among biochemistry, immunocytochemistry, and autoradiography for VIP by Lorén et al. (182) and for GABA by Bélin et al. (23) and Taniyama et al. (302). In addition, there are several neuroactive compounds that have only been detected by biochemical means, e.g., acetylcholine (5–12 pmole/μg protein) in all raphe nuclei by Kobayashi et al. (152), glutamate (5–9 mg/kg body wt), and aspartate (3 mg/kg body wt) in both the nucleus raphe dorsalis and the nucleus centralis superior by Taniyama et al. (302).

Within the raphe nuclei, several transmitter-specified fibers and terminals have been described. A summary of the literature is presented in Table 5. However, until now, no systematic attempt has been made to detect the cells of origin of these fibers and terminals. Combining immunofluorescence with retrograde transport of fluorescent tracers, a technique that has recently been described by Steinbusch et al. (287,288) and Van Der Kooy and Steinbusch (323), or lesion experiments could solve this matter.

Three kinds of monoaminergic fibers have been demonstrated in all seven raphe nuclei: serotoninergic, noradrenergic, and adrenergic. Serotonin immunoreactive fibers and terminals have been recently described by Steinbusch (284). These fibers could play a role in local circuitry within these nuclei or in connecting the raphe nuclei with each other. Fuxe et al. (102), using the FIF method, observed a high degree of noradrenergic innervation of the 5-HT-positive cell bodies in all raphe nuclei, with heaviest concentrations in the nucleus raphe dorsalis. These afferents have been demonstrated by histofluorescence, with immunocytochemistry (118), and biochemically (170). However, the appearance of some fibers within an area containing serotoninergic perikarya does not necessarily imply a direct input. Since the nucleus raphe dorsalis contains serotoninergic as well as nonserotoninergic cell bodies, the noradrenergic afferents may regulate 5-HT cells directly or indirectly. The study of Baraban and Aghajanian (16), using a combination of electron microscopic autoradiography and degeneration, adduced evidence that 67% of the noradrenergic terminals make a synaptic contact with serotoninergic neurons in the nucleus raphe dorsalis. Finally, using an antibody to

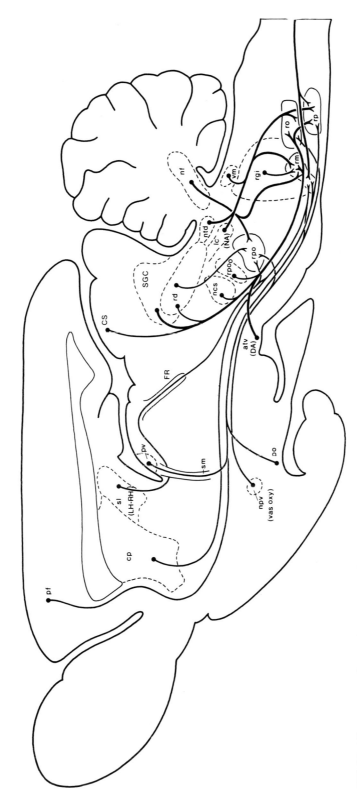

FIG. 34. Afferent connections to the rhombencephalic raphe nuclei. Included are the transmitter-specified afferents (LHRH; vas, vasopressin; oxy, oxytocin; DA, dopamine; NA, norepinephrine). For abbreviations, see Fig. 33.

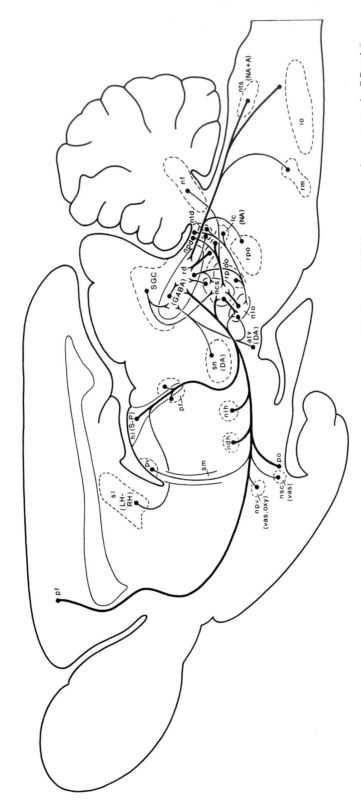

FIG. 35. Afferent connections to the mesencephalic raphe nuclei. Included are the transmitter-specified afferents (LHRH; vas, vasopressin; oxy: oxytocin; S-P, substance P; DA, dopamine; NA, norepinephrine; A, epinephrine; GABA). For abbreviations, see Fig. 33.

TABLE 5. *Transmitter-specified fibers and terminals within the raphe nuclei*

	Nucleus raphe obscurus	Nucleus raphe pallidus	Nucleus raphe magnus	Nucleus raphe pontis	Nucleus raphe dorsalis	Nucleus centralis superior	Nucleus linearis oralis
Serotonin (100,284)	+	+	+	+	+	+	+
Dopamine (100,127)	+	+	+		+	+	+
Norepinephrine (100)	+	+	+	+	+	+	+
Epinephrine (104,126)	+	+	+	+	+	+	+
ACTA (232,277,331)					+		
GABA (23)					+		
APP (134)			+				
CCK (318)			+		+		
β-Endorphin (34)					+		
LHRH (139)			+	+	+	+	+
β-Lipotropin (330)			+		+	+	+
leu-ENK (83,258)		+		+	+	+	
met-ENK (123,258,311)		+		+	+	+	
α-MSH (81,136,328)					+		
γ-MSH (35)					+		
Neurotensin (312)					+	+	+
Oxytocin (51,52,278,281)	+		+	+	+	+	
Vasopressin (51,52,278,281)	+		+	+	+	+	
Substance P (174)	+	+	+	+	+	+	+
VIP (103,182,273)	+				+		

PNMT (see Fig. 1), Hökfelt et al. (126) and Fuxe et al. (104) discovered that epinephrine-positive nerve terminals participate in the innervation of the serotonin-containing cell bodies within the raphe nuclei, suggesting that the raphe nuclei are controlled by both norepinephrine and epinephrine nerve terminals. Besides these three monoaminergic fiber types within the various raphe nuclei, fibers containing numerous other amino acids or peptides have been visualized within the borders of the raphe nuclei, including GABA, ACTH, APP, CCK, β-endorphin, LHRH, β-lipotropin, leu-ENK, met-ENK, α-MSH, γ-MSH, neurotensin, oxytocin, substance P, vasopressin, and vasoactive intestinal polypeptide.

Nucleus raphe obscurus.

Fuxe (100) observed that in this nucleus some dopaminergic fibers occur. Besides the four types of monoaminergic fibers, a moderate density of vasoactive intestinal polypeptide (VIP)-positive fibers were seen by Fuxe et al. (103). However, Lorén et al. (182) and Sims et al. (273) were not able to confirm this finding. Ljungdahl et al. (174) described the presence of a low density of substance P-like immunoreactive fibers in the medial part of this nucleus. Sofroniew and Weindl (281) presented evidence indicating that a few oxytocin- and vasopressin-containing fibers originating from the nucleus paraventricularis terminate in the nucleus raphe obscurus (Fig. 36A,B).

Nucleus raphe pallidus.

Within the confines of the nucleus raphe pallidus, some dopaminergic fibers were described by Fuxe (100). Recent electron microscopic work by Miyakawa and Usui (198) revealed that the catecholaminergic axon terminals in the nucleus were at most 5% of all of the terminals of the neuropil of this region. In addition, leu-ENK-containing fibers were observed in the nucleus raphe pallidus by Sar et al. (258), and met-ENK-positive fibers by Hökfelt et al. (123) and Sar et al. (258); however, Uhl et al. (311), using an antiserum that stains leu-ENK as well as met-ENK, were not able to confirm their findings. This could be because of lower sensitivity of the antibody used by the latter authors. Ljungdahl et al. (174) described a sparse innervation with substance P immunoreactive fibers in the medial part of the nucleus raphe pallidus.

Nucleus raphe magnus.

Within the area of this nucleus, dopaminergic fibers were demonstrated by Fuxe (100) in addition to fibers containing the three other monoamines. A medium density of substance P-like immunoreactive fibers was demonstrated in the nucleus raphe magnus by Ljungdahl et al. (174). The presence of β-lipotropin-positive fibers has been reported by Watson et al. (330). Cholecystokinin-containing fibers are present, according to the work of Vanderhaeghen et al. (318). Jennes and Stumpf (139) reported the presence of LHRH fibers, which arise

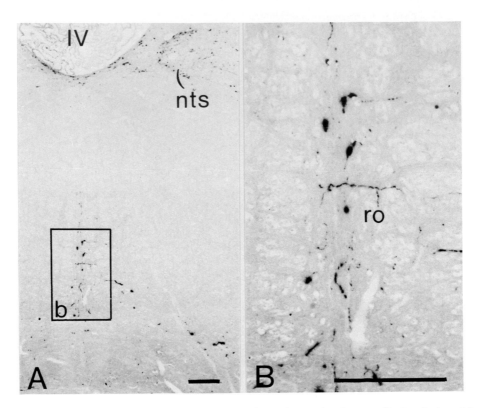

FIG. 36. Photomicrographs of a transverse section through the nucleus raphe obscurus after incubation with neuro-physin antiserum. Neurophysin-like immunoreactive fibers are demonstrated in the nucleus raphe obscurus (ro), the nucleus tractus solitarius (nts), and in the griseum centralis. Some fibers are even distributed close to the fourth ventricle (*Bar*, 75 μm) (Photomicrographs are reproduced by courtesy of M. V. Sofroniew.)

from the septum and continue through the fasciculus retroflexus then caudally along the ventral border of the nucleus interpeduncularis to terminate in the nucleus raphe magnus. The study of Sofroniew and Weindl (281) indicates that in the rat the nucleus contains a low density of vasopressinergic fibers arising from the nucleus paraventricularis and a medium density of oxytocin-containing fibers, also originating from the nucleus paraventricularis. However, these results could not be confirmed by Buys (52).

Nucleus raphe pontis.

Besides containing the three monoamines mentioned above, fibers containing the following six peptides have been demonstrated in the nucleus raphe pontis: LHRH fibers originating from the septum (139), leu-ENK-positive fibers as demonstrated by Elde et al. (83) and Sar et al. (258), met-ENK immunoreactive fibers as visualized by Hökfelt et al. (123) and Sar et al. (258) and con-

firmed by Uhl et al. (311) using an antibody that stains leu-ENK as well as met-ENK, a low density of substance P-like immunoreactive fibers as demonstrated by Ljungdahl et al. (174) in the rostral and medial part of the nucleus (the caudal part receives only single fibers), and, finally, a few vasopressin- and oxytocin-containing fibers, both originating from the nucleus paraventricularis, as those localized by Sofroniew and Weindl (281). Buys (52) remained unable to confirm these findings.

Nucleus raphe dorsalis.

The medium to high serotonergic innervation of this nucleus, according to Mosko et al. (203), originates partly from neurons within the nucleus itself. Dopaminergic and/or noradrenergic fibers have been described by Hökfelt et al. (127) using an antibody to tyrosine hydroxylase. The varicose appearance of these fibers was observed in the midline (Fig. 28A). In the nucleus raphe dorsalis, the presence of a particularly large number of peptides has been demonstrated: leu-ENK fibers have been described by Elde et al. (83) and Sar et al.(258); met-ENK-containing fibers have been visualized by Hökfelt et al. (123) and Sar et al. (258). Uhl et al. (311) confirmed their results using an antibody that stains both leu-ENK and met-ENK. Dubé et al. (81), Jacobowitz and O'Donohue (136), and Watson and Akil (328) adduced evidence for the presence of α-MSH immunoreactive fibers in the nucleus. Bloom et al. (34) demonstrated a low to medium innervation of it with β-endorphin-positive fibers. The same author reported in 1980 the existence of a low reactivity of γ-MSH-positive fibers in the same area.

Ljungdahl et al. (174) showed a medium density of substance P-like immunoreactive fibers. According to the work of Neckers et al. (211), these peptidergic fibers originate from the nucleus habenularis medialis. The study of Ljungdahl et al. (174) showed that in the latter area, indeed, a high pro-

portion of substance P-like immunoreactive neurons was present. A moderate innervation with VIP-positive fibers was mentioned in the studies of Lorén et al. (182) and Sims et al. (273). In the earlier work of Fuxe et al. (101,103), these fibers were not described. Pelletier and Leclerc (232), Sofroniew (277), and Watson et al. (331) visualized a large number of ACTH-containing fibers in this region (Fig. 37A,B). The presence of CCK-positive fibers was reported by Vanderhaeghen (318). Uhl et al. (312) mentioned the presence of neurotensin immunoreactive fibers. Watson et al. (330) adduced evidence for the presence of β-lipotropin-positive fibers. The study of Sofroniew (278) and Sofroniew and Weindl (280,281) revealed that the nucleus under discussion receives a low innervation of vasopressinergic fibers originating from the nucleus suprachiasmaticus. In addition, a few vasopressin- and oxytocin-positive fibers arising from the nucleus paraventricularis were observed (Fig.

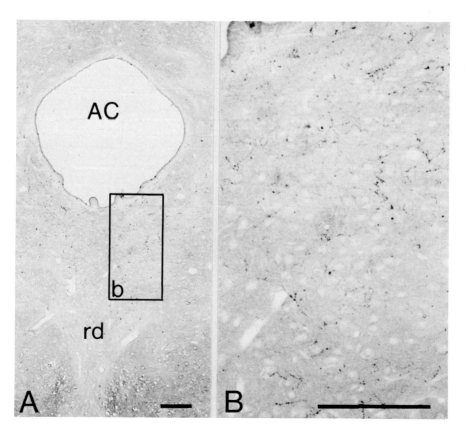

FIG. 37. Transverse section through the nucleus raphe dorsalis after incubation with ACTH antiserum; ACTH-like immunoreactive fibers are demonstrated in the nucleus raphe dorsalis (rd) and in the periaquaductal central gray. (*Bars,* 75 μm) (Photomicrographs are reproduced by courtesy of M. W. Sofroniew.)

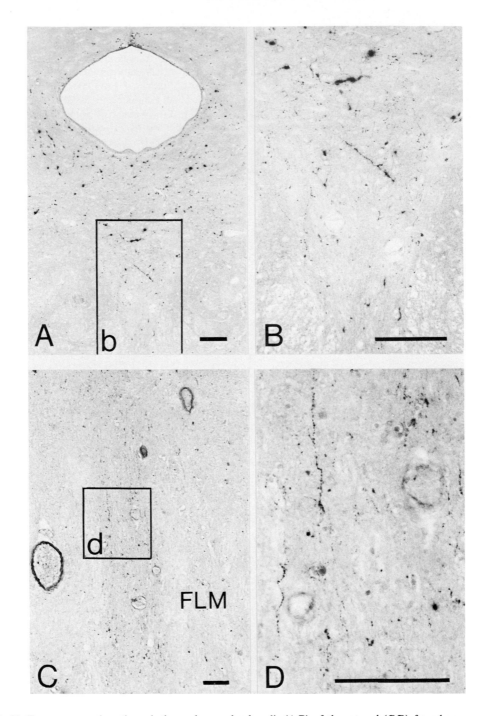

FIG. 38. Transverse sections through the nucleus raphe dorsalis (**A,B**) of the rat and (**C,D**) from human material after immunohistochemistry with neurophysin antiserum. **A, B:** Neurophysin-like immunoreactive fibers are shown in the nucleus raphe dorsalis (**B**) and in the periaqueductal central gray. **C,D:** Neurophysin-positive fibers have also been visualized in the human nucleus raphe dorsalis. (*Bars,* 75 μm) (Photomicrographs are reproduced by courtesy of M. V. Sofroniew.)

38A–D). These results are in conformity with work of Buys (51).

Belin et al. (23), using autoradiography, mentioned the presence of GABA-labeled fibers throughout the whole nucleus. However, according to the work of Forchetti and Meek (95), who measured the 5-HT turnover biochemically, the GABAergic influences might be from afferents arising outside the raphe; for example, a GABAergic habenuloraphe tract was proposed (4) but was not confirmed (113). Alternatively, GABA interneurons in the nucleus raphe dorsalis might mediate extrinsic influences on serotoninergic cells. Finally, Jennes and Stumpf (139) found that LHRH-positive fibers originating from the septum terminate in the nucleus raphe dorsalis.

Nucleus centralis superior.

Massari et al. (191) reported on the basis of lesion experiments that the nucleus centralis superior receives a strong input from noradrenergic as well as adrenergic fibers. These fibers appeared to originate partly from the A1 and A2 groups according to the designations of Dahlström and Fuxe (69) and partly from the locus ceruleus. Hökfelt et al. (127) reported the presence of TH-positive fibers in the nucleus centralis superior. Such fibers may be dopaminergic, noradrenergic, or adrenergic. However, in earlier studies, Hökfelt et al. (126) remained unable to observe any PNMT-positive terminals in this nucleus. Thus, it may be stated that the results of Hökfelt et al. (126) tally only partially with those of Massari et al. (191).

Eight peptide-specific afferents to the nucleus centralis superior have been described: LHRH-positive fibers with their cell bodies situated in the septum were found by Jennes and Stumpf (139); Watson et al. (330) visualized β-lipotropin-containing fibers; leu-ENK and met-ENK immunoreactive fibers and terminals were observed by Sar et al. (258); Uhl et al. (311) showed the presence of neurotensin-positive fibers; oxytocin- and vasopressin-containing fibers were mentioned by Buys (51,52), Sofroniew (278), and Sofroniew and Weindl (280,281); Ljungdahl et al. (174) reported a medium density of substance P-like immunoreactive fibers in the nucleus. However, according to the study of Neckers et al. (211), these substance P-positive fibers, in contrast with those terminating in the nucleus raphe dorsalis, do not originate from the habenular nuclei.

Nucleus linearis oralis.

Besides the 5-HT-, NE-, and EP-positive fibers within the borders of this nucleus (Fig. 21C), the presence of dopaminergic fibers was mentioned by Hökfelt et al. (127). The presence of a number of peptides has been reported for the nucleus linearis oralis. A high density of substance P-positive fibers has been described by Ljungdahl et al. (174). Uhl et al. (312) described neurotensin containing fibers. The existence of β-lipotropin fibers was mentioned by Watson et al. (330). Uhl et al. (311) localized enkephalin fibers; however, this finding is not in accordance with the work of Hökfelt et al. (123) and Sar et al. (258). The study of Vanderhaeghen et al. (318) showed the presence of CCK immunoreactive fibers in the nucleus. Finally LHRH-positive fibers, arising from the septum, were recently observed by Jennes and Stumpf (139).

Non-Transmitter-Specified Connections

The afferents to the raphe nuclei have been investigated with axon degeneration techniques and with the retrograde tracer technique using HRP (45,106,203,253,255,314). The results are discussed separately for the various raphe nuclei (Figs. 28,32).

The nucleus raphe pallidus receives a prominent input from the substantia grisea centralis, the area tegmentalis ventralis, and the nucleus tegmentalis dorsalis (106). Other afferents arise from (a) spinal cord neurons (45), (b) the nucleus vestibularis medialis, the nucleus reticularis pontis oralis, the colliculi superioris and inferioris (106), (c) the nucleus raphe dorsalis, the nucleus centralis superior, the preoptic region, and the prefrontal cortex (45).

The nucleus raphe obscurus receives a substantial number of afferent fibers from the substantia grisea centralis, the area tegmentalis ventralis, and the dorsal tegmental region (106). In addition, some afferents originate from the colliculus superior and inferior, the nucleus reticularis pontis oralis, the nucleus venstibularis medialis, the nucleus raphe dorsalis, and the nucleus centralis superior (106).

The nucleus raphe magnus receives three major and four minor projections. A major ascending projection comes from spinal cord neurons (45). According to these authors, the number of fibers coming from lumbar and sacral segments is apparently small. Another major input is derived from the fastigial nucleus in the cerebellum and the nucleus tegmentalis dorsalis of Gudden (45). This projection also receives some fibers from the nucleus vestibularis medialis (106). Finally, the third major afferent projection to the nucleus raphe magnus consists of fibers descending from the area tegmentalis ventralis (106,270) and the substantia grisea centralis. This projection receives, in addition, some fibers from the colliculus superior and inferior and the nucleus reticularis pontis oralis (106).

Minor afferent projections to the nucleus raphe magnus originate from (a) the nucleus raphe dorsalis and the nucleus centralis superior, (b) the nucleus paragigantocellularis, (c) the prefrontal cortex (45) and preoptic region, and (d) the head of the caudatoputamen. The latter projection has been described by Usunoff et al. (314). According to these authors, the nucleus raphe magnus is the only nucleus of the raphe complex showing degenerating fibers following a selective lesion in the caudatoputamen.

The nucleus raphe pontis receives a major and a minor input. The major input arises from the fastigial nucleus (45). A smaller projection to this nucleus originates from the nucleus raphe dorsalis.

The nucleus raphe dorsalis receives a major ascending projection from the rostral part of the nucleus tractus solitarii (4). In addition, a major input from the nucleus habenulae lateralis has been reported. This projection also receives some fibers from the nucleus parafascicularis (4,227–229, 253). Another major source of fibers terminating in the nucleus raphe dorsalis is the prefrontal cortex and the hippocampus (209). These fibers reach the nucleus raphe dorsalis by way of the medial forebrain bundle. Other fibers that also reach the nucleus raphe dorsalis via the medial forebrain bundle originate from the nucleus dorsalis and lateralis hypothalami and from the preoptic region (4,255).

Finally, a considerable number of afferent fibers to the nucleus have been found to originate from the area dorsolateral to the inferior olivary complex (253). This same area has been designated by Dahlström and Fuxe (69) as the noradrenergic A3 region.

Smaller projections to the dorsal raphe have been observed starting from the area tegmentalis ventralis (255), the substantia nigra (4,228,253), the substantia grisea centralis (253), the nucleus tegmentalis dorsalis (253,255), the locus ceruleus–subceruleus and nucleus tractus solitarii (4,254,255), the nucleus centralis superior (4,203), the nucleus raphe magnus (253,255), and the nucleus raphe pontis and linearis oralis (203, 253,255).

Finally, Mosko et al. (203) observed some HRP-labeled cells in the nucleus raphe dorsalis after injection of HRP into the nucleus raphe dorsalis.

The nucleus centralis superior receives its most prominent input from the nucleus habenulae lateralis, the nucleus parafascicularis (4,229,255), the nucleus linearis oralis (4,255), and the prefrontal cortex. In addition, some fibers originating from the nucleus dorsalis and lateralis hypothalami and the preoptic region enter the medial forebrain bundle and terminate in the nucleus centralis superior (255). Some other fibers terminating in this nucleus are derived from the nucleus periventricularis, the nucleus raphe dorsalis, the substantia grisea centralis (255), the fastigial nucleus (45), the nucleus parabrachialis dorsalis, locus ceruleus and subceruleus (255), and the nucleus tractus solitarii (4).

The nucleus linearis oralis receives most of its afferent fibers from the adjacent nucleus centralis superior. Moreover, several other areas have been observed to give rise to afferents to this nucleus; these include the nucleus raphe dorsalis (255), the nucleus tegmentalis dorsalis, the nucleus parabrachialis dorsalis, the locus ceruleus and subceruleus, the nucleus reticularis pontis oralis, the substantia grisea centralis, the nucleus dorsalis and lateralis hypothalami, and the nucleus habenulae lateralis (255).

The Relationship Between the Raphe Nuclei and the Reticular Formation

The central parts of the brainstem are occupied by cell populations of diverse morphology enmeshed in a complex network of axons which branches in all directions. In this section, we discuss the topography and fiber connections of the grisea present in the central core of the brainstem, with emphasis on the transmitter-specified cell groups.

Topography

The architecture of the central parts of the brainstem and the morphology of its neurons have previously been studied with Nissl, Golgi, and silver stains (43,316). Because of the highly reticular structure, discrete sets of neurons and fiber pathways are not readily delineated by means of these classic neurohistological methods. The term reticular formation refers to the fact that the dendrites of the cells in this area are arranged in bundles that together form a net-like pattern. The reticular formation can be divided in three longitudinal zones: (a) a median zone, which comprises the raphe nuclei, (b) a medial zone, which contains many large cells, and (c) a lateral zone. The median zone, including the raphe nuclei, has been discussed in previous sections.

The medial zone can be subdivided into three areas according to their caudorostral localization: the medullary medial reticular formation, comprising the nucleus reticularis gigantocellularis and the nucleus reticularis paramedianus, the pontine medial reticular formation, consisting of the nucleus reticularis pontis caudalis and the nucleus reticularis pontis oralis, and the tegmental medial reticular formation, including the nucleus reticularis tegmenti pontis and the nucleus cuneiformis.

The lateral zone of the reticular formation can also be divided into three areas: the medullary lateral area, comprising the nucleus reticularis medullae oblongatae, pars dorsalis and ventralis, the pontine lateral area, containing the nucleus reticularis parvocellularis, and the lateral tegmental reticular formation.

Transmitter-Specified Cells in the Reticular Formation

Immunocytochemistry provides us with a tool to characterize neurons on the basis of their chemical individuality and by that to classify them in morphologically and chemically distinct groups.

First, we observed a substantial number of serotoninergic neurons interspersed through the medial and lateral parts of the reticular formation. Moreover, these observations showed us that these serotonin-containing cells do not constitute recognizable cytoarchitectonic subunits (Figs. 14A,C,D; 15; 16A; 18C; and 21A). However, the entities within the confines of which serotoninergic cells do occur may be briefly mentioned. A few 5-HT-positive cells have been found in the nucleus reticularis paramedianus, the nucleus reticularis tegmenti pontis, and the nucleus cuneiformis. A substantial number of serotoninergic neurons were demonstrated in the lateral tegmental reticular formation (Fig. 21A).

Besides the serotoninergic neurons, cells containing one of the following putative transmitters have been demonstrated in the reticular formation: dopamine, NE, histamine, avian pancreatic polypeptide (APP), met-ENK, leu-ENK, CCK, and substance P.

Dopamine-containing cell bodies were described by Hökfelt et al. (127), using an antibody to TH, in the ventrolateral part of the mesencephalic reticular formation. This cell group was previously designated by Dahlström and Fuxe (69) as the A8 cell group.

Norepinephrine-positive cell bodies have been described by histofluorescence (69) and by immunofluorescence, using an antibody to DBH (297). Some of these are situated within the medullary and pontine reticular formation, i.e., the A5 cell group, which is partly situated in the nucleus reticularis parvocellularis, and the A7 cell group, which is situated in the lateral mesencephalic reticular formation. The caudal part of this latter group is identical to the subceruleus NE cell group (172).

The APP-like immunoreactive cell bodies were shown in the lateral medullary reticular formation, especially in the noradrenergic A1 and A3 regions (134). Double-staining experiments demonstrated that 63% of the APP-positive perikarya in the A1 region and 43% in the A3 region are also immunoreactive with a TH antiserum.

The met-ENK-like as well as leu-ENK-like immunoreactive cell bodies were found scattered throughout the reticular formation, with highest concentrations in the nucleus reticularis parvocellularis and the nucleus reticularis medullae oblongatae, pars dorsalis (258). These results have not been confirmed by Hökfelt et al. (123,129), who demonstrated met-ENK-like immunoreactive neurons only in the area medial to the nucleus reticularis lateralis overlying the inferior olive, in the ventromedial parts of the nucleus reticularis gigantocellularis, and in the nucleus reticularis paramedianus.

A few CCK-like immunoreactive neurons have been demonstrated by Vanderhaeghen et al. (318) in the nucleus reticularis medullae oblongatae, pars medialis and ventralis.

A substantial number of substance P-containing cell bodies were found by Ljungdahl et al. (174) in the nucleus reticularis gigantocellularis and in the mesencephalic reticular formation, particularly the nucleus cuneiformis.

Finally, the study of Brownstein (46), who analyzed lesion data biochemically, showed that histaminergic axons projecting to the cerebral cortex might emanate mainly from neurons situated in the mesencephalic reticular formation. These findings have been confirmed by Barbin et al. (17), Pollard et al. (239), and Schwartz et al. (264).

It is worthy of note that, judging from their localization, the groups of neurons containing a transmitter other than serotonin may all enter into dendrodendritic or dendrosomatic contact with serotoninergic elements.

Fiber Connections

We now describe the afferent and efferent connections of the serotonin-containing neurons situated beyond the raphe nuclei. Because the majority of these outlying serotonin-positive neurons are situated in the lateral tegmental reticular formation, we focus mainly on this area. The serotoninergic neurons outside the raphe nuclei do not form discrete nuclei and therefore have resisted neuroanatomical studies involving degeneration experiments or axonal transport techniques. A short review of the efferents from the reticular formation has been presented by Nieuwenhuys et al. (212).

Non-transmitter-specified efferents from the reticular formation.

The lateral tegmental reticular formation gives rise to ascending as well as descending fibers, with the latter being more numerous.

The study of Conrad et al. (65), who injected [³H]proline laterally and ventrally into the tegmental reticular formation, revealed that the ascending projections from this area were ipsilateral. These fibers enter the medial forebrain bundle. They diminish rapidly in number as they continue rostrally. No fibers were seen further rostrally than the level of the anterior hypothalamus. Another major ascending projection spreads rostrally through the anterior mesencephalic reticular formation into the posterior thalamus. Some label also appeared in the zona incerta, a region rich in dopaminergic neurons, and in the subthalamus. Fibers were also observed to project to the nucleus parafascicularis, the nucleus centralis lateralis, and the nucleus dorsomedialis of the thalamus. The studies of Cedarbaum and Aghajanian (58) and Morgane and Jacobs (202), who used HRP injections into the locus ceruleus, demonstrated some labeled cells in the lateral reticular areas of the nucleus reticularis pontis caudalis and oralis.

The descending fibers from the lateral tegmental reticular formation were more dense than the ones emanating from the raphe nuclei. Most of these fibers pass to the medial part of the reticular formation, i.e., the nucleus reticularis pontis oralis, the nucleus reticularis pontis caudalis, and the nucleus reticularis gigantocellularis. However, this same area also gives rise to a substantial number of fibers that descend in the dorsolateral funiculus throughout the spinal cord (18,19,133,158,189).

The study of Tohyama et al. (306), who applied HRP injections in the spinal cord, demonstrated a significant number of HRP-labeled cells in an area ventral to the nucleus cuneiformis. This area has often been mentioned as the mesencephalic locomotor region (283). The pontine reticulospinal tracts originate mainly from the nucleus reticularis gigantocellularis, although the nucleus reticularis pontis oralis, the nucleus reticularis pontis caudalis, the nucleus reticularis parvocellularis, the nucleus reticularis paramedianus, and the nucleus reticularis dorsalis and ventralis also contribute fibers to these tracts. These results were confirmed by Goode et al. (112) who used HRP tracing as well as autoradiography. They also showed that the nucleus reticularis gigantocellularis and the nucleus reticularis pontis oralis innervate only laminae I and II of the spinal cord. However, in addition to the reticulospinal system originating at this level, there exists a major reticulospinal pathway that arises bilaterally from cells located in the caudal reticular formation, just laterally to the decussatio pyramidis (66).

Afferents to the reticular formation.

Transmitter-specified afferents to the serotoninergic reticular nuclei have been described by several authors. It is known that all of the reticular nuclei receive a sparse to moderate innervation with serotoninergic fibers (284). The same holds true for the catecholamines. The major part of the pontine reticular formation contains a low density of uniformly distributed noradrenergic terminals, whereas only a small number of such fibers were found in the mesencephalic reticular formation. A dense terminal field of catecholaminergic axons is present in the area dorsal and dorsolateral to the lemniscus medialis, i.e., the area of the B9 cell group (172,297). Levitt and Moore (170), who studied the catecholamine innervation of the brainstem using a biochemical assay as well as glyoxylic histofluorescence, found that the entire reticular formation received a moderate to dense innervation with catecholaminergic fibers, with highest concentrations in the nucleus reticularis tegmenti pontis. Their study showed in addition that these fibers arise from the locus ceruleus (A6) as well as from the lateral tegmental cell populations, i.e., the A1, A3, and A7 cell groups. Adrenergic fibers have not been described by Hökfelt et al. (125).

In addition to these catecholaminergic terminals, fibers containing one of the following transmitters could be recognized: met-ENK, leu-ENK, α-MSH, substance P, CCK, VIP, and ACTH. The met-ENK-like and leu-ENK-like immunoreactive fibers have been demonstrated by Sar et al. (258) throughout the reticular formation, i.e., with low densities in the nucleus reticularis tegmenti pontis and the nucleus cuneiformis. The α-MSH-positive fibers were demonstrated by Dubé et al. (81) in the dorsolateral part of the mesencephalic formatio reticularis, in the nucleus reticularis tegmenti pontis, and in the nucleus reticularis pontis oralis. A large number of α-MSH-containing fibers were observed by Jacobowitz and O'Donohue (136) in the nucleus cuneiformis. According to them, in the rest of the reticular formation, only a few α-MSH-immunoreactive fibers were present. Substance P-containing fibers have been found by Ljungdahl et al. (174) in many of the reticular nuclei, although their number was relatively small. A moderately dense plexus was present in the nucleus cuneiformis. The ventrolateral mesencephalic reticular formation contained only sparse or low densities of substance P-positive nerve terminals. Vanderhaeghen et al. (318) described thick beaded CCK-positive fibers in the lateral part of the reticular formation. Some VIP-containing axons were demonstrated by Sims et al. (273) in the nucleus reticularis pontis oralis and a sparse number dorsally in the mesencephalic reticular formation. Finally, a moderate density of ACTH immunoreactive fibers was detected throughout the reticular formation (232).

None of the following peptide-containing fibers was observed: APP (134), vasopressin or oxytocin (51,281), LHRH (139), γ-MSH (35), and β-endorphin (34).

Thus, whereas the catecholaminergic fibers were uniformly distributed over the reticular formation, it was observed that the peptide-containing fibers were preferentially located laterally.

Non-transmitter-specified afferents to the serotoninergic reticular nuclei have been described by several authors. First, it was observed that the reticular formation receives a strong input from the raphe nuclei. Bobillier et al. (36) reported that mesencephalic reticular nuclei received some fibers from the nucleus raphe dorsalis and the nucleus centralis superior. Moreover, the autoradiographic study of Bobillier et al. (37,38) revealed that the medullary reticular nuclei, i.e., the nucleus reticularis gigantocellularis, the nucleus reticularis medullae oblongatae, and the nucleus reticularis paramedianus, receive a major input from the nucleus centralis superior, although some fibers also derive from the nucleus raphe magnus and the nucleus raphe pontis. The pontine reticular nuclei receive fibers mainly from the nucleus raphe magnus and the nucleus raphe pontis. Some fibers derive from the nucleus centralis superior. Whereas the mesencephalic reticular formation was observed to receive a substantial number of fibers from the nucleus centralis superior, only a moderate number of fibers arise from the nucleus raphe magnus and pontis, and just a few arise from the nucleus raphe dorsalis.

The study of Kawamura and Chiba (145) employing the retrograde transport of HRP showed the pontine reticular formation receiving fibers from layer V of the ipsilateral cerebral cortex.

The study of Sofroniew and Schrell (279), who applied immunoperoxidase staining of retrogradely transported HRP, revealed that there are no hypothalamic neurons projecting to the reticular formation. This is in contrast with the observations of Wright and Arbuthnott (339), who pretreated rats with 6-hydroxydopamine and observed the presence of nondopaminergic efferent connections of the substantia nigra to the dorsolateral pontine reticular formation. The study of Loewy and Saper (176), using autoradiographic anterograde axonal tracing, showed that the ventral parts of the mesencephalic and pontine reticular formation receive a substantial number of fibers from the nucleus Edinger–Westphal.

Finally, the study of Coulter et al. (66) revealed that the nucleus reticularis gigantocellularis and the neurons adjacent to the decussatio pyramidum receive an ascending spinal input and extensive descending inputs from some rostral structures, i.e., the contralateral tectum and the head and face region of the sensorimotor cerebral cortex.

The Relationship Between Serotonin and the Glia

Glia cells are elements that belong to the CNS, although their function is not directly related to neurotransmission; rather, they have to be considered as supporting cells in the brain. Glia cells are, like neurons, of ectodermal origin, but they differ from them in having only one type of process. They can be divided into macro- and microglia. The macroglia comprise the astrocytes, the oligodendrocytes, and the tanycytes. In this section, we focus on three areas in which we observed glia cells that are serotonin immunoreactive themselves and on one region in which neurons are in close proximity to glia elements.

Serotoninergic Glia Cells

Serotonin-positive glia cells were demonstrated in the following areas: (a) the area postrema, (b) the infundibular stalk, and (c) the extraencephalic area situated immediately ventral to the rhombencephalon.

A compact group of relatively small monopolar serotonin immunoreactive glia cells was found in the area postrema. This observation confirms work of Falck and Owman (86), who used the FIF method, and of Dow and co-workers (78,79), who employed uptake studies of serotonin. However, none of these authors observed serotoninergic glia cells beyond the boundaries of this region.

As mentioned above, specific serotonin immunostaining of glia cells was found in the infundibular stalk. These findings have not been confirmed by other authors. In the medial part of that area, we observed some weakly fluorescent tanycytes with elongated cell bodies that are situated in the vicinity of the ventricular space. Their radially arranged processes extend into the external zone of the median eminence. These observations are in keeping with those of Sladek and Sladek (274). These authors demonstrated by means of microspectrofluorometry the presence of serotonin within tanycytes of the median eminence, although they were unable to show the serotonin-positive glia cells in the infundibular stalk. According to the work of Wittkowski (338), tanycytes are characterized by having only a single process, which either participates in the formation of the membrana limitans gliae externa or extends into the perivascular region (266). Tanycytes in mammals have been encountered mainly in the walls of the third ventricle, particularly ventrally. Each tanycyte can be regarded as consisting of a soma, a neck, and a tail portion. The light microscopic investigations of Kobayashi et al. (153) and Rodriguez (247) demonstrated a substantial uptake and transependymal transport of HRP by "basilar ependymal cells" following injection of that enzyme into the third ventricle and its subsequent transfer to capillaries in the surrounding periventricular neuropil or to the portal capillaries.

The observation of serotonin within tanycytes of the median eminence by Sladek and Sladek (274), which was confirmed by us, and the additional finding of the presence of dopaminergic nerve terminal endings in linear profiles arranged parallel to tanycytes, described by Sladek and Sladek (274) and previously by Hoffman and Sladek (122), suggested that tanycytes may regulate the storage of regulating hormones originating from the cerebrospinal fluid in the third ventricle—and their release into the portal vasculature—by an intracellular mechanism affecting some point along the way from uptake to release. This latter phenomenon, then, could be mediated by a catecholaminergic input.

As previously described, superficial serotonin immunoreactive glia cells were demonstrated in the region adjacent to the rhombencephalic part of the tractus corticospinalis and ventrally to the caudal part of the inferior olive complex (Figs. 14A–D; 15; and 16B). With regard to localization, distribution, and shape, these cells correspond to those recently described by Ross et al. (249). These authors observed that the cells in question give rise to axons that project to the thoracic and lumbar spinal cord. Although these authors identified these cells as neurons, an immuno-electron-microscopic survey using antibodies to serotonin revealed that these cells actually represent glia cells defined on the basis of their morphological appearance, i.e., lack of cell organelles other then mitochondria in their processes and bundling of fibrous elements, consisting of 8- to 9-nm-thick filaments in their processes (L. Leenen, *personal communication*).

It is known that the ventrolateral surface of the brainstem is an important area for the regulation of respiration and cardiovascular activity, and, moreover, it is accepted that serotonin can lead to changes in cardiovascular function. However, combining the results of Ross et al. (249) with ours, we can state that their neurons are not serotoninergic, whereas our serotonin-immunoreactive cells are glia cells. Moreover, these glia cells are in posession of processes that enter the tractus corticospinalis or the area lateral to it. By entering this latter region, these cells could be involved in autonomic and respiratory regulation (246,257).

Serotoninergic Neurons Contacting Glia Cells

Several areas in the rhombencephalon and mesencephalon have been described in which dendrites of serotonin-immunoreactive neurons are in close proximity to tanycyte-like glia cells, i.e., elements with cell bodies forming part of the ependymal ventricular lining and provided with one or a few long, peripherally extending processes (Fig. 39A,B) (67,90,91). These areas, containing high proportions of serotonin-positive neurons correspond to the nucleus raphe pallidus, the nucleus raphe obscurus, the nucleus raphe dorsalis, and the nucleus centralis superior. The glia cells under discussion are nonserotoninergic. However, no direct proof has been found on the ultrastructural level for a direct apposition between serotoninergic dendrites and glia processes. Circumstantial evidence has been presented by Cummings and Felten (67) who used, in different rat brains, either the Golgi–Cox or the histofluorescence method. Our findings are in keeping with theirs, but we remained unable to visualize simultaneously serotoninergic dendrites and Golgi-impregnated tanycytes.

Assuming a direct apposition of serotoninergic dendrites with tanycytes in the medial plane of the brainstem, what functional implications could this lead to? As already pointed out, the dendrites could release serotonin or take up compounds that influence the intraneuronal serotonin levels. Cummings and Felten (67) and Felten et al. (91) sug-

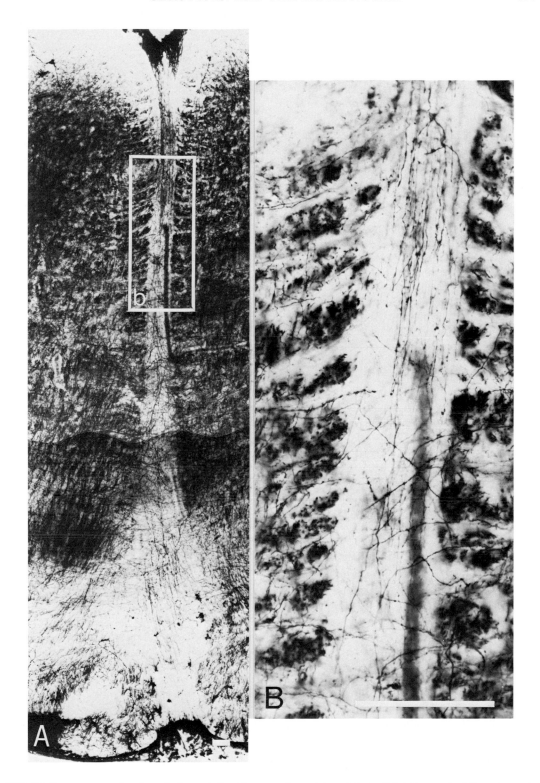

FIG. 39. Transverse section through the medulla oblongata after staining with the Golgi–Cox method. Long tanycyte shafts are seen in the midline, with their somata situated near the ventricular walls. (*Bars,* 75 μm)

gested that the tanycytes represent a communication channel between the cerebrospinal fluid of the fourth ventricle and the raphe nuclei through which a change in the composition of the cerebrospinal fluid could either activate or depress the excitability of the medullary raphe neurons. They suggested furthermore that the raphe neurons in that way might influence blood pressure-regulating centers.

Serotonin and Neuron–CSF and Neuron–Vascular Relationships

Supraependymal Neuronal–CSF Relationships

The presence of supraependymal cells was first reported by Leonhardt and Lindemann (167) using scanning and transmission electron microscopy of the floor of the fourth ventricle. Using the same technique, Jennes et al. (138) and Scott et al. (265) observed a large number of supraependymal cells in the third as well as fourth ventricle. However, the majority of these elements appeared to be glia cells. Jennes et al. (138) reported that the supraependymally situated glia are of two types: small and large.

The presence of supraependymal serotoninergic neuronal elements has been reported by Lorez and Richards (184) using histofluorescence and by Chan-Palay (61) and Parent et al. (225) applying intraventricular injections of [3H]serotonin. However, these authors have only been able to visualize serotoninergic fibers. We were able to confirm their findings and in addition to demonstrate the existence of supraependymal serotoninergic neurons on the lateral walls of the fourth ventricle and in the aqueductus cerebri. These neurons resemble in dimension as well as in number the large neurons described by Jennes et al. (138)

The presence of cerebrospinal fluid-contacting serotonin immunoreactive nerve fibers projecting through or lying on the cerebral ventricular ependyma was observed in all ventricles, although with local differences in intensities. This plexus can be divided into two parts: (a) a dense serotoninergic plexus on the ventricular surface of the rhombencephalon (Fig. 18C), in the aqueductus cerebri (Figs. 19 and 20A), and in the lateral ventricles; (b) a moderately dense serotonin-positive plexus in the dorsal part of the third ventricle (Fig. 24C). No serotonin-containing axons were demonstrated in the ventral part of the third ventricle, i.e., in the zone adjacent to the hypothalamus. The plexus itself consists of thin varicose fibers. The differences between the two plexuses are not related to dispar-

ities in varicosities or intervaricose connections but have to be seen as differences in the absolute number of fibers. Apparently, no correlation exists between the density of these fibers and the density of the serotoninergic innervation in the adjacent brain areas or nuclei.

The appearance of the serotoninergic supraependymal plexus must be later than postnatal day 1 in the rat, since we remained unable to visualize that plexus before or at that time (Fig. 22A,B). These results have been confirmed by J. M. Lauder (personal communication). The observations we made in the adult rat resemble those of Aghajanian et al. (1), Aghajanian and Gallager (2), Calas et al. (55), and Chan-Palay (59), but these authors did not report local differences in density of the plexus. Moreover, Chan-Palay (59) found a positive reaction in the ventral part of the third ventricle. However, our findings are fully in keeping with those of Lorez and Richards (184,185), who studied the 5-HT innervation of the ventricles with fluorescence histochemistry, and those of Cupédo and de Weerd (68), who demonstrated intraventricular axons in the habenular region using both intraventricular injections of 5,7-dihydroxytryptamine and electrolytic midbrain–raphe lesions. In addition to the serotoninergic fibers on the ventricle walls, only one other type of transmitter-specified supraependymal fiber has been described: luteinizing hormone-releasing hormone (LHRH)-like immunoreactive fibers described in the rat by Burchanowski et al. (48) and in the brain of the golden hamster by Jennes and Stumpf (139).

The question arises whether it is possible to determine the site of origin of the supraependymal plexus. Using lesion experiments, Aghajanian and Gallager (2) were able to determine that the serotonin-containing nerve terminals in the cerebral ventricular system are derived from the nucleus raphe dorsalis and the nucleus centralis superior. These results were confirmed by Parent et al. (225), who, using autoradiography, described this periventricular system as one of the two major ascending projections issuing mainly from the rostral pole of the nucleus raphe dorsalis. Cupédo and de Weerd (68), using degeneration experiments, adduced evidence that the supraependymal habenular serotoninergic axons originate from the nucleus centralis superior and the nucleus raphe dorsalis. However, the possibility must be considered that some lesion effects could be caused by damage to serotoninergic axons ascending from rhombencephalic raphe nuclei. Concerning the role of the serotoninergic intraventricular cell bodies and neuronal processes, the following suggestions have been made: (a) secretion of serotonin into the cerebrospinal fluid, (b) regulation of ependymal secretion, (c) absorption of other bioactive compounds from the cerebrospinal fluid, and (d) regulation of ciliary activity.

Secretion in terms of modifying the CSF composition has been suggested by Chan-Palay (59), Leonhardt and Lindemann (167), and Scott et al. (265). Moreover, Leonhardt and Lindemann (167) and Scott et al. (265), all of whom used electron microscopy, observed that most axons are unmyelinated. Secretion of 5-HT into the CSF may be important, since it is not possible for serotonin synthesized outside the brain to reach the ventricular system by way of the choroid plexus (173).

The penetration of the ependyma by neuronal processes is a consistent characteristic of supraependymal neurons, as shown in the electron microscopic study of Mitchell and Card (197). Leonhardt and Prien (168), who studied intraventricular axonal endings in the fourth ventricle of the rat brain electron microscopically, found that the plasmalemma of the bulbs is in synapse-like contact with the ependyma. It has already been mentioned that the ependymal layer contributes directly or indirectly to a significant production of CSF and hormones (245). Taking these findings and our own observations together, we might hypothesize that serotoninergic supraependymal neurons may modulate ependymal activity. It would be interesting to investigate whether there are local differences in the composition of the ependyma, mainly in the ventral part of the third ventricle, an area in which serotoninergic supraependymal fibers are lacking but in which the ependyma is in close apposition to a large number of neuropeptide-secreting endocrine cells.

No direct evidence has been presented for the absorption of compounds from the CSF into the intraventricular axons. However, with regard to this absorption, Westergaard (334) hypothesized, solely on the basis of morphological data, that these axons may be receptors for the regulation of CSF composition.

The last function of the serotoninergic supraependymal plexus suggested is the regulation of the flow of the CSF by modulation of the ciliary activity of ependymal cells. Interestingly, a regulatory role for 5-HT in ciliary movement has been observed on the molluscan epithelium (241). Calas et al. (55) reported in their autoradiographic study that in the third ventricle and the subcommissural region of the rat, the density of cilia is positively correlated with the density of the supraependymally situated serotoninergic fibers. However, according to the study of Ribas (245) in the intracommissural and suprahabenular recesses of the rat epithalamus, a dense serotoninergic innervation was demonstrated in a nonciliated area.

Suprapial Neuronal–CSF Relationships

Extraencephalic serotonin immunoreactive fibers were observed not only on the ventricular walls but also on the entire pial surface of the brain, forming a suprapial plexus there. Highest densities were found in adjacent cortical areas, whereas only a few 5-HT-positive fibers could be demonstrated on the cerebellum and on the basal surface of the brain. It was observed that in the suprapial fibers, the intervaricose distances are much longer than those in the supraependymal fibers. These appeared to be no correlation between the density of the suprapial serotoninergic fibers and that of those present in the adjacent brain areas.

The function of the suprapial serotoninergic fibers is at present unclear. Some fibers are related to the extraencephalic vascularization and are discussed in the next section. The neuronal–CSF relationships resemble those we have described previously, i.e., secretion of serotonin into the CSF and absorption of compounds from the CSF.

Intraencephalic Neuronal–Vascular Relationships

Serotoninergic neurons are strategically located near areas of cardiovascular control. For example, the 5-HT afferents to the sympathetic preganglionic neurons arise from the raphe nuclei (69). The light microscopic study of Scheibel and Scheibel (261) suggested that serotoninergic perikarya and dendrites of the nucleus raphe pontis and the nucleus linearis oralis border on midline blood vessels; however, an electron microscopic survey did not reveal a direct contact between neural and vascular elements in the nucleus raphe pontis. A recent study at the light microscopic level of the nucleus raphe obscurus and the nucleus raphe pallidus (67) revealed a direct neuronal–vascular contact between serotoninergic perikarya and dendrites and blood vessels situated within these nuclei. However, it is not possible to demonstrate conclusively a functional neuron–vascular relationship at the light microscopic level. Only electron microscopy can reveal the presence of direct appositions between neurons and blood vessels. Felten and Crutcher (88), using fluorescence histochemistry and electron microscopy, found perikarya and dendrites abutting on the basement membrane of capillaries and small arteries ranging from 8 to 50 μm in diameter, without evidence of glial interposition. Assuming that all neurons in the nucleus raphe dorsalis are serotoninergic, they considered the neuroactive principle involved in the contact to be serotonin. However, as described above, neurons containing another transmitter than serotonin are present not only in the nucleus raphe dorsalis but also in the other raphe nuclei as well. Hardebo and Owman (120) mentioned that the brain microvascular endothelium contained a large concentration of monoamine oxidase (MAO). The presence of MAO has to be seen as twofold: providing the enzymatic breakdown of amines and thereby fulfilling a simple barrier function against the entrance of circulating monoamines.

It is known that cerebral blood vessels are richly innervated by noradrenergic neurons whose cell bodies are either located within the superior cervical ganglia (324) or in the brainstem locus ceruleus. The ultrastructural study of Swanson et al. (296) revealed that within the nucleus paraventricularis, direct appositions between the noradrenergic terminals and the blood vessels occur. They showed in addition that no astrocytic processes were interposed between the noradrenergic varicosities and the basal laminae of the endothelial cells. The direct noradrenergic innervation of the endothelial cells of blood vessels in the nucleus paraventricularis hypothalami and the presence of amine uptake and enzymatic mechanisms within these cells may influence the activity of these cells. Circumstantial evidence suggesting the presence of similar links between serotoninergic neurons and blood vessels was obtained from pharmacological and biochemical studies (78,79,157).

The question arises whether the neuronal–vascular connections are afferent, efferent, or both. Felten and Crutcher (88) suggested that the neuronal–vascular relationship of serotoninergic raphe nuclei represents an afferent vascular channel for conveying blood-borne substances to receptors on the serotoninergic neurons. However, Reinhard et al. (244), using electric lesions in combinations with radioenzymatic microassays for serotonin, adduced evidence that serotoninergic dendrites can release serotonin into small blood vessels. It was determined that lesions of the nucleus raphe dorsalis and the nucleus linearis oralis resulted in a 70% reduction in microvessel serotonin concentration as compared to controls. Ganglionectomy failed to reduce microvessel serotonin concentrations. Edvinsson et al. (82) brought up the possibility that serotonin present in small brain capillaries originates from mast cells. However, we do not feel that the mast cells contribute substantially

to the blood serotonin because serotonin immunoreactive mast cells appeared to be confined to the area of the median eminence (284).

Smits et al. (276) demonstrated that in rats electric stimulation of either the nucleus raphe dorsalis or the nucleus centralis superior leads to increased blood pressure. This effect in the nucleus centralis superior was abolished when the rats were pretreated with the serotonin depletor *para*-chlorophenylalamine. Presumably, raphe stimulation leads to the release of 5-HT, which activates postsynaptic 5-HT receptors, leading to the observed pressor effect. These results have been confirmed by Kuhn et al. (157) and Fuller (96).

Finally, Reinhard et al. (244) brought up the possibility that other raphe nuclei are also in close proximity to blood vessels, suggesting that serotoninergic neurons receive afferents by way of chemoreceptors that detect changes in blood composition. On the basis of this, they may regulate blood flow and vascular permeability and thereby provide the brain with a mechanism for controlling its own microcirculation. However, direct evidence for a release of serotonin from raphe neurons into the blood is unconvincing. Scheibel and Scheibel (261) and Felten and Crutcher (88) were not able to show synapses or dense-core vesicles within monoaminergic perikarya or dendrites abutting blood vessels.

In summary, there is only circumstantial evidence for the presence of direct appositions of serotoninergic neurons and the neurovascular system. However, pharmacological and electophysiological experiments have conclusively shown that serotonin is involved in the regulation of blood pressure. For this reason, serotonin has frequently been suggested to be implicated in the pathogenesis of a number of vascular disorders, including migraine and ischemia (60,332).

Suprapial Neuronal–Vascular Relationships

The work of Chan-Palay (60), who has used autoradiography, histofluorescence, and immunocytochemistry, revealed that the cerebral blood vessels are innervated not only by serotonin-positive fibers but in addition by norepinephrine-, substance P-like-, and neurotensin-like-positive fibers. A clearly positive reaction with [^{3}H]serotonin was seen not only within the brain parencyma but also in the arachnoid, particularly in the vicinity of the superficial cerebral blood vessels. We were able to confirm these findings and to show in addition that this plexus is much more extensive than was previously thought. The functional significance of this neuronal–vascular relationship may resemble that of the one we have described in the preceding section. Thus, release of serotonin from this plexus could cause elevation of the concentration of serotonin in the CSF surrounding the blood vessel and may even be within the vessel itself. This could lead, in turn, to vasoconstriction, resulting in changes in cerebral blood flow (59).

CONCLUSION

Cytoarchitectonic and immunohistochemical studies revealed that the seven raphe nuclei, which contain the bulk of the serotoninergic cell bodies, represent separate entities. Moreover, it was observed that serotoninergic neurons within the raphe nuclei have no special structural characteristics. Thus, it is not possible to recognize serotonin-positive cells in Nissl or Golgi material.

We consider it likely that the serotoninergic neurons situated within the raphe nuclei differ with regard to both their afferent and efferent connections from those situated beyond these nuclei. In this context, it would be interesting to extend the ontogenetic studies with an analysis of a series of representative vertebrate species.

Because the raphe nuclei are by no means exclusively serotoninergic, their efferents are not exclusively serotoninergic either.

Serotoninergic neurons have been shown to be involved in a number of widely different functions; hence, it would be incorrect to describe the total population of the neurons containing this transmitter as forming a single functional system.

ACKNOWLEDGMENTS

The authors wish to thank Dr. M. Goldstein for the generous gift of tyrosine hydroxylase antiserum, Dr. J. Gribnau for discussions, Mr. H. Joosten for skillful immunocytochemical assistance, Mr. J. de Bekker for the drawings, Mr. C de Bruin and Mr. F. Fransen for the photomicrographs, and Ms. A. Siebring and Ms. M. Sjak Shie for typing the manuscript.

This work was supported in part by the Netherlands Organization for the Advancement of Pure Research (2.W.O.).

REFERENCES

1. Aghajanian, G. K., Bloom, F. E., Lowell, R., Sheard, M., and Freedman, R. E. (1966): The uptake of 5-hydroxytryptamine-³H from the cerebral ventricles: Autoradiographic localization. *Biochem. Pharmacol.*, 15:1401–1403.

2. Aghajanian, G. K., and Gallager, D. W. (1975): Raphe origin of serotonergic nerves terminating in the cerebral ventricles. *Brain Res.*, 88:221–231.

3. Aghajanian, G. K., Kuhar, M. J., and Roth, R. H. (1973): Serotonin-containing neuronal perikarya and terminals: Differential effects of *p*-chlorophenylamine. *Brain Res.* 54:85–101.

4. Aghajanian, G. K., and Wang, R. Y. (1977): Habenular and other midbrain raphe afferents demonstrated by a retrograde tracing technique. *Brain Res.*, 122:229–242.

5. Aghajanian, G. K., Wang, R. Y., and Baraban, J. (1978): Serotonergic and nonserotonergic neurons of the dorsal raphe: Reciprocal changes in firing induced by peripheral nerve stimulation. *Brain Res.*, 153:169–175.

6. Agrawal, H. C., Glisson, S. N., and Himwich, W. A. (1966): Changes in monoamines of rat brain during postnatal ontogeny. *Biochim. Biophys. Acta,* 130:511–513.

7. Ajelis, V., Björklund, A., Falck, B., Lindvall, O., Lorén, I., and Walles, B. (1979): Application of the aluminium–formaldehyhyde (ALFA) histofluorescence method for demonstration of peripheral stores of catecholamines and indolamines in freeze-dried paraffin-embedded tissue, cryostat sections and whole-mounts. *Histochemistry,* 65:1–15.

8. Ajika, K., and Ochi, J. (1978): Serotonergic projections to the suprachiasmatic nucleus and the median eminence of the rat: Identification by fluorescence and electron microscopy. *J. Anat.*, 127:563–576.

9. Anden, N. E., Dahlström, A., Fuxe, K., Larsson, K., Olson, L., and Ungerstedt, U. (1966): Ascending monamine neurons to the telencephalon and diencephalon. *Acta Physiol. Scand.*, 67:313–326.

10. Araneda, S., Gamrani, H., Font, C., Calas, A., Pujol, J.-F., and Bobillier, P. (1980): Retrograde axonal transport following injection of ³H-serotonin into the olfactory bulb. II. Radioautographic study. *Brain Res.*, 196:417–427.

11. Arikuni, T., and Ban, T. (1978): Subcortical afferents to the prefrontal cortex in rabbits. *Exp. Brain Res.*, 32:69–75.

12. Azmitia, E. C. (1978): The serotonin-producing neurons in the midbrain median and dorsal raphe nuclei. In: *Handbook of Psychopharmacology: Chemical Pathways in the Brain,* Vol. 9, edited by L. L. Iversen, S. D. Iversen, and S. H. Snyder, pp. 233–304. Plenum Press, New York.

13. Azmitia, E. C., Buchan, A., and Williams, J. H. (1978): Reorganization of the 5-HT projections to the hippocampus. *Trends Neurosci.*, 3:45–48.

14. Azmitia, E. C., and Henriksen, S. J. (1976): A modification of the Falck–Hillarp technique for 5-HT fluorescence employing hypertonic formaldehyde perfusion. *J. Histochem. Cytochem.*, 24:1286.

15. Azmitia, E. C., and Segal, M. (1978): An autoradiographic analysis of the differential ascending projections of the dorsal and median raphe nuclei in the rat. *J. Comp. Neurol.*, 179:641–668.

16. Baraban, J. H., and Aghajanian, G. K. (1981): Noradrenergic innervation of serotonergic neurons in the dorsal raphe: Demonstration by electronmicroscopic autoradiography. *Brain Res.*, 204:1–11.

17. Barbin, G., Palacios, J. M., Garbarg, M., Schwartz, J. C., Gaspar, P., Javoy-Agid, F., and Agid, Y. (1980): L-Histidine decarboxylase in the human brain: Properties and localization. *J. Neurochem.,* 35:400–406.

18. Basbaum, A. I., Clanton, C. H., and Fields, H. L. (1978): Three bulbospinal pathways from the rostral medulla of the cat: An autoradiographic study of pain modulating systems. *J. Comp. Neurol.,* 178:209–224.

19. Basbaum, A. I., and Fields, H. L. (1979): The origin of descending pathways in the dorsolateral funiculus of the spinal cord of the cat and rat: Further studies on the anatomy of pain modulation. *J. Comp. Neurol.,* 187:513–532.

20. Baumgarten, H. G. (1972): Biogenic amines in the cyclostome and lower vertebrate brain. *Prog. Histochem. Cytochem.,* 4:1–90.

21. Baumgarten, H. G., and Lachenmayer, L. (1972): 5,7-Dihydroxytryptamine: Improvement in chemical lesioning of indolamine neurons in the mammalian brain. *Z. Zellforsch.,* 135:399–414.

22. Beaudet, A., and Descarries, L. (1979): Radioautographic characterization of a serotonin accumulating nerve cell group in adult rat hypothalamus. *Brain Res.,* 160:231–243.

23. Belin, M.-F., Aguera, M., Tappaz, M., Jouvet, M., and Pujol, J.-F. (1978): Identification des neurones accumulant le GABA dans le noyau dorsal du raphé. *C. R. Acad. Sci. [D] (Paris),* 287:865–869.

24. Belin, M. F., Aguera, M., Tappaz, M., McRae-Degueurce, A., Bobillier, P., and Pujol, J.-F. (1979): GABA-accumulating neurons in the nucleus raphe dorsalis and periaqueductal gray in the rat: A biochemical and radioautographic study. *Brain Res.,* 170:279–297.

25. Bentivoglio, M., Macchi, G., Rossini, P., and Tempesta, E. (1978): Brain stem neurons projecting to neocortex: A HRP study in the cat. *Exp. Brain Res.,* 13:489–498.

26. Björklund, A., Axelsson, S., and Falck, B. (1976): Intraneuronal indolamines in the CNS. *Adv. Biochem. Psychopharmacol.,* 15:87–94.

27. Björklund, A., Falck, B., and Steveni, U. (1971): Classification of monoamine neurons in the rat mesencephalon: Distribution of the new indolamine neurone system. *Brain Res.,* 32:269–285.

28. Björklund, A., Falck, B., and Steveni, U. (1971): Microspectrofluorimetric characterization of monoamines in the central nervous system: Evidence for a new neuronal monoamine-like compound. *Brain Res.,* 34:63–72.

29. Björklund, A., Lindvall, O., and Svensson, L.-A. (1972): Mechanisms of fluorophore formation in the histochemical glyoxylic acid method for monoamines. *Histochemie,* 32:113–131.

30. Björklund, A., and Lindvall, O. (1975): Dopamine in dendrites of substantia nigra neurons: Suggestions for a role in dendritic terminals. *Brain Res.,* 83:531–536.

31. Björklund, A., Owman, C., and West, K. A. (1972): Peripheral sympathetic innervation and serotonin cells in the habenular region of the rat brain. *Z. Zellforsch.,* 127:570–579.

32. Björklund, A., and Skagerberg, G. (1979): Simul-

taneous use of retrograde fluorescent tracers and fluorescence histochemistry for convenient and precise mapping of monoaminergic projections and collateral arrangements in the CNS. *J. Neurosci. Methods,* 1:261–277.

33. Bloom, F. E., and Battenberg, E. L. F. (1976): A rapid, simple and sensitive method for the demonstration of central catecholamine-containing neurons and axons by glyoxylic acid-induced fluorescence. II. A detailed description of methodology. *J. Histochem. Cytochem.,* 24:561–571.

34. Bloom, F., Battenberg, E., Rossier, J., Ling, N., and Guillemin, R. (1978): Neurons containing β-endorphin in rat brain exist separately from those containing enkephalin: Immunocytochemical studies. *Proc. Natl. Acad. Sci. U.S.A.,* 75:1591–1595.

35. Bloom, F. E. Battenberg, E. L. F., Shibasaki, T., Benoit, R., Ling, N., and Guillemin, R. (1980): Localization of γ-melanocyte stimulating hormone (γM.S.H.) immunoreactivity in rat brain and pituitary. *Regul. Pept.,* 1:205–222.

36. Bobillier, P., Petitjean, F., Salvert, D., Ligier, M., and Seguin, S. (1975): Differential projections of the nucleus raphe dorsalis and nucleus raphe centralis as revealed by autoradiography. *Brain Res.,* 85:205–210.

37. Bobillier, P., Seguin, S., Petitjean, F., Salvert, D., Touret, M., and Jouvet, M. (1976): The raphe nuclei of the cat brain stem: A topographical atlas of their efferent projections as revealed by autoradiography. *Brain Res.,* 113:449–486.

38. Bobillier, P., Seguin, S., Degueurce, A., Lewis, B. D., and Pujol, J.-F. (1979): The efferent connections of the nucleus raphe centralis superior in the rat as revealed by radioautography. *Brain Res.,* 166:1–8.

39. Bogdansky, D. F., Pletcher, A., Brodie, B. B., and Udenfriend, S. (1956): Identification and assay of serotonin in brain. *J. Pharmacol. Exp. Ther.,* 117:82–88.

40. Bosin, T. R., Jonsson, G., and Beck, O. (1979): On the occurrence of 5-methoxytryptamine in brain. *Brain Res.,* 173:79–88.

41. Braak, H. (1970): Uber die kerngebiete des menschlichen Hirnstammes. II. Die Raphekerne. *Z. Zellforsch.,* 107:123–141.

42. Brammer, M., and Binkley, S. (1979): Daily rhythms of serotonin and N-acetyltransferase in chicks. *Comp. Biochem. Physiol. [B],* 63:305–307.

43. Brodal, A. (1957): *The Reticular Formation of the Brain Stem. Anatomical Aspects and Functional Correlations.* Oliver and Boyd, Edinburgh.

44. Brodal, A., Taber, E., and Walberg, F. (1960): The raphe nuclei of the brain stem in the cat. II. Efferent connections. *J. Comp. Neurol.,* 114:239–259.

45. Brodal, A., Walberg, F., and Taber, E. (1960): The raphe nuclei of the brain stem in the cat. III. Afferent connections. *J. Comp. Neurol.,* 114:261–281.

46. Brownstein, M. (1975): Biogenic amine content of the hypothalamic nuclei. In: *Anatomical Neuroendocrinology,* edited by W. E. Stumpf and L. D. Grant, pp. 393–396. S. Karger, Basel.

47. Buckholtz, N. S. (1980): Neurobiology of tetrahydro-β-carbolines. *Life Sci.,* 27:893–903.

48. Burchanowski, B. J., Knigge, K. M., and Sternber-

ger, L. A. (1979): Rich ependymal investment of lu-liberin (LHRH) fibers revealed immunocytochemically in an image like that from Golgi stain. *Proc. Natl. Acad. Sci. U.S.A.,* 76:6671–6674.

49. Burnstock, G. (1976): Do some nerve cells release more than one transmitter? *Neuroscience,* 1:239–248.

50. Burnstock, G. (1978): Do some sympathetic neurones synthesize and release both noradrenaline and acetylcholine. *Prog. Neurobiol.,* 11:205–222.

51. Buys, R. M. (1978): Intra- and extrahypothalamic vasopressin and oxytocin pathways in the rat. *Cell Tissue Res.,* 192:423–435.

52. Buys, R. (1980): *Vasopressin and Oxytocin Innervation of the Rat Brain. A Light- and Electronmicroscopical Study.* Doctoral thesis, University of Amsterdam, Rodopi, Amsterdam.

53. Cadilhac, J., and Pons, F. (1976): Le développement prénatal des neurones à monoamines chez le rat. *C.R. Soc. Biol. (Paris),* 25–30.

54. Calas, A., Alonso, G., Arnauld, E., and Vincent, J. D. (1974): Demonstration of indolaminergic fibers in the median eminence of the duck, rat and monkey. *Nature,* 250:241–243.

55. Calas, A., Bosler, O., Arluison, M., and Bouchaud, C. (1978): Serotonin as a neurohormone in circumventricular organs and supraependymal fibers. In: *Brain–Endocrine Interaction. III. Neural Hormones and Reproduction,* edited by D. E. Scott, G. P. Kozlowski, and A. Weindl, pp. 238–250. S. Karger, Basel.

56. Calas, A., and Ségu, L. (1976): Radioautographic localization and identification of monoaminergic neurons in the CNS. *J. Microsc. Biol. Cell,* 27:249.

57. Castiglioni, A. J., Gallaway, M. C., and Coulter, J. D. (1978). Spinal projections from the midbrain in monkey. *J. Comp. Neurol.,* 178:329–345.

58. Cedarbaum, J. M., and Aghajanian, G. K. (1978): Afferent projections to the rat locus coeruleus as determined by a retrograde tracing technique. *J. Comp. Neurol.,* 178:1–16.

59. Chan-Palay, V. (1976): Serotonin axons of the supra- and subependymal plexuses and in the leptomeninges: Their roles in local alterations of cerebrospinal fluid and vasomotor activity. *Brain Res.,* 102:103–130.

60. Chan-Palay, V. (1977): Innervation of cerebral blood vessels by norepinephrine, indolamine, substance P and neurotensin fibers and the leptomeningeal indolamine axons: Their roles in vasomotor activity and local alterations of brain blood composition. In: *Neurogenic Control of Brain Circulation,* edited by C. Owman and L. Edvinsson, pp. 39–53. Pergamon Press, Oxford.

61. Chan-Palay, V. (1977): Indolamine neurons and their processes in the normal rat brain and in chronic diet-induced thiamine deficiency demonstrated by uptake of ³H-serotonin. *J. Comp. Neurol.,* 176:467–494.

62. Chan-Palay, V. (1979): Combined immunocytochemistry and autoradiography after *in vivo* injections of monoclonal antibody to substance P and ³H-serotonin: Coexistence of two putative transmitters in single raphe cells and fiber plexuses. *Anat. Embryol.,* 156:241–254.

63. Chan-Palay, V. (1979): Immunocytochemical detection of substance P. Neurons their processes and connections by *in vivo* micro injections of monoclonal antibodies light and electron microscopy. *Anat. Embryol.,* 156:225–240.

64. Chan-Palay, V., Jonsson, G., and Palay, S. L. (1978): Serotonin and substance P coexist in neurons of the rat's central nervous system. *Proc. Natl. Acad. Sci. U.S.A.,* 75:1582–1586.

65. Conrad, L. C. A., Leonard, C. M., and Pfaff, D. W. (1974): Connections of the median and dorsal raphe nuclei in the rat: An autoradiographic and degeneration study. *J. Comp. Neurol.,* 156:179–206.

66. Coulter, J. D., Bowker, R. M., Wise, S. P., Murray, E., Castiglioni, A., and Westlund, K. (1979): Cortical tectal and medullary descending pathways to the cervical spinal cord. *Prog. Brain Res.,* 50:263–279.

67. Cummings, J. P., and Felten, D. L. (1979): A raphe dendrite bundle in the rabbit medulla. *J. Comp. Neurol.,* 183:1–24.

68. Cupédo, R. N. J., and Weerd de, H. (1980): Serotonergic intraventricular axons in the habenular region. Phagocytosis after induced degeneration. *Anat. Embryol.,* 158:213–226.

69. Dahlström, A., and Fuxe, K. (1964): Evidence for the existence of monoamine-containing neurons in the central nervous system. I. Demonstration of monoamines in cell bodies of brain neurons. *Acta Physiol. Scand. [Suppl.],* 232:1–55.

70. Dahlström, A., and Fuxe, K. (1965): Evidence for the existence of monoamine neurons in the central nervous system. II. Experimentally induced changes in the intraneuronal amine levels of bulbospinal neurone systems. *Acta Physiol. Scand. [Suppl. 247],* 64:1–36.

71. Daly, J., Fuxe, K., and Jonsson, G. (1974): 5,7-Dihydroxytryptamine as a tool for the morphological and functional analysis of central 5-hydroxytryptamine neurons. *Res. Commun. Chem. Pathol. Pharmacol.,* 1:175–187.

72. Deitrich, R. (1980): Biogenic amine–aldehyde condensation products: Tetrahydroisoquinolines and tryptolines (β-carbolines). *Annu. Rev. Pharmacol. Toxicol.,* 20:55–80.

73. Descarries, L., Beaudet, A., and Watkins, K. C. (1975): Serotonin nerve terminals in adult rat neocortex. *Brain Res.,* 100:563–588.

74. Descarries, L., Beaudet, A., Watkins, K. C., and Garcia, S. (1979): The serotonin neurons in nucleus raphe dorsalis of adult rat. *Anat. Rec.,* 193:520.

75. Devito, J. L., Anderson, M. E., and Walsh, K. E. (1979): A horseradish peroxidase study of afferent connections of the globus pallidus in *Macaca mulatta. Exp. Brain Res.,* 38:65–73.

76. Dierickx, K., and Vandesande, F. (1979): Immunocytochemical localization of somatostatin containing neurons in the rat hypothalamus. *Cell Tissue Res.,* 201:349–359.

77. Douay, O., and Kamoun, P. (1979): A rapid method for simultaneous estimation of 5-hydroxy-3-indole acetic acid (5-HIAA) and 5-hydroxytryptamine (5-HT) in rat brain. *Microchem. J.,* 24:173–178.

78. Dow, R. C., Laszlo, I., and Ritchie, I. M. (1973):

Cellular localization of the uptake of 5-hydroxy-tryptamine in the area postrema of the rabbit after injection into a lateral ventricle. *Br. J. Pharmacol.*, 49:580–587.

79. Dow, R. C., and Laszlo, I. (1976): Uptake of 5-hydroxytryptamine in different parts of the brain of the rabbit after intraventricular injection. *Br. J. Pharmacol.*, 56:443–447.

80. Dray, A., Gonye, T. J., Oakley, N. R., and Tanner, T. (1976): Evidence for the existence of a raphe projection to the substantia nigra in rat. *Brain Res.*, 113:45–57.

81. Dubé, D., Lissitzki, J. C., Leclerc, R., and Pelletier, G. (1978): Localization of α-melanocyte stimulating hormone in rat brain and pituitary. *Endocrinology*, 102:1283–1291.

82. Edvinsson, L., Cervos-Navarro, J., Larrson, L. I., Owman, C., and Ronnberg, A. L. (1977): Regional distribution of mast cells containing histamine, dopamine, or 5-hydroxytryptamine in the mammalian brain. *Neurology (Minneap.)*, 27:873–878.

83. Elde, R., Hökfelt, T., Johansson, O., and Terenius, L. (1976): Immunohistochemical studies using antibodies to leucine-enkephalin: Initial observations on the nervous system of the rat. *Neuroscience*, 1:349–351.

84. Falck, B. (1962): Observations on the possibilities of the cellular localization of monoamines by a fluorescence method. *Acta Physiol. Scand.* [Suppl. 197], 56:1–25.

85. Falck, B., Hillarp, N. Å., Thieme, G., and Torp, A. (1962): Fluorescence of catecholamines and related compounds with formaldehyde. *J. Histochem. Cytochem.*, 10:348–354.

86. Falck, B., and Owman, C. (1965): A detailed methodological description of the method for the cellular demonstration of biogenic monoamines. *Acta Univ. Lund*, 7:1–23.

87. Falck, B., and Owman, C. (1968): 5-Hydroxytryptamine and related amines in endocrine cell systems. In: *Advances in Pharmacology*, Vol. 6A, edited by I. Garattini and P. A. Those, pp. 211–231. Academic Press, New York.

88. Felten, D. L., and Crutcher, K. A. (1979): Neuronal–vascular relationships in the raphe nuclei, locus coeruleus, and substantia nigra in primates. *Am. J. Anat.*, 155:467–482.

89. Felten, D. L., and Cummings, J. P. (1979): The raphe nuclei of the rabbit brain stem. *J. Comp. Neurol.*, 187:199–244.

90. Felten, D. L., and Harrigan, P. (1980): Dendrite bundles in nuclei raphe dorsalis and centralis superior of the rabbit: A possible substrate for local control of serotonergic neurons. *Neurosci. Lett.*, 16:275–280.

91. Felten, D. L., Harrigan, P., Burnett, B. T., and Cummings, J. P. (1981): Fourth ventricular tanycytes: A possible relationship with monoaminergic nuclei. *Brain Res. Bull.*, 6:427–436.

92. Fibiger, H. C., and Miller, J. J. (1977): An anatomical and electrophysiological investigation of the serotonergic projection from the dorsal raphe nucleus to the substantia nigra in the rat. *Neuroscience*, 2:957–987.

93. Fields, H. L., and Basbaum, A. I. (1978): Brainstem control of spinal of pain-transmission neurons. *Annu. Rev. Physiol.*, 40:217–256.

94. Finley, J. C. W., Grossman, G. H., Dimco, P., and Petrusz, P. (1978): Somatostatin-containing neurons in the rat brain widespread distribution revealed by immunocytochemistry after pretreatment with pronase (1). *Am. J. Anat.*, 153:483–488.

95. Forchetti, C. M., and Meek, J. L. (1981): Evidence for a tonic GABAergic control of serotonin neurons in the median raphe nucleus. *Brain Res.*, 206:208–212.

96. Fuller, R. W. (1980): Pharmacology of central serotonin neurons. *Annu. Rev. Pharmacol. Toxicol.*, 20:111–127.

97. Furness, J. B., and Costa, M. (1975): The use of glyoxylic acid for the fluorescence histochemical demonstration of peripheral stores of NA and 5-hydroxytryptamine in whole mounts. *Histochemistry*, 41:335–352.

98. Furness, J. B., Costa, M., and Blessing, W. W. (1977): Simultaneous fixation and production of CA fluorescence in central nervous tissue by perfusion with aldehydes. *Histochem. J.*, 9:745–750.

99. Furness, J. B., Costa, M., and Wilson, A. J. (1977): Water-stable fluorophores produced by reaction with aldehyde solutions, for the histochemical localization of catechol- and indolethylamines. *Histochemistry*, 52:159–170.

100. Fuxe, K. (1965): Evidence for the existence of monoamine neurons in the central nervous system. IV. Distribution of monoamine nerve terminals in the central nervous system. *Acta Physiol. Scand.* [Suppl.], 247:37–85.

101. Fuxe, K., Andersson, K., Hökfelt, T., Mutt, V., Ferland, L., Agnati, L. F., Ganten, D., Said, S., Eneroth, P., and Gustafsson, J. A. (1979): Localization and possible function of peptidergic neurons and their interactions with central catecholaminergic neurons and their central actions of gut hormones. *Fed. Proc.*, 38:2333–2340.

102. Fuxe, K., Hökfelt, T., and Ungerstedt, U. (1970): Morphological and functional aspects of the central monoamine neurons. *Int. Rev. Neurobiol.*, 13:93–126.

103. Fuxe, K., Hökfelt, T., Said, S. T., and Mutt, V. (1977): Vasoactive intestinal polypeptide and the nervous system: Immunohistochemical evidence for localization in central and peripheral neurons, particularly intracortical neurons of the cerebral cortex. *Neurosci. Lett.*, 5:241–246.

104. Fuxe, K., Hökfelt, T., Agnati, L. F., Johansson, O., Goldstein, M., Perez de la Mora, M., Possani, L., Tapia, R., Teran, L., and Palacios, R. (1978): Mapping out central catecholamine neurons: Immunohistochemical studies on catecholamine-synthesizing enzymes. In: *Psychopharmacology: A Generation of Progress*, edited by M. A. Lipton, A. Di Mascio, and K. F. Killam, pp. 67–94. Raven Press, New York.

105. Fuxe, K., and Jonsson, G. (1974): Further mapping of central 5-hydroxytryptamine neurons: Studies with the neurotoxic dihydroxytryptamines. *Adv. Biochem. Psychopharmacol.*, 10:1–12.

106. Gallager, D. W., and Pert, A. (1978): Afferents to brain stem raphe nuclei (brain stem raphe nucleus reticularis pontis caudalis and nucleus gigantocellularis) in the rat as demonstrated by microiontophoretically applied horseradish peroxidase. *Brain Res.,* 144:257–275.

107. Gamrani, H., Calas, A., Belin, M. F., Aguera, M., and Pujol, J. F. (1979): High resolution radioautographic identification of (^{3}H)GABA labeled neurons in the rat nucleus raphe dorsalis. *Neurosci. Lett.,* 15:43–48.

108. Garattini, S., Consolo, S., and Ladinsky, H. (1980): Neuronal links in the CNS: Focus on dopaminergic and serotonergic regulation of striatal cholinergic neurons. *Pol. J. Pharmacol. Pharm.,* 32:155–164.

109. Gerfen, C. R., and Clavier, R. M. (1979): Neural inputs to the prefrontal agranular insular cortex in the rat: Horseradish peroxidase study. *Brain Res. Bull.,* 4:347–353.

110. Gilbert, R. T. F., Emson, P. C., Hunt, S. P., Bennett, G. W., Marsden, C. A., Sandberg, B. E. B., Steinbusch, H. W. M., and Verhofstad, A. A. J. (1981): The effects of monoamine neurotoxins on peptides in the rat spinal cord. *Neuroscience* 7:69–87.

111. Glazier, E. J., Steinbusch, H. W. M., Verhofstad, A. A. J., and Basbaum, A. J. (1981): Serotonergic neurons of the cat nucleus raphe dorsalis and paragigantocellularis contain encephalin. *J. Physiol. (Paris),* 77:241–245.

112. Goode, G. E., Humbertson, A. O., and Martin, G. F. (1980): Projections from the brain stem reticular formation to laminae I and II of the spinal cord. Studies using light- and electronmicroscopic techniques in the North American opossum. *Brain Res.,* 189:327–342.

113. Gottesfeld, Z., Hoover, D. B., Muth, E. A., and Jacobowitz, D. M. (1978): Lack of biochemical evidence for a direct habenulo–raphe GABAergic pathway. *Brain Res.,* 141:353–356.

114. Green, A. R., Koslow, S. H., and Costa, E. (1972): Identification and quantitation of a new indolealkylamine in rat hypothalamus. *Brain Res.,* 51:371–374.

115. Gribnau, A. A. M., and Geijsberts, L. C. M. (1981): Developmental stages in the rhesus monkey *(Macaca mulatta), Adv. Anat. Embryol. Cell. Biol.,* 68:1–84.

116. Grzanna, R., Molliver, M. E., and Coyle, J. T. (1978): Visualization of central noradrenergic neurons in thick sections by the unlabeled antibody method: A transmitter specific Golgi image. *Proc. Natl. Acad. Sci. U.S.A.,* 75:2502–2506.

117. Grzanna, R., and Molliver, M. E. (1980): The locus coeruleus in the rat: An immunohistochemical delineation. *Neuroscience,* 5:21–41.

118. Grzanna, R., and Molliver, M. E. (1980): Cytoarchitecture and dendritic morphology of central noradrenergic neurons. In: *The Reticular Formation Revisited: Specifying Function for a Nonspecific System,* edited by J. A. Hobson and M. A. B. Brazier, pp. 83–97. Raven Press, New York.

119. Halaris, A. E., Jones, B. E., and Moore, R. Y. (1976): Axonal transport in serotonin neurons of the midbrain raphe. *Brain Res.,* 107:555–574.

120. Hardebo, J. E., and Owman, C. (1980): Barrier mechanisms for neurotransmitter monoamines and their precursors at the blood–brain interface. *Ann. Neurol.,* 8:1–11.

121. Hedner, T., and Lundborg, P. (1980): Serotoninergic development in the postnatal rat brain. *J. Neural Transm.,* 49:257–279.

122. Hoffman, G. E., and Sladek, J. R., Jr. (1980): Age-related changes in dopamine, LHRH and somatostatin in the rat hypothalamus. *Neurobiol. Aging,* 1:27–38.

123. Hökfelt, T., Elde, R., Johansson, O., Terenius, L., and Stein, L. (1977): The distribution of enkephalin-immunoreactive cell bodies in the rat central nervous system. *Neurosci. Lett.,* 5:25–31.

124. Hökfelt, T., Fuxe, K., and Goldstein, M. (1973): Immunohistochemical localization of aromatic-L-aminoacid decarboxylase (DOPA-decarboxylase) in central dopamine and 5-hydroxytryptamine nerve cell bodies of the rat brain. *Brain Res.,* 53:175–180.

125. Hökfelt, T., Fuxe, K., Goldstein, M., and Johansson, O. (1973): Evidence for adrenaline neurons in the rat brain. *Acta Physiol. Scand.,* 89:286–288.

126. Hökfelt, T., Fuxe, K., Goldstein, M., and Johansson, O. (1974): Immunohistochemical evidence for the existence of adrenaline neurons in the rat brain. *Brain Res.,* 66:235–251.

127. Hökfelt, T., Johansson, O., Fuxe, K., Goldstein, M., and Park, D. (1976): Immunohistochemical studies on the localization and distribution of monoamine neuron systems in the rat brain. 1. Tyrosine hydroxylase in the mesencephalon and diencephalon. *Med. Biol.,* 54:427–453.

128. Hökfelt, T., and Ljungdahl, Å. (1972): Modification of the Falck-Hillarp formaldehyde fluorescence method using the vibratome: Simple, rapid and sensitive localization of catecholamines in sections of unfixed or formalin fixed brain tissue. *Histochemie,* 29:325–339.

129. Hökfelt, T., Ljungdahl, Å., Terenius, L., Elde, R., and Nilsson, G. (1977): Immunohistochemical analysis of peptide pathways possibly related to pain and analgesia: Enkephalin and substance P. *Proc. Natl. Acad. Sci. U.S.A.,* 74:3081–3085.

130. Hökfelt, T., Kjungdahl, Å., Steinbusch, H., Verhofstad, A., Nilsson, G., Brodin, E., Pernow, B., and Goldstein, M. (1978): Immunohistochemical evidence of substance-P like immunoreactivity in some 5-hydroxytryptamine containing neurons in the rat central nervous system. *Neuroscience,* 3:517–538.

131. Hökfelt, T., Terenius, L., Kuypers, H. G. J. M., and Dann, O. (1979): Evidence for enkephalin immunoreactive neurons in the medulla oblongata projecting to the spinal cord. *Neurosci. Lett.,* 14:55–60.

132. Hubbard, J., and Di Carlo, V. (1974): Fluorescence histochemistry of monoamine-containing cell bodies in the brain stem of the squirrel monkey *(Saimiri sciureus).* III. Serotonin-containing groups. *J. Comp. Neurol.,* 153:385–398.

133. Huisman, A. M., Kuypers, H. G. J. M., and Ver-

burgh, C. A. (1981): Quantitative differences in collateralization of the descending spinal pathways from red nucleus and other brain stem cell groups in rat as demonstrated with the multiple fluorescent retrograde tracer technique. *Brain Res.*, 209:271–286.

134. Hunt, S. P., Emson, P. C., Gilbert, R., Goldstein, M., and Kimmell, J. R. (1981): Presence of avian pancreatic polypeptide-like immunoreactivity in catecholamine and methionine-enkephalin-containing neurones within the central nervous system. *Neurosci. Lett.*, 21:125–130.

135. Jacobowitz, D. M., and MacLean, P. D. (1978): A brainstem atlas of catecholaminergic neurons and serotonergic perikarya in a pigmy primate *(Cebuella pygmaea)*. *J. Comp. Neurol.*, 177:397–416.

136. Jacobowitz, D. M., and O'Donohue, T. L. (1978): α-Melanocyte stimulating hormone: Immunohistochemical identification and mapping in neurons of rat brain. *Proc. Natl. Acad. Sci. U.S.A.*, 75:6300–6304.

137. Jacobs, B. L., Foote, S. L., and Bloom, F. E. (1978): Differential projections of neurons within the dorsal raphe nucleus of the rat: A horseradish peroxidase (HRP) study. *Brain Res.*, 147:149–153.

138. Jennes, L., Sikora, K., Simonsberger, P., and Adam, H. (1977): Ventrikuläre Topographie des diencephalen Ependyms bei *Rattus rattus* (L.)—eine rasterelektronenmikroskopische Untersuchung. *J. Hirnforsch.*, 18:501–520.

139. Jennes, L., and Stumpf, W. E. (1980): LHRH-systems in the brain of the golden hamster. *Cell Tissue Res.*, 209:239–256.

140. Joh, T. H., Shikimi, T., Pickel, V. M., and Reis, D. J. (1975): Brain tryptophanhydroxylase: Purification of production of antibodies to and cellular and ultrastructural localization in serotonergic neurons of rat midbrain. *Proc. Natl. Acad. Sci. U.S.A.*, 72:3575–3579.

141. Jonsson, G., Einarsson, P., Fuxe, K., and Hallman, H. (1975): Microspectro–fluorimetric analysis of the formaldehyde induced fluorescence in midbrain raphe neurons. *Med. Biol.*, 53:25–39.

142. Jonsson, G., Pollare, T., Hallman, H., and Sachs, C. (1978): Development plasticity of central serotonin neurons after 5,7-dihydroxytryptamine treatment. *Proc. N.Y. Acad. Sci.*, 331:150–167.

143. Kan, J. P., Chouvet, G., Hery, F., Debilly, G., Mermet, A., Glowinsky, J., and Pujol, J. F. (1977): Daily variations of various parameters of serotonin metabolism in the rat brain. I. Circadian variations of tryptophan-5-hydroxylase in the raphe nuclei and the striatum. *Brain Res.*, 123:125–136.

144. Kawa, A., Ariyama, T., Taniguchi, Y., Kamisaki, T., and Kanehisa, T. (1978): Increased sensitivity to 5-HT due to intraventricular administration of 5,6-dihydroxytryptamine. *Acta Endocrinol. (Kbh.)*, 89:432–437.

145. Kawamura, K., and Chiba, M. (1979): Cortical neurons projecting to the pontine nuclei in the cat. An experimental study with the horseradish peroxidase technique. *Exp. Brain Res.*, 35:269–285.

146. Kawasaki, T., and Sato, Y. (1980): Afferent projec-

tion from the dorsal nucleus of the raphe to the flocculus in cats. *Brain Res.*, 197:496–502.

147. Kellar, K. J., Brown, P. A., Madrid, J., Bernstein, M., Vernikos-Danelles, J., and Mehler, W. A. (1977): Origins of serotonin innervation of forebrain structures. *Exp. Neurol.*, 56:52–62.

148. Kellum, J. M., and Jaffe, B. M. (1976): Validation and application of a radioimmunoassay for serotonin. *Gastroenterology*, 70:516–522.

149. Kent, D. L., and Sladek, J. R., Jr. (1978): Histochemical, pharmacological and microspectrofluorometric analysis of new sites of serotonin localization in the rat hypothalamus. *J. Comp. Neurol.*, 180:221–236.

150. Kizer, J. S., Zivin, J. A., Saavedra, J. M., and Brownstein, M. J. (1975): A sensitive microassay for tryptophan hydroxylase in brain. *J. Neurochem.*, 24:779–785.

151. Kneisley, L. W., Biber, M. P., and Lavail, J. H. (1978): A study of the origin of brain stem projections to monkey spinal cord using the retrograde transport method. *Exp. Neurol.*, 60:116–139.

152. Kobayashi, R. M., Brownstein, M., Saavedra, J. M., and Palkovits, M. (1975): Choline acetyltransferase content in discrete regions of the rat brain stem. *J. Neurochem.*, 24:637–640.

153. Kobayashi, H., Wada, M., and Uemura, H. (1972): Uptake of peroxidase from the third ventricle by ependymal cells of the median eminence. *Z. Zellforsch.*, 127:545–551.

154. Köhler, C., and Lorens, S. A. (1978): Open field activity and avoidance behavior following serotonin depletion: A comparison of the effects of parachlorophenylalamine and electrolytic midbrain raphe lesions. *Pharmacol. Biochem. Behav.*, 8:223–233.

155. Komulainen, H., Tuomisto, J., Airaksinen, M. M., Kari, I., Peura, P., and Pollari, L. (1980): Tetrahydro-β-carbolines and corresponding tryptamines: *In vitro* inhabitation of serotonin, dopamine and noradrenaline uptake in rat brain synaptosomes. *Acta Pharmacol. Toxicol. (Kbh.)*, 46:299–307.

156. König, J. F. R., and Klippel, R. A. (1963): *The Rat Brain, A Stereotaxic Atlas.* Williams & Wilkins, Baltimore.

157. Kuhn, D. M., Wolf, W. A., and Lovenberg, W. (1980): Review of the role of the central serotonergic neuronal system in blood pressure regulation. *Hypertension*, 2:243–255.

158. Kuypers, H. G., and Maisky, V. A. (1977): Funicular trajectories of descending brain stem pathways in cat. *Brain Res.*, 136:159–165.

159. Lackner, K. J. (1980): Mapping of monoamine neurones and fibres in the cat lower brain stem and spinal cord. *Anat. Embryol.*, 161:169–195.

160. Lauder, J. M., and Krebs, H. (1978): Serotonin as a differentiation signal in early neurogenesis. *Dev. Neucosci.*, 1:15–30.

161. Lauder, J. M., Wallace, J. A., and Krebs, H. (1981): Roles for serotonin in neuroembryogenesis. *Adv. Exp. Med. Biol.*, 133:477–506.

162. Léger, L., and Descarries, L. (1978): Serotonin nerve terminals in the locus coeruleus of adult rat: A radioautographic study. *Brain Res.*, 145:1–13.

163. Léger, L., McRae-Degueurce, A., and Pujol, J. F. (1980): Anatomie animale. Origine de l'innervation sérotoninergique du locus coeruleus chez le rat. *C. R. Acad. Sci. [D.] (Paris),* 290:807–810.

164. Léger, L., Mouren-Mathieu, A. M., and Descarries, L. (1978): Identification radioautographique de neurones monoaminergiques centraux par micro-instillation locale de serotonine ou de noradrénaline tritiée chez le chat. *C. R. Acad. Sci. [D.] (Paris),* 286:1523–1526.

165. Leichnetz, G. R., Watkins, L., Griffin, G., Murfin, R., and Mayer, D. J. (1978): The projections from nucleus raphe magnus and other brain stem nuclei to the spinal cord in the rat: A study using the HRP-blue reaction. *Neurosci. Lett.,* 8:119–124.

166. Lemberger, L., Rowe, H., Carmichael, R., Crabtree, R., Horng, J. S., Bymaster, F., and Wong, D. (1978): Fluoxetine, a selective serotonin uptake inhibitor. *Clin. Pharmacol. Ther.,* 23:421–429.

167. Leonhardt, H., and Lindemann, B. (1973): Uber ein supraependymales Nervenzell-, Axon- und Gliazellsystem. Eine Raster- und transmissions elektronenmikroskopische Untersuchung am IV Ventrikel (Apertura lateralis) des Kaninchengehirns. *Z. Zellforsch.,* 139:285–302.

168. Leonhardt, H., and Prien, H. (1968): Eine weitere Art intraventrikulärer kolbenförmiger Azonendigungen aus dem IV Ventrikel des Kaninchengehirns. *Z. Zellforsch.,* 92:394–399.

169. Levitt, P., and Moore, R. Y. (1978): Developmental organization of raphe serotonin neuron groups in the rat. *Anat. Embryol.,* 154:241–251.

170. Levitt, P., and Moore, R. Y. (1979): Origin and organization of brain stem catecholamine innervation in the rat *J. Comp. Neurol.,* 186;505–528.

171. Lindvall, O., and Björklund, A. (1974): The glyoxylic acid fluorescence histochemical method: A detailed account of the methodology for the visualization of central catecholamine neurons. *Histochemistry,* 39:97–127.

172. Lindvall, O., and Björklund, A. (1978): Organization of catecholamine neurons in the rat central nervous system. In: *Handbook of Psychopharmacology,* Vol. 9, edited by L. L. Iversen, S. D. Iversen, and S. H. Snyder, pp. 139–231. Plenum Press, New York.

173. Lindvall, M., Hardebo, J. E., and Owman, C. (1980): Barrier mechanisms for neurotransmitter monoamines in the choroid plexus. *Acta Phsyiol. Scand.,* 108:215–221.

174. Ljungdahl, Å., Hökfelt, T., and Nilsson, G. (1978): Distribution of substance P-like immunoreactivity in the central nervous system of the rat. I. Cell bodies and terminals. *Neuroscience,* 3:861–943.

175. Llamas, A., Reinoso-Suárez, F., and Martinez-Moreno, E. (1975): Projections to the gyrus proreus from the brain stem tegmentum (locus coeruleus, raphe nuclei) in the cat, demonstrated by retrograde transport of horseradish peroxidase. *Brain Res.,* 89:331–336.

176. Loewy, A. D., and Saper, C. B. (1978): Edinger-Westphal nucleus: Projections to the brain stem and spinal cord in the cat. *Brain Res.,* 150:1–27.

177. Loizou, L. A. (1972): The postnatal otogeny of monoamine-containing neurones in the central nervous system of the albino rat. *Brain. Res.,* 40:395–418.

178. Lorén, I., Björklund, A., Falck, B., and Lindvall, O. (1976): An improved histofluorescence procedure for freezedried paraffin-embedded tissue based on combined formaldehydeglyoxylic acid perfusion with high magnesium content and acid pH. *Histochemistry,* 49:177–192.

179. Lorén, I., Björklund, A., Falck, B., and Lindvall, O. (1977): The use of magnesium ions for sensitive visualization of catecholamines and serotonin in the CNS. *Acta Physiol. Scand. [Suppl.],* 452:15–19.

180. Lorén, I., Björklund, A., and Lindvall, O. (1977): Magnesium ions in catecholamine fluorescence histochemistry. Application to the cryostat and vibratome techniques. *Histochemistry,* 52:223–239.

181. Lorén, I., Björklund, A., Falck, B., and Lindvall, O. (1980): The aluminium–formaldehyde (ALFA) method for improved visualization of catecholamines and indolamines. 1. A detailed account of the methodology for central nervous tissue using paraffin, cryostat or vibratome sections. *J. Neurosci. Methods,* 2:277–300.

182. Lorén, I., Emson, P. C., Fahrenkrug, J., Björklund, A., Alumets, J., Håkanson, R., and Sundler, F. (1979): Distribution of vasoactive intestinal polypeptide in the rat and mouse brain. *Neuroscience,* 4:1953–1976.

183. Lorén, I., Schwandt, P., Alumets, J., Hakanson, R., Neureuther, G., Richter, W., and Sundler, F. (1980): Evidence that lipolytic peptide B occurs in the ACTH/MSH-cells of the pituitary and in the brain. *Cell Tissue Res.,* 205:349–359.

184. Lorez, H. P., and Richards, J. G. (1973): Distribution of indolealkylamine nerve terminals in the ventricles of the rat brain. *Z. Zellforsch.,* 144:511–522.

185. Lorez, H. P., and Richards, J. G. (1975): 5-HT nerve terminals in the fourth ventricle of the rat brain: Their identification and distribution studied by fluorescence histochemistry and electron microscopy. *Cell Tissue Res.,* 165:37–48.

186. Maeda, T., Nagai, T., Imamoto, K., and Satoh, K. (1979): A glyoxylic acid freeze-drying histofluorescence method for central serotonin neuron. *Acta Histochem. Cytochem.,* 1:572.

187. Marini, J. L., Williams, S. P., and Sheard, M. H. (1979): Simultaneous assay for L-tryptophan, serotonin, 5-hydroxyindoleacetic acid, norepinephrine and dopamine in brain. *Pharmacol. Biochem. Behav.,* 11:183–187.

188. Marschall, C. (1980): Hypothalamic monoamines in lizards *(Lacerta). Cell Tissue Res.,* 205:95–105.

189. Martin, R. F., Jordan, L. H., and Willis, W. D. (1978): Differential projections of cat medullary raphe neurons demonstrated by retrograde labelling following spinal cord lesions. *J. Comp. Neurol.,* 182:77–88.

190. Massari, V. J., Tizabi, Y., Gottesfeld, Z., and Jacobowitz, D. M. (1978): A fluorescence histochemical and biochemical evaluation of the effect of *p-*

chloroamphetamine on individual serotonergic nuclei in the rat brain. *Neuroscience,* 3:339–344.

191. Massari, V. J., Tizabi, Y., and Jacobowitz, D. M. (1979): Potential noradrenergic regulation of serotonergic neurons in the median raphe nucleus. *Exp. Brain Res.,* 34:177–182.

192. McCreery, D. B., Bloedel, J. R., and Hames, E. G. (1979): Effects of stimulating in raphe nuclei and in reticular formation on response of spinothalamic neurons to mechanical stimuli. *J. Neurophysiol.,* 42:166–182.

193. McRae-Degueurce, A., and Pujol, J. F. (1979): Correlation between the increase in tyrosine hydroxylase activity and the decrease in serotonin content in the rat locus coeruleus after 5,6-dihydroxytryptamine. *Eur. J. Pharmacol.,* 59:131–135.

194. Meessen, H., and Olszewski, J. (1949): *A Cytoarchitectonic Atlas of the Rhombencephalon of the Rabbit.* S. Karger, Basel.

195. Metcalf, G. (1974): A rapid for the simultaneous determination of noradrenaline, dopamine and 5-hydroxytryptamine in small samples of brain tissue. *Anal. Biochem.,* 57:316–320.

196. Miller, J. J., Richardson, T. L., Fibiger, H. C., and McLennan, H. (1975): Anatomical and electrophysiological identification of a projection from the mesencephalic raphe to the caudate-putamen in the rat. *Brain Res.,* 97:133–138.

197. Mitchell, J. A., and Card, J. P. (1978): Supraependymal neurons overlying the periventricular region of the third ventricle of the guinea pig: A correlative scanning–transmission electron microscopic study. *Anat. Rec.,* 192:441–458.

198. Miyakawa, M., and Usui, T. (1979): Nucleus raphe pallidus of rat medulla oblongata. A possible contact point of serotonergic and catecholaminergic systems. *Proc. Jpn. Acad. Biol.,* 55:407–412.

199. Møllgård, K., Lundberg, J. J., Wiklund, L., Lachenmayer, L., and Baumgarten, H. G. (1978): Morphological consequences of serotonin neurotoxin administration: Neuron-target cell interaction in the rat subcommissural organ. *Ann. N.Y. Acad. Sci.,* 305:262–288.

200. Møllgård, K., and Wiklund, L. (1979): Serotoninergic synapses on ependymal and hypendymal cells of the rat subcommissural organ. *J. Neurocytol.,* 8:445–467.

201. Moore, R. Y., Halaris, A. E., and Jones, B. E. (1978): Serotonin neurons of the midbrain raphe: Ascending projections. *J. Comp. Neurol.,* 180:417–438.

202. Morgane, P. J., and Jacobs, M. S. (1979): Raphe projections to the locus coeruleus in the rat. *Brain Res. Bull.,* 4:519–534.

203. Mosko, S. S., Haubrich, D., and Jacobs, B. L. (1977): Serotonergic afferents to the dorsal raphe nucleus: Evidence from HRP and synaptosomal uptake studies. *Brain Res.,* 119:269–290.

204. Moss, M. S., Glazer, E. J., and Basbaum, A. I. (1981): Enkephalin-immunoreactive perikarya in the cat raphe dorsalis. *Neurosci. Lett.,* 21:33–37.

205. Nagatsu, I., Inagaki, S., Kondo, Y., Karasawa, N., and Nagatsu, T. (1979): Immunofluorescent studies on the localization of tyrosine hydroxylase and dopamine-β-hydroxylase in the mes-, di-, and telencephalon of the rat using unperfused fresh frozen sections. *Acta Histochem. Cytochem.,* 12:20–37.

206. Nakamura, M., and Fukushima, H. (1978): Effects of reserpine, *para*-chlorophenylalanine, 5,6-dihydroxytryptamine or 5-methoxytryptamine in mice. *J. Pharm. Pharmacol.,* 30:254–256.

207. Nakasimhachari, N., Kempster, E., and Anbar, M. (1980): 5-Methoxytryptamine in rat hypothalamus and human CSF. A fact or artifact? *Biomed. Mass. Spectrom.,* 7:231–235.

208. Nanopoulos, D., Belin, M.-F., Maitre, M., and Pujol, J.-F. (1980): Immunocytochemie de la glutamata décarboxylase: Mise en evidence neuronaux GABAergiques dans le noyau raphé dorsalis du rat. *C. R. Acad. Sci. [D.] (Paris),* 16:1153–1156.

209. Nauta, W. J. H. (1958): Hippocampal projections and related neural pathways to the midbrain in the cat. *Brain Res.,* 81:319–340.

210. Nauta, W. J. H., and Domesick, V. B. (1978): Crossroads of limbic and striatal circuitry: Hypothalamo–nigral connections. In: *Limbic Mechanisms,* edited by K. E. Livingston and O. Hornykiewicz, pp. 75–93. Plenum Press, New York.

211. Neckers, L. M., Schwartz, J. P., Wyatt, R. J., and Speciale, S. G. (1979): Substance P afferents from the habenula innervate the dorsal raphe nucleus. *Exp. Brain Res.,* 37:619–623.

212. Nieuwenhuys, R., Voogd, J., and van Huijzen, C. (1978): Ascending reticular system and descending reticular systems. In: *The Human Central Nervous System. A Synopsis and Atlas,* pp. 142–148, 177–180. Springer Verlag, Berlin.

213. Nobin, A., and Björklund, A. (1973): Topography of the monoamine neuron systems in the human brain as revealed in fetuses. *Acta Physiol. Scand. [Suppl.,]* 388:1–40.

214. Nygren, L. G. (1976): On the visualization of central dopamine and noradrenaline nerve terminals in cryostat sections. *Med. Biol.,* 54:278–285.

215. Nyström, B., Olson, L., and Ungerstedt, U. (1972): Noradrenaline nerve terminals in human cerebral cortices: First histochemical evidence. *Science,* 176:924–926.

216. Ochi, J., and Shimizu, K. (1978): Occurence of dopamine-containing neurons in the midbrain raphe nuclei of the rat. *Neuroscience,* 8:317–320.

217. Oliveras, J., Bourgoin, S., Hery, F., Besson, J. M., and Hamon, M. (1977): The topographical distribution of serotoninergic terminals in the spinal cord of the cat: Biochemical mapping by the combined use of microdissection and microassay procedures. *Brain Res.,* 138:393–406.

218. de Olmos, J., and Heimer, L. (1980): Double and triple labeling of neurons with fluorescent substances: The study of collateral pathways in the ascending raphe system. *Neurosci. Lett.,* 19:7–12.

219. Olson, L., Boréus, L. O., and Seiger, Å. (1973): Histochemical demonstration and mapping of 5-hydroxytryptamine- and catecholamine-containing neuron systems in the human fetal brain. *Z. Anat. Entwickl. Gesch.,* 139:259–282.

220. Olson, L., and Seiger, Å. (1972): Early prenatal ontogeny of central monoamine neurons in the rat: Fluorescence histochemical observations. *Z. Anat. Entwickl. Gesch.*, 137:301–316.

221. Overdijk, J., Uylings, H. B. M., Kuypers, K., and Kamstra, A. W. (1978): An economical, semi-automatic system for measuring cellular tree structures in three dimensions, with special emphasis on Golgi-impregnated neurons. *J. Microscop.*, 114: 271–284.

222. Palkovits, M., Saavedra, J., Jacobowits, D., Kizer, J., Záborsky, L., and Brownstein, M. (1977): Serotonergic innervation of the forebrain: Effect of lesions on serotonin and tryptophan hydroxylase levels. *Brain Res.*, 130:121–134.

223. Pandey, A., and Habibulla, M. (1980): Serotonin in the central nervous system of the cockroach, *Periplaneta americana. J. Insect Physiol.*, 26:1–6.

224. Parent, A. (1979): Anatomical organization of monoamine- and acetylcholinesterase-containing neuronal systems in the vertebrate hypothalamus. In: *Handbook of the Hypothalamus, Vol. 1: Anatomy of the Hypothalamus*, edited by P. J. Morgane and J. Panksepp, pp. 511–554. Marcel Dekker, New York.

225. Parent, A., Descarries, L., and Beaudet, A. (1981): Organization of ascending serotonin systems in the adult rat brain. A radioautographic study after intraventricular administration of (^{3}H)-5-hydroxytryptamine. *Neuroscience*, 6:115–138.

226. Parent, A., O'Reilly-Fromentin, J., and Boucher, R. (1980): Acetylcholinesterase-containing neurons in cat neostriatum: A morphological and quantitative analysis. *Neurosci. Lett.*, 20:271–276.

227. Pasquier, D. A., Anderson, C., Forbes, W. B., and Morgane, P. J. (1976): Horseradish peroxidase tracing of the lateral habenular midbrain raphe nuclei connections in the rat. *Brain Res. Bull.*, 1:443–451.

228. Pasquier, D. A., Kemper, T. L., Forbes, W. B., and Morgane, P. J. (1977): Dorsal raphe, substantia nigra and locus coeruleus interconnections with each other and the neostriatum. *Brain Res. Bull.*, 2:323–339.

229. Pasquier, D. A., Reinoso-Suarez, F., and Morgane, P. J. (1976): Effect of raphe lesions on brain serotonin in the cat. *Brain Res. Bull.*, 1:279–283.

230. Pasquier, D. A., and Reinoso-Suarez, F. (1977): Differential efferent connections of the brain stem to the hippocampus in the cat. *Brain Res.*, 120:540–548.

231. Pasquier, D. A., and Reinoso-Suarez, F. (1978): The topographic organization of hypothalamic and brain stem projections to the hippocampus. *Brain Res. Bull.*, 3:373–389.

232. Pelletier, G., and Leclerc, R. (1979): Immunohistochemical localization of adrenocorticotrophin in the rat brain. *Endocrine Soc.*, 104:1426–1433.

233. Pelletier, G., Steinbusch, H. W. M., and Verhofstad, A. A. J. (1981): Immunoreactive substance P and serotonin are contained in the same dense core vesicles. *Nature*, 293:71–72.

234. Pfister, C., Hölzel, B., and Danner, H. (1981): GABA-containing neurons in the nucleus raphe dorsalis of the rat. *Acta Histochem.*, 68:117–124.

235. Pickel, V. M., Joh, T. H., and Reis, D. J. (1977): A serotonergic innervation of noradrenergic neurons in nucleus locus coeruleus: Demonstration by immunocytochemical localization of the transmitter specific enzymes tyrosine and tryptophan hydroxylase. *Brain Res.*, 131:197–214.

236. Pilc, A., and Nowak, J. Z. (1979): Influence of histamine on the serotonergic system of rat brain. *Eur. J. Pharmacol.*, 55:269–272.

237. Pin, C., Jones, B., and Jouvet, M. (1968): Topographie des neurones monoaminergiques du tronc cérébral du chat: Étude par histofluorescence. *C. R. Soc. Biol. (Paris)*, 162:2136–2141.

238. Poitras, D., and Parent, A. (1978): Atlas of the distribution of monoamine-containing nerve cell bodies in the brain stem of the cat. *J. Comp. Neurol.*, 179:699–718.

239. Pollard, H., Cortes, C. L., Barbin, G., Garbarg, M., and Schwartz, J. C. (1978): Histamine and histidine decarboxylase in brain stem nuclei: Distribution and decrease after lesions. *Brain Res.*, 157:178–181.

240. Prozialeck, W. C., Boehme, D. H., and Vogel, W. H. (1978): The fluorometric determination of 5-methoxytryptamine in mammalian tissues and fluids. *J. Neurochem.*, 30:1471–1477.

241. Quay, W. B. (1979): Biogenic amines in neuroendocrine systems: Multiple sources, messages, targets and controls. *Texas Rep. Biol. Med.*, 38:87–103.

242. Ramón-Moliner, E. (1975): Specialized and generalized dendritic patterns. In: *Golgi Centennial Symposium: Perspectives in Neurobiology*, edited by M. Santini, pp. 87–100. Raven Press, New York.

243. Ramón-Moliner, E., and Nauta, W. J. H. (1966): The isodendritic core of the brain stem. *J. Comp. Neurol.*, 126:311–336.

244. Reinhard, J. F., Jr., Liebmann, J. E., Schlosberg, A. J., and Moskowitz, M. A. (1979): Serotonin neurons project to small blood vessels in the brain. *Science*, 206:85–87.

245. Ribas, J. L. (1977): Morphological evidence for a possible functional role of supra-ependymal nerves on ependyma. *Brain Res.*, 125:362–368.

246. Riche, D., Denavit-Saubie, M., and Champagnat, J. (1979): Pontine afferents to the medullary respiratory system: An anatomico–functional correlation. *Neurosci. Lett.*, 13:151–155.

247. Rodriguez, E. M. (1978): Comparative and functional morphology of the median eminence. In: *Brain Endocrine Interaction. Median Eminence: Structure and Function*, edited by K. M. Knigge, D. E. Scott, and A. Weindl, pp. 319–344. S. Karger, Basel.

248. Roney, K. J., Scheibel, A. B., and Shaw, G. L. (1979): Dendritic bundles: Survey of anatomical experiments and physiological theories. *Brain Res. Rev.*, 1:225–271.

249. Ross, C. A., Ruggiero, D. A., and Reis, D. J. (1981): Projections to the spinal cord from neurons

close to the ventral surface of the hindbrain in the rat. *Neurosci. Lett.,* 21:143–148.

250. Royce, G. J. (1978): Cells of origin of subcortical afferents to the caudate nucleus: A horseradish peroxidase study in the cat. *Brain Res.,* 153:465–475.

251. Saavedra, J. M. (1977): Distribution of serotonin and synthetizing enzymes in discrete areas of the brain. *Fed. Proc.,* 36:2134–2148.

252. Sachs, C., and Jonsson, G. (1975): 5,7-Dihydroxytryptamine induced changes in the postnatal development of central 5-hydroxytryptamine neurons. *Med. Biol.,* 53:156–164.

253. Sakai, K., Salvert, D., Touret, M., and Jouvet, M. (1977): Afferent connections of the nucleus raphe dorsalis in the cat, visualized by the horseradish peroxidase technique. *Brain Res.,* 137:11–35.

254. Sakai, K., Touret, M., Salvert, D., Léger, L., and Jouvet, M. (1977): Afferent projections to the cat locus coeruleus as visualized by the horseradish peroxidase technique. *Brain Res.,* 119:21–41.

255. Sakai, K., Touret, M., Salvert, D., and Jouvet, M. (1978): Afferents to the cat locus coeruleus and rostral raphe nuclei as visualized by the horseradish peroxidase technique. In: *Interactions Between Putative Neurotransmitter in the Brain,* edited by S. Garattini, J. F. Pujol, and R. Samanin, pp. 319–342. Raven Press, New York.

256. Samanin, R., Quattrone, A., Peri, G., Ladinsky, H., and Consolo, S. (1978): Evidence of an interaction between serotoninergic and cholinergic neurons in the corpus striatum and hippocampus of the rat brain. *Brain Res.,* 151:73–82.

257. Saper, C. B., Loewy, A. D., Swanson, L. W., and Cowan, W. M. (1976): Direct hypothalamo–autonomic projections. *Brain Res.,* 117:305–312.

258. Sar, M., Stumpf, W. E., Miller, R. J., Chang, K.-J., and Cuatrecasas, P. (1978): Immunohistochemical localization of enkephalin in rat brain and spinal cord. *J. Comp. Neurol.,* 182:17–38.

259. Sato, M., Itoh, K., and Mizuno, N. (1979): Distribution of thalamo–caudate neurons in the cat as demonstrated by horseradish peroxidase. *Exp. Brain Res.,* 34:143–153.

260. Scheibel, M. E., and Scheibel, A. B. (1970): Organization of spinal motoneuron dendrites in bundles. *Exp. Neurol.,* 28:106–122.

261. Scheibel, M. E., and Scheibel, A. B. (1975): Dendrites as neuronal couplers: The dendrite bundle. In: *Golgi Centennial Symposium: Perspectives in Neurobiology,* edited by M. Santini, pp. 347–354. Raven Press, New York.

262. Schipper, J., Steinbusch, H. W. M., Verhofstad, A. A. J., and Tilders, F. J. H. (1981): Quantitative immunofluorescence of serotonin. *Proceedings of the 22nd Dutch Federation Meeting,* p. 390. Dutch Foundation of Federation of Medical Scientific Societies, Nijmegen, The Netherlands.

263. Schofield, G. C., and Wreford, N. G. M. (1979): Microspectrofluorometric studies on the formaldehyde-induced reaction product of 5-hydroxytryptamine. *J. Microscop.,* 116:185–198.

264. Schwartz, J.-C., Pollard, H., and Quach, T. T. (1980): Histamine as a neurotransmitter in mammalian brain: Neurochemical evidence. *J. Neurochem.,* 35:26–33.

265. Scott, D. E., Kozlowski, G. P., and Krobisch-Dudley, G. (1975): A comparative ultrastructural analysis of the third cerebral ventricle of the North American mink *(Mustela vison). Anat. Rec.,* 175:155–168.

266. Scott, D. E., and Paull, W. K. (1979): The tanycyte of the rat median eminence. *Cell Tissue Res.,* 200:329–334.

267. Segal, M. (1977): Afferents to the entorhinal cortex of the rat studied by the method of retrograde transport of horseradish peroxidase. *Exp. Neurol.,* 57:750–765.

268. Segu, L., and Calas, A. (1978): The topographical distribution of serotoninergic terminals in the spinal cord of the cat: Quantitative radioautographic studies. *Brain Res.,* 153:449–464.

269. Seiler, N. (1977): Chromatography of biogenic amines. I. Generally applicable separation and detection methods. *J. Chromatogr.,* 143:221–246.

270. Shah, Y., and Dostrovsky, J. O. (1980): Electrophysiological evidence for a projection of the periaquaductal gray matter to nucleus raphe magnus in cat and rat. *Brain Res.,* 193:534–538.

271. Shinnar, S., Maciewicz, R. J., and Shofer, R. J. (1975): A raphe projection to cat cerebellar cortex. *Brain Res.,* 97:139–143.

272. Shoemaker, D. W., Cummins, J. T., and Bidder, T. G. (1978): β-Carbolines in rat arcuate nucleus. *Neuroscience,* 3:233–239.

273. Sims, K. B., Hoffman, D. L., Said, S. I., and Zimmerman, E. A. (1980): Vasoactive intestinal polypeptide (VIP) in mouse and rat brain: An immunocytochemical study. *Brain Res.,* 186:165–183.

274. Sladek, J. R., and Sladek, C. D. (1978): Localization of serotonin within tanycytes of the rat median eminence. *Cell Tissue Res.,* 186:465–474.

275. Sladek, J. R., and Walker, P. (1977): Serotonin-containing neuronal perikarya in the primate locus coeruleus and subcoeruleus. *Brain Res.,* 134:354–366.

276. Smits, J. F. M., Van Essen, H., and Struyker-Boudier, H. A. J. (1978): Serotonin-mediated cardiovascular responses to electrical stimulation of the raphe nuclei in the rat. *Life Sci.,* 23:173–178.

277. Sofroniew, M. V. (1979): Immunoreactive β-endorphin and ACTH in the same neurons of the hypothalamic arcuate nucleus in the rat. *Am. J. Anat.,* 154:283–289.

278. Sofroniew, M. V. (1980): Projections from vasopressin, oxytocin and neurophysin neurons to neural targets in the rat and human. *J. Histochem. Cytochem.,* 28:475–478.

279. Sofroniew, M. V., and Schrell, U. (1980): Hypothalamic neurons projecting to the rat caudal medulla oblongata, examined by immunoperoxidase staining of retrogradely transported horseradish peroxidase. *Neurosci. Lett.,* 19:257–263.

280. Sofroniew, M. V., and Weindl, A. (1978): Projections from the parvocellular vasopressin- and neurophysin-containing neurons of the suprachiasmatic nucleus. *Am. J. Anat.,* 153:391–429.

281. Sofroniew, M. V., and Weindl, A. (1982): Central nervous system distribution of vasopressin, oxytocin and neurophysin. In: *Endogenous Peptides and Learning and Memory Processes,* edited by J. L. Martinez, R. A. Jensen, R. B. Messing, H. Rigter, and J. L. McGaugh. Academic Press, New York *(in press).*

282. Solomon, P. R., Nichols, G. L., Kiernan, J. M., III, and Kamer, R. S. (1980): Differential effects of lesions in medial and dorsal raphe of the rat: Latent inhibition and septohippocampal serotonin levels. *J. Comp. Physiol. Psychol.,* 94:145–154.

283. Steeves, J. P., Jordan, L. M., and Lake, N. (1975): The close proximity of catecholamine-containing cells to the mesencephalic locomotor region (MLR). *Brain Res.,* 100:663–670.

284. Steinbusch, H. W. M. (1981): Distribution of serotonin-immunoreactivity in the central nervous system of the rat. Cell bodies and terminals. *Neuroscience,* 6:557–618.

285. Steinbusch, H. W. M., and Nieuwenhuys, R. (1979): Serotonergic neuron systems in the brain of the lamprey *(Lampetra fluviatilis). Anat. Rec.,* 193:693–694.

286. Steinbusch, H. W. M., and Nieuwenhuys, R. (1981): Localization of serotonin-like immunoreactivity in the central nervous system and pituitary of the rat, with special references to the innervation of the hypothalamus. *Adv. Exp. Med. Biol.,* 133:7–36.

287. Steinbusch, H. W. M., Nieuwenhuys, R., Verhofstad, A. A. J., and Van Der Kooy, D. (1981): The nucleus raphe dorsalis of the rat and its projection upon the caudatoputamen. A combined cytoarchitectonic, immunohistochemical and retrograde transport study. *J. Physiol. (Paris),* 77:157–174.

288. Steinbusch, H. W. M., Van Der Kooy, D., Verhofstad, A. A. J., and Pellegrino, A. (1980): Serotonergic and non-serotonergic projections from the nucleus raphe dorsalis to the caudate–putamen complex in the rat, studied by a combined immunofluorescence and fluorescent retrograde axonal labeling technique. *Neurosci. Lett.,* 19:137–142.

289. Steinbusch, H. W. M., and Verhofstad, A. A. J. (1979): Immunofluorescent staining of serotonin in the central nervous system. *Adv. Pharmacol. Ther.,* 2:151–160.

290. Steinbusch, H. W. M., Verhofstad, A. A. J., Penke, B., Varga, J., and Joosten, W. H. J. (1981): Immunohistochemical characterization of monoamine-containing neurons in the central nervous system by antibodies to serotonin and noradrenaline. A study in the rat and the lamprey *(Lampetra fluviatilis). Acta Histochem. [Suppl.],* 24:107–122.

291. Steinbusch, H. W. M., Verhofstad, A. A. J., and Joosten, H. W. J. (1983): Antibodies to serotonin for neuroimmunocytochemical studies on the central nervous system. Methodological aspects and applications. In: *IBRO-Handbook: Neuroimmunocytochemistry,* edited by C. Cuello, pp. 193–214. John Wiley & Sons, New York, Chichester.

292. Steranka, L., Bessent, R., and Sanders-Bush, E. (1977): Reversible and irreversible effects of *p*-chloroamphetamine on brain serotonin in mice. *Commun. Psychopharmacol.,* 1:447–454.

293. Sternberger, L. A., Hardy, P. H., Jr., Cuculis, J. H., and Meyer, H. G. (1970): The unlabeled antibody enzyme method of immunohistochemistry. Preparation and properties of soluble antigen–antibody complex (horseradish peroxidase–antihorseradish peroxidase) and its use in identifications of spirochetes. *J. Histochem. Cytochem.,* 18:315–333.

294. Streit, P., Reubi, J. C., Wolfensberger, M., Henke, H., and Cuénod, M. (1980): Transmitter-specific retrograde tracing of pathways? In: *Progress in Brain Research, Vol. 51: Development and Chemical Specificity of Neurons,* edited by M. Cuénod, G. W. Kreutzberg, and F. E. Bloom, pp. 489–496. Elsevier/North Holland Biomedical Press, Amsterdam.

295. Suzuki, O., Noguchi, E., and Yagi, K. (1977): Tryptophan-5-hydroxylase in developing chick brain. *Brain Res.,* 131:379–382.

296. Swanson, L. W., Conelly, H. A., and Hartman, B. K. (1977): Ultrastructural evidence for central monoaminergic innervation of blood vessels in the paraventricular nucleus of the hypothalamus. *Brain Res.,* 136:166–173.

297. Swanson, L. W., and Hartman, B. K. (1975): The central adrenergic system. An immunofluorescence study of the localization of cell bodies and their efferent connections in the rat utilizing DBH as a marker. *J. Comp. Neurol.,* 163:467.

298. Szabo, J. (1980): Distribution of striatal afferents from the mesencephalon in the cat. *Brain Res.,* 188:3–21.

299. Szabo, J. (1980): Organization of the ascending striatal afferents in monkeys. *J. Comp. Neurol.,* 189:307–321.

300. Taber, E., Brodal, A., and Walberg, F. (1960): The raphe nuclei of the brain stem in the cat. I. Normal topography and cytoarchitecture and general discussion. *J. Comp. Neurol.,* 114:161–187.

301. Taber-Pierce, E., Foote, W. E., and Hobson, J. A. (1976): The efferent connection of the nucleus raphe dorsalis. *Brain Res.,* 107:137–144.

302. Taniyama, K., Nitsch, C., Wagner, A., and Hassler, R. (1980): Aspartate, glutamate and GABA levels in pallidum, substantia nigra, center median and dorsal raphe nuclei after cylindric lesion of caudate nucleus in cat. *Neurosci. Lett.,* 16:155–160.

303. Ternaux, J. P., Héry, F., Bourgoin, S., Adrien, J., Glowinski, J., and Hamon, M. (1977): The topographical distribution of serotoninergic terminals in the neostriatum of the rat and the caudate nucleus of the cat. *Brain Res.,* 121:311–326.

304. Toerk, I., Leventhal, A. G., and Stone, J. (1977): Brain stem afferents to visual cortical areas 17, 18 and 19 in the cat demonstrated by horseradish peroxidase. *Neurosci. Lett.,* 11:247–252.

305. Tohyama, M., Sakai, K., Salvert, D., Touret, M., and Jouvet, M. (1979): Spinal projections from the lower brain stem in the cat as demonstrated by the horseradish peroxidase technique. I. Origins of the reticulospinal tracts and their funicular trajectories. *Brain Res.,* 173:383–403.

306. Tohyama, M., Sakai, K., Touret, M., Salvert, D., and Jouvet, M. (1979): Spinal projections from the lower brain stem in the cat as demonstrated by the horseradish peroxidase technique. II. Projection from the dorsolateral pontine tegmentum and raphe nuclei. *Brain Res.,* 176:215–231.

307. Tohyama, M., Shiosaka, S., Sakanaka, M., Takagi, H., Senba, E., Saitoh, Y., Takahashi, Y., Sakumoto, T., and Shimizu, N. (1980): Detailed pathways of the raphe dorsalis neuron to the cerebral cortex with use of horseradish peroxidase-3,3',5,5' tetramethyl bezidine reaction as a tool for the fibre tracing technique. *Brain Res.,* 181:433–439.

308. Tong, J. H., and Kaufman, S. (1975): Tryptophan hydroxylase purification and some properties of the enzyme from rabbit hindbrain. *J. Biol. Chem.,* 250:4152–4158.

309. de la Torre, J. C., and Surgeon, J. W. (1976): Histochemical fluorescence of tissue and brain monoamines results in 18 minutes using the sucrose-phosphate–glyoxylic acid method. *Neuroscience,* 1:451–453.

310. Twarog, B. H., and Page, I. H. (1953): Serotonin content of some mammalian tissues and urine and a method for its determination. *Am. J. Physiol.,* 175:156–161.

311. Uhl, G. R., Goodman, R. R., Kuhar, M. J., Childers, S. R., and Snyder, S. H. (1979): Immunohistochemical mapping of enkephalin containing cell bodies, fibers and nerve terminals in the brain stem of the rat. *Brain Res.,* 166:75–94.

312. Uhl, G. R., Kuhar, M. J., and Snyder, S. H. (1977): Neurotensin: Immunohistochemical localization in rat central nervous system. *Proc. Natl. Acad. Sci. U.S.A.,* 74:4059–4063.

313. Ungerstedt, U. (1971): Stereotaxic mapping of the monoamine pathways in the rat brain. *Acta Physiol. Scand.* [*Suppl.*], 367:1–48.

314. Usunoff, K. G., Hassler, R., Wagner, A., and Bak, I. J. (1974): The efferent connections of the head of the caudate nucleus in the cat: An experimental morphological study with special reference to a projection to the raphe nuclei. *Brain Res.,* 74:143–148.

315. Uylings, H. B. M. (1977): *A Study on Morphometry and Functional Morphology of Branching Structures, with Applications to Dendrites in Visual Cortex of Adult Rats Under Different Environmental Conditions.* Doctoral thesis, University of Amsterdam. Kaal's Printing House, Amsterdam.

316. Valverde, F. (1962): Reticular formation of the albino rat's brain stem. Cytoarchitecture and corticofugal connections. *J. Comp. Neurol.,* 119:25–54.

317. Van de Kar, L. D., and Lorens, S. A. (1979): Differential serotonergic innervation of individual hypothalamic nuclei and other forebrain regions by the dorsal and median midbrain raphe nuclei. *Brain Res.,* 162:45–54.

318. Vanderhaeghen, J. J., Lotstra, F., De Mey, J., and Gilles, C. (1980): Immunohistochemical localization of cholecystokinin- and gastrin-like peptides in the brain and hypophysis of the rat. *Proc. Natl. Acad. Sci. U.S.A.,* 77:1190–1194.

319. Van Der Kooy, D. (1979): The organization of the thalamic, nigral and raphe cells projecting to the medial vs. lateral caudate–putamen in rat. A fluorescent retrograde double labeling study. *Brain Res.,* 169:381–387.

320. Van Der Kooy, D., and Hattori, T. (1980): Dorsal raphe cells with collateral projections to the caudate–putamen and substantia nigra: A fluorescent retrograde double labeling study in the rat. *Brain Res.,* 186:1–7.

321. Van Der Kooy, D., Hunt, S., Steinbusch, H. W. M., and Verhofstad, A. A. J. (1981): Separate populations of cholecystokinin and 5-HT containing neuronal cells in the rat dorsal raphe and their contribution to its ascending projections. *Neurosci. Lett.,* 26:25–30.

322. Van Der Kooy, D., and Kuypers, H. G. J. M. (1979): Fluorescent retrograde double labeling: Axonal branching in the ascending raphe and nigral projections. *Science,* 204:873–875.

323. Van Der Kooy, D., and Steinbusch, H. W. M. (1980): Simultaneous fluorescent retrograde tracing and immunofluorescent characterization of neurons. *J. Neurosci. Res.,* 5:479–484.

324. Verhofstad, A. A. J., Steinbusch, H. W. M., Penke, B., Varga, J., and Joosten, H. W. J. (1981): Serotonin-immunoreactive cells in the superior cervical ganglion of the rat. Evidence for the existence of separate serotonin- and catecholamine-containing small ganglionic cells. *Brain Res.,* 212:39–49.

325. Wang, R. Y., and Aghajanian, G. K. (1977): Inhibition of neurons in the amygdala by dorsal raphe stimulation mediation through a direct serotonergic pathway. *Brain Res.,* 120:85–102.

326. Wang, R. Y., and Aghajanian, G. K. (1978): Collateral inhibition of serotonergic neurons in the rat dorsal raphe nucleus: Pharmacological evidence. *Neuropharmacology,* 17:819–825.

327. Watkins, L. R., Griffin, G., Leichnetz, G. R., and Mayer, D. J. (1980): The somatotropic organization of the nucleus raphe magnus and surrounding brain stem structures as revealed by HRP slow-release gels. *Brain Res.,* 181:1–15.

328. Watson, S. J., and Skil, H. (1980): α-MSH in rat brain: Occurrence within and outside of β-endorphin neurons. *Brain Res.,* 182:217–223.

329. Watson, S. J., and Barchas, J. D. (1977): Catecholamine histofluorescence using cryostat sectioning and glyoxylic acid in unperfused frozen brain: A detailed description of the technique. *Histochem. J.,* 9:183–195.

330. Watson, S. J., Brachas, J. D., and Hao Li, C. (1977): β-Lipotropin: Localization of cells and axons in rat brain by immunocytochemistry. *Proc. Natl. Acad. Sci. U.S.A.,* 74:5155–5158.

331. Watson, S. J., Richard, C. W., and Barchas, J. D. (1978): Adrenocorticotropin in rat brain: Immunocytochemical localization in cells and axons. *Science,* 200:1180–1182.

332. Welch, K. M. A., Gaudet, R., Wang, T. P. F., and Chabi, E. (1977): Transient cerebral ischemia and brain serotonin: Relevance to migraine. *Headache,* 17:145–147.

333. Welsh, J. H., and Williams, L. D. (1970): Monoamine-containing neurons in planaria. *J. Comp. Neurol.,* 138:103–116.

334. Westergaard, E. (1972): The fine structure of nerve fibers and endings in the lateral cerebral ventricles of the rat. *J. Comp. Neurol.*, 144:345–354.

335. Widmer, F., Mutus, B., Scheckus, A., and Viswanatha, T. (1976): Partial purification of rabbit brain tryptophan hydroxylase by affinity chromatography. *Life Sci.*, 17:1297–1302.

336. Wiklund, L. (1974): Development of serotonin-containing cells and the sympathetic innervation of the habenular region in the rat brain. A fluorescence histochemical study. *Cell Tissue Res.*, 155:231–243.

337. Wiklund, L., Léger, L., and Persson, M. (1980): Monoamine cell distribution in the cat brain stem. A fluorescence histochemical study with quantification of indolaminergic and locus coeruleus cell groups. *J. Comp Neurol.*, 203:613–647.

338. Wittkowski, W. (1968): Zur funktionellen Morphology ependymaler und extraependymaler Glia. Im Rahmen der Neurosekretion. *Z. Zellforsch. Mikrosk. Anat.*, 86:111–128.

339. Wright, A. K., and Arbuthnott, G. W. (1980): Non-dopamine containing efferents of substantia nigra: The pathway to the lower brain stem. *J. Neural Transm.*, 47:221–226.

340. Wünscher, W., Schobler, W., and Werner, L. (1965): *Architektonischer Atlas vom Hirnstamm der Ratte.* S. Hirzel Verlag, Leipzig.

Chemical Neuroanatomy, edited by P.C. Emson,
Raven Press, New York © 1983.

Chemical Neuroanatomy of the Cerebellar Cortex

*Jesse A. Schulman

*MRC Neurochemical Pharmacology Unit, Medical Research Council Medical School,
Cambridge CB2 2QH, England*

The discovery and documentation in the late nineteenth and early twentieth centuries of the dramatic simplicity of cerebellar cytoarchitecture and the elucidation by electron microscopy of the synaptic interconnections of cerebellar neurons have made the cerebellum an attractive object of study for investigators interested in the relationship between structure and function in the central nervous system. The availability of a detailed blueprint of cellular morphology and of synaptic organization has allowed detailed investigation and theoretical analysis of cerebellar transactions ranging in scope from studies of the integration of inputs by dendritic arborizations to the operation of neuronal networks. Considerable progress has been made, although neither a full description of the cellular interactions taking place in the cerebellum nor one of the role of such neuronal interactions in the regulation of motor functions is in immediate prospect.

The great range of histochemical techniques that has become available in recent years has naturally been applied to the cerebellum as to other brain regions. Investigations of localization of neurotransmitters, of their synthetic and degradative enzymes, of receptors, and of other substances involved in the transduction of chemical to electrical signals have enriched our understanding of the mechanics and dynamics of synaptic interactions in the cerebellum. These investigations have also allowed us to begin to superimpose a neurochemical map onto the neuroanatomical map of the cerebellum, and it is this superimposition that is the primary subject of this chapter.

It is fair to ask, however, whether the availability of a neurochemical map and of information regarding the identity and actions of synaptic transmitters is in fact necessary to ensure an understanding of how the cerebellum performs its tasks. One might argue that natural or electrical stimulation of pathways to and within the cerebellus is sufficient to determine the character and duration of synaptically mediated effects and that knowledge of these parameters suffices for an understanding of the computational or signal-processing capabilities that underlie cerebellar regulation of motor function. After all, if one knows whether a given synapse is excitatory or inhibitory, and how long the effects of various patterns of stimulation last, what difference does it make what chemical mediates the effect? One answer is that particular chemicals may be used typically in particular synaptic configurations or to perform particular functions throughout the brain; therefore, insight derived from a study of a chemical system in one region may be applicable to other regions. Analogies based on neurochemical similarity or identity may thereby allow elucidation of types of neuronal interaction that are not apparent in "black box" studies. Another possible answer is that slow variations in parameters of synaptic function may be much more difficult to detect by physiological methods than by neurochemical or histochemical techniques. Consideration of functional implications of chemical data is therefore a secondary purpose in this chapter.

This chapter begins with a brief review of the essentials of cerebellar histology and then proceeds to an examination of the various candidate neurotransmitters that have been proposed for each individual cell type in the cerebellum. The discussion here of transmitter candidates concentrates on neurochemical and histochemical localization of neuroactive substances and their synthetic and degradative enzymes. Electrophysiological investigations are considered only briefly. The chapter

---

Present address: 4, Radnar Walk, London SW3, England.

concludes with a discussion of the role of various neurochemicals in cerebellar operations.

It is necessary before beginning, however, to discuss briefly some questions of the terminology applied to communication between neurons. Some authors have recently insisted that the term *neurotransmitter* is properly applied only to substances released from synaptic specializations and having a rapid effect on the passive ionic conductance of the postsynaptic membrane (4). Recent authors often use the word *neuromodulator* to describe a substance of slow or indirect effect or one that is released other than by conventional synapses. For the purpose of this chapter, a cell's neurotransmitter is defined as a substance whose release mediates the effects of that neuron on the electrical properties of other neurons. Novel modes of neurotransmission, such as the possibility of extrasynaptic release, the colocalization of neuroactive peptides in the same neuron as "conventional" putative transmitters, and others, are discussed as they arise. The term *neurotransmitter* is thus used broadly and is not intended to enforce a narrow view of intercellular neuronal communication.

Following Werman (170) and many other authors, a substance must fulfill four criteria to be termed a neurotransmitter. The substance must be present in the neuron under study; it must be released when the neuron is stimulated; its effect on the postsynaptic cell must mimic the effect of presynaptic stimulation; and the pharmacological properties of the effect of the putative transmitter must mimic those of the effect of presynaptic stimulation.

CYTOARCHITECTURE OF THE CEREBELLAR CORTEX

The major neuronal cell and fiber types of the cerebellum have been known for almost a century and were summarized by Cajal (135). More recent workers have extended and clarified earlier findings and in particular utilized the electron microscope to establish patterns of synaptic connectivity between cell types (48,101,132).

The cerebellum is composed of three major histological divisions: the cortex, the underlying white matter, and the deep nuclei (135). The deep nuclear cell masses form the core of the cerebellum and are surrounded by white matter, which, in turn, is surrounded by the highly involuted cortex. Cells of the deep nuclei provide the output pathways for the cerebellum.

The cortex of the cerebellum is a highly involuted trilaminar structure whose three-dimensional organization may be likened to a crystal lattice. Its organization appears to be histologically uniform in all regions of the cerebellum. Moreover, the basic elements and cytoarchitecture are similar in a broad range of species (101,135). The cerebellar cortex is composed of three layers—the granular, Purkinje cell, and molecular layers—as shown in the accompanying simplified schematic (Fig. 1).

The major cell type of the granular layer is the granule cell, a small neuron whose axon extends into the molecular layer and bifurcates, running parallel to the axis of the folium. Granule cells receive input from mossy fiber afferents and synapse on Purkinje cells. Also in the granular layer is the Golgi cell, whose dendrites ramify in the granular and molecular layers, and which receive input from most, if not all, cerebellar neuron types. Golgi cell axons ramify locally in the granular layer and synapse onto granule cell dendrites as part of the mossy fiber glomeruli which are described below.

The Purkinje cell layer is a single cell thick, and the dendrites of the Purkinje cell branch in the molecular layer. Their branching pattern is a highly restricted one in that the dendrites ramify entirely in a plane perpendicular to the long axis of the folium. Thus, in the schematic shown in Fig. 1, the Purkinje cell dendritic tree is seen in its entirety. The arrangement is therefore such that the parallel fibers run perpendicularly to the dendritic array of the Purkinje cells. The Purkinje cells receive synaptic input from parallel fibers as well as from interneurons of the molecular layer. Purkinje cells project to the cells of the deep nuclei.

The molecular layer contains two neuronal cell types, the basket and stellate cells. Both have dendritic arbors in the molecular layer and receive input from the parallel fibers, projecting in turn to the Purkinje cells. The morphology of the two types of cell differs, however. The stellate cells' axons ramify close to the cell body and therefore synapse on nearby Purkinje cells. The basket cells, however, send their axons away from the cell body in a direction perpendicular to the axis of the folium, that is, parallel to the dendritic array of the Purkinje cell. The basket cell axon ramifies and envelops the Purkinje cell body in a "basket" of fibers. In Fig. 1, only two such contacts are diagrammed, but each basket cell may contact as many as 10 Purkinje cells, all more or less coplanar.

The classical histological studies identified two types of input fibers projecting to the cerebellar cortex (135). To these, more recent research has added a third type. [For a thorough review of cerebellar afferents, see Bloedel (12).] One input type identified in early silver-impregnation studies is the

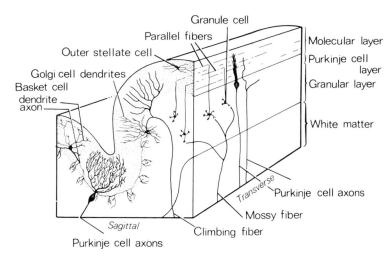

FIG. 1. Organization of the mammalian cerebellum in transverse and sagittal planes.

mossy fiber. Mossy fibers enter the cerebellar cortex from the white matter and ramify extensively in the granular layer, producing large (5–10 μm) terminals and *en passant* profiles of complex shape. Electron microscopy has revealed that these profiles form the core of a complex synaptic structure which is called a glomerulus. The mossy fiber glomeruli consist of a mossy fiber core surrounded by granule cell dendrites and surrounded in turn by axon terminals by Golgi cells. Electrophysiological and anatomical studies (48) indicate that both the mossy fiber core and the Golgi axon terminals are presynaptic to the granule cell dendrites. Thus, input arriving via the mossy fibers is relayed to the Purkinje cells by the granule cells, and the strength of this relay is regulated by the activity of the Golgi cells. Mossy fibers arise from the spinal cord, from nuclei of the reticular formation, and from pontine nuclei which relay signals from primary and associational sensorimotor cerebral cortex.

Another type of input fiber to the cerebellar cortex, called the climbing fiber, synapses directly on the Purkinje cell. The climbing fiber is so named because it branches extensively and winds around the dendrites of the Purkinje cell like climbing strands of ivy. Each Purkinje cell receives a single climbing fiber, and each climbing fiber forms numerous synapses on the Purkinje cell (48,135). Climbing fibers appear to arise mostly or entirely from the inferior olive (165).

The introduction of the monoamine histofluorescence technique (49) allowed the discovery of another class of fibers. These fibers enter the granular layer from the white matter and course up into the molecular layer, often turning to run parallel to the pial surface. Although they appear to synapse on Purkinje cells, their morphology does not resemble that of the climbing fibers (71).

Further morphological details are given where appropriate, as the neurochemical characteristics of the various cell and fiber types are discussed.

CANDIDATE TRANSMITTERS FOR CEREBELLAR NEURON TYPES

Having described the various types of cells and fibers in the cerebellum, I now review the evidence that has led to the identification of certain substances as candidate neurotransmitters for each neuronal element. A discussion of input fibers is first, then intrinsic cerebellar neurons, and finally the output cells.

Cerebellar Afferents: The Mossy Fibers

Among the input types, the mossy fiber has been subjected to the most detailed anatomical and physiological study. Since mossy fibers arise from a wide variety of sources, it might be predicted that mossy fibers from different sources might utilize different transmitters. Several putative transmitters have been identified, but none has been clearly shown to act as transmitter at the mossy fiber–granule cell synapse. This may be in part because of the small size of the granule cells, which makes electrophysiological assessment of the postsynaptic effects of putative mossy fiber transmitters difficult.

Early neurochemical and histochemical studies indicate the presence in the cerebellum of acetylcholine (ACh), acetylcholinesterase (AChE), and choline acetyltransferase (ChAT) activity (21, 50,64,110), suggesting the possibility that ACh might act as a transmitter in the cerebellum. Light microscopic examination of rat tissue stained for AChE suggested the association of AChE with some mossy fiber terminals, particularly in regions receiving primary and secondary vestibular afferents (35,63,87). Interruption of afferent pathways to the cerebellum resulted in build-up of reaction product on the side of the cut away from the cerebellum (154) and loss of both AChE and ChAT in the cerebellar cortex of rat and guinea pig (88), corroborating the association of AChE with cerebellar afferents. Electron microscopic immunohistochemistry of rat brain (152) verified ultrastructurally the association of AChE with some, but not all, mossy fibers.

The reliability of AChE staining as a marker for cholinergic transmission, however, may be questionable (161). Other markers for cholinergic transmission have therefore been developed. Recent investigations using α-bungarotoxin, a marker for nicotinic cholinergic receptors (23,97), indicate the presence in rat cerebellar cortex of cholinergic synapses (77). Immunohistochemical staining of rabbit cerebellum with antiserum against ChAT, the enzyme that synthesizes ACh, reveals ChAT-positive mossy fibers (86). It therefore seems likely that some mossy fibers use ACh as their transmitter. Attempts to corroborate this hypothesis electrophysiologically have generated contradictory reports, however, possibly in part because of the difficulty of recording from granule cells (33,34,36,109).

Studies of catecholamine and serotonin distribution in the cerebellum have indicated the presence of these substances in mossy fibers, but only under special experimental circumstances. If cerebellar tissue is pretreated with norepinephrine and then treated for direct histofluorescence, mossy fibers are stained (71). Likewise, if the tissue is loaded with tritiated serotonin or an analog and prepared for autoradiography, mossy fibers are labeled (5,24,71). However, these terminals are only seen when the tissue is pretreated with the putative transmitter; histofluorescence preparations of untreated cerebellum for norepinephrine and serotonin do not show mossy fibers staining (71). It is possible that these substances are normally present in mossy fibers at very low levels, but it seems more likely that norepinephrine and serotonin can be taken up by mossy fibers in a nonspecific manner

(71) and are not used by mossy fibers as neurotransmitters. The presence of serotonin and norepinephrine in cerebellar afferents that differ from mossy fibers has been demonstrated (71) and is discussed below.

The recent explosive growth of interest in neuroactive peptides has left the cerebellum largely untouched, since only very small amounts of neuroactive peptides have been found in cerebellum. There are, however, reports of immunohistochemical staining of mossy fibers by antisera directed against neuroactive peptides. Korte et al. (92a) found substance P-like immunoreactivity in the cerebellum of the turtle, and Schulman et al. (149) have reported the presence of enkephalin-like immunoreactivity in mossy fibers in the cerebella of fish, frogs, birds, and mammals. Somatostatin-like immunoreactivity is found in the cerebella of very young rats and mice (G. Hoffman, *personal communication*). This staining appears to represent afferent fibers but disappears around 10 days after birth. All of these substances have been shown to affect the electrical properties of neurons in various central nervous system regions (121,128,138). None has been conclusively demonstrated to be a neurotransmitter [although good evidence suggests that substance P may be a transmitter for small-diameter primary afferents (128)]. Moreover, enkephalin (121) and somatostatin (138) have predominantly inhibitory actions, whereas inhibitory mossy fibers have not been reported. The apparent developmental regulation of somatostatin-containing mossy fibers presents a further puzzle. It is likely that more neuroactive peptides will be found in the cerebellum, but for the moment, the role of peptides in cerebellar function is particularly obscure.

Cerebellar Afferents: The Climbing Fibers

Two candidate amino acid neurotransmitters have been suggested as possible mediators for the powerfully excitatory actions of the climbing fibers synapses onto the Purkinje cell. Guidotti et al. (60) suggested that glutamate might be the transmitter; aspartate has also been suggested (117,137). The finding that 3-acetylpyridine (3-AP) produces a fairly selective lesion of the cell bodies of the inferior olive with the consequent degeneration of the climbing fibers (44,47) has allowed neurochemical investigation of this question. Nadi et al. (116) measured the levels of several amino acids in the cerebellum and medulla after 3-AP lesions. They found decreases of both aspartate and glutamate in the medulla. In the cerebellum, however, aspartate levels fell, but glutamate levels did not, suggesting that aspartate, but not glutamate, was present in climbing fibers. Rea et al. (137), however, found that aspartate and glutamate levels both fell in synaptosome preparations of cerebellum after 3-AP treatment. Caution should be used in interpreting all of these results, since the synaptosomal content of taurine, an inhibitory amino acid (56), also fell after 3-AP (137), casting some doubt on the selectivity of the effect. Both aspartate and glutamate are excitatory agents (40), and receptors for both substances have been characterized in cerebellum (55,151). However, the lack of a histochemical method to demonstrate their presence in climbing fibers and the lack of a pharmacological antagonist capable of distinguishing aspartate-from glutamate-mediated effects in cerebellum (163) preclude any but the most tentative conclusion.

Cerebellar Afferents: Catecholamine and Indoleamine Fibers

A third morphological class of cerebellar afferents escaped the notice of the classical neuroanatomists but was discovered through the use of Falck and Hillarp's (49) histofluorescence technique, which demonstrates the presence in tissue of catechol and indole amines. Morphologically, these fibers differ from both mossy and climbing fibers in that they branch and terminate in the molecular layer but do not entwine themselves around the Purkinje cell dendrites in the manner of the climbing fiber. In addition, the manner of termination of the catecholamine and indoleamine fibers in the central nervous system has recently been suggested to differ from classical synaptic terminations (5,45,46). I now summarize the available histological and ultrastructural descriptions of the norepinephrine and serotonin innervation of the cerebellar cortex and discuss evidence regarding the role of norepinephrine and serotonin as transmitters.

Noradrenergic Fibers

Noradrenergic axons ascend through the granular layer as thin varicose fibers and enter the molecular layer where they collateralize (14,71). Many collaterals run in the Purkinje cell layer, but most of the collaterals arise in the proximal part of the molecular layer and ascend towards the pial surface. Just below the pial surface, some fibers bifurcate, sending branches parallel to the surface in the outermost part of the molecular layer. Norad-

renergic fibers in the molecular layer are characterized by regularly spaced round varicosities of 1 to 2 μm in diameter; this configuration is typical of noradrenergic terminal fields (100,115).

The ultrastructural characteristics of noradrenergic terminations in the brain are a controversial subject. Some authors (45,46) have suggested that noradrenergic fibers in the central nervous system may not enter into true synapses and thus may resemble autonomic neuroeffector junctions. This proposal is based on the finding that profiles in cerebral cortex that accumulate tritiated norepinephrine only rarely enter into synapses (45,46). This has been taken to imply a general release of norepinephrine into the extracellular space and to be consistent with a "modulatory" role for norepinephrine.

For methodological reasons, the question is a difficult one to settle at present, since the most widely used marker for the presence of endogenous monoamines, fixation with permanganate, is poor at labeling synaptic thickenings. Positive identification of a labeled profile as a synaptic terminal is therefore difficult. Permanganate-fixed cerebellar tissue shows the presence in synaptic boutons of small granular vesicles (SGV) (96) whose presence has been shown to be a marker for endogenous monoamine in other parts of the nervous system (16,70,140). Close apposition of SGV-containing boutons to the proximal dendrites of Purkinje cells is also seen. In some cases, synaptic thickenings are seen as well. Close apposition of SGV-containing boutons with granule cell dendrites has also been reported (16). Undisputed examples of true synapses containing SGVs are reported to be rare in cerebellum, however (16).

Attempts to use markers that are compatible with conventional osmium staining, which does demonstrate synaptic thickenings, have also been made. Degenerating synaptic terminals were found in cerebellum after animals had been pretreated with 6-OHDA, a neurotoxin specific for catecholaminergic neurons (14).

It is thus clear that at least some noradrenergic terminations in cerebellum do enter into conventional synapses. The proportion of possible release sites that do not, however, is not known. Recently, a report appeared of an ultrastructural examination of cerebral cortex using an antibody that labels the enzyme dopamine-β-hydroxylase (DBH), which synthesizes norepinephrine (126). The authors found that 50% of the terminals labeled, as seen in single thin sections, entered into conventional synapses. Since many terminals were presumably cut in such a manner that synaptic thickenings were out of the plane of section, the proportion of DBH-containing terminals that form synapses may be presumed to be much higher. Application of this technique, including the use of serial thin sections, to cerebellum might clarify the question and is eagerly awaited. The issue is discussed at greater length by Moore and Bloom (115) and by Bloom et al. (16).

Considerable evidence is available to support the notion that ceruleocerebellar fibers use NE as their transmitter. A series of electrophysiological studies (68,69) showed that application of NE to Purkinje cells, or stimulation of LC, inhibited Purkinje cell firing. The effect appears to be mediated by β-adrenergic receptors, and drugs that block the effects of iontophoretic NE also block the effects of stimulation of LC. Uptake and release of tritiated NE from cerebellar slices have been demonstrated (19). β-Adrenergic binding has been demonstrated in cerebellum using neurochemical techniques (113a). Histochemical studies of β-adrenergic receptor binding in cerebellum have produced conflicting results. Atlas and others (2,3) report localization of binding of novel fluorescent β-adrenergic antagonists applied *in vivo* to sites in the Purkinje cell layer. Palacios and Kuhar (130), using *in vitro* autoradiography of tritiated dihydroalprenolol, report binding mostly in the molecular layer. Differences in methodology presumably underlie the discrepant results, but nonetheless, the identity of neurons bearing β-adrenergic receptors in cerebellum remains unknown.

The notion that NE may function as a neuromodulator in the cerebellum has been proposed (57,58,113) and is discussed later in this chapter.

Serotonin Fibers

Histofluorescence methods also indicate the existence of serotonin-containing fibers in cerebellum (71). These fibers arise from the raphe nuclei (17,153). In histofluorescence preparations, the serotonin fibers resemble those containing NE. As with NE, exogenous serotonin is accumulated by mossy fibers (5,24,71). Mossy fibers do not appear in histofluorescence preparations, however, unless exogenous monoamines are added (71). Ultrastructural studies of fibers in cerebellum that take up serotonin have suggested, as for NE, the possibility that serotonin fibers rarely enter into classical synapses (5).

Electrophysiological studies of serotonin's effects on rat Purkinje cells provide results that depend on the anesthetic used (15). In chloral hydrate-anes-

thetized or decerebrate preparations, half of the neurons were consistently excited, and half consistently inhibited. In animals lightly anesthetized with halothane, all cells responded with inhibition. Considerable further research is clearly necessary to establish the role of serotonin in the cerebellum.

Intrinsic Neurons of the Cerebellar Cortex: The Granule Cells

The granule cells are the main neuronal component of the granular layer. They are small cells and serve to relay mossy fiber inputs to the other cell types of the cerebellar cortex which they excite (48). Most of the evidence available regarding candidate transmitters for the granule cell derives from experiments based on the hypothesis of excitatory amino acid involvement. In particular, evidence supporting the possibility that glutamate may be the granule cell transmitter has been presented by several groups, whose work is reviewed below. Final proof has been elusive, however, in large part because of the lack of pharmacological reagents that are sufficiently selective.

The first evidence suggesting that granule cells contain larger amounts of glutamate than other cells (and therefore, presumably, larger amounts than are required for metabolism) was presented by Young et al. (175). They made use of a virus that, if administered to hamsters shortly after birth, inhibits the postnatal proliferation of the granule cells. They found that the levels of glutamate were lower in infected hamsters than in normal animals, suggesting that the granule cells contained glutamate. Also, neurological mutant mice that show loss of granule cells also show depletion of glutamate (76,106,142). Studies in which granule cell proliferation in rats was disrupted by neonatal X-irradiation have, however, produced conflicting results, with some groups (108,143) finding a fall in glutamate levels after neonatal X-irradiation but others not finding it so (146). Patel et al. (133) measured the incorporation of ^{14}C from 2-[^{14}C]-glucose into various amino acids in the cerebellum and found that the proportion of ^{14}C in glutamate was no different in control and X-irradiated animals. The reasons for these discrepancies are not known.

A further problem was noted by Roffler-Tarlov and Sidman (142) who pointed out that the quantitative relationship between granule cell loss and glutamate depletion does not hold well when different types of mutants are compared. In the Weaver heterozygote, they found a 10% to 20%

cell loss as compared with mice not carrying the gene, but no depletion of glutamate. Comparing the Weaver and Reeler homozygotes, however, shows that the same percent depletion of glutamate can be accompanied by differing granule cell depletions. One further problem is posed by the fact that the Weaver mice also show a loss of glutamate in the deep nuclei, where there are no granule cells or even any cells suspected of using glutamate as transmitter (142). It is therefore difficult to be sure that glutamate depletion in cerebellar cortex is, in fact, a result of granule cell loss.

In further support of the candidacy of glutamate, however, is the demonstration of uptake of glutamate (175) and of Ca^{2+}- sensitive release of endogenous glutamate from synaptosomes prepared from cerebellum (146). Synaptosomal release of glutamate was lower in X-ray-degranulated rats than in controls.

Electrophysiological studies have shown repeatedly that Purkinje cells, which are target cells for the granule cell synapses, are excited by glutamate (85,93,163,174). An attempt to block granule cell-mediated excitation of Purkinje cells was made using the glutamate antagonist D-α-aminoadipate (164). Antagonism could only be demonstrated when the excitability of the Purkinje cell was greatly reduced by application to the cell of GABA. The reason for this is not known. Also, it has been demonstrated that D-α aminoadipate does not discriminate between glutamate and aspartate in rat cerebellum (164).

Glutamate is the best available candidate for the granule cell transmitter. However, it does appear that the problem of pharmacological blockade of granule cell-mediated excitation will need to be solved and the discrepancies in the results of the depletion experiments explained before it will be possible to state with assurance that glutamate is the transmitter of the granule cell.

Intrinsic Inhibitory Interneurons

Three major cell types of the cerebellar cortex, the basket, stellate, and Golgi cells, have been ascribed an inhibitory function on the basis of electrophysiological studies (48). As is discussed below, the leading candidate neurotransmitter for all three of these cell types is GABA, and there has been a tendency to treat basket, stellate, and Golgi cells as if they were neurochemically identical. However, there is evidence available that suggests that there may in fact be important differences among them, so that the evidence regarding trans-mitter candidates for each inhibitory interneuron type will be reviewed separately.

The Basket Cell

The basket cells of the cerebellar cortex lie in the molecular layer and are driven by the granule cells via the parallel fibers. The basket cells send their axons perpendicular to the parallel fibers and envelop the cell bodies of the Purkinje cells. They are presumably the major mediator of "off-beam" inhibition of Purkinje cells following parallel fiber stimulation (48). The discovery of GABA in brain (141,167) was followed by the discovery that GABA (66), its synthetic enzyme glutamate decarboxylase (GAD) (1), and its degradative enzyme GABA transaminase (GABA-T) (145) were all present in cerebellum. In particular, all were present in higher levels in gray matter than white. Moreover, all were more abundant in molecular than granular layer. (This latter finding should be treated cautiously, however, as these authors do not always make clear whether the Purkinje cell layer went into their molecular or granular layer fractions.) Subsequent studies have demonstrated high levels of GABA and related enzymes in the Purkinje cells (95).

Localization of GABA to particular interneuronal types in the cerebellum has thus far not proved possible. Several indirect techniques, however, provide evidence suggesting that GABA may be localized to basket cells, *inter alia*.

Immunohistochemical studies performed using antibodies against GAD have demonstrated a pattern of terminal staining distribution of GAD-positive terminals around Purkinje cells somata that closely resembles that of basket cell terminations indicated by study of silver-impregnated material (Fig. 2). This suggestion is consistent with evidence from electron microscopic studies of GAD immunoreactivity (112). Likewise, the pattern of staining shown by autoradiography of sections incubated in radiolabeled GABA, which demonstrates GABA uptake into synaptic terminals, also resembles that of basket cell terminations. Also, basket cell bodies appear to accumulate radiolabeled GABA (72,73), and they are GAD positive in animals in which axoplasmic transport has been blocked with colchicine (139) (Fig. 2).

Release of GABA from cerebellar cortex cannot at present be attributed to particular neuron types. However, uptake and release of tritiated GABA by superfused rat cerebellar cortex has been reported. Release was evoked both by depolarization using

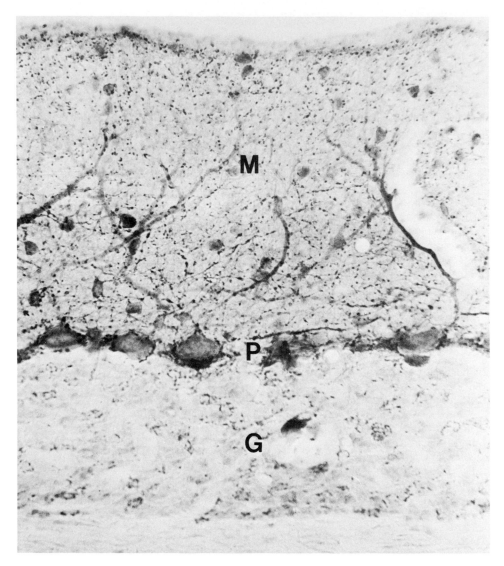

FIG. 2. Localization of glutamic acid decarboxylase immunoreactivity in the cerebellum of the rat. Note the presence of immunoreactivity in the Purkinje cells and in cells of the molecular layer. P, Purkinje cell layer; G, granule cell layer; M, molecular layer.

high potassium concentrations and by veratridine (6,42). Use of veratridine appears to indicate that the evoked release is in fact from neurons rather than from glia (18).

Using the radiolabeled GABA receptor ligand muscimol for autoradiography, Chan-Palay (26) and Chan-Palay and Palay (29) reported significant amounts of GABA receptor on the dendrites, soma, and initial segments of Purkinje cells. This distribution is consistent with the notion that basket cells (or stellate cells; see below) may use

GABA as transmitter. However Palacios et al. (131) found a very different distribution of muscimol binding sites and suggested that earlier results might have been confounded by uptake or metabolism of the muscimol. The similarity of the distribution of radioactivity in the muscimol experiments to that reported by Hökfelt and Ljungdahl (72,73) for GABA uptake is consistent with this contention, but the issue has not been resolved.

Electrophysiological studies indicate that GABA inhibits Purkinje firing (38,89,158). It has been demonstrated in numerous brain regions, including cerebellum and *in vitro* systems, that barbiturates and benzodiazepines potentiate neuronal responses to GABA and the actions of GABA-mediated synapses (41,118,119,125,136). Likewise, off-beam inhibition is greatly strengthened by application of barbiturates (13) or benzodiazepines (114). It has also been shown that off-beam inhibition seen in anesthetized preparations is blocked by the iontophoretic application of the GABA antagonists picrotoxin and bicuculline in several species (11,37,39,172). Pharmacological and electrophysiological evidence therefore favors the identification of GABA as the basket cell transmitter.

The Stellate Cell

The stellate cells are found in the molecular layer of the cerebellar cortex but generally more superficially than the basket cells (135). Like the basket cells, they are driven by the parallel fibers and synapse on Purkinje cells (48). Their axons ramify more locally than those of the basket cells and without obvious directionality (135).

The arguments in favor of the identification of GABA as the stellate cell transmitter follow much the same lines as those for the basket cells. Evidence that stellate cells may contain GABA comes from the autoradiographic demonstration that stellate cells take up tritiated GABA (72,73,148). They also contain GAD immunoreactivity in colchicine-treated rats (139) (Fig. 2).

Since the physiological effects of stellate cells appear to be similar to those of basket cells and to differ only in being confined to a smaller portion of cerebellar cortex, the synaptic physiology and pharmacology of stellate cells have not been studied as thoroughly as those of the basket cells. Electrophysiological corroboration of GABA's role as mediator of stellate cell function is therefore lacking.

Evidence is also available that suggests that the inhibitory amino acid taurine might be the stellate cell transmitter. Taurine is present in cerebellar cortex and is more abundant in the molecular layer than in the granular layer (107,117). Studies in which neonatal rats were exposed to X-rays yielded results consistent with the suggestion that taurine may be present in stellate cells (106). Uptake and release of radiolabeled taurine from superfused cerebellum *in vivo* and *in vitro* have been reported (6,104,125), but the identity of the cells accumulating taurine has not yet been established.

Iontophoresis of taurine onto Purkinje cells results in inhibition that is more marked when the taurine is applied to the dendrites (where stellate cells synapse) than when applied to the soma (where basket cells synapse) (56). Taurine's effects, however, were blocked by the GABA antagonists picrotoxin and bicuculline, suggesting that taurine might be acting via GABA receptors. It will probably be necessary to find antagonists capable of selectively blocking taurine's effects before taurine's candidacy for stellate cell transmitter can be fully evaluated.

The Golgi Cells

The Golgi cells are generally found in the granular layer (135). They receive input from most, if not all, other cerebellar cortical neuron types and appear to act on the dendrites of granule cells, inhibiting the activation of granule cells by mossy fibers (48). As for the basket and stellate cell, the prime candidate for their transmitter is GABA. Levels of GABA and related enzymes are lower in the granular layer than in the molecular layer, consistent with the relatively lower density of inhibitory interneurons in the granular than in the molecular layer. Granular layer GABA and enzyme levels are higher than those of white matter (1,66,134,145).

The autoradiographic studies of GABA uptake in rat also demonstrate staining of cells that appear to be Golgi cells (72,73). One study (90) examined uptake of the tritiated GABA derivative L-2,4-diaminobutyric acid (DABA), suggested to be specifically taken up into neurons and not glia. This study presented electron microscopic evidence of DABA accumulation in Golgi cell terminals. Immunohistochemical studies likewise report the presence of GAD immunoreactivity in cell bodies and terminals of Golgi cells in rat (112) (Fig. 2). The GABA-degrading enzyme GABA transaminase has also been reported to be localized in Golgi cells in rabbit (95,168). An autoradiographic study (131) of the distribution of tritiated muscimol, a marker for GABA receptors, found the highest concentration of label in the granule cell layer, consistent with the possibility that Golgi cells may use GABA as transmitter. However, earlier studies (26,29) yielded quite different results, and the issue remains unresolved.

Electrophysiological examination of Golgi cell actions is difficult since Golgi cells cannot be stimulated selectively and since Golgi cells act on granule cells, which are small and therefore hard to record. Bisti et al. (11) have therefore used the field-potential methodology of Eccles et al. (48) in an attempt to circumvent these problems. They report that effects thought to be mediated by Golgi cells are blocked by GABA antagonists. Although stronger electrophysiological evidence would be reassuring, histochemical and neurochemical evidence does plainly support the role of GABA as Golgi cell transmitter.

Recent immunohistochemical studies, using antibodies directed against enkephalins, have complicated the picture somewhat. Sar et al. (147) reported enkephalin immunoreactivity in Golgi cells of the rat cerebellum, and recently Schulman et al. (149) have extended this finding by demonstrating enkephalin immunoreactivity in Golgi cells of a broad range of species. It is not presently known whether the enkephalin-positive Golgi cells represent a different population than the GAD-positive and GABA-accumulating Golgi cells or whether the Golgi cell may represent another case of colocalization of neuroactive peptides in the same cell as "traditional" neurotransmitters (28,74).

The Purkinje Cells

The Purkinje cells are the output cells of the cerebellar cortex. They project from cerebellar cortex to the deep cerebellar nuclei and the vestibular complex. An elegant series of studies has demonstrated that this pathway is inhibitory and given persuasive evidence that the neurotransmitter of the Purkinje cell is GABA.

The presence of GABA in cerebellar cortex has been repeatedly demonstrated, as discussed earlier in this chapter. Several studies indicate that significant levels of GABA and GAD are found in the Purkinje cells (Fig. 2). In one study, the various layers of rabbit cerebellar cortex were separated from each other by microdissection (95). The Purkinje cells were found to be richer in both GABA and GAD than any other cerebellar region. Otsuka et al. (129) used microdissection and a very sensitive assay for GABA to measure the levels of GABA in single Purkinje cells and lateral vestibular (Dieter's) nuclear cells of cats and rats. The most interesting finding of this study was that the GABA concentration of microdissected Dieter's cells was drastically lower in animals with cerebellar cortical lesions than in normal animals. This was suggested to be a result of the loss of GABA-rich Purkinje cell terminals on the Dieter's cells' somata in lesioned animals. Support for this conclusion comes from the immunohistochemical studies of McLaughlin et al. (112) who found GAD-positive terminals in the deep cerebellar nuclei of rats. Also, it has been shown neurochemi-

cally that the GABA and GAD content of the deep nuclei and Dieter's nuclei in cat and rat are decreased by lesions of the cerebellar cortex (53).

Purkinje cells isolated by bulk fractionation techniques have been shown to accumulate GABA (64). Release of GABA into the cerebrospinal fluid of the fourth ventricle on stimulation of the cerebellar cortex has also been demonstrated (123).

Abundant electrophysiological evidence supports the possibility that GABA is the Purkinje cell transmitter. Administration of GABA to Dieter's and deep nuclear cells in cats mimics the inhibitory effects of cerebellar stimulation (39,41,122,124). The reversal potential of the GABA effect is identical with that of the IPSP generated by cerebellar stimulation (20,124). Also, the inhibition of deep nuclear and Dieter's cells resulting from cerebellar cortical stimulation is blocked by the GABA antagonists picrotoxin and bicuculline (38,41,81, 124). The available evidence therefore seems to demonstrate unambiguously that GABA is the neurotransmitter of the Purkinje cells.

PHYSIOLOGICAL PUZZLES FROM PHARMACOLOGICAL FACTS

As mentioned in the introduction to this chapter, it is not obvious that identification of the chemical agents mediating synaptic transmission is strictly necessary for a complete understanding of the relationship between neuronal activity and cerebellar function. If the relationships between neuronal activity and sensorimotor parameters can be determined, and the responses of neurons to all the various types of synaptic inputs can be measured, it may be possible to generate a complete cellular description of cerebellar function without studying the chemical mediators of synaptic effects. In fact, most physiological research on the cerebellum in recent years has tended to ignore chemical neurotransmitters.

It certainly is obvious, however, that the task of generating a complete, cellular description of cerebellar function is an exceedingly difficult one and that help from any source ought to be welcome. Similarities and analogies between cerebellum and other regions might be predictable on the basis of neurochemical similarities, for example. Also, physiological phenomena of slow onset or long duration, such as one might expect to find underlying long-term functional modifications that could in turn underlie adaptation or learning, may be easier to study neurochemically than electrophysiologically.

Therefore, in the remainder of this chapter, I discuss several lines of research that are based on pharmacological and neurochemical findings and which bear on or suggest physiological problems. The topics to be discussed are the role of norepinephrine in cerebellar function, the findings regarding cyclic GMP in the cerebellar cortex, and a curious paradox arising from the known distribution of enkephalin in cerebellum.

The Ceruleocerebellar Projection

The noradrenergic pathway from the locus ceruleus (LC) to the cerebellum, characterized by Bloom and his colleagues, acts by generating a relatively slow inhibition of Purkinje cell activity (68). Despite the large amount of information available on the anatomy and physiology of the ceruleocerebellar projection, its role in cerebellar function is not well understood by comparison, for example, with that of some of the specific afferents conveying vestibular sensory information to the cerebellar cortex (80). Evidence has been amassed that suggests the possibility that the generation of cyclic AMP in Purkinje cells in response to noradrenergic receptor activation acts to mediate the electrophysiological effects of synaptic stimulation (68). We suggest elsewhere (16) the hypothesis that noradrenergic input may slow Purkinje cell firing rates by acting on their endogenous pacemaker (102) rather than by generating a change in resting membrane potential. Catecholamines and cyclic nucleotides have, in fact, been demonstrated in a variety of neuronal systems (and in heart) to act on pacemakers and on voltage-sensitive conductances (98,166,171).

A possible role for norepinephrine in cerebellar transactions may be deduced from examination of the role of GABA in cerebellar function (58). Eccles and his colleagues (48) demonstrated the role of the basket and stellate cells in so-called off-beam inhibition, wherein activation of a set or "beam" of parallel fibers results not only in excitation of the Purkinje cells to which they project but also in the interneuronal inhibition of other Purkinje cells which are "off the beam." This effect is at least in part mediated by the basket cells, for which the evidence suggests that GABA is the neurotransmitter.

Eccles et al. (48) suggested that off-beam inhibition in the cerebellum might be analogous to lateral inhibition, as demonstrated by Hartline and Ratcliff (62), in the eye. Lateral inhibition is the consequence of a wiring arrangement by which activation of a neuron causes inhibition of that neuron's neighbors and tends to have the effect of restricting the spatial distribution of the effects of an activating signal. In the eye, it is believed to serve a contrast-enhancing effect, allowing the sharp detection of edges. In the cerebellum, a lateral inhibitory effect might similarly serve to restrict the size of a region activated by a given signal, enhance the detection of difference and change, and allow signals to be processed independently by only slightly separated areas of cerebellar cortex.

Available evidence suggests the possibility that the regulation of the strength of a lateral inhibitory effect in cerebellum, by modification of the strength of GABA's actions, may be one role of norepinephrine in cerebellar function. First, norepinephrine increases the resistance of the postsynaptic membrane (156). This has been shown in other systems to increase the voltage amplitude of other incoming postsynaptic potentials (122,150). This should serve to strengthen direct excitation as well as any lateral inhibitory effects. Also, activation and inhibition of Purkinje cells by direct stimulation of cerebellar inputs and of parallel fibers has been shown to be potentiated by LC stimulation and by norepinephrine (57,58,173). Finally, Woodward et al. (173) have presented evidence that suggests that LC stimulation and NE application can increase responses to iontophoretically applied GABA.

These findings suggest that the noradrenergic input to the Purkinje cells from the LC might regulate the strength of lateral inhibition in the cerebellum. The LC might therefore be predicted to be capable of altering such parameters of cerebellar function as the spatial distribution of the activation of cerebellar cortex by an incoming signal, the "sharpness" of somatotopic maps, and the degree of interaction between signals arriving in adjacent areas of cerebellar cortex. Sillito (159,160) has demonstrated that some of the feature-detecting properties of the visual cortex depend critically on the strength of GABA-mediated interneuronal inhibition; in cerebellum, such functions might be regulated in part by the LC. The dependence of LC firing rates on a level of arousal (32,54,67) suggests the further possibility that the character of cerebellar signal processing may vary as a function of behavioral state. Considerable work remains to be done, however, before the validity and utility of this idea can be determined.

Cyclic GMP in the Cerebellum

The role of guanosine 3′,5′-cyclic monophosphate (cyclic GMP) in neuronal function has been the subject of considerable experimentation and speculation. The cerebellum is a region particularly rich in cyclic GMP, and the levels of cyclic GMP are altered by a variety of neuroactive agents and treatments such as ACh, amino acids, apomorphine, harmaline, exposure to cold, and others (51,52,94,105,162). Although cyclic GMP has been suggested to act as an intracellular mediator for certain classes of synaptic events (e.g., 59), no such role has been demonstrated conclusively, and the role of cyclic GMP in the cerebellum remains unknown.

It is known, however, that pharmacological activation of at least two brain regions can elevate cerebellar cyclic GMP, and by different routes. The tremor-causing alkaloid harmaline is known to act by inducing seizure-like activation of the inferior olive (43,103), which gives rise to the climbing fiber projection to Purkinje cells (165). Harmaline also elevates cyclic GMP levels in cerebellum; this effect is reduced by pretreatment with the neurotoxin 3-acetylpyridine (9), which selectively destroys the inferior olive (44,47). It is thus apparent that activation of the climbing fibers results in an increase in cerebellar cyclic GMP. Another pathway appears to exist as well. Administration of the dopamine agonist apomorphine, either systemically or directly to the striatum, also increases cyclic GMP levels in the cerebellum; the dopamine blocker haloperidol decreases cyclic GMP levels and prevents the apomorphine-induced increase (10). The striatally mediated effects are not blocked by 3-acetylpyridine and therefore do not act via climbing fibers (8). The authors conclude that activation of mossy fibers, by some as yet undetermined striatocerebellar route, elevates cerebellar cyclic GMP levels.

The significance of these findings is not yet clear. Guidotti et al. (60) suggest that cyclic GMP might serve as an intracellular second messenger mediating the climbing fiber-induced postsynaptic potential. In support of this proposal, Mao et al. (105) report that a neurological mutant mouse, "nervous," which lacks 90% of its Purkinje cells but whose cerebellum is otherwise intact, is also deficient in cyclic GMP, indicating that cerebellar cyclic GMP may be localized to Purkinje cells. However, it appears unlikely that enzymatically mediated reactions could act swiftly enough to produce synaptic events of the very short latency and duration of the climbing fiber-mediated responses. Also, an immunohistochemical study of cyclic GMP location in the cerebellum suggested a glial localization for cyclic GMP (30). Further work on this subject is clearly necessary, and for the mo-

ment, cyclic GMP in the cerebellum remains a "substance in search of a function." However, the identification of a chemical in cerebellum subject to regulation by certain classes of synaptic inputs remains an intriguing finding, raising as it does the possibility of selective neurochemical alteration of function in response to certain type of inputs.

Neuropeptides in the Cerebellum

The cerebellum, in contrast to most other brain regions, contains only trace amounts of the various neuroactive peptides so far discovered. However, the small amounts of peptide present pose some interesting physiological problems. Two peptides, substance P and somatostatin, are present in significant amounts only during early development and are present only in trace amounts in the adult cerebellum (78,79). These observations suggest that the peptides substance P and somatostatin may have important roles in influencing cerebellar development.

Apart from substance P and somatostatin, which are present in early cerebellar development, two other peptides have been reported to be present in cerebellar neurons. These are motilin and enkephalin-like immunoreactivities. Motilin is a 22-amino-acid peptide that influences gastric motility and emptying (111). Although there are only small amounts of motilin immunoreactivity in the cerebellum, immunohistochemistry reveals that motilin-like immunoreactivity is found in some of the Purkinje cells (31) (Fig. 3). Whether this material is authentic motilin or some cross-reacting material remains to be seen. If this result is substantiated, it may provide a further example of the coexistence within a neuron of a classical transmitter, in this case GABA, and a neuroactive peptide, motilin, or it may be that there are different classes of Purkinje cell, some containing only GABA and others only motilin.

Careful histochemical observations have also revealed the presence of enkephalin immunoreactivity in some Golgi cells and mossy fibers in several species (147,149).

Enkephalin has been shown to be released from synaptic terminals in a variety of systems (65,84,99), and, by analogy, it is therefore likely that some Golgi cells and mossy fibers also release enkephalin. A curious problem thereby presents itself, however. Both Golgi cells and mossy fibers synapse on granule cells. Golgi cells, however, are considered to be inhibitory, and mossy fibers excitatory (48). How can terminals secrete the same

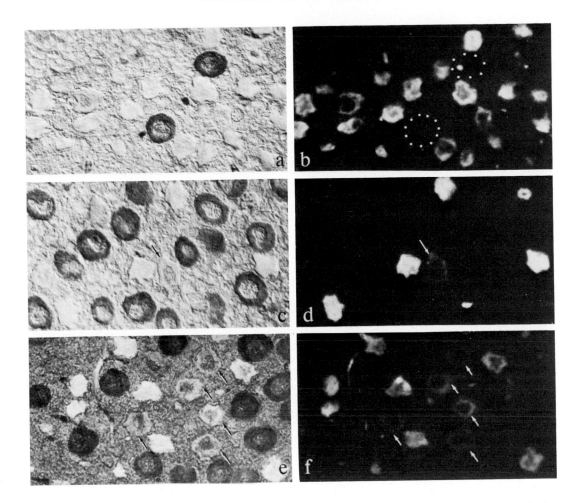

FIG. 3. a,b: Purkinje cell field rich in GAD immunoreactivity (GAD-i) cells. A pair of photomicrographs showing the same field of Purkinje cells in which two of the largest neurons are labeled with motilin-like immunoreactivity (motilin-i) (**a**), and two of the remaining Purkinje cells are labeled with GAD-i (**b**). Note the variable intensity of GAD-i in these cells. The outlines of the two motilin-i cells not visualized by fluorescence are indicated by *dots*. Mouse cerebellum lobule V, vermis, immunoperoxidase; Nomarski interference optics (**a**), immunofluorescence (**b**); both × 200. **c,d:** Purkinje cell field rich in motilin-i cells. A pair of photomicrographs showing the same field of Purkinje cells in which 17 large neurons are labeled with motilin-i (**c**), and five of the remaining Purkinje cells are labeled with GAD-i (**d**). Note again the lower-intensity of GAD-i in one of these cells *(arrow)*. Mouse cerebellum, lobule V, vermis, immunoperoxidase; Nomarski interference optics (**c**), immunofluorescence (**d**); both × 200. **e,f:** Photomicrograph made by combining immunofluorescence and Nomarski interference optics on the same negative to show a Purkinje cell field with motilin-i cells (**e**, dark), GAD-i cells (**e**, light), and some neurons with both motilin-i and GAD-i (**e**, gray, *arrows*). The same field appears in **f** with fluorescence optics to show only GAD-i cells. Note that the neurons with lower levels of fluorescence *(arrows)* are those that contain both motilin-i and GAD-i *(arrows)*. Mouse cerebellum; × 160.

chemical on the same cell type with opposite effects?

Several possibilities suggest themselves. For example, the enkephalin-containing mossy fibers might terminate on a different class of granule cells from those on which the enkephalin-containing Golgi cells terminate. One of these classes might

thus respond to enkephalin with excitation and the other with inhibition. Another possibility is that a small number of inhibitory mossy fibers exist but have escaped detection. A third possibility is that the enkephalin-containing Golgi cells and mossy fibers each contain other neuroactive substances, for example, "classical" neurotransmitters such as

GABA and ACh, and that it is the classical transmitters that determine the polarity of the effect. Colocalization of neuroactive peptides in the same cell as conventional transmitters has been demonstrated in many systems and may include the coexistence of GABA and motilin in the Purkinje cells (27,28,61,74,75). What function the enkephalin in this case might have and exactly why the conventional transmitter and not the peptide would determine the type of effect generated are not known.

The resolution of the puzzle presented by the presence of enkephalin in the cerebellum will thus apparently have interesting consequences for our knowledge of cerebellar function and perhaps for our understanding of synaptic physiology. Further information on the role of enkephalin, and the other peptides, in cerebellar function is therefore eagerly awaited.

CODA

The orderly architecture of the cerebellum and the great store of knowledge of its connections and constituents have made it the great hope of researchers who seek to understand how the properties of single neurons and groups of neurons give rise to the global functions of the brain. Despite the availability of vast amounts of information and serious efforts at synthesis, the relationship between microscopic properties and macroscopic function remains as obscure in the cerebellum as elsewhere in the brain. In this chapter, I have attempted to add to the existing blueprint of cerebellar neuronal interconnections a review of the available information on the identification of chemical agents used by those connections. Also, in an attempt to justify the notion that neurochemical knowledge can inform and help organize the quest for the unification of cellular facts with systemic function, I have offered several physiological puzzles that arise from neurochemical and pharmacological research. A satisfactory description of cerebellar function at all levels will not soon follow from such studies, but studies of cerebellar neurotransmitters will perhaps make the road to such a description easier and shorter.

ACKNOWLEDGMENTS

I am grateful to Mrs. Mary Wynn and Mrs. Jan Ditheridge for typing the manuscript. Particular thanks are due to Dr. E. Mugnaini and Dr. Victoria Chan-Palay for provision of Figs. 2 and 3, respectively.

REFERENCES

1. Albers, R. W., and Brady, R. O. (1959): The distribution of glutamate decarboxylase in the nervous system of the rhesus monkey. *J. Biol. Chem.,* 234:926–928.
2. Atlas, D., and Melamed, E. (1978): Direct mapping of β-adrenergic receptors in the rat central nervous system by a novel fluorescent β-blocker. *Brain Res.,* 150:377–385.
3. Atlas, D., Teichberg, V. I., and Changeux, J. P. (1977): Direct evidence for beta-adrenoreceptors in the Purkinje cells of mouse cerebellum. *Brain Res.,* 128:532–536.
4. Barker, J. L., and Smith, T. G., Jr. (1979): Three modes of communication in the nervous system. In: *Modulators Mediators and Specifiers in Brain Function,* edited by Y. H. Erlich, J. Volavka, L. G. Davis, and E. G. Brunngraber, pp. 109–192. Plenum Press, New York.
5. Beaudet, A., and Sotelo, C. (1980): Synaptic remodeling of serotonin axon terminals in rat agranular cerebellum. *Brain Res.,* 206:305–330.
6. Bernardi, N., Dacke, C. G., Davidson, N., and Fawcett, M. (1978): Veratridine stimulates release of [^{14}C]GABA from the *in vivo* superfused rat cerebellar cortex. *J. Physiol. (Lond.),* 278:25–26P.
7. Bernardo, L. S., and Prince, D. A. (1981): Acetylcholine induced modulation of hippocampal pyramidal neurons. *Brain Res.,* 211:227–234.
8. Biggio, G., Costa, E., and Guidotti, A. (1977): Pharmacologically induced changes in the 3':5'-cyclic guanosine monophosphate content of rat cerebellar cortex: Difference between apomorphine, haloperidol and harmaline. *J. Pharmacol. Exp. Ther.,* 200:207–215.
9. Biggio, G., and Guidotti, A. (1976): Climbing fiber activation and 3',5'-cyclic guanosine monophosphate (cGMP) content in cortex and deep nuclei of cerebellum. *Brain Res.,* 107:365–373.
10. Biggio, G., and Guidotti, A. (1977): Regulation of cyclic GMP in cerebellum by a striatal dopaminergic mechanism. *Nature,* 265:240–242.
11. Bisti, S., Iosif, G., Marchesi, G. F., and Strata, P. (1971): Pharmacological properties of inhibitions in the cerebellar cortex. *Exp. Brain Res.,* 14:24–37.
12. Bloedel, J. (1973): Cerebellar afferent systems: A review. *Prog. Neurobiol.,* 2:1–68.
13. Bloedel, J. R., Gregory, R. S., and Martin, S. H. (1972): Action of interneurons and axon collaterals in cerebellar cortex of a primate. *J. Neurophysiol.,* 35:847–863.
14. Bloom, F. E., Hoffer, B. J., and Siggins, G. R. (1971): Studies on norepinephrine-containing afferents to Purkinje cells of rat cerebellum. I. Localization of the fibers and their synapses. *Brain Res.,* 25:501–521.
15. Bloom, F. E., Hoffer, B. J., Siggins, G. R., Barker, J. L., and Nicoll, R. A. (1972): Effects of serotonin

on central neurons: Microiontophoretic administration. *Fed. Proc.*, 31:97–106.

16. Bloom, F. E., Koob, G. F., and Schulman, J. A. (1982): *Catecholamines and behaviour.* In: *Handbook of Pharmacology,* edited by N. Weiner.

17. Bobillier, P., Seguin, S., Peptitjean, F., Salvent, D., Touret, M., and Jouvet, M. (1976): The raphe nuclei of the cat brain stem: A topographical atlas of their efferent projections as revealed by autoradiography. *Brain Res.*, 113:449–486.

18. Bowery, N. G., and Neal, M. J. (1978): Differential effects of veratridine and potassium depolarization on [^{3}H]GABA release from neurones and glia. *J. Physiol. (Lond.),* 275:58P.

19. Bowery, N. G., Hill, D. R., Hudson, A. L., Doble, A., Middlemiss, D. N., Shaw, J., and Turnbull, M. (1980): (-)Baclofen decreases neurotransmitter release in the mammalian CNS by an action at a novel GABA receptor. *Nature,* 283:92–94.

20. Bruggencate, G. Ten, and Engberg, I. (1971): Iontophretic studies in Deiter's nucleus of the inhibitory actions of GABA and related amino acids and the interactions of strychnine and picrotoxin. *Brain Res.*, 25:431–448.

21. Burgen, A. S. V., and Chipman, L. M. (1951): Cholinesterase and succinic dehydrogenase in the central nervous system of the dog. *J. Physiol. (Lond.),* 114:296–305.

22. Carew, T. J., and Kandel, E. R. (1977): Inking in *Aplysia californica.* III. Two different synaptic conductance mechanisms for triggering central program for inking. *J. Neurophysiol.*, 40:721–734.

23. Changeux, J. P., Kasai, M., and Lee, C. Y. (1970): Use of a snake venom toxin to characterize the cholinergic receptor protein. *Proc. Natl. Acad. Sci. U.S.A.,* 67:1241–1247.

24. Chan-Palay, V. (1975): Fine structure of labelled axons in the cerebellar cortex and nuclei of rodents and primates after intraventricular infusions with tritiated serotonin. *Anat. Embryol.*, 148:235–265.

25. Chan-Palay, V. (1977): *Cerebellar Dentate Nucleus. Organization, Cytology and Transmitters.* Springer, Berlin.

26. Chan-Palay, V. (1978): Autoradiographic localization of γ-aminobutyric acid receptors in the rat central nervous system by using [^{3}H]muscimol. *Proc. Natl. Acad. Sci. U.S.A.,* 75:1024–1028.

27. Chan-Palay, V. (1982): Coexistence of traditional neurotransmitters with peptides in the mammalian brain: Serotonin and substance P in the raphe and GABA and motilin in the cerebellum. In: *Co-Transmission,* edited by A. C. Cuello, pp. 1–24. MacMillan, London.

28. Chan-Palay, V., Jonsson, G., and Palay, S. L. (1978): On the coexistence of serotonin and substance P in neurons of the rat's central nervous system. *Proc. Natl. Acad. Sci. U.S.A.,* 75:1582–1586.

29. Chan-Palay, V., and Palay, S. L. (1978): Ultrastructural localization of γ-aminobutyric acid receptors in the mammalian central nervous system by means of [^{3}H]muscimol binding. *Proc. Natl. Acad. Sci. U.S.A.,* 75:2977–2980.

30. Chan-Palay, V., and Palay, S. L. (1979): Immunocytochemical localization of cyclic GMP: Light and electron microscope evidence for involvement of neuroglia. *Proc. Natl. Acad. Sci. U.S.A.,* 76:1485–1488.

31. Chan-Palay, V., Nilaver, G., Palay, S. L., Beinfeld, M. C., Zimmerman, E. A., Wu, J.-Y., and O'Donohue, T. L. (1981): Chemical heterogeneity in cerebellar Purkinje cells: Existence and coexistence of glutamic acid decarboxylase-like and motilin-like immunoreactivities. *Proc. Natl. Acad. Sci. U.S.A.,* 78:7787–7791.

32. Chu, N.-S., and Bloom, F. E. (1973): Norepinephrine-containing neurons: Changes in spontaneous discharge patterns during sleeping and waking. *Science,* 179:908–910.

33. Crawford, J. M., Curtis, D. R., Voohoeve, P. E., and Wilson, V. J. (1963): Excitation of cerebellar neurones by acetylcholine. *Nature,* 200:579–580.

34. Crawford, J. M., Curtis, D. R., Voorhoeve, P. E., and Wilson, V. J. (1966): Acetylcholine sensitivity of cerebellar neurones in the cat. *J. Physiol. (Lond.),* 186:139–165.

35. Csillik, B., Joo, F., and Kasa, P. (1963): Cholinesterase activity of archicerebellar mossy fibre apparatuses. *J. Histochem. Cytochem.*, 11:103–113.

36. Curtis, D. R., and Crawford, J. M. (1965): Acetylcholine sensitivity of cerebellar neurones. *Nature,* 206:516–517.

37. Curtis, D. R., Duggan, A. W., Felix, D., and Johnston, G. A. R. (1970): GABA, bicuculline and central inhibition. *Nature,* 226:1222–1224.

38. Curtis, D. R., Duggan, A. W., Felix, D., Johnston, G. A. R., and McLennan, H. (1971): Antagonism between bicuculline and GABA in the cat brain. *Brain Res.,* 33:57–73.

39. Curtis, D. R., and Felix, D. (1971): The effect of bicuculline upon synaptic inhibition in the cerebral and cerebellar cortices of the cat. *Brain Res.,* 34:391–421.

40. Curtis, D. R., and Johnston, G. A. R. (1973): Amino acid neurotransmitters in the mammalian central nervous system. *Engeb. Physiol.*, 69:97–188.

41. Curtis, D. R., Lodge, D., Johnston, G. A. R., and Brand, S. J. (1976): Central actions of benzodiazepines. *Brain Res.,* 118:344–347.

42. Davidson, N., Beruardi, N., Fawcett, M., Wong, E., Assumpcao, J. A., and Dacke, C. G. (1979): A possible neuronal release of [^{14}-C] GABA from the rat cerebellum *in vivo. Pfluegers Arch.*, 379:149–155.

43. DeMontigny, C., and Lamarrey, Y. (1973): Rhythmic activity induced by harmaline in the olivo–cerebellar bulbar system of the cat. *Brain Res.,* 53:81–95.

44. Denk, H., Haider, M., Kovak, W., and Studynka, G. (1968): Verhaltensänderlung und Neuropathologie bei der 3-Acetylpyridinvergiftung der Ratte. *Acta Neuropathol. (Berl.),* 10:34–44.

45. Descarries, L., and Lapierre, Y. (1973): Noradrenergic axon terminals in the cerebral cortex of rat I. Radioautographic visualization after topical application of DL-[^{3}H]noreponephrine. *Brain Res.,* 51:141–160.

46. Descarries, L., Watkins, K. C., and Lapierre, Y. (1977): Noradrenergic axon terminals in the cerebral cortex of the rat. III. Topometric ultrastructural analysis. *Brain Res.*, 133:197–222.

47. Desclin, J. C., and Escubi, J. (1974): Effect of 3-acetyl-pyridine on the central nervous system of the rat, as demonstrated by silver methods. *Brain Res.*, 77:365–384.

48. Eccles, J. C., Ito, M., and Szenthagothai, J. (1967): *The Cerebellum as a Neuronal Machine.* Springer-Verlag, New York.

49. Falck, B., Hillarp, N. A., Thieme, G., and Thorp, A. (1962): Fluorescence of catecholamines and related compounds with formaldehyde. *J. Histochem. Cytochem.*, 10:348–354.

50. Feldberg, W., and Vogt, M. (1948): Acetylcholine synthesis in different regions of the central nervous system. *J. Physiol. (Lond.)*, 107:372–381.

51. Ferrendelli, J. A., Chang, M. M., and Kinscherf, D. A. (1974): Elevation of cyclic GMP levels in central nervous system by excitatory and inhibitory amino acids. *J. Neurochem.*, 22:535–540.

52. Ferrendelli, J. A., Kinscherf, D. A., and Chang, M. M. (1973): Regulation of levels of guanosine 3'-5'-monophosphate in the central nervous system. Effects of depolarizing agents. *Mol. Pharmacol.*, 9:445–454.

53. Fonnum, F., Storm-Mathisen, J., and Walberg, F. (1970): Glutamate decarboxylase in inhibitory neurons. A study of the enzyme in the Purkinje cells axons and boutons in the cat. *Brain Res.*, 20:259–275.

54. Foote, S. L., Aston-Jones, G., and Bloom, F. E. (1980): Impulse activity of locus coeruleus neurons in awake rats and monkeys is a function of sensory stimulation and arousal. *Proc. Natl. Acad. Sci. U.S.A.*, 77:3033–3037.

55. Foster, A. C., and Roberts, P. J. (1978): High affinity L-[^{3}H]glutamate binding to postsynaptic receptor sites on rat cerebellar membranes. *J. Neurochem.*, 31:1467–1477.

56. Frederickson, R. C. A., Neuss, M., Morzorati, S. L., and McBride, W. J. (1978): A comparison of the inhibitory effects of taurine and GABA on identified Purkinje cells and other neurons in the cerebellar cortex of the rat. *Brain Res.*, 145:117–126.

57. Freedman, R., and Hoffer, B. J. (1976): Noradrenaline modulation of the responses of the cerebellar Purkinje cell to afferent synaptic activity. *Br. J. Pharmacol.*, 57:603–605.

58. Freedman, R., Hoffer, B. J., Woodward, D. J., and Puro, D. (1977): Interaction of norepinephrine with cerebellar activity evoked by mossy and climbing fibers. *Exp. Neurol.*, 55:269–288.

59. Greengard, P. (1976): Possible role for cyclic nucleotides and phosphorylated membrane proteins in post-synaptic actions of transmitters. *Nature*, 260:101–108.

60. Guidotti, A., Biggio, G., and Costa, E. (1975): 3-Acetylpyridine: A tool to inhibit the tremor and the increase of cGMP content in cerebellar cortex elicited by harmaline. *Brain Res.*, 96:201–205.

61. Hanley, M. R., Cottrell, G. A., Emson, P. C., and Fonnum, F. (1974): Enymataic synthesis of acetyl-choline by a serotonin-containing neurone from *Helix. Nature (New Biol.)*, 251:631–633.

62. Hartline, H. K., and Ratcliff, F. (1957): Inhibitory interaction of receptor units in the eye of *Limulus. J. Gen. Physiol.*, 40:357–376.

63. Hebb, C. O. (1959): Chemical agents of the nervous system. *Int. Rev. Neurobiol.*, 1:165–193.

64. Hebb, C. O., and Silver, A. (1956): Choline acetylase in the central nervous system of man and some other mammals. *J. Physiol. (Lond.)*, 134:718–728.

65. Henderson, G., Hughes, J., and Kosterlitz, H. (1978): *In vitro* release of Leu- and Met-enkephalin from the corpus striatum. *Nature*, 271:677–679.

66. Hirsch, H. E., and Robins, E. (1962): Distribution of γ-aminobutyric acid in the layers of the cerebral and cerebellar cortex. Implications for a physiological role. *J. Neurochem.*, 9:63–70.

67. Hobson, J. A., McCarley, R. W., and Wyzinski, P. W. (1975): Sleep cycle oscillation: Reciprocal discharge by two brainstem neuronal groups. *Science*, 189:55–58.

68. Hoffer, B. J., Siggins, G. R., Oliver, A. P., and Bloom, F. E. (1971): Cyclic AMP mediation of norepinephrine inhibition in rat cerebellar cortex: A unique class of synaptic responses. *Ann. N.Y. Acad. Sci.*, 185:531–549.

69. Hoffer, B. J., Siggins, G. R., Oliver, A. P., and Bloom, F. E. (1973):Activation of the pathway from locus coeruleus to rat cerebellar Purkinje neurons: Pharmacological evidence of noradrenergic central inhibition. *J. Pharmacol. Exp. Ther.*, 184:553–569.

70. Hökfelt, T. (1968): *In vitro* studies on central and peripheral monoamine neurons at the ultrastructural level. *Z. Zellforsch.*, 91:1–74.

71. Hökfelt, T., and Fuxe, K. (1969): Cerebellar monoamine nerve terminals a new type of afferent fibers to the cortex cerebelli. *Exp. Brain Res.*, 9:63–72.

72. Hökfelt, T., and Ljungdahl, A. (1970): Cellular localization of labeled gamma-aminobutyric acid (^{3}H-GABA) in rat cerebellar cortex: An autoradiographic study. *Brain Res.*, 22:391–396.

73. Hökfelt, T., and Ljungdahl, A. (1972): Autoradiographic identification of cerebral cerebellar cortical neurons accumulating labeled gamma-aminobutyric acid (^{3}H-GABA). *Exp. Brain Res.*, 14:354–362.

74. Hökfelt, T., Ljungdahl, A., Steinbusch, H., Verhofstad, A., Nilsson, G., Brodin, E., Pernow, B., and Goldstein, M. (1978): Immunohistochemical evidence for substance P-like immunoreactivity in some 5-hydroxytryptamine-containing neurons in the rat central nervous system. *Neuroscience*, 3:517–538.

75. Hökfelt, T., Rehfeld, J., Skirboll, L., Ivemark, B., Goldstein, M., and Markey, K. (1980): Evidence for coexistence of dopamine and CCK in mesolimbic neurons. *Nature*, 285:476–477.

76. Hudson, D., Valcana, T., Bean, G., and Timiras, P. S. (1976): Glutamic acid: A strong candidate as the neurotransmitter of the cerebellar granule cell. *Neurochem. Res.*, 1:73–81.

77. Hunt, S. P., and Schmidt, J. (1978): Some observations of the binding patterns of β-bungarotoxin in

the central nervous system of the rat. *Brain Res.,* 157:213–232.

78. Inagaki, S., Sakanaka, M., Shiosaka, S., Senba, E., Takagi, H., Takatsuki, K., Kawai, Y., Matsuzaki, T., Iida, H., Hara, Y., and Tohyama, M. (1982): Experimental and immunohistochemical studies on the cerebellar substance P of the rat: Localization, postnatal ontogeny and ways of entry to the cerebellum. *Neuroscience* 7:639–646.

79. Inagaki, S., Shiosaka, S., Takatsuki, K., Iida, H., Sakanaka, M., Senba, E., Hara, Y., Matsuzaki, T., Kaway, Y., and Tohyama, M., (1982): Ontogeny of somatostatin-containing neuron system of the rat cerebellum including its fiber connections: An experimental and immunohistochemical analysis. *Dev. Brain Res.,* 3: 509–529.

80. Ito, M. (1977): Neuronal events in the cerebellar flocculus associated with an adaptive modification of the vestibulo–ocular reflex of the rabbit. In: *Control of Gaze by Brainstem Neurons,* edited by R. Baker and A. Berthoz, pp. 391–398. Elsevier, Amsterdam.

81. Ito, M., Highstein, S. M., and Fukuda, J. (1970): Cerebellar inhibition of the vestibulo–ocular reflex in rabbit and cat and its blockage by picrotoxin. *Brain Res.,* 17:524–526.

82. Ito, M., Nisimaru, N., and Gamamoto, M. (1977): Specific patterns of neuronal connections involved in the control of the rabbit's vestibulo–ocular reflexes by the cerebellar flocculus. *J. Physiol. (Lond.),* 265:833–854.

83. Ito, M., and Yoshida, M. (1966): The origin of cerebellar-induced inhibition of Deiters' neurons. I. Monosynaptic initiation of the inhibitory postsynaptic potentials. *Exp. Brain Res.,* 2:330–349.

84. Iversen, L. L., Iversen, S. D., Bloom, F. E., Vargo, T., and Guillemin, R. (1978): Release of enkephalin from rat globus pallidus *in vitro. Nature,* 271:679–681.

85. Johnson, J. L. (1972): Glutamic acid as a synaptic transmitter in the nervous system. A review. *Brain Res.,* 37:1–19.

86. Kan, K.-S. K., Chao, L. P., and Eng, L. F. (1978): Immunohistochemical localization of choline acetyltransferase in rabbit spinal cord and cerebellum. *Brain Res.,* 146:221–229.

87. Kasa, P., Joo, F., and Csillik, B. (1965): Histochemical localization of acetylcholinesterase in the cat cerebellar cortex. *J. Neurochem.,* 12:31–35.

88. Kasa, P., and Silver, A. (1969): The correlation between choline acetyltransferase and acetylcholinesterase activity in different areas of the cerebellum of rat and guinea pig. *J. Neurochem.,* 16:389–396.

89. Kawamura, H., and Provini, L. (1970): Depression of cerebellar Purkinje cells by microiontophoretic application of GABA and related amino acids. *Brain Res.,* 24:293–304.

90. Kelly, J. S., Dick, F., and Schon, F. (1975): The autoradiographic localization of the GABA-releasing nerve terminals in cerebellar glomeruli. *Brain Res.,* 85:255–259.

91. Kimoto, Y., Tohyama, M., Satoh, K., Sakumoto, T., Takahashi, Y., and Shimizy, N. (1981): Fine structure of rat cerebellar noradrenaline terminals as visualized by potassium *"in situ* perfusion" fixation method. *Neuroscience,* 6:47–58.

92. Koda, L. Y., Schulman, J. A., and Bloom, F. E. (1978): Ultrastructural identification of noradrenergic terminals in rat hippocampus: Unilateral destruction of the locus coeruleus with 6-hydroxydopamine. *Brain Res.,* 145:190–195.

92a. Korte, G .E., Reiner, A., and Karten, H. J. (1980): Substance P-like immunoreactivity in cerebellar mossy fibres and terminals in the red-eared turtle *Chrysemys scripta elegans. Neuroscience,* 5:903–914.

93. Krnjevic, K. (1964): Micro-iontophoretic studies on cortical neurons. *Int. Rev. Neurobiol.,* 7:41–98.

94. Kuo, J. F., Lee, T. P., Reyes, P. L., Walton, K. G., Donnelly, T. E., and Greengard, P. (1972): Cyclic nucleotide dependent protein kinases: An assay method for the measurement of guanosine $3',5'$-monophosphate in various biological materials and a study of agents regulating its levels in heart and brain. *J. Biol. Chem.,* 247:16–22.

95. Kuriyama, K., Haber, B., Sisken, B., and Roberts, E. (1966): The GABA system in rabbit crebellum. *Proc. Natl. Acad. Sci. U.S.A.,* 55:846.

96. Landis, S., and Bloom, F. E. (1975): Ultrastructural identification of noradrenaline boutons in mutant and normal mouse cerebellar cortex. *Brain Res.,* 96:299–305.

97. Lee, C. Y. (1970): Elapid neurotoxins and their mode of action. *Clin. Toxicol.,* 3:457–472.

98. Levitan, I. B., Harmar, A. J., and Adams, W. B. (1979): Synaptic and hormonal modulation of a neuronal oscillator: A search for molecular mechanisms. *J. Exp. Biol.,* 81:131–151.

99. Lindberg, I., and Dahl, J. (1981): Characterization of enkephalin release from rat striatum. *J. Neuro chem.,* 36:506–512.

100. Lindvall, O., and Björklund, A. (1974): The organization of the ascending catecholamine neuron systems in the rat brain, as revealed by the glyoxylic acid fluorescence method. *Acta Physiol. Scand.,* 421:1–48.

101. Llinas, R., and Hillman, D. E. (1969): Physiological and morphological organization of the cerebellar circuits in various vertebrates. In: *Neurobiology of Cerebellar Evolution and Development,* edited by R. Llinas, pp. 43–73. AMA–ERF Institute for Biomedical Research, Chicago.

102. Llinas, R., and Sugimori, M. (1980): Electrophysiological properties of *in vitro* Purkinje cell somata in mammalian cerebellar slices. *J. Physiol. (Lond.)* 305:171–195.

103. Llinas, R., and Volkind, R. A. (1973): The olivocerebellar system: Functional properties as revealed by harmaline-induced tremor. *Exp. Brain Res.,* 18:69–87.

104. Lopez-Colome, A., Tapia, R., Salceda, R., and Pasantes-Morales, H. (1978): K^+-stimulated release of labelled γ-aminobutyrate, glycine and taurine in slices of several regions of rat central nervous system. *Neuroscience,* 3:1069–1074.

105. Mao, C. C., Guidotti, A., and Landis, S. (1975): Cyclic GMP: Reduction of cerebellar concentra-

tions in nervous mutant mice. *Brain Res.*, 90:335–339.

106. McBride, W. J., Aprison, M. H., and Kusano, K. (1976): Contents of several amino acids in the cerebellum, brainstem and cerebram of the "staggerer," "weaver" and "nervous" neurological mutant mice. *J. Neurochem.*, 26:867–870.

107. McBride, W. J., and Frederickson, R. C. A. (1980): Taurine as a possible inhibitory transmitter in the cerebellum. *Fed. Proc.*, 39:2701–2705.

108. McBride, W. J., Nadi, N. S., Altman, J., and Aprison, M. H. (1976): Effects of selective doses of X-irradiation on the levels of several amino acids in the cerebellum of the rat. *Neurochem. Res.*, 7:141–152.

109. McCance, I., and Phillis, J. W. (1964): Discharge patterns of elements in cat cerebellar cortex and their responses to iontophoretically applied drugs. *Nature*, 204:844–846.

110. McIntosh, F. C. (1941): The distribution of acetylcholine in the peripheral and central nervous system. *J. Physiol. (Lond.)*, 99:436–442.

111. McIntosh, C. H. S., and Brown, J. C. (1980): Motlin: Isolation, structure and basic function. In: *Gastrointestinal Hormones*, edited by I. Glass, pp. 233–244. Raven Press, New York.

112. McLauglin, B. J., Wood, J. G., Saita, K., Barber, R., Vaugh, J. E., Roberts, E., and Wu, J. Y. (1974): The fine structural localization of glutamate decarboxylase in synaptic terminals of rodent cerebellum. *Brain Res.*, 76:377–392.

113. Meunier, J.-C., and Zajac, J.-M. (1979): Cerebellar opiate receptors in lagomorphs. Demonstration, characterisation and regional distribution. *Brain Res.*, 168:311–321.

113a. Molinoff, P. B., and Minneman, K. P. (1980): Biochemical and functional aspects of the interactions of agonists and antagonists with β-adrenergic receptors. In: *Psychopharmacology and Biochemistry of Neurotransmitter Receptors*, edited by H. Yamamura, R. Olsen, and E. Usdin, pp. 171–182. Elsevier North Holland, Amsterdam.

114. Montarolo, P. G., Raschi, F., and Strata, P. (1979): Interactions between benzodiazepines and GABA in the cerebellar cortex. *Brain Res.*, 162:358–362.

115. Moore, R. Y., and Bloom, F. E. (1979): Control catecholamine neuron systems: Anatomy and physiology of the norepinephrine and epinephrine systems. *Annu. Rev. Neurosci.*, 2:113–168.

116. Nadi, N. S., Kanter, D., McBride, W. J., and Aprison, M. H. (1977): Effects of 3-acetylpyridine on several putative neurotransmitter amino acids in the cerebellum and medulla of the rat. *J. Neurochem.*, 28:661–662.

117. Nadi, N. S., McBridge, W. J., and Aprison, M. H. (1977): Distribution of several amino acids in regions of the cerebellum of the rat. *J. Neurochem.*, 28:453–455.

118. Nicoll, R. A. (1972): The effects of anaesthetics on synaptic excitation and inhibition in the olfactory bulb. *J. Physiol. (Lond.)*, 223:803–814.

119. Nicoll, R. A. (1975): Pentobarbital: Action on frog motoneurons. *Brain Res.*, 96:119–123.

120. Nicoll, R. A. (1978): Pentobarbital: Differential

postsynaptic actions on sympathetic ganglion cells. *Science*, 199:451–452.

121. Nicoll, R. A., Siggins, G. R., Ling, N., Bloom, F. E., and Guillemin, R. (1977): Neuronal actions of endorphins and enkephalins among brain regions: A microiontophoretic study. *Proc. Natl. Acad. Sci. U.S.A.*, 74:2584–2588.

122. Obata, K., Ito, M., Ochi, R., and Sato, N. (1967): Pharmacological properties of the postsynaptic inhibition by Purkinje cell axons and the action of γ-aminobutyric acid on Deiters' neurones. *Exp. Brain Res.*, 4:43–57.

123. Obata, K., and Takeda, K. (1969): Release of γ-aminobutyric acid into the fourth ventricle induced by stimulation of the cat's cerebellum. *J. Neurochem.*, 16:1043–1047.

124. Obata, K., Takeda, K., and Shinozaki, H. (1970): Further study on pharmacological properties of the cerebellar-induced inhibition of Deiters' neurones. *Exp. Brain Res.*, 11:327–342.

125. Okamoto, K., and Sakai, Y. (1979): Augmentation by chlordiazepoxide of the inhibitory effects of taurine, β-alanine and γ-aminobutyric acid on spike discharges in guinea-pig cerebellar slices. *Br. J. Pharmacol.*, 65:277–285.

126. Olschowka, J. A., Grzanna, R., and Molliver, M. E. (1980): The distribution and incidence of synaptic contacts of noradrenergic varicosities in the rat neocortex: An immunocytochemical study. *Soc. Neurosci. Abstr.*, 6:352P.

127. Olson, L., and Fuxe, K. (1971): On the projections from the locus coeruleus noradrenaline neurones: The cerebellar innervation. *Brain Res.*, 28:165–171.

128. Otsuka, M., and Konishi, S. (1975): Substance P and excitatory transmitter of primary sensory neurons. *Cold Spring Harbor Symp. Quant. Biol.*, 40:135–143.

129. Otsuka, M., Obata, K., Miyata, Y., and Tanaka, Y. (1971): Measurement of γ-aminobutyric acid in isolated nerve cells of cat central nervous system. *J. Neurochem.*, 18:287–295.

130. Palacios, J. M., and Kuhar, M. J. (1980): Beta-adrenergic receptor localization by light microscopic autoradiography. *Science*, 208:1378–1380.

131. Palacios, J. M., Scott Young, W. III, and Kuhar, M. J. (1980): Autoradiographic localization of γ-aminobutyric acid (GABA) receptors in the rat cerebellum. *Proc. Natl. Acad. Sci. U.S.A.*, 77:670–674.

132. Palay, S. L., and Chan-Palay, V. (1974): *Cerebellar Cortex: Cytology and Organization.* Springer-Verlag, Berlin, Heidelberg, New York.

133. Patel, A. J., Balazs, R., Altman, J., and Anderson, W. J. (1975): Effect of X-irradiation on the biochemical maturation of rat cerebellum: Postnatal cell formation. *Radiat. Res.*, 62:470–477.

134. Pitts, F. N., Jr., Quick, C., and Robins, E. (1965): The enzymic measurement of γ-aminobutyric–α-oxoglutaric transaminase. *J. Neurochem.*, 12:93–101.

135. Ramon y Cajal, S. (1909): *Histologie du System Nerveux de l'Homme et des Vertebres.* A. Maloine, Paris.

136. Ransom, B. R., and Barker, J. L. (1975): Pentobarbital modulates transmitter effects on mouse spinal neurones grown in tissue culture. *Nature*, 254:703–705.

137. Rea, M. W., McBride, W. J., and Rohde, B. H. (1980): Regional and synaptosomal levels of amino acid neurotransmitters in the 3-acetylpyridine deafferented rat cerebellum. *J. Neurochem.*, 34:1106–1108.

138. Renaud, L. P., Martin, J. B., and Brazeau, P. (1975): Depressant action of TRH, LH-RH and somatostatin on activity of central neurones. *Nature*, 255:233–235.

139. Ribak, C. E., Vaughn, J. E., and Saito, K. (1978): Immunocytochemical localization of glutamic acid decarboxylase in neuronal somata following colchicine inhibition of axonal transport. *Brain Res.*, 140:315–332.

140. Richardson, K. C. (1966): Electron microscopic identification of autonomic nerve endings. *Nature*, 210:756.

141. Roberts, E., and Frankel, S. (1950): γ-Aminobutyric acid in brain: Its formation from glutamic acid. *J. Biol. Chem.*, 187:55–63.

142. Roffler-Tarlov, S., and Sidman, R. L. (1978): Concentrations of glutamic acid in cerebellar cortex and deep nuclei of normal mice and weaver, staggerer and nervous mutants. *Brain Res.*, 142:269–283.

143. Rohde, B. H., Rea, M. A., Simon, J. R., and McBride, W. J. (1979): Effects of X-irradiation induced loss of cerebellar granule cells on the synaptosomal levels and the high affinity uptake of amino acids. *J. Neurochem.*, 32:1431–1435.

144. Saito, K., Barber, R., Wu, J. Y., Matsuda, T., Roberts, E., and Vaugh, J. E. (1974): Immunohistochemical localization of glutamate decarboxylase in rat cerebellum. *Proc. Natl. Acad. Sci. U.S.A.*, 71:269–277.

145. Salvador, R. A., and Albers, R. W. (1959): The distribution of glutamic-γ-aminobutyric transaminase in the nervous system of the rhesus monkey. *J. Biol. Chem.*, 234:922–925.

146. Sandoval, M. E., and Cotman, C. W. (1978): Evaluation of glutamate as a neurotransmitter of cerebellar parallel fibers. *Neuroscience*, 3:199–206.

147. Sar, M., Stumpf, W. E., Miller, R. J., Chang, K. J., and Cuatrecasas, P. (1978): Immunohistochemical localization of enkephalin in rat brain and spinal cord. *J. Comp. Neurol.*, 182:17–38.

148. Schon, F., and Iversen, L. (1972): Selective accumulation of [^{3}H]GABA by stellate cells in rat cerebellar cortex *in vitro*. *Brain Res*, 42:503–507.

149. Schulman, J. A., Finger, T. E., Brecha, N. C., and Karten, H. J. (1981): Enkephalin immunoreactivity in Golgi cells and mossy fibers of the mammalian, avian, amphibian and teleost cerebellum. *Neuroscience*, 6:2407–2416.

150. Sculman, J. A., and Weight, F. F. (1976): Synaptic transmission—long-lasting potentiation by a postsynaptic mechanism. *Science*, 194:1437–1439.

151. Sharif, N. A., and Roberts, P. J. (1981): L-Aspartate binding sites in rat cerebellum: A comparison of the binding of L-[^{3}H]aspartate and L-[^{3}H]glutamate. *Brain Res.*, 211:293–304.

152. Shimizu, N., and Ishii, S. (1966): Electron microscope histochemistry of acetylcholinesterase of rat brain by Karnovsky's method. *Histochemie*, 6:24–33.

153. Shinnar, S., Maciewicz, R. J., and Shoter, R. J. (1973): A raphe projection to cat cerebellar cortex. *Brain Res.*, 97:139–143.

154. Shute, C. C., and Lewis, P. R. (1969): Cholinesterase-containing pathways of the hindbrain: Afferent cerebellar and centrifugal cochlear fibres. *Nature*, 205:242–246.

155. Siggins, G. R. (1979): Neurotransmitters and neuromodulators and their mediation by cyclic nucleotides. In: *Modulators, Mediators and Specifiers in Brain Function*, edited by Y. H. Erhlich, J. Volavka, L. G. Davis, and E. G. Brunngraber, pp. 41–64. Plenum Press, New York.

156. Siggins, G. R., Hoffer, B. R., and Bloom, F. R. (1971): Studies on norepinephrine-containing afferents to Purkinje cells of rat cerebellum: III. Evidence for mediation of norepinephrine effects by cyclic 3′,5′adenosine monophosphate. *Brain Res.*, 25:535–553.

157. Siggins, G. R., Hoffer, B. J., Oliver, A. P., and Bloom, F. E. (1971): Activation of a central noradrenergic projection to cerebellum. *Nature*, 233:481–483.

158. Siggins, G. R., Oliver, A. P., Hoffer, B. J., and Bloom, F. E. (1971): Cyclic adenosine monophosphate and norepinephrine: Effects on transmembrane properties of cerebellar Purkinje cells. *Science*, 171:192–194.

159. Sillito, A. M. (1975): The contribution of inhibitory mechanism to the receptive field properties of neurones in the striate cortex of the cat. *J. Physiol. (Lond.)*, 250:305–329.

160. Sillito, A. M. (1979): Inhibitory mechanisms influencing complex cell orientation selectivity and their modification at high resting discharge levels. *J. Physiol. (Lond.)*, 289:33–53.

161. Silver, A. (1974): *The Biology of Cholinesterases*. Elsevier North-Holland, Amsterdam.

162. Steiner, A. L., Ferrendelli, J. A., and Kipnis, D. M. (1972): Radioimmunoassay in cyclic nucleotides. III. Effect of ischemia, changes during development and regional distribution of adenosine 3′,5′-monophosphate and guanosine 3′,5′-monophosphate in mouse brain. *J. Biol. Chem.*, 247:1121–1124.

163. Stone, T. W. (1979): Selective antagonism of amino acids by aminoadipate on pyramidal tract neurones but not Purkinje cells. *Brain Res.*, 166:217–220.

164. Stone, T. W. (1979): Glutamate as the neurotransmitter of cerebellar granule cells in the rat: Electrophysiological evidence. *Br. J. Pharmacol.*, 66:291–296.

165. Szenthagothai, J., and Rajkovits, U. (1959): Uber den Ursprung der Keltterfasern des Kleinhirns. *Z. Anat. Entwickl. Gesch.*, 121:130–141.

166. Tsien, R. W. (1973): Adrenaline-like effects of intracellular iontophoresis of cyclic AMP in cardiac Purkinje fibers. *Nature (New Biol.)*, 245:120–122.

167. Udenfriend, S. (1950): Identification of γ-aminobutyric acid in brain by the isotope derivative method. *J. Biol. Chem.*, 187:65–69.

168. Van Gelder, N. M. (1965): The histochemical demonstration of γ-aminobutyric acid metabolism by reduction of a tetrazolium salt. *J. Neurochem.*, 12:231–237.

169. Weight, F. F., Schulman, J. A., Smith, P. A., and Busis, N. A. (1979): Long-lasting synaptic potentials and modulation of synaptic transmission. *Fed. Proc.*, 38:2084–2094.

170. Werman, R. (1966): A review—criteria for identification of a central nervous system transmitter. *Comp. Biochem. Physiol.*, 18:745–766.

171. Wilson, W. A., and Wachtel, H. (1978): Prolonged inhibition in burst firing neurons: Synaptic inactivation of the slow regenerative inward current. *Science*, 202:772–775.

172. Woodward, D. J., Hoffer, B. J., Siggins, G. R., and Oliver, A. P. (1971): Inhibition of Purkinje cells in the frog cerebellum. II. Evidence for GABA as in the inhibitory transmitter. *Brain Res.*, 33:91–100.

173. Woodward, D. J., Moises, H. C., Waterhouse, B. D., Hoffere, B. J., and Freedman, R. (1979): Modulatory actions of norepinephrine in the central nervous system. *Fed. Proc.*, 38:2109–2116.

174. Yamamoto, C. (1967): Pharmacological studies of norepinephrine, acetylcholine and related compounds on neurons in Dieters' nucleus and the cerebellum. *J. Pharmacol. Exp. Ther.*, 156:39–47.

175. Young, A. B., Oster-Granite, M. L., Herndon, R. M., and Snyder, S. H. (1974): Glutamic acid: Selective depletion by viral induced granule cell loss in hamster cerebellum. *Brain Res.*, 73.1–2.

Chemical Neuroanatomy, edited by P.C. Emson,
Raven Press, New York © 1983.

Dopamine- and Norepinephrine-Containing Neuron Systems: Their Anatomy in the Rat Brain

Olle Lindvall and Anders Björklund

Departments of Histology and Neurology, University of Lund, S-223 62 Lund, Sweden

During the two decades that have passed since the pioneering studies of Carlsson et al. (28) and Dahlström and Fuxe (39,59), our knowledge of the anatomy of the catecholamine (CA)-containing neurons in the CNS has undergone continuous development. Although the framework that was laid out in these early studies is still valid, we know today considerably more about the detailed organization and projections of the dopamine (DA)- and norepinephrine (NE)-containing systems, particularly in the CNS of the rat.

In recent years, the most important contributions have come from the application of the modern anterograde and retrograde tracing methods. This has meant a new era in the study of CA neuroanatomy. The present chapter is intended primarily as an update of our previous knowledge, with particular emphasis on the new data that have emerged from studies made over the last few years. For more extensive descriptions of the earlier literature, the reader is referred to our own previous reviews (94,95) and to the reviews by Moore and Bloom (121,122).

CENTRAL DOPAMINE-CONTAINING NEURON SYSTEMS

The majority of DA cells in the CNS are localized in the mesencephalon. Such cells are also found in the diencephalon, olfactory bulb, and possibly in the medulla oblongata. In addition, the retina contains a system of DA neurons. Table 1 lists the major dopaminergic projection systems in the rat brain. The following description focuses on the projections of the mesencephalic DA cells and the recently discovered diencephalospinal system. For information about the other DA systems, the reader is referred, e.g., to Lindvall and Björklund (94,95) and Moore and Bloom (121).

Mesotelencephalic System

Dahlström and Fuxe (39) introduced the currently used terminology of the subdivisions of the DA-containing cell system in the mesencephalon. They distinguished three groups, A8, A9 (corresponding to the substantia nigra, SN), and A10 (partly located in the ventral tegmental area, VTA). Their axonal projections were subsequently separated into two systems, the nigrostriatal system (originating in A9) and the mesolimbic system (originating in A10) (4,191). It now seems well established that the DA neurons in the mesencephalon constitute a single system projecting in at least a crude topographic order to cortical, limbic, and striatal telencephalic regions.

Fallon and Moore (52) have proposed several general topographical principles for the organization of the projections from mesencephalic DA cells to basal forebrain and neostriatum: (a) *inverted dorsal–ventral topography,* i.e., that ventral cells tend to project to more dorsal structures such as septum, nc. accumbens, and neostriatum, and dorsal cells tend to project to more ventral structures, e.g., olfactory tubercle and amygdala (see also ref. 53); (b) *medial–lateral topography* with medially localized cells projecting to more medially located terminal areas, and neurons in lateral sectors of the mesencephalic cell groups projecting to more laterally located areas in the forebrain; (c) *anterior–posterior topography,* i.e., anterior cells projecting more anteriorly, and posterior cells to more posterior areas of the forebrain. From these studies, the projections to neocortical areas

TABLE 1. *Central dopamine-containing neuron systems*

System	Cells of origin	Projections
1. Mesostriatal system	Substantia nigra (A9), ventral tegmental area (A10), retrorubral nucleus (A8)	Nc. caudatus–putamen, globus pallidus, nc. accumbens
2. Mesocortical system (Meso–limbo–cortical system)	Ventral tegmental area, substantia nigra, retrorubral nucleus	Forebrain limbic and cortical areas as indicated in Table 2
3. Mesodiencephalic system	Substantia nigra, ventral tegmental area	Subthalamic nucleus, lateral habenula
4. Mesopontine system	Substantia nigra, ventral tegmental area	Locus ceruleus
5. Diencephalospinal system	Dorsal and posterior hypothalamus, zona incerta, caudal thalamus (A11)	Spinal cord
6. Periventricular system	Mesencephalic periaqueductal gray, periventricular gray of caudal thalamus (A11)	Periaqueductal gray, medial thalamus and hypothalamus
7. Incertohypothalamic system	Zona incerta, periventricular hypothalamus (A11, A13, A14)	Zona incerta, anterior, medial preoptic and periventricular hypothalamus, septum
8. Tuberohypophyseal system	Arcuate and periventricular hypothalamic nuclei (A12, A14)	Median eminence, pars nervosa and pars intermedia of the pituitary
9. Periglomerular dopamine neurons	Olfactory bulb (A15)	Dendritic processes into olfactory glomeruli
10. Retinal dopamine system	Mainly in the inner nuclear layer of the retina	Local dendritic projections

seemed, at least partly, to be organized according to similar topographical principles. From the description below, it will be clear, however, that there is at present no general agreement about all aspects of the topographical arrangements of mesencephalic DA neurons as suggested by Fallon and Moore (52).

According to our terminology, the *mesotelencephalic system* refers to the entire ascending projection to telencephalic areas from the DA neurons in the mesencephalon. This system has been divided into two major subsystems: the *mesostriatal system,* which includes the projections to nc. accumbens, globus pallidus, and nc. caudatus–putamen, and the *mesocortical system* (or mesolimbocortical system), which comprises projections both to allocortical and neocortical areas.

Before the different projections are described in further detail, some general features of the mesotelencephalic system should be mentioned. First, it must be emphasized that most of our present knowledge of the topographical organization of the mesotelencephalic system has been obtained with anterograde and retrograde tracers but that very few of the available studies have differentiated between DA and non-DA neurons. Since several recent observations have indicated the existence of nondopaminergic mesostriatal (10,56,67,70,102, 180,193,194) and mesocortical (43,180,186) sys-

tems, it seems possible that some of the topographical principles described here are unrelated to the DA-containing systems.

The vast majority of neurons in the mesostriatal system are, however, dopaminergic. It has thus been estimated that 5% or fewer of cells in SN or VTA projecting to the nc. caudatus–putamen are non-DA-containing (193). Similarly, Swanson (180) has found that the projection to nc. accumbens from SN comprises 10%, and that from VTA 15%, nondopaminergic neurons. In contrast, the proportion of the non-DA-containing component within the mesocortical system seems to differ considerably between various projections (180). For example, the dopaminergic component of the VTA projection to the lateral septum has been calculated to constitute 72%, whereas the VTA projection to the pregenual frontal cortex comprises only 33% DA-containing neurons. It thus seems that the identification of the cells as dopaminergic is most critical in studies on the topography of the mesocortical system. However, as has been pointed out by Swanson (180), dopaminergic and nondopaminergic cells seem to be essentially intermixed at least with regard to the projections of the VTA.

Our findings (93) that some DA axons running into the frontal cortex send collaterals into the septum and that axons ascending in the MFB give off collaterals towards the amygdaloid–piriform lobe suggested that individual DA cells in the mesencephalon can project to more than one terminal area. There is now convincing evidence that single cells in both VTA and SN innervate separate regions via collateral branches, although the dopaminergic nature of such branching neurons has not been definitely established. In an electrophysiological study (43), some single, presumed DA neurons in the VTA were found to have the following branching patterns: septum–nc. accumbens, septum–nc. caudatus–putamen, and possibly also septum–frontal cortex. After injections of fluorescent retrograde tracers into various combinations of known DA terminal areas, Swanson (180) observed very few double-labeled cells in the mesencephalon. Nevertheless, a minor portion of the labeled VTA cells were labeled concomitantly from injections in different terminal sites, namely, in nc. accumbens and frontal cortex, lateral septum and frontal cortex, frontal cortex and entorhinal cortex, and habenula and nc. accumbens. This suggests that some few VTA neurons may be widely collateralized, although one should keep in mind that labeling of axons-of-passage may yield erroneous results in double-label studies with retrograde tracers.

In Swanson's study (180), no evidence for the existence of mesencephalic neurons with one ascending and one descending axon collateral was obtained. The only projection with a more extensive collateralization was found to be the one from VTA to locus ceruleus, in which 15% of the neurons innervated both sides. It should be pointed out that in this study, no attempt was made to distinguish DA- from non-DA-containing cells. Swanson (180) concluded that, with the exception of the projection to the locus ceruleus, essentially separate populations of neurons in the VTA (and adjacent regions including the SN) project to each of the terminal fields. However, seemingly in discordance with these findings, Fallon and Loughlin (50) have reported from a similar study that as many as 50% to 70% of medial SN cells and 5% to 15% of cells in VTA are doubly labeled after injections into various forebrain areas. Thus, their data indicate that collateralization could be a more important organizational principle for the mesencephalic DA neurons.

The mesotelencephalic system has been believed to project only ipsilaterally (see, e.g., ref. 94). However, there is now some evidence that part of the mesencephalic DA cells may also innervate contralateral forebrain areas. After injections of HRP (152,195) or Evans blue (55) into the nc. caudatus–putamen, a significant but minor population of labeled neurons were found in the contralateral SN and/or VTA. The recent study by Swanson (180) using retrograde fluorescent tracers in combination with tyrosine hydroxylase immunohistochemistry has even indicated that virtually all of the dopaminergic as well as nondopaminergic projections from the VTA are partially crossed.

In the following section, the organization of the subsystems in the mesotelencephalic DA system is described in more detail. Emphasis is put on the localization of cell bodies of origin (Table 2) and on the regional organization of each terminal area (Fig. 1), whereas the reader is referred to the work by Lindvall and Björklund (93) for a detailed account of axonal pathways and branching patterns.

Mesostriatal System

The nc. caudatus–putamen and nc. accumbens are densely supplied with DA fibers (59). In the globus pallidus, a sparse plexus of DA-containing terminal axons is distributed throughout the gray matter (96). These fibers are collaterals from axons running in the nigrostriatal bundle and originate in SN (52,96).

The majority of cells projecting to nc. accumbens belong to the A10 group, but a significant portion is localized in the medial SN (29,52, 129,170,180,197). In addition, there is a minor projection from cells in the A8 group (129,180). The DA cells projecting to the nc. accumbens have a medial–lateral topographical organization in relation to their terminal area (52,101).

The DA innervation in the nc. caudatus–putamen of the rat originates not only in group A9 (for references, see ref. 94) but also in the A8 (52,129,191,192) and A10 cell groups (9,29,52, 170,171,185,192). Many studies have been performed recently on the relationship between the mesencephalic DA cells and the area of termination in the striatum. The projection area of the A8 cell group, which can be regarded as a caudal extension of the SN, has been located in the ventral putamen (9,52,129). Several topographical principles have been proposed for the nigrostriatal system (see also above). It has a medial-to-medial and lateral-to-lateral topography (9,29,45,52, 66,177), although considerable overlap has been found between nigral cells projecting to the medial and lateral parts of the nc. caudatus–putamen (192). Some investigators have also found an anterior–posterior topography with anterior nigral cells projecting anteriorly and caudal cells posteriorly in the striatum (52,183). In contrast, Beckstead and co-workers (9) observed no topographical organi-

TABLE 2. *Origins of different projections from the mesencephalic dopamine neuron system*

Terminal area	Origin[a]
Globus pallidus	A9
Nc. accumbens	A10, medial A9, (A8)
Nc. caudatus–putamen	A9
Ventral part	A8
Anteromedial part	A10 [lateral part]
Olfactory bulb	A10, medial A9
Anterior olfactory nuclei	A10, medial A9
Olfactory tubercle	A10 [lateral part]
Islands of Calleja	A9, (A10)
Lateral septal nucleus	A10 [medial part]
Interstitial nucleus of the stria terminalis	A10
Piriform cortex	A10, medial A9
Amygdala	A10, medial A9
Ventral entorhinal cortex	A10 [lateral part], (A8)
Hippocampus	A10, A9
Suprarhinal cortex	Dorsolateral A10
Pregenual anteromedial cortex	A10 [medial part]
Supragenual anteromedial cortex	A9
Perirhinal cortex	Lateral A10, A9
Temporal association cortex	
Lateral habenular nucleus	Medial A10
Subthalamic nucleus	A9
Locus ceruleus	A10, A9

[a]Brackets denote the predominant localization of cells of origin within a nucleus; parentheses denote minor projection.

zation along the sagittal axis but found that the nigrostriatal fibers originating in each part of the SN are distributed over the entire length of the striatum. The only exception noted in their study was that the projection from the most lateral nigra avoided the anterior pole of the striatum.

An additional topographical principle for the organization of the nigrostriatal system has been suggested by Veening and co-workers (195). From their HRP data, they concluded that this projection is organized along an oblique longitudinal neostriatal axis: from rostromedial and dorsal to caudolateral and ventral. Injections of HRP into the nc. caudatus–putamen along this axis resulted in a gradual shift from a labeling of the medial part of the SN and the ventral VTA to a labeling of the lateral and dorsal parts of the SN–VTA complex.

Several studies have indicated that the neostriatal projection from the A10 group (mainly its lateral part) is confined to the antero–medial part of the head of the nc. caudatus–putamen (29,52,171). However, other experiments have implied that the afferents from VTA are much more widely distributed, reaching the entire ventro–medial half of the nc. caudatus–putamen (9,192).

Mesocortical System

Apart from its periglomerular DA cells (68), the olfactory bulb contains scattered DA terminals in all layers, particularly in its caudal half (51). In the anterior olfactory nuclei, a sparse to moderately dense DA innervation has been observed (51). The density is higher in the medial and dorsal anterior olfactory nucleus than in the lateral nucleus. These innervations have been proposed to originate in A10 and medial A9 (51).

The olfactory tubercle receives a very dense DA input (59) originating in the A10 cell group (4,9,51,52,101,170,171,191), mainly in its lateral part (101). Part of the fibers probably arise in the medial SN (51). A medial–lateral topographical arrangement of the projection has been established (52,101).

The islands of Calleja (IC) are surrounded by a dense plexus of DA terminal axons. Within each island, the central core of neuropil has a moderately dense DA innervation, whereas only a few scattered DA fibers are found between the granule cells (for details, see ref. 54; cf. refs. 51,75,95). The localization of the cell bodies of origin has not

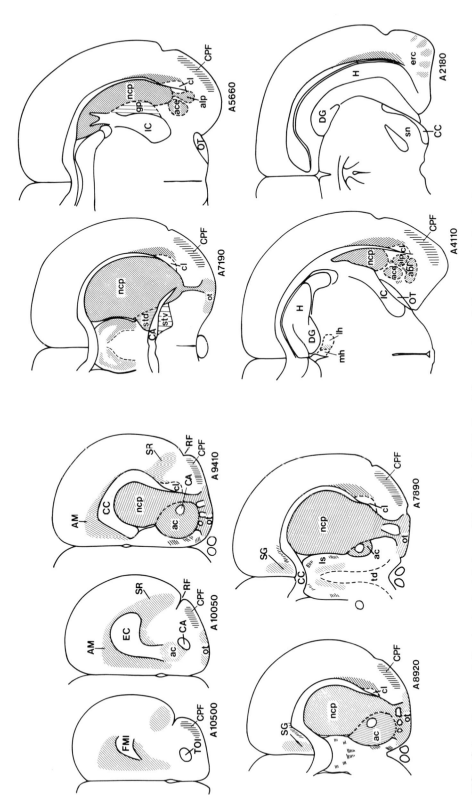

FIG. 1. Schematic representation, in nine frontal planes, of the terminal distribution of the mesotelencephalic and mesohabenular DA systems. Areas of termination are indicated (*hatching*). abl, basal amygdaloid nucleus, lateral part; ac, nc. accumbens; ace, central amygdaloid nucleus; alp, lateral amygdaloid nucleus, posterior part; cl, claustrum; erc, entorhinal cortex; gp, globus pallidus; lh, lateral habenular nucleus; ls, lateral septal nucleus; mh, medial habenular nucleus; ncp, nc. caudatus–putamen; ot, olfactory tubercle; sn, substantia nigra; st, interstitial nucleus of the stria terminalis; std, dorsal part; stv, ventral part; td, nucleus of the diagonal band; AM, anteromedial system; CA, anterior commissure; CC, corpus callosum; CPF, piriform cortex; DG, dentate gyrus; EC, external capsule; FMI, forceps minor; H, hippocampus; IC, internal capsule; OT, optic tract; RF, rhinal fissure; SG, supragenual system; SR, suprarhinal system; TOI, intermediary olfactory tract.

been definitely established. On the basis of lesions and injections of radioactive amino acids, Fallon and co-workers (54) concluded that VTA innervates medial IC, and the SN innervates the lateral IC. However, after similar tracer injections into VTA, Beckstead and co-workers (9) found labeling over the entire olfactory tubercle with the exception of the IC. This is at variance with the results of Fallon and co-workers (54) and would indicate that the DA cells projecting to the IC are separated from those connected with the olfactory tubercle, an arrangement that finds some support in our own lesion data. Thus, an electrolytic lesion of the A10 cell group, which removes the majority of DA fibers in the olfactory tubercle, spared the innervation in the IC *(unpublished observations)*.

Almost the entire mesencephalic DA innervation in the septum is localized in the lateral septal nucleus (for detailed description, see refs. 101,120). It originates in the A10 cell group, mainly in its medial part (5,29,52,92,97,101,120,171,180). The HRP data of Fallon and Moore (52) indicate a rostral–caudal topography in this projection.

The interstitial nucleus of the stria terminalis contains a very dense DA innervation in its dorsal part (59) and a DA terminal plexus of lower density in the ventral part (69,75,101). The fibers have been found to originate in the VTA (9,120,171).

The piriform cortex receives a minor DA input (51,93). Rather scattered DA-containing fibers are distributed through layers II and III, and in layer II, small clusters of cells are innervated by a DA terminal plexus. At the junction between the medial piriform cortex and cortical amygdaloid nucleus, a rich DA innervation has been described (51).

In the amygdala, the DA fibers are concentrated in the central, basolateral, and intercalated nuclei and in the posterior nucleus of the lateral nuclear complex (49,59,61,191). Sparse to moderate DA innervations are found in the cortical and medial nuclei and in the anterior amygdaloid area (49).

The DA innervations of the piriform cortex and the amygdala originate in the VTA and medial SN (9,29,49,52,61,135,136,171,180). The projection is arranged topographically both in anterior–posterior and medial–lateral directions (52). The majority of DA afferents reach the amygdaloid–piriform region via the ansa lenticularis and, as a loosely arranged system of fibers, via the ventral amygdalofugal pathway (46,52,93). No significant population of DA fibers seems to follow the stria terminalis (46,49).

It should be mentioned that Meibach and Katzman (117) recently presented evidence for a different organization of the mesoamygdaloid DA pro-

jection in the cat (cf. 82). According to their findings, the DA innervation in the central nucleus originates in the lateral and dorsal VTA and in the most dorsal portion of the pars compacta of the SN, whereas that in the lateral nucleus originates in the pars lateralis of the SN. The latter projection system does not join the other ascending axons from the mesencephalic DA cells but has its own course, occupying a lateral position adjacent to the cerebral peduncle and joining the ventral amygdalofugal pathway. So far, these organizational features seem to be unique for the cat (117).

The DA innervation of the ventral entorhinal cortex is confined to its anterior part, where the fibers form a series of clusters localized mainly in the second and third layers (11,33,49,61,73,99). The cell bodies of origin are distributed in the VTA, principally in its lateral part (8,9,49,52,61,99,171,180). In addition, Swanson (180) has found evidence for a minor projection from the A8 DA cell group to the entorhinal cortex.

Evidence has recently been provided for a minor DA innervation of the hippocampus. First, bilateral 6-hydroxydopamine injections in the ascending noradrenergic pathways, which gave rise to an almost complete depletion of hippocampal NE, reduced DA to a markedly less degree and failed to affect hippocampal DOPAC level (13). If these injections were combined with lesions in the A9–A10 area, further reductions in hippocampal DA and DOPAC content were observed (162). Second, Simon and co-workers (171) found some labeled terminals in the gyrus dentatus region and at the internal edge of the hippocampus after injections of tritiated leucine into the posterior part of the VTA. No such labeling was, however, observed in another study after injections of anterograde tracers into the VTA or SN (9). After injection of HRP (200) or labeled wheat germ agglutinin (163), labeled neurons have been found both in the VTA and in the SN. In contrast, Riley and Moore (149) found no such labeling in VTA or SN after hippocampal HRP injections. However, Swanson (180) has reported that after injections into the dorsal hippocampus, the fluorescent tracer True Blue labeled cells both in the VTA and SN. A small number of these cells were identified as dopaminergic using tyrosine hydroxylase immunohistochemistry. Third, the effect of drugs on hippocampal HVA and DOPAC levels is similar to that observed in other limbic areas innervated by DA neurons (13,78). Fourth, several papers indicate the existence of DA-sensitive receptor sites in the hippocampus (for references, see ref. 162).

On the basis of these findings, it has been postulated (162,180) that the hippocampus receives a sparse DA input from the A9 and A10 cell groups. However, microscopic techniques have, so far, not shown any well-defined terminal plexus in the hippocampus that could correspond to the proposed DA innervation. Hökfelt and co-workers (76), using the glyoxylic acid method, described a previously unknown minor CA input to the hippocampus, which, on the basis of its reaction to various pharmacological manipulations, was considered to be dopaminergic. However, in a subsequent immunohistochemical study (75), only a few possibly DA-containing terminals were observed in the hilus area dentatae immediately below the granular cells. No systematic studies using the new, more sensitive histofluorescence techniques for CAs have hitherto been performed on the hippocampus from brains with complete lesions of the NE pathways.

In the frontal lobe, three different DA terminal systems have been distinguished: the anteromedial, suprarhinal, and supragenual systems (for detailed description and references, see 98). The anteromedial system originates principally in the medial part (7,9,29,47,52,98,99,170,171,180), and the suprarhinal system in the dorsolateral part of the A10 cell group (49,52,64,98,99). Since lesions of the SN leave the suprarhinal system unaffected (98), and restricted HRP injections into the terminal area only label cells in the A10 area (64), it seems unlikely that SN significantly contributes to this fiber system. The supragenual system, which gives rise to a dense innervation of the second and third layers of the anterior cingulate cortex, has been found to originate in the SN (29,47,52, 98,99,180), and the lesion experiments indicate that the cell bodies are distributed along the mediolateral extent of the pars compacta (98). A contribution from the A10 group is possible (see, e.g., ref. 180), but the labeling in this area after tracer injections into the anterior cingulate cortex probably results from uptake into fibers belonging to the caudal extension of the anteromedial system in the basal (fifth and sixth) layers.

The suprarhinal DA system continues caudally along the rhinal sulcus in close relationship to the claustrum and is then called the perirhinal system (49,98). We have recently observed that this system reaches more dorsally (about 1.6–2 mm above the rhinal sulcus) than has previously been reported. At caudal levels, the DA terminal system extends into the temporal association cortex, where a fiber plexus of low density is found, mainly in the basal layers (I. Divac, A. Björklund, and O. Lindvall, *unpublished data*). This is consistent with biochemical findings in the monkey (14) that have suggested the presence of a more extensive DA in-

nervation to the temporal lobe in the primate. The perirhinal system of the rat seems to originate both in the lateral A10 and in the SN (49,52,98). The exact localization of the mesencephalic DA cells projecting to the temporal association cortex is not known at present.

It should be mentioned that in a recent study in the cat (111), labeled neurons were found in the VTA after HRP injections into many neocortical areas (including posterior regions) where no DA terminal axons have so far been observed in the rat. Although this might indicate species differences, it is also possible, as was pointed out by Markowitsch and Irle themselves, that the projections to areas outside the boundaries of the established DA innervations largely comprise nondopaminergic VTA neurons. However, with HRP tracing in combination with CA histofluorescence, evidence has been obtained (190) for a dopaminergic projection from A10 to the visual cortex in the cat. So far, no such system has been observed in the rat brain.

Mesodiencephalic System

During the last few years, evidence has accumulated for diencephalic projections of the mesencephalic DA neurons. Three main projection areas have been discussed: lateral habenula, subthalamic nucleus, and hypothalamus.

Lateral Habenula

The medial part of the lateral habenular nucleus contains a very dense aggregation of delicate CA axons (100). The dopaminergic nature of this innervation can be inferred from several observations: (a) the habenula contains significant amounts of DA (84,196); (b) tyrosine hydroxylase immunohistochemistry, which preferentially demonstrates DA neurons, has shown a fiber system with identical distribution (74); (c) the uptake of DA into these fibers is unaffected by desipramine, which is a potent inhibitor of the uptake into noradrenergic axons (95; G. Skagerberg, A. Björklund, and O. Lindvall, *unpublished data*); (d) manipulation of DA receptors leads to prominent changes in glucose consumption in the lateral habenula (113).

There is substantial evidence that the DA innervation of the lateral habenula originates in the A10 group. First, large electrolytic lesions comprising the A8, A9, and A10 cell groups markedly reduce its DA content (84), and 6-hydroxydopamine injections in the VTA remove the DA input to the lateral habenula completely (G. Skagerberg, A. Björklund, and O. Lindvall, *unpublished data*).

Second, retrograde tracers injected into the lateral habenula labels cell bodies in the VTA (71,143, 146,180; G. Skagerberg, A. Björklund, and O. Lindvall, *unpublished data*). Third, radioactive amino acids injected into VTA are transported to the lateral habenular nucleus (9,171).

The cells labeled after injections of retrograde tracers into the lateral habenula are localized at and near the midline in the VTA (146,180; G. Skagerberg, A. Björklund, and O. Lindvall, *unpublished data*). However, only a minor portion of these cells are DA containing, which indicates that the mesohabenular projection system is largely nondopaminergic (180; G. Skagerberg, A. Björklund, and O. Lindvall, *unpublished data*). Anterograde tracer studies have indicated that the VTA neurons may project to the habenula both via the fasciculus retroflexus (9,171) and the stria medullaris (171). Both these tracts have previously been shown to carry CA axons (93). Recent experiments from our laboratory with microknife lesions of either of these bundles indicate that the majority of preterminal fibers in the mesohabenular DA system reach the habenula via the fasciculus retroflexus (G. Skagerberg, A. Björklund, and O. Lindvall, *unpublished data*).

Subthalamic Nucleus

The subthalamic nucleus contains significant amounts of DA (196), and the DA agonist apomorphine induces a marked increase of its glucose consumption (27), which indicates that dopaminergic mechanisms are importantly involved in subthalamic functions. Histochemical studies have shown a loose plexus of CA fibers in the subthalamic nucleus of the rat and cat (26,116) and of human fetuses (130). No CA cell bodies were found in the rat, but in the cat, DA cells were observed in the posterior part of the nucleus. It has not, as yet, been clarified whether the CA fiber plexus originates from the nigrostriatal bundle (possibly via collaterals) or from separate DA cells, e.g., in the pars reticulata of the SN or, in the cat, the subthalamic nucleus.

Hypothalamus

Hypothalamic DA has been considered to be associated exclusively with the periventricular, tuberohypophyseal, and incertohypothalamic systems (for references, see ref. 94). However, Kizer and co-workers (84) found significant reductions of DA levels in hypothalamus after large electrolytic lesions of the A8, A9, and A10 cell groups. Palkovits and co-workers (140) found axonal degeneration in the median eminence after such lesions and

after 6-hydroxydopamine injections into the same areas in the mesencephalon. It was therefore suggested (84) that the mesencephalic cell groups contribute to the DA innervation of the hypothalamus.

Other data, however, do not support this hypothesis. Weiner and co-workers (198) found no significant change in hypothalamic DA levels after complete hypothalamic deafferentation. Although Palkovits and co-workers (138) measured a slight decrease of mean DA level in the median eminence after total deafferentiation of the medial hypothalamus, this change did not reach statistical significance. In addition, unilateral 6-hydroxydopamine injections into the SN, which reached also neurons in the VTA, caused no change in hypothalamic DA levels (153). It could be argued, however, on basis of lack of denervation effects, e.g., in the septal area, that some A10 neurons were unaffected by that lesion. Tracer studies have also given conflicting results. Thus, Fallon and Moore (52), Day et al. (42), Wiegand and Price (199), and Berk and Finkelstein (12) found no evidence for a mesohypothalamic DA pathway, and Beckstead and co-workers (9) found only some labeled fibers in the posterior hypothalamus after injections of tritiated leucine and proline into VTA. In contrast, Simon and co-workers (171) observed significant labeling in the medial hypothalamus, including the median eminence, after injection of tritiated leucine into the VTA. The reason for this discrepancy is at present unclear. However, it illustrates that the existence of a mesohypothalamic DA pathway is far from being definitely established. Small injections of retrograde tracers into hypothalamic nuclei combined with transmitter histochemistry to identify any labeled DA cell bodies in the mesencephalon would be desirable in order to solve this problem.

Descending Projections from Mesencephalic Dopamine Cell Groups

Studies with anterograde and retrograde tracers have indicated that neurons in the VTA and SN innervate areas in the lower brainstem, cerebellum, and spinal cord. However, more experimentation is required before the DA nature of these projection systems can be established. In the following section, available data on some possible descending connections of the mesencephalic DA neurons are briefly discussed.

Dorsal Raphe Nucleus

Tritiated leucine and proline injected into VTA (9,45,171) and SN (9) are transported to the dorsal raphe nucleus (DRN). In the cat, a projection from the SN is also supported by the labeling after HRP injection into the DRN (155). Since DRN contains high levels of DA (see, e.g., refs. 91,196), it has been suggested (171) that the afferents originating in VTA and SN are DA containing. At present, this possibility cannot be excluded, but it should be remembered that DRN contains dopaminergic cell bodies (74,93,128,132), which should account for at least part of its DA content.

Locus Ceruleus

Several findings now indicate the existence of a dopaminergic projection from mesencephalon to locus ceruleus (LC). First, LC has been reported to contain significant amounts of DA (196), but no DA-producing cell bodies have been found in this nucleus. Second, studies using the Fink–Heimer technique after lesions (169) and anterograde tracers after injections (9,171,172) in the VTA have indicated that VTA projects bilaterally to the LC. Third, Swanson (180) has identified labeled dopaminergic cells in A10 and A9 after injections of a retrograde fluorescent tracer in the LC. The mesoceruleal DA system has both ipsilateral and contralateral projections, and some individual DA neurons seem to innervate the LC on both sides via collateral branches.

Lateral Parabrachial Nucleus

Hedreen (69) proposed that part of the CA innervation of the lateral parabrachial nucleus is dopaminergic. He found degenerating terminals in the ventrolateral part of the nucleus after intraventricular 6-OHDA with the Fink–Heimer technique, a method that has been reported to stain only degenerating DA and not NE terminals after this treatment (69,70). The existence of a dopaminergic input to the lateral parabrachial nucleus finds some support in recent findings with retrograde tracers combined with tyrosine hydroxylase immunohistochemistry (180), which showed some scattered, presumed DA cells in the VTA. However, it cannot at present be excluded that after the injections the tracer was taken up by axons just passing through the nucleus and, in fact, innervating the LC.

Cerebellum

The CA afferents to the cerebellum in the rat have been considered to be exclusively noradrenergic (for references, see ref. 94). However, Kizer and co-workers (84) reported a 50% de-crease of cerebellar DA level after lesions of the A8–A9–A10 cell groups, suggesting that some afferents to the cerebellum might be dopaminergic and originate in the mesencephalon. So far, the existence of such a system has not been established. Thus, although Simon and co-workers (171) have reported anterograde transport of tritiated leucine to the cerebellum after injection into the VTA, similar experiments by Beckstead and co-workers (9) showed no such labeling. Furthermore, large injections of HRP or a fluorescent tracer into the cerebellum did not label any presumed DA cells in the mesencephalon (158,180).

Spinal Cord

Commissiong and co-workers (36) have shown a decrease of DA in the spinal cord after lesion of the SN, suggesting the existence of a nigrospinal DA system. However, no labeled DA cell bodies have so far been found in the SN after tracer injections into the spinal cord of the rat (see, e.g., ref. 173). It seems possible that the lesions performed by Commissiong and co-workers (36) severed fibers of passage from the more rostrally located hypothalamic sites of origin for the DA innervation in the spinal cord (see below).

Diencephalospinal System

Biochemical studies have provided evidence that DA in the spinal cord is not only a precursor of NE, as previously believed, but serves an independent transmitter role in a separate DA neuron system (35,38,58,109). This has been corroborated with transmitter-specific retrograde tracing techniques, showing that DA-containing neurons in the diencephalon can be retrogradely labeled from injections into the spinal cord in the rat and rabbit (17,19,77,182). From biochemical determinations of DA and NE levels, terminal density of the NE innervation in the spinal cord can be estimated to be at least 10 times higher than that of the DA projection. Therefore, it is not possible to identify microscopically the sparse DA innervation in the presence of the rich NE fiber system.

We have recently developed a procedure using combined neonatal subcutaneous 6-hydroxydopamine and adult intraventricular 5,7-dihydroxytryptamine treatment, which reduces NE levels by 94% to 99% in all parts of the spinal cord (173). In such lesioned animals, the DA levels are only marginally affected in the dorsal horn (at all levels) and in the intermediate zone (at thoraco–lumbar levels). In agreement with these biochemical data, we have observed remaining presumed DA fibers in

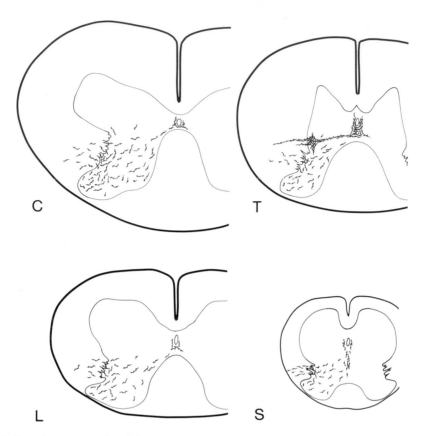

FIG. 2. Semischematic representation of the distribution of presumed DA fibers at four representative levels through the spinal cord. C, cervical; T, thoracic; L, lumbar; S, sacral level.

the dorsal gray of the cervical, thoracic, lumbar, and sacral cord, and in the intermediate gray of the thoracic cord (Fig. 2). The DA axons represent only a minor portion of the total CA innervation, and they are fairly evenly distributed along the cord.

In the dorsal horn, the presumed DA fibers are most abundant in the lateral parts of the superficial layers and in the adjoining reticular nucleus (Fig. 2). The highest density of presumed DA fibers is found in the intermediolateral cell column and in the area surrounding the central canal at thoracic and upper lumbar levels. The presumed DA innervation is not uniform along the intermediolateral column but forms clusters or patches of varicose fibers. These are connected with each other and with the innervation along the central canal by thinner strands of parallel running fibers (Fig. 2). The fiber patches probably correspond to the clustering of preganglionic sympathetic neurons along the intermediolateral column.

With use of CA fluorescence histochemistry or immunohistochemistry in combination with flu-

orescent retrograde tracers, the spinal DA projection system has been found to be entirely uncrossed and to originate exclusively in the A11 group (17,77,173). The labeled DA cell bodies are located in the dorsal and posterior hypothalamus, zona incerta, and caudal thalamus (Fig. 3). According to Swanson and co-workers (182), labeled cells are also found in the paraventricular hypothalamic nucleus. In the rabbit, Blessing and Chalmers (19) found labeling of the A13 cell group in the dorsal hypothalamus after tracer injections into the spinal cord, but these cells are unlabeled in the rat (17,77,173). The reason for this discrepancy is at present unclear: it might be the result of species differences in the topography of the A11–A13 cell groups.

The A11 cell group is known to be a major source of fibers running in the periventricular CA projection system, which innervates, e.g., medial and midline thalamus and several hypothalamic nuclei (93). This fiber system is a component of the dorsal longitudinal fasciculus of Schütz, which is a bidirectional tract interconnecting the lower brain-

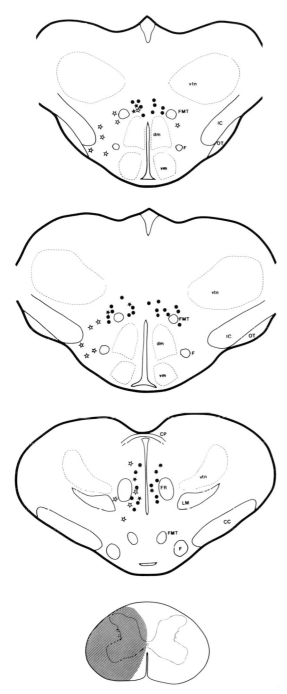

stem and spinal cord with the periaqueductal gray and hypothalamic and thalamic areas.

The diencephalospinal DA system represents the first known descending projection of the A11 neurons and the periventricular CA system. Interestingly, Lindvall and co-workers (100) have observed that the axons of some A11 cells bifurcate in a T-shaped manner, giving rise to one ascending and one descending branch, thus suggesting that the intradiencephalic and the spinal cord projections could be established by collateral axonal branches of the same neurons. Although the projection route of the diencephalospinal system in the brainstem is not yet known, the axons to the spinal cord could possibly descend within the dorsal longitudinal fasciculus. In the spinal cord, the axons appear to descend partly within lamina I of the dorsal horn and in the adjoining parts of the dorsolateral funiculus and partly along the central canal (Fig. 4).

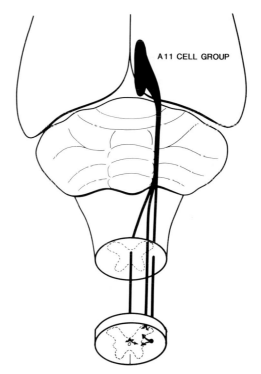

FIG. 4. Proposed arrangement of the diencephalospinal DA system.

FIG. 3. Distribution of DA-containing and True Blue-labeled cells in the diencephalon after unilateral cervical tracer injection. The *shaded area* in the cervical cord section represents the extension of the area of intense True Blue fluorescence at the injection site. *Filled circles* represent nonlabeled CA cells. *Open stars* represent cells labeled with True Blue alone. *Filled stars* represent CA cells labeled with True Blue. CC, crus cerebri; CP, commissura posterior; dm, dorsomedial hypothalamic nucleus; F, fornix; FMT, fasciculus mammillo–thalamicus; FR, fasciculus retroflexus; IC, internal capsule; OT, optic tract; vm, ventromedial hypothalamic nucleus; vtn, ventral thalamic nucleus.

CENTRAL NOREPINEPHRINE-CONTAINING NEURON SYSTEMS

The NE-producing cells of the brain are almost exclusively confined to the medulla oblongata and pons. On basis of topography, they can be divided into three major cell systems (cf. refs. 39,94): *the locus ceruleus–subceruleus complex, the lateral tegmental cell system* (which has one medullary and one pontine part), and *the dorsal medullary cell group.*

The nucleus LC is usually divided into a dorsal part, composed of densely packed fusiform cells, and a ventral part containing somewhat larger multipolar neurons (179). These latter neurons are morphologically similar to the NE neurons in the subceruleus (SC) area; they are topographically continuous with the more ventrally located SC cells and have similar projection patterns. This makes a sharp distinction between LC and SC difficult (see ref. 3 for further discussion). The LC complex has also a dorsolateral extension of cells along the medial aspect of the superior cerebellar peduncle into the roof of the fourth ventricle [the so-called A4 cell group of Dahlström and Fuxe (39)].

The cells of the lateral tegmental cell system are located in the ventrolateral tegmentum, from the caudal pole of the medulla oblongata up to the level of the motor nucleus of the trigeminal nerve in the pons (39,139,181). Topographically, and on basis of its ontogenetic development (167), this rather disseminated cell system can be divided into a medullary part and a pontine part.

The cells in the medullary part (groups A1 and A3) extend from the pyramidal decussation up to the rostral part of the inferior olivary nucleus. They occur mainly scattered around and partly within the lateral reticular nucleus (39). In the rat, the A3 cells are difficult to distinguish from those of the A1 group. In the following description, all the cells in the medullary part of the lateral tegmental system are therefore referred to as the A1 cell group. The cells in the pontine part (groups A5 and A7) are distributed from the level of the rostral part of the facial nucleus up to the level of the trigeminal motor nucleus. Caudally, the cells occur caudal and medial to the outgoing fibers of the facial nerve, close to the superior olivary complex. This cell cluster is the A5 group of Dahlström and Fuxe (39). Further rostrally, the cells extend into the area between the ventrolateral border of the superior cerebellar peduncle and the lateral lemniscus, forming the A7 group. The border between A7 and the SC cell group is not well defined.

The cells of the dorsal medullary cell group, des-ignated A2, occur in the nucleus of the solitary tract and the commissural nucleus, wtih some cells also in the dorsal motor nucleus of the vagus (39).

On the basis of this topography of the NE cells in the lower brainstem, three projection systems have been distinguished: the locus ceruleus system, the lateral tegmental system, and the dorsal medullary system. The following description deals mainly with recent findings on the topographical organization of these systems. For information on axonal pathways and a more detailed review of the earlier literature, see, e.g., Lindvall and Björklund (94) and Moore and Bloom (122).

Locus Ceruleus System

The nucleus LC of the rat has been estimated to comprise about 1,500 cells (179), which are all probably NE producing. Despite the relatively small number of neurons, this nucleus has projections to practically all regions of the CNS. This is accomplished by an extensive collateralization of the LC neurons. The LC system has long been considered to be a homogeneous nucleus, with each individual neuron projecting to most terminal areas. However, in recent years, this opinion has been challenged, primarily through the work of Mason and Fibiger (112). They have reported that the distribution of HRP-positive cells in the LC is markedly different depending on the location of the HRP injection. The patterns of labeling suggested the following topographical principles for the origins of the LC projections to various terminal areas (Table 3). (a) Along the dorsoventral axis. The innervation in the septum originates in the dorsal half of the dorsal LC, the hippocampal NE projection (at least to the dorsal–anterior hippocampus) in the dorsal LC (cf. ref. 149), and the innervation in the spinal cord in the ventral tip of the LC (cf. refs. 65,160). (b) Along the antero–posterior axis. The hypothalamic innervation originates mainly in the anterior pole, and that in the thalamus in the posterior pole of the LC. (c) Diffusely within the nucleus. Both the projections to the neocortex and those to the amygdala–piriform cortex seem to originate in scattered cells located throughout the LC except in the ventral tip. The ceruleo–cerebellar projection originates from throughout the LC including the ventral tip. Corresponding results have since been obtained by Room et al. (150) with fluorescent tracers for the LC projections to hippocampus, thalamus, neocortex, and cerebellum. It thus seems fairly well established that the LC system comprises a number of subsystems. However, more work is needed be-

TABLE 3. *Origins of different projections from noradrenergic neurons in the principal locus ceruleus*

Terminal area	Origin within the nucleus[a]
Hippocampus	Intermediate–dorsal
Septum	Dorsal
Cerebellum	All regions
Hypothalamus	Anterior–(posterior)–intermediate–dorsal
Thalamus	(Anterior)–posterior–intermediate–dorsal
Neocortex	Intermediate–dorsal
Amygdala–piriform cortex	Intermediate–dorsal
Spinal cord	Ventral

[a]Parentheses denote minor projection. Anterior part comprises one intermediate and one dorsal portion. Posterior part consists of ventral, intermediate and dorsal portions.
Data from Mason and Fibiger (112) and Satoh et al. (160).

fore the details of the regional topography within the LC are known.

Although it now seems that part of the LC neurons have more restricted projection areas than was previously believed, there is convincing evidence that some individual cells innervate widely different regions in the brain and spinal cord via collateral branches. This collateralization of the LC neurons was suggested by early fluorescence histochemical observations (see, e.g., refs. 93, 133,191) but has not been well studied until the recent introduction by Kuypers and collaborators of the use of multiple fluorescent retrograde tracers. This methodology has provided evidence for a number of branching patterns for individual LC neurons (127,150; cf. ref. 176), e.g., divergent axonal projections to the ipsilateral neocortex and hippocampus, neocortex and thalamus, hippocampus and thalamus, neocortex and cerebellum, cerebellum and spinal cord, hippocampus and spinal cord, and thalamus and spinal cord. It was estimated by Nagai et al. (127) that after combinations of injections into neocortex and cerebellum, the number of double-labeled neurons was 10% to 30% that of the single-labeled ones. Fallon and Loughlin (50) have distinguished two subdivisions of the LC based on the relative degree of axonal collateralization to the forebrain. In particular, medium-sized multipolar neurons in the dorsal compact part are often (50–70%) doubly labeled after multiple injections in the forebrain, whereas neurons of the extreme dorsal, ventral, or anterior regions of the LC as well as of the SC are less highly (5–20%) collateralized (cf. 150).

It is well known that the LC also has contralateral projections. For the ascending part of the LC system, at least five commissures have been described (for details and references, see 94,122). All

terminal areas for the LC neurons seem also to receive projections from the contralateral nucleus (2,80,150). Jones and co-workers (80) suggested that 20% of LC cells may project contralaterally, whereas the results of Room and co-workers (150) indicated a percentage of only 5% to 10%. Using homotopic bilateral tracer injections, Adèr et al. (2) and Room and co-workers (150) have shown that the axons of some LC neurons bifurcate to project bilaterally to the thalamus, hippocampus, and cortex via collateral branches. The ratio between double- and single-labeled cells in the LC varied from 1:20 in the thalamus and 1:30 in the cortex to 1:40 in the hippocampus (150). It has also been found after heterotopic bilateral tracer injections that an individual LC neuron can innervate one region on the ipsilateral side and another on the contralateral side, e.g., hippocampus and thalamus, cortex and thalamus, hippocampus and cortex (2,150). Whether any of these cells innervate more than two terminal areas is at present not known.

Again, when one is interpreting these data obtained with the double-labeling technique, it is important to realize that erroneous results can in some cases be obtained through labeling of axons passing through the area of one injection on their way to the area of the other injection. This can easily be the case, e.g., with two cortical injections.

In the section that follows the organization of the different terminal projections of the LC system is described in more detail.

Spinal Cord

The ceruleospinal NE system bilaterally innervates the ventral horn, the intermediate gray, and the ventral part of the dorsal horn at all levels of the cord. Thus, bilateral lesion of the LC–SC complex has been shown to cause an almost complete disappearance of the NE innervation in these parts of the spinal cord (131). Furthermore, bilateral LC lesions (whose encroachment upon the SC area is unclear) have been reported to cause 30% to 40% reductions in total NE or DA-β-hydroxylase content in the rat spinal cord (1,37,151) and about 80% reduction of NE in the ventral horn in the cat (57). According to Karoum and co-workers (83) and Commissiong (34), the ceruleospinal projection is 50% crossed, the crossing most probably taking place at the segmental level.

The projection to the spinal cord originates in the ventral LC and in the SC. Injections of HRP into the spinal cord in the rat predominantly label multipolar cells in the ventral subdivision of the LC and in the SC area and only a few of the smaller fusiform cells in the dorsal subdivision (1,65, 159,160). The study of Zemlan et al. (203) using restricted unilateral HRP injections into the white matter of the thoracic cord indicates that the axons from the LC–SC neurons descend ipsilaterally in the ventral and ventrolateral funiculi (Fig. 5). This is consistent with the findings of Basbaum and Fields (6) using HRP injections in combination

with partial lesions of the cord and with the fluorescence histochemical observations of Nygren and Olsson (131) in rats with bilateral LC–SC lesions.

Guyenet (65) has provided electrophysiological evidence that a significant proportion of the ceruleospinal neurons give collaterals that ascend in the dorsal tegmental bundle. Double-labeling studies with fluorescent retrograde tracers support the existence of such collateral arrangements (see also above). Thus, a small portion (perhaps some 10%) of the cells labeled by tracers injected into the spinal cord become doubly labeled with a second tracer injected into cerebral cortex, hippocampus, or thalamus (150) or into the cerebellum (127).

Lower Brainstem

The distribution of CA axons in the lower brainstem of the rat has been dealt with in several papers (59,139,181), but the recent investigation by Levitt and Moore (91) has provided the first detailed analysis of the organization of the CA innervation in the mesencephalon, pons, and medulla oblongata. The following brief account of the topography of the LC projection system in the lower brainstem is based primarily on their description (for details, see 91). The dorsal, compact part of the LC cell group seems to be the only source of the moderately dense NE innervations in the superior and inferior colliculi (cf. 85,93,181), the cochlear nuclei (86,87), and the interpeduncular nucleus (110). Together with the SC, the LC gives rise to the major part of the moderately rich NE fiber patterns in the pontine gray nuclei and the principal sensory trigeminal nucleus. In the spinal sensory trigeminal nucleus, the LC fibers are mixed with afferents from other NE cell groups. The LC innervation has been reported to emanate from both the ipsilateral and the contralateral nucleus (168). The reticular formation at all levels and the central gray contain a small to moderate number of axons probably originating in the LC (91). In conclusion, the LC system mainly innervates primary sensory and association nuclei (91).

The NE innervations in other brainstem nuclei, some of which have previously been considered to have major origins in the LC, are unaffected by bilateral LC lesions (comprising also the SC area), as determined by NE levels and terminal densities (91). This is the case, e.g., for the dense innervations in nc. tractus solitarius, dorsal motor nucleus of the vagus, and nc. commissuralis (cf. 105,134). However, in the HRP study of Takahashi and coworkers (184), a minor portion of the innervation

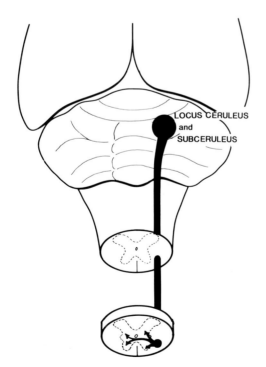

FIG. 5. Proposed arrangement of the ceruleospinal NE system.

in nc. tractus solitarius was found to originate in the ventral part of the LC. Bilateral LC lesions (91) reveal no significant input to the trigeminal and facial (cf. 147) motor nuclei or, in agreement with the HRP study of Brown and co-workers (25), to the inferior olive (cf. 85,181). Several raphe nuclei have previously been proposed to have significant inputs from the LC (see, e.g., 31,105). However, in the study of Levitt and Moore (91), only a minor contribution to the innervation of the dorsal raphe nucleus (see also 155) could be verified, although some LC afferents to medullary raphe nuclei could not be excluded.

Cerebellum

The CA innervation of the cerebellum (for details on the terminal arrangements, see refs. 23,24,72,89,126,133) is probably exclusively noradrenergic and originates primarily in the LC, where the cells of origin are distributed over the entire nucleus (see also above; 112,127,133, 144,150,191). Recently, a minor contribution from the SC group to the innervation of the cerebellar cortex has been reported by Pasquier and co-workers (144). In their study, some evidence was also obtained for the existence of sparse cerebellar afferents from the A5 and A7 cell groups of the LT system (cf. ref. 187). The LC neurons as well as the other possible sources of the cerebellar NE innervation have both ipsilateral and contralateral projections (85,144). It has been estimated (144) that the contralateral projection from the LC amounts to about 50% to 75% of that going to the ipsilateral side.

Thalamus

The dorsal thalamus is richly supplied with NE terminal axons originating in the LC (for references and details on the regional arrangements, see 94). The most dense innervation is found in the anterior nuclei, and particularly in the anteroventral nucleus, but practically all areas of the thalamus receive afferents from the LC (see also 122). In the study of Lindvall and co-workers (100), it was concluded that the specific, or principal, thalamic nuclei (as well as the geniculate bodies) are innervated exclusively by LC neurons, whereas medial and midline nuclei (as well as the habenula) receive NE fibers from several different sources including the LC. The LC terminals in these latter regions were found particularly in the medial and gelatinous nuclei.

Hypothalamus

The LC system gives rise to a minor part of the NE innervation of the hypothalamus. The projections to the periventricular and paraventricular nuclei are the best established ones (12,81,85,105, 115,161,189,201). From autoradiographic studies after injections of radiolabeled amino acids, the LC seems to project only to certain subnuclei within the paraventricular nucleus (for details, see 115,161). In addition, there is now good evidence that LC also has significant projections to some other hypothalamic regions, notably the supraoptic and dorsomedial nuclei (12,81,161,201). However, as described below, the major part of the hypothalamic NE innervation originates in the LT and DM systems.

Hippocampus

The hippocampal NE innervation seems to originate exclusively from the LC (81,100,105,107, 108,112,145,147,149,150,163,164,191,200). The projection has been found to be 75% to 93% ipsilateral (107,150,200). The terminal distribution of NE fibers in the hippocampal formation has been described by Blackstad and co-workers (18), Swanson and Hartman (181), Moore (119), Björklund et al. (16), and Loy and co-workers (107).

The LC NE axons gain access to the hippocampus along three routes: (a) through the septal area to enter hippocampus rostrally, partly through the most caudal septum along the postcommissural fornix and partly through the rostral and dorsal septum along the fornix superior (62,81,93,107); (b) above the corpus callosum along the cingulum bundle and/or the supracallosal striae, sweeping around the splenium of the corpus callosum to enter the hippocampal formation from the dorsal and caudal side (81,93,107,147,181); (c) from the medial forebrain bundle along the ventral amygdalofugal pathway–ansa peduncularis fiber system, through the piriform and entorhinal cortices, to enter the hippocampal formation at its temporal pole (the ventral path; 93,107,181). Judging from the biochemical estimations of Storm-Mathisen and Guldberg (178) and Gage et al. (63), the first two routes account for about 40% of the hippocampal NE, whereas the ventral path contributes the rest. According to the recent study by Loy and co-workers (107), using biochemical and histochemical analyses of the NE innervation after lesions of the various pathways, the supracallosal and the ventral routes are quantitatively the most important ones for the hippocampal NE innervation, whereas the fornix–fimbria route is of relatively minor importance. Their study also indicates that Ammon's horn receives its NE input principally through the ventral path, with smaller contributions from the fornix and the ipsilateral supracallosal route. The innervation of the area dentata is to a larger extent bilateral, with the greatest contribution arising from the ipsilateral supracallosal route and approximately equal proportions of fibers entering via contralateral supracallosal route, fornix, and the ventral path.

Septum

There is a widespread projection from the LC to the septal area in the rat (for details, see 101,120; cf. 81,105,147,165,191). The axons form a moderately dense innervation in the hippocampal rudiment, the medial septal nucleus, and the interstitial nucleus of the stria terminalis and a sparse innervation in the lateral septal nucleus and the septofimbrial nucleus (101). Except in the hippocampal rudiment, the LC fibers in all areas are mixed with NE axons originating in cell groups in the medulla oblongata.

Amygdala and Piriform Cortex

The NE innervation in the amygdala originates partly in the LC (49,81,93,105,112,135,147, 166,202). The LC terminals are found in the entire amygdala and form a moderately dense innervation in the central and basolateral nuclei and a less dense innervation in other areas (for details, see 49). Scattered fibers originating in the LC are found also in the piriform cortex (51; see also 81,147).

Olfactory Bulb, Anterior Olfactory Nuclei, and Olfactory Tubercle

The olfactory bulb contains a moderately dense NE innervation mainly originating in the LC (41,44,48,51,93,118,181,191). In the anterior olfactory nuclei, the NE innervation is denser in the medial and dorsal anterior olfactory nucleus than in the lateral nucleus (51). Fallon and Moore (51) have reported a significant reduction of NE levels in the olfactory tubercle after bilateral LC lesions, indicating a possible LC projection to this region as well.

Neocortex

It is well established that LC gives rise to the NE innervation of the entire neocortex (for references, see 94). During recent years, the distribution of NE fibers and their terminal arrangements in the neocortex of the rat have been studied extensively with the more sensitive fluorescence histochemical and immunohistochemical techniques (for details, see 90,98,123,124,181).

Several routes of entry for the LC axons to the neocortex have been proposed: (a) via the rostral septum and the cingulum (62,81,93,191); (b) via the internal capsule, passing through the nc. caudatus–putamen (79,81,154,188); (c) via the ventral amygdaloid bundle and ansa peduncularis (81,93). However, a recent study by Morrison and co-workers (125), using cortical and subcortical lesions, indicated that the cingulum bundle is not a major intracortical noradrenergic pathway. Thus, only a marginal contribution to the medial cortex from this bundle could be detected, and the dorsal and lateral cortex did not seem to be innervated via the cingulum bundle at all. Instead, the medial cortex was found to be innervated by NE fibers that ascend through the septum, curve over the genu of the corpus callosum, and then run caudally in the supracallosal stria (i.e., medial to the cingulum bundle). Their results further indicate that the dorsal and lateral cortices are innervated chiefly by NE fibers running through the striatum to reach the frontal pole. From here, the axons turn dorsally over the anterior portion of the forceps minor and continue caudally within the deep layers of frontal and dorsolateral cortex. No substantial contribution from the ventral amygdaloid bundle–ansa peduncularis to the innervation of the neocortex was observed.

So far, no distinct subsystems within the ceruleocortical projection system have been distinguished, although it has been reported (106) that a slightly more dorsal distribution of LC cells was labeled by injections of retrograde tracers in medial cortical areas, whereas more lateral cortical injections resulted in somewhat more ventral distributions. However, these distributions overlapped extensively. Double-label studies with fluorescent tracers have suggested that one LC cell may innervate different parts of the neocortex via collateral branches (106,127). From the results of Loughlin and co-workers (106), it appears that the axons of individual LC cells collateralize extensively in the anterior to posterior dimension but only to a limited extent in the medial-to-lateral dimension. This is supported by the lesion data of Morrison and co-workers (125), and it may be hypothesized that one individual LC cell may innervate a longitudinal slice of the neocortex, extending from the frontal areas all the way back to the occipital cortex.

TABLE 4. *Origins of different projections from the noradrenergic lateral tegmental and dorsal medullary neurons*

Terminal area	Origin
Spinal cord	A5, A7
Nc. tractus solitarius and dorsal vagal complex	A1, A2
Spinal sensory trigeminal nucleus	A1, A5
Locus ceruleus	A1, A2, A7
Parabrachial nucleus	A1
Dorsal raphe nucleus	A1
Medial preoptic area	A1, A2
Paraventricular hypothalamic nucleus	A1, A2
Supraoptic nucleus	A1, A2
Dorsomedial hypothalamic nucleus	A1, A2
Ventromedial hypothalamic nucleus	A1, A2
Anterior, lateral, and posterior hypothalamic areas	A1, A2
Median eminence	A1, A2
Arcuate nucleus	A1, A2
Septum	A1, A2
Amygdala	A1, A2

Lateral Tegmental and Dorsal Medullary Systems

The topographical organization of the lateral tegmental (LT) and dorsal medullary (DM) NE systems is less well known than that of the LC system. This is largely explained by the difficulties in interpreting results after lesions of the various LT and DM cell groups or their projection pathways. These cells are found rather scattered in the pons and medulla oblongata, which makes selective ablations virtually impossible, and transections of the axon bundles from individual nuclei can easily sever also other projection systems. However, the new retrograde tracing methods in combination with techniques for identification of labeled CA cells have greatly expanded the possibilities for distinguishing the various subsystems within the DM and LT systems. In the following, the projections of these two systems are described together, but when more detailed knowledge exists about the origin of a certain projection (Table 4), this is mentioned in the text.

Spinal Cord

The LC system is responsible for about 30% to 40% of the spinal NE innervation in the rat. Remaining afferents, primarily going to (a) the intermediolateral column, the area around the central canal, and the fiber strands interconnecting these two areas and (b) the outer layers of the dorsal horn originate in the LT cell system and possibly—to a minor extent—also in the DM cell group. Observations of retrograde cell changes after spinal transection led Dahlström and Fuxe (40) to emphasize the medullary part of the LT cell system, i.e., the A1 group, as the source of NE fibers to the spinal cord. However, later retrograde tracing studies (21,103,114,159,160; G. Skagerberg and A. Björklund, *unpublished observations*) indicate that the NE neurons of the LT cell system projecting to the spinal cord of the rat are primarily confined to the pontine groups (A5 and A7).

The exact contribution of the A2 neurons is unclear. Cells in this area are retrogradely labeled after tracer injections into the cord (88,160). However, combined techniques, using HRP or fluorescent retrograde tracers in combination with CA histofluorescence, have failed to demonstrate any CA-containing spinal cord-projecting neurons in this area (21,114,174; G. Skagerberg and A. Björklund, *unpublished observations*). Fleetwood-Walker and Coote (57) have reported a small (18%) reduction of NE in the region of the intermediolateral column after bilateral lesions of the A2 area in the cat. It seems possible, however, that this effect could have resulted from lesions of fibers of passage, e.g., of axons coming from neurons located in the pons.

Some information is available about the trajectory of the tegmentospinal NE pathway (Fig. 6). Thus, Nygren and Olsson (131) reported that the CA-containing axons remaining after a bilateral lesion of the LC–SC complex, i.e., the axons of the tegmentospinal system, were confined to the dorsolateral funiculus. This is consistent with the observations of Basbaum and Fields (6) that retrograde labeling of cells in the A1 and A5 areas remained in animals with sparing of the dorsolat-

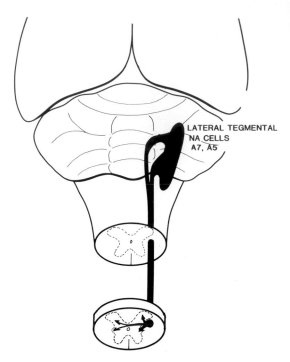

LATERAL TEGMENTAL
NA CELLS
A7, A5

FIG. 6. Proposed arrangement of the tegmentospinal NE system.

eral funiculus but not after sparing of the ventral quadrant. Finally, Loewy et al. (103) have autoradiographically traced axons from the pontine A5 area predominantly ipsilaterally in the medial part of the lateral funiculus. These axons terminated bilaterally in the intermediolateral column and adjoining parts of the intermediate zone.

Lower Brainstem

The distribution of NE fibers in the brainstem was first described by Fuxe (59) and has later been studied with more sensitive histochemical methods by Swanson and Hartman (181) and in more detail by Levitt and Moore (91). The predominant part of the noradrenergic input to the lower brainstem originates in the LT and DM cell groups, and only a minor portion in the LC (see above). The following gives a brief account of the major projection areas of the LT and DM systems. For a more detailed description, the reader is referred to the paper of Levitt and Moore (91). The LT and DM NE neurons innervate mainly primary motor and visceral nuclei, i.e., areas that do not receive any LC afferents. Some cranial nerve nuclei are heavily innervated by NE fibers of nonlocus origin, such as the motor trigeminal, facial, hypoglossal, and ambiguus nuclei, the dorsal motor nucleus of the

vagus, nc. tractus solitarius, and nc. commissuralis. The LT and DM systems also give rise to dense terminal patterns in the ventral mesencephalic central gray, the medial pontine nucleus, the parabrachial nuclei, the ventral tegmental nucleus, and the principal inferior olivary nucleus.

The raphe nuclei, which are distributed in medulla oblongata, pons, and mesencephalon, are richly supplied with NE fibers which (with the possible exception of some termials in the nc. raphe dorsalis which derive from the LC, see above) originate in the LT and DM systems. Raphe pallidus, obscurus, magnus, and dorsalis are the most heavily innervated nuclei, whereas nc. raphe pontis and the rest of the raphe nuclear complex contain low to moderate densities of NE terminals (59,91,181). It should be mentioned that the nc. LC itself is another area with a moderately rich NE innervation of nonlocus origin.

Very little is known at present about the exact localization of the neurons of origin, within the LT and DM cell groups, for the different brainstem NE innervations. Several different sources for the dense NE terminal patterns in the nc. tractus solitarius have previously been proposed on the basis of lesion studies, but it was recently reported in a combined lesion and HRP study (in which labeled CA cells were identified) that the A2 cell group in the nc. commissuralis is the main source of this innervation (184; cf. 137,181). The projection from A2 seemed to be bilateral but with a slight ipsilateral predominance. The A1 cell group in the ventrolateral medulla also innervates the nc. tractus solitarius as well as other parts of the dorsal vagal complex (20,104,161,191). It has been reported that there is a reciprocal projection from the nc. tractus solitarius towards the area of the A1 cells, but this connection seems to be almost exclusively nonnoradrenergic (20,161; cf. 141).

Several studies of interest for the further understanding of the anatomy of NE systems in the lower brainstem have appeared in which the HRP method was used without any attempt to identify the transmitter of the labeled cells. Thus, in the following quoted reports, the catecholaminergic nature of the connections remains to be established.

Injections of HRP into the spinal sensory trigeminal nucleus have been reported to label neurons in the ipsilateral A1 area and also some cells in contralateral A5 area (168). Similarly, HRP injected into the LC has been reported to label neurons in the A1, A2, A6, and A7 (30,32) areas. A projection from the A1 group to the LC nucleus is also supported by results obtained with anterograde tracers (161). Neurons in the A1 area are labeled after injection of retrograde tracers into the parabrachial nucleus (104). Finally, Sakai and co-workers (155) have found labeling in the A1 area after HRP injections into the dorsal raphe nucleus of the cat.

Hypothalamus

The CA innervation of the hypothalamus has been extensively studied, and for details on the distribution and arrangement of the NE axons in this region, the reader is referred to the reviews by Fuxe and Hökfelt (60), Björklund et al. (15), and Moore and Bloom (122). The relative distributions of the different NE afferent systems in the hypothalamic–preoptic region have been a matter of some controversy, mainly because of difficulties in the interpretation of lesion data. These problems have, however, been largely resolved with the introduction of the transmitter-specific retrograde tracing methods. Recent studies based on the use of such methods have established that the bulk of the NE innervation in hypothalamus and the preoptic region can be referred to the LT and DM systems, whereas the contribution of the LC, as mentioned above, is only minor. In the following, the current knowledge on the origins of the hypothalamic NE innervation is described with special emphasis on recent findings.

The NE innervation of the medial preoptic area seems to be derived almost exclusively from A1 and A2 cell groups (12,42,148,157), where most HRP-labeled cells were found on the ipsilateral side, but a substantial number also on the contralateral side. There is also some evidence for a minor contribution from LC (12). Previous lesion studies have indicated that A5 and A7 would contribute to the NE innervation of the medial preoptic area (134,175). On the basis of the HRP data of Day and co-workers (42), it seems likely, however, that the reported lesion effects were caused by transection of fibers ascending from the more caudally located A1 and A2 NE cell groups.

The paraventricular nucleus (PVH) is innervated both by the A1 (12,22,104,115,142,161,189) and A2 (12,22,104,148,161,189) NE cell groups and, in addition, receives a minor input from the LC (see above). According to the estimations of Sawchenko and Swanson (161), 68% of the labeled CA neurons are found in the A1, 26% in A2, and only 6% in LC after tracer injections into PVH. All of the brainstem projections to PVH are partially crossed. Based on results with the anterograde autoradiographic tracing technique, the A1 seems to project densely to those portions of the magnocellular divisions of the PVH in which vasopressin-containing cells are concentrated as well as to the

parvicellular part of the PVH (161; see also ref. 115). In the latter region, the A1 projection is mixed with that originating in A2, which distributes substantially to the periventricular, medial, and dorsal parts of the parvicellular division of the PVH but does not seem to innervate the magnocellular division (161).

The NE innervation in the supraoptic nucleus (SO) originates mainly in A1 (22,115,161), with less extensive contributions from A2 (161) and LC (see above). All projections to SO are partially crossed. Sawchenko and Swanson (161) have reported that following tracer injections into SO, 74% of labeled CA neurons were found in the A1, 15% in A2, and 11% in the LC. The A1 projection seems to be massive in those portions of the SO in which vasopressin-containing cells are concentrated (161).

In addition, there is now some evidence from tracer studies for A1 and A2 projections to the dorsomedial (12,148) and ventromedial (12) nuclei and to the anterior, lateral, and posterior hypothalamic areas (12,157). Using biochemical determinations of NE levels and electron microscopic identification of nerve terminal degeneration after lesions, Palkovits et al. (142) have obtained evidence that the NE afferents to the median eminence and the arcuate nucleus originate in the A1 and A2 cell groups. The projection to the arcuate nucleus from A2 is further supported by studies with both anterograde and retrograde tracers (148). In contrast, it has so far not been possible to label A1 and A2 neurons after injections of HRP into the median eminence (199).

Earlier fluorescence histochemical work has emphasized the pontine part of the LT system as a source for the hypothalamic NE innervation. It is remarkable, therefore, that in studies with retrograde tracers performed during recent years no labeling of A5 and A7 cells has been reported after injections into hypothalamic nuclei. It could be argued that possible hypothalamic projections from these cell groups take up the tracer less efficiently than the other NE systems. However, this seems unlikely since A5 and A7 cells innervating the spinal cord are easily labeled after tracer injections. At present, the most reasonable explanation is that the pontine part of the LT system contributes very few or no fibers to the NE innervations in the hypothalamus.

Thalamus, Septum, and Amygdala

In the thalamus, the LT and DM projections seem to be confined to the nc. paraventricularis, where they constitute the major part of the dense

NE innervation (100). The septal area receives a substantial noradrenergic input from the medullary part of the LT and DM systems (for details, see 101,120). The axons form a very dense innervation in the ventral part of the interstitial nucleus of the stria terminalis (see also 148), a moderately dense innervation in the nucleus of the diagonal band and lateral septal nucleus, and a sparse innervation in the medial septal nucleus, the septofimbrial nucleus, and the dorsal part of the interstitial nucleus of the stria terminalis. The NE fibers of nonlocus origin in the amygdala (for details, see 49) are concentrated in the central nucleus (see also ref. 202) but can also be found in the basolateral nucleus and scattered in the lateral nuclei and anterior amygdaloid area. Although no attempt was made to identify labeled cells as catecholaminergic, the recent HRP study of Ottersen (135) suggests that the nonlocus NE fibers in the amygdala originate in the medulla oblongata. Thus, A1 cells seem to project to the contralateral and A2 cells to the ipsilateral amygdala (see also 148).

CONCLUDING COMMENTS

The study of the chemically specified systems in the CNS has provided an entirely new viewpoint on the organization and function of the brain. The insights we have today into the anatomy, biochemistry, pharmacology, and physiology of the CA-containing neurons represent a unique combination of knowledge, making the CA neurons probably the best known single system in the mammalian CNS. Despite this, the continuous rapid development of CA research demonstrates that our knowledge is far from complete. In fact, it is only recently that we, thanks to the introduction of the transmitter-specific retrograde tracing methods in particular, have been able to start the attack on some of the central issues related to the exact topography and collateralization patterns of the DA- and NE-containing projection systems. This new knowledge brings us rapidly away from the earlier notion of the CA system as a diffuse, "nonspecific" component in the brain. Both the DA and NE neurons are obviously highly organized topographically. Each of the mesencephalic DA neurons appears to have a relatively restricted projection area in the forebrain, which provides at least a crude representation of the limbic and striatal forebrain in the mesencephalon. Likewise, in the LT NE system, each of the subcomponents seems to have a different projection area, suggesting a functional subdivision of the system. Even in the case of the richly collateralized NE neurons in the LC, it may be misleading to speak of a diffuse and "nonspecific" system. The anatomical organization of this nucleus may very well reflect a divergence principle whereby specific control functions are spread in an orderly fashion over wider areas of the forebrain, brainstem, or spinal cord. We are still only at the beginning of the understanding of the central CA neuron systems. Progress in chemical neuroanatomy will undoubtedly continue to play a central role in the future development of this exciting field of neuroscience.

ACKNOWLEDGMENTS

This work was supported by grants from the National Institutes of Health, the Swedish MRC, and the Magnus Bergvall Foundation.

REFERENCES

1. Adèr, J.-P., Postema, F., and Korf, J. (1979): Contribution of the locus coeruleus to the adrenergic innervation of the rat spinal cord: A biochemical study. *J. Neural Transm.*, 44:159–173.
2. Adèr, J.-P., Room, P., Postema, F., and Korf, J. (1980): Bilaterally diverging axon collaterals and contralateral projections from rat locus coeruleus neurons, demonstrated by fluorescent retrograde double labeling and norepinephrine metabolism. *J. Neural Transm.*, 49:207–218.
3. Amaral, D. G., and Sinnamon, H. M. (1977): The locus coeruleus: Neurobiology of a central noradrenergic nucleus. *Prog. Neurobiol.*, 9:147–196.
4. Andén, N.-E., Dahlström, A., Fuxe, K., Larsson, K., Olson, L., and Ungerstedt, U. (1966): Ascending monoamine neurons to the telencephalon and diencephalon. *Acta Physiol. Scand.*, 67:313–326.
5. Assaf, S. Y., and Miller, J. J. (1977): Excitatory action of the mesolimbic dopamine system on septal neurones. *Brain Res.*, 129:353–360.
6. Basbaum, A. I., and Fields, H. L. (1979): The origin of descending pathways in the dorsolateral funiculus of the spinal cord of the cat and rat: Further studies on the anatomy of pain modulation. *J. Comp. Neurol.*, 187:513–532.
7. Beckstead, R. M. (1976): Convergent thalamic and mesencephalic projections to the anterior medial cortex in the rat. *J. Comp. Neurol.*, 166:403–416.
8. Beckstead, R. M. (1978): Afferent connections of the entorhinal area in the rat as demonstrated by retrograde cell-labeling with horseradish peroxidase. *Brain Res.*, 152:249–264.
9. Beckstead, R. M., Domesick, V. B., and Nauta, W. J. H. (1979): Efferent connections of the substantia nigra and ventral tegmental area in the rat. *Brain Res.*, 175:191–217.
10. Berger, B., Nguyen-Legros, J., and Thierry, A. M. (1978): Demonstration of horseradish peroxidase and fluorescent catecholamines in the same neuron. *Neurosci. Lett.*, 9:297–302.

11. Berger, B., Tassin, J. P., Blanc, B., Moyne, M. A., and Thierry, A. M. (1974): Histochemical confirmation for dopaminergic innervation of the rat cerebral cortex after destruction of the noradrenergic ascending pathways. *Brain Res.*, 81:332–337.

12. Berk, M. L., and Finkelstein, J.A. (1981): Afferent projections to the preoptic area and hypothalamic regions in the rat brain. *Neuroscience*, 6:1601–1624.

13. Bischoff, S., Scatton, B., and Korf, J. (1979): Biochemical evidence for a transmitter role of dopamine in the rat hippocampus. *Brain Res.*, 165:161–165.

14. Björklund, A., Divac, I., and Lindvall, O. (1978): Regional distribution of catecholamines in monkey cerebral cortex, evidence for a dopaminergic innervation of the primate prefrontal cortex. *Neurosci. Lett.*, 7:115–119.

15. Björklund, A., Falck, B., Nobin, A., and Stenevi, U. (1974): Organization of the dopamine and noradrenaline innervations of the median eminence–pituitary region in the rat. In: *Neurosecretion—The Final Neuroendocrine Pathway, VIth International Symposium on Neurosecretion, London, 1973.* pp. 209–222. Springer-Verlag, Berlin, Heidelberg, New York.

16. Björklund, A., Segal, M., and Stenevi, U. (1979): Functional reinnervation of rat hippocampus by locus coeruleus implants. *Brain Res.*, 170:409–426.

17. Björklund, A., and Skagerberg, G. (1979): Evidence for a major spinal cord projection from the diencephalic A11 dopamine cell group in the rat using transmitter-specific fluorescent retrograde tracing. *Brain Res.*, 177:170–175.

18. Blackstad, T. W., Fuxe, K., and Hökfelt, T. (1967): Noradrenaline nerve terminals in the hippocampal region of the rat and the guinea pig. *Z. Zellforsch.*, 78:463–473.

19. Blessing, W. W., and Chalmers, J. P. (1979): Direct projection of catecholamine (presumably dopamine)-containing neurons from hypothalamus to spinal cord. *Neurosci. Lett.*, 11:35–40.

20. Blessing, W. W., Furness, J. B., Costa, M., West, M. J., and Chalmers, J. P. (1981): Projection of ventrolateral medullary (A1) catecholamine neurons toward nucleus tractus solitarii. *Cell Tissue Res.*, 220:27–40.

21. Blessing, W. W., Goodchild, A. K., Dampney, R. A. L., and Chalmers, J. P. (1981): Cell groups in the lower brain stem of the rabbit projecting to the spinal cord, with special reference to catecholamine-containing neurons. *Brain Res.*, 221:35–55.

22. Blessing, W. W., Jaeger, C. B., Ruggiero, D. A., and Reis, D. J. (1982): Hypothalamic projections of medullary catecholamine neurons in the rabbit: A combined catecholamine fluorescence and HRP transport study. *Brain Res. Bull.*, 9:279–286.

23. Bloom, F. E., and Battenberg, E. L. F. (1976): A rapid, simple and more sensitive method for the demonstration of central catecholamine-containing neurons and axons by glyoxylic acid induced fluorescence. II. A detailed description of methodology. *J. Histochem. Cytochem.*, 24:561–571.

24. Bloom, F. E., Hoffer, B. J., and Siggins, G. R.

(1971): Studies on norepinephrine-containing afferents to Purkinje cells of rat cerebellum. I. Localization of the fibers and their synapses. *Brain Res.*, 25:501–521.

25. Brown, J. T., Chan-Palay, V., and Palay, S. L. (1977): A study of afferent input to the inferior olivary complex in the rat by retrograde axonal transport of horseradish peroxidase. *J. Comp. Neurol.*, 176:1–22.

26. Brown, L. L., Makman, M. H., Wolfson, L. I., Dvorkin, B., Warner, C., and Katzman, R. (1979): A direct role of dopamine in the rat subthalamic nucleus and an adjacent intrapeduncular area. *Science*, 206:1416–1418.

27. Brown, L. L., and Wolfson, L. I. (1978): Apomorphine increases glucose utilization in the substantia nigra, subthalamic nucleus and corpus striatum of rat. *Brain Res.*, 140:188–193.

28. Carlsson, A., Falck, B., and Hillarp, N.-Å. (1962): Cellular localization of brain monoamines. *Acta Physiol. Scand. [Suppl.]*, 196:1–27.

29. Carter, D. A., and Fibiger, H. C. (1977): Ascending projections of presumed dopamine-containing neurons in the ventral tegmentum of the rat as demonstrated by horseradish peroxidase. *Neuroscience*, 2:569–576.

30. Cedarbaum, J. M., and Aghajanian, G. K. (1978): Afferent projections to the rat locus coeruleus as determined by a retrograde tracing technique. *J. Comp. Neurol.*, 178:1–16.

31. Chu, N.-S., and Bloom, F. E. (1974): The catecholamine-containing neurons in the cat dorsolateral pontine tegmentum: Distribution of the cell bodies and some axonal projections. *Brain Res.*, 66:1–21.

32. Clavier, R. M. (1979): Afferent projections to the self-stimulation regions of the dorsal pons, including the locus coeruleus, in the rat as demonstrated by the horseradish peroxidase technique. *Brain Res. Bull.*, 4:497–504.

33. Collier, T. J., and Routtenberg, A. (1976): Entorhinal cortex: Catecholamine fluorescence and Nissl staining of identical sections. *Neurosci. Abstr.*, 2:43.

34. Commissiong, J. W. (1981): Evidence that the noradrenergic coerulospinal projection decussates at the spinal level. *Brain Res.*, 212:145–151.

35. Commissiong, J. W., Galli, C. L., and Neff, N. H. (1978): Differentiation of dopaminergic and noradrenergic neurons in rat spinal cord. *J. Neurochem.*, 30:1095–1099.

36. Commissiong, J. W., Gentleman, S., and Neff, N. H. (1979): Spinal cord dopaminergic neurons: Evidence for an uncrossed nigrospinal pathway. *Neuropharmacology*, 18:565–568.

37. Commissiong, J. W., Hellström, S. O., and Neff, N. H. (1978): A new projection from locus coeruleus to the spinal ventral columns: Histochemical and biochemical evidence. *Brain Res.*, 148:297–213.

38. Commissiong, J. W., and Neff, N. H. (1979): Current status of dopamine in the mammalian spinal cord. *Biochem. Pharmacol.*, 28:1569–1573.

39. Dahlström, A., and Fuxe, K. (1964): Evidence for the existence of monoamine-containing neurons in

the central nervous system. I. Demonstration of monoamines in the cell bodies of brain stem neurones. *Acta Physiol. Scand.* [*Suppl.*], 232:1–55.

40. Dahlström, A., and Fuxe, K. (1965): Evidence for the existence of monoamine neurons in the central nervous system. II. Experimentally induced changes in the intraneuronal amine levels of bulbospinal neuron systems. *Acta Physiol. Scand.* [*Suppl.*], 247:1–36.

41. Dahlström, A., Fuxe, K., Olson, L., and Ungerstedt, U. (1965): On the distribution and possible function of monoamine nerve terminals in the olfactory bulb of the rabbit. *Life Sci.*, 4:2071–2074.

42. Day, T. A., Blessing, W., and Willoughby, J. O. (1980): Noradrenergic and dopaminergic projections to the medial preoptic area of the rat. A combined horseradish peroxidase/catecholamine fluorescence study. *Brain Res.*, 193:543–548.

43. Deniau, J. M., Thierry, A. M., and Feger, J. (1980): Electrophysiological identification of mesencephalic ventromedial tegmental (VMT) neurons projecting to the frontal cortex, septum and nucleus accumbens. *Brain Res.*, 189:315–326.

44. de Olmos, J., Hardy, H., and Heimer, L. (1978): The afferent connections of the main and the accessory olfactory bulb formations in the rat: An experimental HRP study. *J. Comp. Neurol.*, 181:213–244.

45. Domesick, V. B., Beckstead, R. M., and Nauta, W. J. H. (1976): Some ascending and descending projections of the substantia nigra and ventral tegmental area in the rat. *Neurosci. Abstr.*, II:61.

46. Emson, P. C., Björklund, A., Lindvall, O., and Paxinos, G. (1979): Contributions of different afferent pathways to the catecholamine and 5-hydroxytryptamine-innervation of the amygdala: A neurochemical and histochemical study. *Neuroscience*, 4:1347–1357.

47. Emson, P. C., and Koob, G. F. (1978): The origin and distribution of dopamine-containing afferents to the rat frontal cortex. *Brain Res.*, 142:249–267.

48. Faiers, A. A., and Mogenson, G. J. (1976): Electrophysiological identification of neurons in the locus coeruleus. *Exp. Neurol.*, 53:254–266.

49. Fallon, J. H., Koziell, D. A., and Moore, R. Y. (1978): Catecholamine innervation of the basal forebrain. II. Amygdala, suprarhinal cortex and entorhinal cortex. *J. Comp. Neurol.*, 180:509–532.

50. Fallon, J. H., and Loughlin, S. E. (1982): Monoamine innervation of the forebrain: Collateralization. *Brain Res. Bull.*, 9:295–307.

51. Fallon, J. H., and Moore, R. Y. (1978): Catecholamine innervation of the basal forebrain. III. Olfactory bulb, anterior olfactory nuclei, olfactory tubercle and piriform cortex. *J. Comp. Neurol.*, 180:533–544.

52. Fallon, J. H., and Moore, R. Y. (1978): Catecholamine innervation of the basal forebrain. IV. Topography of the dopamine projection to the basal forebrain and neostriatum. *J. Comp. Neurol.*, 180:545–580.

53. Fallon, J. H., Riley, J. N., and Moore, R. Y. (1978): Substantia nigra dopamine neurons: Separate populations project to neostriatum and allocortex. *Neurosci. Lett.*, 7:157–162.

54. Fallon, J. H., Riley, J. N., Sipe, J. C., and Moore, R. Y. (1978): The islands of Calleja: Organization and connections. *J. Comp. Neurol.*, 181:375–396.

55. Fass, B., and Butcher, L. L. (1981): Evidence for a crossed nigrostriatal pathway in rats. *Neurosci. Lett.*, 22:109–113.

56. Fibiger, H. C., Pudritz, R. E., McGeer, P. L., and McGeer, E. G. (1972): Axonal transport in nigrostriatal and nigrothalamic neurons: Effects of medial forebrain bundle lesions and 6-hydroxydopamine. *J. Neurochem.*, 19:1697–1708.

57. Fleetwood-Walker, S. M., and Coote, J. H. (1981): The contribution of brain stem catecholamine cell groups to the innervation of the sympathetic lateral cell column. *Brain Res.*, 205:141–155.

58. Fleetwood-Walker, S. M., and Coote, J. H. (1981): Contribution of noradrenaline-, dopamine-, and adrenaline-containing axons to the innervation of different regions of the spinal cord of the cat. *Brain Res.*, 206:95–106.

59. Fuxe, K. (1965): Evidence for the existence of monoamine neurons in the central nervous system. IV. Distribution of monoamine nerve terminals in the central nervous system. *Acta Physiol. Scand.* [*Suppl.*], 247:39–85.

60. Fuxe, K., and Hökfelt, T. (1969): Catecholamines in the hypothalamus and the pituitary gland. In: *Frontiers in Neuroendocrinology,* edited by W. F. Ganong and L. Martini, pp. 47–96. Oxford University Press, London.

61. Fuxe, K., Hökfelt, T., Johansson, O., Jonsson, G., Lidbrink, P., and Ljungdahl, Å. (1974): The origin of the dopamine nerve terminals in limbic and frontal cortex. Evidence for mesocortico dopamine neurons. *Brain Res.*, 82:349–355.

62. Fuxe, K., Hökfelt, T., and Ungerstedt, U. (1969): Distribution of monoamines in the mammalian central nervous system by histochemical studies. In: *Metabolism of Amines in the Brain,* edited by G. Hooper, pp. 10–22. Macmillan, London.

63. Gage, F. H., Björklund, A., and Stenevi, U. (1983): Reinnervation of the partially deafferented hippocampus by compensatory collateral sprouting from spared cholinergic and adrenergic afferents. *Brain Res. (in press).*

64. Gerfen, C. R., and Clavier, R. M. (1979): Neural inputs to the prefrontal agranular insular cortex in the rat: Horseradish peroxidase study. *Brain Res. Bull.*, 4:347–353.

65. Guyenet, P. G. (1980): The coeruleospinal noradrenergic neurons: Anatomical and electrophysiological studies in the rat. *Brain Res.*, 189:121–133.

66. Guyenet, P. G., and Aghajanian, G. K. (1978): Antidromic identification of dopaminergic and other output neurons of the rat substantia nigra. *Brain Res.*, 150:69–84.

67. Guyenet, P. G., and Crane, J. K. (1981): Non-dopaminergic nigrostriatal pathway. *Brain Res.*, 213:291–305.

68. Halász, N., Ljungdahl, Å., Hökfelt, T., Johansson, O., Goldstein, M., Park, D., and Biberfeld, P.

(1977): Transmitter-histochemistry of the rat olfactory bulb. I. Immunohistochemical localization of monoamine synthesizing enzymes: Support for intrabulbar, periglomerular dopamine neurons. *Brain Res.,* 126:455–474.

69. Hedreen, J. (1980): Terminal degeneration demonstrated by the Fink–Heimer method following lateral ventricular injection of 6-hydroxydopamine. *Brain Res. Bull.,* 5:425–463.

70. Hedreen, J. C., and Chalmers, J. P. (1972): Neuronal degeneration in rat brain induced by 6-hydroxydopamine: A histological and biochemical study. *Brain Res.,* 47:1–36.

71. Herkenham, M., and Nauta, W. J. H. (1977): Afferent connections of the habenular nuclei in the rat. A horseradish peroxidase study, with a note on the fiber-of-passage problem. *J. Comp. Neurol.,* 173:123–146.

72. Hökfelt, T., and Fuxe, K. (1969): Cerebellar monoamine nerve terminals, a new type of afferent fibers to the cortex cerebelli. *Exp. Brain Res.,* 9:63–72.

73. Hökfelt, T., Fuxe, K., Johansson, O., and Ljungdahl, Å. (1974): Pharmacohistochemical evidence of the existence of dopamine nerve terminals in the limbic cortex. *Eur. J. Pharmacol.,* 25:108–112.

74. Hökfelt, T., Johansson, O., Fuxe, K., Goldstein, M., and Park, D. (1976): Immunohistochemical studies on the localization and distribution of monoamine neuron systems in the rat brain. I. Tyrosine hydroxylase in the mes- and diencephalon. *Med. Biol.,* 54:427–453.

75. Hökfelt, T., Johansson, O., Fuxe, K., Goldstein, M., and Park, D. (1977): Immunohistochemical studies on the localization and distribution of monoamine neuron systems in the rat brain. II. Tyrosine hydroxylase in the telencephalon. *Med. Biol.,* 55:21–40.

76. Hökfelt, T., Ljungdahl, Å., Fuxe, K., and Johansson, O. (1974): Dopamine nerve terminals in the rat limbic cortex: Aspects of the dopamine hypothesis of schizophrenia. *Science,* 184:177–179.

77. Hökfelt, T., Phillipson, O., and Goldstein, M. (1979): Evidence for a dopaminergic pathway in the rat descending from the A11 cell group to the spinal cord. *Acta Physiol. Scand.,* 107:393–395.

78. Ishikawa, K., Ott, T., and McGaugh, J. L. (1982): Evidence for dopamine as a transmitter in dorsal hippocampus. *Brain Res.,* 232:222–226.

79. Jacobowitz, D. M. (1973): Effects of 6-hydroxydopa. In: *Frontiers in Catecholamine Research,* edited by E. Usdin and S. Snyder, pp. 729–739. Pergamon Press, Oxford.

80. Jones, B. E., Halaris, A. E., McIlhany, M., and Moore, R. Y. (1977): Ascending projections of the locus coeruleus in the rat. I. Axonal transport in central noradrenaline neurons. *Brain Res.,* 127:1–21.

81. Jones, B. E., and Moore, R. Y. (1977): Ascending projections of the locus coeruleus in the rat. II. Autoradiographic study. *Brain Res.,* 127:23–53.

82. Kaelber, W. W., and Afifi, A. K. (1977): Nigroamygdaloid fiber connections in the cat. *Am. J. Anat.,* 148:129–135.

83. Karoum, F., Commissiong, J. W., Neff, N. F., and Wyatt, R. J. (1980): Biochemical evidence for uncrossed and crossed locus coeruleus projections to the spinal cord. *Brain Res.,* 196:237–241.

84. Kizer, J. S., Palkovits, M., and Brownstein, M. J. (1976): The projections of the A8, A9, A10 dopaminergic cell bodies: Evidence for a nigral–hypothalamic–median eminence dopaminergic pathway. *Brain Res.,* 108:363–370.

85. Kobayashi, R. M., Palkovits, M., Kopin, I. J., and Jacobowitz, D. M. (1974): Biochemical mapping of noradrenergic nerves arising from the rat locus coeruleus. *Brain Res.,* 77:269–279.

86. Kromer, L. F., and Moore, R. Y. (1976): Cochlear nucleus innervation by central norepinephrine neurons in the rat. *Brain Res.,* 118:531–537.

87. Kromer, L. F., and Moore, R. Y. (1980): Norepinephrine innervation of the cochlear nuclei by locus coeruleus neurons in the rat. *Anat. Embryol.,* 158:227–244.

88. Kuypers, H. G. J. M., and Maisky, V. A. (1975): Retrograde axonal transport of horseradish peroxidase from spinal cord to brain stem cell groups in the cat. *Neurosci. Lett.,* 1:9–14.

89. Landis, S., Shoemaker, W. J., Bloom, F. E., and Schlumpf, M. (1975): Catecholamines in mutant mouse cerebellum. Fluorescence microscopic and chemical studies. *Brain Res.,* 93:253–266.

90. Levitt, P., and Moore, R. Y. (1978): Noradrenaline neuron innervation of the neocortex in the rat. *Brain Res.,* 139:219–231.

91. Levitt, P., and Moore, R. Y. (1979): Origin and organization of brainstem catecholamine innervation in the rat. *J. Comp. Neurol.* 186:505–528.

92. Lindvall, O. (1975): Mesencephalic dopaminergic afferents to the lateral septal nucleus of the rat. *Brain Res.,* 87:89–95.

93. Lindvall, O., and Björklund, A. (1974): The organization of the ascending catecholamine neuron systems in the rat brain as revealed by the glyoxylic acid fluorescence method. *Acta Physiol. Scand.* [*Suppl.*], 412:1–48.

94. Lindvall, O., and Björklund, A. (1978): Organization of catecholamine neurons in the rat central nervous system. In: *Handbook of Psychopharmacology,* Vol. 9, edited by L. L. Iversen, S. D. Iversen, and S. H. Snyder, pp. 139–231. Plenum Press, New York.

95. Lindvall, O., and Björklund, A. (1978): Anatomy of the dopaminergic neuron systems in the rat brain. *Adv. Biochem. Psychopharmacol.,* 19:1–23.

96. Lindvall, O., and Björklund, A. (1979): Dopaminergic innervation of the globus pallidus by collaterals from the nigrostriatal pathway. *Brain Res.,* 172:169–173.

97. Lindvall, O., Björklund, A., and Divac, I. (1977): Organization of mesencephalic dopamine neurons projecting to neocortex and septum. *Adv. Biochem. Psychopharmacol.,* 16:39–46.

98. Lindvall, O., Björklund, A., and Divac, I. (1978): Organization of catecholamine neurons projecting to the frontal cortex in the rat. *Brain Res.,* 142:1–24.

99. Lindvall, O., Björklund, A., Moore, R. Y., and Stenevi, U. (1974): Mesencephalic dopamine neurons projecting to neocortex. *Brain Res.*, 81:325–331.

100. Lindvall, O., Björklund, A., Nobin, A., and Stenevi, U. (1974): The adrenergic innervation of the rat thalamus as revealed by the glyoxylic acid fluorescence method. *J. Comp. Neurol.*, 154:317–348.

101. Lindvall, O., and Stenevi, U. (1978): Dopamine and noradrenaline neurons projecting to the septal area in the rat. *Cell Tissue Res.*, 190:383–407.

102. Ljungdahl, Å., Hökfelt, T., Goldstein, M., and Park, D. (1975): Retrograde peroxidase tracing of neurons combined with transmitter histochemistry. *Brain Res.*, 84:313–319.

103. Loewy, A. D., McKellar, S., and Saper, C. B. (1979): Direct projections from the A5 catecholamine cell group to the intermediolateral cell column. *Brain Res.*, 174:309–314.

104. Loewy, A. D., Wallach, J. H., and McKellar, S. (1981): Efferent connections of the ventral medulla oblongata in the rat. *Brain Res. Rev.*, 3:63–80.

105. Loizou, L. A. (1969): Projections of the nucleus locus coeruleus in the albino rat. *Brain Res.*, 15:563–566.

106. Loughlin, S. E., Foote, S. L., and Fallon, J. H. (1982): Locus coeruleus projections to cortex: Topography, morphology, and collateralization. *Brain Res. Bull.*, 9:287–294.

107. Loy, R., Koziell, D. A., Lindsey, J. D., and Moore, R. Y. (1980): Noradrenergic innervation of the adult rat hippocampal formation. *J. Comp. Neurol.*, 189:699–710.

108. Maeda, T., and Shimizu, N. (1972): Projections ascendantes du locus coeruleus et d'autres neurones aminergiques pontiques au niveau du prosencéphale de rat. *Brain Res.*, 36:19–35.

109. Magnusson, T. (1973): Effect of chronic transection on dopamine, noradrenaline and 5-hydroxytryptamine in the rat spinal cord. *Naunyn Schmiedebergs Arch. Pharmacol.*, 278:13–22.

110. Marchand, E. R., Riley, J. N., and Moore, R. Y. (1980): Interpeduncular nucleus afferents in the rat. *Brain Res.*, 193:339–352.

111. Markowitsch, H. J., and Irle, E. (1981): Widespread cortical projections of the ventral tegmental area and of other brain stem structures in the cat. *Exp. Brain Res.*, 41:233–246.

112. Mason, S. T., and Fibiger, H. C. (1979): Regional topography within noradrenergic locus coeruleus as revealed by retrograde transport of horseradish peroxidase. *J. Comp. Neurol.*, 187:703–724.

113. McCulloch, J., Savaki, H. E., and Sokoloff, L. (1980): Influence of dopaminergic systems on the lateral habenular nucleus of the rat. *Brain Res.*, 194:117–124.

114. McKellar, S., and Loewy, A. D. (1979): Spinal projections of norepinephrine-containing neurons in the rat. *Soc. Neurosci. Abstr.*, 5:344.

115. McKellar, S., and Loewy, A. D. (1981): Organization of some brain stem afferents to the paraventricular nucleus of the hypothalamus in the rat. *Brain Res.*, 217:351–357.

116. Meibach, R. C., and Katzman, R. (1979): Cate-cholaminergic innervation of the subthalamic nucleus: Evidence for a rostral continuation of the A9 (substantia nigra) dopaminergic cell group. *Brain Res.*, 173:364–368.

117. Meibach, R. C., and Katzman, R. (1981): Origin, course and termination of dopaminergic substantia nigra neurons projecting to the amygdaloid complex in the cat. *Neuroscience*, 6:2159–2171.

118. Moore, R. Y. (1973): Telencephalic distribution of terminals of brainstem norepinephrine neurons. In: *Frontiers in Catecholamine Research*, edited by E. Usdin and S. H. Snyder, pp. 767–769. Pergamon Press, New York.

119. Moore, R. Y. (1975): Monoamine neurons innervating the hippocampal formation and septum: Organization and response to injury. In: *The Hippocampus*, Vol. 1, edited by L. Isaacson and K. H. Pribam, pp. 215–237. Plenum Press, New York.

120. Moore, R. Y. (1978): Catecholamine innervation of the basal forebrain. I. The septal area. *J. Comp. Neurol.*, 177:665–684.

121. Moore, R. Y., and Bloom, F. E. (1978): Central catecholamine neuron systems: Anatomy and physiology of the dopamine systems. *Annu. Rev. Neurosci.*, 1:129–169.

122. Moore, R. Y., and Bloom, F. E. (1979): Central catecholamine neuron systems: Anatomy and physiology of the norepinephrine and epinephrine systems. *Annu. Rev. Neurosci.* 2:113–168.

123. Morrison, J. H., Grzanna, R., Molliver, M. E., and Coyle, J. T. (1978): The distribution and orientation of noradrenergic fibers in neocortex of the rat: An immunofluorescence study. *J. Comp. Neurol.* 181:17–40.

124. Morrison, J. H., Molliver, M. E., Grzanna, R., and Coyle, J. T. (1979): Noradrenergic innervation patterns in three regions of medial cortex: An immunofluorescence characterization. *Brain Res. Bull.*, 4:849–857.

125. Morrison, J. H., Molliver, M. E., Grzanna, R., and Coyle, J. T. (1981): The intra-cortical trajectory of the coeruleo-cortical projection in the rat: A tangentially organized cortical afferent. *Neuroscience*, 6:139–158.

126. Mugnaini, E., and Dahl, A.-L. (1975): Mode of distribution of aminergic fibers in the cerebellar cortex of the chicken. *J. Comp. Neurol.*, 162:417–432.

127. Nagai, T., Satoh, K., Imamoto, K., and Maeda, T. (1981): Divergent projections of catecholamine neurons of the locus coeruleus as revealed by fluorescent retrograde double labeling technique. *Neurosci. Lett.*, 23:117–123.

128. Nagatsu, I., Inagaki, S., Kondo, Y., Karasawa, N., and Nagatsu, T. (1979): Immunofluorescent studies on the localization of tyrosine hydroxlyase and dopamine-β-hydroxylase in the mes-, di-, and telencephalon of the rat using unperfused fresh frozen sections. *Acta Histochem. Cytochem.*, 12:20–37.

129. Nauta, W. J. H., Smith, G. P., Faull, R. L. M., and Domesick, V. B. (1978): Efferent connections and nigral afferents of the nucleus accumbens septi in the rat. *Neuroscience*, 3:385–401.

130. Nobin, A., and Björklund, A. (1973): Topography

of the monoamine neuron systems in the human brain as revealed in fetuses. *Acta Physiol. Scand.* [*Suppl.*], 388:1–40.

131. Nygren, L.-G., and Olson, L. (1977): A new major projection from locus coeruleus: The main source of noradrenergic nerve terminals in the ventral and dorsal columns of the spinal cord. *Brain Res.*, 132:85–93.

132. Ochi, J., and Shimizu, K. (1978): Occurrence of dopamine-containing neurons in the midbrain raphe nuclei of the rat. *Neurosci. Lett.*, 8:317–320.

133. Olson, L., and Fuxe, K. (1971): On the projections from the locus coeruleus noradrenaline neurons: The cerebellar innervation. *Brain Res.*, 28:165–171.

134. Olson, L., and Fuxe, K. (1972): Further mapping out of central noradrenaline neuron systems: Projections of the "subcoeruleus" area. *Brain Res.*, 43:289–295.

135. Ottersen, O. P. (1981): Afferent connections to the amygdaloid complex of the rat with some observations in the cat. III. Afferents from the lower brain stem. *J. Comp. Neurol.*, 202:335–356.

136. Ottersen, O. P., and Ben-Ari, Y. (1978): Pontine and mesencephalic afferents to the central nucleus of the amygdala of the rat. *Neurosci. Lett.*, 8:329–334.

137. Palkovits, M., de Jong, W., Zandberg, P., Versteeg, D. H. G., van der Gugten, J., and Léránth, C. (1977): Central hypertension and nucleus tractus solitarii catecholamines after surgical lesions in the medulla oblongata of the rat. *Brain Res.*, 127:307–312.

138. Palkovits, M., Fekete, M., Makara, G. B., and Herman, J. P. (1977): Total and partial hypothalamic deafferentations for topographical identification of catecholaminergic innervations of certain preoptic and hypothalamic nuclei. *Brain Res.*, 127:127–136.

139. Palkovits, M., and Jacobowitz, D. M. (1974): Topographic atlas of catecholamine and acetylcholinesterase-containing neurons in the rat brain. II. Hindbrain (mesencephalon, rhombencephalon). *J. Comp. Neurol.*, 157:29–42.

140. Palkovits, M., Léranth, C., Záborszky, L., and Brownstein, M. J. (1977): Electron microscopic evidence of direct neuronal connections from the lower brain stem to the median eminence. *Brain Res.*, 136:339–344.

141. Palkovits, M., and Záborszky, L. (1977): Neuroanatomy of central cardiovascular control. Nucleus tractus solitarius: Afferent and efferent neuronal connections in relation to the baroreceptor reflex arc. *Prog. Brain Res.*, 47:9–34.

142. Palkovits, M., Záborszky, L., Feminger, A., Mezey, E., Fekete, M. I. K., Herman, J. P., Kanyicska, B., and Szabó, D. (1980): Noradrenergic innervation of the rat hypothalamus: Experimental biochemical and electron microscopic studies. *Brain Res.*, 191:161–171.

143. Parent, A., Gravel, S., and Boucher, R. (1981): The origin of forebrain afferents to the habenula in rat, cat and monkey. *Brain Res. Bull.*, 6:23–38.

144. Pasquier, D. A., Gold, M. A., and Jacobowitz, D.

M. (1980): Noradrenergic perikarya (A5–A7, subcoeruleus) projections to the rat cerebellum. *Brain Res.*, 196:270–275.

145. Pasquier, D. A., and Reinoso-Suarez, F. (1978): The topographic organization of hypothalamic and brain stem projections to the hippocampus. *Brain Res. Bull.*, 3:373–389.

146. Phillipson, O. T., and Griffith, A. C. (1980): The neurones of origin for the mesohabenular dopamine pathway. *Brain Res.*, 197:213–218.

147. Pickel, V. M., Segal, M., and Bloom, F. E. (1974): A radioautographic study of the efferent pathways of the nucleus locus coeruleus. *J. Comp. Neurol.*, 155:15–42.

148. Ricardo, J. A., and Koh, E. T. (1978): Anatomical evidence of direct projections from the nucleus of the solitary tract to the hypothalamus, amygdala, and other forebrain structures in the rat. *Brain Res.*, 153:1–26.

149. Riley, J. N., and Moore, R. Y. (1981): Diencephalic and brainstem afferents to the hippocampal formation of the rat. *Brain Res. Bull.*, 6:437–444.

150. Room, P., Postema, F., and Korf, J. (1981): Divergent axon collaterals of rat locus coeruleus neurons: Demonstration by a fluorescent double labeling technique. *Brain Res.*, 221:219–230.

151. Ross, R. A., and Reis, D. J. (1974): Effects of lesions of locus coeruleus on regional distribution of dopamine-beta-hydroxylase activity in rat brain. *Brain Res.*, 73:161–166.

152. Royce, G. J. (1978): Cells of origin of subcortical afferents to the caudate nucleus: A horseradish peroxidase study in the cat. *Brain Res.*, 153:465–475.

153. Saavedra, J. M., Setler, P. E., and Kebabian, J. W. (1978): Biochemical changes accompanying unilateral 6-hydroxydopamine lesions in the rat substantia nigra. *Brain Res.*, 151:339–352.

154. Sachs, C., Jönsson, G., and Fuxe, K. (1973): Mapping of central noradrenaline pathways with 6-hydroxy-dopa. *Brain Res.*, 63:249–261.

155. Sakai, K., Salvert, D., Touret, M., and Jouvet, M. (1977): Afferent connections of the nucleus raphe dorsalis in the cat as visualized by the horseradish peroxidase technique. *Brain Res.*, 137:11–35.

156. Sakai, K., Touret, M., Salvert, D., Leger, L., and Jouvet, M. (1977): Afferent projections to the cat locus coeruleus as visualized by the horseradish peroxidase technique. *Brain Res.*, 119:21–41.

157. Sakumoto, T., Tohyama, M., Satoh, K., Kimoto, Y., Kinugasa, T., Tanizawa, O., Kurachi, K., and Shimizu, N. (1978): Afferent fiber connections from lower brain stem to hypothalamus studied by the horseradish peroxidase method with special reference to noradrenaline innervation. *Exp. Brain Res.*, 31:81–94.

158. Sapawi, R. R., and Divac, I. (1979): Absence of evidence for the nigro–cerebellar projection in the rat. *Neurosci. Lett.* [*Suppl.*], 3:S234.

159. Satoh, K. (1979): The origin of reticulospinal fibers in the rat: A HRP study. *J. Hirnforsch.*, 20:313–332.

160. Satoh, K., Tohyama, M., Yamamoto, K., Sakumoto, T., and Shimizu, N. (1977): Noradrenaline

innervation of the spinal cord studied by the horse-radish peroxidase method combined with mono-amine oxidase staining. *Exp. Brain Res., 30*:175–186.

161. Sawchenko, P. E., and Swanson, L. W. (1981): Central noradrenergic pathways for the integration of hypothalamic neuroendocrine and autonomic responses. *Science, 214*:685–687.

162. Scatton, B., Simon, H., Le Moal, M., and Bischoff, S. (1980): Origin of dopaminergic innervation of the rat hippocampal formation. *Neurosci. Lett., 18*:125–131.

163. Schwab, M. E., Javoy-Agid, F., and Agid, Y. (1978): Labeled wheat germ agglutinin (WGA) as a new, highly sensitive retrograde tracer in the rat brain hippocampal system. *Brain Res., 152*:145–150.

164. Segal, M., and Landis, S. C. (1974): Afferents to the hippocampus of the rat studied with the method of retrograde transport of horseradish peroxidase. *Brain Res., 78*:1–15.

165. Segal, M., and Landis, S. C. (1974): Afferents to the septal area of the rat studied with the method of retrograde axonal transport of horseradish peroxidase. *Brain Res., 82*:263–268.

166. Segal, M., Pickel, V., and Bloom, F. (1973): The projections of the nucleus locus coeruleus: An autoradiographic study. *Life Sci., 13*:817–821.

167. Seiger, Å., and Olson, L. (1973): Late prenatal ontogeny of central monoamine neurons in the rat: Fluorescence histochemical observations. *Z. Anat. Entwickl. Gesch., 140*:281–318.

168. Senba, E., Tohyama, M., Shiosaka, S., Takagi, H., Sakanaka, M., Matsuzaki, T., Takahashi, Y., and Shimizu, N. (1981): Experimental and morphological studies of the noradrenaline innervations in the nucleus tractus spinalis nervi trigemini of the rat with special reference to their fine structures. *Brain Res., 206*:39–50.

169. Simon, H., and Le Moal, M. (1977): Demonstration by the Fink–Heimer impregnating method of a ventral mesencephalic–locus coeruleus projection in the rat. *Experientia., 33*:614–616.

170. Simon, H., Le Moal, M., Galey, D., and Cardo, B. (1976): Silver impregnation of dopaminergic systems after radiofrequency and 6-OHDA lesions of the rat ventral tegmentum. *Brain Res., 115*:215–231.

171. Simon, H., Le Moal, M., and Calas, A. (1979): Efferents and afferents of the ventral tegmental–A10 region studied after local injection of (^{3}H)leucine and horseradish peroxidase. *Brain Res., 178*:17–40.

172. Simon, H., Le Moal, M., Stinus, L., and Calas, A. (1979): Anatomical relationships between the ventral mesencephalic tegmentum–A10 region and the locus coeruleus as demonstrated by anterograde and retrograde tracing techniques. *J. Neural Trans., 44*:77–86.

173. Skagerberg, G., Björklund, A., Lindvall, O., and Schmidt, R. H. (1982): Origin and termination of the diencephalo–spinal dopamine system in the rat. *Brain Res. Bull., 9*:237–244.

174. Smolen, A. J., Glazer, E. J., and Ross, L. L. (1979): Horseradish peroxidase histochemistry combined with glyoxylic acid-induced fluorescence used to identify brain stem catecholaminergic neurons which project to the chick thoracic spinal cord. *Brain Res., 160*:353–357.

175. Speciale, S. G., Crowley, W. R., O'Donohue, T. L., and Jacobowitz, D. M. (1978): Forebrain catecholamine projections of the A5 cell group. *Brain Res., 154*:128–133.

176. Steindler, D. A. (1981): Locus coeruleus neurons have axons that branch to the forebrain and cerebellum. *Brain Res., 223*:367–373.

177. Steindler, D. A., and Deniau, J. M. (1980): Anatomical evidence for collateral branching of substantia nigra neurons: A combined horseradish peroxidase and (^{3}H)wheat germ agglutinin axonal transport study in the rat. *Brain Res., 196*:228–236.

178. Storm-Mathisen, J., and Guldberg, H. C. (1974): 5-Hydroxytryptamine and noradrenaline in the hippocampal region: Effect of transection of afferent pathways on endogenous levels, high affinity uptake and some transmitter-related enzymes. *J. Neurochem., 22*:793–803.

179. Swanson, L. W. (1976): The locus coeruleus: A cytoarchitectonic, Golgi and immunohistochemical study in the albino rat. *Brain Res., 110*:39–56.

180. Swanson, L. W. (1982): The projections of the ventral tegmental area and adjacent regions: A combined fluorescent retrograde tracer and immunofluorescence study in the rat. *Brain Res. Bull., 9*:321–353.

181. Swanson, L. W., and Hartman, B. K. (1975): The central adrenergic system. An immunofluorescence study of the location of cell bodies and their efferent connections in the rat utilizing dopamine-β-hydroxylase as a marker. *J. Comp. Neurol., 163*:467–506.

182. Swanson, L. W., Sawchenko, P. E., Bérod, A., Hartman, B. K., Helle, K. B., and Vanorden, D. E. (1981): An immunohistochemical study of the organization of catecholaminergic cells and terminal fields in the paraventricular and supraoptic nuclei of the hypothalamus. *J. Comp. Neurol., 196*:271–285.

183. Szabo, J. (1980): Distribution of striatal afferents from the mesencephalon in the cat. *Brain Res., 188*:3–21.

184. Takahashi, Y., Satoh, K., Sakumoto, T., Tohyama, M., and Shimizu, N. (1979): A major source of catecholamine terminals in the nucleus tractus solitarii. *Brain Res., 172*:372–377.

185. Tassin, J. P., Chéramy, A., Blanc, G., Thierry, A. M., and Glowinski, J. (1976): Topographical distribution of dopaminergic innervation and of dopaminergic receptors in the rat striatum. I. Microestimation of (^{3}H)dopamine uptake and dopamine content in microdiscs. *Brain Res., 107*:291–301.

186. Thierry, A. M., Deniau, J. M., Herve, D., and Chevalier, G. (1980): Electrophysiological evidence for non-dopaminergic mesocortical and mesolimbic neurons in the rat. *Brain Res., 201*:210–214.

187. Tohyama, M. (1976): Comparative anatomy of cerebellar catecholamine innervation from teleosts to mammals. *J. Hirnforsch., 17*:43–60.

188. Tohyama, M., Maeda, T., and Shimizu, N. (1974): Detailed noradrenaline pathways of locus coeruleus neuron to the cerebral cortex with use of 6-hydroxydopa. *Brain Res.,* 79:139–144.

189. Tribollet, E., and Dreifuss, J. J. (1981): Localization of neurones projecting to the hypothalamic paraventricular nucleus area of the rat: A horseradish peroxidase study. *Neuroscience,* 7:1315–1328.

190. Törk, I., and Turner, S. (1981): Histochemical evidence for a catecholaminergic (presumably dopaminergic) projection from the ventral mesencephalic tegmentum to visual cortex in the cat. *Neurosci. Lett.,* 24:215–219.

191. Ungerstedt, U. (1971): Stereotaxic mapping of the monoamine pathways in the rat brain. *Acta Physiol. Scand. [Suppl.],* 367:1–48.

192. Van der Kooy, D. (1979): The organization of the thalamic, nigral and raphe cells projecting to the medial vs lateral caudate–putamen in rat. A fluorescent retrograde double labeling study. *Brain Res.,* 169:381–387.

193. Van der Kooy, D., Coscina, D. V., and Hattori, T. (1981): Is there a nondopaminergic nigrostriatal pathway? *Neuroscience,* 6:345–357.

194. Van der Kooy, D., and Wise, R. A. (1980): Retrograde fluorescent tracing of substantia nigra neurons combined with catecholamine histofluorescence. *Brain Res.,* 183:447–452.

195. Veening, J. G., Cornelissen, F. M., and Lieven, P. A. J. M. (1980): The topical organization of the afferents to the caudatoputamen of the rat. A horseradish peroxidase study. *Neuroscience,* 5:1253–1268.

196. Versteeg, D. H. G., Van der Gugten, J., de Jong, W., and Palkovits, M. (1976): Regional concentrations of noradrenaline and dopamine in rat brain. *Brain Res.,* 113:563–574.

197. Wang, R. Y. (1981): Dopaminergic neurons in the rat ventral tegmental area. I. Identification and characterization. *Brain Res. Rev.,* 3:123–140.

198. Weiner, R. I., Shryne, J. E., Gorski, R. A., and Sawyer, C. H. (1972): Changes in the catecholamine content of the rat hypothalamus following deafferentation. *Endocrinology,* 90:867–873.

199. Wiegand, S. J., and Price, J. L. (1980): Cells of origin of the afferent fibers to the median eminence in the rat. *J. Comp. Neurol.,* 192:1–19.

200. Wyss, J. M., Swanson, L. W., and Cowan, W. M. (1979): A study of subcortical afferents to the hippocampal formation in the rat. *Neuroscience,* 4:463–476.

201. Záborszky, L., Brownstein, M. J., and Palkovits, M. (1979): Ascending projections to the hypothalamus and limbic nuclei from the dorsolateral pontine tegmentum: A biochemical and electron microscopic study. *Acta Morphol. Acad. Sci. Hung.,* 25:175–188.

202. Záborszky, L., Feminger, A., and Palkovits, M. (1979): Afferent brain stem connections of the central amygdaloid nucleus. *Verh. Anat. Ges.,* 73:1117–1120.

203. Zemlan, F. P., Kow, L.-M., Morell, J. I., and Pfaff, D. W. (1979): Descending tracts of the lateral columns of the rat spinal cord: A study using the horseradish peroxidase and silver impregnation techniques. *J. Anat.,* 128:489–512.

Chemical Neuroanatomy, edited by P.C. Emson,
Raven Press, New York © 1983.

The Thalamus

E. G. Jones

Department of Anatomy and Neurobiology and McDonnell Center for Studies of Higher Brain Function, Washington University School of Medicine, St. Louis, Missouri 63110

The thalamus of even the most generalized mammal is a complex of many nuclei. Some of these nuclei are components of pathways with established functions, whereas others have unknown functional relationships. Together, they present a bewildering array of input–output connections. The functional role of any thalamic nucleus is best assessed in terms of the particular system of which it forms a part, but it is also true that there are some principles of organization that are common to all thalamic nuclei. In what follows, it is these common principles that are emphasized, and, unless particularly relevant, little attempt is made to consider any particular nucleus in detail. The choice of references cited herein is selective. Other lengthy reviews of this topic from different perspectives and with fuller bibliographies may be found in Berman and Jones (17) and in Jones (113).

THE ORGANIZATIONAL PLAN OF THE THALAMUS

Basic Divisions

From the earliest comparative studies, it has been customary to divide the mammalian thalamus into three parts (Fig. 1): (a) the dorsal thalamus, having close affinities with the cerebral cortex; (b) the ventral thalamus (the reticular nucleus, ventral lateral geniculate nucleus, and zona incerta), having less close affinities with the cortex and with a different ontogenetic derivation; and (c) the epithalamus, composed of the paraventricular and habenular nuclei, having close affinities with the hypothalamus and from which the pretectum develops (33,204). There is still no reason to question this useful primary division into three parts. Of the three, only the dorsal thalamus provides input to the cerebral cortex. Although the ventral thalamus may receive inputs from the cortex and although one of its components has very intimate connections with the dorsal thalamus, unlike the latter, its cells do not send axons to the cortex. The epithalamus is connected neither with the cortex nor with the striatum, another principal target of the dorsal thalamus.

Not only the neocortex but also the paleocortex of the pyriform lobule and even the archicortex of the hippocampal formation have now been shown to receive inputs from the dorsal thalamus (91,124,135,268). Probably every dorsal thalamic nucleus sends a projection to the cortex. An old controversy over whether the intralaminar nuclei, unlike the other nuclei of the dorsal thalamus, projected only to the cortex or only to the striatum (caudate nucleus and putamen) has also been resolved in favor of their projecting to both (119). No other nuclei, however, project to the striatum.

Specific and Nonspecific Projections

The nature of the thalamocortical projection can vary depending on the nucleus of origin. The thalamocortical axons emanating from some nuclei can be called specific in the sense that they terminate within the confines of a particular cytoarchitectonic field, in a topographically ordered fashion, and within the middle layers (usually III and IV) of the cortex. Those emanating from other nuclei, however, can be called nonspecific, for, though tending to have favored cortical regions of projection, they spread rather diffusely over several architectonic fields and terminate commonly in layer I (Fig. 2). There had always been some reason to believe that fibers from the intralaminar nuclei did this, and their diffuse projection has been confirmed (92,119,159). Other nuclei now shown to have diffuse projections include the principal ventral medial nucleus (92), the anteromedial nucleus

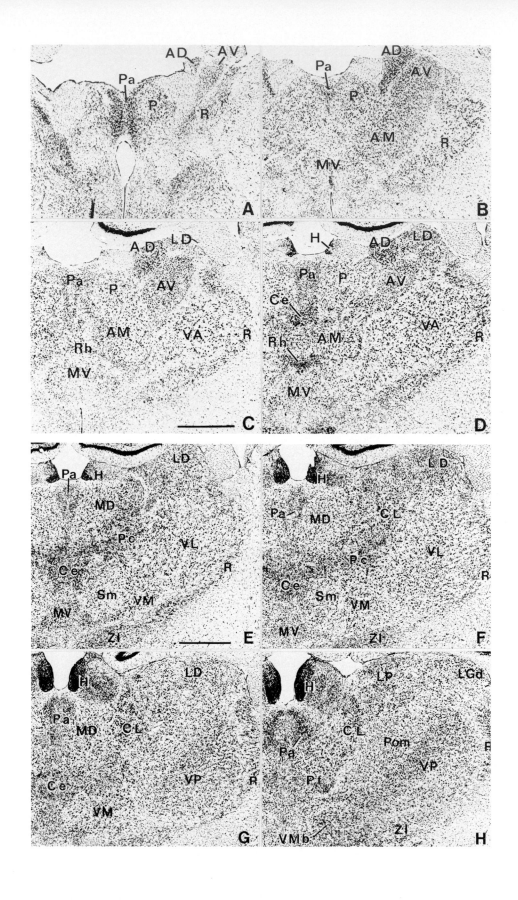

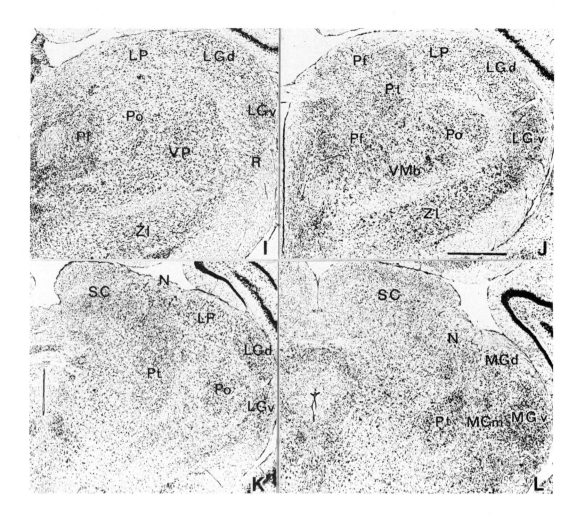

FIG. 1. Nissl-stained frontal sections through the thalamus of a rat. The sections are arranged in anterior (**A**) to posterior (**L**) order. *Bars,* 1 mm.

(The following abbreviations are used in the illustrations of this chapter: AD, anterodorsal nucleus; AM, anteromedial nucleus; AV, anteroventral nucleus; Ce, central medial nucleus; CL, central lateral nucleus; CM, centre médian nucleus; GP, globus pallidus; H, habenular nuclei; LD, laterodorsal nucleus; LGd, dorsal lateral geniculate nucleus; LGv, ventral lateral geniculate nucleus; LP, lateroposterior nucleus; MD, mediodorsal nucleus; MGd, dorsal division, medial geniculate nucleus; MGm, medial division, medial geniculate nucleus; MGv, ventral division, medial geniculate nucleus; MV, medioventral (reuniens) nucleus; N, nucleus of optic tract; P, parataenial nucleus; Pa, paraventricular nuclei; Pc, paracentral nucleus; Pf, parafascicular nucleus; Pla, anterior pulvinar nucleus; Pli, inferior pulvinar nucleus; Pll, lateral pulvinar nucleus; Plm, medial pulvinar nucleus; Po, posterior complex; Pom, posterior complex, medial division; Pt, pretectal nuclei; R, reticular nucleus; Rh, rhomboid nucleus; SC, superior colliculus; Sm, submedial (gelatinosus) nucleus; VA, ventroanterior nucleus; VL, ventrolateral nucleus; VLo, ventrolateral nucleus, oral division; VM, principal ventromedial nucleus; VMb, basal ventromedial nucleus; VPLc, ventroposterior nucleus, caudal division; VPLo, ventroposterior nucleus, oral division; ZI, zona incerta; I–VI, numbered layers of cerebral cortex.)

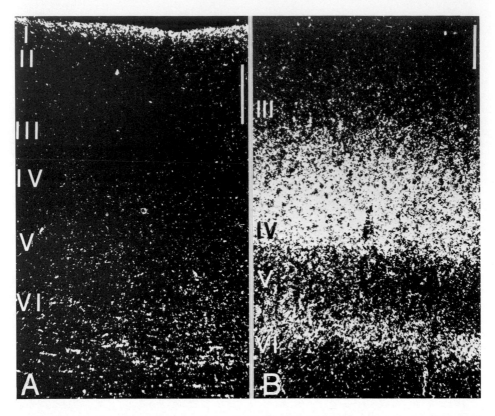

FIG. 2. Autoradiographs from the cerebral cortex photographed in dark field and demonstrating terminal ramifications of thalamocortical fibers by axoplasmic transport following injections of tritiated amino acids in the thalamus. **A:** "Nonspecific" projections to layers I and VI in a cat. **B:** "Specific" projections to adjacent parts of layers III and IV and of layers V and VI in a monkey. *Bars,* 100 μm. (Figure 2B from Jones and Burton, ref. 116, with permission.)

(48,135), parts of the medial and lateral geniculate nuclei (116,145,210), and possibly several others (92,177,198).

Changing Concepts

As work on thalamic connections has progressed, it has forced the revision of two other time-honored, though not always universally accepted, principles. It is clear that we can no longer assert that all inputs to the cerebral cortex must make an obligatory synaptic relay in the thalamus. Several afferent systems to the cortex are now known to reach it directly, bypassing the thalamus altogether. These include afferents from certain of the nuclei of the amygdaloid complex (109,134); from the serotoninergic, noradrenergic, dopaminergic, and certain other cell groups of the brainstem (4,14,16,36,150,190,213); from the cholinergic cell groups of the basal forebrain (46,117,128, 142,163); and from the claustrum (27,128,

146,158,181,200). For the present, it seems rather disappointing that we know far more about the transmitter substances involved in these pathways than about those in the classic thalamocortical pathways.

The second concept that we have been forced to discard is that of relay and association nuclei in the thalamus. Relay nuclei were generally held to be the only nuclei receiving well-defined extrinsic afferent pathways, such as the optic tract or medial lemniscus, whereas association nuclei, though known to project to the cortex, were considered to receive their inputs only from other thalamic nuclei. With the exception of the intralaminar nuclei, which show fairly extensive interconnections among themselves, and the reticular nucleus (described below), we now know that there are few if any internuclear connections in the thalamus. In addition, it seems probable that every thalamic nucleus does, indeed, receive an extrinsic input from a brainstem or other subcortical source. Large parts of the pulvinar, for example, are the targets of the superficial layers of the superior colliculus and pretectum (18,77,79,86,184,257), and the mediodorsal nucleus receives substantial inputs from the basal forebrain (134,172,193). Therefore, every thalamic nucleus can be considered a relay nucleus.

Thalamostriate Projections

The other major target of the dorsal thalamus is the striatum, i.e., the caudate nucleus, putamen, nucleus accumbens, and groups of cells of identical character linking these together around the anterior limb of the internal capsule [the "fundus striati" of Heimer (89)]. The nuclei giving rise to the thalamostriate projections are those of the rostral and caudal components of the intralaminar system: the central medial, central lateral, and paracentral nuclei (rostral group); and the centre médian and parafascicular nuclei (caudal group) (119,124,138,171,209). There have been no other positively identified sources.

Few other extrinsic targets of the thalamus have been demonstrated. One is a portion of the lateral amygdaloid nucleus that receives fibers from the medial nucleus of the pulvinar (115). The functional significance of this is not known.

In the foregoing, nothing has been said of the so-called midline nuclei of the thalamus. The nuclei commonly mentioned under this term include representatives of the epithalamus and of the intralaminar system as well as nuclei that give rise to specific projections and others that give rise to diffuse or nonspecific projections. Therefore, the term has little organizational value and is probably better dropped from the scientific lexicon. It seems likely that the well-known effects, such as cortical recruiting responses, that can be demonstrated by stimulating the "midline nuclei" stem from stimulation of the intralaminar system and possibly of the principal ventromedial nucleus (113).

NATURE OF THALAMIC INPUTS

Specific and Nonspecific Inputs

For the purposes of description, it seems appropriate to divide the subcortical inputs to the dorsal thalamus into two general categories. The first of these are the classic pathways, such as the optic tract, the medial lemniscus, and the brachium of the inferior colliculus, which have an obvious information-bearing function, arise in well-defined nuclei, and terminate with a coherent, topographic ordering within the confines of the appropriate thalamic relay nucleus. The other category is that in which the thalamic input is part of a seemingly rather diffusely organized pathway that distributes to a number of diencephalic and other basal forebrain centers en route to the cerebral cortex. The most obvious representative of this category is the ascending noradrenergic system (110,244) (Fig. 3).

Specificity is the hallmark of the classic system. Not only do the afferent fibers terminate within the confines of a particular thalamic nucleus, but there is also a systematic distribution of the input fibers that forms the basis of the topographic ordering and the mapping of the particular receptor sheet that they represent. Within this ordered system there is further specificity, for fibers with different physiological characteristics appear to relay on distinct classes of thalamocortical relay cell. This seems to have been conclusively demonstrated for at least two of the three categories of retinal ganglion cell axon in the lateral geniculate nucleus of the cat and other species (35,51,96,216,223,262).

Topographic ordering of inputs within the borders of a defined thalamic relay nucleus can be demonstrated in the three major sensory relay nuclei, but it can also be seen in the distribution of fibers from the deep cerebellar nuclei to the thalamic relay to motor cortex (248) and in the distribution of fibers from the superficial layers of the superior colliculus to the lateral posterior nucleus (77) or inferior pulvinar nucleus (86). In each of these cases, a representation of the appropriate half of the body or of the visual field has been correspondingly demonstrated in the nucleus (3,71,161,240).

The second category of input system seems to be organized without the topographic finesse described above. The two obvious representatives of this system are the ascending noradrenergic system arising principally in the locus ceruleus (110,149,190,244,251) and the ascending serotoninergic system arising principally in the dorsal nucleus of the midbrain raphe (21,36,42). Though each of these systems may show localized concentrations of presumed terminal ramifications in certain thalamic nuclei, unlike in the classically ordered system, the terminations are by no means confined to particular nuclei. For example, though they show a very dense concentration in the anteroventral nucleus, noradrenergic fibers can be demonstrated in many other nuclei as they ascend through and around the thalamus (149,244). In these nuclei, the noradrenergic fibers would converge on the territory of distribution of some of the

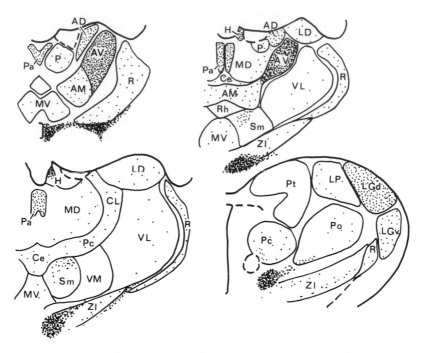

FIG. 3. Schematic figures, redrawn from Swanson and Hartman (244), showing the distribution of noradrenergic fibers in the rat thalamus. The fibers are localized by dopamine-β-hydroxylase immunohistochemistry. Note high concentrations of fibers only in anteroventral and medial habenular nuclei and moderate concentrations in certain others. (For abbreviations, see Fig. 1, legend)

classic pathways. Similarly, though there has been much emphasis on the lateral geniculate complex as a major site of termination of the ascending serotoninergic system (141), the parent cells of the system in the dorsal raphe nucleus can be retrogradely labeled by horseradish peroxidase injected in other thalamic nuclei as well (73,250).

The Amine-Containing Pathways

Apart from the noradrenergic and serotoninergic systems just mentioned, none of the major input pathways to the thalamus has been correlated with any identified neurotransmitter agent or transmitter-related enzyme. The studies of regional distributions of such substances, reviewed in the last section of this chapter, at the present time do not correlate at all well with the distributions of the better known thalamic input pathways. The other widely studied amine, dopamine, seems not to be a major thalamic neurotransmitter, since the dopamine–containing fibers arising in the pars compacta of the substantia nigra and in adjacent cell groups of the ventral tegmental area largely bypass the thalamus as they project forward to the basal ganglia (251). The large nigrothalamic

pathway, which terminates primarily in the principal ventromedial nucleus of the thalamus (14,28,60,90), arises from cells of the pars reticulata of the substantia nigra (60,201) that do not contain dopamine (167). This nigrothalamic pathway has, however, been interpreted as being GABAergic (45).

THE RETICULAR NUCLEUS AND RELATED STRUCTURES

New Observations

After a period in which it was regarded rather vaguely as a rostral continuation of the brainstem reticular formation, the reticular nucleus has in recent years become fairly well understood. Recent anatomical work shows that the thalamocortical and corticothalamic fiber systems, and probably the thalamostriate and pallidothalamic systems, distribute a heavy density of terminals in the reticular nucleus as they traverse it (111) (Fig. 4). It is probable that the axons terminating in the reticular nucleus are collateral branches of those traversing it (26,215). There is a predictable topography in the system such that thalamocortical fibers leaving and corticothalamic fibers returning to a particular dorsal thalamic nucleus always give terminals to the same constant part of the reticular nucleus. This leads to some parts of the nucleus being dominated by a particular system (111,164). Consequently, unit responses to appropriate stimuli can often be recorded in a given part of the nucleus (241,242). In the part connected with the lateral geniculate nucleus, there may even be some degree of retinotopic organization (164). It is doubtful, however, that the organization can be too specific, for the cells of the nucleus are very large, with extremely long dendrites that spread widely over the surface of the dorsal thalamus, and, inevitably, there must be a good deal of convergence of different systems onto a single cell.

The output of the reticular nucleus is not to the cortex as was once suggested (32,205) but into the dorsal thalamus itself (26,111,215). The projection passes to both principal and intralaminar nuclei, and a portion of the reticular nucleus traversed by the thalamocortical and corticothalamic fiber sys-

tems related to a particular dorsal thalamic nucleus includes that nucleus in its somewhat diffuse projection field (111). Other brainstem projections of the reticular nucleus, though described by some, could not be identified by Jones (111).

GABA Transmission

The cells of the reticular nucleus can be labeled immunocytochemically with antiserum to glutamic acid decarboxylase (GAD) (100) (Fig. 5). In the dorsal thalamus, the terminals of the reticular nucleus axons have the morphological characteristics of inhibitory synapses (165,179) and presumably correspond to GAD-positive puncta that can also be demonstrated immunocytochemically in the dorsal thalamus. The morphological and immunocytochemical evidence is, therefore, strong that the reticular nucleus is the source of an inhibitory input to the underlying dorsal thalamus that uses the transmitter, γ-aminobutyric acid (GABA). Further details of this system are taken up below.

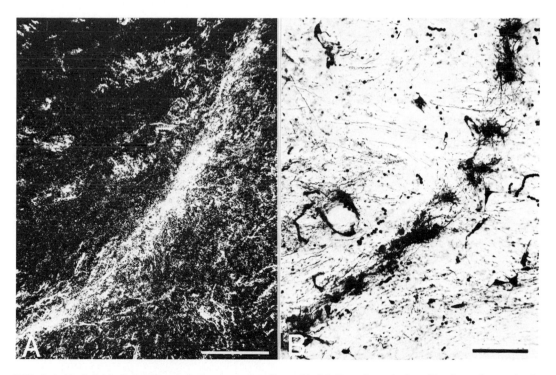

FIG. 4. A: Dark-field photomicrograph showing autoradiographic labeling of terminal ramifications of axons in the reticular nucleus of a monkey following injection of tritiated amino acids at a more posterior level in one of the principal nuclei of the dorsal thalamus. Bundles of labeled thalamocortical axons can be seen entering from the left and entering the internal capsule on the right. *Bar*, 200 μm. **B:** Retrograde labeling of cell bodies in the reticular nucleus of a rat following injection of horseradish peroxidase in the dorsal thalamus. *Bar*, 100 μm. (From Jones, ref. 111, with permission.)

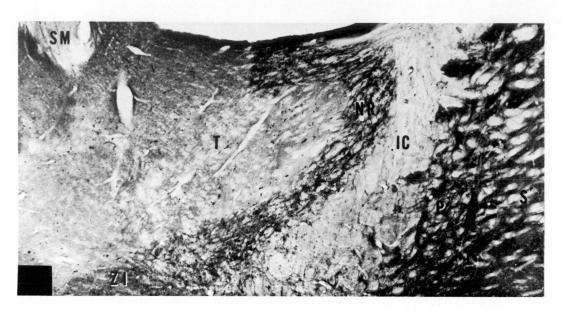

FIG. 5. Immunocytochemical labeling of thalamic cell somata only in the reticular nucleus of a rat by antiserum to the GABA-related enzyme glutamic acid decarboxylase. *Bar,* 500 μm. IC, internal capsule; P, globus pallidus; S, striatum; SM, stria medullaris; T, thalamus. (From Houser et al., ref. 100, with permission.)

Apart from its thalamic, cortical, and presumed basal ganglia inputs, the only other known afferent connections of the reticular nucleus come from certain of the deeper-seated nuclei of the pretectum (18). Descriptions of inputs from the mesencephalic reticular formation may result from involvement of the pretectal nuclei rather than the reticular formation proper (55,67,270). The other components of the ventral thalamus (the ventral lateral geniculate nucleus and the zona incerta), though closely related to the reticular nucleus, have different patterns of connectivity (113), and neither seems to project into the dorsal thalamus. The tiny perigeniculate nucleus of the cat has been described as having connections and electrophysiological properties comparable to those of adjacent parts of the reticular nucleus (1,52,61).

NATURE OF THALAMOCORTICAL PROJECTIONS

At present, virtually nothing is known of the transmitter characteristics of the "specific" and "nonspecific" thalamocortical projections mentioned above. Nuclei with specific projections project within the confines of one or at most a few cortical cytoarchitectonic fields. The projection of the dorsal lateral geniculate nucleus to area 17 of the monkey or of the ventroposterior nucleus to the first and second somatic sensory areas are exam-

ples of this type of projection. Nuclei with nonspecific projections are not constrained by cortical architectonic boundaries and project widely and seemingly rather diffusely over relatively large regional zones of cortex.

Laminar Patterns

Within each of these two patterns, there are further and finer differences of organization. The most obvious of these are the variations in laminar distributions of thalamocortical fibers arising in different nuclei. Within the specific system, it has become evident that, despite a long-held belief, layer IV of the cortex in the primate receives the principal thalamocortical input in only a minority of areas (116). Outside the primary sensory areas, which represent little more than about 20% of the primate cortex, the principal thalamocortical projection terminates primarily among the large pyramidal cells of the deeper half of layer III, not among the small granule cells of layer IV.

Columnar Patterns

As well as being focused on one or a few architectonic fields and on a limited number of cortical layers, a specific projection is focused in a further sense. The horizontal lamina of terminations is composed of focal patches of terminations derived from small groups of thalamic cells. The first indication of this was given by Hubel and Wiesel (103) when they showed that thalamocortical fibers arising in laminae of the dorsal lateral geniculate nucleus related to one eye terminated in layer IV in strips of terminal ramifications that alternated with similar strips formed by the terminal ramifications of fibers arising in laminae of the geniculate related to the other eye. This observation has subsequently been confirmed many times with a variety of techniques (105). At any region along the length of a pair of left-eye–plus–right-eye strips, the thalamic input to the region comes from a restricted grouping of geniculate cells that extends like a narrow rod through the full thickness of the geniculate and across all its layers. Such a rod represents the input from homonymous parts of the two retinae and, thus, a particular region of the visual field. In physiological terms it is referred to as a projection column (211).

The focusing of the cortical projection of the bundle of axons arising from the relay cells along a projection column ensures that the topography of the visual field representation is preserved in the input to the visual cortex. The relative lack of precision in topographic organization when studied at the single-unit level in the visual cortex (104) may stem from the overlapping distributions of axons within an input bundle on single cortical neurons. Despite this caveat, the groupings of thalamic relay cells into organized clusters and the projection of their bundled axons onto focal zones of cortex are characteristic of all the major relay nuclei (64,123) (Fig. 6). The aggregations of relay neurons in the somatic sensory relay nucleus represent not only a place on the body surface but also a particular constellation of receptors related to a single submodality of somatic sensation, e.g., hair movement, light touch, deep pressure, joint movement (191). The organizing principle for this appears to be the bundling of incoming lemniscal axons into groups that run along the aggregations (113) (Fig. 7). A similar organizational pattern is present in the medial geniculate nucleus and in the thalamic nuclei receiving cerebellar inputs and projecting to motor cortex (9,11,169,248), though in neither of these cases is the feature known that is comparable to "modality."

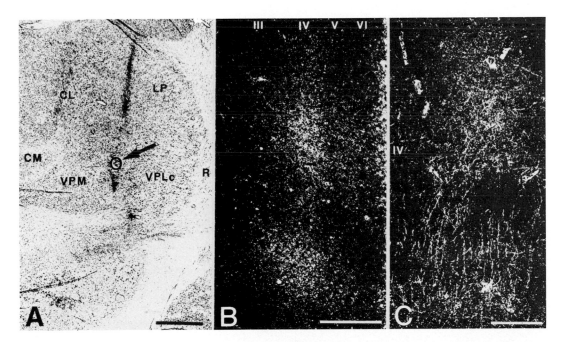

FIG. 6. A: Microelectrode track in the ventroposterior nucleus of a monkey. A small injection of tritiated amino acids, made at a site from which units responding to cutaneous stimulation of part of a finger were recorded *(circled area)*, led to transported label (**B**) in two foci in the somatic sensory cortex. Each focus is composed of a bundle of axons and their terminations such as that illustrated (**C**) by axonal degeneration following a microlesion in the same thalamic nucleus. *Bars:* 1 mm (**A**), 250 μm (**B**), 100 μm (**C**). (For abbreviations, see Fig. 1, legend.) (From Friedman and Jones, ref. 64, with permission.)

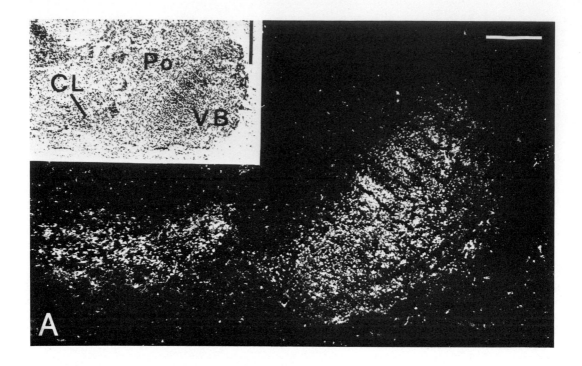

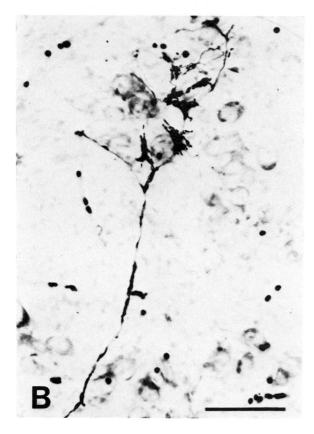

FIG. 7. A: Retrograde labeling of thalamocortical relay cells in clusters in the ventroposterior nucleus (VB) following injection of horseradish peroxidase in the somatic sensory cortex of a young rat. Additional labeling of cells appears in the central lateral nucleus (CL) of the intralaminar complex. *Bars:* 250 μm, 500 μm (**inset**). (From Wise and Jones, ref. 266, with permission.) **B:** Terminal portion of a medial lemniscal axon anterogradely labeled by injection of horseradish peroxidase in the medial lemniscus of a cat. Bundles of terminal ramifications of this type constitute the input to clusters of relay cells of the type seen in **A** which then project to focal zones in the cortex. *Bar,* 100 μm. (From unpublished work of W. T. Rainey and E. G. Jones.)

Collateral Projection to Deep Layers

In every area, in addition to the concentrated, focused input to the middle layers of the cortex, a smaller lamina of terminations is found at the junction of layers V and VI (101,116,202,206,266) (Fig. 2). It is made up of collaterals of the thalamocortical axons terminating in layer IV (61). In the cat visual cortex, there is some evidence that the deep zone of terminations represents a direct monosynaptic input to certain classes of output cell, i.e., the corticotectal (182) and corticothalamic (22,87) cells, though the latter is not completely accepted by all workers (72).

Other Laminar Patterns

Other variations in laminar distribution patterns may well reflect preferential inputs to different classes of cortical neuron from specific classes of thalamic relay cell. In the cat, for example, the inputs from X and Y retinal ganglion cells are relayed directly to the visual cortex, with little transformation of the characteristic electrophysiological properties in the dorsal lateral geniculate nucleus (34,35,68,96,238,261,262). Thalamocortical axons probably arising from the morphological equivalents of Y-type geniculate relay cells terminate in the superficial two-thirds of layer IV and in the overlying part of layer III, whereas those probably arising from the morphological equivalents of X-type geniculate relay cells terminate beneath them in the deepest one-third of layer IV (61). There is also evidence that the distributions of the two classes of thalamocortical axon correspond to the laminar positions of cortical cells with different categories of receptive field (72,74,102).

A third type of thalamocortical projection arising from the dorsal lateral geniculate nucleus of the cat arises in laminae of the nucleus (the C laminae) separate from those (the A laminae) in which the X and Y classes of retinal ganglion cell axon relay. The relay cells of the C laminae project in the visual cortex to parts of layers III and V superficial and deep to the terminations of axons arising in the A laminae as well as sending branches to terminate in layer I (61,145). The cells of the C laminae probably correspond to those receiving inputs from a class of retinal ganglion cells with a third type of discharge property (W cells) (35,261,262). The projection from the C laminae is also a diffuse one: the projections of the A laminae are focused on areas 17 and 18, but that from the C laminae spreads from these areas into adjacent cortical areas as well (145).

Summary

There seems to be no simple principle whereby we can rationalize the organization of the specific and nonspecific (diffuse) projections to a single cortical area. In many instances, the specific and diffuse projections arise from different thalamic nuclei. Different fields of the auditory cortex, for example, receive their specific inputs from separate subnuclei of the medial geniculate complex and a diffuse or nonspecific layer I input from the magnocellular nucleus of the complex (116,263). But there may be several sources of nonspecific input, including those from nuclei generally classified as principal nuclei (31,49,66,92). In the cat, for example, part of the lateral posterior nucleus, like the C laminae of the lateral geniculate, may also furnish a diffuse cortical input to the striate and adjacent cortical areas (73). It is certainly not simply a distinction between the intralaminar nuclei providing the diffuse and a principal relay nucleus the specific.

THE INTRALAMINAR NUCLEI

The Striatal Projection

The five major nuclear components of the intralaminar system are distinguished by a rather heavy projection to the striatum and a lighter, more diffuse projection to the cerebral cortex (112,119). It has not yet been determined whether or not the axons directed to the cortex are collaterals of those directed toward the striatum, and there is still some disagreement as to whether the axons reaching the cortex terminate in layer I (27,112) or only in the deeper layers (92).

A topographic organization in the thalamostriate projection such that different intralaminar nuclei project to different parts of the striatum was demonstrated some years ago by Powell and Cowan (192). Recently, a finer organization has also been discovered. Axons arising from a part of the intralaminar system end in a series of dissociated burst-like clusters (124,209) that resemble similar burst-like terminations of corticostriatal (76,118) fibers and burst-like clusters of acetylcholinesterase activity (80) and of opiate receptor binding (93). The extent to which the different terminations converge or alternate is not yet clear.

The Transmitter Agent

There is no firm evidence as to the nature of the transmitter in the thalamostriate pathway. However, Streit (239) has noted that intralaminar thalamic cells are retrogradely labeled following injection of [³H]-D-aspartate in the striatum of rats. There was comparable retrograde labeling of cells in layer V of the cerebral cortex, the source of corticostriatal projections (118,265) which are thought to be glutaminergic (19,47,156,197). Since aspartate shares the same uptake system as glutamate (43,153), the possibility is raised that the retrograde labeling experiments might imply use of one or another of these amino acids as a transmitter in the thalamostriate projection.

Certain other transmitter-related compounds have relatively high concentrations within the intralaminar nuclei. Rather high concentrations of acetylcholinesterase (see Fig. 15) have been known for some years (109,180,183,225). More recently, opiate receptors and enkephalin-containing fibers have been shown to have their highest thalamic concentrations in the intralaminar nuclei, though there is some discrepancy among the descriptions of different authors (56,185,186,214,226,256).

The Cortical Projection

The cortical projection of the intralaminar system is diffuse and may spread over the whole cortex, but there are clearly regional zones of higher concentrations, as judged by the number of cells retrogradely labeled in the intralaminar nuclei following injections of horseradish peroxidase in different cortical areas (16,90,119,175) (Fig. 8). The central medial nucleus seems to project primarily to cingulate and anterior limbic areas, the paracentral and central lateral to parietal fields, the centre

médian to motor and premotor areas, and the parafascicular to lateral frontal areas. The primary sensory areas appear to receive relatively fewer intralaminar connections. All projections to the cortex are reciprocated by returning corticointralaminar projections.

Subcortical Afferents

Although for many years they were regarded as rather diffuse and displaying a great deal of convergence, the inputs to the intralaminar system of nuclei now appear to be a little more discrete. The principal input is not from the brainstem reticular formation but from the deep cerebellar nuclei that distribute axons through all the nuclei except the parafascicular or the small part of the central lateral nucleus that receives spinal fibers (90). Some other inputs are more restricted: the internal segment of the globus pallidus, for example, sends fibers only to the centre médian nucleus (90,130,140). Other sources of rather weak inputs, mostly to the central lateral and paracentral nuclei, include the perihypoglossal nuclei (133), the pontine parabrachial nuclei (213), the substantia nigra (14,60,90), the deep layers of the superior colliculus (77), and certain of the deeper nuclei of the pretectum (18,257). The latter two sources have sometimes been interpreted as belonging to the mesencephalic reticular formation (55). Older reports of inputs from more caudally situated parts of the reticular formation (173) have not yet been confirmed to any great extent (78). The only described input to the parafascicular nucleus in large mammals is from the central gray matter of the

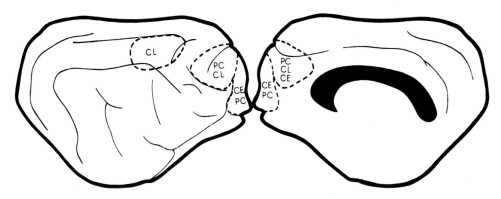

FIG. 8. Schematic drawings of a cat brain showing regional zones of heaviest input from the intralaminar nuclei, based on the distribution of cellular degeneration following regional cortical ablations. More recent work with retrograde labeling techniques indicates intralaminar projections to more widespread areas of cortex, but the zones indicated still represent the principal input regions of the nuclei. (From Macchi et al., ref. 159, with permission.)

midbrain (84). In rats (152) and certain other small mammals (162,203), the spinal cord seems to project to it.

With the exception of the spinothalamic system of fibers, no sensory pathway furnishes a particularly direct input to the intralaminar nuclei. The parts of the superior colliculus and pretectum that provide input do not receive direct retinal projections (18). The spinothalamic input is rather small in comparison with the cerebellar. In the cat, it is restricted to a small number of large cells situated at the caudal end of the central lateral nucleus (114,162). In the monkey, these cells are often included in the paralamellar part of the mediodorsal nucleus (70). Given the predominance of inputs from motor-related sources and the paucity of direct sensory inputs, it is hard to see the intralaminar system as a major sensory relay center, though this concept has prevailed in the past. More recently, there have been some attempts to implicate the intralaminar nuclei in motor function, especially in the control of gaze (217,218). This may turn out to be a more profitable approach to determining their significance. It is even possible that the spinal inputs may be more involved with motor than sensory behavior. They seem to arise from cells in deeper layers of the spinal central gray, where neurons with proprioceptive rather than thermal and nociceptive responses are found (10,29,258).

BASIC SYNAPTOLOGY IN THE THALAMUS

Relay Neurons and Interneurons

There is reason to believe that all thalamic nuclei, including those of the intralaminar system (83,85,88), have similar patterns of synaptic organization. Cajal (26) described the two principal forms of thalamic neuron. The principal or relay cell (Fig. 9) is rather symmetrical in shape with many equally radiating dendrites carrying a moderate number of stout protrusions. The second cell is small and has a thin, locally ramifying axon and relatively few sparsely branched dendrites with bulbous protrusions and dilatations resembling axon terminals (Fig. 9).

In 1966, Guillery (81) drew attention to the two types again and, in the cat lateral geniculate nucleus, divided the principal type into three subclasses. These have subsequently been linked to the cell types that receive the X-, Y-, and W-type ganglion cell inputs and project differentially to the visual cortex (61). Similar subclasses have not yet

been detected in other nuclei. The interneuron has been redescribed in detail by Szentágothai et al. (245), Famiglietti and Peters (59), and Morest (170). Certain forms of cell seemingly intermediate between principal neurons and interneurons have also been described (59,253).

There are further descriptions of interneurons with either long or short axons (178,249). According to Tömböl (249), in the lateral geniculate nucleus, those with the longer axons provide for interlaminar inhibitory effects, whereas those with the short axons act locally.

There is still some controversy over the proportion of interneurons in a thalamic relay nucleus. Many of the earlier studies that examined retrograde labeling with horseradish peroxidase after injecting the material in the cerebral cortex remarked that every neuron in the affected thalamic nucleus appeared labeled. Some workers felt, therefore, that all thalamic neurons might project to the cortex (148,176). Others contested this, indicating that unlabeled cells, presumably interneurons, account for as much as 25% of the population and escape detection because of their small size (143,144,264).

Synaptic Islands

A particularly striking electron microscopic feature of the thalami of some mammals (e.g., cats and rats), though not so obvious in others (e.g., monkeys), is the presence of large aggregations of synaptic terminations that are often unsheathed by astroglia. Some workers have called these "glomeruli" (120,245), though they are not totally segregated from one another and may spread, sheet-like, for considerable distances.

The central elements in these synaptic aggregations (Fig. 10) are one or more protrusions from the proximal dendrite(s) of a principal cell and one or two large axon terminals derived from the major afferent source to the nucleus. The terminals contain spherical synaptic vesicles and end in asymmetric synapses on the dendrite(s). Surrounding the dendritic and axonal elements and usually considerably outnumbering them are a number of apparent axon terminals that are, in fact, presynaptic dendrites, almost certainly belonging to the interneurons. These terminals contain pleomorphic or flattened synaptic vesicles and terminate in symmetric synapses on the dendrites of the principal cell and to some extent on one another. In addition, they are themselves postsynaptic to the principal afferent axon terminal. Finally, at the periphery of

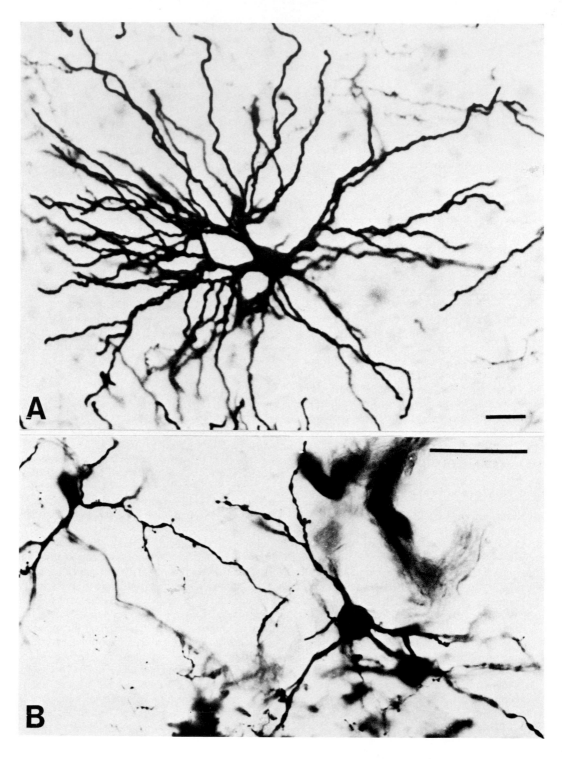

FIG. 9. A: Golgi-impregnated principal neuron from the ventroposterior nucleus of a rat, showing the symmetrically radiating dendrites. **B:** Parts of three Golgi-impregnated interneurons from the ventroposterior nucleus of a cat showing the beaded dendritic processes that are probably the presynaptic dendrites of electron microscopy. *Bars,* 50 μm. Note different magnifications.

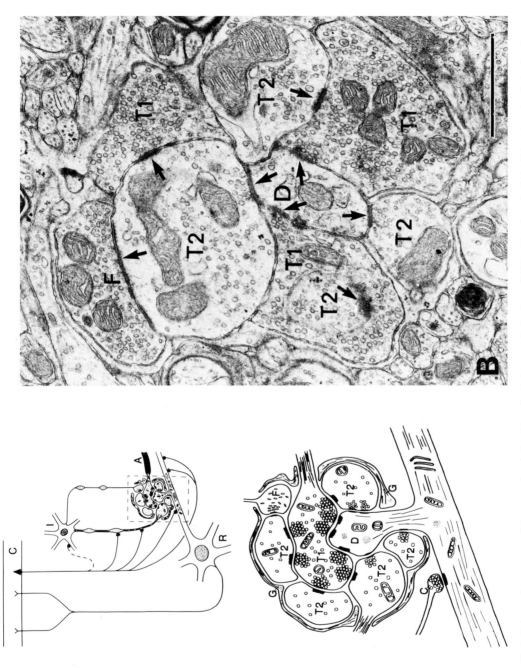

FIG. 10. A: Schematic summary of the synaptic relationships of a thalamocortical relay cell (R) with subcortical (A, T_1) and corticothalamic afferents (C) and with presynaptic dendrites (T_2) and conventional axon terminals (F) of interneurons. Not shown are the terminals of reticular nucleus axons (165,179). G indicates astroglial processes. See text for description. (From Jones et al., ref. 113, with permission.) **B:** Electron micrograph from the ventroposterior nucleus of a cat showing some of the features illustrated in **A.** *Bar,* 1 μm.

the aggregation, an axon terminal containing flattened vesicles and terminating in a symmetric synapse may also be seen. These end on the presynaptic dendrites and probably belong to the true axons of the interneurons. [For complete references, see Jones (113).]

Other elements in the neuropil include many small terminals containing spherical vesicles and ending in asymmetric contacts on the dendrites of principal cells and interneurons, usually distally. Most of these are the terminals of corticothalamic axons (121,178). The terminals of reticular nucleus axons make symmetric membrane contacts and contain synaptic vesicles that flatten. Montero and Scott (165) describe them only on dendrites outside the synaptic islands. O'Hara et al. (179) describe them on cell somata as well. The terminals of noradrenergic and other amine-containing pathways that end in certain thalamic nuclei have not yet been described at the fine structure level.

The Nature of Synaptic Events

Stimulation of the major afferent pathway to a dorsal thalamic nucleus leads to activation of thalamocortical relay cells followed by a profound and often quite prolonged inhibition of the cells, lasting as long as 150 msec and followed by a period of enhanced excitability (2,6,8,25,157,174,230). The postexcitatory depression is said not to occur in the ventral lateral geniculate nucleus (part of the ventral thalamus) (83).

Perhaps the classic study of synaptic events in the dorsal thalamus is that of Andersen et al. (6) in the cat somatic sensory relay nucleus. The inhibitory postsynaptic potentials (IPSPs) in the relay cells commence about 2 msec subsequent to the excitory postsynaptic potentials (EPSPs) induced by the afferent volley and have a rather prolonged rise time. This temporal sequence suggested to Andersen et al. (6,8) that interneurons responsible for this postsynaptic inhibition should be activated by collaterals of thalamocortical axons and that the interneurons' axons should end on the relay cells. Repetitive firing of the interneurons would account for the slow rise of the IPSPs in the relay cells. A second class of interneuron, tentatively identified by Andersen et al. (6), was considered to receive direct lemniscal inputs rather than collateral inputs from thalamocortical axons. The EPSPs generated in it by afferent volleys were not succeeded by the characteristic prolonged IPSPs of the relay neurons, and the experimenters, for reasons that need not concern us here, felt that its axon should effect presynaptic inhibition of the relay neurons

by forming axoaxonic contacts on the lemniscal terminals. Similar circuitry has been proposed to account for presynaptic inhibition in the lateral geniculate nucleus, but in no case has an appropriate morphological correlate been observed (24,228).

The lateral geniculate nucleus has in recent years become the principal site for studying synaptic transmission in the thalamus. Several types of interlaminar and intralaminar inhibitory phenomena, presumed to be mediated by inhibitory interneurons, have been described (96,212,229–231). Most workers now seem to consider that all the interneurons are activated monosynaptically by afferent fibers. Dubin and Cleland (52), for example, have described interneurons selectively activated, like geniculate relay cells, by X or Y retinal ganglion cell inputs and found that some Y interneurons are activated by branches of Y ganglion cell axons terminating on Y relay cells; however, later activation of interneurons via collaterals of thalamocortical axons have not been ruled out (58).

Most of the effects mentioned in the preceding are probably mediated by inhibitory interneurons with local axons (126,166). Long-range interneurons exerting inhibitory effects on geniculocortical relay cells in other laminae of the lateral geniculate nucleus have also been described (228). They may correspond to the long-axoned interneuron of Tömböl (249). No excitatory interneurons seem to have been discovered in the thalamus.

Correlating the synaptic events mentioned above with the finer morphology described earlier still remains an exercise in conjecture (113). The synaptic contacts made by afferent fibers on relay cell dendrites and on the presynaptic dendrites of interneurons have the morphological features usually associated with excitatory synapses, and it is probably safe to assume that they lead to excitation of the relay cell. From the physiological studies, we may also tentatively assume that the presynaptic dendritic terminals exert an inhibitory effect on the relay cells. The prolonged, deep nature of the IPSP generated following excitation of a relay cell might be a result of the large numbers of presynaptic dendritic terminals on the relay cell.

What are difficult to predict are the circumstances under which the dendritic terminals may release their transmitter agent. Possibly this could be a local phenomenon occurring as an immediate consequence of depolarization by afferent terminals situated on the dendrite of the interneuron near a dendritic terminal. But, equally, transmitter release from the presynaptic dendrites might occur only after an action potential that was set up in the interneuron by the afferent terminals secondarily invaded the presynaptic dendrites. Or, the slow buildup of the IPSP might indicate initial local release followed by a more general, synchronous release from the interneuron, provided that an action potential generated in the soma can invade the thin presynaptic dendrites. As a final speculation, it is possible that the release of the relay cell from inhibition may occur by inhibition of the interneuron via synapses between the true axons of the interneurons and their presynaptic dendrites or even via the synapses between the presynaptic dendrites themselves.

Where recurrent axon collaterals of thalamocortical relay cells might fit into this scheme is uncertain. Such collaterals have rarely been described in Golgi studies (26,170,249) and are only just beginning to be recognized in studies in which relay neurons are directly injected with a histological marker (1,259) (Fig. 11).

The Potential Transmitters

Acetylcholine

The excitatory transmitter agent in the principal afferent pathway to a relay nucleus of the thalamus has not yet been identified. Acetylcholine, when applied iontophoretically, has a predominantly inhibitory effect on relay cells in some nuclei (75,246), but excitation may be more common in others (5,155,189). Excitatory effects have been attributed to pathways such as those from the brainstem reticular formation because the facilitatory effect of reticular formation stimulation on thalamic neurons, but not the excitatory effect of peripheral nerve stimulation, is abolished by antagonists of acetylcholine (188,246). Inhibitory effects have been attributed to presynaptic action (53,160); the inhibitory effect is relatively weak and has a very slow rise time (up to 1 min). It seems unlikely that acetylcholine can be a major transmitter in the thalamus, since the number of nicotinic (107) and muscarinic (207,269) cholinergic receptor sites in most of its nuclei is relatively low. *In vitro* studies in man, rat, and some other species show that the thalamus has a concentration of muscarinic sites approximately one-fourth that of the caudate nucleus (which has the highest concentration) and approximately one-half that of the cerebral cortex (44,94,131). In a detailed histological study of the binding of [³H]propylbenzilycholine mustard, Rotter et al. (207) found the highest concentration of thalamic muscarinic

receptor sites in the anterior nuclei (Fig. 12). There seem to be slight discrepancies between the distributions reported by Rotter et al. and that reported by Wamsley et al. (254), who localized the receptors by the binding of [³H]-*N*-methylscopolamine. This may have something to do with the different nature of the preparative techniques used or the relative capacities of the different antagonists to recognize high- and low-affinity agonist binding sites.

The demonstration of nicotinic cholinergic sites in the thalamus by [¹²⁵I]-α-bungarotoxin binding indicates heavy concentrations only in the ventral lateral geniculate nucleus (107,222) and reticular nucleus (Fig. 12). Moderate concentrations occur in the rhomboid, parataenial, and "medial" nuclei (107). There is a reasonable correspondence between the collective distribution of the muscarinic and nicotinic receptor sites and that of acetylcholinesterase (see below). Muscarinic and nicotinic receptor sites have not been localized electron microscopically in the thalamus.

Glutamate

Of other potential excitatory amino acids, glutamate, when iontophoretically applied, has been found to excite relay neurons in a number of nuclei (40). The excitatory effect of glutamate on relay neurons in the ventroposterior nucleus is similar to that elicited by threshold stimulation of peripheral nerves, and both effects are said to be enhanced by the application of substances, such as L-glutamic acid dimethylester, that compete for the uptake of glutamate and other excitatory amino acids (82). There is some reason for suggesting that glutamate may be the transmitter released at corticothalamic and thalamostriate synapses, as mentioned elsewhere in this chapter.

GABA

When applied iontophoretically, GABA depresses the firing of relay cells in the ventroposterior and lateral geniculate nuclei (38,41). Glycine and taurine are relatively ineffective (41). The depressant effect of GABA and the inhibition that succeeds stimulation of peripheral nerves or of the visual cortex is suppressed by the application of the GABA antagonist bicuculline (39,41,54). It has usually been assumed that GABA is released from thalamic interneurons that lie within the relay nucleus itself. The recent observations of Houser et al. (100) on the immunocytochemical localization of GAD cast some doubt on this. As mentioned

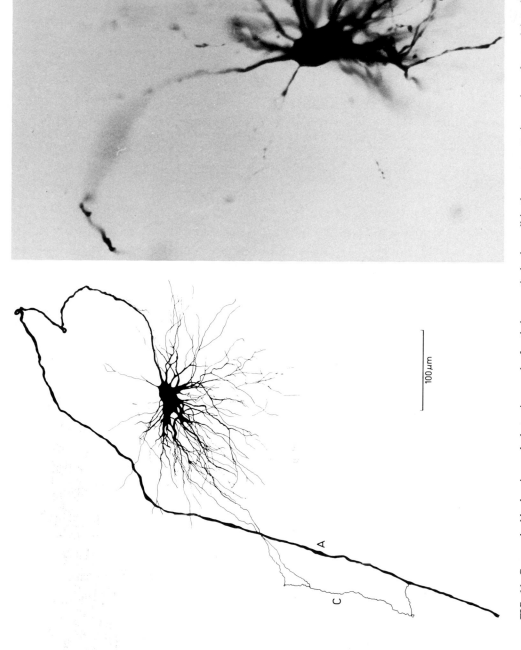

FIG. 11. Camera lucida drawing and photomicrograph of a thalamocortical relay cell in the ventroposterior nucleus of a cat injected directly with horseradish peroxidase. Note the axon collaterals. (Kindly supplied by Dr. B. Walmsley, Australian National University.)

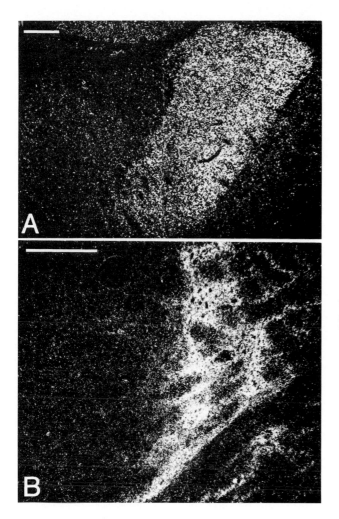

FIG. 12. A: Autoradiographic demonstration of muscarinic cholinergic receptor sites in the anteroventral nucleus of a rat thalamus by binding of [^{3}H]propylbenzilylcholine mustard. (From Rotter et al., ref. 207, with permission.) **B:** Autoradiographic demonstration of presumed nicotinic cholinergic receptor sites in the reticular nucleus of a monkey thalamus by binding of [^{125}I]-α-bungarotoxin. *Bars,* 200 μm. (From unpublished work of S. H. C. Hendry, N. Schechter, and E. G. Jones.)

earlier, Houser et al. found that the only GAD-positive neuronal cell bodies in the rat thalamus lie in the reticular nucleus (Fig. 5). The dorsal thalamic nuclei are filled with small GAD-positive structures that probably represent GABAergic axon terminals, but these presumably are the terminals of the reticular nucleus axons rather than of the local interneurons. On the other hand, Sterling and Davis (237) have shown by electron microscopic autoradiography that [^{3}H]-GABA injected into the dorsal lateral geniculate nucleus of the cat is selectively accumulated by small cell somata and flattened vesicle-containing profiles, which they regard as belonging to the local interneurons. They obtained similar results following the injection of tritiated forms of the GABA analog diaminobutyric acid and of the GABA agonist muscimol. It is conceivable that intrinsic GABAergic neurons

were not detected by Houser et al. (100) on account of the relative insensitivity of the immunocytochemical technique toward small concentrations of GAD. They did, however, pretreat their animals with colchicine which, in most circumstances, by blocking axoplasmic transport, enhances the immunocytochemical labeling of cell somata. For the moment, it would seem that both reticular neurons and at least one population of thalamic interneurons may be GABAergic.

The Amines

The distributions of noradrenergic and serotoninergic fibers in the thalamus have already been described. The paraventricular nuclei of the epithalamus, unlike the dorsal thalamus, receive noradrenergic innervation from caudal brainstem cell groups as well as from the locus ceruleus (168). And the paraventricular nuclei contain the only significant adrenergic innervation in the thalamus (98).

A modest dopaminergic innervation reaches only the intralaminar nuclei. It comes not from the substantia nigra but from the periventricular system of fibers (150). None of the amines seems to have particularly strong effects when applied iontophoretically to thalamic neurons (247).

Thalamocortical Transmitters

The transmitter agent or agents synthesized by thalamocortical relay cells and used at their synapses in the cerebral cortex have not been positively identified. Iontophoretic studies have indicated that acetylcholine can excite certain populations of neurons in the cerebral cortex. The effect seems to be greatest on those of layer V, including pyramidal tract cells (37,137). Neurons in other layers are unaffected or may even be inhibited by the application of acetylcholine (188). The excitatory amino acids such as glutamate, aspartate, and certain others seem to have a nonspecific excitatory effect on all cortical neurons (40). There is no compelling reason for assuming that these or acetylcholine may be the transmitter released by thalamocortical relay cells.

In the visual cortex and in some other areas as well, acetylcholinesterase is concentrated in the middle layers in a laminar pattern that may be coextensive with that of the main zone of termination of thalamocortical axons (62,136). The enzymatic activity, however, does not disappear after thalamic lesions, perhaps implying that it is not directly associated with the thalamocortical axon terminals (62). Nicotinic cholinergic receptor sites are found in a moderate concentration in layers I, V, and VI of the rat cortex (107). The distribution does not coincide with the terminations of thalamocortical fibers (266). Muscarinic sites, perhaps present in greater numbers, are found in two strata (208,254) in a pattern that does resemble the distribution of thalamocortical fibers. In the experiments of Wamsley et al. (254), the presumed high-affinity sites in layer IV disappeared after pretreatment with carbachol which blocked the binding of the antagonist [³H]-*N*-methylscopolamine. In the other study, Rotter et al. (208) described binding of [³H]propylbenzilylcholine mustard in layers II and III rather than in layer IV, but their photomicrographs suggest localization in layer IV as well. However, apart from similarities of this sort, there is again no particularly compelling evidence to suggest that the cholinergic input to the cerebral cortex arises in the thalamus.

Role of the Reticular Nucleus

The connectional organization and the GABAergic neurons of the reticular nucleus have already been mentioned. The significance of the high density of acetylcholinesterase staining and α-bungarotoxin binding in the reticular nucleus, also mentioned above, has not been determined, although it has been reported that iontophoretically applied acetylcholine will inhibit reticular nucleus cells (15).

For many years, the reticular nucleus has been assumed to play a major role in modulating the activities of thalamocortical relay cells. Low-frequency electrical stimulation of a number of forebrain structures, e.g., the caudate nucleus, subcortical white matter, or certain dorsal thalamic nuclei, leads at very short latency to prolonged, high-frequency burst discharges in the neurons of the dorsal thalamic nuclei; the temporal characteristics of these IPSPs are very similar to those of the EPSPs in the reticular nucleus neurons (65,194,219). Rhythmic burst discharges occur naturally in the dorsal thalamus, either spontaneously or following peripheral stimulation, under barbiturate anesthesia and during certain phases of the sleep cycle (235). Many, though not all (8), workers consider that rhythmic inhibition emanating from the reticular nucleus in response to thalamocortical and/or corticothalamic excitation of the reticular nucleus may be the cause of the rhythmicity of the discharges. From the effects of iontophoretically applied bicuculline, there is reason to believe that GABA may be involved in the generation of the prolonged IPSPs that occur in the thalamic neurons following their excitation by afferent volleys or by cortical stimulation (41).

The recent anatomical and immunocytochemical findings on the reticular nucleus are all in keeping with a scheme that envisages GABAergic reticular nucleus cells activated by collaterals of thalamocortical, thalamostriate, corticothalamic, or pallidothalamic axons passing through the nucleus, followed by an inhibitory effect by the reticular axons on relay cells of the underlying dorsal thalamic nuclei. This may serve as a gate in the traffic between dorsal thalamus and the rest of the forebrain. The nature of the interactions that the reticulothalamic terminals might have with the intrinsic dorsal thalamic interneurons (126) has not been elucidated.

The Role of Corticothalamic Fibers

Organization

Corticothalamic axons return to every thalamic nucleus. Any thalamic nucleus projecting to a particular cortical area or areas will receive fibers back from that area or areas. This means that most cortical areas will return corticothalamic fibers to at least two thalamic nuclei: to the principal relay nucleus and to the nucleus or nuclei providing diffuse thalamocortical projections. In the cat visual system, for example, corticothalamic axons to the A laminae of the lateral geniculate nucleus come only from areas 17 and 18, whereas those to the C laminae and to the lateral posterior nucleus come from areas 17, 18, and 19 (252). Corticothalamic fibers from the somatic sensory cortex return to both the ventroposterior nucleus and the intralaminar nuclei (123). Even the hippocampal formation can be brought into this reciprocal scheme, for those thalamic nuclei such as the anterodorsal and the medioventral (reuniens) that project to the hippocampal formation receive fibers from it via the fornix (91,224,243,268).

Corticothalamic axons arise from pyramidal or modified pyramidal cells in layers V and VI of the cerebral cortex (73,122,151). Those arising in layer VI (Fig. 13) project to the principal relay nucleus, and, in the case of the monkey lateral geniculate nucleus, deeper layer VI cells project to the magnocellular laminae, and more superficial layer VI cells to the parvocellular laminae (151). The corticothalamic projection to the principal relay nucleus exactly reciprocates the thalamocortical (Fig. 13). So precise is the organization that the distribution of corticothalamic fibers can be used to map the topography in the thalamocortical projection (123). The layer V corticothalamic cells project to the intralaminar nuclei or to another nucleus of origin of the diffuse projection (30,73,151).

In the thalamus, corticothalamic axons end on the more distal parts of the dendrites of relay cells and interneurons (121,178) (Fig. 10). The synapses, of which there are large numbers, have the morphological features of excitatory synapses in

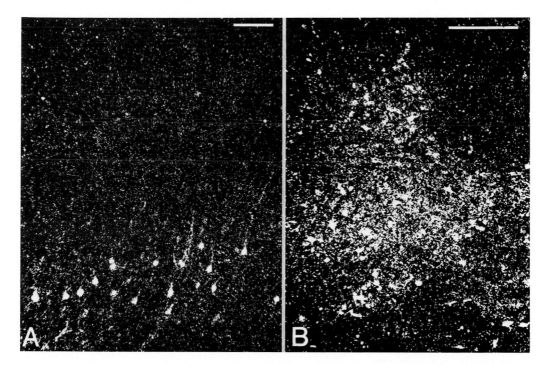

FIG. 13. A: Retrograde labeling of corticothalamic cell somata in layer VI of the cerebral cortex of a monkey following injection of [³H]-ᴅ-aspartate in the ventroposterior nucleus of the thalamus. (From unpublished work of S. H. C. Hendry and E. G. Jones.) **B:** Exact correspondence of corticothalamic axon terminations *(fine dots)* and thalamocortical projection cells *(large dots)* demonstrated by a combined injection of ³H-amino acids and horseradish peroxidase at the same small focus in the cerebral cortex of a rat. *Bars,* 100 μm. (From Jones, ref. 113, with permission.)

other sites: spherical synaptic vesicles and asymmetric membrane contacts. The parent axons are rather thin, though the latency of antidromic response of corticothalamic cells to stimulation in the vicinity of the lateral geniculate nucleus can vary considerably (72,87,228).

Function

Corticothalamic cells in the visual cortex have been described as receiving monosynaptic inputs from the thalamus and having simple receptive fields (87). They have also been described as having large, complex receptive fields (72), implying convergent input from other cortical neurons. Possibly, both types of input occur.

Corticothalamic stimulation has been variously described as causing facilitation or inhibition of the passage of an afferent volley through a relay nucleus, and both EPSPs and IPSPs have been described in relay neurons following cortical stimulation (7,23,106,125,199,228,255). Some workers have reported the effect as weak and best demonstrated when synaptic transmission is impaired by fatigue; others have regarded it as powerful and long-lasting.

Given the terminations of corticothalamic axons on relay neurons and on interneurons, as well as on the inhibitory cells of the reticular nucleus, it is not surprising that such varied electrophysiological effects have been described. The net behavioral effect of corticothalamic axons is even less clear, though in the visual system there have been some interesting recent speculations about their role in mechanisms of stereoscopic vision (187,220,228).

The Transmitters

The transmitter substance involved in corticothalamic transmission has not been positively identified, but there have been a number of interesting observations regarding the possible role of glutamate or aspartate. A number of workers have suggested, mainly on biochemical grounds, that glutamate or aspartate might serve as the transmitter agent at corticostriatal and corticospinal synapses (40). Lund-Karlsson and Fonnum (153) showed that within 3 days of destruction of the visual cortex in rats, the high-affinity uptake of L-glutamate and of D-aspartate was substantially reduced in the ipsilateral dorsal lateral geniculate nucleus and superior colliculus. The reductions particularly affected synaptosomal fractions. There were no obvious changes in high-affinity uptake of GABA, nor could changes in choline acetyltransferase or in

glutamic acid decarboxylase activities be detected. The effect was greatest on the high-affinity uptake of D-aspartate. However, the intrinic levels of only L-glutamate, not of L-aspartate, fell in the nucleus or colliculus following the cortical ablation, suggesting that glutamate is the transmitter at the corticothalamic and corticotectal synapses.

The D-isomer of aspartic acid is concentrated in nerve terminals by the same high-affinity uptake system as the L-forms of glutamate and aspartate. But because D-aspartate is metabolically inactive, it remains in the tissue for a relatively long period. This makes it amenable to autoradiographic localization. Other workers have now made use of this phenomenon to show that [^{3}H]-D-aspartate injected into the visual or sensory–motor cortex is particularly concentrated in pyramidal cell somata of layer VI (234). And when injected into the thalamus, it is retrogradely transported to the somata of corticothalamic neurons in layer VI (13) (Fig. 13). Though these observations by no means prove that either glutamate or aspartate is the transmitter at corticothalamic synapses, the remarkable specificity of the phenomenon deserves further study from this point of view.

Recent observations of Fitzpatrick and Diamond (62) raise some intriguing questions about the relationship of acetylcholinesterase to some but not all corticothalamic projections in the lateral geniculate nucleus. These workers showed particularly high concentrations of the enzyme in two of the seven cellular layers of the lateral geniculate nucleus of the bush baby. (Comparably high levels were observed in the parvocellular but not in the magnocellular layers of the owl monkey lateral geniculate.) The high level of enzymatic activity in these layers was unchanged following total destruction of geniculate neurons by kainic acid injections or severe transneuronal atrophy of the neurons by longstanding eye enucleation. But destruction of part of the visual cortex led to loss of the cholinesterase staining in relevant parts of the two layers (Fig. 14). These findings not only imply that the enzyme is associated with the terminals of corticothalamic axons rather than with the relay cells but also, because all layers of the lateral geniculate nucleus receive corticothalamic fibers, that the cholinesterase is associated with only one population of corticothalamic cells.

The Role of the Brainstem Reticular Formation

Electrical stimulation of the brainstem reticular formation, particularly in the vicinity of the midbrain, leads to facilitation of transmission in the

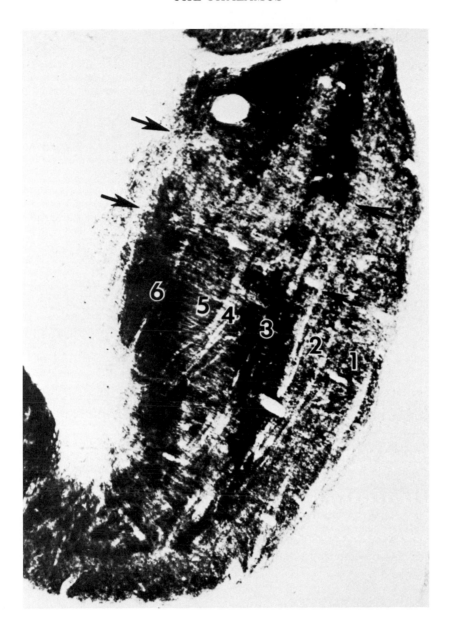

FIG. 14. Disappearance of acetylcholinesterase staining from topographically related parts of two laminae (3 and 6) of the lateral geniculate nucleus of a bush baby following a lesion of a part of the visual cortex. *Bar,* 500 μm. (From Fitzpatrick and Diamond, ref. 62, with permission.)

thalamic relay nuclei (24,50,63,227,228,260). The effect has been particularly well studied in the dorsal lateral geniculate nucleus (24,228), but comparable effects are seen elsewhere (195,236). The effect, which occurs at rather long latency (60–100 msec), seems to be brought about by a reduction of intranuclear inhibition (228). It is associated with field potentials that resemble very closely the so-

called PGO waves occuring in the pontine and mesencephalic reticular formation, the lateral geniculate nucleus, and the occipital cortex during the rapid eye movements of paradoxical sleep (24,228).

There seems to be every reason to believe that these effects on thalamic transmission during sleep and arousal are correlated with levels of neuronal activity in the brainstem reticular formation. However, identifying the pathways involved and the mode of action of presumed brainstem afferents is difficult. Routes that have been suggested include direct projections, relay via the intralaminar or reticular nuclei, and relays via the cerebral cortex. Direct projections are not particularly obvious. A small number of neurons may be retrogradely labeled in the aminergic cell groups of the dorsal nucleus of the raphe and locus ceruleus and in the parabrachial region following injections of horseradish peroxidase in various thalamic nuclei (21,141), but it is not clear whether these results indicate direct projections or merely involvement of fibers of passage destined for selected thalamic nuclei or even other sites such as the striatum and cortex (213,250). Among the sensory relay nuclei, only the gustatory relay seems to receive a dense parabrachial projection, and the ventral lateral geniculate nucleus receives a heavier projection of catecholaminergic and serotoninergic fibers than the dorsal (36,154,213,244).

Brainstem reticular effects can be demonstrated on the intralaminar nuclei, but these do not project to the relay nuclei. It is possible that the intralaminar nuclei could exert an indirect effect on the relay nuclei via their projections to the cerebral cortex and/or thalamic reticular nucleus or even via the striatum and reticular nucleus. There have been plausible suggestions in favor of all these routes [reviewed by Singer (228) and Burke and Cole (24)]. An involvement of the thalamic reticular nucleus is appealing in view of its inhibitory projection to the dorsal thalamus and because it is inhibited by brainstem reticular stimulation. However, whether the reticular nucleus is recruited by direct projections from the brainstem reticular formation or indirectly via other structures remains an open question.

LOCALIZATION OF SOME OTHER COMPOUNDS IN THE THALAMUS

Where possible in the foregoing account, I have sought to incorporate the distribution of relevant transmitter-related compounds into the morphological description. There remain a number of other transmitter candidates and transmitter-related substances that, though localized within the thalamus, cannot for the present be provided with obvious functional correlates.

Acetylcholinesterase

The association of acetylcholinesterase staining with the distribution of some corticothalamic axons in the lateral geniculate nucleus was described above. Although, as is well known, there are strong grounds for denying that the presence of acetylcholinesterase at a site necessarily implies the existence of cholinergic transmission at that site, the differences in cholinesterase staining among the thalamic nuclei have continued to attract attention (Fig. 15). In their papers on the cholinergic reticular system of the rat forebrain, Shute and Lewis (147,225) demonstrated a dorsal tegmental system of cholinesterase-positive fibers extending from the midbrain reticular formation up through the tectum to the thalamus and possibly other forebrain areas. No cholinesterase-positive cell somata were observed in the thalamus, but dense neuropil staining was demonstrated in the ventral lateral geniculate nucleus, in the whole intralaminar system, and in the anteroventral nucleus, with less dense staining in the reticular nucleus, dorsal lateral, and medial geniculate nuclei, and in certain nuclei of the lateral and ventral complexes. Most of the staining of the thalamus disappeared after destruction of the midbrain reticular formation (the so-called nucleus cuneiformis). Lewis and Shute (147) considered that the anterior thalamic nuclei, in receiving inputs from the hippocampus and projecting to cortex on the medial surface of the cerebral hemisphere, completed a cholinergic limbic circuit.

In 1974, Jacobowitz and Palkovits (108) confirmed the observations of Shute and Lewis in the rat but, again, found no cholinesterase-positive cell bodies in the thalamus. Parent and Butcher (183), though agreeing in most respects with the other authors, reported that the anterodorsal, not the anteroventral, thalamic nucleus contained the highest concentration of stain and that cholinesterase-positive cell bodies were present in this and in several other thalamic nuclei. Heavier staining in the anterodorsal nuclei in the monkey was reported by Olivier et al. (180), and it appears in the rat in Fig. 15. After the anterodorsal nucleus, the anteroventral, intralaminar, reticular, and ventral lateral geniculate nuclei show the strongest staining.

The significance of these patterns of acetylcholinesterase distribution is still elusive. However, as shown recently by Graybiel and Berson (79), it may be possible to correlate them with the patterns of distribution of certain afferent fiber systems. These workers have shown that, in the lateral posterior nucleus of the cat, zones of termination of fibers from the superficial layers of the superior colliculus and pretectum are cholinesterase positive, whereas zones of termination of fibers from the visual areas of the cortex are cholinesterase negative. These observations, together with those

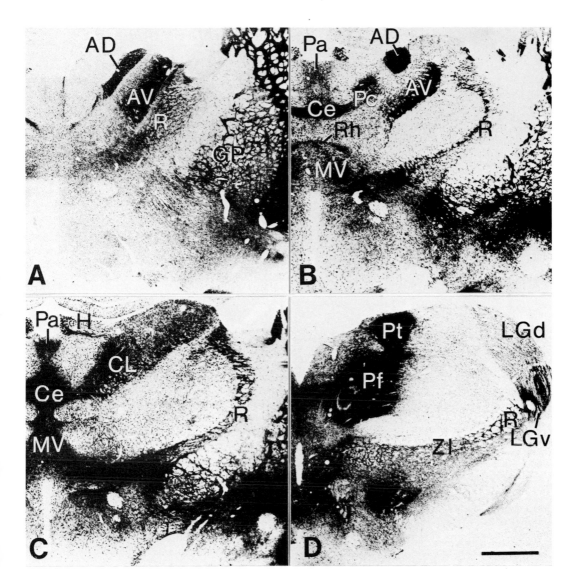

FIG. 15. A series of frontal sections in anterior (**A**) to posterior (**D**) sequence through the thalamus of a rat showing the distribution of acetylcholinesterase activity. *Bar,* 1 mm. (For abbreviations, see Fig. 1, legend.) (Photographed from material prepared by Dr. S. P. Wise.)

of Fitzpatrick and Diamond (62) on the relationship of cholinesterase staining to certain groups of corticogeniculate fibers, suggest greater specificity than has up to now been considered.

Enkephalins and Opiate Receptors

The principal concentrations of enkephalins and opiate receptors in the thalami of a number of species are in the ventral lateral geniculate nucleus and intralaminar nuclei (Fig. 16); there are also concentrations in the paraventricular nuclei of the

epithalamus, which are the only nuclei known to contain β-endorphin fibers (10,12,139,185, 214,226,256). High concentrations of enkephalins and opiate receptors reported in the "nucleus posterior thalami" of König and Klippel's atlas (132) are best regarded as being in the pretectum (cf. Fig. 1). Reports vary regarding dorsal thalamic nuclei other than the intralaminar: the mediodorsal nucleus is emphasized by some workers and parts of the ventral and anterior nuclei by others. The paratenial nucleus is said to have the highest concentration of enkephalinergic fibers (56), but no

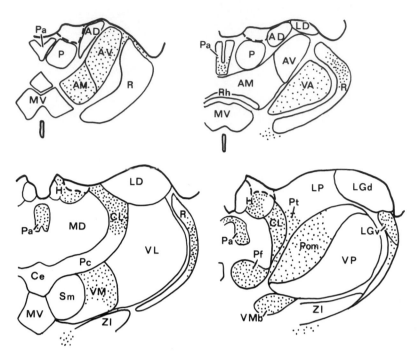

FIG. 16. Schematic figures showing immunocytochemical localization of leu- and met-enkephalin-containing fibers in the thalamus of the rat. (For abbreviations, see Fig. 1, legend.) (Redrawn from Sar et al., ref. 214.)

enkephalinergic cell bodies have been reported in any thalamic nucleus (97). None of the lesion studies carried out to demonstrate the presence or absence of enkephalins in different pathways of the forebrain and brainstem have reported effects on the thalamus. Therefore, the cells of origin of the thalamic enkephalinergic fibers remain uncertain.

The subcellular distribution of enkephalins in the thalamus is also unknown. When applied iontophoretically to thalamic neurons, enkephalin has been found to depress both spontaneous discharges and discharges in response to nociceptive stimuli. This effect is reversed by the application of the opiate antagonist naloxone (95). Whether enkephalin acts as a transmitter in its own right (233) or serves as a modulator of the actions of other transmitters remains to be determined.

Though seemingly implicated in pain pathways elsewhere in the brain, it is hard to relate the thalamic distribution of enkephalins to any of the conventional nociceptive pathways. Although fibers arising in the spinal cord and periaqueductal gray matter terminate in the intralaminar nuclei, their numbers are relatively modest and their distribution more restricted than that of enkephalin. Far more spinal fibers terminate in the ventral nuclei,

which contain neurons with receptive fields far more characteristic of spinothalamic neurons than do the intralaminar nuclei (10). Paradoxically, however, the ventral nuclei seem to contain few or no enkephalinergic fibers or opiate receptors. As Snyder and Childers (233) have pointed out, it may be necessary to view the high concentration of opiate receptors and opioid peptides in the intralaminar and mediodorsal nuclei as reflections of a role of these nuclei in affective aspects of pain appreciation. The high concentrations in the intralaminar nuclei plus the seeming involvement of these nuclei in some aspects of motor behavior and their close relationship with other motor centers, such as the globus pallidus (which contains one of the highest brain concentrations of enkephalins), might in some way also relate to the effects of opiates on motility (20).

Other Peptides

To date, virtually none of the other known neuronal or brain–gut peptides has been reported in significant amounts in the thalamus. There seems good reason to believe that some, such as substance P, which appear to exert a powerful effect in the spinal cord and peripheral nervous system and those, such as vasoactive intestinal polypeptide and cholecystokinin, which occur in neurons of the cerebral cortex are absent from the dorsal thalamus. [For recent reviews, see Emson (57), Hökfelt et al. (99), and Synder (232).] Others, such as angiotensin II, are present in a few thalamic fibers (69,196).

"Metabolic Markers"

As might be expected, increased metabolic activity has been detected with the 2-deoxy-D-glucose method in a number of thalamic nuclei under appropriate stimulus conditions (e.g., 127,221). Two other metabolic markers that have attracted some attention recently are the mitochondrial enzymes succinic acid dehydrogenase and cytochrome oxidase, which may be localized by simple histochemical techniques. To date, use of the former seems to have been mainly restricted to an examination of the maturation of the trigeminal representation in the rat ventroposterior nucleus (129). There, the enzyme clearly outlines the terminal bundles of trigeminal axons related to the mystacial vibrissae (Fig. 17).

Cytochrome oxidase shows a high resting level in many principal thalamic nuclei but appears to be much reduced in others and in the intralaminar system (Fig. 18). In the lateral geniculate nucleus of the kitten, the level of cytochrome oxidase activity declines in appropriate laminae after monocular visual deprivation (267). Each of these markers, then, seems to be associated with the terminal ram-

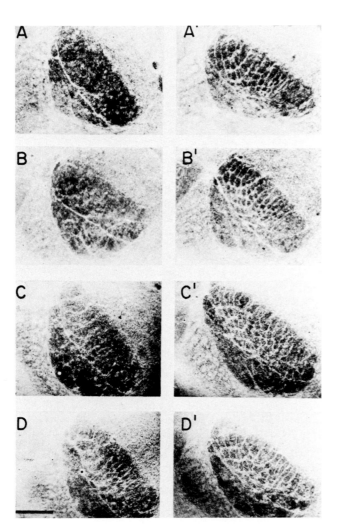

FIG. 17. Localization of succinic acid dehydrogenase activity, probably in axonal ramifications around the cell clusters (see Fig. 7) of the ventroposterior nuclei of a series of rats at 5 days of age. **Right column** is normal; **left column** is contralateral to the side of the body on which the trigeminal nerve was divided at different postnatal ages (0–3 days). *Bar,* 500 μm. (From H. Killackey and A. Shinder, ref. 129, with permission.)

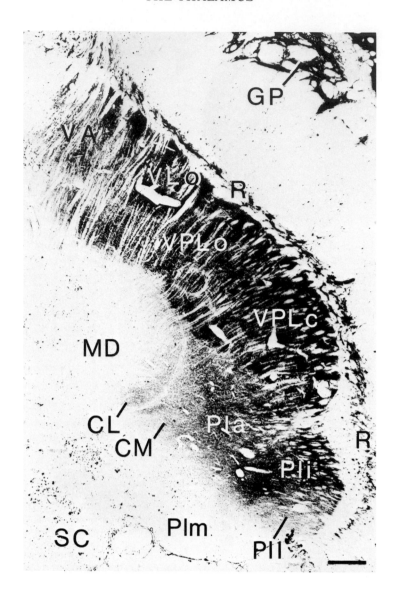

FIG. 18. Horizontal section through the thalamus of a normal monkey showing concentrations of cytochrome oxidase activity in the reticular nucleus, ventral nuclei, and inferior pulvinar nucleus, reduced activity in the intralaminar nuclei and in the anterior and lateral pulvinar nuclei, and lack of activity in other nuclei. *Bar,* 1 mm. (For abbreviations, see Fig. 1 legend.) (From unpublished work of S. H. C. Hendry and E. G. Jones.)

ifications of afferent axons, and they may prove to be useful experimental tools in the future.

ACKNOWLEDGMENTS

Personal work reported here was supported by Grant NS10526 from the National Institutes of Health, United States Public Health Service.

REFERENCES

1. Ahlsén, G., Lindström, S., and Sybirska, E. (1978): Subcortical axon collaterals of principal cells in the lateral geniculate body of the cat. *Brain Res.,* 156:106–109.
2. Aitkin, L. M., and Dunlop, C. W. (1969): Inhibition in the medial geniculate body of the cat. *Exp. Brain Res.,* 7:68–83.

3. Allman, J. M., Kaas, J. H., Lane, R. H., and Miezin, F. M. (1972): A representation of the visual field in the inferior nucleus of the pulvinar in the owl monkey *(Aotus trivirgatus). Brain Res.,* 40:291–302.

4. Andén, N. E., Dahlström, A., Fuxe, K., Larsson, K., Olsson, L., and Ungerstedt, U. (1966): Ascending monoamine neurons to the telencephalon and diencephalon. *Acta Physiol. Scand.,* 67:313–326.

5. Andersen, P., and Curtis, D. R. (1964): The excitation of thalamic neurones by acetylcholine. *Acta Physiol. Scand.,* 61:85–99.

6. Andersen, P., Eccles, J. C., and Sears, T. A. (1964): The ventro-basal nucleus of the thalamus: Types of cells, their responses and their functional organization. *J. Physiol. (Lond.),* 174:370–399.

7. Andersen, P., Junge, K., and Sveen, O. (1967): Cortico–thalamic facilitation of somatosensory impulses. *Nature,* 214:1011–1012.

8. Andersen, P., and Sears, T. A. (1964): The role of inhibition in the phasing of spontaneous thalamocortical discharge. *J. Physiol. (Lond.),* 173:459–480.

9. Andersen, R. A., Roth, G. L., Aitkin, L. M., and Merzenich, M. M. (1980): The efferent projections of the central nucleus and the pericentral nucleus of the inferior colliculus in the cat. *J. Comp. Neurol.,* 194:649–662.

10. Appelbaum, A. E., Leonard, R. B., Kenshalo, D. R., Jr., Martin, R. F., and Willis, W. D. (1979): Nuclei in which functionally identified spinothalamic tract neurons terminate. *J. Comp. Neurol.,* 188:575–585.

11. Asanuma, C., Thach, W. T., and Jones, E. G. (1980). Patterns of termination of the cerebello-thalamic pathway in the monkey. *Neurosci. Abstr.,* 6:512.

12. Atweh, S., and Kuhar, M. (1977): Autoradiographic localization of opiate receptors in rat brain. II. The brain stem. *Brain Res.,* 129:1–12.

13. Baughman, R. W., and Gilbert, C. D. (1980): Possible neurotransmitter of cells in layer 6 of the visual cortex. *Neurosci. Abstr.,* 6:671.

14. Beckstead, R. M., Domesick, V. B., and Nauta, W. J. H. (1979): Efferent connections of the substantia nigra and ventral tegmental area in the rat. *Brain Res.,* 175:191–218.

15. Ben-Ari, Y., Dingledine, R., Kanazawa, I., and Kelly, J. S. (1976): Inhibitory effects of acetylcholine on neurones in the feline nucleus reticularis thalami. *J. Physiol. (Lond.),* 261:647–671.

16. Bentivoglio, M., Macchi, G., Rossini, P., and Tempestra, E. (1978): Brain stem neurons projecting to neocortex: An HRP study in the cat. *Exp. Brain Res.,* 31:489–498.

17. Berman, A. L., and Jones, E. G. (1982): *The Thalamus and Basal Telencephalon of the Cat. A Cytoarchitectonic Atlas with Stereotaxic Coordinates.* University of Wisconsin Press, Madison.

18. Berman, N. (1977): Connections of the pretectum in the cat. *J. Comp. Neurol.,* 174:227–254.

19. Biziere, K., and Coyle, J. T. (1978): Influence of cortico–striatal afferents on striatal kainic acid neurotoxicity. *Neurosci. Lett.,* 8:303–310.

20. Bloom, F. E., Rossier, J., Battenburg, E. L. F., Bayon, A., French, E., Henriksen, S. J., Siggins, G. R., Segal, D., Browne, R., Ling, N., and Guillemin, R. (1978): β-Endorphin: Cellular localization, electrophysiological, and behavioral effects. In: *Advances in Biochemical Psychopharmacology, Vol. 1: The Endorphins,* edited by E. Costa and M. Trabucchi, pp. 89–110. Raven Press, New York.

21. Bobillier, P., Seguin, S., Petitjean, F., Salvert, D., Touret, M., and Jouvet, M. (1976): The raphe nuclei of the cat brain stem: A topographical atlas of their efferent projections as revealed by autoradiography. *Brain Res.,* 113:449–486.

22. Bullier, J., and Henry, G. H. (1980): Ordinal position and afferent input of neurons in monkey striate cortex. *J. Comp. Neurol.,* 193:913–936.

23. Burchfiel, J. L., and Duffy, F. H. (1974): Corticofugal influence upon cat thalamic ventrobasal complex. *Brain Res.,* 70:395–411.

24. Burke, W., and Cole, A. M. (1978): Extraretinal influences on the lateral geniculate nucleus. *Rev. Physiol. Biochem. Pharmacol.,* 80:106–166.

25. Burke, W., and Sefton, A. J. (1966): Discharge patterns of principal cells and interneurones in lateral geniculate nucleus of rat. *J. Physiol. (Lond.),* 187:201–212.

26. Cajal, S. Rámon y (1909–1911): *Histologie du Système Nerveux de l'Homme et des Vertébrés, Vols. 1 and 2,* translated by L. Azoulay. Maloine, Paris.

27. Carey, R. G., Fitzpatrick, D., and Diamond, I. T. (1979): Layer I of striate cortex of *Tupaia glis* and *Galago senegalensis:* Projections from thalamus and claustrum revealed by retrograde transport of horseradish peroxidase. *J. Comp. Neurol.,* 186:393–438.

28. Carpenter, M. B., Nakano, K., and Kim, R. (1976): Nigrothalamic projections in the monkey demonstrated by autoradiographic techniques. *J. Comp. Neurol.,* 165:401–415.

29. Carstens, E., and Trevino, D. L. (1978): Laminar origins of spinothalamic projections in the cat as determined by the retrograde transport of horseradish peroxidase. *J. Comp. Neurol.,* 182:151–165.

30. Catsman-Berrevoets, C. E., and Kuypers, H. G. J. M. (1978): Differential laminar distribution of corticothalamic neurons projecting to the VL and the center median. An HRP study in the cynomolgus monkey. *Brain Res.,* 154:359–365.

31. Caviness, V. S., Jr., and Frost, D. O. (1980): Tangential organizations of thalamic projections to the neocortex in the mouse. *J. Comp. Neurol.,* 194:335–368.

32. Chow, K. L. (1952): Regional degneration of the thalamic reticular nucleus following cortical ablations in monkeys. *J. Comp. Neurol.,* 92:227–240.

33. Clark, W. E. LeGros (1932): The structure and connections of the thalamus. *Brain,* 55:406–470.

34. Cleland, B. G., Dubin, M. W., and Levick, W. R. (1971): Sustained and transient neurones in the cat's retina and lateral geniculate nucleus. *J. Physiol. (Lond.),* 217:473–496.

35. Cleland, B. G., Morstyn, R., Wagner, H. G., and Levick, W. R. (1975): Long-latency retinal input to

lateral geniculate neurons of the cat. *Brain Res.*, 91:306–310.

36. Conrad, L. C. A., Leonard, C. M., and Pfaff, D. W. (1974): Connections of the median and dorsal raphe nuclei in the rat: An autoradiographic and degeneration study. *J. Comp. Neurol.*, 156:179–206.

37. Crawford, J. M. (1970): The sensitivity of cortical neurones to acidic amino acids and acetylcholine. *Brain Res.*, 17:287–296.

38. Curtis, D. R., Duggan, A. W., Felix, D., and Johnston, G. A. R. (1970): GABA, bicuculline and thalamic inhibition. *Nature*, 226:1222–1224.

39. Curtis, D. R., Duggan, A. W., Felix, D., Johnston, G. A. R., and McLennan, H. (1971): Antagonism between bicuculline and GABA in the cat brain. *Brain Res.*, 33:57–73.

40. Curtis, D. R., and Johnston, G. A. R. (1974): Amino acid transmitters in the mammalian central nervous system. *Ergeb. Physiol.*, 69:97–188.

41. Curtis, D. R., and Tebécis, A. K. (1972): Bicuculline and thalamic inhibition. *Exp. Brain Res.*, 16:210–218.

42. Dahlström, A., and Fuxe, K. (1964): Evidence for the existence of monoamine-containing neurons in the central nervous system. I. Demonstration of monoamines in the cell bodies of brainstem neurons. *Acta Physiol. Scand. [Suppl.]*, 232:1–55.

43. Davies, L. P., and Johnston, G. A. R. (1976): Uptake and release of D- and L-aspartate by rat brain. *J. Neurochem.*, 26:1007–1014.

44. Davies, P., and Verth, A. H. (1978): Regional distribution of muscarinic acetylcholine receptor in normal and Alzheimer's-type dementia brains. *Brain Res.*, 138:385–392.

45. DiChiara, G., Porceddu, M. L., Morelli, M., Mulas, M. L., and Gessa, G. L. (1979): Evidence for a GABAergic projection from the substantia nigra to the ventromedial thalamus and to the superior colliculus of the rat. *Brain Res.*, 176:273–284.

46. Divac, I. (1975): Magnocellular nuclei of the basal forebrain project to neocortex, brainstem, and olfactory bulb: Review of some functional correlates. *Brain Res.*, 93:385–398.

47. Divac, I., Fonnum, F., and Storm-Mathisen, J. (1977): High affinity uptake of glutamate in terminals of corticostriatal axons. *Nature*, 266:377–378.

48. Domesick, V. B. (1969): Projections from the cingulate cortex in the rat. *Brain Res.*, 12:296–320.

49. Donoghue, J. P., Kerman, K. L., and Ebner, F. E. (1979): Evidence for two organizational plans within the somatic sensory–motor cortex of the rat. *J. Comp. Neurol.*, 183:647–664.

50. Doty, R. W., Wilson, P. D., Bartlett, J. R., and Pecci-Saavedra, J. (1973): Mesencephalic control of lateral geniculate nucleus in primates. I. Electrophysiology. *Exp. Brain Res.*, 18:189–203.

51. Dreher, B., Fukada, Y., and Rodieck, R. W. (1976): Identification, classification and anatomical segregation of cells with x-like and y-like properties in the lateral geniculate nucleus of Old World primates. *J. Physiol. (Lond.)*, 258:433–452.

52. Dubin, M. W., and Cleland, B. G. (1977): The organization of visual inputs to interneurons of the lateral geniculate nucleus of the cat. *J. Neurophysiol.*, 40:410–427.

53. Duggan, A. W., and Hall, J. G. (1975): Inhibition of thalamic neurones by acetylcholine. *Brain Res.*, 100:445–449.

54. Duggan, A. W., and McLennan, H. (1971): Bicuculline and inhibition in the thalamus. *Brain Res.*, 25:188–191.

55. Edwards, S. B., and deOlmos, J. S. (1976): Autoradiographic studies of the projections of the midbrain reticular formation: Ascending projections of nucleus cuneiformis. *J. Comp. Neurol.*, 165:417–432.

56. Elde, R., Hökfelt, T., Johansson, O., and Terenius, L. (1976): Immunohistochemical studies using antibodies to leucine-enkephalin: Initial observations on the nervous system of the rat. *Neuroscience*, 1:349–351.

57. Emson, P. C. (1979): Peptides as neurotransmitter candidates in the mammalian CNS. *Prog. Neurobiol.*, 13:61–116.

58. Eysel, V. T. (1976): Quantitative studies of intracellular postsynaptic potentials in the lateral geniculate nucleus of the cat with respect to optic tract stimulus response latencies. *Exp. Brain Res.*, 25:469–486.

59. Famiglietti, E. V., Jr., and Peters, A. (1972): The synaptic glomerulus and the intrinsic neuron in the dorsal lateral geniculate nucleus of the cat. *J. Comp. Neurol.*, 144:285–334.

60. Faull, R. L. M., and Mehler, W. R. (1978): The cells of origin of nigrotectal, nigrothalamic and nigrostriatal projections in the rat. *Neuroscience*, 3:989–1002.

61. Ferster, D., and LeVay, S. (1978): The axonal arborizations of lateral geniculate neurons in the striate cortex of the cat. *J. Comp. Neurol.*, 182:923–944.

62. Fitzpatrick, D., and Diamond, I. T. (1980): Distribution of acetylcholinesterase in the geniculo striate system of *Galago senegalensis* and *Aotus trivirgatus*: Evidence for the origin of the reaction product in the lateral geniculate body. *J. Comp. Neurol.*, 194:703–720.

63. Foote, W. E., Maciewicz, R. J., and Mordes, J. P. (1974): Effect of midbrain raphe and lateral mesencephalic stimulation on spontaneous and evoked activity in the lateral geniculate of the cat. *Exp. Brain Res.*, 19:124–130.

64. Friedman, D. P., and Jones, E. G. (1980): Focal projection of electrophysiologically defined groupings of thalamic cells on the monkey somatic sensory cortex. *Brain Res.*, 191:249–252.

65. Frigyesi, T. L., and Schwartz, R. (1972): Cortical control of thalamic sensorimotor relay activities in the cat and the squirrel monkey. In: *Corticothalamic Projections and Sensorimotor Activities*, edited by T. L. Frigyesi, E. Rinvik, and M. D. Yahr, pp. 161–195. Raven Press, New York.

66. Frost, D. O., and Caviness, V. S., Jr. (1980): Radial organization of thalamic projections to the neocortex in the mouse. *J. Comp. Neurol.*, 194:369–394.

67. Fukuda, Y., and Iwama, K. (1971): Reticular inhibition of internuncial cells in the rat lateral geniculate body. *Brain Res.*, 35:107–118.

68. Fukuda, Y., and Stone, J. (1974): Retinal distribution and central projections of Y-, X- and W-cells of the cat's retina. *J. Neurophysiol.*, 37:749–772.

69. Fuxe, K., Ganten, D., Hökfelt, T., and Bohne, P. (1976): Immunohistochemical evidence for the existence of angiotensin II-containing nerve terminals in the brain and spinal cord in the rat. *Neurosci. Lett.*, 2:229–234.

70. Ganchrow, D. (1978): Intratrigeminal and thalamic projections of nucleus caudalis in the squirrel monkey *(Saimiri sciureus):* A degeneration and autoradiographic study. *J. Comp. Neurol.*, 178:281–312.

71. Gatass, R., Oswaldo-Cruz, E., and Sousa, A. P. B. (1978): Visuotopic organization of the cebus pulvinar: A double representation of the contralateral hemifield. *Brain Res.*, 152:1–16.

72. Gilbert, C. D. (1977): Laminar differences in receptive field properties of cells in cat primary visual cortex. *J. Physiol. (Lond.)*, 268:391–422.

73. Gilbert, C. D., and Kelly, J. P. (1975): The projections of cells in different layers of the cat's visual cortex. *J. Comp. Neurol.*, 163:81–105.

74. Gilbert, C. D., and Wiesel, T. N. (1979): Morphology and intracortical projections of functionally characterized neurones in the cat visual cortex. *Nature*, 280:120–125.

75. Godfraind, J.-M. (1975): Micro-electrophoretic studies in the cat pulvinar region: Effect of acetylcholine. *Exp. Brain Res.*, 22:243–254.

76. Goldman, P. S., and Nauta, W. J. H. (1977): An intricately patterned prefronto–caudate projection in the rhesus moneky. *J. Comp. Neurol.*, 171:369–386.

77. Graham, J. (1977): An autoradiographic study of the efferent connections of the superior colliculus in the cat. *J. Comp. Neurol.*, 173:629–654.

78. Graybiel, A. M. (1977): Direct and indirect preoculomotor pathways of the brainstem: An autoradiographic study of the pontine reticular formation in the cat. *J. Comp. Neurol.*, 175:37–78.

79. Graybiel, A. M., and Berson, D. M. (1980): Histochemical identification and afferent connections of subdivisions in the lateralis posterior–pulvinar complex and related thalamic nuclei in the cat. *Neuroscience*, 5:1175–1238.

80. Graybiel, A. M., and Ragsdale, C. W., Jr. (1978): Histochemically distinct compartments in the striatum of human, monkey and cat demonstrated by acetylthiocholinesterase staining. *Proc. Natl. Acad. Sci. U.S.A.*, 75:5723–5726.

81. Guillery, R. W. (1966): A study of Golgi preparations from the dorsal lateral geniculate nucleus of the adult cat. *J. Comp. Neurol.*, 128:21–50..

82. Haldeman, S., and McLennan, H. (1973): The action of two inhibitors of glutamic acid uptake upon amino acid-induced and synaptic excitations of thalamic neurones. *Brain Res.*, 63:123–130.

83. Hale, P. T., and Sefton, A. J. (1978): A comparison of the visual and electrical response properties of cells in dorsal and ventral lateral geniculate nuclei. *Brain Res.*, 153:591–595.

84. Hamilton, B. L. (1973): Projections of the nuclei of the periaqueductal gray matter in the cat. *J. Comp. Neurol.*, 152:45–58.

85. Harding, B. N., and Powell, T. P. S. (1977): An electron microscopic study of the centre-median and ventrolateral nuclei of the thalamus in the monkey. *Phil. Trans. R. Soc. Lond. [Biol.]*, 279:357–412.

86. Harting, J. K., Huerta, M. F., Frankfurter, A. J., Strominger, N. L., and Royce, J. G. (1980): Ascending pathways from the monkey superior colliculus: An autoradiographic analysis. *J. Comp. Neurol.*, 192:853–882.

87. Harvey, A. R. (1978): Characteristics of corticothalamic neurons in area 17 of the cat. *Neurosci. Lett.*, 7:177–181.

88. Hazlett, J. C., Dutta, C. R., and Fox, C. A. (1976): The neurons in the centromedian-parafascicular complex of the monkey *(Macaca mulatta):* A Golgi study. *J. Comp. Neurol.*, 168:41–74.

89. Heimer, L. (1972): The olfactory connections of the diencephalon in the rat: An experimental light- and electron-microscopic study with special emphasis on the problem of terminal degeneration. *Brain Behav. Evol.*, 6:484–523.

90. Hendry, S. H. C., Jones, E. G., and Graham, J. (1979): Thalamic relay nuclei for cerebellar and certain related fiber systems in the cat. *J. Comp. Neurol.*, 185:679–714.

91. Herkenham, M. (1978): The connections of the nucleus reuniens thalami: Evidence for a direct thalamo–hippocampal pathway in the rat. *J. Comp. Neurol.*, 177:589–610.

92. Herkenham, M. (1980): Laminar organization of thalamic projections to the rat neocortex. *Science*, 207:532–534.

93. Herkenham, M., and Pert, C. (1980): *In vitro* autoradiography of opiate receptors in rat brain suggests loci of "opiatergic" pathways. *Proc. Natl. Acad. Sci. U.S.A.*, 77:5532–5536.

94. Hiley, C. R., and Burgen, A. S. V. (1974): The distribution of muscarinic receptor sites in the nervous system of the dog. *J. Neurochem.*, 22:159–162.

95. Hill, R. G., Pepper, C. M., and Mitchell, J. F. (1976): Depression of nociceptive and other neurones in the brain by iontophoretically applied met-enkephalin. *Nature*, 262:604–606.

96. Hoffman, K.-P., Stone, J., and Sherman, S. M. (1972): Relay of receptive-field properties in dorsal lateral geniculate nucleus of the cat. *J. Neurophysiol.*, 35:518–531.

97. Hökfelt, T., Elde, R., Johansson, O., Terenius, L., and Stein, L. (1977): The distribution of enkephalin-immunoreactive cell bodies in the rat central nervous system. *Neurosci. Lett.*, 5:25–31.

98. Hökfelt, T., Fuxe, K., Goldstein, M., and Johansson, O. (1974): Immunohistochemical evidence for the existence of adrenaline neurons in the rat brain. *Brain Res.*, 66:235–251.

99. Hökfelt, T., Johansson, O., Ljungdahl, Å., Lund-

berg, J. M., and Schultzberg, M. (1980): Peptidergic neurones. *Nature* 284:515–521.

100. Houser, C. R., Vaughn, J. E., Barber, R. P., and Roberts, E. (1980): GABA neurons are the major cell type of the nucleus reticularis thalami. *Brain Res.,* 200:341–354.

101. Hubel, D. H. (1975): An autoradiographic study of the retino–cortical projections in the tree shrew *(Tupaia glis). Brain Res.,* 96:41–50.

102. Hubel, D. H., and Wiesel, T. N. (1962): Receptive fields, binocular interaction and functional architecture in the cat's visual cortex. *J. Physiol. (Lond.),* 160:106–154.

103. Hubel, D. H., and Wiesel, T. N. (1972): Laminar and columnar distribution of geniculo–cortical fibers in the macaque monkey. *J. Comp. Neurol.,* 146:421–450.

104. Hubel, D. H., and Wiesel, T. N. (1974): Uniformity of monkey striate cortex: A parallel relationship between field size, scatter and magnification factor. *J. Comp. Neurol.,* 158:295–306.

105. Hubel, D. H., and Wiesel, T. N. (1977): Functional architecture of macaque monkey visual cortex. *Proc. R. Soc. Lond. [Biol.],* 198:1–59.

106. Hull, E. M. (1968): Corticofugal influence in the macaque lateral geniculate nucleus. *Vis. Res.* 8:1285–1298.

107. Hunt, S. P., and Schmidt, J. (1978): Some observations on the binding patterns of α-bungarotoxin in the central nervous system of the rat. *Brain Res.,* 157:213–232.

108. Jacobowitz, D. M., and Palkovits, M. (1974): Topographic atlas of catecholamine- and acetylcholinesterase-containing neurons in the rat brain. I. Forebrain (telencephalon, diencephalon). *J. Comp. Neurol.,* 157:13–28.

109. Jacobson, S., and Trojanowski, J. Q. (1975): Amygdaloid projections to the prefrontal granular cortex in rhesus monkey demonstrated with horseradish peroxidase. *Brain Res.,* 100:132–139.

110. Jones, B. E., and Moore, R. Y. (1977): Ascending projections of the locus coeruleus in the rat. II. Autoradiographic study. *Brain Res.,* 127:23–53.

111. Jones, E. G. (1975): Some aspects of the organization of the thalamic reticular complex. *J. Comp. Neurol.,* 162:285–308.

112. Jones, E. G. (1975): Possible determinants of the degree of retrograde neuronal labeling with horseradish peroxidase. *Brain Res.,* 85:249–253.

113. Jones, E. G. (1981): Functional subdivision and synaptic organization of the mammalian thalamus. In: *International Review of Physiology; Neurophysiology IV,* edited by R. Porter, pp. 173–245. University Park Press, Baltimore.

114. Jones, E. G., and Burton, H. (1974): Cytoarchitecture and somatic sensory connectivity of thalamic nuclei other than the ventrobasal complex in the cat. *J. Comp. Neurol.,* 154:395–432.

115. Jones, E. G., and Burton, H. (1976): A projection from the medial pulvinar to the amygdala in primates. *Brain Res.,* 194:142–147.

116. Jones, E. G., and Burton, H. (1976): Areal differences in the distribution of thalamo–cortical fibers in cortical fields of the insular, parietal and temporal regions of primates. *J. Comp. Neurol.,* 168:197–248.

117. Jones, E. G., Burton, H., Saper, C. B., and Swanson, L. (1976): Midbrain, diencephalic and cortical relationships of the basal nucleus of Meynert and related structures in primates. *J. Comp. Neurol.,* 167:385–420.

118. Jones, E. G., Coulter, J. D., Burton, H., and Porter, R. (1977): Cells of origin and terminal distribution of corticostriatal fibers arising in the sensory–motor cortex of monkeys. *J. Comp. Neurol.,* 173:53–80.

119. Jones, E. G., and Leavitt, R. Y. (1974): Retrograde axonal transport and the demonstration of non-specific projections to the cerebral cortex and striatum from thalamic intralaminar nuclei in the rat, cat and monkey. *J. Comp. Neurol.,* 154:349–378.

120. Jones, E. G., and Powell, T. P. S. (1969): Electron microscopy of synaptic glomeruli in the thalamic relay nuclei of the cat. *Proc. R. Soc. Lond. [Biol.],* 172:153–171.

121. Jones, E. G., and Powell, T. P. S. (1969): An electron microscopic study of the mode of termination of corticothalamic fibers in the thalamic relay nuclei of the cat. *Proc. R. Soc. Lond. [Biol.],* 172:173–185.

122. Jones, E. G., and Wise, S. P. (1977): Size, laminar and columnar distribution of efferent cells in the sensory–motor cortex of primates. *J. Comp. Neurol.,* 175:391–438.

123. Jones, E. G., Wise, S. P., and Coulter, J. D. (1979): Differential thalamic relationships of sensory–motor and parietal cortical fields in monkeys. *J. Comp. Neurol.,* 183:833–882.

124. Kalil, K. (1978): Patch-like termination of thalamic fibers in the putamen of the rhesus monkey: An autoradiographic study. *Brain Res.,* 140:333–339.

125. Kalil, R. E., and Chase, R. (1970): Corticofugal influence on activity of lateral geniculate neurons in the cat. *J. Neurophysiol.,* 33:459–474.

126. Kelly, J. S., Godfraind, J. M., and Maruyama, S. (1979): The presence and nature of inhibition in small slices of the dorsal lateral geniculate nucleus of the rat and cat incubated *in vitro. Brain Res.,* 168:388–392.

127. Kennedy, C., Des Rosiers, M. H., Jehle, J. W., Reivich, M., Sharp, F., and Sokoloff, L. (1975): Mapping of functional neural pathways by autoradiographic survey of local metabolic rate with [^{14}C]deoxyglucose. *Science,* 187:850–853.

128. Kievit, J., and Kuypers, H. G. J. M. (1975): Basal forebrain and hypothalamic connections to frontal and parietal cortex in the rhesus monkey. *Science,* 187:660–662.

129. Killackey, H., and Shinder, A. (1981): Central correlates of peripheral pattern alterations in the trigeminal system of the rat. II. The effect of nerve section. *Dev. Brain Res.,* 1:121–126.

130. Kim, R., Nakano, K., Jayaraman, A., and Carpenter, M. B. (1976): Projections of the globus pallidus and adjacent structures: An autoradiographic study in the monkey. *J. Comp. Neurol.,* 169:263–290.

131. Kobayashi, R. M., Palkovits, M., Hruska, R. E.,

Rothschild, R., and Yamamura, H. I. (1978): Regional distribution of muscarinic cholinergic receptors in the rat brain. *Brain Res.*, 154:13–23.

132. König, J. F. R., and Kippel, R. M. (1963): *The Rat Brain.* Williams & Wilkins, Baltimore.

133. Kotchabhakdi, N., Rinvik, E., Yingcharoen, Y., and Walberg, F. (1980): Afferent projections to the thalamus from the perihypoglossal nuclei. *Brain Res.*, 187:457–461.

134. Krettek, J. E., and Price, J. L. (1977): Projections from the amygdaloid complex to the cerebral cortex and thalamus in the rat and cat. *J. Comp. Neurol.*, 172:687–722.

135. Krettek, J. E., and Price, J. L. (1977): The cortical projections of the mediodorsal nucleus and adjacent thalamic nuclei in the rat. *J. Comp. Neurol.*, 171:157–191.

136. Kristt, D. A. (1979): Development of neocortical circuitry: Histochemical localization of acetylcholinesterase in relation to the cell layers of rat somatosensory cortex. *J. Comp. Neurol.*, 186:1–16.

137. Krnjević, K., and Phillis, J. W. (1963): Acetyl choline-sensitive cells in the cerebral cortex. *J. Physiol. (Lond.)*, 166:296–327.

138. Kuypers, H. G. J. M., Kievit, J., and Groen-Klevant, A. C. (1974): Retrograde axonal transport of horseradish peroxidase in rat's forebrain. *Brain Res.*, 67:211–218.

139. LaMotte, C. C., Snowman, A., Pert, C. B., and Snyder, S. N. (1978): Opiate receptor binding in rhesus monkey brain: Association with limbic structures. *Brain Res.*, 155:374–379.

140. Larsen, K. D., and McBride, R. L. (1979): The organization of feline entopeduncular nucleus projections: Anatomical studies. *J. Comp. Neurol.*, 184:293–308.

141. Leger, L., Skai, K., Salvert, D., Touret, M., and Jouvet, M. (1975): Delineation of dorsal lateral geniculate afferents from the cat brain stem as visualized by the horseradish peroxidase technique. *Brain Res.*, 93:490–496.

142. Lehmann, J., Nagy, J. I., Atmadja, S., and Fibiger, H. C. (1980): The nucleus basalis magnocellularis: The origin of a cholinergic projection to the neocortex of the rat. *Neuroscience*, 5:1161–1174.

143. LeVay, S., and Ferster, D. (1977): Relay cell classes in the lateral geniculate nucleus of the cat and the effects of visual deprivation. *J. Comp. Neurol.*, 172:563–584.

144. LeVay, S., and Ferster, D. (1979): Proportion of interneurons in the cat's lateral geniculate nucleus. *Brain Res.*, 164:304–308.

145. LeVay, S., and Gilbert, C. D. (1976): Laminar patterns of geniculocortical projection in the cat. *Brain Res.*, 113:1–20.

146. LeVay, S., and Sherk, H. (1980): Visual area in cat claustrum: Structure, receptive fields and outputs. *Neurosci. Abstr.*, 6:482.

147. Lewis, P. R., and Shute, C. C. D. (1967): The cholinergic limbic system: Projection to hippocampal formation, medial cortex, nuclei of the ascending cholinergic reticular system, and the subfornical organ and supra-optic crest. *Brain*, 90:521–540.

148. Lin, C.-S., Katz, K. E., and Sherman, S. M. (1978): Percentage of relay cells in the cat's lateral geniculate nucleus. *Brain Res.*, 131:167–173.

149. Lindvall, O., and Björklund, A. (1974): The organization of the ascending catecholamine neuron systems in the rat brain as revealed by the glyoxylic acid fluorescence method. *Acta Physiol. Scand. [Suppl.]*, 412:1–48.

150. Lindvall, O., Björklund, A., Moore, R. Y., and Stenevi, U. (1974): Mesencephalic dopamine neurons projecting to neocortex. *Brain Res.*, 81:325–331.

151. Lund, J. S., Lund, R. D., Hendrickson, A. E., Bunt, A. H., and Fuchs, A. F. (1975): The origin of efferent pathways from the primary visual cortex, area 17, of the macaque monkey as shown by retrograde transport of horseradish peroxidase. *J. Comp. Neurol.*, 164:287–304.

152. Lund, R. D., and Webster, K. E. (1967): Thalamic afferents from the spinal cord and trigeminal nuclei: An experimental anatomical study in the rat. *J. Comp. Neurol.*, 130:313–328.

153. Lund-Karlsen, R., and Fonnum, F. (1978): Evidence for glutamate as a neurotransmitter in the corticofugal fibres to the dorsal lateral geniculate body and the superior colliculus in rats. *Brain Res.*, 151:457–468.

154. McBride, R. L., and Sutin, J. (1975): Projections of the locus coeruleus and adjacent pontine tegmentum in the cat. *J. Comp. Neurol.*, 165:265–284.

155. McCance, I., Phillis, J. W., and Westerman, R. A. (1968): The pharmacology of acetylcholine excitation of thalamic neurones. *Br. J. Pharmacol. Chemother.*, 32:652–662.

156. McGeer, P. L., McGeer, E. G., Scherer, U., and Singh, K. (1977): A glutamatergic cortico–striatal path? *Brain Res.*, 128:369–373.

157. McIlwain, J. T., and Creutzfeldt, O. D. (1967): Microelectrode study of synaptic excitation and inhibition in the lateral geniculate nucleus of the cat. *J. Neurophysiol.*, 30:1–21.

158. Macchi, G., Bentivoglio, M., Miniciacchi, D., and Molinari, M. (1981): The organization of claustro-neocortical projections in the cat studied by means of the HRP retrograde axonal transport. *J. Comp. Neurol.*, 195:681–695.

159. Macchi, G., Quattrini, A., Chinzari, P., Marchesi, G., and Capocchi, G. (1975) Quantitative data on cell loss and cellular atrophy of intralaminar nuclei following cortical and subcortical lesions. *Brain Res.*, 89:43–59.

160. Marshall, K. C., and McLennan, H. (1972): The synaptic activation of neurones of the feline ventrolateral thalamic nucleus: Possible cholinergic mechanisms. *Exp. Brain Res.*, 15:472–483.

161. Mason, R. (1978): Functional organization in the cat's pulvinar complex. *Exp. Brain Res.*, 31:51–66.

162. Mehler, W. R. (1966): Further notes on the center median nucleus of Luys. In: *The Thalamus*, edited by D. P. Purpura and M. D. Yahr, pp. 109–122. Columbia University Press, New York.

163. Mesulam, M.-M., and Van Hoesen, G. W. (1976): Acetylcholinesterase-rich projections from the

basal forebrain of the rhesus monkey to neocortex. *Brain Res.*, 109:152–157.

164. Montero, V. M., Guilllery, R. W., and Woolsey, C. N. (1977): Retinotopic organization within the thalamic reticular nucleus demonstrated by a double label autoradiographic technique. *Brain Res.*, 138:407–421.

165. Montero, V. M., and Scott, G. L. (1980): Synaptic terminals in dorsal lateral geniculate nucleus from neurons of the thalamic reticular nucleus: An electron microscope autoradiographic study. *Neurosci. Abstr.*, 6:838.

166. Mooney, R. D., Dubin, M. W., and Rusoff, A. C. (1979): Interneuron circuits in the lateral geniculate nucleus of monocularly deprived cats. *J. Comp. Neurol.*, 187:533–543.

167. Moore, R. Y., and Bloom, F. E. (1978): Central catecholamine neuron systems: Anatomy and physiology of the dopamine systems. *Annu. Rev. Neurosci.*, 1:129–169.

168. Moore, R. Y., and Bloom, F. E. (1979): Central catecholamine neuron systems: Anatomy and physiology of the norepinephrine and epinephrine systems. *Annu. Rev. Neurosci.*, 2:113–168.

169. Morest, D. K. (1964): The neuronal architecture of the medial geniculate body of the cat. *J. Anat*, 98:611–630.

170. Morest, D. K. (1975): Synaptic relationships of Golgi type II cells in the medial geniculate body of the cat. *J. Comp. Neurol.*, 162:157–194.

171. Nauta, H. J. W., Pritz, M. B., and Lasek, R. J. (1974): Afferents to the rat caudatoputamen studied with horseradish peroxidase: An evaluation of a retrograde neuroanatomical research method. *Brain Res.*, 67:219–238.

172. Nauta, W. J. H. (1962): Neural associations of the amygdaloid complex in the monkey. *Brain Res.*, 85:505–520.

173. Nauta, W. J. H., and Kuypers, H. G. J. M. (1958): Some ascending pathways in the brain stem reticular formation. In: *Reticular Formation of the Brain,* edited by H. H. Jasper, L. D. Proctor, R. S. Knighton, W. C. Noshay, and R. T. Costello, pp. 3–30. Little, Brown, Boston.

174. Nelson, P. G., and Erulkar, S. D. (1963): Synaptic mechanisms of excitation and inhibition in the central auditory pathway. *J. Neurophysiol.*, 26:908–923.

175. Niimi, K., Niimi, M., and Okada, Y. (1978): Thalamic afferents to the limbic cortex in the cat studied with the method of retrograde axonal transport of horseradish peroxidase. *Brain Res.*, 145:225–238.

176. Norden, J. J., and Kaas, J. H. (1978): The identification of relay neurons in the dorsal lateral geniculate nucleus of monkeys using horseradish peroxidase. *J. Comp. Neurol.*, 182:707–725.

177. Ogren, M. P., and Hendrickson, A. E. (1977): The distribution of pulvinar terminasl in visual areas 17 and 18 of the moneky. *Brain Res.*, 137:343–350.

178. Ogren, M. P., and Hendrickson, A. E. (1979): The morphology and distribution of striate cortex terminals in the inferior and lateral subdivisions of the *Macaca* monkey pulvinar. *J. Comp. Neurol.*, 188:179–197.

179. O'Hara, P. T. Sefton, A. J., and Lieberman, A. R. (1980): Mode of termination of afferents from the thalamic reticular nucleus in the dorsal lateral geniculate nucleus of the rat. *Brain Res.*, 197:503–506.

180. Olivier, A., Parent, A., and Poirier, L. J. (1970): Identification of the thalamic nuclei on the basis of their cholinesterase content in the monkey. *J. Anat.*, 106:37–50.

181. Olson, C. R., and Graybiel, A. M. (1980): Sensory maps in the claustrum of the cat. *Nature*, 288:479–480.

182. Palmer, L. A., and Rosenquist, A. C. (1974): Visual receptive fields of single striate cortical units projecting to the superior colliculus in the cat. *Brain Res.*, 67:27–42.

183. Parent, A., and Butcher, L. L. (1977): Organization and morphologies of acetylcholinesterase-containing neurons in the thalamus and hypothalamus of the rat. *J. Comp. Neurol.*, 170:205–226.

184. Partlow, G. D., Colonnier, M., and Szabo, J. (1977): Thalamic projections of the superior colliculus in the rhesus monkey, *Macaca mulatta*. A light and electron microscopic study. *J. Comp. Neurol.*, 171:285–318.

185. Pert, C. B., Aposhian, D., and Snyder, S. H. (1974): Phylogenetic distribution of opiate receptor binding. *Brain Res.*, 75:356–361.

186. Pert, C. B., Kuhar, M. J., and Snyder, S. H. (1976): Autoradiographic localization of opiate receptor in rat brain. *Proc. Natl. Acad. Sci. U.S.A.*, 73:3729–3733.

187. Pettigrew, J. D. (1972): The importance of early visual experience for neurons of the developing geniculostriate system. *Invest. Ophthalmol.*, 11:386–393.

188. Phillis, J. W. (1970): *The Pharmacology of Synapses*. Pergamon Press, Oxford.

189. Phillis, J. W., Tébecis, A. K., and York, D. H. (1967): A study of cholinoceptive cells in the lateral geniculate nucleus. *J. Physiol. (Lond.)*, 192:695–713.

190. Pickel, V. M., Segal, M., and Bloom, F. E. (1974): A radioautographic study of the efferent pathways of the nucleus locus coeruleus. *J. Comp. Neurol.*, 155:15–41.

191. Poggio, G. F., and Mountcastle, V. B. (1963): The functional properties of ventrobasal thalamic neurons studied in unanesthetized monkeys. *J. Neurophysiol.*, 26:775–806.

192. Powell, T. P. S., and Cowan, W. M. (1956): A study of thalamostriate relations in the monkey. *Brain*, 79:364–390.

193. Powell, T. P. S., Cowan, W. M., and Raisman, G. (1965): The central olfactory connexions. *J. Anat.*, 99:791–813.

194. Purpura, D. P., and Cohen, B. (1962): Intracellular recording from thalamic neurons during recruiting responses. *J. Neurophysiol.*, 25:621–635.

195. Purpura, D. P., McMurtry, J. G., and Maekawa, K. (1966): Synaptic events in ventrolateral thalamic neurons during suppression of recruiting responses

by brain stem reticular stimulation. *Brain Res.,* 1:63–76.

196. Quinlan, J. T., and Phillips, M. I. (1981): Immunoreactivity for an angiotensin II-like peptide in the human brain. *Brain Res.,* 205:212–218.

197. Reubi, J. C., and Cuénod, M. (1979): Glutamate release *in vitro* from corticostriatal terminals. *Brain Res.,* 176:185–188.

198. Rezak, M., and Benevento, L. A. (1979): A comparision of the organization of the projections of the dorsal lateral geniculate nucleus, the inferior pulvinar and adjacent lateral pulvinar to primary visual cortex (area 17) in the macaque monkey. *Brain Res.,* 167:19–40.

199. Richard, D., Gioanni, Y., Kitsikis, A., and Buser, P. (1975): A study of geniculate unit activity during cryogenic blockade of the primary visual cortex in the cat. *Exp. Brain Res.,* 22:235–242.

200. Riche, D., and Lanoir, J. (1978): Some claustro-cortical connections in the cat and baboon as studied by retrograde horseradish peroxidase transport. *J. Comp. Neurol.,* 177:435–444.

201. Rinvik, E. (1975): Demonstration of nigrothalamic connections in the cat by retrograde axonal transport of horseradish peroxidase. *Brain Res.,* 90:313–318.

202. Robson, J. A., and Hall, W. C. (1975): Connections of layer VI in striate cortex of the grey squirrel *(Sciureus carolinensis). Brain Res.,* 93:133–139.

203. Rockel, A. J., Heath, C. J., and Jones, E. G. (1972): Afferent connections to the diencephalon in the marsupial phalanger and the question of sensory convergence in the "posterior group" of the thalamus. *J. Comp. Neurol.,* 145:105–130.

204. Rose, J. E. (1942): The ontogenetic development of the rabbit's diencephalon. *J. Comp. Neurol.,* 77:61–129.

205. Rose, J. E. (1952): The cortical connections of the reticular complex of the thalamus. *Res. Publ. Assoc. Nerv. Ment. Dis.,* 30:454–479.

206. Rosenquist, A. C., Edwards, S. B., and Palmer, L. A. (1974): An autoradiographic study of the projections of the dorsal lateral geniculate nucleus and the posterior nucleus in the cat. *Brain Res.,* 80:71–93.

207. Rotter, A., Birdsall, N. J. M., Burgen, A. S. V., Field, P. M., Hulme, E. C., and Raisman, G. (1979): Muscarinic receptors in the central nervous system of the rat. I. Technique for autoradiographic localization of the binding of [^{3}H]propyl-benzilylcholine mustard and its distribution in the forebrain. *Brain Res.,* 1:141–166.

208. Rotter, A., Field, P. M., and Raisman, G. (1979): Muscarinic receptors in the central nervous system of the rat. III. Postnatal development of binding of [^{3}H]propylbenzilylcholine mustard. *Brain Res. Rev.,* 1:185–206.

209. Royce, G. J. (1978): Autoradiographic evidence for a discontinuous projection to the caudate nucleus from the centromedian nucleus in the cat. *Brain Res.,* 146:145–150.

210. Ryugo, D. K., and Killackey, H. P. (1974): Differential telencephalic projections of the medial and ventral divisions of the medial geniculate body of the rat. *Brain Res.,* 82:173–177.

211. Sanderson, K. J. (1971): The projection of the visual field to the lateral geniculate and medial interlaminar nuclei in the cat. *J. Comp. Neurol.,* 143:101–117.

212. Sanderson, K. J., Bishop, P. O., and Darian-Smith, I. (1971): The properties of binocular receptive fields of lateral geniculate neurons. *Exp. Brain Res.,* 13:178–207.

213. Saper, C. B., and Loewy, A. F. (1980): Efferent connections of the parabrachial nucleus in the rat. *Brain Res.,* 197:291–318.

214. Sar, M., Stumpf, W. E., Miller, R. J., Chang, K.-J., and Cuatrecasas, P. (1978): Immunohistochemical localization of enkephalin in rat brain and spinal cord. *J. Comp. Neurol.,* 182:17–38.

215. Scheibel, M. E., and Scheibel, A. B. (1966): The organization of the nucleus reticularis thalami: A Golgi study. *Brain Res.,* 1:43–62.

216. Schiller, P. H., and Malpeli, J. G. (1978): Functional specificity of lateral geniculate nucleus laminae of the rhesus monkey. *J. Neurophysiol.,* 41:788–797.

217. Schlag, J., Lethinen, I., and Schlag-Rey, M. (1974): Neuronal activity before and during eye movements in thalamic internal medullary lamina of the cat. *J. Neurophysiol.,* 37:982–995.

218. Schlag, J., Schlag-Rey, J., Peck, C. K., and Joseph, J. P. (1980): Visual responses of thalamic neurons depending on the direction of gaze and the position of targets in space. *Exp. Brain Res.,* 40:170–184.

219. Schlag, J., and Waszak, M. (1970): Characteristics of unit responses in nucleus reticularis thalami. *Brain Res.,* 21:286–288.

220. Schmielau, F., and Singer, W. (1977): The role of visual cortex for binocular interactions in the cat lateral geniculate nucleus. *Brain Res.,* 120:359–361.

221. Schwartz, W. J., and Sharp, F. R. (1978): Autoradiographic maps of regional brain glucose consumption in resting, awake rats using [^{14}C]2-deoxyglucose. *J. Comp. Neurol.,* 177:335–359.

222. Segal, M., Dudai, Y., and Amsterdam, A. (1978): Distribution of an α-bungarotoxin-binding cholinergic nicotinic receptor in rat brain. *Brain Res.,* 148:105–120.

223. Sherman, S. M., Wilson, J. R., Kaas, J. H., and Webb, S. V. (1976): *X*- and *Y*-cells in the dorsal lateral geniculate nucleus of the owl monkey *(Actus trivirgatus). Science,* 192:475–477.

224. Shipley, M. T., and Sørenson, K. E. (1975): On the laminar organization of the anterior thalamus projections to the presubiculum in the guinea pig. *Brain Res.,* 86:473–477.

225. Shute, C. C. D., and Lewis, P. R. (1967): The ascending cholinergic reticular system: Neocortical, olfactory and subcortical projections. *Brain,* 90:497–520.

226. Simantov, R., Snowman, A. M., and Snyder, S. H. (1976): A morphine-like factor "enkephalin" in rat brain: Subcellular localization. *Brain Res.,* 107:650–657.

227. Singer, W. (1973): The effect of mesencephalic reticular stimulation on intracellular potentials of cat lateral geniculate neurones. *Brain Res.*, 61:35–54.

228. Singer, W. (1977): Control of thalamic transmission by corticofugal and ascending reticular pathways in the visual system. *Physiol. Rev.*, 57:386–420.

229. Singer, W. (1973): Inhibitory interaction between *X* and *Y* units in the cat lateral geniculate nucleus. *Brain Res.*, 49:291–307.

230. Singer, W., and Creutzfeldt, O. (1970): Reciprocal lateral inhibition of on- and off-centre neurones in the lateral geniculate body of the cat. *Exp. Brain Res.*, 10:311–330.

231. Singer, W., Pöppel, E., and Creutzfeldt, O. (1972): Inhibitory interaction in the cat's lateral geniculate nucleus. *Exp. Brain Res.*, 14:210–226.

232. Snyder, S. H. (1980): Brain peptides as neurotransmitters. *Science*, 209:976–983.

233. Snyder, S. H., and Childers, S. R. (1979): Opiate receptors and opioid peptides. *Annu. Rev. Neurosci.*, 2:35–64.

234. Søreide, A. J., and Fonnum, F. (1980): High affinity uptake of D-aspartate in the barrel subfield of the mouse somatic sensory cortex. *Brain Res.*, 201:427–430.

235. Steriade, M., Deschênes, M., Wyzinski, P., and Hallé, J. Y. (1974): Input–output organization of the motor cortex and its alterations during sleep and waking. In: *Basic Sleep Mechanisms*, edited by O. Petre-Quadens and J. Schlag, pp. 144–200. Academic Press, New York.

236. Steriade, M., Oakson, G., and Diallo, A. (1977): Reticular influences on lateralis posterior thalamic neurons. *Brain Res.*, 131:55–71.

237. Sterling, P., and Davis, T. L. (1980): Neurons in cat lateral geniculate nucleus that concentrate exogenous [^{3}H]-γ-aminobutyric acid (GABA). *J. Comp. Neurol.*, 192:737–750.

238. Stone, J., and Dreher, B. (1973): Projection of *X*- and *Y*-cells of the cat's lateral geniculate nucleus to areas 17 and 18 of visual cortex. *J. Neurophysiol.*, 36:551–567.

239. Streit, P. (1980): Selective retrograde labeling indicating the transmitter of neuronal pathways. *J. Comp. Neurol.*, 191:429–464.

240. Strick, P. L. (1976): Anatomical analysis of ventrolateral thalamic input in primate motor cortex. *J. Neurophysiol.*, 39:1020–1031.

241. Sugitani, M. (1979): Electrophysiological and sensory properties of the thalamic reticular neurones related to somatic sensation in rats. *J. Physiol. (Lond.)*, 290:79–95.

242. Sumitomo, I., Nakamura, M., and Iwana, K. (1976): Location and function of the so-called interneurons of rat lateral geniculate body. *Exp. Neurol.*, 51:110–123.

243. Swanson, L. W., and Cowan, W. M. (1977): An autoradiographic study of the organization of the efferent connections of the hippocampal formation in the rat. *J. Comp. Neurol.*, 172:49–84.

244. Swanson, L. W., and Hartman, B. K. (1975): The central adrenergic system: An immunofluorescence

245. Szentágothai, J., Hámori, J., and Tömböl, T. (1966): Degeneration and electron microscope analysis of the synaptic glomeruli in the lateral geniculate body. *Exp. Brain Res.*, 2:283–301.

246. Tebécis, A. K. (1972): Cholinergic and non-cholinergic transmission in the medial geniculate nucleus of the cat. *J. Physiol. (Lond.)*, 226:153–172.

247. Tebécis, A. K., and DiMaria, A. (1972): A re-evaluation of the mode of action of 5-hydroxytryptamine on lateral geniculate neurones: Comparison with catecholamines and LSD. *Exp. Brain Res.*, 14:480–493.

248. Thach, W. T., and Jones, E. G. (1979): The cerebellar dentatothalamic connection: Terminal field, lamellae, rods and somatotopy. *Brain Res.*, 169:168–172.

249. Tömböl, T. (1969): Two types of short axon (Golgi 2nd) interneurones in the specific thalamic nuclei. *Acta. Morphol. Acad. Sci. Hung.*, 17:285–297.

250. Tracey, D. J., Asanuma, C., Jones, E. G., and Porter, R. (1980): Thalamic relay to motor cortex: Afferent pathways from brain stem, cerebellum and spinal cord in monkeys. *J. Neurophysiol.*, 44:532–554.

251. Ungerstedt, U. (1971): Stereotaxic mapping of the monoamine pathways in the rat brain. *Acta Physiol. Scand. [Suppl.]*, 367:1–48.

252. Updyke, B. V. (1975): The patterns of projection of cortical areas 17, 18 and 19 onto the laminae of the dorsal lateral geniculate nucleus in the cat. *J. Comp. Neurol.*, 4:377–395.

253. Updyke, B. V. (1979): A Golgi study of the class V cell in the visual thalamus of the cat. *J. Comp. Neurol.*, 186:603–619.

254. Wamsley, J. K., Zarbin, M., Birdsall, N., and Kuhar, M. J. (1980): Muscarinic cholinergic receptors: Autoradiographic localization of high and low affinity agonist binding sites. *Brain Res.*, 200:1–12.

255. Watanabe, T., Yanagisawa, K., Kanzaki, J., and Katsuki, Y. (1966): Cortical efferent flow influencing unit responses of medial geniculate body to sound stimulation. *Exp. Brain Res.*, 2:302–317.

256. Watson, S., Akil, H., Sullivan, S., and Barchas, J. (1977): Immunocytochemical localization of methionine enkephalin: Preliminary observations. *Life Sci.*, 21:733–738.

257. Weber, J. T., and Harting, J. K. (1980): The efferent projections of the pretectal complex: An autoradiographic and horseradish peroxidase analysis. *Brain Res.*, 194:1–28.

258. Willis, W. D., Kenshalo, D. R., Jr., and Leonard, R. B. (1979): The cells of origin of the primate spinothalamic tract. *J. Comp. Neurol.*, 188:543–573.

259. Wilson, J. R., Friedlander, M. J., and Sherman, S. M. (1980): Synaptic morphology of X- and Y-cells in the cat's dorsal lateral geniculate nucleus. *Neurosci. Abstr.*, 6:583.

260. Wilson, P. D., Pecci-Saavedra, J., and Doty, R. W. (1973): Mesencephalic control of lateral geniculate

study of the location of cell bodies and their efferent connections in the rat utilizing dopamine-β-hydroxylase as a marker. *J. Comp. Neurol.*, 163:467–506.

nucleus in primates. II. Effective loci. *Exp. Brain Res.,* 18:204–213.

261. Wilson, P. D., Rowe, M. H., and Stone, J. (1976): Properties of relay cells in cat's lateral geniculate nucleus: A comparison of W-cells with X- and Y-cells. *J. Neurophysiol.,* 39:1193–1209.

262. Wilson, P. D., and Stone, J. (1975): Evidence of W-cell input to the cat's visual cortex via the C laminae of the lateral geniculate nucleus. *Brain Res.,* 92:472–478.

263. Winer, J. A., Diamond, I. T., and Raczkowski, D. (1977): Subdivisions of the auditory cortex of the cat: The retrograde transport of horseradish peroxidase to the medial geniculate body and posterior thalamic nuclei. *J. Comp. Neurol.,* 176:387–418.

264. Winfield, D. A., Gatter, K. C., and Powell, T. P. S. (1975): An electron microscopic study of retrograde and orthograde transport of horseradish peroxidase to the lateral geniculate nucleus of the monkey. *Brain Res.,* 92:462–467.

265. Wise, S. P., and Jones, E. G. (1977): Cells of origin and terminal distribution of descending projections of the rat somatic sensory cortex. *J. Comp. Neurol.,* 175:129–158.

266. Wise, S. P., and Jones, E. G. (1978): Developmental studies of thalamocortical and commissural connections in the rat somatic sensory cortex. *J. Comp. Neurol.,* 178:187–208.

267. Wong-Riley, M. (1979): Changes in the visual system of monocularly sutured or enucleated cats demonstrable with cytochrome oxidase histochemistry. *Brain Res.,* 171:11–28.

268. Wyss, J. M., Swanson, L. W., and Cowan, W. M. (1979): A study of subcortical afferents to the hippocampal formation in the rat. *Neuroscience,* 4:463–476.

269. Yamamura, H. I., Kuhar, M. J., Greenberg, D., and Snyder, S. H. (1974): Muscarinic cholinergic receptor binding: Regional distribution in monkey brain. *Brain Res.,* 66:541–546.

270. Yingling, C. D., and Skinner, J. E. (1976): Selective regulation of thalamic sensory relay nuclei by nucleus reticularis thalami. *Electroencephalogr. Clin. Neurophysiol.,* 41:476–482.

Chemical Neuroanatomy, edited by P.C. Emson, Raven Press, New York © 1983.

The Hypothalamus

Ann-Judith Silverman and Gary E. Pickard

Department of Anatomy, Columbia University College of Physicians & Surgeons, New York, New York 10032

The study of the chemical neuroanatomy of the hypothalamus began with the descriptions of Scharrer and Scharrer and Bargmann of neurosecretory neurons using the Gomori chrome alum hematoxylin stain (13,14,276,277). Although the functions of the hypothalamus extend far beyond neurosecretion, it has been the interest in this class of cells that has spurred much of the chemical neuroanatomical research in this region of the brain. In the 40 years since the initial descriptions of neurosecretory material, we have gained a great deal of knowledge about the distribution of peptidergic and monoaminergic cells and their processes. Less is known, especially in the hypothalamus, about cells that use acetylcholine or amino acids as transmitters. Until recently, research has concentrated on the hypophysiotropins and posterior pituitary hormones. In the past few years, descriptions of nonneurosecretory cell types within the hypothalamus, the non-neural-hemal efferent projections of neurosecretory neurons (i.e., extrahypothalamic), and the chemical nature of the afferent synaptic input to identified cells within the hypothalamus have given us some insight into the wiring diagram of this region.

Of equal importance to our understanding of the regulation of hypothalamic function is knowledge of the distribution of specific receptor systems. The most extensively studied receptors have been those for gonadal steroids. Again, interest has focused on neuroendocrine problems. In the past year or two, investigators have also approached the problems of the distribution of receptors for putative transmitters.

In this chapter. we concentrate on certain cell groups within the hypothalamus, either well-defined nuclear clusters or more diffuse neuronal systems, about which detailed chemical information is available. A discussion of cytoarchitectonics can be found in Bleier et al. (35) and of hodology in Palkovits and Zaborszky (227)

THE MAGNOCELLULAR NEUROSECRETORY SYSTEM

The study of both neurosecretion and neuropeptides begins with the magnocellular neurosecretory system formed by the large neurons of the supraoptic (SON) and paraventricular (PVN) nuclei. The axons of these neurons form the hypothalamo–hypophyseal tract, and their terminals are in the posterior pituitary. The peptides specific for these large neurons, oxytocin and vasopressin, were the first hypothalamic peptides, indeed, the first brain peptides, to be isolated and characterized by DuVigneaud and colleagues (85,246,249). These peptides are always present in conjunction with a class of larger peptides, the neurophysins (72,73). For many years, the neurophysins were thought to be "carrier proteins" for the peptides. From the early work of Sachs and collaborators (265) and from the more recent work of Gainer and Brownstein (48,98,99), it has become clear that the neurophysins are part of the precursor molecules that contain the peptides. A specific precursor exists for each of the neurohormones.

Cysteine-rich neurophysins react with Gomori's chrome alum hematoxylin and the aldehyde fuchsin stains (276,277). This fortuitous circumstance allowed the Scharrers and Bargmann (14,276,277) to elucidate the relationships among the cell bodies in the SON (and PVN), the axons of the hypothalamo–neurohypophyseal tract, and the neurosecretory material in the posterior pituitary. Furthermore, these authors showed that transection of the pituitary stalk results in an accumulation of Gomori-positive material in the neurosecretory axons proximal to the cut. These experiments demonstrated that neurosecretory material was synthesized in the cell body and transported down the axon to the terminal.

Since that time, numerous immunohistochemical papers have appeared on the distribution of the neurohormones and their neurophysins at both the light and electron microscopic levels in a variety of species. The first localization studies were carried out by Livett et al. (172) using an antiserum to porcine neurophysin. These and subsequent studies (3,89,171) established the presence of neurophysin immunoreactivity within the cell bodies, axons, and terminals of the magnocellular neurosecretory system and confirmed that the direction of flow of the neurosecretory material (neurophysin) was from the cell body to the neural lobe (3).

It had already been noted by biochemical assay (72,73) that there were specific neurophysins for each of the hormones. Using antisera generated against specific neurophysins (neurophysin I = oxytocin neurophysin; neurophysin II = vasopressin neurophysin), Zimmerman and colleagues demonstrated by both immunocytochemistry (372,373) and radioimmunoassay (375) that both neurophysins were present within both the SON and PVN. Using antisera to the neurohormones as well as to the neurophysins, Vandesande, DeMey, and Dierickx (76,77,344) described the separate distribution of NP I and oxytocin and NP II and vasopressin within the bovine hypothalamus. They also showed, as had Zimmerman, that both proteins are present within the SON and PVN, with NP II predominating in the SON of this species (77). The dorsal aspect of the pars supraoptica of the SON contains primarily NP I neurons, and the ventral aspect NP II. The two neuron types are intermingled at the border of the two regions. These authors further reported that NP I neurons are larger than NP II neurons in the SON. The postoptic (or retrochiasmatic) portion of the SON was shown to contain mostly NP II cells except at its most caudal extent.

Using antisera to vasopressin and oxytocin, these authors extended their findings and confirmed anatomically that NP I is associated with oxytocin and NP II with vasopressin (345). A similar distribution of oxytocin and vasopressin cells has also been observed in the rat (259,309,343). It is well established in these and numerous other species, including human, that both oxytocin and vasopressin are present in separate neurons of the supraoptic and paraventricular nuclei (see 75,79,308, 343,353,355,371) (Fig. 1). In the case of the supraoptic nucleus, both Vandesande et al. (345) and Sokol et al. (309) stated that all cells in the supraoptic nucleus of the rat were neurophysin positive; this statement should be remembered when we discuss the presence of other biologically active peptides in the supraoptic nucleus. However, the distribution of vasopressin and oxytocin cells does show some species variability. In the guinea pig, for example, the vasopressin cells in the SON outnumber the oxytocin cells 5:1 (308).

The subcellular localization of the neurohormones has been studied by cell fractionation (72) and electron microscopic immunocytochemistry. In the neural lobe, neurophysin (233,295) and vasopressin (167,299) are found in large, 120- to 200-nm granules in axons, Herring bodies, and nerve terminals. Oxytocin is also localized in similarly sized large granules in the neural lobe (8,288,347). Differential absorption experiments clearly indicated that oxytocin and vasopressin were present in separate axon profiles, further extending the one-cell/one-hormone theory (8). At the level of the neurons, neurophysin and associated peptides are present within the neurosecretory granules (57,150,288) as well as in the organelles associated with protein synthesis (43). There has been discussion concerning the possibility of extragranular neurohormone (160,288), but this question has not been resolved.

The tenets of neurosecretion that were first postulated in reference to the magnocellular system have been largely confirmed in that system. Recently, it has been suggested that other biologically active substances are present within the neurons of the supraoptic nucleus. In both rat (262,272) and cat (197), some cells in this nucleus (and paraventricular nucleus; see below) contain enkephalin immunoreactivity. These cells project to the posterior pituitary where opiate receptors have been demonstrated (10,235). Recent work indicates that in some neurons at least this enkephalin immunoreactivity is related to dynorphin, and dynorphin and vasopressin have been shown to coexist in magnocellular neurons (358a), much as enkephalin coexists with monoamines in the adrenal medulla (278).

Similarly, glucagon (326), cholecystokinin (CCK-8) (27), dynorphin (358), and angiotensin II (142,241,374) have all been found in supraoptic (and PVN) neurons (see Fig. 1A). In the case of the latter compound, it is severely depleted, if not absent, in Brattleboro rats, which also lack the ability to synthesize vasopressin (374). Data in this latest study suggest that angiotensin II may be part of the precursor for vasopressin or that its biosynthesis may be regulated in a similar manner (see Fig. 1). Studies at the electron microscopic level are necessary to determine the relationship among the various axons containing these different peptides. The possibility exists that two peptides can be stored in the same granule (229).

Of the two major nuclear groups of the magnocellular system, the supraoptic is more simply or-

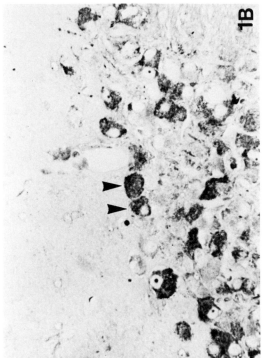

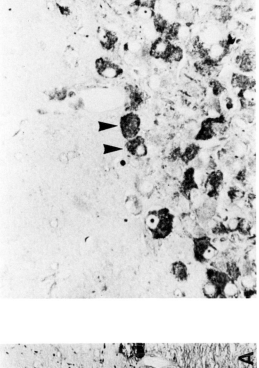

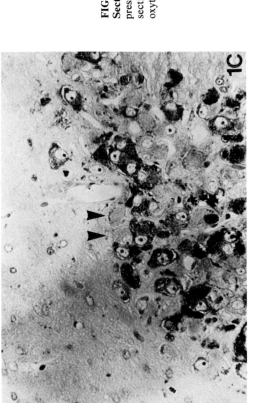

FIG. 1. Serial 6-μm paraffin sections through the supraoptic nucleus of the rat. **Section A** was reacted with an antiserum to angiotensin II; **section B,** to vasopressin; and **section C,** to oxytocin. *Arrowheads* indicate the same cell in each section. The same cell is reactive for angiotensin II and for vasopressin but not for oxytocin. (From Zimmerman et al., ref. 374, with permission.)

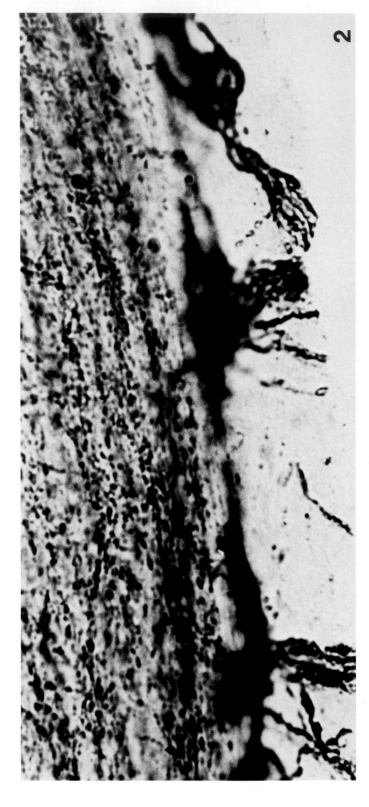

FIG. 2. A 50-µm vibratome section from a mouse brain reacted with rabbit antiserum to bovine neurophysin I. The immunoreactive cells are part of the retrochiasmatic portion of the supraoptic nucleus. Note the thick, ventrally oriented dendrites that extend to the pial surface. Dendrites that course laterally are out of the plane of focus. Beaded structures are axons of the hypothalamo–neurohypophyseal tract. (From Silverman et al., ref. 292, with permission.)

ganized. The supraoptic nucleus was first mentioned by Meynert in 1872 and hence is the oldest recognized structure within the hypothalamus (196). The cells of this nucleus appear as a lateral and dorsal cap on the optic chiasm and extend dorsally, medially, and ventrally around the optic tract as the latter leaves the chiasm. Cells associated with the nucleus are found in the retrochiasmatic area as far caudal as the tuber cinereum.

Cytoarchitectonics of the SON indicate that the nucleus is relatively uniform; the vast majority of cells are magnocellular, measuring 22 to 28 μm in diameter in the rat (343). The presence of another population of small cells in the SON, presumably interneurons, has been argued for many years. Their existence, at least in the rat, appears to be confirmed in Golgi-impregnated material (92). These authors estimated that they comprise 5% of the total cell population of the nucleus.

In vibratome sections and Golgi-impregnated material, it has been shown that SON neurons have dendritic processes that extend toward the pial surface of the brain (292) (see Fig. 2). Cell groups lying just dorsal to the primary SON frequently have long dendritic processes that radiate for several hundred micrometers and can have spinous processes (Figs. 3 and 4). It is not certain at this time if the presence of neurosecretory material in these dendrites (or in those of other peptidergic neurons) is artifactual or real; it is also unclear if the immunoreactivity in the dendrites is associated with neurosecretory granules, rough endoplasmic reticulum, or is found free in the cytoplasm. Further immunocytochemical studies at the ultrastructural level are required.

Among the known chemical afferents to the SON, a substantial noradrenergic innervation (96,170,335) exists. This input is apparently inhibitory, at least to the vasopressin neurons (15,16), and its activation results in a decrease in vasopressin secretion (367). In a recent study using combined immunocytochemistry and catecholamine histofluorescence, the highest density of CA varicosities was found ventral to the neurophysin-positive soma (181), the region of numerous dendrites (see above). Apparent axosomatic contacts are also present in varying degrees at all rostral–caudal levels of the nucleus. The exact nature of the synaptic contacts between catecholamine (presumably noradrenergic) terminals and the vasopressin/oxytocin cells awaits electron microscopic studies.

An acetylcholine (ACh) input to the supraoptic

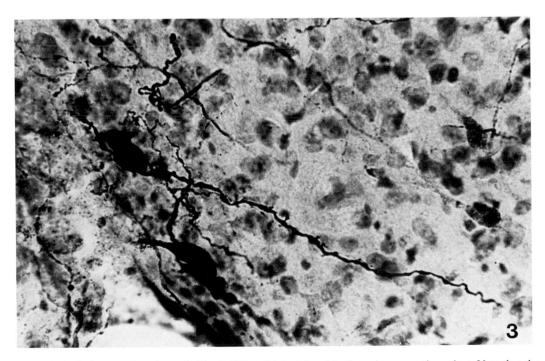

FIG. 3. A similarly reacted section as in Fig. 2. This cell is just dorsal to the main supraoptic nucleus. Note that the spines on the dendrite are also immunoreactive.

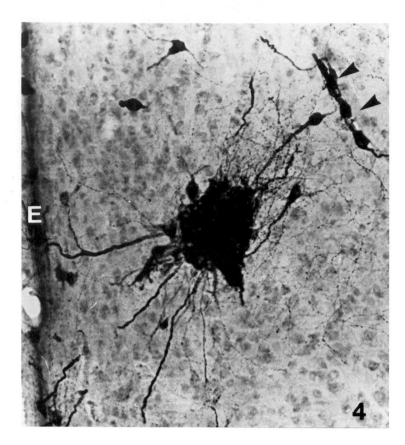

FIG. 4. An accessory magnocellular group in the mouse hypothalamus as visualized with antiserum to bovine neurophysin I. The cluster lies on midline (E, ependymal cells of the third ventricle) and contains at least 50 neurons. Also shown *(arrowheads)* are scattered magnocellular neurons in close proximity to blood vessels.

nucleus, using either a nicotinic (164) or muscarinic (266) receptor, has long been suspected. Application of ACh onto supraoptic neurons *in vitro* definitely increases vasopressin release (302). However, no immunocytochemical studies for the localization of choline acetyltransferase (CAT) have been carried out in the hypothalamus. The identification of such terminals and their relationship to catecholamine terminals on identified neurons would greatly increase our understanding of CNS regulation of vasopressin secretion.

Histamine (328) and histamine receptors (223) are very high (as judged by autoradiographic procedures) in the supraoptic nucleus. The presumptive terminals are thought to originate from cells rich in histidine decarboxylase in the "upper midbrain" (280). Histamine injected into the region of the SON increases antidiuresis (28), presumably through an activation of VP cells.

Other possible afferents to the supraoptic nu-

cleus include GABAergic terminals (327); these terminals are thought to originate, in part, from the nucleus accumbens septi and, in part, from nearby hypothalamic tissue (195). GABA's role is unknown, though it does decrease firing rates in cultured SON neurons (266). Recently Zingg et al. (376) have reported that GABA might act directly on the neurosecretory axons. The effects of the compound applied to axonal processes in the posterior pituitary were inhibitory.

The efferent projections of the supraoptic nucleus are predominantly to the posterior pituitary and possibly the median eminence (see discussion below of the paraventricular nucleus). Injections of horseradish peroxidase into the neural lobe (7) or into the circulation (42) result in the retrograde labeling of almost all of the SON cells. Some neurons, however, may project to the paraventricular nucleus (293). These latter cells are present mostly in the oxytocin-containing region of the nucleus

(293), but their identity with oxytocin cells has not yet been determined. The primacy of the projection to the neural lobe for cells of this nucleus is also suggested by the fact that the majority of the cells degenerate following hypophysectomy (251). However, a careful [³H]-amino-acid anterograde study should be carried out to further elucidate the efferent connections of this nucleus.

The paraventricular nucleus of the hypothalamus, although classically a portion of the magnocellular neurosecretory system, has recently been recognized to be a considerably more complex nuclear group than its counterpart, the supraoptic nucleus. This complexity is reflected in its cytoarchitectural configuration (see Fig. 5), neuropeptide content, afferent inputs, and, especially, efferent projections. The division of the nucleus into various subnuclei has been suggested by several investigators based on one or more of these grounds (7,149,332). Originally described by Gurdjian (106) as being divided into medial, parvocellular and lateral magnocellular components, the above authors have suggested that the nucleus be divided into 5 to 10 divisions. We shall adopt the nomenclature of Armstrong et al. (7) since it is the simplest and the subnuclei are easy to recognize in Nissl-stained sections (see Fig. 5). These divisions have been described only for the laboratory rat; other animals have not been investigated in such detail. Wherever possible, however, comparisons across species will be made.

The first of the subnuclei is the anterior commissural nucleus (ac). This appears as a clump of cells lying below and slightly medial to the descending columns of the fornix, in the dorsal preoptic area. As one proceeds caudally, the cells assume a position more medial to the fornix. Some of these cells and those of other accessory magnocellular groups scattered in the hypothalamus (237) (to be discussed below) appear to project to the neural lobe (7), although Rhodes et al. (259) have suggested that some neurophysin-positive axons extend from this cell cluster into the stria terminalis. The majority of cells in this nucleus are oxytocinergic (259).

The main body of the PVN is divided into four portions: (a) a more medial, predominately parvocellular group, pvm, (b) the main lateral wing, pvl, (c) a dorsal cap, pvdc, over the pvl, and (d) a posterior group, pvpo. The pvm appears (in Nissl stain) as a band of darkly staining cells lying at approximately a 45° angle to the wall of the third ventricle. More posteriorly, the pvm extends laterally and somewhat dorsally, forming a stripe between the anterior hypothalamus and the ball of cells composing the pvl. The cells of the pvm, when immunoreactive for either neurohypophyseal peptide, are more likely to contain oxytocin than vasopressin (259). Many of the cells in the pvm are parvocellular; similarly, there are smaller cells intermixed within the other subnuclei. Many of the pvm parvocellular neurons may contain neurotensin (135) or enkephalin (350), although this latter peptide is usually described as being present in the lateral aspect of the nucleus (262,272). Cholecystokinin is also present in the PVN, but its precise location has not yet been described (27). The recently described corticotropin-releasing factor (CRF) (338) is also present in this region (51a).

The pvl is the most prominent of the subnuclei, composed of a cluster of magno- and parvocellular elements extending laterally towards the fornix. Its most posterior aspect appears in the same coronal plane as the rostral limit of the dorsomedial nucleus. The pvl is separated from the adjacent hypothalamic tissue by a relatively cell-free, myelinfree zone. The distribution of neurohypophyseal peptides in this subnucleus has been well described by numerous authors [see Zimmerman et al. (374)]. There is a core of vasopressin cells surrounded by a rim of oxytocin cells; this distribution has been confirmed in the Brattleboro rat [(see Sokol et al. (309)]. In the guinea pig, however, the distribution is very different: vasopressin cells fill the equivalent of the pvl and pvm, whereas oxytocin cells occupy a thin strip immediately adjacent to the ventricular wall (308).

Along the dorsomedial edge of the pvl, there is a cap of neurons (pvdc) composed of small to medium-sized cells. We shall return to the importance of these cells when we discuss the efferent projections of the nucleus. The final subnucleus (pvpo) occupies the most posterior aspect of the nucleus. In coronal section, the cells form a triangular grouping. Many of the medium-sized cells in this region are neurophysin positive and are predominantly oxytocinergic (259).

The determination of the projections of the paraventricular nucleus has been carried out in three ways: (a) by immunocytochemical studies; (b) by anterograde tracing using [³H]-amino acids; (c) by retrograde tracing using HRP histochemistry or with the newer fluorescent dyes [see Zimmerman (370) for review]. Some cells within the PVN project, of course, to the neural lobe. With the use of various retrograde tracers (7,126,321,365), the hypophyseal projecting neurons are seen in the anterior commissural nucleus, large portions of the pvl, parts of pvm, and in a cluster of cells overlying the fornix. The heaviest concentration of neurohypo-

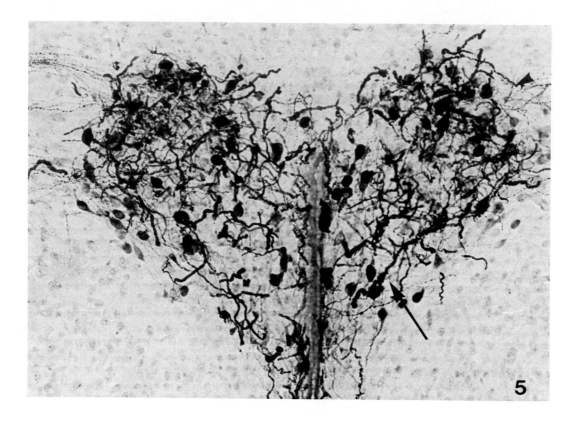

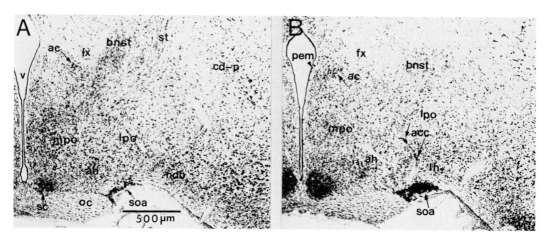

FIG. 5. Top: Paraventricular nucleus of the mouse hypothalamus. Section was reacted as in Figs. 2–4. The regions corresponding to the pvl *(arrowhead)* and pvm *(arrow)* of the rat (7) are indicated. Both dendritic and axonal processes are seen to cross over the ventricle. **Bottom and facing page:** Photomicrographs (A–H) of thionine-stained, celloidin-embedded coronal sections through the major divisions of the anterior commissural and paraventricular nuclei with surrounding hypothalamus. *Abbreviations:* ac, anterior commissural nucleus; acc, accessory neurosecretory nuclei; ah, anterior hypothalamus; ar, arcuate nucleus; bnst, bed nucleus of the stria terminalis; cd-p, caudate putamen; cp, cerebral peduncle; dm, dorsomedial hypothalamic nuclei; fx, fornix; hnt, hypothalamo–neurohypophyseal tract; ic, internal capsule, lh, lateral hypothalamic area; lpo, lateral preoptic area; me, median eminence; mpo, medial preoptic area; nc, nucleus circularis; ndb, nucleus of the diagonal band of Broca; oc, optic chiasm; ot, optic tract; pem, magnocellular periventricular cells; pvdc, dorsomedial cap of the paraventricular nucleus; pvl, lateral magnocellular paraventricular

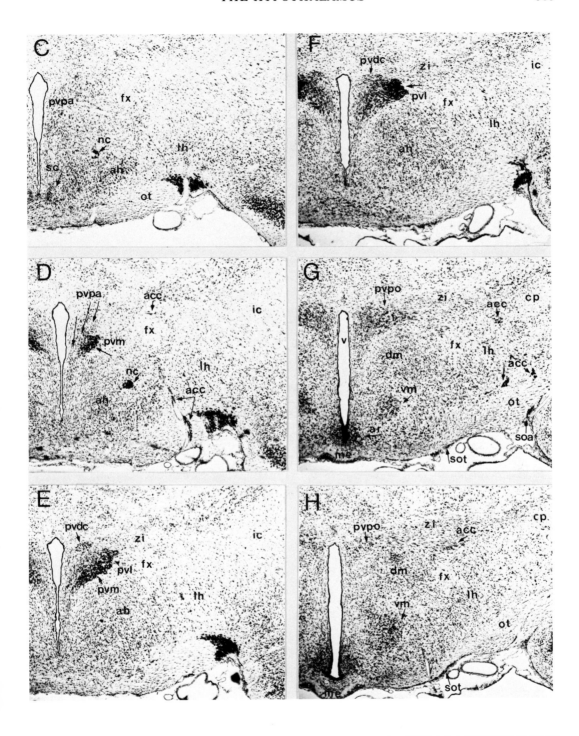

nucleus; pvm, medial magnocellular paraventricular nucleus; pvpa, parvocellular portion of the paraventricular nucleus; pvpo, posterior portion of the paraventricular nucleus; sc, suprachiasmatic nucleus; sm, stria medullaris; soa, anterior portion of the supraoptic nucleus; sot, tuberal portion of the supraoptic nucleus; st, stria terminalis; v, third ventricle; vm, ventromedial hypothalamic nucleus; zi, zona incerta (7).

physeal projecting neurons resides in the pvl. The cells that project to the neural lobe obviously include oxytocinergic and vasopressinergic neurons. In addition, however, it is likely that the enkephalinergic neurons and those containing CCK-8 also send axons to the neural lobe. In the case of the former, it has been noted that morphine can stimulate vasopressin release (74) and that there are high levels of opiate receptors in the gland (300). This has led Rossier et al. (262) to suggest that the enkephalin terminals are involved in regulating vasopressin release within the neural lobe.

The second efferent projection of the magnocellular system to be described was the neurophysin-positive projection to the external zone of the median eminence (Figs. 6,7). This projection was first described in Scrapie-infected sheep by Parry and Livett (228) and in the rhesus monkey by Zimmerman and co-workers (373). At the same time, the latter investigators demonstrated that there were very high levels of vasopressin in the portal blood. This pathway was then demonstrated in the bovine hypothalamus (76,345), the rat (342,356), and the guinea pig (287).

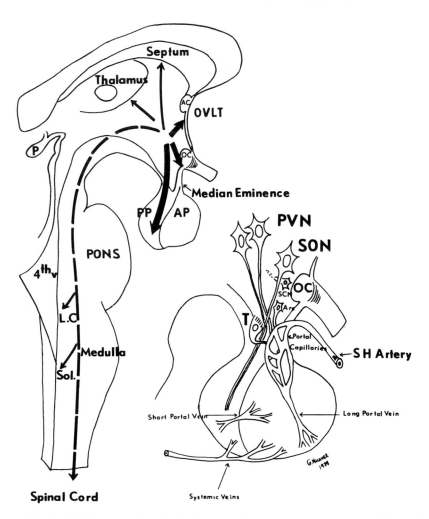

FIG. 6. Lower right: Sagittal diagram of the classical magnocellular neurosecretory system of the rat. Both paraventricular (PVN) and supraoptic (SON) nuclei project to the posterior pituitary gland. Vasopressin neurons of the PVN also project to the primary portal plexus in the median eminence. Vasopressin neurons are also found in the suprachiasmatic nucleus (SCN). Arc, arcuate nucleus; SH, superior hypophyseal artery; OC, optic chiasm. **Left:** Neurosecretory projections of the magnocellular system *(bold arrows)* to the blood vessels of the posterior pituitary, median eminence, and organum vasculosum of the lamina terminalis (ovlt). *Smaller arrows* represent some of the extrahypothalamic projections of the PVN. (Drawn by G. Nilaver; from Sar and Stumpf, ref. 270, with permission.)

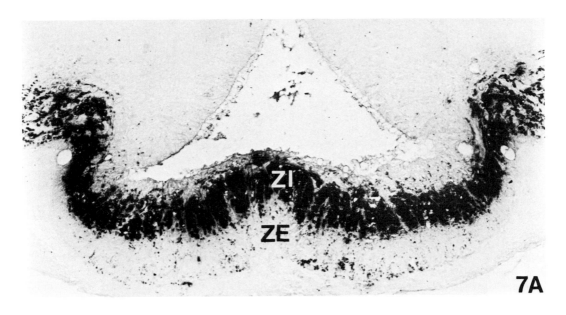

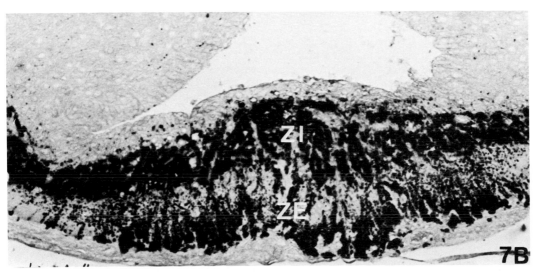

FIG. 7. A: A 6-μm section through the normal rat median eminence reacted with antiserum to rat neurophysin. The fibers of the hypothalamo–neurohypophyseal tract are evident in the zona interna (ZI). A few positive axons are seen in the zona externa (ZE). **B:** A section at approximately the same level as that shown in **A** but from a rat that had been bilaterally adrenalectomized for 2 weeks. The increase in neurophysin immunoreactivity is in vasopressin axons. (From Silverman et al., ref. 292, with permission.)

The fact that most of these fibers are vasopressinergic was first demonstrated in bovine tissue using specific neurophysins (344); the termination of vasopressin-containing fibers on the primary portal capillaries was confirmed at the ultrastructural level by Silverman and Zimmerman (299). The fact that these PVN cells might represent a class different from those projecting to the neurohypophysis was suggested by the observation that the neurosecretory granules in the two terminal types are different (289,299). The origin of these terminals was first suggested to be the PVN (228), but the discovery of vasopressin neurons in the suprachiasmatic nucleus (SCN) focused attention on these parvocellular neurons (342,345). Later, it was conclusively demonstrated by Vandesande et al. (346) in the rat and Antunes et al. (6) in the rhesus monkey that the PVN and not the SCN projected to the external zone. These conclusions were based on lesions of the PVN and the subsequent disappearance of fibers in the median eminence on the side ipsilateral to the lesion.

Recently Wiegand and Price (365) have applied HRP or [^{125}I]-wheat germ agglutinin to the median eminence in an effort to precisely localize the neurons projecting to this structure. In their experiments, many parvocellular neurons in the pvm were labeled, and these may be in part neurotensin containing (135). In addition, magnocellular neurons are found in the pvl and the border region between the pvl and pvm. This location of median eminence afferents has been confirmed in our laboratory using anterograde HRP tracing (A.-J. Silverman, *unpublished observations*). However, Weigand and Price also consistently labeled some magnocellular neurons in the supraoptic and accessory nuclei. The ipsilateral nature of this projection has been suggested in the rhesus monkey study cited above (6), by a deafferentiation study employing histochemical analysis (39), and with anterograde tracing (2a, 299a).

The role of the vasopressin in the zona externa is still unresolved. However, vasopressin immunoreactivity increases dramatically following bilateral adrenalectomy (81,314) (see Fig. 7), and this increase can be prevented by treating the animal with glucocorticoids (314) [also see Silverman et al. (294)] or by lesioning the PVN but not the SCN (346). Dehydration, however, appears not to influence the amount of immunoreactivity in this system (314). This has led several investigators to conclude that vasopressin in the zona externa may be a regulator of ACTH release.

Vasopressin is released into the portal vasculature as mentioned above. Oliver et al. (221) have suggested that the vasopressin in these capillaries originates from the neural lobe. However, Recht et al. (254) have reexamined this question in acutely posterior lobectomized rats in which blood was collected from individual portal veins. These authors found no diminution in vasopressin concentration in the portal blood following this surgery and concluded that vasopressin in this microcirculation originates primarily from the terminals on the zona externa.

Recently, Bock et al. (38), using both immunocytochemistry and aldehyde–fuchsin histochemistry, suggested that more vasopressin is released from these zona externa terminals in adrenalecto-mized, non-sodium-replaced animals, whereas less is released in animals with adequate sodium replacement. They suggested that vasopressin might be involved in mineralocorticoid feedback. However, in salt-replaced animals, glucocorticoids are more effective in inhibiting the response to adrenalectomy than mineralocorticoids (294). In this latter study, only deoxycorticosterone and not aldosterone was tested. The effectiveness of gluco- versus mineralocorticoid replacement might also reflect differences in the number of steroid receptors or the K_d for different steroids.

The next set of projections of the paraventricular nucleus to be investigated was the descending projections to the brainstem and spinal cord (Fig. 6). These studies have been carried out with immunocytochemical and standard tracing techniques. Kuypers and Maisky (165), using retrograde tracers, demonstrated that hypothalamic neurons project to the spinal cord. Conrad and Pfaff (65) and Saper et al. (269) confirmed this finding with anterograde [^{3}H]-amino-acid autoradiography. The descending PVN projections (which form part but not all of the hypothalamic input to caudal structures) contain both oxytocin and vasopressin (322). The descending neurophysin-positive axons course primarily in the medial forebrain bundle, ventral and lateral to the fornix, through the supramammillary region into the ventral tegmental area. There they ascend posterodorsolaterally to terminate in the parabrachial nucleus and locus ceruleus. Most fibers continue through the lateral tegmental field; at the level of the inferior olive, fibers arch dorsomedially to the solitary tract, dorsal motor nucleus of the vagus, nucleus intermedius, and commissural and intercalated nuclei. Other fibers proceed into the dorsolateral funiculus to innervate all levels of the spinal cord. Terminal fields are found in Rexed's lamina I (substantia gelatinosa), diffusely in laminae II and III, and in the central gray (Rexed's lamina X). An innervation of the intermediolateral cell column is also prominent. In all cases, however, electron microscopic observations must be carried out to determine if these structures are really presynaptic elements. There is some indication that oxytocin fibers may innervate cerebral blood vessels (G. Nilaver, *personal communication*).

The relative contribution of oxytocin versus vasopressin to these descending fiber systems is not known for certain. Both fiber types are present in all regions cited above in both normal and Brattleboro rats (219). One major problem in deciding on the predominance of a fiber type (as opposed to the cells of origin) is that the detectability of both nonapeptides is considerably lower than that of the neurophysins. Indeed, the quality of antisera used in the studies cited above varies considerably from laboratory to laboratory.

The distribution of the cells in the PVN with descending projections is different from the distribution of cells that project to the posterior pituitary. However, to date, this problem has only been studied with large injections into the caudal medulla or spinal cord (7,126,321). Armstrong et al. (7) report brainstem afferents originating from regions bordering the pvl, especially the dorsal cap, the pvm, and, predominantly, the pvpo. It should be remembered that these include both magno- and parvocellular elements and that cells outside the PVN project to the brainstem and spinal cord. The spinal cord efferent cells have a similar distribution (126). Swanson and Kuypers (321) used fluorescent tracers to determine whether or not individual PVN neurons project to both the vagal complex and spinal cord. They estimate that 10 to 15% do so. However, caution is urged, since these small molecules can pass through gap junctions or out of the retrogradely filled cell into the extracellular space to be taken up by neighboring cells. Andrew et al. (5) have shown that some cells in the PVN are electrically coupled, can pass Lucifer yellow, and have gap junctions as seen in freeze–fracture.

Ascending pathways, especially to limbic structures, have also been described by various investigators. However, in this case, there has been some controversy on the contributions of paraventricular and suprachiasmatic neurons. Sofroniew and Weindl (307) have attempted to distinguish fibers from the two nuclei based on fiber diameter and by tracing individual fibers. Clearly, lesion studies are necessary to distinguish between possible inputs to limbic structures from the vasopressin cells of these two nuclei. Anterograde tracing studies suggest that the efferent projections of the SCN are limited (29,317) (see section on SCN).

Peptidergic projections (oxytocin and vasopressin) that apparently originate from the PVN project into the stria meullaris and from there into the lateral habenular nuclei (52). Additional fibers follow the fornix dorsorostrally into the dorsal hippocampus and subiculum; they continue into the ventral hippocampus via the fimbria. Axons are also observed in the stria terminalis from whence they project to numerous amygdaloid nuclei (52). In the case of the ascending projections, electron microscopic observations have indicated that these axons form presynaptic elements (53).

The function of these various extrahypothalamic PVN projections is not known. However, in many instances, there is a substantial reciprocal connection between the PVN and other CNS sites. The best substantiated of these is between the PVN and the vagal complex (261,293). This suggests a strong functional relationship, perhaps for the homeostatic regulation of blood pressure and blood volume. Indeed, Swanson and Hartman (320) have suggested that the descending projections of the PVN and the reciprocal innervation from these regions might function as a "central autonomic system" that regulates the microcirculation of the brain. These remain areas for fruitful investigation in the future.

The accessory magnocellular groups are small clusters of neurons first described in detail by Peterson (237) (see Fig. 4). They actually make up about one-half of the oxytocin/vasopressin cells in the hypothalamus. These groups frequently lie along the path of the axons from the paraventricular nucleus. The groups described by Peterson for the rat include: (a) anterior commissural nucleus (discussed previously as a part of the PVN); (b) nucleus circularis [also mentioned in Bodian (40)] whose cells are intimately associated with a capillary network (331); (c) anterior and posterior fornical nuclei; the former is found at the level of the anterior part of the PVN, whereas the latter is located caudal and dorsal to the medial forebrain bundle; (d) nucleus of the medial forebrain bundle which, like the nucleus circularis, has cells that are associated with blood vessels; and (e) the retrochiasmatic group which we have included with the SON.

Oxytocin predominates in the accessory groups as a whole, although in the nucleus circularis, there is a more even mixture of cell types (259). In the cat, similar accessory groups have been described and appear to have a relatively equal mixture of oxytocin and vasopressin cells (253). Additional groups may occur in other species.

The majority of accessory cells appear to project to the neural lobe (7). Efferent projections to the median eminence (365), the PVN proper (293), and the caudal medulla (306) have also been reported.

THE PARVOCELLULAR NEUROSECRETORY SYSTEM

The parvocellular neurosecretory system (also referred to as tuberoinfundibular) consists of those neurons whose nerve terminals reside in the median eminence and whose neurosecretory product is carried via the portal circulation to the anterior pituitary. The neurons that comprise this system would therefore synthesize and release the hypo-physiotropic substances and other modulating molecules. We discuss the components of this system under several headings. The first of these concerns the distribution of the known releasing/release-inhibiting hormones: luteinizing hormone-releasing hormone (LHRH), thyrotropin-releasing hormone (TRH), and somatostatin or growth hormone release-inhibiting hormone (SRIF). The second concerns afferents to the median eminence that have not clearly been defined as hypophysiotropic. Both the vasopressin input (see section under paraventricular nucleus) and the noradrenergic input (see section on hypothalamic monoaminergic innervation) fall into this category. Finally, afferents to the median eminence have been studied using both anterograde and retrograde tracing techniques, and these papers are referred to in the appropriate sections. For a discussion of the organization of the median eminence itself, see Knigge and Silverman (148).

Thyrotropin-Releasing Hormone

Thyrotropin-releasing hormone was the first hypophysiotropin to be isolated and characterized (55). Like the other releasing factors, it is widely distributed in the nervous system [see Brownstein et al. (46)]. Although terminals immunoreactive for this peptide are present in the median eminence (61,121), the localization of the cell bodies is uncertain. Recently, Johansson et al. (130) reported TRH-positive cells at the electron microscopic level in the area dorsal to the optic chiasm and in the dorsomedial nucleus. Immunoreactive terminals were observed in this latter study in the median eminence and suprachiasmatic, dorsomedial, and parvocellular paraventricular nuclei. High-pressure liquid chromatography has confirmed the identity of the TRH immunoreactivity throughout the CNS (127,310). Until the distribution of cell bodies is more carefully analyzed, perhaps with the aid of colchicine or other conditions that would maximize perikaryal staining, it is not possible to determine the origin of the terminals in the median eminence.

Clearly, the main function of the TRH in the median eminence is the regulation of TSH release. Additionally, this neurohormone also releases prolactin [see Vale et al. (337)].

Luteinizing Hormone-Releasing Hormone

Luteinizing hormone-releasing hormone (also called GnRH—gonadotropin-releasing hormone)

was the second hypophysiotropic substance to be isolated and identified from hypothalamic tissue. It is a decapeptide that regulates both LH (luteinizing hormone) and FSH (follicle-stimulating hormone) release from the anterior pituitary (4, 273). The distribution of this substance has been extensively studied in mammalian and, to a lesser extent, nonmammalian species. As with many other peptides that were first characterized as releasing or release-inhibiting factors, LHRH has an extensive distribution outside of the hypothalamus.

The first question that must be addressed is the equivalence of the LHRH immunoreactivity with the decapeptide. Identity has only been shown for the LH-releasing material in the hypothalamus of the mammal and amphibian (144). In birds, reptiles, teleosts, and elasmobranchs, the gonadotropin-releasing material in the hypothalamus is related to, but not identical with, the LHRH decapeptide (144). Even within those vertebrate groups in which identity between the biologically active material and the decapeptide has been shown, there are still questions as to the identity of the LHRH immunoreactivity in nonhypothalamic regions. Recently, Jan et al. (128) reported the presence of LHRH immunoreactivity in frog sympathetic ganglia and suggested that it was a preganglionic neurotransmitter resulting in the late, slow excitatory postsynaptic potential (EPSP) recorded from ganglion cells. This material has now been shown to migrate differently than LHRH in high-pressure liquid chromatography (HPLC) (86). This underscores the necessity for careful analysis of immunoreactive material. Therefore, the descriptions presented below, even though confined to the mammal, are qualified by referring to them as LHRH-like immunoreactivity. This should continue to be the practice until rigorous separation procedures have been applied.

It is now well recognized that the LHRH-containing neurons are not organized into a discrete nuclear group. Instead, both within the hypothalamus and in many extrahypothalamic areas, LHRH cells are scattered through a variety of structures with relatively little reference to anatomical boundaries. The only exception to date is the ganglionic arrangement of LHRH-positive and -negative cell bodies within the nervus terminalis (279) [also see Jennes and Stumpf (129)]. The precise distribution of LHRH-containing neurons within the preoptic area and hypothalamus has been somewhat controversial.

The primary disagreement in the literature has centered around the presence or absence of LHRH neurons in the medial basal hypothalamus (MBH), the region of the classical hypophysiotropic area (108,109,325). Such neurons have now been demonstrated unequivocally in guinea pigs (22,288), hamsters (129,243), and several primate species (20,186,290,297) including human (17,49). Their presence in the MBH of some rodents—rats, mice—still remains a matter of doubt [however, see Silverman et al. (297)]. The possibility exists that the decapeptide is "buried" in the middle of the precursor protein (198) as has been hypothesized for vasopressin and oxytocin (48). This would make the peptide unavailable to the antibody molecules until it is uncovered during degradation. It is also possible that the rate of degradation of the precursor to the active form varies among LHRH cell bodies or that the precursor itself is not identical from cell group to cell group.

Such speculations must await the purification of the precursor molecule (198). It does appear to be true that in some rodents but not in primates (297), the detectability of LHRH neurons in the MBH varies with the antiserum preparation used [see Sternberger and Hoffman (313)]. Whether this reflects differences in the structure of the LHRH or of the precursor is not known. We do know, however, that different physiological conditions (21,23,24,159) and developmental ages (22,222) can influence the detectability of LHRH neurons in this region [see Barry (18) for review].

In those animals in which LHRH cells have been demonstrated in arcuate nucleus, these cells have also been shown by either lesion studies (153,288) or direct tracing of axons (186,290) to project to the primary portal plexus. Furthermore, this projection has been shown in some species such as guinea pig (288,329) and rhesus monkey (152) to be essential and sufficient for both tonic and cyclic gonadotropin release.

In all species studied, many more LHRH neurons are present rostrally in a diffuse continuum that begins in the bed nucleus of the stria terminalis, surrounds the anterior commissure, and continues ventrally in the medial preoptic area, including the suprachiasmatic preoptic region, and caudally to the periventricular anterior hypothalamic area [see reviews by Barry (18), Silverman et al. (297), Sternberger and Hoffman (313)]. In the rat (93,145,151,282), cell bodies have only been observed consistently in these rostral regions. The initial demonstration (115) of cell bodies in the arcuate nucleus of the rat may have resulted in large part from contamination of the antiserum used with ACTH antibodies (63). In the guinea pig (22,24,153), hamster (129), and primates (20,186,290), some rostral cells have been shown

to project to the median eminence (ME). Certainly, in the rat the majority of LHRH fibers terminating in the ME originate from the medial preoptic cells (45,136.282,362). There is circumstantial evidence for the existence of LHRH cell bodies in the rat arcuate nucleus since some (though little) LHRH is still present in the median eminence after the surgical isolation of the medial basal hypothalamus from the remainder of the CNS (45,282,362) [however, see Mickvych and Elde (197)]. Jennes and Stumpf (129) suggested that there merely exists a continuum from very few to many LHRH cells in the arcuate nucleus among species.

Another important consideration is the actual number of cells involved in the entire LHRH-containing neuronal network that projects to the median eminence. Studies in rats (145,222), hamster (129), and guinea pig (296) indicate that the numbers are very low. The possibility that this small number is accurate rather than a false negative result of the immunocytochemistry is suggested by the recent findings of Wiegand and Price (365). These authors traced afferents to the median eminence by applying the horseradish peroxidase method. The number of cells in the medial preoptic area that corresponds with the location of LHRH neurons (an inverted Y over the most anterior tip of the third ventricle) contained very few filled neurons (approximately 30). In primates, as mentioned above, the number of LHRH neurons in the entire medial preoptic–periventricular–infundibular continuum appears to be much greater than that found in rodents (186).

The neuronal circuits, both LHRH-secreting and otherwise, that are critical to the regulation of gonadotropin secretions remain a matter of debate. It would appear that there are major differences among species. In the guinea pig (329) and the rhesus monkey (152), complete isolation of the MBH is compatible with both tonic and cyclic gonadotropin secretion. Similarly, ovulatory cycles continue in animals of these species with lesions of the suprachiasmatic nucleus or medial preoptic area (154).

This is not true for the rat. Lesions of the SCN result in persistent estrus, vaginal cornification, and polyfollicular ovaries (44,366), but gonadotropin surges and/or ovulation can be induced either by copulation (44) or by estrogen–progesterone treatment (366). The effect of the SCN lesion is thought to result from the destruction of the timing mechanism for the daily surge of LHRH (252). Such keying of ovulation to a time-keeping mechanism is apparently absent in guinea pigs and rhesus monkeys (252). Additionally, in the rat, lesions of a small group of cells anterior to the SCN proper (called the medial preoptic nucleus) not only result in persistent estrus but also in a blockade of progesterone-induced surges (366). Finally, large medial preoptic–anterior hypothalamic area lesions that do not affect this small medial preoptic nucleus or the suprachiasmatic nucleus result in pseudopregnancy—long periods of diestrus with brief periods of vaginal cornification and the presence of corpora lutea.

In contrast, such lesions have no effect on ovulation in the guinea pig (154). These results suggest that there are multiple intrahypothalamic connections that regulate gonadotropin secretion as well as important extrahypothalamic inputs. In some species, the medial basal hypothalamus can act independently; in others, especially the rat, it cannot.

The distribution of LHRH fibers has been studied as extensively as the cell bodies. Some of the debate concerning the origin of LHRH terminals in the median eminence may be settled by the finding in the guinea pig that both the preoptic cell group and the arcuate nucleus cells terminate on the primary portal vasculature. The terminal fields for each cell group are somewhat different (153). In both the rat (102) and guinea pig (291), the peptide has been demonstrated by ultrastructural immunocytochemistry within granules in axons and terminals within the median eminence. Interestingly, very few neurosecretory terminals positive for LHRH actually abut on the capillaries of the primary portal plexus. This led to the speculation that one aspect of regulation of the release of LHRH might be changes in the position of these terminals at the perivascular space (291). Such a change in the dynamics of neurosecretory terminals and surrounding glial or ependymal elements has been proposed for other neurosecretory systems (275) including the neural lobe (173,174,333).

In addition to the terminal field in the median eminence, LHRH axons and terminals are found in many other areas. In all species studied to date, it appears that cell bodies extending from the pericommissural region to the lamina terminalis contribute to terminals in the vascular organ of the lamina terminalis (ovlt), although the concentration of fibers in this region varies among species [see Barry (18)]. In the guinea pig (296) and hamster (129), it has also been shown that fibers originating from the medial preoptic area and septal regions project via the stria medullaris into the medial habenula and from there through the fasciculus retroflexus into the interpeduncular nucleus. In addition, there are scattered fibers that enter the superior colliculus. The medial preoptic group also appears to project diffusely through the dorsal hypothalamus over and under the mammillary bodies to the midbrain tegmentum. Neurons containing LHRH are present in a variety of other brain regions including main olfactory and accessory olfactory bulbs, anterior hippocampus, and nervus terminalis (129,279,297,366a). A discussion of these groups is beyond the scope of this chapter. Figure 8 indicates the distribution of LHRH neurons and fibers in the guinea pig CNS.

These widespread extrahypothalamic projections of the medial preoptic and hypothalamic cell groups as well as the extrahypothalamic cell bodies appear to be much less common in primates [see Barry and Carette (20) and Marshall and Goldsmith (186)] including prosimians (19). However, the presence of LHRH in the intracranial portions of the nervus terminalis appears to be common, although the structure is usually not named by the investigators but referred to as LHRH cells and fibers along the blood vessels in the "parolfactory area."

Very recently, a number of laboratories have begun to utilize thick vibratome sections for immunocytochemical demonstration of LHRH and various other peptides. This has led not only to more complete visualization of LHRH cell bodies in terms of numbers (129,279,297) but also to a visualization of more of the cell body, in particular of the dendritic processes. An example of the long, minimally branched dendrites of LHRH neurons is shown in Fig. 9. These dendrites are quite long (250 μm in rat, 1 mm in rhesus monkey) and may enter other nuclear regions adjacent to that containing the perikaryon. Therefore, any studies on the synaptic input to LHRH neurons should take this into account.

Somatostatin

The existence of a growth hormone release-inhibiting factor was discovered by Krulich et al. (161,162). The factor, somatostatin, a tetradecapeptide, was isolated from ovine (41) and porcine (274) hypothalamic tissue. Physiological studies in mammals have shown that it inhibits the release of growth hormone (GH) from the anterior pituitary both *in vivo* and *in vitro* (41,188). The secretions of TSH and prolactin (336) as well as ACTH (334) are also inhibited by this compound under some circumstances. Somatostatin has a very wide

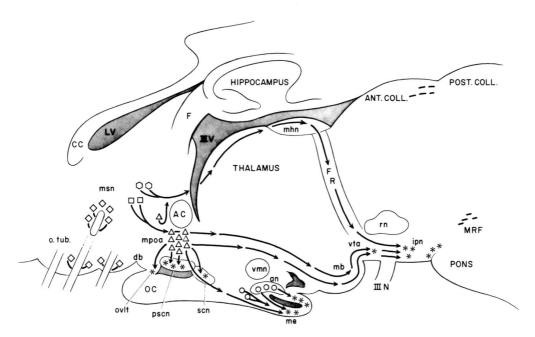

FIG. 8. Diagrammatic representation of the distribution of LHRH neuronal elements in the guinea pig brain. Terminal fields are indicated with an asterisk (∗). Positive neurons of the medial basal hypothalamus (○) project to the zona externa of the median eminence (me). Others in the medial preoptic area (mpoa; △) project to the organum vasculosum of the lamina terminalis (ovlt), preoptic portion of the suprachiasmatic nucleus (pscn), and hypothalamic portion of the suprachiasmatic nucleus (scn). The LHRH neurons in this region also project to the ventral tegmental area (vta), where they appear to terminate. Finally, these neurons also innervate the median eminence. both in the internal and external zones. The scattered neurons in the medial septal nucleus (msn; ◯) project into and under the stria medularis, into the medial habenular nucleus (mhn), and down the fasciculus retroflexus (FR) to terminate in two regions of the interpeduncular and nucleus (ipn). Other LHRH neurons (◇) are seen in close proximity to the blood vessels of the anterior perforated substance; these represent the intracranial portion of the nervus terminalis (279). O. tub, olfactory tubercle; db, diagonal band; AC, anterior commissure; F, fornix; rn, red nucleus; an, arcuate nucleus; vmn, ventromedial nucleus; CC, corpus callosum; LV, lateral ventricle; III V, third ventricle. (From Silverman and Krey, ref. 296, with permission.)

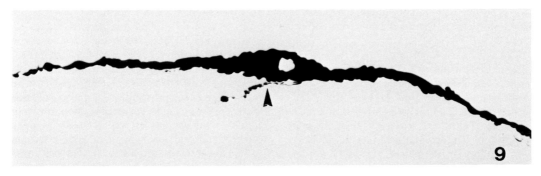

FIG. 9. Camera lucida drawing of an LHRH neuron in the arcuate nucleus of a rhesus monkey. Neuron was drawn from a 75-μm frozen section that had been reacted with an antiserum against LHRH [RbIII] (154). *Arrowhead* points at the axon. (Magnification, × 820)

distribution in the CNS, PNS, and in endocrine tissues, and the SRIF-like immunoreactivity in hypothalamus as well as in these other structures has been studied in several vertebrate groups including rat, pigeon, tortoise, frog, teleost (cichlid), elasmobranch (dogfish), and cyclostome (hagfish, brain only). The immunoreactivity coelutes in cation-exchange chromatography with authentic SRIF (143).

After the purification of the tetradecapeptide, immunocytochemical studies demonstrated positive fibers in the median eminence at both the light (117) and electron (231) microscopic level. The peptide is present in 110-nm granules in terminals and in the perikaryon (230).

Since these early studies, the distribution of SRIF within the hypothalamus has proven to be complex in nature and to have both an intra- and extrahypothalamic origin. The intrahypothalamic cell group in the rat (87,116,158) and other mammals (51,114) is concentrated in the periventricular zone beginning at the level of the suprachiasmatic nucleus and extending through the anterior aspect of the median eminence, a distance of 0.5 mm (in rat). Outside this zone, they are fairly rare. They are particularly prominent at the level of the paraventricular nucleus. Some authors (51,83,87) have found SRIF cells dispersed among the magnocellular elements of the paraventricular nucleus; these are parvocellular elements. Dubois and Kolodziejczyk (83) also reported that substantial numbers of magnocellular neurosecretory neurons, especially in the supraoptic nucleus, were somatostatin containing. Dierickx and Vandesande (80) investigated this problem in normal rats and rats treated to maximize neurophysin content. The SRIF cells were present in the parvocellular aspect of the paraventricular nucleus as well as the other levels of the periventricular zone. These authors concluded that the staining in magnocellular elements was caused by nonspecific reaction with neurophysin.

The evidence is fairly strong that these periventricular SRIF neurons project to the portal capillaries of the median eminence and, in some species, to the neural lobe as well. Lesions of this region reduce the SRIF immunoreactivity in the median eminence (67,88) and seriously impair the inhibitory control of growth hormone regulation (67).

In addition, in the guinea pig, SRIF terminals are abundant in the arcuate, ventromedial, and suprachiasmatic nuclei as well as the ovlt (117). The origin of some of these terminals was thought to be the amygdaloid complex (88). In a recent study, small lesions of the periventricular zone of the hypothalamus were followed by assay for SRIF in microdissected brain regions (68). These lesions resulted in significant decreases in SRIF immunoreactivity in the median eminence and in the arcuate and medial preoptic nuclei. No changes are seen in the ventromedial nucleus or other telencephalic or mesencephalic structures. On the other hand, lesions of the medial–basal amygdaloid nucleus or stria terminalis also result in a decline in median eminence SRIF content, although the decrease was less than with the hypothalamic lesions (36% versus 72%). Surprisingly, neither of these latter two lesions decreased the levels of SRIF in the other hypothalamic areas (e.g., the ventromedial nucleus). These discrepancies in the literature require further investigation. Another note of caution should also be added; that concerns the assumption that decreases in radioimmunoassayable peptide result from loss of fibers [see Krey and Silverman (153)]. It is known, however, that both the medial preoptic–periventricular region (88,188, 189) and the medial amygdala (187) influence GH secretion in similar manners.

Somatostatin, like LHRH, is present in terminals of circumventricular organs such as ovlt, subfornical, and subcommissural (82,224). The distribution of SRIF cells and fibers in the dog diencephalon are shown in Fig. 10.

LOCALIZATION OF HORMONE RECEPTORS

Of equal importance to the localization of neurotransmitter/neuromodulator/neurohormonal substances in the hypothalamus is the distribution of neurons that concentrate peripheral hormones. In general, steroid hormones and thyroid hormones have ready access to brain tissue, and both bind to putative intracellular receptor molecules [see McEwen (180)]. Steroid hormones have been the most extensively studied. Numerous studies indicate that gonadal steroids are critical in the expression of certain behaviors as well as in the development of sexually dimorphic characteristics of the central nervous system [see Gorski (103)]. In the rodent, the effects of steroids on gonadotropin secretion are also mediated via the action of gonadal steroids with nervous as well as pituitary tissue. Neuroanatomical localization of cells containing steroid receptor molecules is carried out by radioautographic procedures in which castrated animals are injected with radioactive steroid and tissue is processed to prevent or minimize translocation of material (238,315).

The distribution of cells whose nuclei are radio-

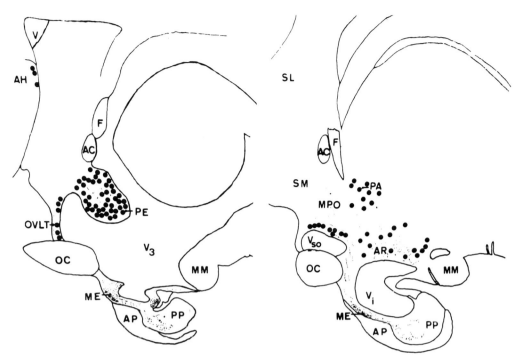

FIG. 10. Distribution of somatostatin-reactive elements in the dog diencephalon shown diagramatically in the mid-sagittal plane. *Filled circles* are cell bodies; *dotted processes* are axonal processes. (From Hoffman and Hayes, ref. 114, with permission.)

active after injection of ^{3}H estradiol has been extensively studied in a variety of vertebrate species [see Morrell et al. (213) and Stumpf and Sar (316) for reviews]. In the brains of rodents such as mice (351), rats (213,238,315,316), guinea pig (352), and hamster (157) as well as rhesus monkey (100), the distribution of estrogen-concentrating cells is remarkably similar, although some small species differences exist. These differences appear to be ones of intensity and numbers of positive cells rather than an absolute qualitative difference. The distribution of labeled cells in mink brain is shown in Fig. 11. Heavily labeled cells are present in large numbers in: (a) the medial preoptic area at levels close to the lamina terminalis, with the largest numbers in the posterior, ventral, and medial portions; (b) the dorsal aspect of the anterior hypothalamic area, with labeled cells extending laterally to the medial forebrain bundle and dorsolaterally toward the fornix and stria terminalis; and (c) in the medial basal hypothalamus, with cells particularly concentrated in the arcuate nucleus throughout its anterior–posterior extent, in the lateral subdivision of the ventromedial nucleus, and in the ventral premammillary nucleus. Labeled cells are either ab-

sent or very low in numbers in other hypothalamic regions.

Outside of the hypothalamic–preoptic continuum, there are several important regions for steroid concentration. These include a few cells in the olfactory bulb (both granule and mitral cells), nucleus accumbens septi, lateral septal nucleus, and the bed nucleus of the stria terminalis at both preoptic and hypothalamic levels. In other portions of the limbic system, labeled cells are found in the medial and cortical amygdaloid nuclei as well as the ventral subiculum. Scattered cells may be found in other hippocampal areas, but in small numbers. In the mesencephalon, labeled cells are concentrated in the ventral lateral quadrant of the central gray. Other areas of steroid concentration have been noted but are beyond the scope of this chapter.

Recently, workers have tried to obtain other kinds of information regarding estrogen-concentrating neurons by using double-labeling procedures. Keefer et al. (139) showed that estrogen is concentrated primarily in gonadotropin cells of the anterior pituitary by a combined autoradiographic–immunocytochemical procedure [see also

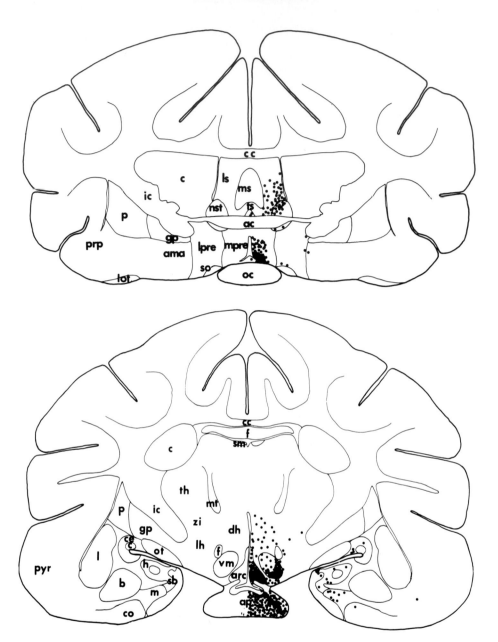

FIG. 11. These are two representative transverse sections of the mink brain and pituitary which contained the greatest number of estradiol concentrating cells. The right side of each section shows the position of estradiol concentrating cells *(solid circles)*. Each *solid circle* equals approximately *two* estradiol concentrating cells. The left side of each section gives the anatomical structures. Both sections are taken from one estrous animal, although they are equally representative of the anestrous pattern of labeled cells. (From Morrell et al., ref. 214, with permission.)

Abbreviations: ac, anterior commissure; ama, anterior amygdaloid area; ap, anterior pituitary; arc, arcuate nucleus; b, basal nucleus of the amygdala; C, caudate nucleus; CC, corpus callosum; ce, external capsule, proper; co, cortical nucleus of the amygdala; dh, dorsal hypothalamus; f, fornix; gp, globus pallidus; h, hippocampus; ic, internal capsule; l, lateral nucleus of the amygdala; lh, lateral hypothalamus; lot, nucleus of the lateral olfactory tract; lpre, lateral preoptic area; ls, lateral septum; m, medial nucleus of the amygdala; mpre, medial preoptic area; ms, medial septum; mt, mammillothalamic tract; nst, bed nucleus of the stria terminalis; OC, optic chiasm; OT, optic tract; P, putamen; prp, prepyriform cortex; pyr, pyriform cortex; sb, subiculum; sm, stria medullaris; SO, supraoptic nucleus; th, thalamus; ts, nucleus triangularis septi; vm, ventromedial nucleus; zi, zona incerta.

Sar and Stumpf (271)]. Similarly, Rhodes et al. (258) have demonstrated the presence of estrogen radioactivity in neurophysin-positive cells primarily in the paraventricular nucleus. Their location in the nucleus suggests that they may be oxytocin cells (Fig. 12). Furthermore, Morrell and Pfaff (212) have combined retrograde tracing with primuline, granular blue, or true blue and estrogen autoradiography. In this study, they have shown that (a) about 30% of the cells (combined neurons and glia) in the ventrolateral division of the ventromedial nucleus concentrate estrogen and (b) of these, 30% to 50% project to the mesencephalic gray. This connection has been shown to be important in modulating female lordosis behavior (70,239,240,267).

Although the action of estrogen on the CNS is commonly thought to be mediated via binding of estrogen to the cytoplasmic receptor and the translocation of receptor complex into the nucleus, this might not be the only mechanism of action. Using a hypothalamic slice preparation and intracellular electrodes, Kelly et al. (140) have shown that the addition of 10^{-10} M estradiol caused hyperpolarization of the resting membrane potential of arcuate neurons; estrone at 10^{-8} M had no effect. Subsequent filling of these cells with procion yellow showed them to be small and fusiform, with few dendritic processes. The larger cells in this region showed no response to estradiol. The response to estradiol was rapid and reversible in a manner similar to a neurotransmitter effect. These findings, if confirmed, may lead to a rethinking of the mechanism of steroid action on neural tissue.

In addition to estradiol receptors [see McEwen (180) for reviews of biochemistry of estradiol receptors in neuroendocrine tissue], separate androgen receptors also exist in some neurons. The ability to determine the distribution of such cells is complicated by the fact that testosterone (T) is either aromatized to estradiol (E) within brain tissue (169,216,281,364) or undergoes 5α reduction to 5α-dihydrotestosterone (see refs. 58,62,90 for review).

This problem has been approached in two ways—by using the nonaromatizable androgen 5α-dihydrotestosterone (5-DHT) (270) or by using testosterone with the ^{3}H in different parts of the molecule (284). In the case of [^{3}H]-DHT or of [^{3}H]-testosterone with the label in the α positions, the distribution of labeled cells is similar in the limbic system and hypothalamus to that seen with estrogen except that the number of labeled cells in the ventromedial nucleus of the hypothalamus is

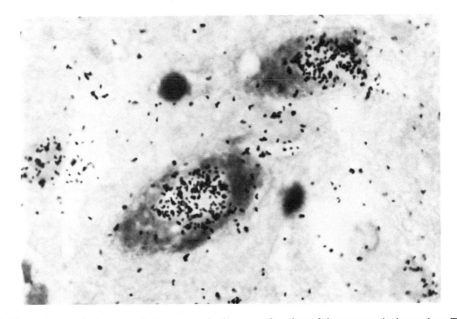

FIG. 12. Photomicrograph of magnocellular neurons in the pvpo subnucleus of the paraventricular nucleus. The tissue is from a Brattleboro rat with hereditary diabetes insipidus; the animal therefore cannot synthesize vasopressin. The tissue was processed to show both estradiol (black silver grains over the nucleus) and neurophysin (DAB reaction product in the cytoplasm). Since these rats do not synthesize vasopressin, this must be an oxytocin cell. (From Rhodes et al., ref. 259, with permission.)

much greater and their distribution broader. By using [³H]-T labeled in the beta positions, Sheridan (283) could examine regions in which label was either bound as T or as 5-DHT, since for any material aromatized to E, the ³H would have been lost. In these experiments, labeled cells were seen in the bed nucleus of the stria terminalis and in the medial amygdaloid nucleus, especially in the region just bordering the optic tract. This would suggest that in the hypothalamus and preoptic area, the majority of circulating T is converted to E. Estradiol receptors per se (191) are present in male rat brain, and E has been recovered from male brain nuclei (168). However, the autoradiographic data cited above as well as biochemical data (134,138,201,215) indicate the presence of a separate androgen-binding molecule. In the hypothalamus, amygdala, and preoptic areas, the androgen receptor, which has a K_d for 5-DHT and T of about 1×10^{-9} M, also binds E (K_d 2×10^{-8} M) (59). In both rats and mice (9,94), the amount of androgen receptor is reduced in testicular-feminized individuals.

The degree to which specific androgen receptors play a significant role in producing the sexually dimorphic characteristics of the adult is still not known [see Gorski (103)]. Furthermore, the degree to which aromatization is or is not necessary for displays of various behaviors in males differs among species. For example, estrogens and aromatizable androgens together, but not alone, will restore sexual behavior in castrated male rats. 5-Dihydrotestosterone has no effect (90,368). In other species such as the mouse, hamster, rabbit, rhesus monkey, and guinea pig, however, 5α-reduced androgens will restore sexual behavior [see Luttge (177) for review]. Interestingly 5α-DHT will activate aggressive behavior in castrated female guinea pigs although it has no influence on inducing mounting behavior in these animals (101). These studies indicate that the hormone sensitivity of the neural systems mediating the two behaviors are different and that androgen receptors are present in the female brain.

Progesterone, like testosterone, undergoes several metabolic transformations in the body. Therefore, the distribution of progestin receptors in brain and the roles progestins might have in modulating behavioral events are still not certain. Injection of [³H]progesterone (P) or [³H]-20-OH-progesterone results in the concentration of label in midbrain, hypothalamus, cerebral cortex, and hippocampus, in that order (348,349). Both the guinea pig midbrain and hypothalamus are sites in which implantation of P exerts behavioral effects similar to those of systemic injection [see Feder and Marrone (91)]. Recently, Blaustein and Feder (34) have used a synthetic progestin, R5020, to determine the characteristics of the P receptor. It is still uncertain, however, that the binding of P to the cytoplasmic receptor is a mechanism by which P facilitates sexual behavior.

THE SUPRACHIASMATIC NUCLEUS

The suprachiasmatic nucleus (SCN) is located immediately dorsal to the optic chiasm at its caudal aspect (Fig. 13). Anteriorly, the SCN is bounded by the anterior hypothalamic area and posteriorly by the supraoptic commissure. The paired suprachiasmatic nuclei are separated in their dorsal aspect by the third ventricle. The SCN is characterized by tightly packed small neurons (5–15 μm) with a relative paucity of axonal processes in comparison to the surrounding hypothalamic tissue (340). Although the packing density of the entire SCN sets it apart from the surrounding hypothalamic tissue, the SCN can also be subdivided on the basis of cell size and intranuclear packing density. The dorsomedial SCN tends to have smaller, more tightly packed neurons than the ventrolateral region, although the cell populations in any region are not homogenous (330,340).

In Golgi material, SCN neurons demonstrate a variety of relatively simple dendritic forms. The simplest SCN neurons have only two primary dendrites which branch very little, and the most differentiated SCN neurons usually have no more than five primary dendrites. Dendritic spines are a common feature of SCN neurons, although the lack of spines on some neurons serves to illustrate the morphological heterogeneity of this hypothalamic nucleus (340). This heterogeneity of the SCN cellular morphology has been suggested by some to imply functional specificity within the nucleus (178). The distribution of afferent fibers to discrete regions of the SCN (202,206,319) supports the suggestion of intranuclear specificity of function.

The most frequently described afferent to the SCN is that from the retina (208), and because of its functional importance, we describe it in detail. Each eye projects bilaterally to the SCN, and in most species the retinal innervation to the contralateral SCN appears about twice that of the ipsilateral input [see Moore (203)]. However, the retinal input to the SCN has been described as being relatively equal to both nuclei in the hamster (95,245) (see Fig. 14), the chimpanzee (330), and the pig-tailed macaque (G. E. Pickard, *unpub-*

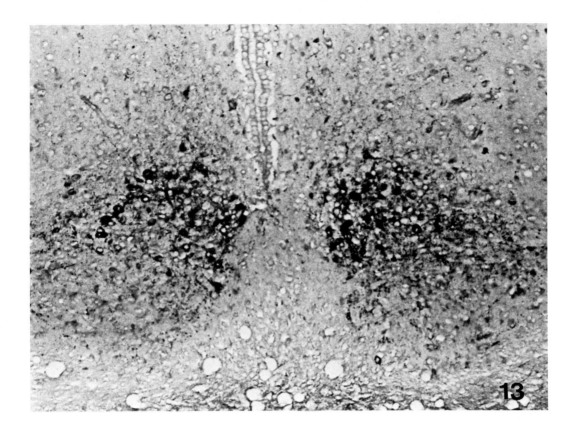

FIG. 13. Neurophysin-positive elements in the rat suprachiasmatic nuclei. These cells are exclusively vasopressinergic. (From Silverman et al., ref. 294, with permission.)

lished observation). The significance of these species variations is unknown at present.

The morphological characteristics of the retinal ganglion cells that innervate the SCN have been described to date only in the hamster; the cells are large (11–17 μm diameter), and their dendritic spread indicates a large receptive field (242,244). Interestingly, in the rat, retinal ganglion cells form both symmetrical and asymmetrical synapses in the SCN (105). Additionally, the axonal fibers from the retina that innervate the SCN may arise as collateral branches from optic fibers that continue caudally in the optic tracts (190,199). In many species, the retinal innervation of the SCN is generally heaviest in the ventrolateral aspect (110), although distinct species differences clearly exist (202,245). Unfortunately, the ganglion cell neurotransmitter(s) is not known.

In addition to direct retinal signals, the SCN receives an indirect input from the retina via the ventral nucleus of the lateral geniculate body (vLGN) (319). Like the input from the retina, the afferents

from the vLGN are bilateral, although unlike the retina, the ipsilateral projection predominates (244,260,319). Recently, it has been shown that the vLGN afferents to the SCN arise from cells located almost exclusively in the dorsal lamina of the internal division of the vLGN (244).

The SCN receives many extrahypothalamic afferents in addition to those from structures in the optic system. The paraventricular nucleus of the thalamus sends a moderately heavy projection to the SCN (244). The hippocampal formation may also innervate SCN neurons. Meibach and Siegel (192) have reported that the anteroventral subiculum projects to the "region of the SCN" via the medial corticohypothalamic tract, whereas Swanson and Cowan (318) describe a projection from the ventral subiculum that merely skirts over the dorsal border of the SCN. Pickard and Silverman (244) have recently demonstrated that HRP iontophoresed into the SCN or just dorsal to it will label cells in the ventral subiculum. In view of the fact that SCN neurons often have dendrites that

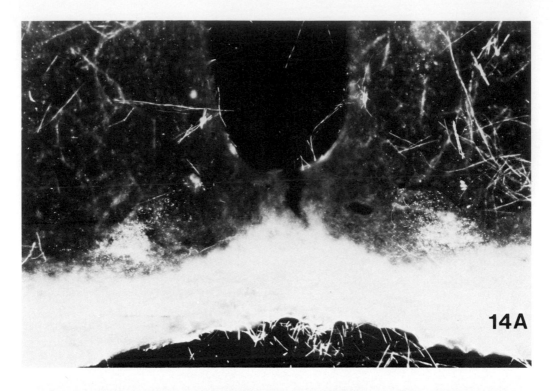

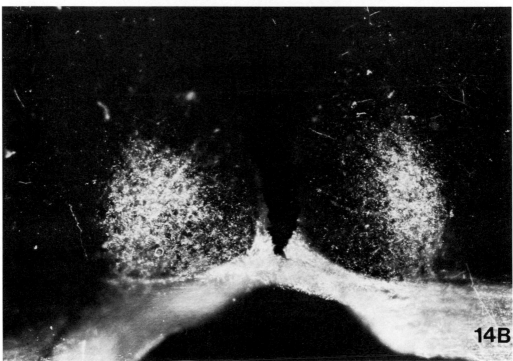

FIG. 14. **A:** A dark-field photomicrograph through the caudal SCN of the rat following monocular HRP injection. Note the paucity of labeled fibers compared to the hamster. **B:** A dark-field photomicrograph of the caudal SCN of the hamster. The HRP reaction product appears to be more evenly distributed over the ipsilateral nucleus, leaving only a dorsomedial quadrant relatively label-free. On the contralateral side, label is much more concentrated in the lateral aspect of the nucleus. (From Pickard and Silverman, ref. 245, with permission.)

extend dorsally beyond the boundaries of the nucleus (155,286,325,340), the ventral subiculum could, in effect, innervate the SCN without sending fibers directly into the nucleus.

The SCN may also receive a noradrenergic (NE) input. Although only a few scattered immunoreactive dopamine-β-hydroxylase fibers pass through the dorsal aspect of the SCN (320), Moore and Bloom (204) indicate that the SCN is surrounded by a dense shell of NE fibers. These NE fibers arise from the lateral tegmental NE cell groups (204).

Serotonergic terminals in the SCN were first described by Fuxe (96) and subsequently by many others (1,2,220). The dense 5-HT innervation originates from neurons in the midbrain nucleus centralis superior (median raphe) and the dorsal raphe nucleus (11,37,206). van de Kar and Lorens (339) have reported that the nucleus centralis superior is the primary source of 5-HT terminals in the SCN, although further verification would be valuable.

It has been reported that the SCN contains significant levels of dopamine as determined by biochemical assay (225) and that the level of dopamine is reduced following lesions of the nigral A8, A9, and A10 dopamine cell bodies (146). However, morphological studies by the glyoxylic acid histochemical method have not demonstrated dopamine in the SCN (32).

The SCN receives many afferents from neighboring hypothalamic structures. Most of these inputs are minor and arise from neurons scattered throughout the afferent nuclei. The ventromedial nucleus, the arcuate nucleus, and the periventricular nucleus have all been reported to innervate the SCN (65,209,244). The medial preoptic area also sends a minor projection to the SCN (66,244). The most significant intrahypothalamic connection to the SCN is from the contralateral SCN (244,340). The discovery of the reciprocal innervation of the SCN may provide valuable insights into the understanding of the physiology of this nucleus (247).

Information on the efferent projections of the SCN is limited. Krieg (155) initially described axons that leave the SCN dorsally to course through the tractus periventricularis. Since that original descriptive study on normal material, several experimental studies have been completed. Using orthograde tracing procedures, Swanson and Cowan (317) described a short ipsilateral projection to the periventricular area of the hypothalamus, the internal lamina of the median eminence, and the lateral tuberal region of the hypothalamus. Recently, these findings have been confirmed and extended (29). The SCN was shown to innervate

the paraventricular thalamic nucleus, the dorsomedial and ventromedial nuclei of the hypothalamus, the ventrolateral border of the hypothalamic paraventricular nucleus (PVN), the posterior hypothalamic nucleus, and the external layer of the median eminence. Some labeled fibers were also described continuing caudally into the periventricular gray of the midbrain (29). Many of these efferent projections have been confirmed by retrograde tracing experiments. Injections of HRP into the PVN (293), dorsomedial and ventromedial nuclei (176), and the mesencephalic central gray (163) label neurons in the SCN in a retrograde manner. However, a projection to the median eminence arising from the SCN was not observed following HRP injection into the median eminence (166,363).

Immunocytochemical procedures have been applied to identify specific functional components of the SCN efferent system. Neurons containing vasoactive intestinal polypeptide (VIP) have been identified in the ventrocaudal and medial aspects of the SCN (175,301). The efferent projection pattern described for these VIP neurons is in accordance with the previously described efferent projections of the SCN; labeled VIP fibers were traced into the PVN, dorsomedial, ventromedial, and possibly the premammillary nucleus (301).

Vasopressin-neurophysin (VP-NP)-positive cells have been identified in the SCN in the mouse, rat (see Fig. 13), guinea pig, and human (79,307,314,346). The VP-NP neurons are located in the medial and dorsomedial regions of the SCN, with a heavier concentration in the rostral aspect of the nucleus. Axons from the VP-NP cells have been reported to project to a number of hypothalamic and extrahypothalamic loci (54,307). However, the pattern of SCN VP-NP efferents reported differs substantially from the results obtained for SCN efferent pathways by other tracing techniques (29,111,185,317). Further substantiation of the SCN VP-NP projections will be valuable.

The well-defined physiological role of the SCN is that of a biological clock [see Rusak and Zucker (264)]. This neural region functions as an endogenous oscillator maintaining behavioral and physiological rhythms. The destruction of the SCN abolishes the normal circadian pattern of a number of biological rhythms including locomotor activity (311), adrenal corticosteroid release (205), sleep–wake cycle (126a), and pineal enzyme activity (207). An intact SCN is also required for seasonal breeders to regulate their reproductive system in response to a changing environment (263).

In addition to maintaining internal temporal

homeostasis, the SCN timekeeper functions to co-ordinate internal physiological rhythms to the environmental day/night cycle. The retinohypothalamic projection to the SCN provides the anatomical link between the cyclic environment and the internal clock. Under normal light/dark (L/D) conditions, the SCN clock is synchronized or entrained to the external cyclic photoperiod by the retinohypothalamic projections even in the absence of all other central retinal projections (147). If the retinal input is removed, the SCN will produce an oscillating signal of its own circadian frequency of around 24 hr. Under these conditions, behavioral and endocrine rhythms free run with periods of little more or little less than 24 hr.

The neurotransmitter released at the retinal ganglion cell synapses of the SCN, responsible for entrainment, is unknown. Recently, Zatz and Brownstein (369) have demonstrated that carbachol, a cholinergic agonist, infused into the hypothalamus adjacent to the SCN will mimic the acute effect of light on pineal serotonin N-acetyltransferase (SNAT) enzyme activity. These findings are suggestive of a transmitter role for ACh in the SCN. Serotonin, dopamine, glycine, and GABA had no effect on pineal enzyme activity. However, the site of action of carbachol cannot be stated unambiguously from these experiments, nor can it be stated with certainty that the cholinergic agonist mimicked the effect of light rather than directly altering the SCN circadian oscillator. Additional neuropharmacological studies of this type are needed to dissect the chemistry of the SCN clock.

The absence of significant chemical effects (anesthetics, hallucinogens, poisons, protein synthesis inhibitors, neurotransmitter depleters) on the period of free-running rhythms has greatly hindered progress in understanding the chemical basis for circadian periodicity (264). The ingestion of heavy water (D_2O) has been shown to consistently alter the periodicity of free-running circadian rhythms (377), although its mode of action is unclear. More interestingly from a physiological perspective, gonadal steroids have also been shown to affect the normal circadian pattern of locomotor activity (107,210,211). The role of estradiol and testosterone in facilitating integrated circadian rhythmicity may be subtle. The implications are, however, far reaching and require further investigation.

Roles for the endogenous SCN peptides and neurotransmitters in circadian rhythm generation are still being sought. Studies on the Brattleboro rat, genetically deficient for vasopressin, have indicated that the presence of VP-NP within SCN neurons is not required for the normal maintenance of circadian rhythmicity (236,312). The function of VIP in the SCN has not been examined.

As described previously, the SCN receives a serotonergic input from the midbrain raphe, and fluctuations in the 5-HT uptake capacity of the SCN demonstrate a circadian pattern (194). However, all attempts to disrupt circadian rhythms by eliminating the raphe 5-HT innervation of the SCN have been surprisingly ineffective. Circadian rhythms of corticosterone secretion (12), body temperature (84), locomotor activity (137), plasma TSH (133), and gonadotropin secretion (112) persist after destruction of the dorsal and/or median raphe nuclei. However, conclusions concerning the role of 5-HT in the SCN from these ablation studies can not be made because even large lesions do not entirely deplete the 5-HT content of the SCN (226,339).

The findings from pharmacological studies have also been difficult to interpret because global depletion of all brain 5-HT has been employed as a means of assessing the role of 5-HT in the SCN. Honma and co-workers (125), using para-chlorophenylalanine (PCPA) to deplete brain 5-HT, have suggested that the treatment affects the circadian clock directly. However, other investigators using PCPA have indicated that serotonin plays a permissive function in the control of circadian hormonal rhythms; 5-HT in the SCN modulates the amplitude of daily hormonal secretions but does not affect the clock itself (64,112,323). There is some indication that NE may also play a role in the circadian oscillation of hormonal secretion (124).

THE ARCUATE NUCLEUS

The arcuate (infundibular) nucleus surrounds the infundibular recess of the third ventricle throughout its length. Caudally, it continues along the lateral walls of the mammillary recess of the third ventricle. The neurons of the arcuate nucleus have been described in Golgi preparations as unipolar or bipolar (200), with one to four primary dendrites that usually have spines (200,341).

The efferent projections of the arcuate nucleus are of great interest because of the importance of this neural region to adenohypophyseal function. Szentagothai and colleagues (324), using Golgi-stained material, were the first to trace axons from neuronal perikarya in the arcuate nucleus to the external layer or palisade zone of the median eminence. This initial observation has subsequently been corroborated by numerous investigators using a variety of techniques (250,255,257). More recently, unequivocal anatomical evidence demonstrating arcuate neuron projections to the median eminence has been presented by two independent laboratories using retrograde HRP-tracing procedures. Horseradish peroxidase injected into the median eminence from either a dorsal (166) or ventral approach (365) labeled neurons throughout the arcuate nucleus, with the heaviest concentration in the rostral aspect.

Dopamine was one of the first of many substances that have been identified in the arcuate nucleus. Dopamine cells of the arcuate nucleus and adjacent periventricular nucleus correspond to the A12 group of Dahlstrom and Fuxe (69). It is known that these dopaminergic cells innervate the external layer of the median eminence and intermediate and posterior lobes of the pituitary (31,33,96,220). However, it is not clear whether all of the dopamine terminals in the median eminence arise from the A12 group.

Kizer et al. (146) have suggested that dopaminergic cells in the ventral tegmentum also innervate the median eminence. These findings are in accordance with the findings from studies of monosodium glutamate (MSG)-treated animals. Given neonatally, MSG destroys 80% to 90% of all arcuate neurons, but median eminence dopamine content is only reduced about 50% (217). However, Holzwarth-McBride et al. (123) have indicated that many dopaminergic arcuate neurons remain in MSG-treated animals. Furthermore, complete hypothalamic deafferentation produces little change in the dopamine innervation pattern (132,333) or the dopamine content of the median eminence (363). The available morphological data do not support an extrahypothalamic dopamine median eminence pathway (166,365). In view of the existing data, the major source of dopamine found in the portal vasculature is believed to be derived from the A12 dopamine cell group.

It is now generally accepted that dopamine released into the portal capillaries from the arcuate nucleus tonically inhibits the release of prolactin from the anterior pituitary (182). A short-loop feedback has been suggested whereby prolactin inhibits dopamine release from the median eminence (118,234). This hypothesis is consistent with the findings of prolactin (presumably of pituitary origin) in hypophyseal portal blood (221). Further evidence in support of this theory of a short-loop negative feedback has recently been presented (104). Interestingly, there are also limited data suggesting that prolactin may be synthesized in central nervous system structures of the hypothalamus (92). However, conclusions at this time regarding the source of prolactin in portal blood would seem premature.

In addition to dopamine, other putative neurotransmitters have been attributed to arcuate cell bodies. Serotonergic fibers and terminals are abundant throughout the hypothalamus but arise from serotonergic neurons in the lower brainstem (335). However, an intrinsic hypothalamic 5-HT system has been suggested from deafferentation studies (361). Arcuate cells containing 5-HT have also been reported in the rat (141,303), but these findings require further verification in other species.

A substantial literature now exists describing cholinergic systems in the CNS. Acetylcholine (ACh) has been identified in the arcuate nucleus by many indirect procedures (56), but these are not considered to be totally specific for ACh [see Silver (285)]. Therefore, the neuroendocrine role attributed to the putative arcuate cholinergic system must also remain tentative (217).

In the past few years, there have been numerous reports of peptides in the arcuate nucleus that are similar to the hormones in the intermediate and anterior lobes of the pituitary [see Fuxe et al. (97) and Krieger and Liotta (156)]. Adrenocorticotropic hormone (ACTH), α-melanoctye-stimulating hormone (α-MSH), β-lipotropic hormone (β-LPH), and β-endorphin have all been identified in the hypothalamus in intact and hypophysectomized animals (36,50,218,232,259,260).

Immunocytochemical reports have indicated that arcuate neurons positive for ACTH also contain β-LPH (36,218,359,360). Others have shown both β-endorphin and ACTH in the same arcuate neurons (36,305). Arcuate cell bodies containing both α-MSH and β-endorphin have also been reported (357). It is now known that these peptides are derived from a common precursor molecule in the pituitary gland referred to as 31 K or "proopiocortin" (183), and a similar glycoprotein precursor and subsequent processing are suspected in the hypothalamus (156). Although it has recently been shown that substance P and serotonin can be demonstrated in the same neurons (122), Bloch et al. (36) have shown that ACTH/β-endorphin neurons are different from dopamine neurons in the arcuate nucleus.

Arcuate neurons appear to be the only perikaryal source of ACTH, β-LPH, and β-endorphin. No other cell groups have been consistently reported to be immunoreactive for these peptides (232,354). However, immunoreactive fibers with these peptides have a much larger distribution throughout the brain, including the hypothalamus, amygdala, preoptic area, septum, thalamus, periaqueductal gray, and reticular formation (156). These findings suggest that the efferent projection of arcuate cells extends far beyond the well-known projection to the median eminence. In accordance with these morphological findings, Renaud and colleagues [see Renaud (256)] have provided electrophysiological data indicating that arcuate neurons have widely distributed axon collaterals to areas including the medial basal hypothalamus, anterior hypothalamic area, medial preoptic area, thalamus, and amygdala. The extensive axonal collateralization described by Renaud and colleagues suggests that these cells perform a very complex integrative role in brain function. This complex circuitry must be considered before functional roles are ascribed to these peptides. It is beyond the scope of this discussion to categorize the many and diverse effects reported for these peptides on neuronal activity and behavior [see reviews by deWied and Gispen (78) and Snyder and Childers (304)].

The arcuate nucleus receives many intrahypothalamic afferents from structures including the ventromedial medial nucleus (184,268), the medial and periventricular preoptic area (65), and the anterior hypothalamic area (66).

The arcuate nucleus, in addition to the remaining hypothalamus, receives an extensive noradrenergic innervation. The great majority of the NE terminals in the hypothalamus arise from lateral tegmental NE cell groups, with only a minor NE input from the locus ceruleus [see Moore and Bloom (204) for review]. Moreover, the NE terminals noted in the ME are also derived from brainstem catecholaminergic neurons (30). These data are supported by the deafferentation study of Weiner (361); after isolation from the rest of the brain, NE in the hypothalamic island was undetectable.

The heterogeneity of substances found in the arcuate nucleus precludes a simple description of the role of this hypothalamic structure. The arcuate nucleus undoubtedly plays a major role in the regulation of anterior pituitary function. However, the presence of some releasing/release-inhibiting substances outside of this area suggests that it is not the hypophysiotrophic region envisioned by Halasz and co-workers (108,109).

MONOAMINERGIC INPUT

A considerable body of evidence exists on the role of noradrenergic, dopaminergic, and/or serotonergic control of neurosecretory events, especially of ovulation [see McCann and Ojeda (179)].

From an anatomical point of view, however, many of these experiments are difficult to interpret since the site of action of these widespread neuronal systems is not known. Two anatomical approaches to this problem will be of considerable importance in the future: (a) retrograde tracing combined with procedures to identify the filled cell (71) and (b) immunocytochemistry combined with autoradiographic procedures at the electron microscopic level. The latter could be used to identify general afferents to known cell types as well as monoaminergic terminals (25,26). The first technique has been used to identify NE and DA input to the medial preoptic area (a region containing LHRH neurons). Horseradish perioxidase-filled cells were found in the nucleus of the solitary tract (nts) and the dorsal or cortical borders of the lateral reticular nucleus (lrn). In the nts, most but not all HRP-filled cells were positive for catecholamines (A2); all filled cells in the lrn (A1) were positive. Dopaminergic input appeared to arise from the A14 group of the periventricular hypothalamus, although this observation was less conclusive. Similar types of experiments are likely to reveal more precise organization of synaptic input to specific hypothalamic nuclei than attempts to trace axons with histofluorescence or immunocytochemistry for synthetic enzymes (298).

The anatomy and physiology of central catecholaminergic systems has recently been reviewed by Moore and Bloom (204). The locus ceruleus sends noradrenergic fibers via the periaqueductal gray into the dorsal longitudinal fasciculus. These cells innervate the dorsomedial, paraventricular, and supraoptic nuclei (170). These findings have been confirmed by anterograde tracing procedures (131). The remainder of the noradrenergic innervation to the hypothalamus appears to originate from the lateral tegmental system (A1, A3, A5, A7) (69) and probably from the nucleus of the solitary tract (see above) (261). There is also a direct noradrenergic input to the median eminence (30). The distribution of terminals in the rat hypothalamus as originally determined by histofluorescence (96) has been confirmed using immunocytochemistry for dopamine-β-hydroxylase (320). Similar patterns have been reported for the cat (60,248) and the primate (113).

Epinephrine terminals also innervate hypothalamic structures as determined by immunocytochemical localization of PMNT, the rate-limiting enzyme (119,120). The cell bodies reside in the caudal medulla (C1, C2), and terminals are found in the periventricular hypothalamus, ventrolateral arcuate nucleus, and posterolateral hypothalamus.

REFERENCES

1. Aghajanian, G. K., Bloom, F. E., and Sheard, M. H. (1969): Electron microscopy of degeneration within the serotonin pathway of rat brain. *Brain Res.,* 13:266–273.
2. Ajika, K., and Ochi, J. (1978): Serotonergic projections to the SCN of the median eminence of the rat: Identification by fluorescence and electron microscopy. *J. Anat.,* 127:563–576.
2a. Alonso, G., and Assenmacher. I. (1981): Radioautographic studies in the neurohypophyseal projections of the SON and PVN in the rat. *Cell Tiss. Res.,* 219:525–534.
3. Alvarez-Buylla, R., Livett, B. G., Uttenthal, L. O., Hope, D. B., and Milton, S. H. (1973): Immunological evidence for the transport of neurophysin in the hypothalamo–neurohypophysial system of the dog. *Z. Zellforsch.,* 137:435–450.
4. Amoss, M., Burgus, R., Blackwell, R., Vale, W., Fellows, R., and Guillemin, R. (1971): Purification, amino acid composition and *N*-terminal of the hypothalamic luteinizing hormone releasing factor, LRF, of ovine origin. *Biochem. Biophys. Res. Commun.,* 44:205–210.
5. Andrew, R. D., Macvicar, B. A., Dudek, F. E., and Hatton, G. I. (1980): Dye-coupling by gap junctions in magnocellular neuroendocrine cells of rat hypothalamus: Evidence for electrotonic coupling. *Soc. Neurosci.,* 6:456.
6. Antunes, J. L., Carmel, P. W., and Zimmerman, E. A. (1977): Projections from the paraventricular nucleus to the zona externa of the median eminence of the rhesus monkey: An immunohistochemical study. *Brain Res.,* 137:1–10.
7. Armstrong, W. E., Warach, S., Hatton, G. I., and McNeill, T. H. (1980): Subnuclei in the rat hypothalamic paraventricular nucleus: A cytoarchitectural, HRP and immunocytochemical analysis. *Neuroscience,* 5:1931–1958.
8. Aspeslagh, M.-R., Vandesande, F., and Dierickx, K. (1976): Electron microscopic immunocytochemical demonstration of separate neurophysin–vasopressinergic and neurophysin–oxytocinergic nerve fibers in the neural lobe of the rat hypophysis. *Cell Tissue Res.,* 171:31–37.
9. Attardi, B., Geller, L. N., and Ohno, S. (1976): Androgen and estrogen receptors in brain cytosol from male, female and testicular feminized (tfm/y ♂) mice. *Endocrinology,* 98:864–874.
10. Atweh, S. F., and Kuhar, M. I. (1977): Autoradiographic localization of opiate receptors in rat brain. II. The brain stem. *Brain Res.,* 129:1–12.
11. Azmitia, E. C., and Segal, M. (1978): An autoradiographic analysis of the differential ascending projections of the dorsal and median raphe nuclei in the rat. *J. Comp. Neurol.,* 179:641–668.
12. Balestrery, F. G., and Moberg, G. P. (1976): Effect of midbrain raphe nuclei lesions on the circadian rhythm of plasma corticosterone in the rat. *Brain Res.,* 118:503–508.
13. Bargmann, B. (1949): Uber die Neurosekretorische Verknupfung von Hypothalamus und Neurohypophyse. *Z. Zellforsch.,* 34:610–634

14. Bargmann, W., and Scharrer, E. (1951): The site of origin of the hormones of the posterior pituitary. *Am. Sci.,* 39:255–259.
15. Barker, J. L., Crayton, J. W., and Nicole, R. A. (1971): Supraoptic neurosecretory cells: Adrenergic and cholinergic sensitivity. *Science,* 171:208–209.
16. Barker, J. L., Crayton, J. W., and Nicole, R. A. (1971): Noradrenalin and acetylcholine responses of supraoptic neurosecretory cells. *J. Physiol.* (Lond.), 218:19–32.
17. Barry, J. (1976): Characterization and topography of LHRH neurons in the human brain. *Neurosci. Lett.,* 3:287–291.
18. Barry, J. (1979): Immunohistochemistry of luteinizing hormone-releasing hormone-producing neurons of the vertebrates. *Int. Rev. Cytol.,* 60:179–221.
19. Barry, J. (1980): Immunofluorescence study of LRH-producing neurons in prosimians (*Tupaia* and *Galago*). *Cell Tissue Res.,* 206:355–365.
20. Barry, J., and Carette, B. (1975): Immunofluorescence study of LRF neurons in primates. *Cell Tissue Res.,* 164:163–178.
21. Barry, J., and Croix, D. (1978): Immunofluorescence study of the hypothalamo-infundibular LHRH tract and serum gonadotropin levels in the female squirrel monkey during the estrous cycle. *Cell Tissue Res.,* 192:215–226.
22. Barry, J., and Dubois, M. P. (1974): Etude en immunofluorescence de la differentiation prenatale des cellules hypothalamiques elaboratrices de LH RF et de la maturation de la voie neurosectretice preoptico–infundibulaire chez le cobaye. *Brain Res.,* 67:103–113.
23. Barry, J., and Dubois, M. P. (1974): Immunofluorescence study of the preoptic infundibular LH–RH neurosecretory pathway of the guinea pig during the estrous cycle. *Neuroendocrinology,* 15:200–208.
24. Barry, J., Dubois, M. P., and Carrette, B. (1974): Immunofluorescence study of the preoptic–infundibular LRF neurosecretory pathway in the normal, castrated or testosterone-treated male guinea pig. *Endocrinology,* 95:1416–1423.
25. Beaudet, A., and Descarries, L. (1978): The monoamine innervation of rat cerebral cortex: Synaptic and nonsynaptic axon terminals. *Neuroscience,* 3:851–860.
26. Beaudet. A., and Descarries, L. (1979): Radioautographic characterization of a serotonin-accumulating nerve cell group in adult rat hypothalamus. *Brain Res.,* 160,231–243.
27. Beinfeld. M. C., Meyer, D. K., and Brownstein, M. J. (1980): Cholecystokinin octapeptide in the rat hypothalamo–neurohypophysial system. *Nature,* 288:376–378.
28. Bennett, C. T., and Pert, A. (1974): Antidiuresis produced by injections of histamine into the cat supraoptic nucleus. *Brain Res.,* 28:151–156.
29. Berk, M. L., and Finkelstein, J. A. (1980): An autoradiographic analysis of the efferent connections of the suprachiasmatic nucleus. *Soc. Neurosci.,* 6:521.

30. Bjorklund, A., Falck, B., Hromek, F., Owman. C., and West, K. A. (1970): Identification and terminal distribution of the tubero–hypophyseal monoamine systems in the rat by means of stereotaxic and microspectrofluorimetric techniques. *Brain Res.,* 17:1–23.

31. Bjorklund, A.. Falck, B., Nobin, A., and Stenevi, U. (1973): Organization of the dopamine and noradrenaline innervations of the median eminence pituitary region in the rat. In: *Neurosecretion—The Final Neuroendocrine Pathway,* edited by F. Knowles and L. Vollrath, pp. 209–222. Springer, New York.

32. Bjorklund, A., Lindvall, O., and Nobin, A. (1975): Evidence for an incertohypothalamic dopamine neurone system in the rat. *Brain Res.,* 89:29–42.

33. Bjorklund, A.. Moore, R. Y., Nobin, A.. and Stenevi, U. (1973): The organization of tubero–hypophyseal and reticulo–infundibular catecholamine neuron systems in the rat brain. *Brain Res.,* 51:171–191.

34. Blaustein, J. D., and Feder, H. H. (1979): Cytoplasmic progestin receptors in guinea pig brain: Characteristics and relationship to the induction of sexual behavior. *Brain Res.,* 169:481–497.

35. Bleier, R., Cohn, P., and Siggelkow, I. R. (1979): A cytoarchitectonic atlas of the hypothalamus and hypothalamic third ventricle of the rat. In: *Anatomy of the Hypothalamus,* Vol. 1. edited by P. J. Morgane and J. Panksepp, pp. 137–220. Marcel Dekker, New York.

36. Bloch, B., Bugnon, C., Fellman, D., and Lenys, D. (1978): Immunocytochemical evidence that the same neurons in the human infundibular nucleus are stained with anti-endorphins and antisera of other related peptides. *Neurosci. Lett.,* 10:147–152.

37. Bobillier, P., Seguin, S., Degueurce, A., Lewis, B. D., and Pujol, J. F. (1979): The efferent connections of the nucleus raphe centralis superior in the rat as revealed by radioautography. *Brain Res.,* 166:1–8.

38. Bock, R., Detzer, K., Leicht, E., and Roder, R. (1980): Functional difference between "classical" neurosecretory material and vasopressin-like substances of the outer layer of the median eminence. *Cell Tissue Res.,* 212:257–277.

39. Bock, R., and Jurna, I. (1977): Ipsilateral diminution of CRF-granules after unilateral hypothalamic lesions. *Cell Tissue Res.,* 185:215–229.

40. Bodian, D. (1951): Nerve endings, neurosecretory substance and lobular organization of the neurohypophysis. *Johns Hopkins Hosp. Bull.,* 89:354.

41. Brazeau, P., Vale, N., Burgus, R., Ling, N., Butcher, M., Rivier, J.. and Guillemin, R. (1973): Hypothalamic polypeptide that inhibits the secretion of immunoreactive pituitary growth hormone. *Science,* 179:77–79.

42. Broadwell, R. D., and Brightman, M. W. (1976): Entry of peroxidase into neurons of the central and peripheral nervous systems from extracerebral and cerebral blood. *J. Comp. Neurol.,* 166:257–284.

43. Broadwell, R. D., Oliver, C., and Brightman, M. W. (1979): Localization of neurophysin within organelles associated with protein synthesis and packaging in the hypothalamo–neurohypophysial system: An immunocytochemical study. *Proc. Natl. Acad. Sci. U.S.A.,* 76:5999–6003.

44. Brown-Grant, K., and Raisman, G. (1977): Abnormalities in reproductive function associated with the destruction of the suprachiasmatic nuclei in female rats. *Proc. R. Soc. Lond. [Biol.],* 198:279–296.

45. Brownstein, M., Arimura, A., Schally, A. V., Palkovits, M., and Kizer, J. S. (1976): The effect of surgical isolation of the hypothalamus on its luteinizing hormone-releasing hormone content. *Endocrinology,* 98:662–665.

46. Brownstein, M. J., Palkovits, M., Saavedra, J. M., Bassiri, R. M., and Utiger, R. D. (1974): Thyrotropin-releasing hormone in specific nuclei of rat brain. *Science,* 185:267–269.

47. Brownstein, M. J., Palkovits, M., Tappaz, M. L., Saavedra, I. M., and Kizer, J. S. (1976): Effect of surgical isolation of the hypothalamus on its neurotransmitter content. *Brain Res.,* 117:287–295.

48. Brownstein, M. J., Russell, J. T., and Gainer, H. (1980): Synthesis, transport and release of posterior pituitary hormones. *Science,* 207:373–378.

49. Bugnon, C.. Bloch, B., and Fellman, D. (1976): Immunocytological studies of LH–RH neurons in the human fetus. *C. R. Acad. Sci. [D] (Paris),* 282:1625–1628.

50. Bugnon, C., Bloch, B., Lenys, D., Gouget, A., and Fellman, D. (1979), Comparative study of the neuronal populations containing β-endorphin, corticotropin and dopamine in the arcuate nucleus of the rat hypothalamus. *Neurosci. Lett.,* 14:43–48.

51. Bugnon, C., Fellman, D., and Bloch, B. (1977): Immunocytochemical study of the ontogenesis of the hypothalamic somatostatin-containing neurons in the human fetus. *Cell Tissue Res.,* 183:319–328.

51a. Bugnon, C., Fellman, D., Gouget, A., and Cardot, J. (1982): Corticoliberin in rat brain: Immunocytochemical identification and localization of a novel neuroglandular system. *Neruosci. Lett.,* 30:25–30.

52. Buijs, R. M. (1978): Intra- and extrahypothalamic vasopressin and oxytocin pathways in the rat. *Cell Tissue Res.,* 192:423–436.

53. Buijs, R. M., and Swaab, D. F. (1979): Immunoelectron microscopical demonstration of vasopressin and oxytocin synapses in the limbic system of the rat. *Cell Tissue Res.,* 204:335–365.

54. Buijs, R. M., Swaab, D. F., Dogsterom, J., and van Leeuwen, F. W. (1978): Intra- and extrahypothalamic vasopressin and oxytocin pathways in the rat. *Cell Tissue Res.,* 186:423–433.

55. Burgus, R., Dunn, T. F., Desidero, D., Ward. D. N., Vale, W., and Guillemin, R. (1970): Characterization of ovine hypothalamic hypophysiotropic TSH-releasing factor. *Nature,* 226,321.

56. Carson. K. A., Nemeroff, C. B., Rone, M. S., Nicholson, G. F., Kizer, J. S., and Hanker, J. S.

(1978): Experimental studies on the ultrastructural localization of acetylcholinesterase in the mediobasal hypothalamus of the rat. *J. Comp. Neurol.*, 182:201–220.

57. Castel, M., and Hochman, J. (1976): Ultrastructural immunohistochemical localization of vasopressin in the hypothalamic–neurohypophyseal system of three murides. *Cell Tissue Res.*, 174:69–81.

58. Celotti, F., Massa, R., and Martini, L. (1979): Metabolism of sex steroids in the central nervous system. In: *Endocrinology*, Vol. 1, edited by L. J. DeGroot, pp. 41–53. Grune & Stratton, New York.

59. Chamness, G. C., King, T. W., and Sheridan. P. J. (1979): Androgen receptor in the rat brain—assays and properties. *Brain Res.*, 161:267–276.

60. Cheung, Y., and Sladek, J. R., Jr. (1975): Catecholamine distribution in feline hypothalamus. *J. Comp. Neurol.*, 164:339–360.

61. Choy, V. J., and Watkins, W. B. (1977): Immunohistochemical localization of thyrotropin-releasing factor in the rat median eminence. *Cell Tissue Res.*, 177:371–374.

62. Christensen, L. W., and Clemens, L. G. (1974): Intrahypothalamic implants of testosterone or estradiol and resumption of masculine sexual behavior in long-term castrated male rats. *Endocrinology*, 95:984–990.

63. Clayton, C. J., and Hoffman, G. E. (1979): Immunocytochemical evidence for anti-LHRH and anti-ACTH activity in the "F" antiserum. *Am. J. Anat.*, 165:139–145.

64. Coen, C. W., and MacKinnon, P. C. B. (1979): Serotonin involvement in the control of phasic luteinizing hormone release in the rat: Evidence for a critical period. *J. Endocrinol.*, 82:105–113.

65. Conrad, L. C., and Pfaff, D. W. (1976): Efferents from medial basal forebrain and hypothalamus in the rat. I. An autoradiographic study of the medial preoptic area. *J. Comp. Neurol.*, 169:185–220.

66. Conrad, L. C., and Pfaff. D. W. (1976): Efferents from medial basal forebrain and hypothalamus in the rat. II. An autoradiographic study of the anterior hypothalamus. *J. Comp. Neurol.*, 169:221–262.

67. Critchlow, V., Rice, R. W., Abe, K., and Vale, W. (1978): Somatostatin content of the median eminence in female rats with lesion-induced disruption of the inhibitory control of growth hormone secretion. *Endocrinology*, 103:817–825.

68. Crowley, W. R., and Terry, L. C. (1980): Biochemical mapping of somatostatinergic systems in rat brain. Effects of periventricular hypothalamic and medial basal amygdaloid lesions on somatostatin-like immunoreactivity in discrete brain nuclei. *Brain Res.*, 200:283–291.

69. Dahlstrom, A., and Fuxe, K. (1964): Evidence for the existence of monoamine-containing neurons in the central nervous system. I. Demonstration of monoamines with cell bodies of brain stem neurons. *Acta Physiol. Scand.*, 232:1–55.

70. Davis, P. G., and Barfield, R. J. (1979): Activation of feminine sexual behavior in castrated male rats by intrahypothalamic implants of estradiol benzoate. *Neuroendocrinology*, 28:228–233.

71. Day, T. A., Blessing, W., and Willoughby, J. O. (1980): Noradrenergic and dopaminergic projections to the medial preoptic area of the rat. A combined horseradish perioxidase/catecholamine fluorescence study. *Brain Res.*, 193:543–548.

72. Dean. C. R., Hope, D. B., and Kazic, T. (1968): Evidence for the storage of oxytocin with neurophysin I and of vasopressin with neurophysin II in separate neurosecretory granules. *Br. J. Pharmacol.*, 34:192–193.

73. Dean. C. R., and Hope, D. B. (1968): The isolation of neurophysin I and II from bovine pituitary neurosecretory granules separated on a large scale from other subcellular organelles. Demonstration of slow equilibrium of neurosecretory granules during centrifugation in a sucrose density gradient. *Biochem. J.*, 106:565–573.

74. DeBrodo, R. C. (1944): The antidiuretic action of morphine and its mechanism. *J. Pharmacol. Exp. Ther.*, 82:74–85.

75. Defindini, R., and Zimmerman, E. A. (1978): The magnocellular neurosecretory system of the mammalian hypothalamus. In: *The Hypothalamus*, edited by S. Reichlin, R. J. Baldessarini, and J. B. Martin, pp. 137–152. Raven Press, New York.

76. DeMey, J., Dierickx, K., and Vandesande, F. (1975): Immunohistochemical demonstration of neurophysin I- and Neurophysin II-containing nerve fibers in the external region of the bovine median eminence. *Cell Tissue Res.*, 157:517–519.

77. DeMey, J., Vandesande, F., and Dierickx, K. (1974): Identification of neurophysin producing cells. II. Identification of the neurophysin I and neurophysin II producing neurons in the bovine hypothalamus. *Cell Tissue Res.*, 153:531–543.

78. deWied, D., and Gispen, W. H. (1977): Behavioral effects of peptides. In: *Peptides in Neurobiology*, edited by H. Gainer. Plenum Press, New York.

79. Dierickx, K., and Vandesande, F. (1977): Immunocytochemical localization of the vasopressinergic and the oxytocinergic neurons in the human hypothalamus. *Cell Tissue Res.*, 184:15–27.

80. Dierickx, K., and Vandesande, F. (1979): Immunocytochemical localization of somatostatin-containing neurons in the rat hypothalamus. *Cell Tissue Res.*, 201:349–359.

81. Dierickx, K., Vandesande, F., and DeMey, J. (1976): Identification in the external region of the rat median eminence of separate neurophysin-vasopressin and neurophysin-oxytocin containing nerve fibers. *Cell Tissue Res.*, 168:141–151.

82. Dube, D., LeClerc, R., and Pelletier, G. (1975): Immunohistochemical detection of growth hormone-release inhibiting hormone (somatostatin) in the guinea pig brain. *Cell Tissue Res.*, 161:385–392.

83. Dubois, M. P., and Kolodziejczyk, E. (1975):

Centres hypothalamiques du rat, secretant la somatostatine: Repartition, des pericaryons en deux systemes magno- et parvocellulaires (etude immunocytologique). *C. R. Acad. Sci. [D] (Paris),* 281:1737–1740.

84. Dunn, J. D., Castro, A. J., and McNulty, J. A. (1978): Effect of suprachiasmatic ablation on the daily temperature rhythm. *Neurosci. Lett.,* 6:345–348.

85. DuVigneaud, V. (1956): Hormones of the posterior pituitary gland: Oxytocin and vasopressin. In: *The Harvey Lectures, 1954–1955,* pp. 1–26. Academic Press, New York.

86. Eiden, L. E., and Eskay, R. L. (1980): Characterization of LRF-like immunoreactivity in the frog sympathetic ganglia: Non-identity with LRF decapeptide. *Neuropeptides,* 1:29–37.

87. Elde, R. P., and Parsons, J. A. (1975): Immunocytochemical localization of somatostatin in cell bodies of the rat hypothalamus. *Am. J. Anat.,* 144:541–548.

88. Epelbaum, J., Willoughby, J. O., Brazeau, P., and Martin, J. B. (1977): Effects of brain lesions and hypothalamic deafferentation on somatostatin distribution in the rat brain. *Endocrinology,* 101:1495–1502.

89. Evans, J. J., and Watkins. W. N. (1973): Localization of neurophysin in the neurosecretory elements of the hypothalamus and neurohypophysis of the normal osmotically stimulated guinea pig as demonstrated by immunofluorescence. *Z. Zellforsch.,* 145:39–55.

90. Feder. H. H. (1971): The comparative actions of testosterone proprionate and 5-androstan-17β-ol-3-one proprionate on the reproductive behavior, physiology and morphology of male rats. *J. Endocrinol.,* 51:241–252.

91. Feder, H. H., and Marrone, B. L. (1977): Progesterone: Its role in the central nervous system as a facilitator and inhibitor of sexual behavior and gonadotropin release. *Ann. N.Y. Acad. Sci.,* 286:331–354.

92. Felten, D. L., and Cashner, K. A. (1979): Cytoarchitecture of the supraoptic nucleus. *Neuroendocrinology,* 29:221–230.

93. Flerko, B., Setalo, G., Vigh, S., Arimura, A., and Schally, A. V. (1978): The luteinizing hormone-releasing hormone (LHRH) neuron system in the rat and rabbit. In: *Brain–Endocrine Interaction III, Neural Hormones and Reproduction,* edited by D. E. Scott, G. P. Kozlowski, and A. Weindl, pp. 108–116. S. Karger, Basel.

94. Fox, T. O. (1975): Androgen- and estrogen-binding macromolecules in developing mouse brain: Biochemical and genetic evidence. *Proc. Natl. Acad. Sci. U.S.A.,* 72:4303–4307.

95. Frost, D. O., So, K.-F., and Schneider, G. E. (1979): Postnatal development of retinal projections in Syrian hamsters: A study using autoradiographic and anterograde degeneration techniques. *Neuroscience,* 4:1649–1677.

96. Fuxe, K. (1965): Evidence for the existence of monoamine neurons in the central nervous system. IV. The distribution of monoamine nerve terminals in the central nervous system. *Acta Physiol. Scand. [Suppl.],* 247:37–85.

97. Fuxe, K., Hokfelt, T., Eneroth, P., Gustafsson, M., and Skett, P. (1977): Prolactin-like immunoreactivity: Localization in nerve terminals of rat hypothalamus. *Science,* 196:899–900.

98. Gainer, H., and Saine, Y. (1977): Neurophysin biosynthesis: Conversion of a putative precursor during axonal transport. *Science,* 195:1354–1355.

99. Gainer, H., Saine, Y., and Brownstein, M. J. (1977): Biosynthesis and axonal transport of rat neurohypophysial proteins and peptides. *J. Cell Biol.,* 73:366–381.

100. Gerlach, J. L., McEwen, B. S., Pfaff, D. W., Moskowitz, S., Ferin, M., Carmel, P. N., and Zimmerman, E. A. (1976): Cells in regions of rhesus monkey brain and pituitary retain radioactive estradiol, corticosterone and cortisol differentially. *Brain Res.,* 103:603–612.

101. Goldfoot, D. A. (1979): Sex-specific, behavior-specific actions of dihydrotestosterone: Activation of aggression, but not mounting in ovariectomized guinea pigs. *Hormones Behav.,* 13:241–255.

102. Goldsmith, P. C., and Ganong, W. F. (1975): Ultrastructural localization of luteinizing hormone-releasing hormone in the median eminence of the rat. *Brain Res..* 97:181–193.

103. Gorski, R. A. (1980): Sexual differentiation of the brain. In: *Neuroendocrinology,* edited by D. T. Krieger and J. C. Hughes, pp. 215–222. Sinauer, Sunderland, Massachusetts.

104. Gudelsky, G. A., and Porter, J. C. (1980): Release of dopamine from tuberoinfundibular neurons into pituitary stalk blood after prolactin or haloperidol administration. *Endocrinology,* 106:526–529.

105. Guldner, F. H., and Wolff, J. R. (1978): Retinal afferents from Gray-type-I and type-II synapses in the suprachiasmatic nucleus (rat). *Exp. Brain Res.,* 32:83–89.

106. Gurdjian, E. S. (1927): The diencephalon of the albino rat. Studies in the brain of the rat. *J. Comp. Neurol.,* 43:1–114.

107. Gwinner, E. (1974): Testosterone induces splitting of circadian locomotor activity rhythms in birds. *Science,* 185:72–74.

108. Halasz, B., and Gorski, R. A. (1967): Gonadotrophic hormone secretion in female rats after partial or total interruption of neural afferents to the medial basal hypothalamus. *Endocrinology,* 80,608–622.

109. Halasz, B., and Pupp, L. (1965): Hormone secretion of the anterior pituitary gland after physical interruption of all nervous pathways to the hypophysiotrophic area. *Endocrinology,* 77:553–562.

110. Hendrickson, A. E., Wagoner, N.. and Cowan. W. M. (1972): An autoradiographic and electron microscopic study of retino–hypothalamic connections. *Z. Zellforsch.,* 135:1–26.

111. Herkenham, M.. and Nauta, W. J. (1977): Afferent connections of the habenular nuclei in the rat. A horseradish peroxidase study with a note on the fiber of passage problem. *J. Comp. Neurol..* 173:123–146.

112. Hery, M., Laplante, E., and Kordon, C. (1978): Participation of serotonin in the phasic release of luteinizing hormone. II. Effects of lesions of serotonin-containing pathways in the central nervous system. *Endocrinology,* 102:1019–1025.

113. Hoffman, G. E., Felten, D. L., and Sladek, J. R., Jr. (1976): Monoamine distribution in primate brain. III. Catecholamine-containing varicosities in the hypothalamus of *Macaca mulatta. Am. J. Anat.,* 147:501–514.

114. Hoffman, G. E., and Hayes, T. A. (1979): Somatostatin neurons and their projections in dog diencephalon. *J. Comp. Neurol.,* 186:371–392.

115. Hoffman, G. E., Knigge, K. M., Moyniban. J. A., Melnyk, V. and Arimura, A. (1978): Neuronal fields containing luteinizing hormone releasing hormone (LHRH) in mouse brain. *Neuroscience,* 3:219–231.

116. Hokfelt, T., Efendic, S., Hellerstrom, C., Johansson. O.. Luft, R., and Arimura, A. (1975): Cellular localization of somatostatin in endocrine-like cells and neurons of the rat with special reference to the A_1-cells of the pancreatic islets and to the hypothalamus. *Acta Endocrinol. (Kbh.),* 80:5–41.

117. Hokfelt, T., Efendic, S.. Johansson, O., Luft. R., and Arimura, A. (1974): Immunohistochemical localization of somatostatin (growth hormone release–inhibiting factor) in the guinea pig brain. *Brain Res.,* 80:165–169.

118. Hokfelt, T., and Fuxe, K. (1972): Effects of prolactin and ergot alkaloids on the tuberoinfundibular dopamine (DA) neurons. *Neuroendocrinology,* 9:100–122.

119. Hokfelt, T., Fuxe, K.. and Goldstein. M. (1973): Immunohistochemical studies on monoamine-containing cell systems. *Brain Res.,* 62:461–469.

120. Hokfelt, T., Fuxe, K.. Goldstein, M., and Johansson, O. (1974): Immunohistochemical evidence for the existence of adrenaline neurons in the rat brain. *Brain Res.,* 66:233–251.

121. Hokfelt, T., Fuxe, K., Johansson, O., Jeffcoate, S., and White, N. (1975): Distribution of thyrotropin-releasing hormone (TRH) in the central nervous system as revealed with immunohistochemistry. *Eur. J. Pharmacol.,* 34:389–392.

122. Hokfelt, T., Ljungdahl, A., Steinbusch, H., Verhofstad, A., Nilsson, G., Brodin, E., Pernow, B., and Goldstein, M. (1978): Immunohistochemical evidence of substance P-like immunoreactivity in some 5-hydroxytryptamine-containing neurons in the rat central nervous system. *Neuroscience,* 3:517–538.

123. Holzwarth-McBride, M. A., Sladek, J. R., and Knigge. K. M. (1976): Monosodium glutamate induced lesions of the arcuate nucleus. II. Fluorescence histochemistry of catecholamines. *Anat. Rec.,* 186:197–206.

124. Honma, K., and Hiroshige, T. (1979): Participation of brain catecholaminergic neurons in a self-sustained circadian oscillation of plasma corticosterone in the rat. *Brain Res.,* 169:519–529.

125. Honma, K., Watanabe, K., and Hiroshige. T. (1979): Effects of *para*-chlorophenylalanine and 5,6-dihydroxytryptamine on the free-running rhythms of locomotor activity and plasma corticosterone in the rat exposed to continuous light. *Brain Res.,* 169:531–544.

126. Hosoya, Y., and Matsushita, M. (1979): Identification and distribution of the spinal and hypophyseal projection neurons in the paraventricular nucleus of the rat. A light and electron microscopic study with the HRP method. *Exp. Brain Res.,* 35:315–331.

126a. Ibuka, N., and Kawamura. H. (1975): Loss of circadian rhythm in sleep–wakefulness cycle in the rat by suprachiasmatic nucleus lesions. *Brain Res.,* 96:76–81.

127. Jackson, I. M. D. (1980): TRH in the rat nervous system: Identity with synthetic TRH on high performance liquid chromatography following affinity chromatography. *Brain Res.,* 201:245–248.

128. Jan, Y. N., Jan L. Y., and Kuffler, S. W. (1979): A peptide as a possible transmitter in sympathetic ganglia of the frog. *Proc. Natl. Acad. Sci. U.S.A.,* 76:1501–1505.

129. Jennes, L., and Stumpf, W. E. (1980): LHRH-systems in the brain of the golden hamster. *Cell Tissue Res..* 209:239–256.

130. Johansson, O., Hokfelt, T., Jeffcoate, S. L., White, N., and Sternberger, L. A. (1980): Ultrastructural localization of TRH-like immunoreactivity. *Exp. Brain Res.,* 38:1–10.

131. Jones, B. E., and Moore, R. Y. (1977): Ascending projections of the locus coeruleus in the rat. II. Autoradiographic study. *Brain Res.,* 127:23–53.

132. Jonsson, G., Fuxe, K., and Hokfelt, T. (1972): On the catecholamine innervation of the hypothalamus with special reference to the median eminence. *Brain Res.,* 40:271–281.

133. Jordan, D., Pigeon, P., McRae-Degueurce, A., Pujol, J. F., and Mornex, R. (1979): Participation of serotonin in thyrotropin release. II. Evidence for the action of serotonin on the phasic release of thyrotropin. *Endocrinology,* 105:975–979.

134. Jouan, P., Samperez, S., and Thieulant, M. L. (1973): Testosterone "receptors" in purified nuclei of rat anterior hypophysis. *J. Steroid Biochem.,* 4:65–74.

135. Kahn, D., Abrams, G. M., Zimmerman, E. A., Carraway, R., and Leeman, S. (1980): Neurotensin neurons in the rat hypothalamus: An immunocytochemical study. *Endocrinology,* 107:47–51.

136. Kalra, S. P., Kalra, P. S., and Mitchell, E. O. (1977): Differential response of luteinizing hormone–releasing hormone in the basal hypothalamus and the preoptic area following anterior hypothalamic deafferentation and/or castration in male rats. *Endocrinology,* 100:201–204.

137. Kam, L. M., and Moberg, G. P. (1977): Effect of raphe lesions on the circadian pattern of wheel running in the rat. *Physiol. Behav.,* 18:213–217.

138. Kato. J., and Onouchi, T. (1973): 5α-Dihydrotestosterone "receptor" in the rat hypothalamus. *Endocrinol. Jpn.,* 20:429–432.

139. Keefer, D. A., Stumpf, W. E., Petrusz, P., and

Sar, M. (1975): Simultaneous autoradiographic and immunohistochemical localization of estrogen and gonadotropin in the rat pituitary. *Am. J. Anat.*, 142:129–135.

140. Kelly, M. J., Kuhnt, V., and Wuttke, W. (1980): Hyperpolarization of hypothalamic parvocellular neurons by 17β-estradiol and their identification through intracellular staining with procion yellow. *Exp. Brain Res.*. 40:440–447.

141. Kent, D. L., and Sladek, J. R., Jr. (1978): Histochemical, pharmacological and microspectrofluorometric analysis of new sites of serotonin localization in the rat hypothalamus. *J. Comp. Neurol.*. 180:221–236.

142. Kilcoyne, M., Hoffman, D. L., and Zimmerman, E. A. (1980): Immunocytochemical localization of angiotensin II and vasopressin in rat hypothalamus: Evidence for production in the same neuron. *Clin. Sci.*, 59:575–605.

143. King, J. A., and Millar, R. P. (1979), Phylogenetic and anatomical distribution of somatostatin in vertebrates. *Endocrinology*, 105:1322–1329.

144. King, J. A., and Millar, R. P. (1980): Comparative aspects of luteinizing hormone–releasing hormone structure and function in vertebrate phylogeny. *Endocrinology*, 106:707–717.

145. King, J. C., Tobet. S. A., Snavely, F. L., and Arimura, A. A. (1980): The LHRH system in normal and neonatally androgenized female rats. *Peptides*, 1(Suppl. 1):85–100.

146. Kizer, J. S., Palkovits, M., and Brownstein, M. J. (1976): The projections of the A8, A9 and A10 dopaminergic cell bodies: Evidence for a nigral–hypothalamic–median eminence dopaminergic pathway. *Brain Res.*, 108:363–370.

147. Klein, D. C., and Moore. R. Y. (1979): Pineal *N*-acetyltransferase and hydroxyindole-*O*-methyltransferase: Control by the retinohypothalamic tract and the suprachiasmatic nucleus. *Brain Res.*, 174:245–262.

148. Knigge, K. M., and Silverman, A. J. (1974): Anatomy of the endocrine hypothalamus. In: *Handbook of Physiology*, edited by S. R. Geiger, pp. 1–32. Academic Press, New York.

149. Koh, E. T., and Ricardo, J. A. (1980): Paraventricular nucleus of the hypothalamus: Anatomical evidence of ten functional discrete subdivisions. *Soc. Neurosci.*, 6:521.

150. Kozlowski, G. P., Frenk, S.. and Brownfield, M. S. (1977): Localization of neurophysin in the rat supraoptic nucleus. *Cell Tissue Res.*, 179:467–473.

151. Kozlowski, G. P., and Hostetter, G. (1978): Cellular and subcellular localization and behavioral effects of gonadotropin releasing hormone (GnRH) in the rat. In: *Brain Endocrine Interactions III: Neural Hormones and Reproduction*, edited by D. E. Scott, G. P. Kozlowski. and A. Windl, pp. 138–153. S. Karger, Basel.

152. Krey, L. C., Butler, W. R.. and Knobil, E. (1975): Surgical disconnection of the medial basal hypothalamus and pituitary function in the rhesus monkey. I. Gonadotropin secretion. *Endocrinology*, 96:1073–1987.

153. Krey, L. C., and Silverman, A. J. (1978): The luteinizing hormone–releasing hormone (LH–RH) neuronal networks of the guinea pig brain. II. The regulation of gonadotropin secretion and the origin of terminals in the median eminence. *Brain Res.*, 157:247–255.

154. Krey, L. C., and Silverman, A. J. (1981): The luteinizing hormone–releasing hormone neuronal networks of the guinea pig brain: III. Regulation of cyclic gonadotropin secretion. *Brain Res.*, 229:429–444.

155. Krieg. W. J. S. (1932): The hypothalamus of the albino rat. *J. Comp. Neurol.*, 55:19–89.

156. Krieger, D. T., and Liotta, A. S. (1979): Pituitary hormones in brain: Where, how and why? *Science*, 205:366–372.

157. Krieger, M. S., Morrell, J. I., and Pfaff, D. W. (1976): Autoradiographic localization of estradiol-concentrating cells in the female hamster brain. *Neuroendocrinology*, 22:193–205.

158. Krisch, B. (1977): Morphological equivalent of the bifunctional role of somatostatin. *Cell Tissue Res.*, 179:211–224.

159. Krisch, B. (1978): The distribution of LHRH in the hypothalamus of the thirsty rat. *Cell Tissue Res.*, 186:135–148.

160. Krisch, B. (1980): Nongranular vasopressin synthesis and transport in early stages of rehydration. *Cell Tissue Res.*, 207:89–107.

161. Krulich, L. (1979): Central neurotransmitters and the secretion of prolactin, GH, LH and TSH. *Annu. Rev. Physiol.*, 41:603–615.

162. Krulich, L., Dhariwal, A. P. S., and McCann, S. M. (1968): Stimulatory and inhibitory effects of purified hypothalamic extracts on growth hormone release from rat pituitary *in vitro*. *Endocrinology*, 83:783–790.

163. Kucera, P., and Favrod, P. (1979): Suprachiasmatic nucleus projection to mesencephalic central grey in the woodmouse *(Apodemus sylvaticus* L.). *Neuroscience*, 4:1705–1715.

164. Kuhn, E. R. (1974): Cholinergic and adrenergic release mechanism for vasopressin in the male rat: A study with injection of neurotransmitters and blocking agents into the third ventricle *Neuroendocrinology*, 16:255–264.

165. Kuypers, H. G. J. M., and Maisky, V. A. (1975): Retrograde axonal transport of horseradish peroxidase from spinal cord to brain stem cell groups in the cat. *Neurosci. Lett.*. 1:9–14.

166. Lechan, R. M., Nestler, J. L., Jacobson, S., and Reichlin, S. (1980): The hypothalamic tuberoinfundibular system of the rat as demonstrated by horseradish peroxidase (HRP) microiontophoresis. *Brain Res.*, 195:1–27.

167. LeClerc, R., and Pelletier, G. (1974): Electron microscope immunohistochemical localization of vasopressin in the hypothalamus and neurohypophysis of the normal and Brattleboro rat. *Am. J. Anat.*, 140:583–587.

168. Lieberburg, I., and McEwen, B. S. (1975): Estradiol-17b: A metabolite of testosterone recovered in cell nuclei from limbic areas of neonatal rat brain. *Brain Res.*, 85:165–170.

169. Lieberburg, I.. and McEwen, B. S. (1977): Brain cell nuclear retention of testosterone metabolites, 5-dihydrotestosterone and estradiol 17B in adult rats. *Endocrinology,* 100:588–597.

170. Lindvall, O., and Bjorklund, A. (1974): The glyoxylic acid fluorescence histochemical method: A detailed account of the methodology for the visualization of central catecholamine neurons. *Histochemistry,* 39:97–127.

171. Livett, B. G. (1975): Immunocytochemical studies on the storage and axonal transport of neurophysin in the hypothalamo–neurohypophyseal system. *Ann. N.Y. Acad. Sci.,* 248:112–133.

172. Livett, B. G., Uttenthal, L. O., and Hope, D. B. (1971): Localization of neurophysin II in the hypothalamo–neurophyseal system of the pig by immunofluorescence histology. *Phil. Trans. R. Soc. Lond. [Biol.],* 261:371–378.

173. Livingston, A. (1975): Morphology of the perivascular regions of the rat neural lobe in relation to hormone release. *Cell Tissue Res.,* 159:551–561.

174. Livingston, A. (1978): Effects of hormone-releasing stimuli on the area of the perivascular space in the neural lobe of the rat. *Cell Tissue Res.,* 191:501–506.

175. Loren, I., Emson, P. C., Fahrenkrug, J., Bjorklund, A. Alumets, J., Hakanson, R., and Sundler, F. (1979): Distribution of vasoactive intestinal polypeptide in the rat and mouse brain. *Neuroscience,* 4:1953–1976.

176. Luiten, P. G. M., and Room, P. (1980): Interrelations between lateral, dorsomedial and ventromedial hypothalamic nuclei in the rat. *Brain Res.,* 190:321–332.

177. Luttge, W. G., Hall, N. R., and Wallis, C. J. (1974): Studies on the neuroendocrine, somatic and behavioral effectiveness of testosterone and its 5-alpha-reduced metabolites in Swiss–Wistar mice. *Physiol. Behav.,* 13:553–561.

178. Lydic, R., and Moore-Ede, M. C. (1980): Three dimensional structure of the suprachiasmatic nuclei in the diurnal squirrel monkey *(Saimiri sciureus). Neurosci. Lett.,* 17:295–299.

179. McCann, S. M., and Ojeda, S. R. (1979): The role of brain monoamines, acetylcholine and prostaglandins in the control of anterior pituitary function. In: *Endocrinology,* edited by L. J. deGroot, pp. 41–54. Grune & Stratton, New York.

180. McEwen, B. S. (1979): Distribution and binding of hormones in different CNS areas. In: *Endocrinology,* edited by L. J. deGroot, pp. 35–40. Grune & Stratton, New York.

181. McNeill, T. H.. and Sladek, J. R., Jr. (1981): Simultaneous monoamine histofluorescence and neuropeptide immunocytochemistry. *J. Comp. Neurol.,* 193:1023–1033.

182. Macleod, R. M., and Lehmeyer, J. E. (1974): Studies on the mechanism of the dopamine-mediated inhibition of prolactin secretion. *Endocrinology,* 94:1077–1085.

183. Mains, R. E., Eipper, B. A., and Zing, N. (1977): Common precursor to corticotropins and endorphins. *Proc. Natl. Acad. Sci. U.S.A.,* 74:3014–3018.

184. Makara, G. B., and Hodacs, L. (1975), Rostral projections from the hypothalamic arcuate nucleus. *Brain Res.,* 84:23–29.

185. Marchand, E. R., Riley, J. N., and Moore, R. Y. (1980): Interpeduncular nucleus afferents in the rat. *Brain Res.,* 193:339–352.

186. Marshall, P. E., and Goldsmith, P. C. (1980): Neuroregulatory and neuroendocrine GnRH pathways in the hypothalamus and forebrain of the baboon. *Brain Res.,* 193:353–372.

187. Martin, J. B., Kontor, J., and Mead, P. (1973): Plasma GH responses to hypothalamic, hippocampal and amygdaloid electrical stimulation. Effects of variation in stimulus parameters and treatment with alpha-methyl-*p*-tyrosine (alphaMT). *Endocrinology,* 92:1354–1361.

188. Martin. J. B., Renaud, L. P., and Brazeau, P. (1974): Pulsatile growth hormone secretion: Suppression by hypothalamic ventromedial lesions and by long-acting somatostatin. *Science,* 186:538–540.

189. Martin, J. B., Tannenbaum, G., Willoughby, J. O., Renaud, L. P., and Brazeau, P. (1975): Functions of the central nervous system in regulation of pituitary GH secretion. In: *Hypothalamic Hormones,* edited by M. Motta, P. G. Crosignani, and L. Martini, pp. 217–236. Academic Press, New York.

190. Mason, C. A., Sparrow, N., and Lincoln, D. W. (1977): Structural features of the retinohypothalamic projection in the rat during normal development. *Brain Res.,* 132:141–148.

191. Maurer, R. A., and Woolley, D. E. (1974): Demonstration of nuclear ³H-estradiol binding in hypothalamus and amygdala of female, androgenized female and male rats. *Neuroendocrinology,* 16:137–147.

192. Meibach, R. C., and Siegel, A. (1977): Efferent connections of the hippocampal formation in the rat. *Brain Res.,* 124:197–224.

193. Merchenthaler, I., Kovacs, G., Lovasz, G., and Setalo, G. (1980): The preoptico–infundibular LH–RH tract of the rat. *Brain Res.,* 198:63–74.

194. Meyer, D. C., and Quay, W. B. (1976): Hypothalamic and suprachiasmatic uptake of serotonin *in vitro:* Twenty-four-hour changes in male and proestrous rats. *Endocrinology,* 98:1160–1165.

195. Meyer, D. K., Oertel, W. H., and Brownstein. M. J. (1980): Deafferentation studies on the glutamic acid decarboxylase of the supraoptic nucleus of the rat. *Brain Res.,* 200:165–168.

196. Meynert, T. (1872): Vom Gehirne der Saugetiere. In: *Handbuch der Genebelehre,* Vol. 2, edited by S. Stricker, pp. 953–1066. W. Wood and Co., New York.

197. Mickvych, P., and Elde, R. (1980): Relationship between enkephalinergic neurons and the vasopressin–oxytocin neuroendocrine system of the cat: An immunohistochemical study. *J. Comp. Neurol..* 190:135–146.

198. Millar, R. P., Aehnelt, C., and Rossier, G. (1977): Higher molecular weight immunoreactive

species of luteinizing hormone releasing hormone: Possible precursors of the hormone. *Biochem. Biophys. Res. Commun.,* 74:720–731.

199. Millhouse, O. E. (1977): Optic chiasm collaterals afferent to the suprachiasmatic nucleus. *Brain Res.,* 137:351–355.

200. Millhouse, O. E. (1979): A Golgi anatomy of the rodent hypothalamus. In: *Handbook of the Hypothalamus,* Vol. 1, edited by P. J. Morgane and J. Panksepp, pp. 221–266. Marrel Dekker, New York.

201. Monbon, M., Loras, B., Reboud, J. P., and Bertrand, J. (1973): Uptake, binding, and metabolism of testosterone in rat brain tissues. *Brain Res.,* 53:139–150.

202. Moore, R. Y. (1973): Retinohypothalamic projection in mammals: A comparative study. *Brain Res..* 49:403–409.

203. Moore, R. Y. (1978): Central neural control of circadian rhythms. In: *Frontiers in Neuroendocrinology.* Vol. 5, edited by W. F. Ganong and L. Martini, pp. 186–206. Raven Press. New York.

204. Moore, R. Y., and Bloom, F. E. (1979): Central catecholamine neuron systems: Anatomy and physiology of the norepinephrine and epinephrine systems. *Annu. Rev. Neurosci.,* 2:113–168.

205. Moore, R. Y., and Eichler. V. B. (1972): Loss of circadian adrenal corticosterone rhythm following suprachiasmatic lesions in the rat. *Brain Res.,* 42:201–206.

206. Moore, R. Y., Halaris, A. E., and Jones, B. F. (1978): Serotonin neurons of the midbrain raphe: Ascending projections. *J. Comp. Neurol.,* 180:417–438.

207. Moore, R. Y. and Klein, D. C. (1974): Visual pathways and the central neural control of a circadian rhythm in pineal serotonin *N*-acetyltransferase activity. *Brain Res.,* 71:17–33.

208. Moore, R. Y., and Lenn, N. J. (1972): A retinohypothalamic projection in the rat. *J. Comp. Neurol.,* 146:1–14.

209. Moore, R. Y., Marchand, E. R., and Riley, J. N. (1979): Suprachiasmatic nucleus afferents in the rat: An HRP-retrograde transport study. *Soc. Neurosci..* 5:232.

210. Morin, L. P. (1980): Effect of ovarian hormones on synchrony of hamster circadian rhythms. *Physiol. Behav.,* 24:741–749.

211. Morin, L. P., Fitzgerald, K. M., and Zucker. I. (1977): Estradiol shortens the period of hamster circadian rhythms. *Science,* 196:305–307.

212. Morrell, J. I., and Pfaff, D. W. (1982): Characterization of estrogen-concentrating hypothalmic neurons by their axonal projections. *Science,* 217:1273–1276.

213. Morrell, J. I., Kelley, D. B., and Pfaff, D. W. (1975): Sex steroid binding in the brains of vertebrates: Studies with light microscopic autoradiography. In: *The Ventricular System in Neuroendocrine Mechanisms,* edited by K. M. Knigge and D. E. Scott, pp. 230–256. Karger, Basel.

214. Morrell. J. I., Ballin, A., and Pfaff, D. W. (1977): Autoradiographic demonstration of the pattern of

[3]H-estradiol concentrating cells in the brain of a carnivore the mink, *Mustela vison. Anat. Rec.,* 189:609–624.

215. Naess, O., Attramadal, A., and Askvaag, A. (1975): Androgen binding proteins in the anterior pituitary, hypothalamus. preoptic area and brain cortex of the rat. *Endocrinology,* 96:1–9.

216. Naftolin, F., Ryan, K. J., Davies, I. J., Reddy. V. V., Flores, F.. Petro, Z., and Kuhn, M. (1975): The formation of estrogens by central neuroendocrine tissue. *Recent Prog. Horm. Res.,* 31:295–315.

217. Nemeroff, C. B., Konkol, R. J.. Bissette, G., Youngblood, W., Martin, J. B., Brazeau, P., Rone, M. S., Prange, A. J., Breese, G., and Kizer, J. S. (1977): Analysis of the disruption in hypothalamic–pituitary regulation in rats treated neonatally with monosodium L-glutamate (MSG). *Endocrinology,* 101:613–622.

218. Nilaver, G., Zimmerman, E. A., Defendini, R., Liotta, A. S., Krieger, D. T., and Brownstein, M. J. (1979): Adrenocorticotropin and β-lipotropin in the hypothalamus. *J. Cell Biol.,* 81:50–58.

219. Nilaver. G., Zimmerman, E. A., Wilkins, J., Michaels, J., Hoffman, D. L.. and Silverman, A. J. (1980): Magnocellular hypothalamic projections to the lower brainstem and spinal cord of the rat: Immunocytochemical evidence for the predominance of oxytocin–neurophysin system compared to a vasopressin–neurophysin system. *Neuroendocrinology,* 30:150–158.

220. Nojyo, Y., and Sano, Y. (1978): Ultrastructure of the serotonergic nerve terminals in the suprachiasmatic and interpeduncular nuclei of rat brains. *Brain Res.,* 149:482–488.

221. Oliver, C., Mical, R. S., and Porter, J. C. (1977): Hypothalamic–pituitary vasculature: Evidence for retrograde blood flow in the pituitary stalk. *Endocrinology,* 101:598–604.

222. Paden, C. M., and Silverman, A. J. (1979): The ontogeny of the LHRH neurosecretory system in the albino rat: An immunocytochemical study. *Soc. Neurosci.,* 5:454.

223. Palacios, J. M., Wamsley, J. K., and Kuhar, M. J. (1981): The distribution of histamine H_1-receptors in the rat brain: An autoradiographic study. *Neuroscience,* 6:15–38.

224. Palkovits, M., Brownstein, M. J., Arimura. A., Sato, H., Schally, A. V.. and Kizer, J. S. (1976): Somatostatin content of the hypothalamic ventromedial and arcuate nuclei and the circumventricular organs in the rat. *Brain Res.,* 109:430–434.

225. Palkovits, M.. Brownstein, M., Saavedra, J. M., and Axelrod, J. (1974): Norepinephrine and dopamine content of hypothalamic nuclei of the rat. *Brain Res.,* 77:137–149.

226. Palkovits, M., Saavedra, J. M., Jacobowitz, D. M., Kizer, J. S., Zaborszky. L., and Brownstein, M. (1977): Serotonergic innervation of the forebrain: Effect of lesions on serotonin and tryptophan hydroxylase levels. *Brain Res..* 130:121–134.

227. Palkovits, M., and Zaborszky, L. (1979): Neural connections of the hypothalamus. In: *Anatomy of*

the Hypothalamus, Vol. 1, edited by P. J. Morgane and J. Panksepp, pp. 379–510. Marcel Dekker, New York.

228. Parry, H. B., and Livett, B. G. (1973): A new hypothalamic pathway to the median eminence containing neurophysin and its hypertrophy in sheep with natural scrapie. Nature, 242:63–65.

229. Pelletier, G. (1980): Ultrastructural localization of a fragment (16K) of the common precursor for adrenocorticotropin (ACTH) and β-lipotropin (β-LPH) in the rat hypothalamus. Neurosci. Lett., 16:85–90.

230. Pelletier, G., Dube, D., and Puviani, R. (1977): Somatostatin: Electron microscope immunohistochemical localization in secretory neurons of rat hypothalamus. Science, 196:1469–1470.

231. Pelletier, G., Labrie, F., Arimura, A., and Schally, A. V. (1974): Electron microscopic immunohistochemical localization of growth hormone–release inhibitng hormone (somatostatin) in the rat median eminence. Am. J. Anat., 140:445–450.

232. Pelletier, G., and Leclerc, R. (1979): Immunohistochemical localization of adrenocorticotropin in the rat brain. Endocrinology, 104:1426–1433.

233. Pelletier, G., LeClerc, R., LaBrie, F., and Puviani, R. (1974): Electron microscopic immunohistochemical localization of neurophysin in the rat hypothalamus and pituitary. Mol. Cell. Endocrinol., 1:157–166.

234. Perkins, N. A.. Westfall, T. C., Paul, C. V., MacLeod, R., and Rogol. A. (1979): Effect of prolactin on dopamine synthesis in medial basal hypothalamus: Evidence for a short loop feedback. Brain Res., 160:431–437.

235. Pert, C. B., Kuhar, M. J., and Snyder, S. H. (1976): The opiate receptor: Autoradiographic localization in rat brain. Proc. Natl. Acad. Sci. U.S.A., 73:3729–3733.

236. Peterson, G. M., Watkins, W. B., and Moore, R. Y. (1980): The suprachiasmatic hypothalamic nuclei of the rat. VI. Vasopressin neurons and circadian rhythmicity. Behav. Neurol. Biol., 29:236–245.

237. Peterson, R. P. (1966): Magnocellular neurosecretory centers in the rat hypothalamus. J. Comp. Neurol., 128:181–190.

238. Pfaff, D., and Keiner, M. (1974): Atlas of estradiol-concentrating cells in the central nervous system of the female rat. J. Comp. Neurol., 151:121–158.

239. Pfaff, D. W., and Sakuma, Y. (1979): Facilitation of the lordosis reflex of female rats from the ventromedial nucleus of the hypothalamus. J. Physiol. (Lond.), 288:189–202.

240. Pfaff. D. W., and Sakuma, Y. (1979): Deficit in the lordosis reflex of female rats caused by lesions in the ventromedial nucleus of the hypothalamus. J. Physiol. (Lond.), 288:203–210.

241. Phillips, M. I., Weyhenmeyer, J., Felix, J., Gouten, D., and Hoffman, W. E. (1979): Evidence for an endogenous brain renin-angiotensin system. Fed. Proc., 38:2260–2266.

242. Pickard, G. E. (1980): Morphological characteristics of retinal ganglion cells projecting to the suprachiasmatic nucleus: A horseradish peroxidase study. Brain Res., 183:458–465.

243. Pickard, G. E., and Silverman, A. J. (1976): Distribution of luteinizing hormone–releasing hormone (LH–RH) in the brain of the adult golden hamster. Soc. Neurosci., 2:975.

244. Pickard, G. E., and Silverman, A. J. (1979): The hypothalamic suprachiasmatic nucleus of the golden hamster: Afferent connections. Soc. Neurosci., 2:975.

245. Pickard, G. E., and Silverman, A. J. (1981): Direct retinal projections to the hypothalamus. piriform cortex and accessory optic nuclei in the golden hamster as demonstrated by a sensitive anterograde horseradish perioxidase technique. J. Comp. Neurol., 196:155–172.

246. Pierce, J. G., and DuVigneaud, V. (1950): Preliminary studies on amino acid content of a high potency preparation of the oxytoxic hormone of the posterior pituitary gland. J. Cell Biol., 182:359–366.

247. Pittendrigh, C. S., and Dann, S. (1976): A functional analysis of circadian pacemakers in nocturnal rodents. V. Pacemaker structure: A clock for all seasons. J. Comp. Physiol., 106:333–355.

248. Poitras, D., and Parent, A. (1975): A fluorescence microscopic study of the distribution of monoamines in the hypothalamus of the cat. J. Morphol., 145:387–408.

249. Poperoe, N. A., and DuVigneaud, V. (1954): A partial sequence of amino acids in performic-oxidized vasopressin. J. Biol. Chem., 206:353–360.

250. Raisman, G. (1972): A second look at the parvicellular neurosecretory system. In Brain–Endocrine Interaction. Median Eminence: Structure and Function, edited by K. M. Knigge, D. E. Scott, and A. Weindl, pp. 109–118. Karger, Basel.

251. Raisman, G. (1973): An ultrastructural study of the effects of hypophysectomy on the supraoptic nucleus of the rat. J. Comp. Neurol., 147:181–208.

252. Raisman, G. (1980): The neural trigger for ovulation—a safety catch. In: Development of Responsiveness to Steroids, edited by A. M. Kaye and M. Kaye, pp. 415–422. Pergamon Press, Oxford.

253. Reaves, T. A., Jr., and Hayward, J. N. (1979): Immunocytochemical identification of enkephalinergic neurons in the hypothalamic magnocellular preoptic nucleus of the goldfish, Carassius auratus. Cell Tissue Res., 200:147–151.

254. Recht, L. D., Hoffman, D. L., Haldar, J., Silverman, A. J., and Zimmerman, E. A. (1981): Vasopressin concentrations in hypophysial portal plasma: Insignificant reduction following removal of the posterior pituitary gland. Neuroendocrinology, 33,88–90.

255. Renaud, L. P. (1976): Tuberoinfundibular neurons in the basomedial hypothalamus of the rat: Electrophysiological evidence for axon collaterals to hypothalamic and extrahypothalamic areas. Brain Res.. 105:59–72.

256. Renaud, L. P. (1979): Neurophysiology and neuropharmacology of medial hypothalamic neurons
and their extrahypothalamic connections. In:
Handbook of the Hypothalamus, Vol. 1, edited
by P. J. Morgane and J. Panksepp, pp. 593–694.
Marcel Dekker, New York.

257. Rethelyi, M., and Halasz, B. (1970): Origin of
the nerve endings in the surface zone of the median eminence of the rat hypothalamus. Exp.
Brain Res., 11:145–158.

258. Rhodes, C. H., Morrell, J. I., and Pfaff, D. W.
(1981): Distribution of estrogen-concentrating,
neurophysin-containing magnocellular neurons in
the rat hypothalamus as demonstrated by a technique combining steroid autoradiography and immunohistology in the same tissue. Neuroendocrinology, 33:18–23.

259. Rhodes, C. H., Morrell, J. I., and Pfaff, D. W.
(1981): Immunohistochemical analysis of magnocellular elements in rat hypothalamus: Distribution and numbers of neurophysin, oxytocin, and
vasopressin containing cells. J. Comp. Neurol.,
198:45–64.

260. Ribak, C. E., and Peters, A. (1975): An autoradiographic study of the projections from the lateral geniculate body of the rat. Brain Res.,
92:341–368.

261. Ricardo, J. A., and Koh, E. T. (1978): Anatomical evidence of direct projections from the nucleus
of the solitary tract to the hypothalamus. amygdala and other forebrain structures in the rat.
Brain Res., 153:1–26.

262. Rossier, J., Battenberg, E., Pittman, Q., Bayon,
A., Koda, L., Miller, R., Guillemin, R., and
Bloom, F. (1979): Hypothalamic enkephalin neurones may regulate the neurohypophysis. Nature,
277:653–655.

263. Rusak, B., and Morin, L. P. (1976): Testicular responses to photoperiod are blocked by lesions of
the suprachiasmatic nuclei in golden hamsters.
Biol. Reprod., 15:366–374.

264. Rusak, B.. and Zucker, I. (1979): Neural regulation of circadian rhythms. Physiol. Rev.,
59:449–526.

265. Sachs, H., Fawcett, P., Takabatake, Y., and Por-
tanova, R. (1969): Biosynthesis and release of vasopressin and neurophysin. Recent Prog. Horm.
Res., 25:447–484.

266. Sakai, K. K., Marks, B. H., George, J. M., and
Koestner, A. (1974): The isolated organ-cultured
supraoptic nucleus as a neuropharmacological
test system. J. Pharmacol. Exp. Ther., 190:482–
491.

267. Sakuma, Y., and Pfaff, D. C. (1981): Mesencephalic mechanism for integration of female reproductive behavior in the rat. Am. J. Physiol.,
237:R285–R290.

268. Saper, C. B., Swanson, L. W., and Cowan, W. M.
(1976): The efferent connections of the ventromedial nucleus of the hypothalamus of the rat. J.
Comp. Neurol., 169:409–442.

269. Saper, C. B., Swanson, L. W., and Cowan, W. M.
(1978): The efferent connections of the anterior

hypothalamic area of the rat, cat and monkey. J.
Comp. Neurol., 182:575–600.

270. Sar, M., and Stumpf, W. E. (1977): Distribution
of androgen target cells in rat forebrain and pituitary after ^{3}H-dihydrotestosterone administration. J. Steroid Biochem., 8:1131–1135.

271. Sar, M., and Stumpf, W. E. (1979): Simultaneous localization of steroid and peptide hormones
in rat pituitary by combined thaw-mount autoradiography and immunohistochemistry: Localization of dihydrotestosterone in gonadotropes, thy-
rotropes and pituicytes. Cell Tissue Res., 203:1–
7.

272. Sar, M., Stumpf, W. E., Miller, R. J., Chang, K.-
J., and Cuatrecasas, P. (1978): Immunohistochemical localization of enkephalin in rat brain
and spinal cord. J. Comp. Neurol., 182:17–38.

273. Schally, A. V., Arimura, A., Baba, Y., Nair, R.
M. G., Matsuo, H., Redding, T. W., Debeljuk. L.,
and White, W. F. (1971): Isolation and properties
of the FSH and LH-releasing hormone. Biochem.
Biophys. Res. Commun.. 43:393–399.

274. Schally, A. V., Dupont, T. A., Arimura, A., Redding, T. W., Nishi, N., Linthicum, G., and
Schlesinger, D. H. (1976): Isolation and structure
of somatostatin from porcine hypothalami. Biochemistry, 15:509–514.

275. Scharrer, B., and Kater, St. B. (1969): Neurosecretion. XV. An electron microscopic study of the
corpus cardiaca of Periplaneta americana after
experimentally induced hormone release. Z. Zellforsch., 95:177–186.

276. Scharrer, E., and Scharrer, B. (1954): Hormones
produced in neurosecretory cells. Recent Prog.
Horm. Res., 10:183–240.

277. Scharrer, E.. and Scharrer, B. (1954): Neurosekretion. In: Handbuch der Mikroskopischen
Anatomie des Menschen, edited by R. Backmann
and E. B. Scharrer, pp. 953–1006. Springer-Verlag, Berlin-Gottingen-Heidelberg.

278. Schultzberg, M., Lundberg, I. M., Hokfelt, T.,
Terenus, L., Brandt, J., Elde, R. P., and Goldstein, M. (1978): Enkephalin-like immunoreactivity in gland cells and nerve terminals of the adrenal medulla. Neuroscience, 3:1169–1186.

279. Schwanzel-Fukuda, M., and Silverman, A. J.
(1980): The nervus terminalis of the guinea pig:
A new luteinizing hormone–releasing hormone
(LH–RH) neuronal system. J. Comp. Neurol.,
191:213–226.

280. Schwartz, J. C., Barbin, G., Garbarg, M., Llo-
rens, C., Palacios, J. M., and Pollard, H. (1978):
Histaminergic systems in brain. In Advances in
Pharmacology and Therapeutics, Vol. 2. Neuro-
transmitters, edited by P. Simon, pp. 171–180.
Pergamon Press, Oxford.

281. Selmanoff, M. K., Brodkin, L. D., Weiner, R. I.,
and Siiteri, P. K. (1977): Aromatization and 5-
alpha-reduction of androgens in discrete hypothalamic and limbic regions of the male and female
rat. Endocrinology, 101:841–848.

282. Setalo, G., Vigh, S., Schally, A. V., Arimura, A.,
and Flerko, B. (1976): Immunohistochemical

study of the origin of LH–RH-containing nerve fibers in the rat hypothalamus. *Brain Res.,* 103:597–602.

283. Sheridan, P. J. (1979): The nucleus interstitialis striae terminalis and the nucleus amygdaloideus medialis: Prime targets for androgen in the rat forebrain. *Endocrinology,* 104:130–136.

284. Sheridan, P. J., Sar, M., and Stumpf, W. E. (1974): Autoradiographic localization of ^{3}H-testosterone or its metabolites in the neonatal rat brain. *Am. J. Anat.,* 140:589–594.

285. Silver, A. (1974): The biology of cholinesterases. In: *Frontiers of Biology,* Vol. 36, edited by A. Neuberger and E. L. Tatum, pp. 1–596. North Holland, Amsterdam.

286. Silver, J., and Brand, S. (1979): A route for direct retinal input to the preoptic hypothalamus: Dendritic projections into the optic chiasm. *Am. J. Anat.,* 155:391–402.

287. Silverman, A. J. (1975): The hypothalamic magnocellular neurosecretory system of the guinea pig. I. Immunohistochemical localization of neurophysin in the adult. *Am. J. Anat..* 144:433–444.

288. Silverman, A. J. (1976): Distribution of luteinizing hormone-releasing hormone (LH-RH) in the guinea pig brain. *Endocrinology,* 99:30–41.

289. Silverman, A. J. (1976): Ultrastructural studies on the localization of neurohypophysial hormones and their carrier proteins. *J. Histochem. Cytochem.,* 24:816–827.

290. Silverman, A. J., Antunes, J. L., Ferin, M., and Zimmerman. E. A. (1977): The distribution of luteinizing hormone-releasing hormone in the hypothalamus of the rhesus monkey. *Endocrinology,* 101:134–142.

291. Silverman, A. J., and Desnoyers, P. (1976): Ultrastructural immunocytochemical localization of luteinizing hormone-releasing hormone (LH-RH) in the median eminence of the guinea pig. *Cell Tissue Res ,* 169:157–166.

292. Silverman, A. J., Goldstein, R., and Gadde, C. A. (1980): The ontogenesis of neurophysin-containing neurons in the mouse hypothalamus. *Peptides,* 1 (Suppl. 1):27–44.

293. Silverman, A. J., Hoffman, D. L., and Zimmerman. E. A. (1981): The descending afferent connections of the paraventricular nucleus of the hypothalamus. *Brain Res. Bull.,* 6:47–61.

294. Silverman, A. J., Hoffman, D., Gadde, C. A., Krey, L. C., and Zimmerman, E. A. (1981): Adrenal steroid inhibition of the vasopressin–neurophysin neurosecretory system to the median eminence of the rat: Differential effects of corticosterone and deoxycorticosterone administration after adrenalectomy. *Neuroendocrinology,* 32:129–133.

295. Silverman, A. J., Knigge, K. M., and Zimmerman, E. A. (1975): Electron microscopic localization of neurophysin in freeze-substituted posterior pituitary. *Am. J. Anat.,* 142:265–271.

296. Silverman, A. J., and Krey, L. C. (1978): The luteinizing hormone-releasing hormone (LHRH) neuronal networks of the guinea pig brain. I.

Intra- and extra-hypothalamic projections. *Brain Res.,* 157:233–246.

297. Silverman, A. J., Krey, L. C., and Zimmerman, E. A. (1979): A comparative study of the luteinizing hormone releasing hormone (LHRH) neuronal networks in mammals. *Biol. Reprod.,* 20:98–110.

298. Silverman, A. J., and Sladek, J. R. (1978): Simultaneous visualization of luteinizing hormone-releasing hormone (LHRH) and catecholamines in the guinea pig brain. *Soc. Neurosci. Abstr.,* 4:589.

299. Silverman, A. J., and Zimmerman, E. A. (1975): Ultrastructural immunocytochemical localization of neurophysin and vasopressin in the median eminence and posterior pituitary of the guinea pig. *Cell Tissue Res.,* 159:291–301.

299a. Silverman, A. J., and Zimmerman, E. A. (1982): Adrenalectomy increase neurosecretory system. *Neuroscience,* 7:2705–2710.

300. Simantov, R., and Synder, S. (1977): Opiate receptor binding in the pituitary gland. *Brain Res.,* 124:178–184.

301. Sims, K. B., Hoffman, D. L., Said, S. I., and Zimmerman, E. A. (1980): Vasoactive intestinal polypeptide (VIP) in mouse and rat brain: An immunocytochemical study. *Brain Res.,* 186:165–183.

302. Sladek, C. D., and Knigge, K. M. (1977): Cholinergic stimulation of vasopressin release from the rat hypothalamo–neurohypophyseal system in organ culture. *Endocrinology,* 101:411–420.

303. Smith, A. R., and Kappers, J. A. (1975): Effect of pinealectomy, gonadectomy, pCPA and pineal extracts on the rat parvocellular neurosecretory hypothalamic system; a fluorescence histochemical investigation. *Brain Res.,* 86:353–371.

304. Snyder, S. H., and Childers, S. R. (1979): Opiate receptors and opioid peptides. *Annu. Rev. Neurosci..* 2:35–64.

305. Sofroniew, M. V. (1979): Immunoreactive β-endorphin and ACTH in the same neurons of the hypothalamic arcuate nucleus in the rat. *Am. J. Anat.,* 154:283–289.

306. Sofroniew, M. V., and Schrell, V. (1980): Hypothalamic neurons projecting to the rat caudal medulla oblongata, examined by immunoperoxidase staining of retrogradely transported horseradish peroxidase. *Neurosci. Lett.,* 19:257–263.

307. Sofroniew, M. V., and Weindl, A. (1978): Projections from the parvocellular vasopressin- and neurophysin-containing neurons of the suprachiasmatic nucleus. *Am. J. Anat.,* 153:391–430.

308. Sofroniew. M. V., Weindl, A., Schinko, I., and Wetzstein, R. (1979): The distribution of vasopressin, oxytocin and neurophysin-producing neurons in the guinea pig brain. I. The classical hypothalamo-neurohypophyseal system. *Cell Tissue Res.,* 196:367–384.

309. Sokol, H. W., Zimmerman, E. A., Sawyer, W. H., and Robinson, A. G. (1976): The hypothalamo–neurohypophyseal system of the rat: Localization and quantitation of neurophysin by light microscopic immunocytochemistry in normal rat

and in Brattleboro rats deficient in vasopressin and a neurophysin. *Endocrinology,* 98:1176–1188.

310. Spindel, E.. and Wurtman, R. J. (1980): TRH immunoreactivity in rat brain regions, spinal cord and pancreas: Validation by high-pressure liquid chromatography and thin-layer chromatography. *Brain Res.,* 201:279–288.

311. Stephan, F. K., and Zucker, I. (1972): Circadian rhythms in drinking behavior and locomotor activity of rats are eliminated by hypothalamic lesions. *Proc. Natl. Acad. Sci. U.S.A.,* 69:1583–1586.

312. Stephan, F. K., and Zucker, I. (1974): Endocrine and neural mediation of the effects of constant light on water intake of rats. *Neuroendocrinology,* 14:44–60.

313. Sternberger, L. A., and Hoffman, G. E. (1978): Immunocytology of luteinizing hormone-releasing hormone. *Neuroendocrinology,* 25:111–128.

314. Stillman, M. A., Recht, L. D., Rosario, S. L., Seif, S. M.. Robinson, A. G., and Zimmerman, E. A. (1977): The effects of adrenalectomy and glucocorticoid replacement on vasopressin and vasopressin-neurophysin in the zona externa of the rat. *Endocrinology,* 101:42–49.

315. Stumpf, W. E. (1968): Cellular and subcellular ³H-estradiol localization in the pituitary by autoradiography. *Z. Zellforsch.,* 92:23–45.

316. Stumpf, W. E., and Sar, M. (1977): Steroid hormone target cells in the periventricular brain: Relationship to peptide producing cells. *Fed. Proc.,* 36:1973–1977.

317. Swanson, L. W., and Cowan, W. M. (1975): The efferent connections of the suprachiasmatic nucleus of the guinea pig. *J. Comp. Neurol.,* 160:1–12.

318. Swanson, L. W., and Cowan, W. M. (1977): An autoradiographic study of the organization of the efferent connections of the hippocampal formation in the rat. *J. Comp. Neurol.,* 172:49–84.

319. Swanson, L. W., Cowan, W. M., and Jones, E. G. (1974): An autoradiographic study of the efferent connections of the ventral lateral geniculate nucleus in the albino rat and the cat. *J. Comp. Neurol.,* 156:143–163.

320. Swanson, L. W., and Hartman, B. K. (1975): The central adrenergic system. An immunofluorescence study of the location of cell bodies and their efferent connections in the rat utilizing dopamine-β-hydroxylase as a marker. *J. Comp. Neurol..* 163:467–505.

321. Swanson, L. W., and Kuypers, A. G. J. M. (1980): The paraventricular nucleus of the hypothalamus: Cytoarchitectonic subdivisions and organization of projections to the pituitary, dorsal vagal complex, and spinal cord as demonstrated by retrograde fluorescence double labeling method. *J. Comp. Neurol.,* 194:555–570.

322. Swanson, L. W., and Sawchenko, P. E. (1980): Paraventricular nucleus: A site for the integration of neuroendocrine and autonomic mechanisms. *Neuroendocrinology,* 31:410–417.

323. Szafarczyk, A., Ixart, G., Malaval, F., Nouguier-Soule, J., and Assenmacher, I. (1979): Effects of lesions of the suprachiasmatic nuclei and of p-chlorophenylalanine on the circadian rhythms of adrenocorticotrophic hormone and corticosterone in the plasma, and on locomotor activity of rats. *J. Endocrinol.,* 83:1–16.

324. Szentagothai, J. (1964): The parvicellular neurosecretory system. In: *Lectures on the Diencephalon,* edited by W. Bargmann and J. P. Schade, pp. 135–146. Elsevier, Amsterdam.

325. Szentagothai, J., Flerko, B., Mess, B., and Halasz, B. (1968): *Hypothalamic Control of the Anterior Pituitary.* Akademiai Kiado, Budapest.

326. Tager, A., Hohenboken, M., Markese, J., and Dinerstein, R. J. (1981): Identification and localization of glucagon-related peptides in rat brain. *Proc. Natl. Acad. Sci. U.S.A.,* 77:6229–6233.

327. Tappaz, M. L., Brownstein, M. J., and Kopin, I. J. (1977): Glutamate decarboxylase (GAD) and γ-aminobutyric acid (GABA) in discrete nuclei of the hypothalamus and substantia nigra. *Brain Res.,* 125:109–121.

328. Taylor, K. M., Gfeller, E.. and Snyder, S. H. (1972): Regional localization of histamine and histadine in the brain of the rhesus monkey. *Brain Res.,* 41:171–176.

329. Terasawa, E., and Wiegand, S. G. (1978): Effects of hypothalamic deafferentation on ovulation and estrous cyclicity in the female guinea pig. *Neuroendocrinology,* 26:229–237.

330. Tigges, J., Bos, J., and Tigges, M. (1977): An autoradiographic investigation of the subcortical visual system in chimpanzee. *J. Comp. Neurol.,* 172:367–380.

331. Tweedle, C. D., and Hatton, G. I. (1976): Ultrastructural comparisons of neurons of supraoptic and circularis nuclei in normal and dehydrated rats. *Brain Res. Bull.,* 1:103–121.

332. Tweedle, C. D., and Hatton, G. I. (1980): Evidence for dynamic interactions between pituicytes and neurosecretory axons in the rat. *Neuroscience,* 5:661–667.

333. Turpen, C., and Sladek, J. R., Jr. (1978): Localization of glyoxylic acid-induced histofluorescence in surgically isolated medial basal hypothalamus of the rat. *Cell Tissue Res.,* 187:449–456.

334. Tyrell, J. B., Lorenzi, M., Gerich, J. E., and Forsham, P. H. (1971): Inhibition by somatostatin of ACTH secretion in Nelson's syndrome. *J. Clin. Endocrinol. Metab..* 285:443–448.

335. Ungerstedt, U. (1971): Stereotaxic mapping of the monoamine pathways in the rat brain. *Acta Physiol. Scand.,* 367:1–48.

336. Vale, W., Rivier. C., Brazeau. P., and Guillemin, R. (1974): Effects of somatostatin on the secretion of thyrotropin and prolactin. *Endocrinology,* 95:968–977.

337. Vale, W., Rivier, C., and Brown, M. (1977): Regulatory peptides of the hypothalamus. *Physiol. Rev.* 39:473–527.

338. Vale, W., Spiess, J., Rivier, C., and Rivier, J.

(1981): Characterization of a 41-residue ovine hypothalamic peptide that stimulates secretion of corticotropin and B-endorphin. *Science*, 213:1394–1357.

339. van de Kar, L. D., and Lorens, S. A. (1979): Differential serotonergic innervation of individual hypothalamic nuclei and other forebrain regions by the dorsal and median midbrain raphe nuclei. *Brain Res.*, 162:45–54.

340. van den Pol, A. N. (1980): The hypothalamic suprachiasmatic nucleus of rat: Intrinsic anatomy. *J. Comp. Neurol.*, 191:661–702.

341. van den Pol, A. N., and Cassidy, J. R. (1980): The hypothalamic arcuate nucleus of rat: A quantitative Golgi analysis. *Soc. Neurosci.*, 6:456.

342. Vandesande, F., DeMey, J., and Dierickx, K. (1974): Identification of neurophysin producing cells. I. The origin of the neurophysin-like substance-containing nerve fibers of the external region of the median eminence of the rat. *Cell Tissue Res.*, 151:187–200.

343. Vandesande, F., and Dierickx, K. (1975): Identification of the vasopressin producing and oxytocin producing neurons in the hypothalamic magnocellular neurosecretory system of the rat. *Cell Tissue Res.*, 164:153–162.

344. Vandesande, F., Dierickx, K., and DeMey, J. (1975): Identification of separate vasopressin-neurophysin II and oxytocin-neurophysin I containing nerve fibres in the external region of the bovine median eminence. *Cell Tissue Res.*, 158:509–516.

345. Vandesande, F., Dierickx, K.. and DeMey, J. (1975): Identification of the vasopressin-neurophysin II and the oxytocin-neurophysin I producing neurons in the bovine hypothalamus. *Cell Tissue Res.*, 156:189–200.

346. Vandesande, F., Dierickx, K., and DeMey, J. (1977): The origin of the vasopressinergic and oxytocinergic fibers of the external region of the median eminence of the rat hypophysis. *Cell Tissue Res.*, 180:443–452.

347. van Leeuvan, F. W., and Swaab, D. F. (1977): Specific immunoelectronmicroscopic localization of vasopressin and oxytocin in the neurohypophysis of the rat. *Cell Tissue Res.*, 177:493–501.

348. Wade, G. N., and Feder, H. H. (1972): Uptake of $(1,2,^3H)$-20-hydroxypregn-4-ene-3-one, $(1,2,^3H)$ corticosterone and $(6,7,^3H)$ estradiol 17β by guinea pig brain and uterus: Comparison with uptake of $1,2^3H$ progesterone. *Brain Res.*, 45:545–555.

349. Wade, G. N., Harding, C. F., and Feder, H. H. (1973): Neural uptake of $[1,2-^3H]$ progesterone in ovariectomized rats, guinea pigs and hamsters: Correlation with species differences in behavioral responsiveness. *Brain Res.*, 61:357–367.

350. Wamsley, J. K., Young, W. S. III, and Kuhar, M. J. (1980): Immunohistochemical localization of enkephalin in rat forebrain. *Brain Res.*, 190: 153–174.

351. Warembourg, M. (1970): Fixation de l'oestradiol ^3H au niveau des noyaux amygdaliens, septaux, et du systeme hypothalamo–hypophysaire chez la souris femelle. *C. R. Acad. Sci. [D] (Paris)*, 270:152–154.

352. Warembourg, M. (1977): Radioautographic localization of estrogen-concentrating cells in the brain and pituitary of the guinea pig. *Brain Res.*, 23:357–362.

353. Watkins, W. B. (1976): Immunocytochemical study of the hypothalamo-neurohypophyseal system. I. Localization of neurosecretory neurons containing neurophysin I or neurophysin II in the domestic pig. *Cell Tissue Res.*, 175:165–181.

354. Watkins, W. B. (1980): Presence of adrenocorticotropin and β-endorphin immunoreactivities in the magnocellular neurosecretory system of the rat hypothalamus. *Cell Tissue Res.*, 207:65–80.

355. Watkins, W. B., and Choy, V. R. (1977): Immunohistochemical demonstration of a CRF-associated neurophysin in the external zone of the rat median eminence. *Cell Tissue Res.*, 100:491–503.

356. Watkins, W. B., Schwabedal, P., and Bock, R. (1974): Immunohistochemical demonstration of a CRF-associated neurophysin in the external zone of the rat median eminence. *Cell Tissue Res.*, 152:411–421.

357. Watson, S. J., and Akil, H. (1980): α-MSH in rat brain: Occurrence within and outside of β-endorphin neurons. *Brain Res.*, 182:217–223.

358. Watson, S. J., Akil, H., and Walker, J. M. (1980): Anatomical and biochemical studies of the opioid peptides and related substances in the brain. *Peptides*, 1(Suppl. 1):11–20.

358a. Watson, S. J., Akil, H., Fischli, W., Goldstein, A., Zimmerman, E., Nilaver, G. and Van Wimersma Greidarius, T. B. (1982): Dynorphin and vasopressin: Common localization in magnocellular neurones. *Science*, 216:85–87.

359. Watson, S. J., Barchas, J. D., and Li, C. H. (1977): B-lipotropin: Localization of cells and axons in rat brain by immunocytochemistry. *Proc. Natl. Acad. Sci. U.S.A.*, 74:5155–5158.

360. Watson, S. J., Richard. C. W., and Barchas, J. D. (1978): Adrenocorticotropin in rat brain: Immunocytochemical localization in cells and axons. *Science*. 200:1180–1181.

361. Weiner, R. I. (1973): Hypothalamic monoamine levels and gonadotropin secretion following deafferentation of the medial basal hypothalamus. *Prog. Brain Res.*, 39:165–170.

362. Weiner, R. I., Pattou, E., Kerdelhue. B., and Kordon, C. (1975): Differential effects of hypothalamic deafferentation upon luteinizing hormone-releasing hormone in the median eminence and organum vasculosum of the lamina terminalis. *Endocrinology*, 97:1597–1600.

363. Weiner, R. I., Shryne, J. E., Gorski, R. A., and Sawyer, C. H. (1972): Changes in the catecholamine content of the rat hypothalamus following deafferentation. *Endocrinology*, 90:867–873.

364. Weiss, J., and Gibbs, C. (1974): Conversion of testosterone and androstenedione to estrogen *in*

vitro by the brain of female rats. *Endocrinology,* 94:616–624.

365. Wiegand, S. J., and Price, J. L. (1980): Cells of origin of the afferent fibers to the median eminence in the rat. *J. Comp. Neurol.,* 192:1–19.

366. Wiegand, S. J., Terasawa, E., Bridson, W. E., and Goy, R. W. (1980): Effects of discrete lesions of preoptic and suprachiasmatic structures in the female rat. *Neuroendocrinology,* 31:147–157.

366a. Witkin, J., Paden, C., and Silverman, A. J. (1982): The luteinizing hormone-releasing hormone (LHRH) systems in the rat brain. *Neuroendocrinology,* 35:429–438.

367. Wolny, H. L., Plech, A , and Herman, Z. S. (1974): Diuretic effects of intraventricularly injected noradrenaline and dopamine in rats. *Experientia,* 30:1062–1063.

368. Young, W. C. (1961): The hormone and mating behavior. In: *Sex and Internal Secretion,* Vol. 2, edited by W. C. Young, p. 1196. Williams & Wilkins, Baltimore.

369. Zatz, M., and Brownstein, M. J. (1979): Intraventricular carbachol mimics the effects of light on the circadian rhythm in the rat pineal gland. *Science,* 203:358–361.

370. Zimmerman, E. A. (1981): The organization of oxytocin and vasopressin pathways. In: *Neurosecretion and Brain Peptides,* edited by J. B. Martin, S. Reichlen, and K. L. Bick, pp. 63–75. Raven Press, New York.

371. Zimmerman, E. A., and Antunes, J. L. (1976): Organization of the hypothalamic–pituitary system: Current concepts from immunohistochemi-

cal studies. *J. Histochem. Cytochem..* 24:807–815.

372. Zimmerman, E. A., Carmel, P. W., Husain, M. K., Ferin, M., Tannenbaum, M., Frantz, A. G., and Robinson, A. G. (1973): Vasopressin and neurophysin: High concentration in monkey hypophyseal portal blood. *Science,* 182:925–927.

373. Zimmerman, E. A., Hsu, K. C., Robinson, A. G., Carmel, P. W., Frantz, A. G., and Tannenbaum, M. (1973): Studies on neurophysin secreting neurons with immunoperoxidase techniques employing antibody to bovine neurophysin. I. Light microscopic findings in monkey and bovine tissue. *Endocrinology,* 92:931–940.

374. Zimmerman, E. A., Krupp, L., Hoffman, D. L., Matthew. E., and Nilaver, G. (1980): Exploration of peptidergic pathways in brain by immunocytochemistry: A ten year perspective. *Peptides,* 1:3–10.

375. Zimmerman, E. A., Robinson, A. G., Husain, M. K., Acosta, A., Frantz, A., and Sawyer, W. H. (1974): Neurohypophyseal peptides in the bovine hypothalamus: The relationship of neurophysin I to oxytocin and neurophysin II to vasopressin in supraoptic and paraventricular regions. *Endocrinology,* 95:931–938.

376. Zingg, H. H.. Baertschi, A. J., and Dreifuss, J. J. (1979): Action of gamma-aminobutyric acid on hypothalamo–neurohypophysial axons. *Brain Res.,* 171:453–459.

377. Zucker, I., Rusak, B., and King, R. G., Jr. (1976): Neural bases for circadian rhythms in rodent behavior. *Adv. Psychobiol.,* 3:35–74.

Chemical Neuroanatomy, edited by P.C. Emson,
Raven Press, New York © 1983.

The Hippocampus

Ivar Walaas

Department of Pharmacology, Yale University School of Medicine, New Haven, Connecticut 06510

The hippocampal formation is a simplified, phylogenetically old part of the cerebral cortex (25) with a unique structural organization. The major fiber connections are located in sharply demarcated regions; the hippocampal cells and fibers are segregated in clearly demarcated laminae, which also are displayed after visualization of oxidative enzymes (132) or of heavy metals (79), and the afferent fibers and intrinsic circuits are organized in transverse lamellae (13). Recent studies have also pointed to the hippocampus as a model system for the study of anatomical (35) and physiological (30) plasticity in the central nervous system (CNS) (5,34). The anatomy, physiology, neurochemistry, and behavioral characteristics of the hippocampal neurons have therefore been investigated in some detail, and these subjects have recently been discussed in a comprehensive review (95), a monograph (147), and a symposium (33).

The present chapter gives a short description of the anatomical organization of the hippocampal formation and then describes the current knowledge of the neurotransmitter identity of the neuronal elements present in the region. No complete coverage of the literature is attempted; in particular, studies on receptor–ligand binding and electrophysiology are only mentioned where they have a direct bearing on the problem discussed. The methods used for neurotransmitter identification are only briefly described, and the reader is referred to a comprehensive recent review (191) for a more detailed discussion of these aspects.

ANATOMY

In the rodent brain, the hippocampal formation is located on the posteromedial border of the hemisphere, where it extends from the rostromedially located septum to the ventrolaterally located amygdaloid area. In cross section, it has a C-shaped form with a deep convex surface (the fiber-rich alveus) bordering on the lateral ventricle and a superficial surface represented by the obliterated fissura hippocampi. A frontal section through the septal parts displays some of the major subdivisions of the structure (Fig. 1). Following Blackstad's description (23), the present review divides the hippocampal region into the area dentata and the hippocampus proper, followed caudally by the subicular region, the retrosplenial area, and the entorhinal cortex. These regions are all parts of the hippocampal formation (23), but this chapter focuses on the area dentata and the hippocampus proper, as most neurochemical studies have centered on these regions.

The area dentata is the major entrance to the hippocampus (4,24,155). A massive excitatory fiber tract, the perforant path, originates in the entorhinal cortex, perforates the subiculum and hippocampal fissure, and terminates in the superficial parts of the area dentata, i.e., the outer parts of the stratum moleculare (9,10,24,86,88,118). The principal neurons in the area dentata, the granule cells, have cell bodies arranged in a dense layer beneath the molecular layer, where they surround the hilus fasciae dentate [the CA4 region of Lorente de Nó (121)], and they extend their dendrites out through the stratum moleculare. Local interneurons are also present both in the molecular layer and close to the granule cells. The hilus is a complex region with a number of different cell types, some of them projection neurons (2,72).

The granule cells propagate the impulses from the perforant path through their excitatory axons, the mossy fibers, to the cells in the hilus (27). Some of the hilar cells then send their excitatory axons both ipsi- and contralaterally back to a sharply delimited lamina in the area dentata, deep to the perforant path and above the granule cells (73,90,112,204,223).

The mossy fibers penetrate further into the hippocampus proper where they make contact with

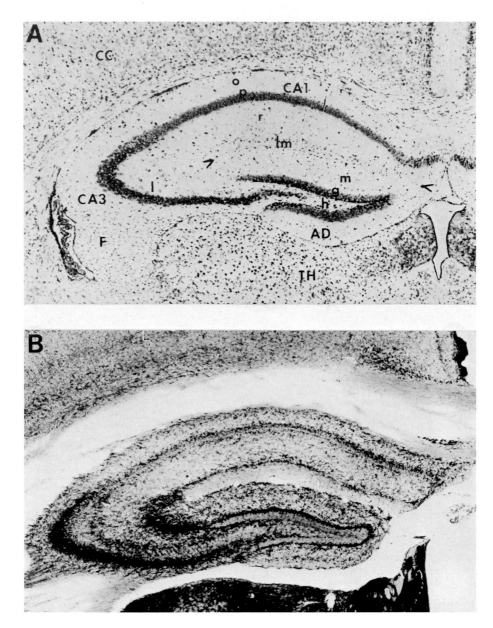

FIG. 1. A: Mouse brain, frontal section through the dorsal hippocampal region, toluidine-blue stained. *Abbreviations:* AD, area dentata; CA1 and CA3, subfields of hippocampus; m, stratum moleculare; g, granule cells; h, hilus fasciae dentatae; F, fimbria; l, stratum lucidum of CA3; lm, stratum lacunosum moleculare; o, stratum oriens; p, stratum pyramidale; r, stratum radiatum; TH, thalamus; CC, cerebral cortex. *Arrowheads* indicate fissura hippocampi. **B:** Acetylcholinesterase-stained frontal section of mouse dorsal hippocampus.

the principal hippocampal neurons, the pyramidal cells, in the CA3 region (27,70,204). Both the CA3 and the following hippocampal subfield, the CA1, are very similarly organized [the CA2 subfield is considered, in this chapter, to be included in CA3 (23)]. The pyramidal cells are arranged in a dense, continuous layer, the stratum pyramidale, which divides both CA3 and CA1 into the deep stratum oriens, which abuts on the alveus and contains the basal dendrites of the pyramidal cells, and the stratum radiatum and the superficial stratum lacunosum moleculare, which contain the apical pyr-

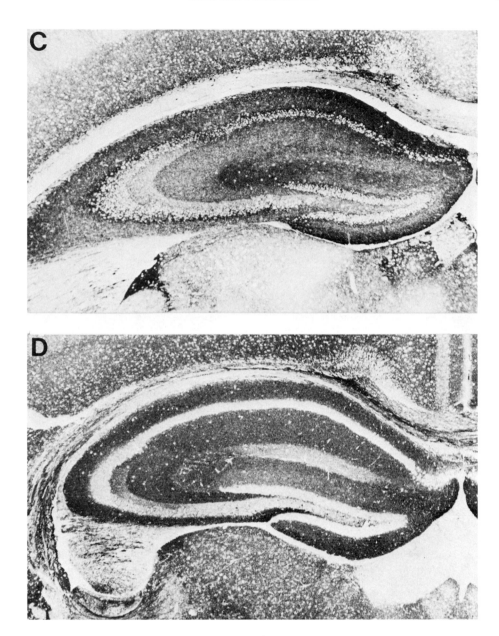

FIG. 1. (*continued*) **C:** Autoradiographic demonstration of [³H]-GABA uptake in mouse dorsal hippocampus. Mouse brain slices incubated with 1 μM [³H]-GABA and 2 mM β-alanine to inhibit glial uptake for 20 min. **D:** Autoradiographic demonstration of [³H]-D-aspartate uptake in mouse dorsal hippocampus. Mouse brain slices incubated with 2 μM [³H]-D-aspartate for 20 min.

amidal dendrites. Similarly to the area dentata, the hippocampus has a restricted number of interneurons outside the stratum pyramidale, some of which are called basket cells because of their dense, basket-like terminal plexus around the pyramidal cell perikarya and proximal dendrites (121,154).

The mossy fibers, which distribute strictly ipsilaterally (27), penetrate into CA3 in a thin, suprapyramidal zone, the stratum lucidum, where they innervate the apical dendrites of the pyramidal cells with peculiar giant boutons and *en passage* synapses (26,27,70). The CA3 pyramidal cells then propagate these impulses further. The excitatory CA3 axons distribute to both the ipsi- and contralateral hippocampus, where they terminate densely in both strata oriens and radiatum, but not in stratum pyramidale, of CA3 and CA1 (11,23,73,87,204). They do not, however, send fibers back into the area dentata (90,112). Some CA3 axons also terminate in the lateral septal nucleus on both sides, and some go to the subiculum and entorhinal cortex (12,85,87,201). The fibers going into the CA1 region are the major link between the CA3 and CA1. They appear to terminate more densely in the ipsilateral stratum radiatum (112) as the so-called Schaffer collaterals (161), whereas the contralateral projection, the commissural fibers, are more dense in the stratum oriens (112).

As the last neuronal link in the hippocampus, the excitatory CA1 pyramids send most of their axons caudally into the subicular complex (12,87,201). Some fibers may also go to the lateral septum (131,201), but there are apparently no fibers from CA1 to CA3 (4). Thus, impulses originating in the entorhinal cortex and sent through the perforant path into the area dentata are processed through the hippocampal formation by a three-membered neuronal chain, i.e., the mossy fibers, the CA3 axons, and the CA1 axons. All of these excitatory pathways appear to be monosynaptically connected (4), but they are also influenced by recurrent inhibition at each step. Thus, local inhibitory axosomatic synapses probably belonging to interneurons have been identified in the hippocampus (7,8), and similar arrangements are probably present in both the area dentata (117) and subiculum (59).

Another striking characteristic of the hippocampal formation is the lamellar organization of the structure. Thus, both the perforant path input and, particularly, the mossy fiber projection are localized in thin lamellae oriented approximately transversely to the septotemporal axis of the hippocampal formation (13,27,70,204). The CA3–CA1 axons are more divergent, but most of the ipsilateral CA3 axons also appear to terminate in the same lamella (112), as do the CA1 fibers to the subiculum (12,13). This organization has led to the development of the hippocampal slice preparation (179,206,219), which has allowed *in vitro* studies on viable well-defined excitatory or inhibitory neurons from mammalian brain (6,47,122).

The connections reviewed above undoubtedly represent the quantitatively important parts of the hippocampal circuitry. However, other projections also exist; e.g., some fibers in the perforant path do terminate in the stratum lacunosum moleculare of the ipsilateral CA1 and CA3 regions (24,86,186),

and other fibers cross the midline and constitute a small crossed perforant path (89). Other afferents include fibers from the cingulum (50), the thalamus (82,218), and the lateral hypothalamus and supramammillary region (148,218). However, other pathways have received more attention from neurochemists. The most important of these is probably the septohippocampal projection, which originates in the medial septum and diagonal band nucleus and distributes to the whole hippocampal formation and adjacent cortical areas (171,202). Inputs from the ventral tegmental area, the substantia nigra, and the raphe nuclei and locus ceruleus have also been described (15,103,150,218). The transmitter chemistry of these connections is discussed below.

NEUROTRANSMITTERS IN THE HIPPOCAMPUS

Because of the orderly and specific organization of the hippocampal formation described above, neurochemists were early attracted to this structure in an effort to identify and localize central neurotransmitters. Today it is known that the hippocampal formation contains the classic transmitter candidates, e.g., acetylcholine (ACh) and the catecholamines norepinephrine and dopamine, which together with serotonin and histamine might function as hippocampal transmitters. Three amino acid transmitter candidates, i.e., γ-aminobutyrate (GABA), L-glutamate, and L-aspartate, are probably also important in the hippocampal region, and recent studies have also shown the presence of some of the neuropeptides.

Besides being present in the hippocampal formation, all of these compounds apparently have the capacity to influence the excitability of hippocampal neurons (22,29,42,47,52,74,166,169,172,184). However, a completely convincing demonstration of identity of action (212) between exogenously applied transmitter candidate and endogenously released compound has apparently not yet been achieved (4). The electrophysiological and pharmacological evidence seems to be most convincing in the case of GABA (42), followed by glutamate and aspartate (36). The present chapter begins, however, with ACh, which was the first transmitter studied in detail, and then discusses the amino acids, which probably are the major transmitters. The data on monoamines, which are probably quantitatively less important, are then discussed, and some recent results on peptides are finally mentioned.

Acetylcholine

The early work on cholinergic structures in the brain gained major impetus from the histochemical demonstration of acetylcholinesterase (AChE) activity (104). The presence of this enzyme was taken as evidence for cholinergic neurotransmission (175), and it was therefore deemed of great interest that the enzyme was found in several well-defined fiber systems in the brain (113). In the hippocampus, a dense staining was observed, organized in a strikingly laminated fashion (175, 191,195). Some characteristics of this staining are seen in Fig. 1. The stain is concentrated in zones above and below the cellular layers but is also concentrated in the hilus and deep in the hippocampal molecular layers. In contrast, the staining intensity is low in the fields most heavily innervated by the mossy fibers and the ipsi- and contralateral hilus and CA3 pyramidal cell axons. High-power microscopy has further disclosed that most of the stain is present in the neuropil, but some scattered perikarya in the hilus and stratum oriens of the hippocampus are also stained (123,176). The latter cells have been stated to resemble basket cells (191). Electron microscopic studies indicate that AChE-positive boutons innervate pyramidal and granule cell dendrites (176). This laminated distribution of AChE was confirmed in a detailed quantitative histochemical and biochemical study by Storm-Mathisen (187).

However, AChE is not a specific cholinergic marker [for review, see Silver (178)]; the enzyme has also been found, e.g., in a number of noncholinergic, monoamine-containing tracts (57), some of which belong to the suggested "cholinergic ascending reticular systems" of Shute and Lewis (177). In contrast, the biosynthetic enzyme choline acetyltransferase (ChAT) appears to be specifically localized in cholinergic neurons (for reviews, see refs. 61,62,191). Choline acetyltransferase activity was therefore also studied in the hippocampus. A detailed biochemical distribution study with microdissection techniques showed the same distribution as AChE (60), and subcellular fractionation indicated that nearly 80% of the enzyme was present in nerve ending particles. Also, most of the activity sedimented together with AChE (60,141). Thus, in the hippocampal formation, most of AChE and ChAT appeared to be present in the same neuronal system. The anatomical origin of this system has been defined by the seminal experiments of Lewis and Shute (113), who traced the origin of the hippocampal AChE rostrally to cells in the medial septum and diagonal band nucleus and showed that an interruption of the septohippocampal fibers abolished most of the AChE staining in the hippocampus (175). Similar results were reported for ChAT activity (114).

Later work has amply supported these results, and it is now generally accepted that this was the first demonstration of a major cholinergic tract in the mammalian brain (191 and references therein). The present knowledge on this system can be summarized as follows. Most of the fibers originate in AChE-positive cells in the anterior diagonal band nucleus, with a minor component coming from the medial septum (123,127). They course through the fimbria and fornix superior and enter the hippocampal formation via the alveus. Large lesions in the medial septum irreversibly decrease hippocampal ChAT activity by approximately 90% and AChE activity by 80% to 85% (191) without affecting other hippocampal enzymes. After a fimbrial transection, AChE staining and ChAT activity accumulate on the septal side but disappear on the hippocampal side of the lesion (64,114). The biochemical changes appear only ipsilaterally; an increase in contralateral AChE activity (145) has not been confirmed (198).

The rapid and massive decreases in hippocampal ChAT after septal lesions or complete deafferentations (188) suggest that any intrinsic hippocampal cholinergic system must be very small. Histochemical AChE studies, as mentioned above, show staining of intrinsic cells, but these cells are probably cholinoceptive (123). Further, destruction of hippocampal neurons, but not of afferent fibers, by local injection of kainic acid (37,140,163) does not decrease ChAT activity or AChE staining significantly (64,164). However, both AChE staining and the ChAT activity in a small part of the molecular layer of subiculum are apparently resistant to deafferentation procedures (183). The region may therefore contain intrinsic cholinergic neurons, which might be responsible for 5% to 10% of the total hippocampal ChAT activity (64,191).

The concept of a unilateral cholinergic septohippocampal fiber tract was initially not supported by anatomical evidence. Rather, silver staining studies after septal lesions indicated that degenerating structures presumed to represent septal axons and terminals were diffusely distributed and not organized in the striking laminae seen in AChE preparations (87,133,138,153). However, recent studies with anterogradely transported ³H-labeled protein are apparently in better agreement with AChE histochemistry even if some discrepancies still remain (202). Some septohippocampal fibers could conceivably be noncholinergic.

The quantitative importance of the AChE-containing septohippocampal fibers in the hippocampal formation has been estimated to represent 6% of all hippocampal nerve terminals (107). The existence of this rather modest input has for the first time presented investigators with a system in which the behavior of the transmitter (ACh) and the synthetic machinery could be studied in a cholinergic CNS pathway. Some of the important results from these studies include the following. Most of the hippocampal ACh is located in a bound, nerve terminal-associated fraction (152), and this ACh pool increases dramatically immediately after interruption of septal axons, probably because of continued synthesis combined with interrupted ACh release (152,173). Thereafter, ACh levels decrease to the same extent as ChAT (111,174). Further, ACh is released from the septohippocampal fibers (180), and this release is apparently increased by septal stimulation (53). Similarly, ACh turnover in the hippocampus has been reported to increase after septal stimulation and to decrease after septal lesions (137).

Following degradation of the synaptically released ACh by AChE, the formed choline is apparently taken up again by cholinergic terminals through a specific, sodium-dependent high-affinity uptake system (76,220). This choline uptake is also present in the septohippocampal fibers (111), where it may serve as a part of the mechanism regulating ACh synthesis and release (109,139). Finally, both "muscarinic" and "nicotinic" ACh receptors have been tentatively identified by ligand-binding and autoradiographic techniques in the hippocampus, using [^{3}H]quinuclidinyl benzilate and ^{125}I-α-bungarotoxin, respectively (21, 108,151,221). Lesion studies indicate that most of these binding sites are located on hippocampal neurons (51,221). However, the distribution of these binding sites does not correlate completely with the known distribution of the ACh fibers, and their possible physiological and pharmacological importance has not yet been defined.

γ-Aminobutyrate

GABA is at present probably the best documented neurotransmitter candidate in the mammalian brain (158). The role of this amino acid as an inhibitory transmitter at several well-defined central synapses is strongly supported by electrophysiological and pharmacological studies (for reviews, see refs. 38,40,105). Also, localization studies have demonstrated GABA markers distributed in relation to these synapses [for review, see Fon-

num and Storm-Mathisen (63)], and GABA has in some cases also been found to be released from such regions simultaneously with inhibitory synaptic activity (100).

A number of "markers" have been investigated in localization studies on the GABA system. The level of endogenous GABA, the presumed inactivation mechanism for synaptically released GABA through a high-affinity uptake system (96,128), and the activity or presence of the biosynthetic enzyme L-glutamate decarboxylase (GAD) appear to be the most suitable (63). In particular, GAD appears to be almost exclusively located in alleged GABA neurons, where it is concentrated in terminals. Further, it disappears rapidly and almost completely after degeneration of the presumed GABA fiber, it is stable post mortem, and it does not diffuse or redistribute during tissue preparation (61,191). Purification of GAD has also allowed antibody production, and high- and low-resolution immunocytochemical studies on GABA neurons have been performed (157).

The level of endogenous GABA appears less useful. It has repeatedly been shown that post-mortem GABA levels in the rodent brain are unstable, increasing rapidly if the tissue is not adequately fixed (1,17). GABA is also more liable to diffuse during tissue preparation, and it is technically more difficult to measure GABA at a high level of resolution. The high-affinity uptake of GABA, which appears to occur into most GABA neurons (128,190), is more accessible for post-mortem study and has the advantage of being amenable to both quantitative biochemical and histochemical analysis. However, different GABA neurons may accumulate GABA with different avidities (190), and there is also a fairly active uptake of GABA into glial cells (97). GABA uptake studies should therefore be interpreted with some caution and preferably be performed with specific blockers of the neuronal or glial uptake systems (211).

The known inhibitory action of GABA, together with the demonstration of segregated inhibitory axosomatic (7,8) and excitatory axodendritic (11) synapses in the hippocampus, led Storm-Mathisen and Fonnum (196,197) to investigate the distribution of GAD activity in the rat hippocampal region. In both area dentata, CA1 and CA3, GAD was concentrated near the pyramidal/granular cell bodies, but it also showed a peak in the outer molecular layers (188,191,196). Similar results were later reported from guinea pig brain (146), and those authors also reported that the level of endogenous GABA coincided with the GAD activity. Putative GABA receptors also display a similar distribution (31). Thus, some of the GABA nerve terminals in the hippocampal region are concentrated near the somata of the pyramidal and granular cells, i.e., where the terminals of the inhibitory basket cells are concentrated. Histochemical studies on GABA uptake in slices (91,98) or immunochemical staining of GAD (156) further confirmed this localization, and pharmacological studies also support GABA as the transmitter responsible for inhibition at these synapses (42,172).

An autoradiogram prepared after incubation of a slice from mouse forebrain with 10^{-6} M [^{3}H]-GABA is shown in Fig. 1, where the dense network of silver grains surrounding and penetrating between the pyramidal cells can be seen. However, the GAD activity in the cellular layers accounts for only one-third of the total GAD in the hippocampus (191). Appreciable amounts are also found in the superficial stratum moleculare in both area dentata and the hippocampus proper.

In extensive studies, Storm-Mathisen has demonstrated that both of these populations of GABA terminals originate inside the hippocampal region. Thus, lesions of the perforant path did not decrease GAD activity in the molecular layers of area dentata or hippocampus (188,189). Further, lesions of ipsilateral or contralateral CA3 or hilus cell axons left GAD unchanged in the target zones in the strata oriens and radiatum of CA3/CA1 or in the inner molecular layer of area dentata, respectively (188,192), and lesions of the mossy fibers left GAD unchanged in the stratum lucidum of CA3. Also, both GAD and GABA uptake, when assayed in the whole hippocampal formation, were unchanged after complete interruption of fibers entering from the septum and forebrain through fornix, cingulum or the supracallosal striae, or through the amygdaloid area (64,111,190,198). It is therefore clear that the hippocampal formation contains only intrinsic GABA neurons. This conclusion is supported by studies with kainic acid-induced necrosis of local hippocampal cells, which led to a 76% decrease in GAD and a 49% decrease in GABA content in a coronal hippocampal slice (64). Similar results were also reported by other workers (164).

The origin and functional role of GABA in the superficial dendritic layers were originally uncertain. However, recent immunohistochemical studies, with colchicine injection given to increase the amount of enzyme in the cell bodies (156), have conclusively shown that GAD-containing perikarya are present in all hippocampal layers, with a morphology similar to the short-axon neurons and basket cells originally described in Golgi-stained material (121). Pyramidal and granular cells, together with glial structures, were unstained. Recent physiological studies have also indicated that the superficial GABA synapses may play a distinct role in a local regulation of dendritic excitability (14). Thus, the GABA neurons in the hippocampal formation are typical examples of local neurons probably involved in both recurrent inhibition of the principal projection neurons in the region and regulation of local excitability in the dendritic tree that receives the major excitatory inputs. Similar arrangements may also be present in neocortex, where the evidence for an intrinsic GABA system is strong (214).

Acidic Amino Acids

After identification of the cholinergic septohippocampal fibers, the intrinsic GABA neurons, and the afferent monoamine systems, it became clear that the transmitter chemistry of the major excitatory afferent, local, and efferent fiber projections in the hippocampal formation remained unknown (191,196). Work in the 1960s had, however, shown that the naturally occurring acidic amino acids L-glutamate and L-aspartate exhibited powerful excitatory effects on central neurons (41,106). These effects were also seen in the hippocampus (22), suggesting (60) that one of these amino acids could be involved in excitatory transmission in the hippocampus.

However, the neurotransmitter role of these compounds proved to be difficult to substantiate, as both glutamate and aspartate are important metabolites in brain (45). The concentrations of the free endogenous aspartate and, particularly, glutamate in the brain are very high (45), but the differences in regional concentration of these amino acids are not very marked (18) and do not indicate a correlation with any particular neuronal system. Further, no antagonist with the specificity necessary for identifying glutamate or aspartate synapses was available (39). However, a multitude of independent observations now support a major transmitter role for these compounds (36,39,40). Even so, no specific, rate-limiting enzymes responsible for synthesis of the transmitter pool of these amino acids have been identified (129,143). Thus, no specific enzyme marker of glutamate or aspartate neurons, similar to ChAT or GAD, is available, and hodological studies have therefore employed other parameters [for review, see Fonnum et al. (65)].

Early work indicated that the sodium-dependent high-affinity uptake of glutamate or aspartate into nerve terminals or depolarization-induced calcium-dependent release of the amino acids could represent chemical events specifically restricted to putative glutamate/aspartate neurons (for reviews, see refs. 36,65,77,78). However, the uptake mechanism does not distinguish between the naturally occurring L-glutamate and L-aspartate and the false transmitter analog D-aspartate (16,44,216), and it is also present on glial cells (81), which makes this system less suited as a specific marker.

Other workers have studied the changes in amino acid concentration after lesion of specific pathways or neuronal populations, particularly in the spinal cord [for review, see Johnson (101,102)]. All of these approaches have been used in studies on the hippocampal formation. Indeed, the hippocampal studies have represented major advances in our knowledge of the properties of central glutamate or aspartate neurons (36,193). In the early studies, the topographical distribution of high-affinity L-glutamate uptake in hippocampal slices was analyzed by autoradiography (99), or changes in the depolarization-induced calcium-dependent release of endogenous glutamate or aspartate were studied after lesions of specific pathways (142). These studies indicated that most, and possibly all, major hippocampal projections could be glutamate or aspartate pathways.

Area Dentata

The target zones for the perforant path in the area dentata and the hippocampal molecular layers contain uptake sites for L-glutamate, L-aspartate, and D-aspartate (192,200,205). The uptake activity of these axons is probably less than that of the hilus cell axons or CA3 pyramidal cell axons (193), but electron microscopic, autoradiographic studies from the molecular layer of area dentata showed that most of the labeled amino acid had been taken up by nerve endings and axons, and these structures probably accounted for 80% of the total radioactivity in the tissue (194,200). Transection of perforant path axons decreased this uptake activity selectively when analyzed both biochemically and histochemically (192). Further, endogenous glutamate and aspartate were released from dentate nerve terminals by depolarization in a calcium-dependent manner, and a perforant path lesion decreased the release of glutamate selectively. Release of labeled glutamate synthesized *in situ* from exogenous glutamine showed the same characteristics (77,78). Finally, pharmacological studies showed a preferential blockade of both perforant path-induced and glutamate-induced excitation of granule cells by glutamate diethylester or by 2-

amino-4-phosphonobutyrate (84). These results make the entorhinal perforant path axons to the area dentata the best documented glutamate pathway in the mammalian brain to date (36,194).

Similar studies have shown that the ipsi- and contralateral inputs from the cells in the hilus to the proximal part of the granule cell dendrites behave somewhat similarly. The target zones for these axons display very active glutamate/aspartate uptake (192,205), and this uptake is reduced after axotomy (194; and A. Aamodt, F. Fonnum, and I. Walaas, *unpublished data*). However, these neurons might release aspartate and not glutamate, at least from their contralateral terminals, as sectioning the hippocampal commissure, significantly decreased aspartate, but not glutamate, release from the dentate area (142,143). Further, both synaptic transmission in the commissural fiber–granule cell synapses and aspartate application to the granule cell dendrites were preferentially blocked by DL-α-aminoadipate or 2-amino-3-phosphonopropionate, antagonists more specific for aspartate receptors (84,213).

The Hippocampus

The identity of the transmitter released from the granule cell axons, the mossy fibers, has not been determined. Autoradiographic studies show that these fibers have an active high-affinity glutamate/aspartate uptake (200). Further, they rapidly transport D-aspartate from their cell bodies anterogradely into their terminals in the hippocampus (194). However, neither content nor release of glutamate or aspartate is changed in the CA3 region when the mossy fibers are lesioned (143). This could be due to the small proportion of mossy fiber terminals compared to the number of other terminals in the CA3 region. However, the pharmacological data are also inconclusive, as neither 2-amino-4-phosphonobutyrate nor 2-amino-3-phosphonopropionate (see above) blocked the synaptic transmission in the mossy fiber synapses (213). Instead, the mossy fiber transmitter appears to bind to a particular type of receptor, which has higher affinity for the heterocyclic, neurotoxic glutamate analog kainic acid (67). Thus, the role of acidic amino acids in the hippocampal mossy fibers is as yet uncertain.

In contrast, the evidence for glutamate/aspartate as transmitters in CA3-derived axons is strong. The target zones for the fibers, the strata radiatum and oriens of CA3 and CA1 and the lateral septal nucleus, all display active glutamate/aspartate uptake, with the hippocampal regions being particularly active (199). The uptake in these regions is probably responsible for most of the glutamate/aspartate uptake in the hippocampal formation (Fig. 1). Chemical destruction of the CA3 pyramidal cells with low doses of kainic acid (without any visible damage to the mossy fibers, the granule cells, or the CA1 pyramidal cells) greatly decreased the glutamate/aspartate uptake in the whole CA3 and in the CA1 stratum radiatum without affecting ACh or GABA markers in CA1 (A. Aamodt, F. Fonnum, and I. Walaas, *unpublished data*). The results from CA1 after this treatment are similar to the results after surgical interruption of ipsilateral and commissural CA3 axons (192).

Commissural denervations alone also decreased the glutamate/aspartate uptake in CA1, but less dramatically (193) and, in addition, led to a decrease in both glutamate and aspartate release from CA1 (142). Specific electric stimulation of CA3 axons in stratum radiatum of CA1, which induced monosynaptic activation of the Schaffer collateral–CA1 pyramidal cell synapse, also released preloaded D-aspartate and L-glutamate from the CA3 axons when tested in the hippocampal slice *in vitro* (125,215). Similarly, the axon collaterals from these cells going into the lateral septum were also found to have glutamate/aspartate uptake (64,199) and to release preloaded D-aspartate when stimulated *in vitro* (126).

Thus, all types of axon collaterals from the CA3 pyramidal cells are putative glutamate/aspartate fibers. However, it is not clear which of the amino acids the fibers utilize as the natural transmitter. Complete destruction of CA3 cells together with CA1 cells, hilus cells, and some granule cells by means of intrahippocampal kainic acid decreased the levels of endogenous glutamate and aspartate by 35% to 40% in a frontal hippocampal slice (64,162), and both glutamate and aspartate release from CA1 decreased after a commissurotomy (142).

However, surgical or chemical lesions reduce the content of glutamate alone in the lateral septum, although aspartate and other amino acids remain normal (64,144,209,217,222). The CA3 cells might therefore project intra- and interhippocampal glutamate and aspartate fibers, although the evidence favors a glutamate projection to the lateral septum.

The major projection from the CA1 pyramidal cells is directed toward the subiculum (12,204). The subiculum, which also receives fibers from CA3 (87), has less active glutamate/aspartate uptake than the CA1, but transection of the CA1/ CA3 fibers decreases this uptake in this region also (193). Thus, these excitatory fibers may also use glutamate or aspartate as transmitter.

Hippocampal Efferents

It thus seems clear that most of the fibers in the major afferent and intrinsic excitatory projection systems in the hippocampal formation might be glutamate or aspartate fibers. The hippocampus influences other brain regions by means of extensive cortical and subcortical projections, which have been mapped in some detail by modern anatomical techniques. Except for a bilateral input to the lateral septum noted above, which originates in CA3 and in some CA1 cells (12,201), most of the hippocampal efferents are now known to arise in the subicular complex (32,131,201). In the rat, this region sends most of its subcortical fibers through the fimbria into the fornix and the medial corticohypothalamic tract and distributes terminals ipsilaterally to, e.g., the lateral septum, nucleus accumbens, diagonal band nucleus, bed nucleus of the stria terminalis, basal periventricular hypothalamus, and the mammillary body (32,131,201). Most of these fibers are apparently excitatory (46,124,130), and recent evidence indicates that they may use glutamate as their transmitter. Thus fimbria/fornix transections selectively decreased the glutamate/aspartate uptake and the concentration of endogenous glutamate in these regions (64,208,209)—results supported by workers studying the effects of hippocampal extirpation (144). These data therefore suggest that the subicular efferent fibers could also use glutamate as transmitter. This would be in line with other corticofugal projections (66).

Monoamines

Catecholamines

The demonstration of a specific neuronal localization of the catecholamines norepinephrine (NE) and dopamine (DA) and of the indoleamine serotonin with a histofluorescence technique (43,58,68) was strong support for their proposed neurotransmitter role in the CNS. The catecholamine systems have been investigated in great detail (115,116,134,135,207). It is now clear that the major NE fiber system in the brain arises in the brainstem locus ceruleus and distributes fibers widely into the forebrain, cerebellum, brainstem, and spinal cord (103,116,150). Other, less dense

NE cell groups are also present in the brainstem, with projection patterns partly different from the locus ceruleus fibers (207). In contrast, the major DA system arises in mesencephalic cells located in the pars compacta of substantia nigra, the A9 cell groups, and in the adjacent ventral tegmental area, the A10 cell group (43). These cells project densely to the basal ganglia, septum, and amygdala, but they also give rise to a restricted cortical innervation (116). Other DA cells and projections exist but are of less importance in this context.

The distribution of catecholamine histofluorescence in the hippocampal formation was investigated early (28). A diffuse pattern was observed, with fibers concentrated in the hilus, in the stratum radiatum of CA3, and in the stratum moleculare of CA1. These fibers were initially assumed to be NE fibers. However, later immunocytochemical studies on dopamine-β-hydroxylase, a specific enzyme marker for NE neurons (159), showed a different distribution of immunoreactive fibers (203). A plexus was seen in the hilus, but these workers also observed immunoreactive fibers in the mossy fiber layer and a superficial plexus in CA3/CA1. The reasons for these discrepancies are not clear [see Storm-Mathisen (191,193) for discussion]. They may, however, be partly explained if some of the fibers observed by histofluorescence are DA fibers. Such fibers would not be displayed by dopamine-β-hydroxylase immunostaining. Recent work has indeed suggested that a restricted dopamine input to the hippocampus and area dentata exists (160).

The histofluorescent catecholamine fibers enter the hippocampal region both through the fimbria, fornix superior, and cingulum and through the amygdaloid region (28). In contrast, the dopamine-β-hydroxylase immunoreactive fibers are stated to penetrate the septum and follow only a supracallosal path to the retrosplenial cortex, from where they enter the hippocampus (203). The pathways through the fimbria and amygdaloid area may therefore be predominantly composed of DA fibers.

Biochemical studies have also mapped the monoamine fibers. Endogenous NE was found to decrease by 60% to 70% after medial forebrain bundle lesions (80), and a transection of the supracallosal, fimbrial, and fornix superior afferents decreased the NE content by 70% and the high-affinity NE uptake by 50%, whereas a complete transection of all brain stem afferents abolished the hippocampal NE uptake completely (198). This uptake activity would measure both the NE and DA terminals (181). A lesion of locus ceruleus decreased the dopamine-β-hydroxylase activity by 80% (159). Kainic acid-induced local cell necrosis, in contrast, did not decrease the activities of the other catecholamine marker enzymes tyrosine hydroxylase (164) and DOPA decarboxylase (64).

Thus, it is clear that the hippocampal formation does not contain intrinsic catecholamine neurons; rather, the NE input originates in the locus ceruleus, whereas the proposed dopamine input apparently arises in both the A9 and A10 cells (160). The catecholamine fibers enter either through the "dorsal" pathways—i.e., after following the medial forebrain bundle, they project through the supracallosal striae, the fimbria, and the fornix superior—or through a "ventral" pathway which penetrates the amygdala. The relative contributions of NE and DA in the two pathways are not clear. The catecholamine fibers distribute most densely to the hilus but are also present in parts of the hippocampus proper.

Quantitative estimates indicate that the catecholamine terminals are few and probably represent less than 1% of all terminals (28,198). However, physiological studies have demonstrated that the locus ceruleus–hippocampal pathway may be functionally important *in vivo* and that it works by releasing NE onto β-adrenergic receptors which induce a depression of hippocampal pyramidal cells (169,170).

Serotonin

Serotonin fibers in the mammalian brain are known to arise from the complex of midline raphe nuclei in the brainstem, from which they distribute wide-ranging projections into most brain regions (3,69). In the hippocampus, the presence of serotonin, its biosynthetic enzyme tryptophan hydroxylase, and a high-affinity uptake system for serotonin was early demonstrated by biochemical methods; these parameters all decreased after raphe lesions, particularly following lesions of the median raphe nucleus (110,120). Selective lesions indicated that most of these serotonin fibers entered through fimbria and other dorsal pathways, and transections of both dorsal and ventral pathways essentially abolished the serotonin uptake (198). Thus, it seems clear that no intrinsic serotonin system is present in the hippocampus or area dentata.

The intrahippocampal distribution of serotonin fibers has not been studied as thoroughly as that of the catecholamines. The best descriptions have come from studies in which serotonin fibers from the raphe nuclei have been identified by anterogradely transported ³H-labeled protein combined with use of specific serotonin neurotoxins or by the use of the serotonin-directed antisera (see H. W. M. Steinbusch and R. Nieuwenhuys, *this volume*). Thus, Moore and Halaris (136) demonstrated raphe serotonin fibers in the molecular layers of the hippocampus proper and in an infragranular layer in the area dentata. Azmitia and Segal (15) showed that the major projection arises in the median raphe, projects through the fimbria and supracallosal striae, and terminates in strata oriens and radiatum of CA3, in stratum moleculare of CA1, and in hilus fasciae dentatae. The dorsal raphe nucleus also projects some fibers that enter through the amygdala, entorhinal area, and into the molecular layer of area dentata.

Physiological data also indicate that raphe–hippocampal serotonin fibers exist, with raphe stimulation or serotonin applications depressing the activity of hippocampal pyramidal cells (167,168). Other workers have also observed depressant effects of serotonin in the hippocampus (22,28).

Histamine

No histochemical method is yet available for visualizing histamine in tissues, but recent work strongly supports a transmitter role for this amine in the brain (165). The marker of choice for this transmitter candidate has been histidine decarboxylase, and studies with this enzymatic marker have suggested that the neuronal histamine system in the brain arises in cells from the mesencephalic reticular substance and the hypothalamus (20). In the hippocampus, histidine decarboxylase decreased by more than 95% after transections of both the dorsal and ventral pathways, the dorsal route of entry being responsible for about two-thirds of this decrease (19,193). Further, histidine decarboxylase was more active in the hippocampus proper than in the area dentata (19), suggesting that histamine nerves may be less concentrated in the area dentata, in contrast with the other monoamines. Histamine is known to depress hippocampal neurons (74), thus sharing an apparent inhibitory effect on hippocampal cells with the other monoamines.

Peptides

Compared with the detailed knowledge of the distribution of neuropeptides in some other CNS regions, e.g., the spinal cord (54,92,93), knowledge on the organization of these transmitter candidates in the hippocampus is still fragmentary. From histochemical studies, it seems clear that vasoactive intestinal polypeptide (VIP), cholecystokinin octapeptide (CCK), somatostatin, and enkephalins are present in the hippocampus (54–56) (Figs. 2–4). A VIP-like immunoreactivity is present in a considerable number of interneurons in the area dentata, CA3 and CA1 regions, and in the subiculum (119), and physiological studies indicate that VIP excites pyramidal cells (49) (Fig. 4). Thus, the VIP cells could represent excitatory interneurons. Cholecystokinin-reactive cells have been observed near the hilus or granule cell layers (92), although other workers observed CCK-reactive cells near the pyramidal cell layer in the hippocampus (94) (Fig. 3). Cholecystokinin apparently is also a potent excitant when applied to CA1 pyramidal cells (47). Somatostatin-immunoreactive terminals were observed near a small number of CA1/CA3 pyramidal cells in the dorsal hippocampus (149), and other workers detected some cells in the hilus and in stratum oriens (92) (Fig. 4). Again, physiological studies indicate potent excitatory actions of somatostatin on CA1 cells (48).

Enkephalins are apparently not among the major neuropeptides in the hippocampal formation, but some enkephalin-reactive cells have been seen in the subicular complex (210), and some fibers are probably present in the perforant path to area dentata and in the hippocampal stratum radiatum (210) (Fig. 3). A laminated but sparse distribution of opiate receptors has also been described near the pyramidal cells and in the molecular layer of the hippocampus (83).

Two recent studies have also demonstrated enkephalin-like immunoreactivity in up to 40% of the dentate granule cells and their axons, the mossy fibers (71,185) (Fig. 3). Thus, a number of these fibers could conceivably use these peptides as transmitters. Future studies are required to analyze whether the enkephalins satisfy the criteria of release and of identity of action with the naturally occurring excitatory (4) mossy fiber transmitter. It is interesting also to compare this localization of enkephalin immunoreactivity in excitatory terminals with the similar observation of enkephalin-like immunoreactivity in some cerebellar mossy fibers (see J. A. Schulman, *this volume,* for discussion).

Finally, angiotensin-II–like immunoreactivity may also be present in some granule cells and some CA3 and CA1 pyramidal cells (75). Physiological experiments demonstrated an excitatory effect of this peptide on CA1 cells, but this effect might be the result of disinhibition of the local inhibitory neurons (75).

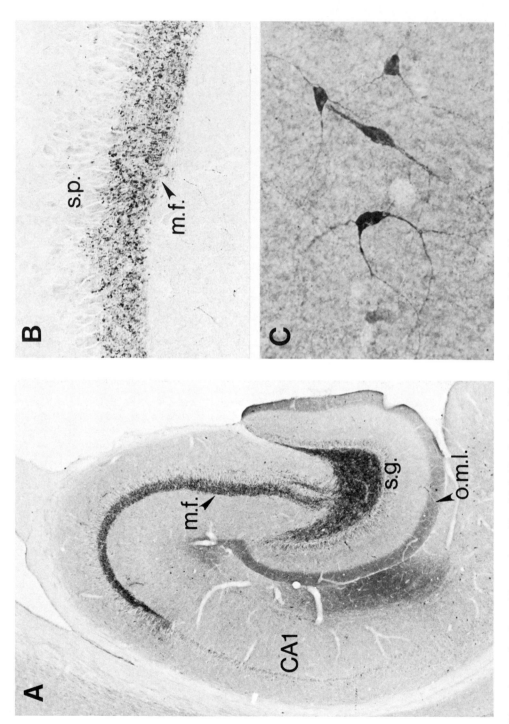

FIG. 2. Photomicrographs of peroxidase–antiperoxidase-labeled leucine-enkephalin-like immunoreactivity in the hippocampal formation of the adult rat. In the low-power photomicrograph (**A**), enkephalin-like immunoreactivity can be seen to be localized to two major axonal systems: the mossy fibers (m.f.) and the lateral entorhinal/perirhinal afferents to the outer molecular layer (o.m.l.) of the dentate gyrus. At higher magnification (**B**), the punctate character of the immunoreactive staining of the mossy fibers indicates that the enkephalin is primarily localized within the large terminal boutons that characterize this system. In addition to this axonal staining, enkephalin-like immunoreactivity is also localized to the perikarya of granule cells of the stratum granulosum and scattered interneurons. A few immunoreactive polymorph neurons of regio inferior stratum radiatum can be seen in micrograph C.

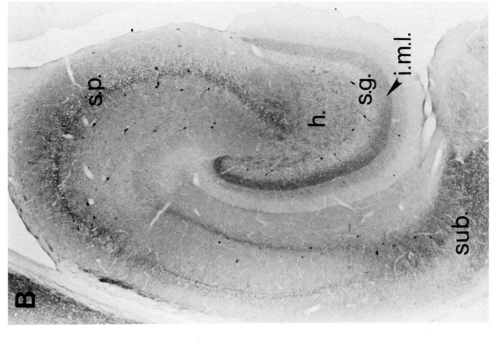

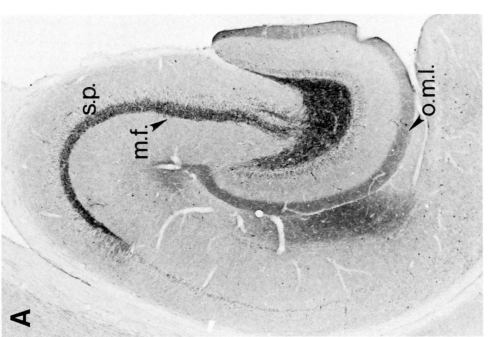

FIG. 3. Horizontal sections through the temporal hippocampal formation of the adult rat processed by the peroxidase technique for the localization of leucine-enkephalin-like (**A**) and cholecystokinin (CCK) (**B**) immunoreactivity. Enkephalin has been found to be localized within two axonal systems, the mossy fibers and afferent axons to the outer molecular layer (o.m.l.) of the dentate gyrus, within granule cells of stratum granulosum (s.g.), and within scattered interneurons. In contrast, CCK can be seen to be localized within the inner molecular layer (i.m.l.) of the dentate gyrus, within axons surrounding the neuronal perikarya of stratum pyramidale (s.p.), and within scattered interneurons. *Abbreviations:* h., hilus; i.m.l., inner molecular layer; m.f., mossy fibers; s.g., stratum granulosum; s.p., stratum pyramidale; sub., subiculum.

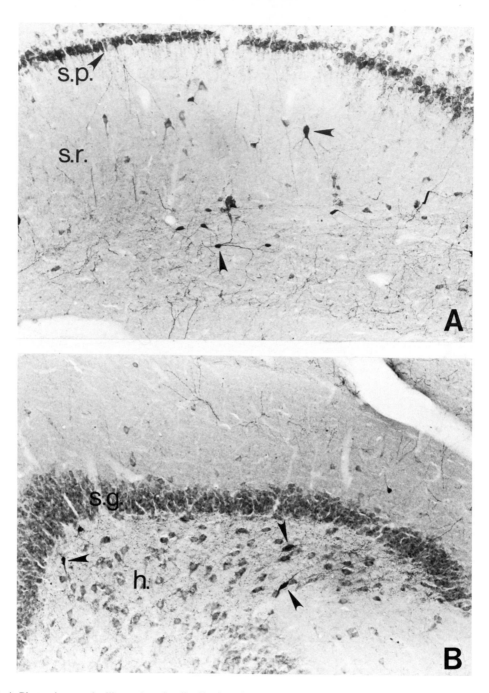

FIG. 4. Photomicrographs illustrating the distribution of vasoactive intestinal peptide (VIP) and somatostatin immunoreactivity in the hippocampal formation. Micrographs **A** and **B** are taken from adult rat tissue processed to localize VIP immunoreactivity. In field CA1 (**A**), VIP immunoreactivity can be seen to be localized within scattered interneuronal perikarya *(arrowheads)* as well as within numerous dendritic (and possibly axonal) processes of the apical dendritic field. In the dentate gyrus (**B**), VIP is mainly seen within occasional interneuronal perikarya *(arrowheads)* and fine puncta within the hilus (h.).

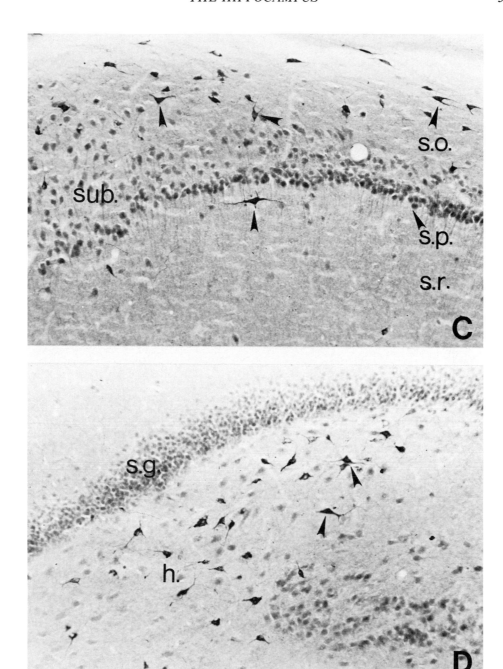

Fig. 4. (*continued*) Somatostatin is similarly localized within interneurons, but, as can be seen in micrograph **C** of the subicular (sub.)/CA1 region of the hippocampus of the cat, the somatostatin interneurons predominantly lie along the alveus and within stratum oriens (s.o.). In the dentate gyrus (**D**), somatostatin, like VIP, is localized within the scattered neurons of the hilus. *Abbreviations:* h., hilus; s.g., stratum granulosum; s.o., stratum oriens; s.p., stratum pyramidale; s.r., stratum radiatum; sub., subiculum.

ACKNOWLEDGMENTS

The author thanks Dr. Arvid Søreide for providing Fig. 1 and extends his particular thanks to Dr. Christine Gall for providing the superb illustrations Figs. 2–4; to Dr. F. Fonnum for help with the manuscript preparation; and to Mrs. T. Thorsen for typing the manuscript. This manuscript was prepared while the author was a recipient of a NATO Science Fellowship from the Royal Norwegian Council for Scientific and Industrial Research.

REFERENCES

1. Alderman, J. L., and Shellenberger, M. K. (1974): γ-Aminobutyric acid (GABA) in the rat brain: Reevaluation of sampling procedures and the postmortem increase. *J. Neurochem.*, 22:937–940.
2. Amaral, D. G. (1978): A Golgi study of cell types in the hilar region of the hippocampus in the rat. *J. Comp. Neurol.*, 182:851–914.
3. Andén, N.-E., Dahlström, A., Fuxe, K., Larsson, K., Olsson, L., and Ungerstedt, U. (1966): Ascending monoamine neurons to the telencephalon and diencephalon. *Acta Physiol. Scand.*, 67:313–326.
4. Andersen, P. (1975): Organization of hippocampal neurons and their interconnections. In: *The Hippocampus*, Vol. 1, edited by R. L. Isaacson and K. H. Pribram, pp. 155–175. Plenum Press, New York.
5. Andersen, P. (1978): Long-lasting facilitation of synaptic transmission. In: *Ciba Foundation Symposium, Vol. 58 (New Series): Functions of the Septo–Hippocampal System*, pp. 87–102. Elsevier/North-Holland, Amsterdam.
6. Andersen, P. (1980): Brain slice preparations as a neurophysiological tool. *Neurosci. Lett. [Suppl.].* 5:7.
7. Andersen, P., Eccles, J. C., and Løyning, Y. (1964): Location of postsynaptic inhibitory synapses on hippocampal pyramids. *J. Neurophysiol.*, 27:592–607.
8. Andersen, P., Eccles, J. C., and Løyning, Y. (1964): Pathway of postsynaptic inhibition in the hippocampus. *J. Neurophysiol.*, 27:608–619.
9. Andersen, P., Holmquist, B., and Voorhoeve, P. E. (1966): Entorhinal activation of dentate granule cells. *Acta Physiol. Scand.*, 66:448–460.
10. Andersen, P., Holmquist, B., and Voorhoeve, P. E. (1966): Excitatory synapses on hippocampal apical dendrites activated by entorhinal stimulation. *Acta Physiol. Scand.*, 66:461–472.
11. Andersen, P., Blackstad, T. W., and Lømo, T. (1966): Location and identification of excitatory synapses on hippocampal pyramidal cells. *Exp. Brain Res.*, 1:236–248.
12. Andersen, P., Bland, B. H., and Dudar, J. D. (1973): Organization of the hippocampal output. *Exp. Brain Res.*, 17:152–168.
13. Andersen, P., Bliss, T. V. P., and Skrede, K. K. (1971): Lamellar organization of hippocampal excitatory pathways. *Exp. Brain Res.*, 13:222–238.

14. Andersen, P., Dingledine, R., Gjerstad, L., Langmoen, J. A., and Mosfeldt Laursen, A. (1980): Two different responses of hippocampal pyramidal cells to application of gamma-amino butyric acid. *J. Physiol. (Lond.)*, 305:279–296.
15. Azmitia, E., and Segal, M. (1978): An autoradiographic analysis of the differential ascending projections of the dorsal and median raphe nuclei in the rat. *J. Comp. Neurol.*, 179:641–668.
16. Balcar, V. J., and Johnston, G. A. R. (1972): The structural specificity of the high affinity uptake of L-glutamate and L-aspartate by rat brain slices. *J. Neurochem.*, 19:2657–2666.
17. Balcom, G. J., Lenox, R. H., and Meyerhoff, J. L. (1975): Regional γ-aminobutyric acid levels in rat brain determined after microwave fixation. *J. Neurochem.*, 24:609–613.
18. Balcom, G. J., Lenox, R. H., and Meyerhoff, J. L. (1976): Regional glutamate levels in rat brain determined after microwave fixation. *J. Neurochem.*, 26:423–425.
19. Barbin, G., Garbarg, M., Schwartz, J.-C., and Storm-Mathisen, J. (1976): Histamine synthesizing afferents to the hippocampal region. *J. Neurochem.*, 26:259–263.
20. Barbin, G., Garbarg, M., Llorens-Cortes, C., Palacios, J. M., Pollard, H., and Schwartz, J.-C. (1977): Biochemical mapping of histaminergic pathways and cell bodies in brain. *Proc. Int. Soc. Neurochem.*, 6:486.
21. Ben-Barak, J., and Dudai, Y. (1979): Cholinergic binding sites in rat hippocampal formation: Properties and ontogenesis. *Brain Res.*, 166:245–257.
22. Biscoe, T. J., and Straughan, D. W. (1966): Microelectrophoretic studies on neurones in the cat hippocampus. *J. Physiol. (Lond.)*, 183:341–359.
23. Blackstad, T. W. (1956): Commissural connections of the hippocampal region in the rat, with special reference to their mode of termination. *J. Comp. Neurol.*, 105:417–537.
24. Blackstad, T. W. (1958): On the termination of some afferents to the hippocampus and fascia dentata. An experimental study in the rat. *Acta Anat. (Basel)*, 35:202–214.
25. Blackstad, T. W. (1967): Cortical gray matter. A correlation of light and electron microscopic data. In: *The Neuron*, edited by H. Hydén, pp. 49–118. Elsevier, Amsterdam.
26. Blackstad, T. W., and Kjaerheim, Å. (1961): Special axodendritic synapses in the hippocampal cortex: Electron and light microscopic studies on the layer of mossy fibers. *J. Comp. Neurol.*, 117:133–160.
27. Blackstad, T. W., Brink, K., Hem, J., and Jeune, B. (1970): Distribution of hippocampal mossy fibers in the rat. An experimental study with silver impregnation methods. *J. Comp. Neurol.*, 138:433–450.
28. Blackstad, T. W., Fuxe, K., and Hökfelt, T. (1967): Noradrenalin nerve terminals in the hippocampal region of the rat and guinea pig. *Z. Zellforsch. Mikrosk. Anat.*, 78:463–473.
29. Bland, B. H., Kostopoulos, G. K., and Phillis, J. W. (1974): Acetylcholine sensitivity of hippocampal formation neurons. *Can. J. Physiol. Pharmacol.*, 52:966–971.

30. Bliss, T. V. P., and Lømo, T. (1973): Long-lasting potentiation of synaptic transmission in the dentate area of the anaesthetized rabbit following stimulation of the perforant path. *J. Physiol. (Lond).*, 232:331–356.

31. Chan-Palay, V. (1978): Quantitative visualization of γ-aminobutyric acid receptors in hippocampus and area dentata demonstrated by ^{3}H-muscimol autoradiography. *Proc. Natl. Acad. Sci. USA*, 75:2516–2520.

32. Chronister, R. B., Sikes, R. W., and White, L. E., Jr. (1976): The septohippocampal system: Significance of the subiculum. In: *The Septal Nuclei*, edited by J. F. DeFrance, pp. 115–132. Plenum Press, New York.

33. Ciba Foundation (1978): *Functions of the Septo–Hippocampal System*. Elsevier/North-Holland, Amsterdam.

34. Cotman, C. W., and Nadler, J. V. (1978): Reactive synaptogenesis in the hippocampus. In: *Neuronal Plasticity*, edited by C. W. Cotman, pp. 227–271. Raven Press, New York.

35. Cotman, C. W., Matthews, D. A., Taylor, D., and Lynch, G. (1973): Synaptic rearrangement in the dentate gyrus: Histochemical evidence of adjustments after lesions in immature and adult rats. *Proc. Natl. Acad. Sci. USA*, 70:3473–3477.

36. Cotman, C. W., Foster, A., and Lanthorn, T. (1981): An overview of glutamate as a neurotransmitter. *Adv. Biochem. Psychopharmacol.*, 2:1–27.

37. Coyle, J. T., Molliver, M. E., and Kuhar, M. J. (1978): *In situ* injection of kainic acid: A new method for selectively lesioning neuronal cell bodies while sparing axons of passage. *J. Comp. Neurol.*, 180:301–324.

38. Curtis, D. R. (1979): Gabergic transmission in the mammalian central nervous system. In: *GABA-Neurotransmitters*, edited by P. Krogsgaard-Larsen, J. Scheel-Krüger, and H. Kofod, pp. 17–27. Munksgaard, Copenhagen.

39. Curtis, D. R. (1979): Problems in the evaluation of glutamate as a central nervous system transmitter. In: *Glutamic Acid: Advances in Biochemistry and Physiology*, edited by L. J. Filer, S. Garattini, M. R. Kare, W. A. Reynolds, and R. J. Wurtman, pp. 163–175. Raven Press, New York.

40. Curtis, D. R., and Johnston, G. A. R. (1974): Amino acid transmitters in the mammalian central nervous system. *Rev. Physiol. Pharmacol.*, 69:97–188.

41. Curtis, D. R., Phillis, J. W., and Watkins, J. C. (1960): The chemical excitation of spinal neurones by certain acidic amino acids. *J. Physiol. (Lond.)*, 150:656–682.

42. Curtis, D. R., Felix, D., and McLennan, H. (1970): GABA and hippocampal inhibition. *Br. J. Pharmacol.*, 40:881–883.

43. Dahlström, A., and Fuxe, K. (1964): Evidence for the existence of monoamine-containing neurons in the central nervous system. I. Demonstration of monoamines in the cell bodies of brainstem neurons. *Acta Physiol. Scand. [Suppl.]*, 232:1–55.

44. Davies, L. P., and Johnston, G. A. R. (1976): Uptake and release of D- and L-aspartate by rat brain slices. *J. Neurochem.*, 26:1007–1014.

45. Davidson, N., (1976): *Neurotransmitter Amino Acids*. Academic Press, New York.

46. DeFrance, J. F., Kitai, S. T., and Shimono, T. (1973): Electrophysiological analysis of the hippocampal–septal projections: II. Functional characteristics. *Exp. Brain Res.*, 17:463–476.

47. Dingledine, R., Dodd, J., and Kelly, J. S. (1980): The *in vitro* brain slice as a useful neurophysiological preparation for intracellular recording. *J. Neurosci. Methods*, 2:323–362.

48. Dodd, J., and Kelly, J. S. (1978): Is somatostatin an excitatory transmitter in hippocampus? *Nature*, 273:674–675.

49. Dodd, J., Kelly, J. S., and Said, S. J. (1979): Excitation of CA I neurons of the rat hippocampus by the octapeptide vasoactive intestinal polypeptide (VIP). *Br. J. Pharmacol.*, 66:125P.

50. Domesick, V. B. (1969): Projections from the cingulate cortex in the rat. *Brain Res.*, 12:296–320.

51. Dudai, Y., and Segal, M. (1978): α-Bungarotoxin binding sites in rat hippocampus: Localization in postsynaptic cells. *Brain Res.*, 154:167–171.

52. Dudar, J. D. (1974): *In vitro* excitation of hippocampal pyramidal cell dendrites by glutamic acid. *Neuropharmacology*, 13:1083–1089.

53. Dudar, J. D. (1975): The effect of septal nuclei stimulation on the release of acetylcholine from the rabbit hippocampus. *Brain Res.*, 83:123–133.

54. Emson, P. C. (1979): Peptides as neurotransmitter candidates in the mammalian CNS. *Prog. Neurobiol.*, 13:61–116.

55. Emson, P. C., and Hunt, S. P. (1981): Anatomical chemistry of the cerebral cortex. In: *The Organization of the Cerebral Cortex*, edited by F. O. Schmitt, F. G. Wardon, G. Adelman, and S. G. Dennis, pp. 325–346. MIT Press, Cambridge, Mass.

56. Emson, P. C., Hunt, S. P., Rehfeld, J. F., Golterman, N., and Fahrenkrug, J. (1980): Cholecystokinin and vasoactive intestinal polypeptide in the mammalian CNS: Distribution and possible physiological roles. In: *Neural Peptides and Neuronal Communication*, edited by E. Costa and M. Trabucchi, pp. 63–74. Raven Press, New York.

57. Emson, P. C., and Lindvall, O. (1979): Distribution of putative neurotransmitters in the neocortex. *Neuroscience*, 4:1–30.

58. Falck, B., Hillarp, N. Å., Thieme, G., and Torp, A. (1962): Fluorescence of catecholamines and related compounds condensed with formaldehyde. *J. Histochem. Cytochem.*, 10:348–354.

59. Finch, D. M., and Babb, T. L. (1980): Inhibition in subicular and entorhinal principal neurons in response to electrical stimulation of the fornix and hippocampus. *Brain Res.*, 196:89–98.

60. Fonnum, F. (1970): Topographical and subcellular localization of choline acetyltransferase in rat hippocampal region. *J. Neurochem.*, 17:1029–1037.

61. Fonnum, F. (1972): Application of microchemical analysis and subcellular fractionation techniques to the study of neurotransmitters in discrete areas of mammalian brain. *Adv. Biochem. Psychopharmacol.*, 6:75–88.

62. Fonnum, F. (1975): Review of recent progress in the synthesis, storage, and release of acetylcholine.

In: *Cholinergic Mechanisms,* edited by P. G. Waser, pp. 145–159. Raven Press, New York.

63. Fonnum, F., and Storm-Mathisen, J. (1978): Localization of GABA-ergic neurons in CNS. In: *Handbook of Psychopharmacology,* Vol. 9, edited by L. L. Iversen, S. D. Iversen, and S. H. Snyder, pp. 357–401. Plenum Press, New York.

64. Fonnum, F., and Walaas, I. (1978): The effect of intrahippocampal kainic acid injections and surgical lesions on neurotransmitters in hippocampus and septum. *J. Neurochem.,* 31:1173–1181.

65. Fonnum, F., Karlsen, R. L., Malthe-Sørenssen, D., Skrede, K. K., and Walaas, I. (1979): Localization of neurotransmitters, particularly glutamate, in hippocampus, septum, nucleus accumbens and superior colliculus. *Prog. Brain Res.,* 51:167–191.

66. Fonnum, F., Søreide, A., Kvale, I., Walker, J., and Walaas, I. (1981): Glutamate in cortical fibers. *Adv. Biochem. Psychopharmacol.,* 27:29–41.

67. Foster, A. C., Mena, E. E., Monaghan, D. T., and Cotman, C. W. (1981): Synaptic localization of kainic acid binding sites. *Nature,* 289:73–75.

68. Fuxe, K. (1965): Evidence for the existence of monoamine neurons in the central nervous system. IV. The distribution of monoamine terminals in the central nervous system. *Acta Physiol. Scand.* [*Suppl.*], 247:37–84.

69. Fuxe, K., and Jonsson, G. (1974): Further mapping of central 5-hydroxytryptamine neurons: Studies with the neurotoxic dihydroxytryptamines. *Adv. Biochem. Psychopharmacol.,* 10:1–12.

70. Gaarskjaer, F. (1978): Organization of the mossy fiber system of the rat studied in extended hippocampi. II. Experimental analysis of fiber distribution with silver impregnation methods. *J. Comp. Neurol.,* 178:73–88.

71. Gall, C., Brecha, N., Karten, H. J., and Chang, K.-J. (1981): Localization of enkephalin-like immunoreactivity to identified axonal and neuronal populations of the rat hippocampus. *J. Comp. Neurol.,* 198:335–350.

72. Geneser-Jensen, F. A. (1972): Distribution of acetyl cholinesterase in the hippocampal region of the guinea pig. III. The dentate area. *Z. Zellforsch. Mikrosk. Anat.,* 131:481–495.

73. Gottlieb, D. I., and Cowan, W. M. (1973): Autoradiographic studies of the commissural and ipsilateral association connections of the hippocampus and dentate gyrus of the rat. I. The commissural connections. *J. Comp. Neurol.,* 149:393–422.

74. Haas, H. L., and Wolf, P. (1977): Central actions of histamine: Microelectrophoretic studies. *Brain Res.,* 122:269–279.

75. Haas, H. L., Felix, D., Celio, M. R., and Inagemi, T. (1980): Angiotensin II in the hippocampus. A histochemical and electrophysiological study. *Experientia,* 36:1394–1395.

76. Haga, T., and Noda, H. (1973): Choline uptake systems of rat brain synaptosomes. *Biochim. Biophys. Acta,* 291:564–575.

77. Hamberger, A., Chiang, G. H., Nylen, E. S., Scheff, S. W., and Cotman, C. W. (1979): Glutamate as a CNS transmitter. I. Evaluation of glucose and glutamine as precursors for the synthesis of preferentially released glutamate. *Brain Res.,* 168:513–530.

78. Hamberger, A., Chiang, G. H., Sandoval, E., and Cotman, C. W. (1979): Glutamate as a CNS transmitter. II. Regulation of synthesis in the releasable pool. *Brain Res.,* 168:531–541.

79. Haug, F.-M. S. (1974): Light microscopical mapping of the hippocampal region, the pyriform cortex and the corticomedial amygdaloid nuclei of the rat with Timm's sulphide silver method. I. Area dentata, hippocampus and subiculum. *Z. Anat. Entwikl. Gesch.,* 145:1–27.

80. Heller, A., and Moore, R. Y. (1968): Control of brain serotonin and norepinephrine by specific neuronal systems. *Adv. Pharmacol.,* 6A:191–209.

81. Henn, F. A., Goldstein, M., and Hamberger, A. (1974): Uptake of the neurotransmitter candidate glutamate by glia. *Nature,* 249:663–664.

82. Herkenham, M. (1978): The connections of the nucleus reuniens thalami: Evidence for a direct thalamo–hippocampal pathway in the rat. *J. Comp. Neurol.,* 177:589–610.

83. Herkenham, M., and Pert, C. B. (1980): *In vitro* autoradiography of opiate receptors in rat brain suggests loci of "opiatergic" pathways. *Proc. Natl. Acad. Sci. USA,* 77:5532–5536.

84. Hicks, T. P., and McLennan, H. (1979): Amino acids and the synaptic pharmacology of granule cells in the dentate gyrus of the rat. *Can. J. Physiol. Pharmacol.,* 57:973–978.

85. Hjort-Simonsen, A. (1971): Hippocampal afferents to the ipsilateral entorhinal area: An experimental study in the rat. *J. Comp. Neurol.,* 142:417–438.

86. Hjort-Simonsen, A. (1972): Projection of the lateral part of the entorhinal area to the hippocampus and fascia dentata. *J. Comp. Neurol.,* 146:219–231.

87. Hjort-Simonsen, A. (1973): Some intrinsic connections of the hippocampus in the rat: An experimental analysis. *J. Comp. Neurol.,* 147:145–162.

88. Hjort-Simonsen, A., and Jeune, B. (1972): Origin and termination of the hippocampal perforant path in the rat studied by silver impregnation. *J. Comp. Neurol.,* 144:215–232.

89. Hjort-Simonsen, A., and Zimmer, J. (1975): Crossed pathways from the entorhinal area to the fascia dentata. I. Normal in rabbits. *J. Comp. Neurol.,* 161:57–70.

90. Hjort-Simonsen, A., and Laurberg, S. (1977): Commissural connections of the dentate area in the rat. *J. Comp. Neurol.,* 174:591–606.

91. Hökfelt, T., and Ljungdahl, Å, (1971): Uptake of (^{3}H) noradrenaline and γ-(^{3}H) aminobutyric acid in isolated tissues of the rat: An autoradiographic and fluorescence microscopic study. *Prog. Brain Res.,* 34:87–102.

92. Hökfelt, T., Elde, R., Johansson, O., Ljungdahl, Å., Schulzberg, M., Fuxe, K., Goldstein, M., Nilsson, G., Pernow, B., Terenius, L., Ganten, D., Jeffcoate, S. L., Rehfeldt, J., and Said, D. (1978): Distribution of peptide-containing neurons. In: *Psychopharmacology: A Generation of Progress,* edited by M. A. Lipton, A. DiMascio, and K. F. Killam, pp. 39–66. Raven Press, New York.

93. Hökfelt, T., Johansson, O., Ljungdahl, Å., Lundberg, J. M., and Schulzberg, M. (1980): Peptidergic neurons. *Nature,* 284:515–521.

94. Innis, R. B., Correa, F. M. A., Uhl, G. R., Schneider, B., and Snyder, S. H. (1979): Cholecystokinin octapeptide-like immunoreactivity: Histochemical localization in rat brain. *Proc. Natl. Acad. Sci. USA,* 76:521–525.

95. Isaacson, R. L., and Pribram, K. H., editors (1975): *The Hippocampus,* Vols. I, II. Plenum Press, New York.

96. Iversen, L. L. (1971): Role of transmitter uptake mechanisms in synaptic neurotransmission. *Br. J. Pharmacol.,* 41:571–591.

97. Iversen, L. L., and Kelly, J. S. (1975): Uptake and metabolism of γ-aminobutyric acid by neurones and glial cells. *Biochem. Pharmacol.,* 24:933–938.

98. Iversen, L. L., and Schon, F. F. (1973): The use of autoradiographic techniques for the identification and mapping of transmitter specific neurones in CNS. In: *New Concepts in Neurotransmitter Regulation,* edited by A. J. Mandel, pp. 153–193. Plenum Press, New York.

99. Iversen, L. L., and Storm-Mathisen, J. (1976): Uptake of ^{3}H-glutamic acid in excitatory nerve endings in the hippocampal formation of the rat. *Acta Physiol. Scand.,* 96:22A–23A.

100. Iversen, L. L., Mitchell, J. F., and Srinivasan, V. (1971): The release of γ-aminobutyric acid during inhibition from the cat visual cortex. *J. Physiol. (Lond.),* 212:519–534.

101. Johnson, J. L. (1972): Glutamic acid as a synaptic transmitter in the nervous system. A review. *Brain Res.,* 37:1–19.

102. Johnson, J. L. (1978): The excitant amino acids glutamic and aspartic acids as transmitter candidates in the vertebrate central nervous system. *Prog. Neurobiol.,* 10:155–202.

103. Jones, B. E., and Moore, R. Y. (1977): Ascending projections of the locus coeruleus in the rat. II. Autoradiographic study. *Brain Res.,* 127:23–53.

104. Koelle, G. B., and Friedenwald, J. S. (1949): A histochemical method for localizing cholinesterase activity. *Proc. Soc. Exp. Biol. Med.,* 70:617–622.

105. Krnjević, K. (1974): Chemical nature of synaptic transmission in vertebrates. *Physiol. Rev.,* 54:418–540.

106. Krnjević, K., and Phillis, J. W. (1963): Iontophoretic studies of neurones in the mammalian cerebral cortex. *J. Physiol. (Lond.),* 165:274–304.

107. Kuhar, M. J., and Rommelspacher, H. (1974): Acetylcholinesterase-staining synaptosomes from rat hippocampus: Relative frequency and tentative estimation of internal concentration of free or 'labile-bound' acetylcholine. *Brain Res.,* 77:85–96.

108. Kuhar, M. J., and Yamamura, H. J. (1975): Light microscopic autoradiographic localization of cholinergic muscarinic receptors in rat brain by specific binding of a potent antagonist. *Nature,* 253:560–561.

109. Kuhar, M. J., and Murrin, L. C. (1978): Sodium-dependent high affinity choline uptake. *J. Neurochem.,* 30:15–21.

110. Kuhar, M. J., Aghajanian, G. K., and Roth, R. H.

(1972): Tryptophan hydroxylase activity and synaptosomal uptake of serotonin in discrete brain regions after midbrain raphe lesions: Correlations with serotonin levels and histochemical fluorescence. *Brain Res.,* 44:165–176.

111. Kuhar, M. J., Sethy, V. H., Roth, R. H., and Aghajanian, G. K. (1973): Choline: Selective accumulation by central cholinergic neurones. *J. Neurochem.,* 20:581–593.

112. Laurberg, S. (1979): Commissural and intrinsic connections of the rat hippocampus. *J. Comp. Neurol.,* 184:685–708.

113. Lewis, P. R., and Shute, C. C. D. (1967): The cholinergic limbic system: Projections to the hippocampal formation, medial cortex, nuclei of the ascending cholinergic reticular system, and the subfornical organ and supraoptic crest. *Brain,* 90:521–540.

114. Lewis, P. R., Shute, C. C. D., and Silver, A. (1967): Confirmation from choline acetylase analyses of a massive cholinergic innervation to the rat hippocampus. *J. Physiol. (Lond.),* 191:215–224.

115. Lindvall, O., and Björklund, A. (1974): The organization of the ascending catecholamine neuron systems in the rat brain. *Acta Physiol. Scand. [Suppl.],* 412:1–48.

116. Lindvall, O., and Björklund, A. (1978): Organisation of catecholamine neurons in the rat central nervous system. *Handbook of Psychopharmacology,* Vol. 9, edited by L. L. Iversen, S. I. Iversen, and S. H. Snyder, pp. 139–231. Plenum Press, New York.

117. Lømo, T. (1968): Nature and distribution of inhibition in a simple cortex (dentate area). *Acta Physiol. Scand.,* 74:8A–9A.

118. Lømo, T. (1971): Patterns of activation in a monosynaptic cortical pathway: The perforant path input to the dentate area of the hippocampal formation. *Exp. Brain Res.,* 12:18–45.

119. Lorén, I., Emson, P. C., Fahrenkrug, J., Björklund, A., Alumets, J., Håkansson, R., and Sundler, F. (1979): Distribution of vasoactive intestinal polypeptide in the rat and mouse brain. *Neuroscience,* 4:1953–1976.

120. Lorens, S. A., and Guldberg, H. C. (1974): Regional 5-hydroxytryptamine following selective midbrain raphe lesions in the rat. *Brain Res.,* 78:45–56.

121. Lorente de Nó, R. (1934): Studies on the structure of the cerebral cortex. II. Continuation of the study of the Ammonic system. *J. Psychol. Neurol.,* 46:113–117.

122. Lynch, G., and Schubert, P. (1980): The use of *in vitro* brain slices for multidisciplinary studies of synaptic function. *Annu. Rev. Neurosci.,* 3:1–22.

123. Lynch, G., Rose, G., and Gall, C. (1978): Anatomical and functional aspects of the septohippocampal projections. In: *Ciba Foundation Symposium, Vol. 58 (New Series): Functions of the Septo–Hippocampal System,* pp. 5–20. Elsevier/North-Holland, Amsterdam.

124. MacLean, P. D. (1975): An ongoing analysis of hippocampal inputs and outputs: Microelectrode and neuroanatomical findings in squirrel monkeys. In: *The Hippocampus,* Vol. I, edited by R. L. Isaacson

and K. H. Pribram, pp. 177–211. Plenum Press, New York.

125. Malthe-Sørenssen, D., Skrede, K. K., and Fonnum, F. (1979): Calcium-dependent release of D-(^{3}H)aspartate evoked by selective electrical stimulation of excitatory afferent fibres to hippocampal pyramidal cells *in vitro. Neuroscience,* 4:1255–1263.

126. Malthe-Sørenssen, D., Skrede, K. K., and Fonnum, F. (1980): Release of D-(^{3}H)aspartate from the dorsolateral septum after electrical stimulation of the fimbria *in vitro. Neuroscience,* 5:127–133.

127. Malthe-Sørenssen, D., Odden, E., and Walaas, I. (1980): Selective destruction by kainic acid of neurons innervated by putative glutamergic afferents in septum and nucleus of the diagonal band. *Brain Res.,* 182:461–465.

128. Martin, D. L. (1976): Carrier-mediated transport and removal of GABA from synaptic regions. In: *Kroc Foundation Series, Vol. 5: GABA in Nervous System Function,* edited by E. Roberts, T. N. Chase, and D. Tower, pp. 347–386. Raven Press, New York.

129. McGeer, E. G., and McGeer, P. L. (1979): Localization of glutaminase in the rat neostriatum *J. Neurochem.,* 32:1071–1075.

130. McLennan, H., and Miller, J. J. (1979): The hippocampal control of neuronal discharges in the septum of the rat. *J. Physiol. (Lond.),* 237:607–624.

131. Meibach, R., and Siegel, A. (1977): Efferent connections of the hippocampal formation in the rat. *Brain Res.,* 124:197–224.

132. Mellgren, S. I., and Blackstad, T. W. (1967): Oxidative enzymes (tetrazolium reductases) in the hippocampal regions of the rat. *Z. Zellforsch. Mikrosk. Anat.,* 78:167–207.

133. Mellgren, S. I., and Srebro, B. (1973): Changes in acetylcholinesterase and distribution of degenerating fibres in the hippocampal region after septal lesions in the rat. *Brain Res.,* 52:19–36.

134. Moore, R. Y., and Bloom, F. E. (1978): Central catecholamine neuron systems: Anatomy and physiology of the dopamine systems. *Annu. Rev. Neurosci.,* 1:129–169.

135. Moore, R. Y., and Bloom, F. E. (1979): Central catecholamine neuron systems: Anatomy and physiology of the norepinephrine and epinephrine systems. *Annu. Rev. Neurosci.,* 2:113–168.

136. Moore, R. Y., and Halaris, A. E. (1975): Hippocampal innervation by serotonin neurons of the midbrain raphe in the rat. *J. Comp. Neurol.,* 164:171–183.

137. Moroni, F., Malthe-Sørenssen, D., Cheney, D. L., and Costa, E. (1978): Modulation of ACh turnover in the septal hippocampal pathway by electrical stimulation and lesioning. *Brain Res.,* 150:333–341.

138. Mosko, S., Lynch, G., and Cotman, C. W. (1973): The distribution of the septal projections to the hippocampus of the rat. *J. Comp. Neurol.,* 152:163–174.

139. Mulder, A. H., Yamamura, H. J., Kuhar, M. J., and Snyder, S. H. (1974): Release of acetylcholine from hippocampal slices by potassium depolariza-

tion: Dependency on high affinity choline uptake. *Brain Res.,* 70:372–376.

140. Nadler, J. V. (1979): Kainic acid: Neurophysiological and neurotoxic actions. *Life Sci.,* 24:289–300.

141. Nadler, J. V., Cotman, C. W., and Lynch, G. S. (1974): Subcellular distribution of transmitter related enzyme activities in discrete areas of the rat dentate gyrus. *Brain Res.,* 79:465–477.

142. Nadler, J. V., Vaca, K. W., White, W. F., Lynch, G. S., and Cotman, C. W. (1976): Aspartate and glutamate as possible transmitters of excitatory hippocampal afferents. *Nature,* 260:538–540.

143. Nadler, J. V., White, W. F., Vaca, K. W., Perry, B. W., and Cotman, C. W. (1978): Biochemical correlates of transmission mediated by glutamate and aspartate. *J. Neurochem.,* 31:147–155.

144. Nitsch, C., Kim, J.-K., Shimada, C., and Okada, Y. (1979): Effect of hippocampus extirpation in the rat on glutamate levels in target structures of hippocampal efferents. *Neurosci. Lett.,* 11:295–299.

145. Oderfeld-Nowak, B., Narkiewicz, O., Dabrowska, J., Wieraszko, A., and Gradkowska, M. (1973): Acetylcholinesterase and choline acetyltransferase in hippocampus after various septal lesions in rats. In: *Central Nervous System—Studies on Metabolic Regulation and Function,* edited by E. Genazzani and H. Herken, pp. 158–163. Springer, Berlin.

146. Okada, Y., and Shimada, C. (1975): Distribution of γ-aminobutyric acid (GABA) and glutamate decarboxylase (GAD) activity in the guinea-pig hippocampus—microassay method for the determination of GAD activity. *Brain Res.,* 98:202–206.

147. O'Keefe, J., and Nadel, L. (1978): *The Hippocampus as a Cognitive Map.* Oxford University Press, New York.

148. Pasquier, D. A., and Reinoso-Suarez, F. (1976): Direct projections from hypothalamus to hippocampus in the rat demonstrated by retrograde transport of horseradish peroxidase. *Brain Res.,* 108:165–169.

149. Petrusz, P., Sar, M., Grossman, G. H., and Kizer, J. S. (1977): Synaptic terminals with somatostatin-like immunoreactivity in the rat brain. *Brain Res.,* 137:181–187.

150. Pickel, V. M., Segal, M., and Bloom, F. E. (1974): A radioautographic study of the efferent pathways of the nucleus locus coeruleus. *J. Comp. Neurol.,* 155:15–42.

151. Polz-Tejera, G., Schmidt, J., and Karten, H. J. (1975): Autoradiographic localization of α-bungarotoxin binding sites in the central nervous system. *Nature,* 285:349–351.

152. Potemska, A., Gradkowska, A. M., and Oderfeld-Nowak, B. (1975): Early changes in acetylcholine pools in the hippocampus of the rat brain after septal lesions. *J. Neurochem.,* 24:787–789.

153. Raisman, G. (1966): The connexions of the septum. *Brain,* 89:317–348.

154. Ramon y Cajal, S. (1893): *The Structure of Ammon's Horn.* Charles C. Thomas, Springfield, Illinois.

155. Ramon y Cajal, S. (1911): *Histologie de Système Nerveux de l'Homme et des Vertebres,* Vol. 2. Maloine, Paris.

156. Ribak, C. E., Vaughn, J. E., and Saito, K. (1978):

Immunocytochemical localization of glutamic acid decarboxylase in neuronal somata following colchicine inhibition of axonal transport. *Brain Res.,* 140:315–332.

157. Roberts, E. (1979): New directions in GABA research. I: Immunocytochemical studies of GABA neurons. In: *GABA-Neurotransmitters,* edited by P. Krogsgaard-Larsen, J. Scheel-Kruger, and H. Kofod, pp. 28–45. Munksgaard, Copenhagen.

158. Roberts, E., Chase, T. N., and Tower, D. B. (1976): *Kroc Foundation Series, Vol. 5: GABA in Nervous System Function.* Raven Press, New York.

159. Ross, R. A., and Reis, D. J. (1974): Effects of lesions of locus coeruleus on regional distribution of dopamine-β-hydroxylase activity in rat brain. *Brain Res.,* 73:161–166.

160. Scatton, B., Simon, H., Le Moal, M., and Bischoff, S. (1980): Origin of dopaminergic innervation of the rat hippocampal formation. *Neurosci. Lett.,* 18:125–131.

161. Schaffer, K. (1892): Beitrag zum Histologie der Ammonshornformation. *Arch. Mikroskop. Anat.,* 39:611–632.

162. Schmid, R., Hong, J. S., Meek, J., and Costa, E. (1980): The effect of kainic acid on the hippocampal content of putative transmitter amino acids. *Brain Res.,* 200:355–362.

163. Schwarcz, R., and Coyle, J. T. (1977): Striatal lesions with kainic acid: Neurochemical characteristics. *Brain Res.,* 127:235–249.

164. Schwarcz, R., Zaczek, R., and Coyle, J. T. (1978): Microinjection of kainic acid into the rat hippocampus. *Eur. J. Pharmacol.,* 50:209–220.

165. Schwartz, J.-C., Barbin, G., Garbarg, M., Pollard, H., Rose, C., and Verdire, M. (1976): Neurochemical evidence for histamine acting as a transmitter in mammalian brain. *Adv. Biochem. Psychopharmacol.,* 15:111–126.

166. Schwartzkroin, P. A., and Andersen, P. (1975): Glutamic acid sensitivity of dendrites in hippocampal slices *in vitro. Adv. Neurol.,* 12:45–51.

167. Segal, M. (1975): Physiological and pharmacological evidence for a serotonergic projection to the hippocampus. *Brain Res.,* 94:115–131.

168. Segal, M. (1976): 5-HT antagonists in rat hippocampus. *Brain Res.,* 103:161–166.

169. Segal, M., and Bloom, F. E. (1974): The action of norepinephrine in the rat hippocampus. I. Iontophoretic studies. *Brain Res.,* 72:79–97.

170. Segal, M., and Bloom, F. E. (1976): The action of norepinephrine in the rat hippocampus. III. Hippocampal cellular responses to locus coeruleus stimulation in the awake rat. *Brain Res.,* 107:499–511.

171. Segal, M., and Landis, S. (1974): Afferents to the hippocampus of the rat studied with the method of retrograde transport of horseradish peroxidase. *Brain Res.,* 78:1–15.

172. Segal, M., Sims, K., and Smissman, E. (1975): Characterization of an inhibitory receptor in rat hippocampus: A microiontophoretic study using conformationally restricted amino acid analogues. *Br. J. Pharmacol.,* 54:181–188.

173. Sethy, V. H., Kuhar, M. J., Roth, R. H., Van Woert, M. H., and Aghajanian, G. K. (1973): Cholinergic neurones: Effect of acute septal lesion on acetylcholine content of rat hippocampus. *Brain Res.,* 55:481–484.

174. Sethy, V. H., Roth, R. H., Kuhar, M. J., and Van Woert, M. H. (1973): Choline and acetylcholine: Regional distribution and effect of degeneration of cholinergic nerve terminals in the rat hippocampus. *Neuropharmacology,* 12:819–823.

175. Shute, C. C. D., and Lewis, P. R. (1961): The use of cholinesterase techniques combined with operative procedures to follow nervous pathways in the brain. *Bibl. Anat.,* 2:34–49.

176. Shute, C. C. D., and Lewis, P. R. (1966): Electron microscopy of cholinergic terminals and acetylcholinesterase containing neurones in the hippocampal formation of the rat. *Z. Zellforsch. Mikrosk. Anat.,* 69:334–343.

177. Shute, C. C. D., and Lewis, P. R. (1967): The ascending cholinergic reticular system: Neocortical, olfactory and subcortical projections. *Brain,* 90:497–520.

178. Silver, A. (1974): *Frontiers in Biology, Vol. 36: The Biology of Cholinesterases.* Elsevier/North-Holland, Amsterdam.

179. Skrede, K. K., and Westgaard, R. (1971): The transverse hippocampal slice: A well-defined cortical structure maintained *in vitro. Brain Res.,* 35:589–593.

180. Smith, C. M. (1974): Acetylcholine release from the cholinergic septo–hippocampal pathway. *Life Sci.,* 14:2159–2166.

181. Snyder, S. H., Kuhar, M. J., Green, A. J., Coyle, J. T., and Shaskan, E. G. (1970): Uptake and subcellular localization of neurotransmitters in the brain. *Int. Rev. Neurobiol.,* 13:127–158.

182. Snyder, S. H., Young, A. B., Bennett, J. P., and Mulder, A. H. (1973): Synaptic biochemistry of amino acids. *Fed. Proc.,* 32:2039–2047.

183. Srebro, B., and Mellgren, S. I. (1974): Changes in postnatal development of acetylcholinesterase in the hippocampal region after early septal lesions in the rat. *Brain Res.,* 79:119–131.

184. Stefanis, C. (1964): Hippocampal neurons: Their responsiveness to microelectrophoretically administered endogenous amines. *Pharmacologist,* 6:171.

185. Stengaard-Pedersen, K., Fredens, K., and Larsson, L.-I. (1981): Enkephalin and zinc in the hippocampal mossy fiber system. *Brain Res.,* 212:230–233.

186. Steward, O., and Scoville, S. A. (1976): Cells of origin of entorhinal cortical afferents to the hippocampus and fascia dentata of the rat. *J. Comp. Neurol.,* 169:347–370.

187. Storm-Mathisen, J. (1970): Quantitative histochemistry of acetylcholinesterase in rat hippocampal region correlated to histochemical staining. *J. Neurochem.,* 17:739–750.

188. Storm-Mathisen, J. (1972): Glutamate decarboxylase in the rat hippocampal region after lesions of the afferent fibre systems. Evidence that the enzyme is localized in intrinsic neurons. *Brain Res.,* 40:215–235.

189. Storm-Mathisen, J. (1974): Choline acetyltransferase and acetylcholinesterase in fascia dentata following lesion of the entorhinal afferents. *Brain Res.,* 80:181–197.

190. Storm-Mathisen, J. (1975): High affinity uptake of

GABA in presumed GABA-ergic nerve endings in rat brain. *Brain Res.,* 84:409–427.

191. Storm-Mathisen, J. (1977): Localization of transmitter candidates in the brain: The hippocampal formation as a model. *Prog. Neurobiol.,* 8:119–181.

192. Storm-Mathisen, J. (1977): Glutamic acid and excitatory nerve endings: Reduction of glutamic acid uptake after axotomy. *Brain Res.,* 120:379–386.

193. Storm-Mathisen, J. (1978): Localization of putative transmitters in the hippocampal formation. In: *Ciba Foundation Symposium, Vol. 58 (New Series): Functions of the Septo–Hippocampal System,* pp. 49–86. Elsevier/North-Holland, Amsterdam.

194. Storm-Mathisen, J. (1981): Glutamate in hippocampal pathways. *Adv. Biochem. Psychopharmacol.,* 27:43–55.

195. Storm-Mathisen, J., and Blackstad, T. W. (1964): Cholinesterase in the hippocampal region. *Acta Anat.,* 56:216–253.

196. Storm-Mathisen, J., and Fonnum, F. (1971): Quantitative histochemistry of glutamate decarboxylase in the rat hippocampal region. *J. Neurochem.,* 18:1105–1111.

197. Storm-Mathisen, J., and Fonnum, F. (1972): Localization of transmitter candidates in the hippocampal region. *Prog. Brain Res.,* 36:41–57.

198. Storm-Mathisen, J., and Guldberg, H. C. (1974): 5-Hydroxytryptamine and noradrenaline in the hippocampal region: Effect of transection of afferent pathways on endogenous levels, high affinity uptake and some transmitter-related enzymes. *J. Neurochem.,* 22:793–803.

199. Storm-Mathisen, J., and Opsahl, M. W. (1978): Aspartate and/or glutamate may be transmitters in hippocampal efferents to septum and hypothalamus. *Neurosci. Lett.,* 9:65–70.

200. Storm-Mathisen, J., and Iversen, L. L. (1979): Uptake of (^{3}H)glutamic acid in excitatory nerve endings: Light and electron microscopic observations in the hippocampal formation of the rat. *Neuroscience,* 4:1237–1253.

201. Swanson, L. W., and Cowan, W. M. (1977): An autoradiographic study of the organization of the efferent connections of the hippocampal formation in the rat. *J. Comp. Neurol.,* 172:49–84.

202. Swanson, L. W., and Cowan, W. M. (1979): The connections of the septal region in the rat. *J. Comp. Neurol.,* 186:621–656.

203. Swanson, L. W., and Hartman, B. K. (1975): The central adrenergic system. An immunofluorescence study of the location of cell bodies and their efferent connections in the rat utilizing dopamine-β-hydroxylase as a marker. *J. Comp. Neurol.,* 163:467–505.

204. Swanson, L. W., Wyss, J. M., and Cowan, W. M. (1978): An autoradiographic study of the organization of intrahippocampal association pathways in the rat. *J. Comp. Neurol.,* 181:681–716.

205. Taxt, T., and Storm-Mathisen, J. (1979): Tentative localization of glutamergic and aspartergic nerve endings in the brain. *J. Physiol. (Paris),* 75:677–684.

206. Teyler, T., and Skrede, K. K. (1973): Preservation of synaptic mechanisms in isolated slices of mammalian hippocampal cortex. *Acta Physiol. Scand. [Suppl.],* 396:109.

207. Ungerstedt, U. (1971): Stereotaxic mapping of the monoamine pathways in the rat brain. *Acta Physiol. Scand. [Suppl.],* 367:1–48.

208. Walaas, I., and Fonnum, F. (1979): The effects of surgical and chemical lesions on neurotransmitter candidates in the nucleus accumbens of the rat. *Neuroscience,* 4:209–216.

209. Walaas, I., and Fonnum, F. (1980): Biochemical evidence for glutamate as a transmitter in hippocampal efferents to the basal forebrain and hypothalamus in the rat brain. *Neuroscience,* 5:1691–1698.

210. Wamsley, J. K., Young, W. S. III, and Kuhar, M. J. (1980): Immunohistochemical localization of enkephalin in rat forebrain. *Brain Res.,* 190:153–174.

211. Weitsch-Dick, F., Jessel, T. M., and Kelly, J. S. (1978): The selective neuronal uptake and release of (^{3}H) DL-2,4-diaminobutyric acid by rat cerebral cortex. *J. Neurochem.,* 30:799–806.

212. Werman, R. (1966): A review—criteria for identification of a central nervous system transmitter. *Comp. Biochem. Physiol.,* 18:745–766.

213. White, W. F., Nadler, J. V., and Cotman, C. W. (1979): The effect of acidic amino acid antagonists on synaptic transmission in the hippocampal formation *in vitro. Brain Res.,* 164:177–194.

214. White, W. F., Snodgrass, S. R., and Dichter, M. (1980): Identification of GABA neurons in rat cortical cultures by GABA uptake autoradiography. *Brain Res.,* 190:139–152.

215. Wieraszko, A., and Lynch, G. S. (1979): Stimulation-dependent release of possible transmitter substances from hippocampal slices studied with localized perfusion. *Brain Res.,* 160:372–376.

216. Wofsey, A. R., Kuhar, M. J., and Snyder, S. H. (1971): A unique synaptosomal fraction which accumulates glutamic and aspartic acids in brain tissue. *Proc. Natl. Acad. Sci. USA,* 68:1102–1106.

217. Wood, P. L., Peralta, E., Cheney, D. L., and Costa, E. (1979): The turnover rate of ACh in the hippocampus after lesion of hippocampal pyramidal cells with kainic acid. *Neuropharmacology,* 18:519–523.

218. Wyss, J. M., Swanson, L. W., and Cowan, W. M. (1979): A study of subcortical afferents to the hippocampal formation in the rat. *Neuroscience,* 4:463–476.

219. Yamamoto, C. (1972): Activation of hippocampal neurons by mossy fiber stimulation in thin brain sections *in vitro. Exp. Brain Res.,* 14:423–435.

220. Yamamura, H. J., and Snyder, S. H. (1972): Choline: High affinity uptake by rat brain synaptosomes. *Science,* 178:626–628.

221. Yamamura, H. J., and Snyder, S. H. (1974): Postsynaptic localization of muscarinic receptor binding in rat hippocampus. *Brain Res.,* 78:320–326.

222. Zaczek, R., Hedreen, J. C., and Coyle, J. T. (1979): Evidence for a hippocampal–septal glutamergic pathway in the rat. *Exp. Neurol.,* 65:145–156.

223. Zimmer, J. (1971): Ipsilateral afferents to the commissural zone of the fascia dentata, demonstration in decommissurated rats by silver impregnation. *J. Comp. Neurol.,* 142:393–416.

Chemical Neuroanatomy, edited by P. C. Emson, Raven Press, New York © 1983.

Putative Neurotransmitters in the Amygdaloid Complex with Special Reference to Peptidergic Pathways

Sadao Shiosaka, Masahiro Sakanaka, Shinobu Inagaki, Emiko Senba, Yoshinobu Hara, Kenichi Takatsuki, Hiroshi Takagi, Yuriko Kawai, and Masaya Tohyama

Department of Neuroanatomy, Institute of Higher Nervous Activity, Osaka University Medical School, Osaka 530, Japan

The amygdala is, as its name implies, an almond-shaped brain area lying between the internal capsule and the hypothalamus. The amygdala has attracted particular interest from the apparent variety of the functions it subsumes. For example, electrical stimulation of different parts of the amygdaloid complex can cause cardiovascular and respiratory changes, produce flight and defense behavior, salivation, chewing, penile erection, changes in gastrointestinal motility, and ovulation (40,41,58). In good agreement with this apparent complexity of function, cytoarchitectural studies have also revealed a complexity of structure, with a number of nuclei and subdivisions within the amygdaloid complex. In addition to classic cytoarchitectural studies carried out with such techniques as Golgi and Nissl staining, recent studies have used histochemical and immunohistochemical techniques to reveal an additional complexity of amygdaloid transmitters. However, before considering recent histochemical studies, we outline the cytoarchitecture of the amygdaloid complex as elucidated by classic anatomical methods and autoradiography.

CYTOARCHITECTURE OF THE AMYGDALOID COMPLEX

The cytoarchitecture of the amygdaloid complex in mammals has been described in detail by a number of authors (10,36,42,69).

The amygdaloid complex is situated lateral to the hypothalamus and ventral to the nucleus caudatus–putamen and nucleus globus pallidus. Rostrally, it extends to the level of the nucleus supra-chiasmaticus and caudally to the level of the mammillary body. The amygdaloid complex is usually divided into two main nuclear masses, a corticomedial nuclear group and a basolateral nuclear group (18,41,69).

Corticomedial Nuclear Group

The corticomedial nuclear group is subdivided into six nuclear groups or areas.

Medial Amygdaloid Nucleus

The medial amygdaloid nucleus (am) is a well-defined cell mass composed of small, relatively tightly packed cells (Fig. 1A–D). Krettek and Price (69) have further divided this nucleus into anterior and posterodorsal subdivisions.

Amygdalohippocampal Area

The amygdalohippocampal area is a nuclear mass forming a thin plate-like structure that is situated in the ventral part of the caudal amygdaloid complex (Fig. 1D–F). This area is readily distinguished from the other amygdaloid regions and is characterized by densely packed, darkly staining fusiform neurons. This nucleus extends medially to fuse with the ventral hippocampus. No clear boundaries between the amygdalohippocampal area and ventral hippocampus are recognized. Moreover, this nucleus extends laterally to merge with the basomedial nucleus at the rostral level and with the ventral part of the lateral entorhinal area.

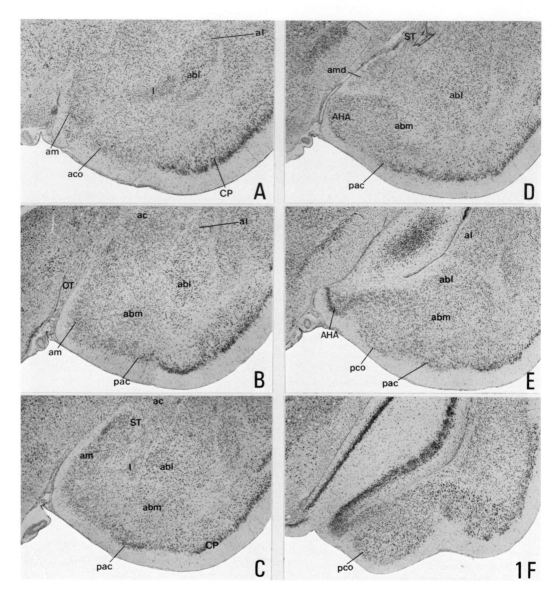

FIG. 1. Photomicrographs illustrating the cytoarchitecture of the amygdaloid complex of the rat, arranged from rostral to caudal (**A–F**). ×20.

The following abbreviations are used in the illustrations of this chapter: AA, anterior amygdaloid area; abl, n. amygdaloideus basolateralis; abm, n. amygdaloideus basomedialis; ac, n. amygdaloideus centralis; ACh, acetylcholinesterase; aco, n. amygdaloideus corticalis; AH, anterior hypothalamic nucleus; AHA, anterior hippocampal area; al, n. amygdaloideus lateralis; ala, al, pars anterior; alp, al, pars posterior; am, n. amygdaloideus medialis; amd, am, pars dorsalis; c, central canal; CA, catecholamine; CCK, cholecystokinin; CP, piriform cortex; ENK, enkephalin; I, massa intercalatus; NT, neurotensin; nXII, hypoglossal nucleus; OT, optic tract; pac, periamygdaloid cortex; pco, posterior cortical area; pm, n. reticularis paramedianus; rd, n. reticularis medullae oblongatae, pars dorsalis; rv, n. reticularis medullae oblongatae, pars ventralis; SOM, somatostatin; SP, substance P; ST, stria terminalis; TOL, tractus olfactorius lateralis; VIP, vasoactive intestinal polypeptide; 5-HT, serotonin.

Anterior Cortical Nucleus

The anterior cortical nucleus (aco) is located in the anteroventral portion of the amygdaloid complex (Fig. 1A) and is composed of small and relatively densely stained cell bodies which are packed tightly in the rostral and caudal parts of the nucleus. The nucleus is limited medially by the nucleus of the olfactory tract and the medial amygdaloid nucleus and dorsally by the neurons of the intercalated nucleus. This nucleus extends laterally and caudally to intermingle with the neurons of the periamygdaloid nucleus and the elongation of the periamygdaloid cortex, where its boundaries are not distinct.

Periamygdaloid Complex

The periamygdaloid complex is a transitional area between the amygdaloid complex and cortical area. This area is rostrally continuous with the anterior cortical region, medially continuous with the posterior cortical area, and laterally with the piriform cortex (Fig. 1B–F).

Posterior Cortical Nucleus

The posterior cortical nucleus (pco) is situated just ventral to the amygdalohippocampal area and occupies the most ventral portion of the caudal amygdaloid complex (Fig. 1E,F). This nucleus is delineated rostrally and laterally by the periamygdaloid cortex and caudally by the lateral entorhinal cortex. The posterior cortical nucleus is characterized by small and lightly stained cells, which form an ovoid mass surmounted by the plexiform layer.

Nucleus of the Lateral Olfactory Tract

This nucleus occupies the most rostromedial portion of the amygdaloid complex. This nucleus is well defined and is composed of three layers: condensed small cells (layer I), large deeply stained cells (layer II), and larger cells corresponding to those of layer II (layer III) as defined by Krettek and Price (69).

Basolateral Nuclear Group

Lateral Amygdaloid Nucleus

The lateral amygdaloid nucleus (al) is situated in the most lateral portion of the amygdaloid complex next to the external capsule (Fig. 1A–F). Dorsally, it is covered by the nucleus caudatus–putamen and caudally by the endopiriform cortex. The lateral amygdaloid nucleus is a well-defined mass of small to medium-sized cells, although these are known to be heterogeneous [for discussion, see Krettek and Price (69)].

Basolateral Amygdaloid Nucleus

The basolateral amygdaloid nucleus (abl) extends over the entire rostrocaudal extent of the complex. This nucleus is easily delineated from the lateral amygdaloid nucleus and the basomedial nuclei (abm) on the basis of the cell size, because abl contains the largest cells in the amygdaloid complex (Fig. 1A–E). It has been suggested that this nucleus can be further subdivided into anterior and posterior divisions, the anterior division being composed of very large round cells, and the posterior division containing smaller round cells (69).

Basomedial Amygdaloid Nucleus

The basomedial amygdaloid nucleus (abm) is a small round nuclear mass situated ventral to the abl and lateral to the am and amygdalohippocampal area. This nucleus comprises sparsely distributed small to medium-sized cells.

Central Amygdaloid Nucleus

The central amygdaloid nucleus (ac) is a spherical nuclear mass which is surrounded by the stria terminalis, al, and abl, and is packed with small densely stained cells (Fig. 1B,C). In the rostral direction, the central amygdaloid nucleus blends into the anterior amygdaloid area; caudally, into the putamen. Thus, at the rostral and caudal end of the central amygdaloid nucleus, it is very difficult to separate the nucleus from its adjacent structures.

Other Nuclear Masses Associated with the Amygdaloid Complex

The Bed Nucleus of the Accessory Olfactory Tract

This nucleus is situated ventral to the am and consists of comparatively large and deeply stained cells (Fig. 1C,D).

The Intercalated Cell Islands

These islands comprise very small, tightly packed cells which are located in the rostral half of the amygdaloid complex.

The Intraamygdaloid Portion of the Bed Nucleus of the Stria Terminalis

This nucleus is located in the area between ac and am and is composed of medium-sized cells. Some of the neurons in this nucleus are contained within the fibers of the stria terminalis. This nucleus seems to correspond to "amc" (the area between ac and am) defined by our previous studies (49,107) (Fig. 1A–C).

FIBER CONNECTIONS OF THE AMYGDALOID COMPLEX

The fiber connections of the amygdaloid complex have been investigated by many authors using a number of anatomical and physiological techniques. In this section, we summarize the main pathways shown by conventional anatomical techniques (i.e., degeneration, autoradiography, and horseradish peroxidase techniques).

Efferent Connections of the Amygdaloid Complex

Stria Terminalis

This is the most prominent efferent pathway from the amygdaloid complex. It has been shown that the majority of stria terminalis (ST) fibers arise from the corticomedial part of the amygdaloid complex (36,72). However, recent autoradiographic studies have revealed that ST fibers also originate from other nuclear masses of the amygdaloid complex such as abl, ac, abm, am, pco, and the amygdalohippocampal area (70). A major part of ST terminates in the bed nucleus of the ST (bst) and hypothalamus (36,70,72). With regard to the hypothalamic termination of ST, it has been reported that both abm and am project to the core of the ventromedial hypothalamic nucleus (VMH) and premammillary nucleus, whereas the amygdalohippocampal area projects to an outer shell of the VMH and the premammillary nucleus, and the pc projects exclusively to the premammillary nucleus (70). In addition, the anterior hypothalamic nucleus (AH) and lateral hypothalamic nucleus (LH) are known to receive dense inputs from the ST (70,77). However, it should be noted that LH receives a denser input from the ac than from the anterior amygdaloid area (AA) (70,80).

Ventral Amygdalofugal Projection

The ventral amygdalofugal fibers have been considered to take their origins in the abl and piriform cortex (17,40,87,118). These fibers pass through the substantia innominata and enter the lateral preoptic area, hypothalamus, nucleus accumbens, septal area, diagonal band, and ventral putamen. Some of the fibers that enter the preoptic area and hypothalamus have also been shown to enter the inferior thalamic peduncle to project to the magnocellular part of the dorsomedial nucleus of the thalamus (37,87). In addition, some authors have reported that abm also projects to the nucleus accumbens and ventral putamen (70).

Olfactory Connection

It is well known that the amygdaloid complex receives a substantial olfactory input. However, there is some evidence that the amygdaloid complex projects to the olfactory bulb [reciprocal connections between the amygdaloid complex and olfactory bulb have been reported (61,62,68)] (for details, see F. Macrides and B. J. Davis, *this volume*).

Amygdalocortical Projection

In addition to the amygdalocortical projection mentioned above, there are efferent connections from abl to the prelimbic (area 32) and infralimbic cortex, from al to the prerhinal area and to the posterior insular cortex, and from aco to the infralimbic and ventral insular cortex (67).

Lower Brainstem Projections from the Amygdaloid Complex

Previous autoradiographic studies have indicated the presence of descending projections from ac to the lateral part of the substantia nigra, ventral tegmental area, mesencephalic reticular formation, periaqueductal gray, parabrachial area, locus ceruleus, lateral tegmental field, solitary nucleus, dorsal motor nucleus of the vagus nerve, and the rhombencephalic reticular formation (70). It seems likely that these fibers reach the lower brainstem by way of both the ST and the ventral amygdalofugal tract (70).

Afferent Connections of the Amygdaloid Complex

Projections from the Thalamus

Ottersen and Ben-Ari (94) have reported precise projection patterns from the thalamus to the amygdaloid complex. Their principal findings were as follows: the paraventricular and paratenial nuclei project to the entire amygdaloid complex; the medial geniculate complex and the basal nucleus of the ventromedial complex (the thalamic taste area) project to the centromedial part of the amygdala; the interanteromedial nucleus projects to the basolateral nucleus; and the parafascicular nucleus projects to the central amygdaloid nucleus. Although Ottersen and Ben-Ari (94) could not demonstrate the existence of a mediodorsal thalamic nucleus–basolateral amygdaloid tract in the cat, Krettek and Price (67) and Siegel et al. (119) have described this pathway in the rat.

Afferent Connections from the Hypothalamus and Basal Telencephalon to the Amygdaloid Complex

In contrast to the thalamic projections to the amygdaloid complex, no obvious species differences in the afferent projections from hypothalamus and basal telencephalon were found. We summarize here the main projections.

From hypothalamus.

The axons from the neurons in the area dorsal and medial to the paraventricular nucleus terminate in the am and the intraamygdaloid part of the bed nucleus of the ST (amc); axons from the VMH, ventral premammillary nucleus, and arcuate nucleus terminate in the am; axons from LH terminate in the ac and also partly in the am and abl; and axons from the dorsal hypothalamic area and supramammillary nucleus terminate in the ac and abl, respectively (71,92,101).

From basal telencephalon.

The axons of the ventral pallium and ventral part of the globus pallidus terminate in the al and abl; axons of the substantia innominata terminate in the entire amygdaloid complex except for the al and the caudal part of the am; axons of the dorsal subdivision of the nucleus of the lateral olfactory tract terminate in the abl. In addition, axons from the ventral subdivision of the nucleus of the lateral olfactory tract terminate in the ac; axons from the nucleus of the horizontal limb of the diagonal band terminate in the ac, am, and anterior cortical nucleus; and axons from the bst terminate in the am, anterior amygdaloid area, and entire amygdaloid complex with the exception of am and al (92).

Afferent Projections from Olfactory Bulb

It is well known that the amygdaloid complex receives numerous afferent fibers from the olfactory bulb. Based on the fiber connections from the olfactory bulb, two separate systems have been proposed in the amygdala, namely, a vomeronasal amygdala and an olfactory amygdala (61, 62,100,140). The am and the posterior cortical amygdaloid nucleus belong to the former category and receive inputs from the accessory olfactory bulb, whereas the anterior cortical and periamygdaloid nuclei belong to the latter category and receive the afferent fibers from the main olfactory bulb (61,62,100).

Afferent Connections from the Lower Brainstem

Afferent connections from the lower brainstem to the amygdaloid complex have been investigated by many authors using various anatomical techniques. A summary of this work is as follows (88,93,108,145): the substantia nigra, pars compacta, ventral tegmental area, peripeduncular nucleus, periaqueductal gray, raphe nuclei group, locus ceruleus, nucleus tractus solitari, and mesencephalic and rhombencephalic reticular formation all project to the ac, and the peripeduncular nucleus, nucleus raphe dorsalis, nucleus centralis superior, parabrachial area, and dorsal nucleus of the lemniscus lateralis all project to the am.

Intraamygdaloid Axonal Connections

In 1978, Krettek and Price (69) reported a detailed study of the connections among the amygdaloid nuclei. They showed that al projects to the abm, the lateral part of the ac, and the periamygdaloid cortex; abl projects to itself, the medial part of the ac, and the nucleus of the lateral olfactory tract; abm projects to the cellular layer of the am; and the amygdalohippocampal area, the periamygdaloid cortex, and the endopiriform cortex project to the molecular layer and the am, the amygdalohippocampal area, and the posterior cortical nucleus, respectively. In addition, they also reported interconnections between the am and the posterior cortical nuclei of the two sides.

PUTATIVE TRANSMITTERS IN THE AMYGDALOID COMPLEX

Peptides

Somatostatin

Distribution.

Somatostatin (SOM) is a tetradecapeptide responsible for the inhibition of growth hormone release from the anterior pituitary (47). Since the original isolation and synthesis of SOM, a wide but uneven regional distribution of SOM in the central nervous system (both in the hypothalamus and extrahypothalamic areas) has been shown by means of radioimmunoassay and immunohistochemistry (9,11,30,115–117,130). In the amygdaloid complex, a number of SOM-positive structures, both neurons and fibers, have been demonstrated (9,104,107,117). The regional distribution of SOM neurons and fibers in the amygdaloid complex is summarized in Fig. 2. Numerous SOM-positive

cells were seen in the ac and in the area between ac and am (amc) (Figs. 2–4). Fewer positive cells were seen in the am and pac, and only a few scattered SOM-positive cells were present in the al, pars anterior (ala); al, pars posterior (alp); abl; and abm (Fig. 2). In addition, numerous SOM cells are also detected in the piriform cortex (Fig. 2) (J. G. Parnavelas and J. K. McDonald, *this volume*). A dense network of SOM-positive fibers is seen in the ac, medial part of the am, and periamygdaloid cor-

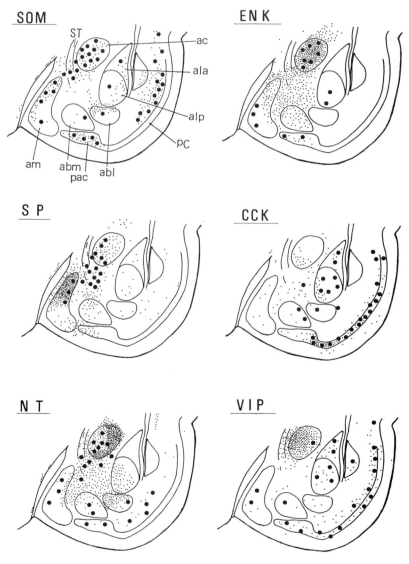

FIG. 2. Schematic drawing of the distribution of various peptides (somatostatin, substance P, neurotensin, leucine-enkephalin, cholecystokinin, and vasoactive intestinal polypeptide) in the amygdaloid complex based on indirect immunofluorescence microscopy. *Large dots* indicate peptidergic cells; *small dots,* terminal fibers. (For abbreviations, see Fig. 1, legend.)

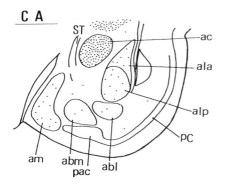

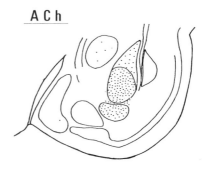

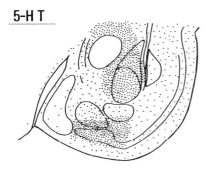

FIG. 3. Schematic drawing of the distribution of catecholamine, serotonin, and acetylcholinesterase activity in the amygdaloid complex. Distribution of CA and 5-HT is based on the histofluorescence method, and that of acetylcholinesterase on enzyme histochemistry. (For abbreviations, see Fig. 1, legend.)

tex (pac). In other subdivisions of the amygdaloid complex, diffuse SOM-positive fibers are found (Fig. 2).

Fiber connections.

There is good evidence for a periventriculo–median eminence SOM-containing tract (47), a cochlearofugal SOM-containing tract (128,129), and a cerebellar SOM tract (54; and J. A. Schulman, *this volume*). In addition, two further amygdalofugal SOM-containing tracts were experimentally demonstrated in the rat; one is an amygdalohypothalamic SOM tract (107), and the other is an amygdalo–lower brainstem SOM tract (50). After destruction of the ac and amc, a substantial decrease in the number of SOM-containing fibers is seen in the ipsilateral hypothalamic nucleus (lateroventral part) (Figs. 5 and 6), in the midbrain and rhombencephalic reticular formation (Fig. 7), and in the hypoglossal nucleus, facial nucleus, and lamina VII of the cervical cord from C1 to C3. Amygdalofugal SOM fibers described above reach the areas mentioned by traveling through the ST, as destruction or transection of the ST caused similar changes in the pattern of SOM fibers to those found after destruction of the amygdaloid complex. After leaving the ST, the amygdalofugal SOM fibers that innervate the lower brainstem and upper cervical cord pass through the medial forebrain

bundle (50). Thus, these experimental immuno-histochemical studies have clearly shown that the amygdalofugal SOM-containing tracts are an important component of the amygdalohypothalamic and amygdalo–lower-brainstem connections, although their exact physiological roles are quite unknown.

With regard to the sources of the SOM fibers in the amygdaloid complex, no clear evidence is yet available. However, it is probable that amygdaloid SOM fibers may originate from intrinsic SOM neurons, because sagittal section between amygdaloid complex and diencephalon failed to produce a decrease in the number of SOM fibers in the amygdaloid complex (S. Inagaki, *unpublished data*).

Ontogeny and phylogeny.

The ontogenic development of the SOM-containing neuronal system of the rat has been reported in some detail (116,117). Somatostatin neurons of the hypothalamus occur in the 10- to 12-mm embryo (day 14 of gestation), whereas those of the amygdaloid complex appear in the 14- to 15-mm embryo (day 16 of gestation). At gestational day 17, a few SOM fibers make their appearance in the developing amygdaloid complex. At gestational days 18 to 19 (17–26-mm embryos),

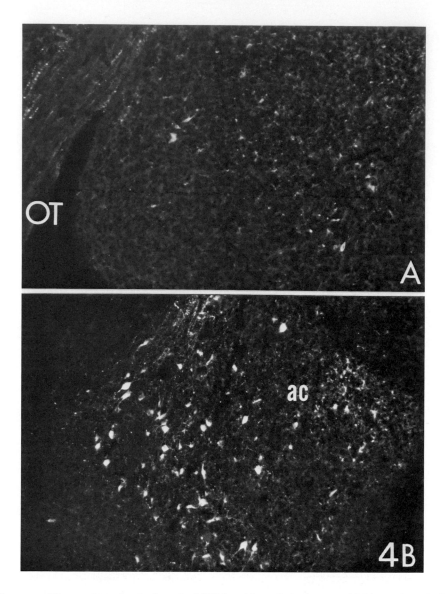

FIG. 4. Ontogeny of immunohistochemically stained SOM-positive cells in the amygdaloid complex. The SOM cells located in the amygdaloid complex appear during the fetal stage (**A**) and reach maximum content at the perinatal stage. Frontal sections. **A:** Gestational day 19. **B:** Postnatal day 30. OT, optic tract; ac, n. amygdaloideus centralis. ×120.

there is a remarkable increase in the number of SOM cells and fibers in the developing amygdaloid complex. The SOM-positive structures in the amygdaloid complex continue to increase in number during the perinatal stage and more or less maintain their immunoreactivity even in the adult rat (114,129) (Fig. 4).

The phylogeny of the SOM-containing neuronal system has also been examined. The existence of SOM neurons and fibers has been reported in the amygdaloid area of a number of lower vertebrates (114,127,129,132,142).

As described above, the SOM-containing neuronal system appears early in vertebrate ontogeny and phylogeny, suggesting that the peptide SOM might play an important role in the development of the vertebrate brain in both the ontogenetic and phylogenetic sense (115–117,128,130).

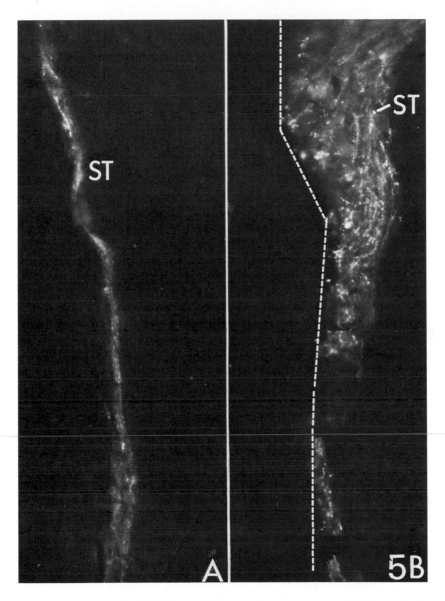

FIG. 5. Transection of the stria terminalis (ST) resulted in a marked accumulation of SOM-positive fibers in the ST caudal to the lesion (on the amygdaloid side), whereas no immunoreactive fibers were seen in the ST rostral to the lesion (on the hypothalamic side) (**B**). One week after operation. **A:** The contralateral side. *Dotted line* indicates the lesion. Frontal sections. ×145.

Substance P

Distribution.

Substance P (SP) was discovered by von Euler and Gaddum (31) and characterized as an undeca-peptide by Chang et al. (15). Since the successful isolation and characterization of SP, the regional distribution of SP in the brain and spinal cord has been studied by both radioimmunoassay and immunohistochemistry (12,46,75). These studies have demonstrated a widespread distribution of SP in the central nervous system (CNS), suggesting that the SP neuron system may be involved in a variety of physiological functions in addition to its proposed transmitter function in some of the primary afferent neurons.

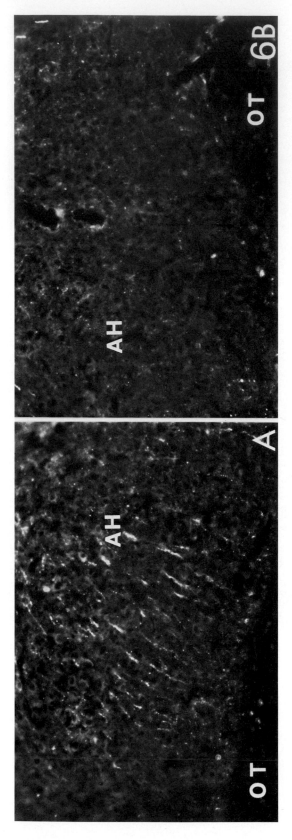

FIG. 6. A: Destruction of the amygdaloid complex results in a marked reduction of SOM fibers in the lateroventral part of the anterior hypothalamic nucleus (AH). **B:** SOM-positive fibers in the same area of the contralateral side. Frontal sections. ×180.

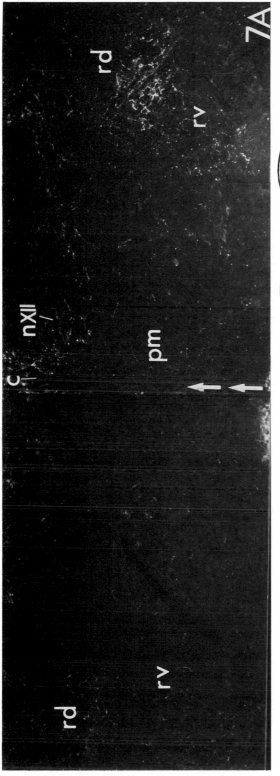

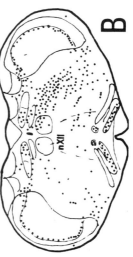

FIG. 7. Fluorescent photomicrograph (**A**) and schematic representation (**B**) of the ipsilateral reduction of SOM fibers in the medulla oblongata at the level of the obex after unilateral destruction of the amygdaloid complex. Seven days after operation. **Left** is operated side; **right** is normal side. Note a marked ipsilateral reduction of SOM-positive fibers in the reticular formation and hypoglossal nucleus. Frontal section. ×70. (For abbreviations, see Fig. 1, legend.)

In the amygdaloid complex, a large number of SP neurons can be visualized, the majority of which are concentrated in the ac and amc (Figs. 2 and 8). In addition, a less numerous but still substantial number of SP neurons are found in the am. A very high concentration of SP fibers is seen in the am, particularly in its dorsal part (Figs. 2 and 9). In this nucleus, it is very difficult to distinguish cell bodies from the numerous SP fibers. In ac, a moderately dense SP fiber plexus is also detected. In addition, all other subdivisions of the amygdaloid complex contain a low to moderate density of SP fibers (Fig. 2).

Fiber connection.

There is evidence for a habenulointerpeduncular SP tract (83), a descending strionigral SP tract (59), a cerebellar SP tract (51), and a nucleus laterodorsalis tegmenti (Castaldi) to septum SP-containing tract (106). In addition, there are SP-containing projections to the frontal cortex, entopeduncular nucleus, and medial preoptic area (96) together with the primary afferent SP neurons (91). In addition, it was also suggested that there was an amygdalofugal SP-containing tract (107). Recent immunohistochemical studies using the rat have clearly revealed the presence of this amygdalofugal SP pathway and have revealed the detailed termination of this pathway (Figs. 10 and 11). After destruction of the amygdaloid complex, there is a disappearance of SP fibers in the lateral hypothalamus on the operated side. The available evidence indicates clearly that amygdalofugal SP fibers reach the bst and lateral hypothalamus by traveling through the ST (107).

On the other hand, little is known of the origins of SP fibers in the amygdaloid complex, although there is evidence suggesting that SP fibers in the amygdaloid complex may originate from intrinsic SP neurons. Thus, SP fibers remain in the amygdaloid complex despite the presence of sagittal cuts between amygdaloid complex and diencephalon [see also Emson et al. (29)].

Ontogeny and phylogeny.

The ontogeny of the SP neuronal system has been examined in detail in the rat (52,105). The SP cells of the amygdaloid complex first appear at gestational day 15 (12–14 mm embryo), whereas those of the epithalamus occur earlier than SP cells of the amygdaloid complex (at gestational day 14, 10–12 mm embryo). In the fetus of gestational day 16, SP fibers are clearly identified in the developing amygdaloid complex. On and after gestational day 16, SP-positive structures in this area increase gradually in number; SP-positive structures continue to increase in number and density during the fetal and perinatal stage and show histochemically a maximum content at the stage between postnatal days 5 and 15. After this time, the SP neurons seem to decrease slightly in number as the rat grows, although SP fibers maintain their strong immunoreactivity even in the adult rats (see Figs. 8 and 9).

The phylogeny of the SP neuron system has also been investigated, and occurrence of SP-positive neuronal systems in lower vertebrate brains have been reported (53). For example, a very high concentration of SP-containing structures (both neurons and fibers) in the amygdaloid complex of the frog brain has been reported using immunohistochemical techniques (Fig. 12).

Neurotensin

Distribution.

Neurotensin (NT) is a tridecapeptide isolated from bovine hypothalamus and characterized by Carraway and Leeman (14). Subsequent radioimmunoassay and immunohistochemical studies have demonstrated a wide but uneven regional distribution of NT in the CNS (65,104,123,134).

In the amygdaloid complex, a large number of NT cells are observed in the ac and amc, a less numerous but still significant number of NT cells in the am and abm, with scattered NT cells in the pac (Figs. 2,13). In addition, it should be noted that in the young rat, numerous NT cells are seen in the anterior amygdaloid area just medial to the medial forebrain bundle and laterally to the piriform cortex; these are very difficult to identify in the adult rat even with colchicine treatment. Abundant NT fibers are found in the amygdaloid complex (Fig. 2). The highest density of NT fibers is detected in the lateral part of the ac and the area that surrounds the ac (Fig. 2), and numerous NT fibers are found in the medial part of the abl (Fig. 2). In addition, a moderate number of NT fibers are detected in the amygdaloid areas that do not correspond to any clear anatomical subdivisions of the amygdaloid complex (Fig. 2).

Fiber connections.

An amygdalofugal NT neuronal system projecting via ST was demonstrated by means of surgical lesions of ST (134,137). According to this study,

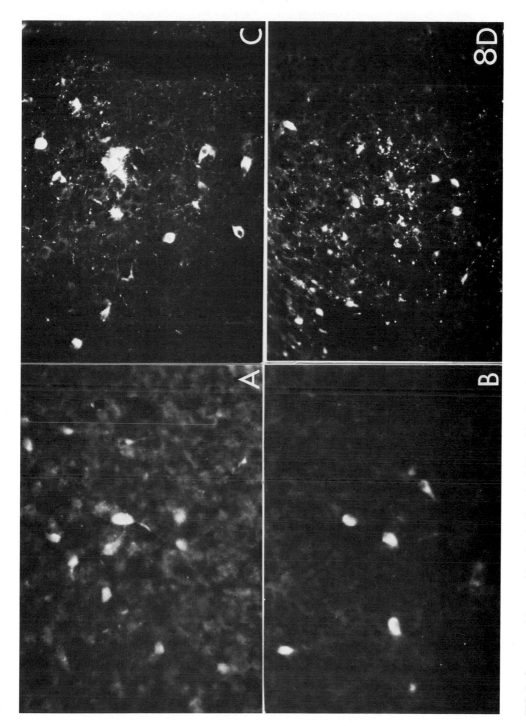

FIG. 8. Ontogeny of immunohistochemically stained SP-positive fibers in the area between ac and am. **A:** Gestational day 15. **B:** Gestational day 17. **C:** Postnatal day 15. **D:** Postnatal day 20. Frontal sections. **A,B** ×340; **C,D** ×180.

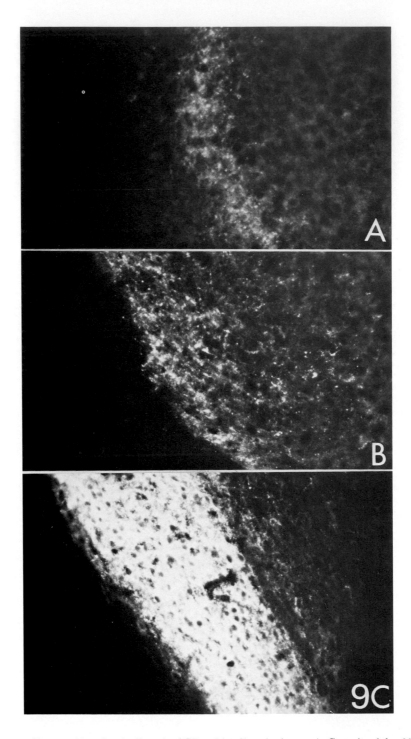

FIG. 9. Ontogeny of immunohistochemically stained SP-positive fibers in the am. **A:** Gestational day 22. **B:** Postnatal day 5. **C:** Adult. Frontal sections. The SP-positive fibers in the amygdaloid complex first appear at gestational day 22. After gestational day 22, SP-positive fibers continued to increase in number and intensity, and, in the amygdaloid complex of the adult, a large number of SP-positive fibers are seen. **A,B** ×370; **C** ×180.

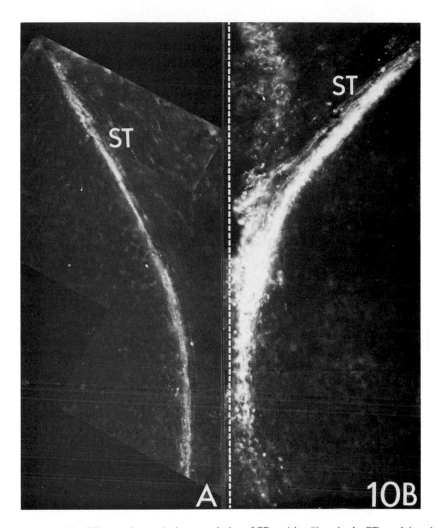

FIG. 10. Transection of the ST caused a marked accumulation of SP-positive fibers in the ST caudal to the lesion (on the amygdaloid side) (**B**), whereas rostral to the lesion (on the hypothalamic side), SP-positive fibers substantially decreased. One week after operation. **A**: Contralateral side. *Dotted line* indicates the lesion. Frontal sections. ×100.

the origin of this fiber pathway is the ac, and its terminal field is the bst. Recently, another NT pathway originating from the amygdaloid complex was demonstrated (49). Destruction of the amygdaloid complex and anterior amygdaloid area resulted in a marked decrease of NT fibers in the ipsilateral olfactory bulb, diagonal band, and medial thalamic nucleus. However, lesions that were restricted to the ac or ST failed to decrease the number of NT fibers in the olfactory bulb and medial thalamic nucleus. These observations suggest that NT neurons located in the amygdaloid complex (with the exception of those in the ac) and anterior amygdaloid area give rise to the axons innervating the areas mentioned above.

Little is known of the origins of NT fibers in the amygdaloid complex. However, it is likely that many of these arise from local intrinsic NT neurons.

Ontogeny and phylogeny.

Neurotensin cells located in the amygdaloid complex and anterior amygdaloid area first appear at gestational day 16 (43,81). Until the perinatal stage, NT-positive structures (both neurons and fibers) in these areas increase progressively in number and in density. As the rat grows, they reach their maximum apparent NT content between postnatal days 1 and 7. On and after that time, NT neurons located in the anterior amygdaloid area

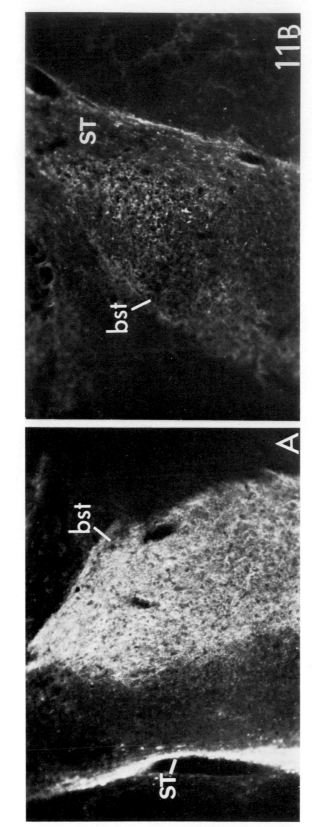

FIG. 11. Destruction of the amygdaloid complex resulted in a marked decrease of SP-positive fibers in the ST and dorsal part of the bed nucleus of the ST (bst) on the operated side (**B**). Frontal sections. Ten days after operation. **A:** Contralateral side. ×100.

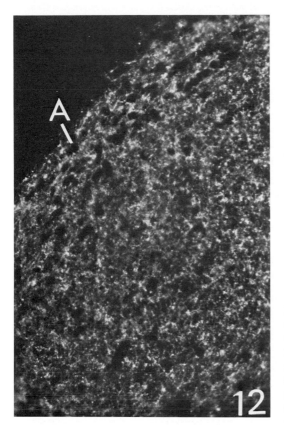

FIG. 12. Fluorescent photomicrograph showing a dense plexus of SP-positive fibers (*A*) in the amygdaloid complex of the frog. ×130.

and various amygdaloid areas except for ac, amc, and am decrease gradually in number, and in the adult rat, it is very difficult to identify NT-positive cells in these regions. On the other hand, in the ac, amc, and am, a less numerous but a still substantial number of NT neurons can be observed even in the adult rat. Recent immunohistochemical studies dealing with the distribution of NT-positive structures failed to demonstrate NT cells in the anterior amygdaloid area and amygdaloid subdivisions except for ac, amc, and am, although they described NT cells in the ac, amc, and am (104,123,135). This discrepancy between the results concerning the distribution of NT cells in the amygdaloid complex and anterior amygdaloid area obtained in our ontogenetic study and previous studies can presumably be best explained by the different ages of the experimental animals.

To date, no results are available on the phylogeny of NT neuron systems in the amygdaloid com-

plex, although it is clear that NT-positive structures occur in the teleost brain.

Enkephalins

Distribution.

The first two enkephalins (ENK) were the endogenous pentapeptides that were isolated by Hughes et al. (48) from the pig brain and identified as methionine-enkephalin (met-ENK) and leucine-enkephalin (leu-ENK). Both of these peptides have been shown to have potent agonist activity at opiate receptor sites. As described for other peptides, radioimmunoassay and immunohistochemistry have shown a widespread but uneven distribution of enkephalins in the CNS. As the distributions of leu-ENK and met-ENK in the brain are nearly identical, we refer to leu-ENK and met-ENK as ENK in this section (35,109,123, 124,146).

In the amygdaloid complex, a large group of ENK cells are found in the ac, and ENK neurons are also dispersed throughout the am, pco, and alp (Fig. 2). A very high concentration of ENK fibers is found in the ac, and a moderate density of ENK fibers is found in the abm, dorsal part of the am, amc, and several areas that do not readily correspond to anatomical subdivisions (see Fig. 1). In addition, scattered ENK fibers are reported in the pac.

Fiber connections.

It has been shown that there are some central ENK pathways such as the caudatus–putamen–globus pallidus ENK tract and the descending ENK tract from the caudal raphe nuclei (19,45). Previously, Uhl et al. reported on the basis of lesion studies that the amygdalofugal ENK tract passed through the ST (134,136). Although the exact terminal field of this tract was not clear, they suggested that these ENK fibers project to the bst.

On the other hand, there is no available description of the origins of ENK fibers in the amygdaloid complex.

Ontogeny and phylogeny.

Enkephalin neurons located in the amygdaloid complex first appear in the fetus at gestational day 18, and ENK fibers appear later (110,111). From that time onward, ENK-positive structures continue to increase in number and in density and reach their maximum content at the perinatal stage. These structures maintain their strong immunoreactivity even in the adult rat (Fig. 14).

The ENK neuronal system has also been investigated phylogenetically (22,86). According to

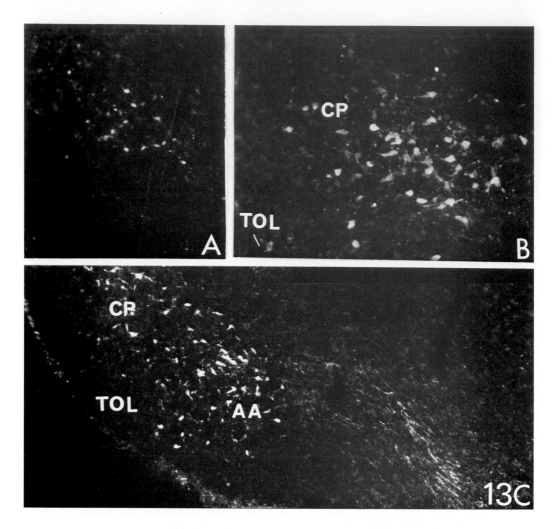

FIG. 13. Ontogeny of immunohistochemically stained NT-positive structures in the anterior amygdaloid area (AA) and piriform cortex (CP). The NT-positive cells first appeared in these areas on gestational day 16 (A) and increased remarkably in number on gestational day 17 (**B**). On gestational day 19 (**C**), two major NT fiber bands were identified. One was located in the lateral olfactory tract (TOL), and the other was situated medial to the NT-positive cells located in the AA and CP. The later fiber band is traced laterally to the NT-positive cell group seen in the AA and CP and medially to the hypothalamic area.

Naik et al., numerous ENK-positive structures were detected in the amygdaloid complex of the lizard (86).

Cholecystokinin

Distribution.

Cholecystokinin octapeptide (CCK-8) was first identified as a gastrin-like peptide in brain extracts by Vanderhaeghen et al. (140). Subsequent studies have shown that this gastrin-like material is distinct from gastrin and identical with or closely re-

lated to CCK-8, the COOH-terminal eight-amino-acid sequence of CCK. Distribution of CCK-8 in the brain has been studied by radioimmunoassay and immunohistochemistry. According to these studies, CCK-8 is particularly concentrated in the hippocampus, cerebral cortex, amygdaloid complex, diencephalon, and ventral tegmental area, whereas the lower brainstem is comparatively poorly innervated by CCK-8 neurons (25,55,73). More recently, the coexistence of CCK-8 and dopamine within the same neurons of the ventral tegmental area has been reported (46).

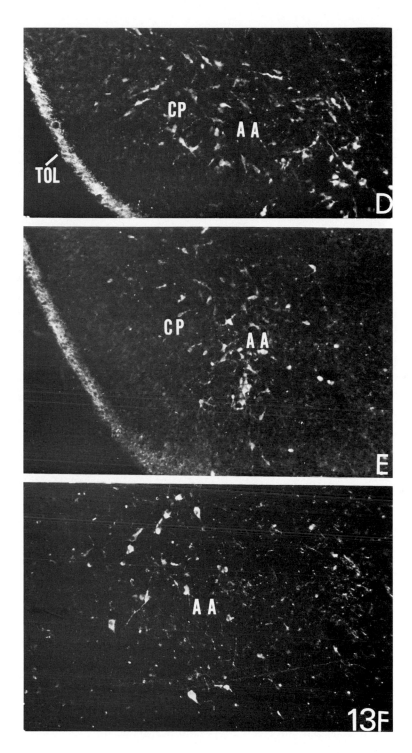

FIG. 13. (*continued*) On gestational day 21 (**D**), NT-positive fibers located in the TOL still continued to increase in number and intensity. However, after that time, NT-positive structures seemed to decrease slightly in number, but still, numerous NT-positive structures are detectable both in the colchicine-treated and nontreated rat. **E:** Newborn without colchicine treatment. **F:** 7-day-old colchicine-treated rat. Frontal sections. **A,C–E** ×110; **B,F** ×170.

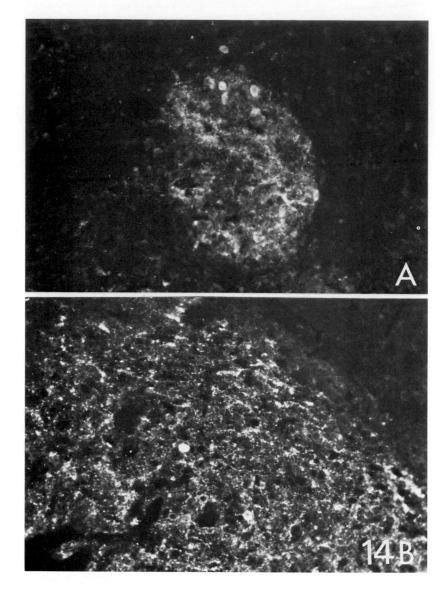

FIG. 14. Ontogeny of immunohistochemically stained leucine-enkephalin-positive structures in the amygdaloid complex. Frontal sections. **A:** postnatal day 5. **B:** Postnatal day 60. ×230.

In the amygdaloid complex, CCK-8-positive neurons are mainly located in the alp and ala, and partly in the pac and abl (Fig. 2). In addition, a few CCK-8 cells are spread throughout the amygdaloid complex. It should be noted that numerous CCK-8 cells are seen in the piriform cortex (see Fig. 2) (J. G. Parnavelas and J. K. McDonald, *this volume*). A significant number of CCK-8 fibers are found in the ventral parts of the ac and alp, and some in the am, abm, abl, and ala (Fig. 2). Scat-tered CCK-8 terminals are seen in the neuropile among the amygdaloid subdivisions (Fig. 2).

Fiber connections.

Recent immunohistochemical studies combined with retrograde tracer techniques have suggested that a CCK-like peptide is localized in the dopamine neurons located in the ventral tegmental area and projecting to limbic area (46). As it is well established that these mesencephalic dopamine neurons project to the amygdaloid complex, particularly ac, it is probable that some of the CCK terminals located in the ac may be provided by the axons of the mesencephalic dopamine/CCK containing neurons.

Ontogeny.

No systematic analysis of the ontogeny of CCK neuronal system in the amygdala has been reported. However, our recent results have shown that CCK-containing structures can be identified in very young rats, suggesting that initial differentiation of the CCK-8 neuron system might occur during the fetal period, as is the case for other peptide systems in the amygdala.

Vasoactive Intestinal Polypeptide

Distribution.

Vasoactive intestinal polypeptide (VIP) is a 28-amino-acid peptide isolated from porcine duodenum by Mutt and Said (84). By means of radioimmunoassay and immunohistochemistry, a wide but uneven distribution of VIP in the CNS has been reported (32,76,121). It has been shown that cerebral cortex contains numerous VIP neurons (J. G. Parnavelas and J. K. McDonald, *this volume*).

In the amygdaloid complex, a significant number of VIP neurons are situated in the am, pac, alp, and ala, and a few cells in the abm and ac (Fig. 2). Moreover, numerous VIP cells are found in the piriform cortex (Fig. 2). A very high density of VIP fibers is found in the ac, whereas the other subdivisions of the amygdaloid complex contain only a low density of VIP fibers (Fig. 2) (102,103).

Fiber connections.

An amygdalofugal VIP tract was reported by Roberts et al. (102,103). They have suggested that VIP neurons located in the amygdaloid complex project through the ST to innervate the bst, preoptic area, and anterior hypothalamic area. In addition, the same authors have suggested a number of intraamygdaloid VIP connections, although direct evidence for these pathways is lacking.

Ontogeny and phylogeny.

In 1979, Emson et al. (28) reported the ontogeny of VIP neuron systems of the rat brain and peripheral system using immunohistochemistry and radioimmunoassay. According to these authors, VIP-containing neuronal systems appear postnatally in the CNS. They suggested that VIP might form a chemical marker for studying the maturation of

cerebral cortical neurons. In reasonable agreement with this study, a subsequent radioimmunoassay study also confirmed this finding (79). Previous studies have not discussed the ontogeny of the VIP neurons in the amygdaloid complex. However, it is probable that the amygdaloid VIP neuron system also develops after birth. It should be stressed that the fact that the VIP neuron system appears postnatally and develops remarkably after birth is in contrast to the ontogenetic findings with the other peptides SOM, SP, NT, and ENK (43,52, 105,110,111,116,117), because these all appear during the fetal life of the rat and develop remarkably at the perinatal stage. This type of difference in ontogenetic history between neuropeptides suggests that they may have different functional roles in the organization of the brain.

No phylogenetic studies concerning the VIP neuron system have been reported.

Vasopressin and Oxytocin

Distribution.

The octapeptide neurohypophyseal hormones vasopressin (VP) and oxytocin (OXY), together with their carrier substances the neurophysins, are localized within the magnocellular neurons of the hypothalamus [for review, see Zimmerman (148) and A.-J. Silverman and G. E. Pickard, *this volume*]. However, recent studies have shown the existence of VP and OXY in extrahypothalamic areas (13).

In the amygdaloid complex, the presence of these peptides has been confirmed. In this area, no VP and OXY neurons are seen; however, a significant number of VP and OXY fibers are seen. They are located in the ac, am, al, abm, and abl. It is believed that most of these fibers contain VP (13).

Fiber connections.

Fiber pathways from magnocellular paraventricular and supraoptic nuclei, which contain VP and OXY, to the median eminence and neurohypophysis are well established (141,143,148). In addition, there is evidence that the parvocellular suprachiasmatic nucleus contains VP, and a VP-containing projection from this nucleus to the septal area has been proposed, although direct evidence is lacking (23).

With respect to the origins and pathways of VP and OXY terminals located in the amygdaloid complex, from observations of serial sections, it has been suggested that these fibers originate from hypothalamic VP- and OXY-containing neurons and reach the amygdaloid area through the ST. In support of this suggestion, the ST has been shown to contain VP and OXY fibers (13). In addition to the tentative VP and OXY pathway from the hypothalamus to the amygdaloid complex mentioned above, it is likely that some of these fibers reach the amygdaloid area by traveling through the so-called ventral amygdalofugal pathway, because some of the VP and OXY fibers are also seen in this area.

Ontogeny and phylogeny.

No systematic ontogenetic and phylogenetic analyses concerning the development of the amygdaloid VP and OXY have been reported. However, several authors have examined the ontogeny of VP and OXY in the hypothalamus (23,60). They report that in the rat, VP and OXY neuron systems first appear after birth and develop markedly postnatally. Thus, it is probable that VP and OXY fibers in the amygdaloid complex appear after birth. In this regard, the ontogeny of VP and OXY neuronal system is very similar to that of VIP but is in contrast to SOM, SP, NT, and ENK (see above).

Luteinizing Hormone-Releasing Hormone

Distribution.

Luteinizing hormone-releasing hormone (LHRH) is a decapeptide that was originally characterized by Amoss et al. (1) and Sétéró et al. (113). Subsequently, numerous reports dealing with the distribution and fiber connections of the LHRH-containing neurons appeared, showing that the hypothalamic area and preoptic area are very rich in LHRH. In addition, the existence of LHRH-containing structures was reported in extrahypothalamic areas (5). In the amygdaloid complex, although no LHRH neurons are seen, sparse LHRH fibers are found, particularly in the

Fiber connections.

The hypothalamic LHRH neuron system has been investigated by many authors (4,5,44,84, 112,120). However, the origins and pathways of the extrahypothalamic LHRH are not completely known, although it is likely that these fibers originate from hypothalamic or preoptic LHRH neurons.

Ontogeny and phylogeny.

Systematic analysis of ontogeny and phylogeny of LHRH in the amygdaloid complex has not been carried out.

Angiotensin

Distribution.

Three types of angiotensin (ANG) have been characterized: ANG I, a decapeptide; ANG II, an octapeptide; and ANG III, a heptapeptide (26,120). Recent radioimmunoassay and immunohistochemical studies have revealed the existence of trace amounts of ANG in the central nervous system, particularly concentrated in the hypothalamus (47). Furthermore, the existence of ANG II immunoreactivity in extrahypothalamic area has been demonstrated (38,99).

According to these studies, ANG II fibers were located in the amygdaloid complex, but no ANG II neurons were found in this region. Furthermore, it was claimed that the spontaneously hypertensive rat apparently contains more ANG II fibers than normal rats (99).

Fiber connections.

The origins and connections of the extrahypothalamic ANG neuronal systems are unknown.

Ontogeny and phylogeny.

No findings concerning the ontogeny and phylogeny of ANG neuronal systems have been presented.

Adrenocorticotropin

Distribution.

Recent radioimmunoassay and immunohistochemical studies have shown the existence of ACTH in the CNS (57,66,97). The ACTH cells are mainly located in the basal hypothalamic area, and no ACTH cells have been detected in other brain regions (57,66,97).

In the amygdaloid complex, previous reports dealing with the distribution of ACTH have shown the existence of numerous ACTH fibers in the amygdaloid complex (57,66,97). The detailed distribution of ACTH fibers in the amygdaloid complex has not been described, although it is clear that a dense ACTH fiber plexus is located in the am (57).

Fiber connections.

The exact origins and pathways of the amygdaloid ACTH fibers are unknown. However, Joseph (57) has supposed that ACTH fibers originate from ACTH neurons located in the hypothalamus and reach the amygdaloid complex through two separate pathways: one pathway running in a ventrolateral direction from the medial hypothalamus through the medial forebrain bundle to project to the anterior part of the amygdaloid complex (57) and the other pathway originating in the ventral hypothalamus and taking a direct horizontal course dorsally along the optic tract to enter the posterior amygdaloid complex (57). Although they denied the existence of an amygdalopetal ACTH tract through the ST, it seems that this possibility cannot be excluded because, as was shown in this study, the ST, which connects hypothalamus and amygdaloid complex, also contains ACTH fibers. In order to explore the fiber pathways of ACTH neuron system further, it will be important to combine both surgical lesions and immunohistochemical procedures.

Ontogeny and phylogeny.

No information is available on this subject to date.

Amino Acids

Gamma-Aminobutyric Acid

Distribution.

The precise regional distribution of the GABA-containing neuronal systems has been investigated by means of immunohistochemistry with the help of antibodies to glutamic acid decarboxylase (GAD) (98).

A recent immunohistochemical study has shown the existence of GABA terminals in the amygdaloid complex (98), although a detailed regional distribution of GABA terminals in this region was not described. The researchers, however, failed to demonstrate GABA neurons in the amygdaloid complex. In contrast to these observations, Le Gal La Salle et al. (74) suggested the existence of GABA neurons in the amygdaloid complex.

Fiber connections.

There is good evidence for a nigrothalamic GABA-containing pathway (78), a strionigral GABA pathway (63), and a Purkinje GABA pathway (89). In 1978, Le Gal La Salle et al. reported on the basis of lesion studies that there was an amygdalofugal GABA pathway that terminated in the bst. The evidence for this pathway came from lesions of the ST which resulted in a marked reduction of GAD activity in the bst. Furthermore they suggested the presence of an amygdalopetal GABA neuronal system projecting to the ac, because destruction of the ST also caused a slight decrease of GAD activity in the ac (74).

Other Amino Acids

The presence of aspartic acid, glycine, glutamate, glutamic acid, and taurine in the amygdaloid complex has been reported (21,24). Among these, it should be noted that a very high content of glutamic acid is found in the amygdaloid complex, particularly in the ac.

Little is known about the projections of these putative amino-acid-containing neuronal systems.

Acetylcholine

Distribution

Many authors have reported (for reviews, see refs. 2,8,56) the mapping of acetylcholinesterase (AChE)-positive neuronal systems. In the amygdaloid complex, intensely stained cholinesterase-positive cell bodies could not be demonstrated. Small intensely labeled AChE islands in the amygdaloid complex were identified as massae intercalatae. In the al, abl, and alp, strong AChE activity was found, whereas in the other subdivisions, only faint activity was detected (see Fig. 3). No AChE-positive cells were observed. In agreement with the previous studies, recent immunohistochemical studies with the help of the antibody to choline acetyltransferase (ChAT) have also showed a dense fiber plexus in the al and abl, and no cholinergic neurons were seen in the amygdaloid complex (64).

Fiber Connections

Ben-Ari et al. suggested that acetylcholine (ACh) terminals in the amygdaloid complex reach the amygdaloid complex via the ventral amygdalofugal pathway (8).

Monoamines

Catecholamines

Distribution.

The regional distribution of catecholamines (CA) in the CNS has been studied by means of the Falck–Hillarp histofluorescence method and its recent modifications (20,39,56).

Although the amygdaloid complex contains no CA neurons, it does contain numerous CA terminals (7). They are particularly concentrated in the ac, and the other subdivisions of amygdala are characterized by a low density of CA terminals.

Fiber connections.

Fallon et al. (33) have suggested that norepinephrine (NE) terminals in the amygdaloid complex originate from the locus ceruleus, since destruction of this nucleus resulted in a marked reduction of NE-type fibers in the amygdaloid complex. Subsequently, this suggestion has been supported by HRP and autoradiographic studies (93,138).

On the other hand, the dopamine (DA) located in the amygdaloid nucleus is provided by axons of DA neurons situated in the ventral tegmental area (34,46,138). It should be noted that, as discussed earlier, these DA-containing neurons are also supposed to contain a CCK-like peptide.

Ontogeny and phylogeny.

It has been reported that the DA fluorescence appeared on gestational day 13 and NE on gestational day 14 (90,124,125), although no systematic analysis of the ontogeny of CA neuron system in the amygdala has been reported. A recent immunohistochemical study using an antibody to tyrosine hydroxylase has reported the existence of CA fibers in the developing amygdaloid complex of the fetus (124).

The CA neuron system has been investigated phylogenetically, and a dense fiber plexus of CA terminals is seen in the amygdaloid complex of the lower vertebrates (95,147). It should be stressed that fiber connections of the CA neuron system in this area of the lower vertebrate are very different from those of the higher vertebrates (birds and mammals), because in the lower vertebrates, such as frogs, CA terminals in the amygdaloid complex originate from forebrain or diencephalic CA neurons, whereas those of the mammals originate from mesencephalic and rhombencephalic CA neurons (133).

Serotonin

Distribution.

Although the mapping of serotonin (5-HT) terminals in the CNS has been performed by histofluorescence method (20), the comprehensive mapping of the 5-HT neuron system is very difficult because of the low sensitivity of the histofluorescence method (see Fig. 3). However, recently Steinbusch has succeeded in producing an antiserum specific to 5-HT and has reported the detailed mapping of 5-HT-containing neuronal sys-

tems in the brain (126). In the amygdaloid complex, a very high density of 5-HT terminals is seen in the nucleus amygdaloideus basalis, al, and am.

Fiber connections.

It has previously been shown by histofluoroescence, HRP, autoradiographic, and biochemical techniques that the 5-HT terminals in the amygdaloid complex originate from the midbrain raphe nuclei, particularly from nucleus raphe dorsalis (3,27,82).

Ontogeny and phylogeny.

Olson and Seiger (90) have reported that 5-HT neurons first appear at gestational day 12 or 13. Thus, it is probable that 5-HT terminals located in the amygdaloid complex first appear during the fetal period.

It is also well known that the 5-HT neuron system is phylogenetically ancient (95,147). As is the case for the catecholamines, fiber connections of 5-HT neuron system are very different between lower vertebrates (amphibia and teleost) and higher vertebrates (bird and mammal) (133).

Histamine

The existence of histamine in the CNS has been shown biochemically. However, no precise information is available as to the regional distribution of histamine. Previously, Ben-Ari et al. have suggested the presence of an amygdalopetal histaminergic pathway projecting through the ST (6).

COMMENTS

The results briefly summarized in this chapter show that the amygdaloid complex is very rich in neuropeptides and other putative transmitters. Recently, Roberts et al. have also reported the distribution of several neuropeptides in the amygdaloid complex (104).

Amygdalofugal Peptidergic Pathways

As mentioned above, the amygdaloid complex contains many peptide-containing neurons including those containing SOM, SP, NT, ENK, CCK, and VIP (Fig. 15). Recent experimental immunohistochemical studies have clearly demonstrated that the axons from SOM, SP, NT, ENK, and VIP neurons reach the bst or hypothalamic area through the ST. It is well known that an amygdalohypothalamic connection may be involved in the

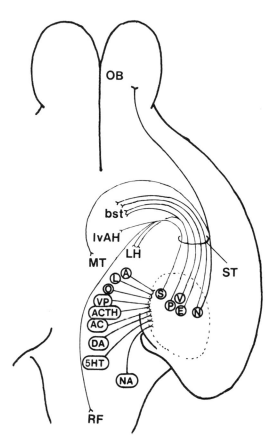

FIG. 15. Schematic drawing showing the amygdalofugal peptidergic and amygdalopetal peptidergic, monoaminergic, and cholinergic systems in the rat. Note that amygdalofugal peptidergic fibers except for amygdalo–olfactory bulb (OB) and amygdalo–medial thalamic (MT) NT tracts mostly leave the amygdaloid complex through the stria terminalis (ST).

Abbreviations: A, angiotensin; AC, acetylcholine; ACTH, adrenocorticotropin; bst, bed nucleus of stria terminalis; DA, dopamine; E, enkephalin; L, luteinizing hormone-releasing hormone; LH, lateral hypothalamus; lvAH, lateroventral part of the anterior hypothalamic nucleus; N, neurotensin; NA, norepinephrine; O, oxytocin; OB, olfactory bulb; P, substance P; RF, reticular formation; S, somatostatin; ST, stria terminalis; V, vasoactive intestinal polypeptide; VP, vasopressin; 5-HT, serotonin.

regulation of autonomic, endocrine, and behavioral functions. Accordingly, these amygdalofugal peptidergic systems, which project to bst or hypothalamic area through ST, may play some role in the regulation of these functions. In the case of SOM, the fibers arising from the amygdaloid complex pass through the ST to reach various areas of the reticular formation such as the hypoglossal nuclei and facial nucleus. These observations suggest that

SOM neurons located in the amygdaloid complex may also be concerned with various functions of the reticular formation such as analgesia, respiration, sleep, locomotion, and branchio- and somatomotor functions. Furthermore, the additional projections from NT-containing neurons located in the amygdaloid complex to the anterior olfactory nucleus, diagonal band, and medial thalamic nucleus suggest that these amygdaloid NT neurons may also influence olfactory or prefrontal cortex functions.

Amygdalopetal Peptidergic Pathways

Recent immunohistochemical studies have shown that the amygdaloid complex receives many peptidergic afferents such as VP, OXY, LHRH, and ACTH, which probably originate from hypothalamic areas in addition to the well-known monoaminergic afferents from the lower brainstem (Fig. 15). As to the functional roles of extrahypothalamic VP and OXY, physiological roles related to water balance, milk ejection, and avoidance behavior have been proposed, but their exact physiological functions are unknown.

Intraamygdaloid Peptidergic Connections

Experimental results obtained from our laboratory have shown that SOM, SP, and NT fibers located in the amygdaloid complex at least partly originate from intrinsic peptidergic neurons, because a significant number of these fibers remain intact after isolation of the amygdaloid complex (including the anterior amygdaloid area and piriform cortex). Thus, it is probable that these intrinsic peptidergic pathways may be involved in numerous behavioral functions ascribed to the amygdaloid complex.

Fine Structure of the Peptidergic Fibers in the Amygdaloid Complex

The fine structure of peptidergic terminals and neurons has recently been demonstrated in various regions of the CNS. Unfortunately, however, no systematic study on the fine structure of the peptidergic fibers in the amygdaloid complex has been attempted. In other brain regions, it is generally agreed that neuropeptides are localized at least partly in large-cored vesicles (131). However, there is evidence that neuropeptides are also localized in the small-cored vesicles, although electron-dense precipitates were observed on the membranes of these small vesicles. It should be noted that peptidergic fibers often show an asymmetrical synapse (possibly excitatory), whereas noradrenergic terminals, for example, seldom show this type of synapse (131).

CONCLUSION

It is well established that the amygdaloid complex is involved in a variety of physiological functions, and this complexity is mirrored by the heterogeneity and complexity of its neuronal populations. Thus, in order to explore amygdaloid function, it will be necessary to analyze this heterogeneous population of neurons and to arrange them in groups based on homology. The experimental histochemical approach of characterizing neurons by their content will be useful for all who are interested in this type of homology.

ACKNOWLEDGMENTS

We are grateful to the following scientists for the kind gift of antisera used in these studies: Dr. N. Yanaihara (VIP), Dr. T. Hamaoka (CCK), Dr. O. Tanizawa (oxytocin), and Dr. T. Aono (LHRH).

REFERENCES

1. Amoss, M., Burgus, R., Blackwell, R., Vale, W., Fellows, K., and Guillemin, R. (1971): Purification, amino acid composition and N-terminus of the hypothalamic luteinizing hormone releasing factor (LRF) of ovine origin. *Biochem. Biophys. Res. Commun.*, 44:205–210.
2. Arimatsu, Y., Seto, A., and Amano, T. (1981): An atlas of α-bungarotoxin binding sites and structures containing acetylcholinesterase in the mouse central nervous system. *J. Comp. Neurol.*, 198:603–631.
3. Azmitia, E. C., and Segal, M. (1978): An autoradiographic analysis of the different ascending projections of the dorsal and median raphe nuclei in the rat. *J. Comp. Neurol.*, 179:641–668.
4. Barry, J., Dubois, M. P., and Carette, B. (1974): Immunofluorescence study of the preoptic–infundibular LRF neurosecretory pathway in the normal, castrated or testosterone-treated male guinea pig. *Endocrinology*, 95:1416–1423.
5. Barry, J., Dubois, M. P., and Poulain, P. (1973): LRF producing cells of the mammalian hypothalamus. A fluorescent antibody study. *Z. Zellforsch.*, 146:351–366.
6. Ben-Ari, Y., Le Gal La Salle, G., Barbin, G., Schwartz, J. C., and Garbarg, M. (1978): Histamine synthesizing afferents within the amygdaloid complex and bed nucleus of stria terminalis of the rat. *Brain Res.*, 138:285–294.
7. Ben-Ari, Y., Zigmond, R. E., and Moore, K. E. (1975): Regional distribution of tyrosine hydroxyl-

8. ase, norepinephrine and dopamine within the amygdaloid complex of the rat. *Brain Res.*, 87:96–101.
8. Ben-Ari, Y., Zigmont, R. E., Shute, C., and Lewis, P. R. (1977): Regional distribution of choline acetyltransferase and acetylcholinesterase within the amygdaloid complex and stria terminalis system. *Brain Res.*, 120:435–445.
9. Bennett-Clarke, C., Romagnano, M. A., and Joseph, S. A. (1980): Distribution of somatostatin in the rat brain: Telencephalon and diencephalon. *Brain Res.*, 188:473–486.
10. Brodal, A. (1947): The amygdaloid nucleus in the rat. *J. Comp. Neurol.*, 87:1–16.
11. Brownstein, M., Arimura, A., Sato, H., Schally, A. V., and Kizer, J. S. (1975): The regional distribution of somatostatin in the rat brain. *Endocrinology*, 96:1456–1461.
12. Brownstein, M. J., Mroz, E. A., Kizer, J. S., Palkovits, M., and Leeman, S. E. (1976): Regional distribution of substance P in the brain of the rat. *Brain Res.*, 116:299–305.
13. Buijs, R. M. (1978): Intra- and extrahypothalamic vasopressin and oxytocin pathway in the rat. *Cell Tissue Res.*, 192:423–435.
14. Carraway, R., and Leeman, S. E. (1973): The isolation of a new hypotensive peptide neurotensin from bovine hypothalami. *J. Biol. Chem.*, 248:6454–6861.
15. Chang, M. M., Leeman, S. E., and Niall, H. D. (1971): Amino acid sequence of substance P. *Nature (New Biol.)*, 232:86–87.
16. Coons, A. H. (1958): Fluorescent antibody methods. In: *General Cytochemical Methods*, edited by J. F. Danielli, pp. 399–422. Academic Press, New York.
17. Cowan, W. M., Raisman, G., and Powell, T. P. S. (1965): The connections of the amygdala. *J. Neurol. Neurosurg. Psychiatry*, 28:137–151.
18. Crosby, S. J., and Humphrey, T. (1941): Studies on the vertebrate telencephalon. II. The nuclear pattern of the anterior olfactory nucleus, tuberculum olfactorium and the amygdaloid complex in adult man. *J. Comp. Neurol.*, 74:309–352.
19. Cuello, A. C., and Paxinos, G. (1978): Evidence for a long leu-enkephalin striopallidal pathway in the rat brain. *Nature*, 271:178–180.
20. Dahlström, A., and Fuxe, K. (1964): Evidence for existence of monoamine containing neurons in the central nervous system. *Acta Physiol. Scand.* [*Suppl.*], 232:1–55.
21. Defeudis, F. V., and Mandel, P. (1981): *Amino Acid Neurotransmitters*. Raven Press, New York.
22. De Lanerolle, N. C., Elde, R. P., Sparber, S. B., and Frich, M. (1980): Distribution of methionine-enkephalin immunoreactivity in the chick brain: An immunohistochemical study. *J. Comp. Neurol.*, 199:513–532.
23. De Vries, G. D., Buijs, R. M., and Swaab, D. K. (1981): Ontogeny of the vasopressinergic neurons and their extrahypothalamic projections in the rat brain. Presence of a sex difference in lateral septum. *Brain Res.*, 218:67–78.
24. DiChiara, G., and Gessa, G. L. (1981): *Glutamate as a Neurotransmitter*. Raven Press, New York.

25. Dockray, G. J. (1976): Immunohistochemical evidence of cholecystokinin-like peptides in the brain. *Nature,* 264:568–570.
26. Elliot, D. F., and Peart, W. S. (1956): Amino acid sequence in a hypertensin. *Nature,* 177:527–528.
27. Emson, P. C., Björklund, A., Lindvall, O., and Paxinos, G. (1979): Contributions of different afferent pathways to the catecholamine and 5-hydroxytryptamine-innervation of the amygdala: A neurochemical and histochemical study. *Neuroscience,* 4:1347–1357.
28. Emson, P. C., Gilbert, R. F. T., Loren, I., Fahrenkrug, J., Sunder, F., and Schaffalitzky de Muckadell, O. B. (1979): Development of vasoactive intestinal polypeptide (VIP) containing neurons in the rat brain. *Brain Res.,* 177:437–444.
29. Emson, P. C., Jessel, T., Paxinos, G., and Cuello, A. C. (1978): Substance P in the amygdaloid complex, bed nucleus and stria terminalis of the rat brain. *Brain Res.,* 149:97–105.
30. Epelbaum, J., Aranciba, L. T., Kordon, C., Ottersen, O. P., and Ben-Ari, Y. (1979): Regional distribution of somatostatin within the amygdaloid complex of the rat brain. *Brain Res.,* 174:172–174.
31. Euler, U. S. von, and Gaddum, J. H. (1931): An identified depressor substance in certain tissue extracts. *J. Physiol. (Lond.),* 72:74–87.
32. Fahrenkrug, J., and Schaffalitzky de Muckadell, O. B. (1978): Distribution of vasoactive intestinal polypeptide (VIP) in the porcine central nervous system. *J. Neurochem.,* 31:1445–1459.
33. Fallon, J. H., Koziell, D. A., and Moore, R. Y. (1978): Catecholamine innervation of the basal forebrain. II. Amygdala, suprarhinal cortex and entorhinal cortex. *J. Comp. Neurol.,* 180:509–532.
34. Fallon, J. H., and Moore, R. Y. (1978): Catecholamine innervation of the basal forebrain. IV. Topology of the dopamine projection to the basal forebrain and neostriatum. *J. Comp. Neurol.,* 180:545–580.
35. Finley, J. C. W., Maderdrut, J. L., and Petrusz, P. (1981): The immunocytochemical localization of enkephalin in the central nervous system of the rat. *J. Comp. Neurol.,* 198:541–565.
36. Fox, C. A. (1940): Certain basal telencephalic centers in the cat. *J. Comp. Neurol.,* 72:1–62.
37. Fox, C. A. (1943): The stria terminalis, longitudinal association bundle and precommissural fornix fibers in the cat. *J. Comp. Neurol.,* 79:277–291.
38. Fuxe, K., Ganten, D., Hökfelt, T., and Bolme, P. (1976): Immunohistochemical evidence for the existence of angiotensin II-containing nerve terminals in the brain and spinal cord in the rat. *Neurosci. Lett.,* 2:229–234.
39. Fuxe, K., Hökfelt, T., Johansson, O., Jonsson, G., Lidbrink, P., and Ljungdahl, A. (1974): The origin of the dopamine nerve terminals in the limbic and frontal cortex. Evidence for mesocortical dopamine neurons. *Brain Res.,* 82:349–355.
40. Gloor, P. (1955): Electrophysiological studies on the connections of the amygdaloid nucleus in the cat. *Electroencephalogr. Clin. Neurophysiol.,* 7:243–264.
41. Gloor, P. (1960): Amygdala. In: *Handbook of Physiology,* Sect. 1, Vol. 2, edited by J. Field, H. W. Magoun, and V. E. Hall, pp. 1395–1420. American Physiological Society, Washington.
42. Gurdjian, E. A. (1928): The corpus striatum of the rat. Studies on the brain of the rat, No. 3. *J. Comp. Neurol.,* 45:249–281.
43. Hara, Y., Shiosaka, S., Senba, E., Sakanaka, M., Inagaki, S., Takagi, H., Kawai, Y., Takatsuki, K., Matsuzaki, T., and Tohyama, M. (1982): Ontogeny of the neurotensin-containing neuron system of the rat: Immunohistochemical analysis. I. Forebrain and diencephalon. *J. Comp. Neurol.,* 208:177–195.
44. Hoffman, G. E., Knigge, K. M., Moynian, J. A., Melnyk, V., and Arimura, A. (1978): Neuronal fields containing luteinizing hormone releasing hormone (LHRH) in mouse brain. *Neuroscience,* 3:219–231.
45. Hökfelt, T., Ljungdahl, A., Terenius, L., Elde, R., and Nilsson, G. (1977): Immunohistochemical analysis of peptide pathways possibly relate to pain and analgesia: Enkephalin and substance P. *Proc. Natl. Acad. Sci. U.S.A.,* 74:3081–3085.
46. Hökfelt, T., Skirboll, L., Rehfeld, J. F., Goldstein, M., Markey, K., and Dann, O. (1980): A subpopulation of mesencephalic dopamine neurons projecting to limbic areas contains a cholecystokinin-like peptide: Evidence from immunohistochemistry combined with retrograde tracing. *Neuroscience,* 5:2093–2124.
47. Hökfelt, T., Elde, R., Fuxe, K., Johansson, D., Ljungdahl, A., Goldstein, M., Lufet, R., Efendic, S., Nilsson, G., Terenius, L., Ganten, D., Jeffecoate, S. L., Rehfeld, J., Said, S., Perez de la Mola, M., Possani, R., Tapia, R., Teran, L., and Palacius, R. (1978): Aminergic and peptidergic pathways in the nervous system with special reference to the hypothalamus. In: *The Hypothalamus,* edited by S. Reichlin, R. J. Baldessarini, and J. B. Martin, pp. 69–136. Raven Press, New York.
48. Hughes, J., Smith, T. W., Kosterlitz, H. W., Fothergill, L., Morgan, B. A., and Morrith, H. R. (1975): Identification of two related pentapeptides from the brain with potent opiate agonist activity. *Nature,* 258:577–579.
49. Inagaki, S., Hara, Y., Shinoda, K., Shiosaka, S., Senba, E., Kawai, Y., Sakanaka, M., Takatsuki, K., Tohyama, M., and Shiotani, Y. (1983): Experimental and immunohistochemical study on neurotensin-containing neuron system in the rat. Limbic system I. *Neurosci. Lett. (in press).*
50. Inagaki, S., Kawai, Y., Shiosaka, S., Matsuzaki, T., and Tohyama, M. (1983): The long descending somatostatin (SRIF) pathways from amygdaloid complex to the lower brain stem in the rat. *J. Hirnforsch. (in press).*
51. Inagaki, S., Sakanaka, M., Shiosaka, S., Senba, E., Takatsuki, K., Kawai, Y., Matsuzaki, T., Iida, H., Hara, Y., and Tohyama, M. (1982): Experimental and immunohistochemical studies on the cerebellar substance P of the rat: Localization, postnatal ontogeny and ways of entry to the cerebellum. *Neuroscience,* 7:639–645.
52. Inagaki, S., Sakanaka, M., Shiosaka, S., Senba, E., Takatsuki, K., Takagi, H., Kawai, Y., Minagawa,

H., and Tohyama, M. (1982): Ontogeny of sub-stance P-containing neuron system of the rat: Im-munohistochemical analysis-I. Forebrain and upper brain stem. *Neuroscience*, 7:251–277.

53. Inagaki, S., Senba, E., Shiosaka, S., Takagi, H., Kawai, Y., Takatsuki, K., Sakanaka, M., Matsu-zaki, T., and Tohyama, M. (1981): Regional distri-bution of substance P in the frog brain. *J. Comp. Neurol.*, 201:243–254.

54. Inagaki, S., Shiosaka, S., Takatsuki, K., Iida, H., Sakanaka, M., Senba, E., Hara, Y., Matsuzaki, T., Kawai, Y., and Tohyama, M. (1982): Ontogeny of somatostatin-containing neuron system of the rat cerebellum including its fiber connections: An ex-perimental and immunohistochemical analysis. *Dev. Brain Res.*, 3:509–527.

55. Innis, R. B., Correa, F. M. A., Uhl, G. R., Schnei-der, B., and Snyder, S. H. (1979): Cholecystokinin octapeptide-like immunoreactivity: Histochemical localization in rat brain. *Proc. Natl. Acad. Sci. U.S.A.*, 76:521–525.

56. Jacobowitz, D. M., and Palkovits, M. (1974): To-pographic atlas of catecholamine and acetylcho-linesterase-containing neurons in the rat brain. I. Forebrain (telencephalon, diencephalon). *J. Comp. Neurol.*, 157:12–28.

57. Joseph, S. A. (1980): Immunoreactive adrenocorti-cotropin in rat brain: A neuroanatomical study using antiserum generated against synthetic ACTH(1–39). *Am J. Anat.*, 158:533–548.

58. Kaada, B. R. (1972): Stimulation and regional ablation of the amygdaloid complex with reference to functional representations. In: *The Neurology of the Amygdala*, edited by B. E. Eleftheriou, pp. 205–281. Plenum Press, New York.

59. Kanazawa, I., Emson, P. C., and Cuello, A. C. (1977): Evidence for the existence of substance P-containing fibers in striatonigral and pallido–nigral pathways in rat brain. *Brain Res.*, 119:447–453.

60. Khachaturian, H., and Sladek, J. R. (1980): Si-multaneous monoamine histofluorescence and neu-ropeptide immunocytochemistry. III. Ontogeny of catecholamine varicosities and neurophysin neurons in the rat supraoptic and paraventricular nuclei. *Peptide*, 1:77–95.

61. Kevetter, G. A., and Winans, S. S. (1981): Connec-tions of the cortico-medial amygdala in the golden hamster. I. Efferents of the "vomeronasal amyg-dala." *J. Comp. Neurol.*, 197:81–98.

62. Kevetter, G. A., and Winans, S. S. (1981): Connec-tions of the cortico-medial amygdala in the golden hamster. II. Efferents of the "olfactory amygdala." *J. Comp. Neurol.*, 197:99–111.

63. Kim, J. S., Bak, I. J., Hassler, R., and Okada, Y. (1971): Role of aminobutyric acid (GABA) in the extrapyramidal motor system. 2. Some evidence for the existence of a type of GABA-rich strionigral neurons. *Exp. Brain Res.*, 14:94–104.

64. Kimura, H., Mcgeer, P. L., Peng, J. H., and Mcgeer, E. G. (1981): The central cholinergic sys-tem studied by cholin acetyltransferase immuno-histochemistry in the cat. *J. Comp. Neurol.*, 200:151–202.

65. Kobayashi, R., Nrown, M., and Vale, W. (1977):

Regional distribution of neurotensin and somato-statin in the rat. *Brain Res.*, 126:584–588.

66. Knigge, K. M., Joseph, S. H., and Nocton, J. (1981): Topography of the ACTH-immunoreactive neurons in the basal hypothalamus of the rat brain. *Brain Res.*, 216:333–341.

67. Krettek, J. E., and Price, J. L. (1977): Projections from the amygdaloid complex to the cerebral cortex and thalamus in the rat and cat. *J. Comp. Neurol.*, 172:687–722.

68. Krettek, J. E., and Price, J. L. (1977): Projections from the amygdaloid complex and adjacent olfac-tory structures to the entorhinal cortex and to the subiculum in the rat and cat. *J. Comp. Neurol.*, 172:723–752.

69. Krettek, J. E., and Price, J. L. (1978): Amygdaloid projections to subcortical structures within the basal forebrain and brainstem in the rat and cat. *J. Comp. Neurol.*, 178:225–254.

70. Krettek, J. E., and Price, J. L. (1978): A description of the amygdaloid complex in the rat and cat, with observations on intra-amygdaloid axonal connec-tions. *J. Comp. Neurol.*, 178:255–280.

71. Krieger, M. S., Conrad, L. C., and Pfaff, D. W. (1979): An autoradiographic study of the efferent connections of the ventromedial nucleus of the hy-pothalamus. *J. Comp. Neurol.*, 183:785–816.

72. Lammer, H. J. (1972): The neural connections of amygdaloid complex in mammals. In: *The Neuro-biology of the Amygdala*, edited by B. E. Eleft-herriou, pp. 123–144. Plenum Press, New York.

73. Larsson, L.-I., and Rehfeld, J. F. (1979): Locali-zation and molecular heterogeneity of cholecysto-kinin in the central and peripheral nervous system. *Brain Res.*, 165:201–218.

74. Le Gal La Salle, G., Paxinos, G., Emson, P., and Ben-Ari, Y. (1978): Neurochemical mapping of GABAergic systems in the amygdaloid complex and bed nucleus of the stria terminalis. *Brain Res.*, 155:397–403.

75. Ljungdahl, A. O., Hökfelt, T., and Nilsson, G. (1978): Distribution of substance P-like immuno-reactivity in the central nervous system of the rat. I. Cell bodies and nerve terminals. *Neuroscience*, 3:861–943.

76. Loren, I., Emson, P. C., Fahrenkrug, J., Björklund, A., Alumets, J., Håkanson, R., and Sundler, F. (1980): Distribution of vasoactive intestinal poly-peptide in the rat and mouse brain. *Neuroscience*, 5:1953–1976.

77. Luiten, P. G. M., and Room, P. (1980): Interrela-tions between lateral, dorsomedial, and ventrome-dial hypothalamic nuclei in the rat, an HRP study. *Brain Res.*, 190:321–332.

78. Macleod, N. K., James, T. A., Kilpatrick, I. C., and Starr, M. S. (1980): Evidence for a GABAergic ni-grothalamic pathways in the rat. II. Electrophysio-logical studies. *Exp. Brain Res.*, 40:55–61.

79. Maletti, M., Bessin, J., Bataille, D., Laburthe, M., and Rosselin, G. (1980): Ontogeny and immuno-reactive forms of vasoactive intestinal peptide (VIP) in rat brain. *Acta Endocrinol. (Kbh.)*, 93:479–487.

80. McBride, R. L., and Sutin, J. (1977): Amygdaloid

and pontine projections to the ventromedial nucleus of the hypothalamus. *J. Comp. Neurol.,* 174:377–396.

81. Minagawa, H., Shiosaka, S., Takatsuki, K., Hara, Y., Inagaki, S., Sakanaka, M., Takagi, H., Senba, E., Matsuzaki, T., Kawai, Y., and Tohyama, M. (1983): Ontogeny of neurotensin-containing neuron system of the rat: Immunohistochemical analysis. II. Lower brain stem *(in press).*

82. Moore, R. Y., Halaris, A. E., and Jones, B. (1978): Serotonin neurons of the midbrain raphe. Ascending projections. *J. Comp. Neurol.,* 180:417–438.

83. Mroz, E. A., Brownstein, M. J., and Leeman, S. E. (1976): Evidence for substance P in the habenulo–interpeduncular tract. *Brain Res.,* 113:597–599.

84. Mutt, V., and Said, S. I. (1974): Structure of the porcine vasoactive intestinal octapeptide. The amino-acid sequence. Use of kallikrein in its determination. *Eur. J. Biochem.,* 42:581–589.

85. Naik, D. V. (1975): Immunoreactive LH-RH neurons in the hypothalamus identified by light and fluorescent microscopy. *Cell Tissue Res.,* 157:423–436.

86. Naik, D. R., Sar, M., and Stumpf, W. E. (1981): Immunohistochemical localization of enkephalin in the central nervous system and pituitary of the lizard, *Anolis carolinensis. J. Comp. Neurol.,* 198:583–602.

87. Nauta, W. J. H. (1961): Fibre degeneration following lesions of the amygdaloid complex in the monkey. *J. Anat.,* 95:515–531.

88. Norgren, R. (1976): Taste pathways to hypothalamus and amygdala. *J. Comp. Neurol.,* 166:17–30.

89. Obata, K., Ito, M., Ochi, R., and Sato, M. (1967): Pharmacological properties of the postsynaptic inhibition by Purkinje cell axons and the action of α-aminobutyric acid on Deiters neurons. *Exp. Brain Res.,* 4:43–57.

90. Olson, L., and Seiger, A. (1972): Early prenatal ontogeny of central monoamine neurons in the rat: Fluorescence histochemical observations. *Z. Anat. Entwickl. Gesch.,* 137:301–316.

91. Otsuka, M., and Konishi, S. (1977): Electrophysiological and neurochemical evidence for substance P as a transmitter of primary sensory neurons. In: *Substance P,* edited by U. S. von Euler and B. Pernow, pp. 207–214. Raven Press, New York.

92. Ottersen, O. P. (1980): Afferent connections to the amygdaloid complex of the rat and cat. II. Afferents from the hypothalamus and basal telencephalon. *J. Comp. Neurol.,* 194:267–289.

93. Ottersen, O. P. (1981): Afferent connections to the amygdaloid complex of the rat with some observations in the cat. III. Afferents from the lower brain stem. *J. Comp. Neurol.,* 202:335–356.

94. Ottersen, O. P., and Ben-Ari, Y. (1979): Afferent connections to the amygdaloid complex of the rat and cat. I. Projections from the thalamus. *J. Comp. Neurol.,* 187:401–424.

95. Parent, A., Dube, L., Braford, M. R., Jr., and Northcutt, R. G. (1978): The organization of monoamine-containing neurons in the brain of the sunfish *(Lepomis gibbosus)* as revealed by fluorescence microscopy. *J. Comp. Neurol.,* 182:495–516.

96. Paxinos, G. P., Emson, P. C., and Coello, A. C. (1978): Some substance P projections in the rat central nervous system. *Neurosci. Lett.,* 7:127–131.

97. Pelletier, G., Leclerc, R., Saavedra, J. M., Brownstein, M. J., Vaudry, H., Ferland, L., and Labrie, F. (1980): Distribution of β-lipotropin (βLPH), adrenocorticotropin (ACTH) and α-melanocyte-stimulating hormone (αMSH) in the rat brain. I. Origin of the extrahypothalamic fibers. *Brain Res.,* 192:433–440.

98. Perez De La Mora, M., Possani, L. D., Tapia, R., Teran, L., Pracios, R., Fuxe, K., Hökfelt, T., and Ljungdahl, A. (1981): Demonstration of central γ-aminobutyrate-containing nerve terminals by means of antibodies against glutamate decarboxylase. *Neuroscience,* 6:875–895.

99. Phillip, M. I., Quinlan, J. T., and Weyhenmeyer, J. (1980): An angiotensin peptide in the brain. *Life Sci.,* 277:2589–2594.

100. Raisman, G. (1972): An experimental study of the projection of the amygdala to the accessory olfactory bulb and its relationship to the concept of a dual olfactory system. *Exp. Brain Res.,* 14:395–408.

101. Renaud, L. P., and Hopkins, D. A. (1977): Amygdala afferents from the mediodorsal hypothalamus: An electrophysiological and neuroanatomical study in the rat. *Brain Res.,* 121:201–213.

102. Roberts, G. W., Woodhams, P. L., Bryant, M. G., Crow, T. J., Bloom, S. R., and Polak, J. M. (1980): VIP in the rat brain: Evidence for a major pathway linking the amygdala and hypothalamus via the stria terminalis. *Histochemistry,* 65:103–119.

103. Roberts, G. W., Woodhams, P. L., Crow, T. J., and Polak, J. M. (1980): Loss of immunoreactive VIP in the bed nucleus following lesions of the stria terminalis. *Brain Res.,* 195:471–475.

104. Roberts, G. W., Woodhams, P. L., Polak, J. M., and Crow, T. J. (1982): Distribution of neuropeptides in the limbic system of the rat: The amygdaloid complex. *Neuroscience,* 7:99–131.

105. Sakanaka, M., Shiosaka, S., Inagaki, S., Takatsuki, K., Takagi, H., Senba, E., Kawai, Y., Matsuzaki, T., and Tohyama, M. (1982): Ontogeny of substance P-containing neuron system of the rat: Immunohistochemical analysis. II. Lower brain stem. *Neuroscience,* 7:1097–1126.

106. Sakanaka, M., Shiosaka, S., Takatsuki, K., Inagaki, S., Takagi, H., Senba, E., Kawai, Y., Hara, Y., Iida, H., Minagawa, H., Matsuzaki, T., and Tohyama, M. (1981): Evidence for the existence of a substance P-containing pathway from the nucleus laterodorsalis tegmenti (Castaldi) to the lateral septal area of the rat. *Brain Res.,* 230:351–355.

107. Sakanaka, M., Shiosaka, S., Takatsuki, K., Inagaki, S., Takagi, H., Senba, E., Kawai, Y., Matsuzaki, T., and Tohyama, M. (1981): Experimental immunohistochemical studies on the amygdalofugal peptidergic (substance P and somatostatin) fibers in the stria terminalis of the rat. *Brain Res.,* 221:231–242.

108. Saper, C. B., and Loewy, A. D. (1980): Efferent connections of the parabrachial nucleus in the rat. *Brain Res.,* 197:291–317.

109. Sar, M., Stumpf, W. E., Miller, R. J., Chung, K.-J., and Cuatrecasas, P. (1978): Immunohistochemical localization of enkephalin in rat brain and spinal cord. *J. Comp. Neurol.,* 182:17–38.

110. Schally, A. V., Arimura, A., Baba, Y., Nair, R. M. G., Matsuo, J., Redding, I. W., Debeljuk, L., and White, W. F. (1971): Isolation and properties of the FSH- and LH-releasing hormone. *Biochem. Biophys. Res. Commun.,* 43:393–399.

111. Senba, E., Shiosaka, S., Hara, Y., Inagaki, S., Kawai, Y., Takatsuki, K., Sakanaka, M., Takagi, H., and Tohyama, M. (1982): Ontogeny of leucine-enkephalin neuron system of the rat: Immunohistochemical analysis. II. Forebrain and upper brain stem. *J. Comp. Neurol.,* 204:211–224.

112. Senba, E., Shiosaka, S., Hara, Y., Inagaki, S., Kawai, Y., Takatsuki, K., Sakanaka, M., Iida, H., Takagi, H., Minagawa, H., and Tohyama, M. (1982): Ontogeny of leucine-enkephalin neuron system of the rat: Immunohistochemical analysis. I. Lower brain stem. *J. Comp. Neurol.,* 205:341–359.

113. Sétéró, G., Vigh, S., Schally, A. V., Arimura, A., and Flerko, B. (1976): Immunohistochemical study of the origin of LH-RH-containing nerve fibers in the rat hypothalamus. *Brain Res.,* 103:597–602.

114. Shiosaka, S., Takatsuki, K., Inagaki, S., Sakanaka, M., Takagi, H., Senba, E., Matsuzaki, T., and Tohyama, M. (1981): Topographic atlas of somatostatin-containing neuron system in the avian brain in relation to catecholamine-containing neuron system. II. Mesencephalon, rhombencephalon, and spinal cord. *J. Comp. Neurol.,* 202:115–124.

115. Shiosaka, S., Takatsuki, K., Sakanaka, M., Inagaki, S., Takagi, H., Senba, E., Kawai, Y., Minagawa, H., and Tohyama, M. (1981): New somatostatin-containing sites in the diencephalon of the neonatal rat. *Neurosci. Lett.,* 25:69–73.

116. Shiosaka, S., Takatsuki, K., Sakanaka, M., Inagaki, S., Takagi, H., Senba, E., Kawai, Y., and Tohyama, M. (1981): Ontogeny of the somatostatin neuron system in the rat central nervous system: Immunohistochemical observations. I. Lower brain stem. *J. Comp. Neurol.,* 203:173–188.

117. Shiosaka, S., Takatsuki, K., Sakanaka, M., Inagaki, S., Takagi, H., Senba, E., Kawai, Y., Iida, H., Minagawa, H., Hara, Y., Matsuzaki, T., and Tohyama, M. (1982): Ontogeny of somatostatin-containing neuron system of the rat: Immunohistochemical analysis. II. Forebrain and diencephalon. *J. Comp. Neurol.,* 204:211–224.

118. Shiosaka, S., Tohyama, M., Takagi, H., Takahashi, Y., Saito, Y., Sakumoto, T., Nakagawa, H., and Shimizu, N. (1980): Ascending and descending components of the medial forebrain bundle in the rat as demonstrated by a horseradish peroxidase-blue reaction. I. Forebrain and upper brain stem. *Exp. Brain Res.,* 39:377–388.

119. Siegel, A., Fukushima, T., Meibach, R., Burke, H., Edinger, H., and Weimer, S. (1977): The origin of afferent supply to the mediodorsal thalamic nucleus: Enhancement of HRP transport by selective lesions. *Brain Res.,* 135:11–23.

120. Silverman, A. J. (1976): Distribution of luteinizing hormone-releasing hormone (LH-RH) in the guinea pig brain. *Endocrinology,* 99:30–41.

121. Sims, K. B., Hoffman, D. L., Said, S. I., and Zimmerman E. A. (1980): Vasoactive intestinal polypeptide (VIP) in mouse and rat brain: An immunocytochemical study. *Brain Res.,* 186:165–183.

122. Skeggs, T. L., Jr., Marsh, W. J., Kaln, J. R., and Shumway, N. P. (1955): Amino acid composition and electrophoretic properties of hypertensin I. *J. Exp. Med.,* 102:435–440.

123. Snyder, S. H., Uhl, G. R., and Kuhar, M. J. (1978): Comparative features of enkephalin and neurotensin in the mammalian central nervous system. In: *Centrally Acting Peptides,* edited by J. Hughes, pp. 85–97. Macmillan, London.

124. Specht, L. A., Pickel, V. M., Joh, T. H., and Reis, D. A. (1981): Light-microscopic immunocytochemical localization of tyrosine hydroxylase in prenatal rat brain. I. Early ontogeny. *J. Comp. Neurol.,* 199:233–253.

125. Specht, L. A., Pickel, V. M., Joh, T. H., and Reis, D. J. (1981): Light-microscopic immunocytochemical localization of tyrosine hydroxylase in prenatal rat brain. II. Late ontogeny. *J. Comp. Neurol.,* 199:255–276.

126. Steinbusch, H. W. M. (1981): Distribution of serotonin-immunoactivity in the central nervous system of the rat. Cell bodies and terminals. *Neuroscience,* 6:557–618.

127. Takagi, H., Shiosaka, S., Sakanaka, M., Senba, E., Takatsuki, K., and Tohyama, M. (1981): Distribution of substance P in the fish (carp). *Acta Histochem. Cytochem.,* 14:69.

128. Takatsuki, K., Sakanaka, M., Shiosaka, S., Inagaki, S., Takagi, H., Senba, E., Hara, Y., Kawai, Y., Minagawa, H., Iida, H., and Tohyama, M. (1982): Pathways and terminal fields of the cochlearofugal somatostatin tract of very young rats. *Dev. Brain Res.,* 3:613–626.

129. Takatsuki, K., Shiosaka, S., Inagaki, S., Sakanaka, M., Takagi, H., Senba, E., Matsuzaki, T., and Tohyama, M. (1981): Topographic atlas of somatostatin-containing neuron system in the avian brain in relation to catecholamine-containing neuron system. I. Telencephalon and diencephalon. *J. Comp. Neurol.,* 202:103–114.

130. Takatsuki, K., Shiosaka, S., Sakanaka, M., Inagaki, S., Senba, E., Takagi, H., and Tohyama, M. (1981): Somatostatin in the auditory system of the rat. *Brain Res.,* 213:211–216.

131. Tohyama, M. (1983): Experimental morphological studies of somatostatinergic system. In: *Central Aminergic and Peptidergic System,* edited by Y. Sano. John Wiley & Sons, New York.

132. Tohyama, M., Shiosaka, S., Takagi, H., Inagaki, S., Takatsuki, K., Sakanaka, M., Senba, E., Kawai, Y., and Minagawa, H. (1981): Somatostatin in the carp gustatory system. *Neurosci. Lett.,* 24:233–236.

133. Tohyama, M., Yamamoto, K., Satoh, K., Sakumoto, T., and Shimizu, N. (1977): Catecholamine innervation of the forebrain in the bull frog, *Rana catesbiana. J. Hirnforsch.,* 18:223–228.

134. Uhl, G. R., Goodman, R. R., Kuhar, M. J., and Snyder, S. M. (1978): Enkephalin and neurotensin: Immunohistochemical localization and identification of amygdalofugal pathway. In: *Advances in Biochemical Psychopharmacology,* Vol. 18, edited by E. Costa and M. Trabucchi, pp. 71–87. Raven Press, New York.

135. Uhl, G. R., Goodman, R. R., and Snyder, S. H. (1979): Neurotensin-containing cell bodies, fibers and nerve terminals in the brain stem of the rat: Immunohistochemical mapping. *Brain Res.,* 167:77–91.

136. Uhl, G. R., Kuhar, M. J., and Snyder, S. H. (1978): Neurotensin: Immunohistochemical localization in rat central nervous system. *Brain Res.,* 149:223–228.

137. Uhl, G. R., and Snyder, S. H. (1979): Neurotensin: A neuronal pathway projecting from amygdala through stria terminalis. *Brain Res.,* 161:522–526.

138. Ungerstedt, U. (1971): Stereotaxic mapping of the monoamine pathways in the rat brain. *Acta Physiol. Scand. [Suppl.],* 364:1–48.

139. Vanderhaegen, J. J., Lostra, F., De May, J., and Gillus, C. (1980): Immunohistochemical localization of cholecystokinin- and gastrin-like peptide in the brain and hypophysis of the rat. *Proc. Natl. Acad. Sci. U.S.A.,* 77:1190–1194.

140. Vanderhaegen, J. J., Signeau, J. C., and Gepts, W. (1975): New peptide in the vertebrate CNS reacting with antigastrin antibodies. *Nature,* 221:557–559.

141. Vandesande, F., and Dierickx, K. (1975): Identification of the vasopressin producing and of the oxytocin producing neurons in the hypothalamus magnocellular neurosecretory system of the rat. *Cell Tissue Res.,* 164:153–162.

142. Vandesande, F., and Dierickx, K. (1980): Immunocytochemical localization of somatostatin-containing neurons in the brain of *Rana temporaria. Cell Tissue Res.,* 205:43–53.

143. Vandesande, F., Dierickx, K., and De May, J. (1975): Identification of separate vasopressin-neurophysin II and oxytocin-neurophysin I containing nerve fibers in the exterminal region of the bovine median eminence. *Cell Tissue Res.,* 158:509–516.

144. Veening, J. G. (1978): Cortical afferents of the amygdaloid complex in the rat: An HRP study. *Neurosci. Lett.,* 8:191–195.

145. Veening, J. G. (1978): Subcortical afferents of the amygdaloid complex in the rat: An HRP study. *Neurosci. Lett.,* 8:197–199.

146. Wamsley, J. K., Young, W. S. III, and Kuhar, J. M. (1980): Immunohistochemical and localization of enkephalin in rat forebrain. *Brain Res.,* 190:153–174.

147. Yamamoto, K., Tohyama, M., and Shimizu, N. (1977): Comparative anatomy of the topography of catecholamine neuron system in the brain stem from birds to teleosts. *J. Hirnforsch.,* 18:229–240.

148. Zimmerman, E. A. (1976): Localization of hypothalamic hormones by immunocytochemical techniques. In: *Frontiers in Neuroendocrinology,* edited by L. Martini and W. F. Ganong, pp. 25–62. Raven Press, New York.

Chemical Neuroanatomy, edited by P.C. Emson,
Raven Press, New York © 1983.

The Olfactory Bulb

Foteos Macrides and Barry J. Davis

Worcester Foundation for Experimental Biology, Shrewsbury, Massachusetts 01545

The olfactory bulbs are cortically organized rostral extensions of the forebrain that contain the second-order neurons of the olfactory system. Until recent years, the olfactory bulbs also could be described as that portion of the central nervous system that is left in the skull when a neurochemist attempts to remove the brain and study the central distributions of putative transmitter or neuromodulatory substances. The tendency to omit the olfactory bulb in such studies has abated, however, and this structure now appears to be a veritable cornucopia of putative transmitters and neuroactive peptides. The list of such substances that have been associated with the olfactory bulb includes acetylcholine, norepinephrine, serotonin, dopamine, luteinizing hormone-releasing hormone (LHRH), substance P, glutamate, aspartate, γ-aminobutyric acid (GABA), methionine-enkephalin, somatostatin, carnosine, cholecystokinin (CCK), thyrotropin-releasing hormone (TRH), vasoactive intestinal polypeptide (VIP), and vasopressin (cf. 16,41,141). Furthermore, a wealth of knowledge now exists concerning the neuronal morphology and synaptic organization of the olfactory bulb, the organization of its interconnections with more central regions of the nervous system, and its involvement in behavioral and hormonal regulation (cf. 129,130,132,135,170,172,176,222,224). Like the hippocampus (I. Walaas, *this volume*), the olfactory bulb is a well-laminated structure whose afferents, intrinsic circuits, and efferents are segregated in manners that are highly advantageous for neurochemical and electrophysiological research. The olfactory bulb therefore is becoming widely recognized as an excellent model system in which to study the neurophysiological actions of these substances and the roles that they play in sensory, behavioral, neuroendocrine, or affective functions.

In this chapter on the morphological and neurochemical organization of the olfactory bulb, we do not attempt a complete coverage of the literature. Emphasis is on recent findings in macrosmatic mammals and on the functional implications of these findings. Also, we try to illustrate the many experimental advantages offered by the olfactory system for neurochemical research.

MORPHOLOGICAL AND FUNCTIONAL OVERVIEW

Stimulus Access and Basic Input–Output Relationships

The olfactory bulb of macrosomatic mammals consists of two distinct structures which receive peripheral inputs from separate populations of primary receptor neurons (4,115,119). The main olfactory bulb (Fig. 1c) receives strictly ipsilateral projections from the olfactory receptor neurons located on the olfactory turbinates and septal wall of the nasal cavity (Fig. 1b). Stimulus access to these receptors is regulated in conjunction with respiration (cf. 131,135,155,156,234). The accessory olfactory bulb (Fig. 2b) receives projections from receptor neurons that are sequestered within the ipsilateral vomeronasal organ (Figs. 1a,2a) and thus are not directly exposed to inhaled air. In different species, the vomeronasal organ opens either into the rostral portion of the nasal cavity or into the nasopalatine canal which connects the nasal and oral cavities (55,148,160). Recent studies in the hamster have demonstrated that stimulus access to the vomeronasal receptors is facilitated by an autonomic pumping mechanism that alters the degree of engorgement of the vomeronasal cavernous tissue (150).

Several lines of evidence suggest that the vomeronasal (i.e., accessory olfactory) system is specialized for the reception of relatively nonvolatile chemical signals excreted in urine or secreted in a viscous medium (55,182,249). However, single

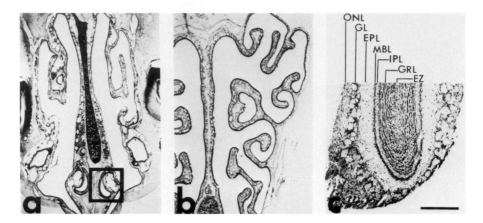

FIG. 1. Coronal sections through the rostral nasal cavity (**a**), caudal nasal cavity (**b**), and main olfactory bulb (**c**) of the hamster. Respiratory epithelium lines the turbinates and septal wall of the rostral nasal cavity. The vomeronasal organ *(boxed)* is embedded in the base of the septal wall and is illustrated at higher magnification in Fig. 2. Olfactory epithelium lines most of the surface in the caudal nasal cavity. The olfactory bulb is organized into six distinct layers which surround the ependymal zone. *Bar,* 1 mm for **a** and **b**; 500 μm for **c**. (Adapted from Burd et al., ref. 23.)

The following abbreviations are used in the illustrations of this chapter: AC, anterior commissure; AOB, accessory olfactory bulb; DPC, dorsal peduncular cortex; EPL external plexiform layer; EZ, ependymal zone; GL, glomerular layer; GRL, granule cell layer; HDB, nucleus of the horizontal limb of the diagonal band; HR$_d$, dorsal hippocampal rudiment; HR$_v$, ventral hippocampal rudiment; IPL, internal plexiform layer; LOT, lateral olfactory tract; MBL, mitral body layer; MS$_a$, anterior pole of the medial septal area; ONL, olfactory nerve layer; OT, olfactory tubercle; PC, piriform cortex; pD, pars dorsalis of the anterior olfactory nucleus; pE$_d$, dorsal sector of pars externa of the anterior olfactory nucleus; pE$_l$, lateral sector of pars externa of the anterior olfactory nucleus; pE$_v$, ventral sector of pars externa of the anterior olfactory nucleus; pL, pars lateralis of the anterior olfactory nucleus; pM, pars medialis of the anterior olfactory nucleus; pmCA, posteromedial division of the cortical amygdaloid nucleus; pP, pars posterior of the anterior olfactory nucleus; pV, pars ventralis of the anterior olfactory nucleus; RS, rhinal sulcus; SAT, sagittal association tract; tD, transitional zone of pars dorsalis of the anterior olfactory nucleus; tL, transitional zone of pars lateralis of the anterior olfactory nucleus; tPC, transitional zone of the piriform cortex; VDB, vertical limb of the diagonal band; VE, vomeronasal epithelium; VNL, vomeronasal nerve layer.

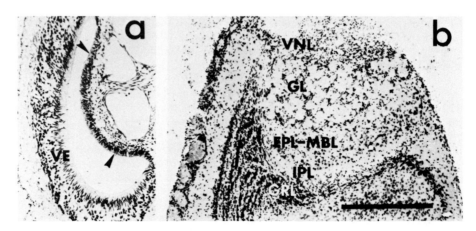

FIG. 2. Coronal sections through the vomeronasal organ (**a**) and accessory olfactory bulb (**b**) of the hamster. Vomeronasal epithelium lines the medial and ventral surface of the vomeronasal organ; respiratory epithelium *(arrowheads)* and cavernous tissue form the lateral wall. The laminae of the accessory olfactory bulb are similar to those in the main olfactory bulb. However, the external plexiform layer is reduced and indistinct. *Bar,* 100 μm for **a**; 500 μm for **b**. (For abbreviations, see Fig. 1, legend.) (Adapted from Burd et al., ref. 23.)

units in the accessory olfactory bulb can respond robustly to odorants presented in the vapor phase if they are inhaled during activation of the autonomic pumping mechanism, and in behaving animals, the pumping mechanism may cycle with the respiratory rhythm (150). The spatial organization of projections from the vomeronasal receptor neurons to the accessory olfactory bulb has not been studied. Contemporary neuroanatomical tracing techniques have demonstrated a topographic organization of projections to the main olfactory bulb from the olfactory receptor neurons, and this organization appears to be more precise in mammalian than in nonmammalian species (35–37, 66,108,114,115).

The main and accessory olfactory bulbs send strictly ipsilateral projections centrally and exhibit no overlap in their projection targets (14,44, 48,75,88,89.111,118,145,207.210–212,218,220, 228,236,237,246). This total segregation of their peripheral inputs and central projections has led to the now popular concept that the main and accessory olfactory pathways comprise a dual olfactory system (cf. 14,44,212,213). The main olfactory bulb has the more extensive central projections, with heavy terminations in all subdivisions of the anterior olfactory nucleus (i.e., pars externa, lateralis, dorsalis, medialis, ventralis, and posterior) (Figs. 3 and 4), the ventral hippocampal rudiment and dorsal peduncular cortex (Fig. 4), the olfactory tubercle (Figs. 4 and 5), the entire rostrocaudal extent of the piriform cortex (Figs. 4 and 5), cortical amygdaloid regions (i.e., the anterior and posterolateral divisions of the cortical nucleus and the nucleus of the lateral olfactory tract), and the entorhinal cortex. The entorhinal projections terminate predominantly in the lateral regions, but a substantial projection to the medial entorhinal cortex has recently been demonstrated in the rat (111). A projection from the main olfactory bulb to neocortex which lines the dorsal bank of the rhinal sulcus has been reported in marsupials (212,220) and has recently been demonstrated in the mouse (M. T. Shipley, *personal communication*) but may not be present in all mammalian species (cf. 44,212).

In contrast to these widespread main olfactory projections, the projections of the accessory olfactory bulb to the piriform lobe are restricted to amygdaloid regions. Terminal fields are present in a small region of the amygdala which has been termed the bed nucleus of the accessory olfactory tract (cf. 213), in the medial nucleus, and in the posteromedial division of the cortical nucleus (Fig. 5). In addition, efferents of the accessory olfactory bulb enter the stria terminalis and proceed to a small region of its bed nucleus near the crossing of the anterior commissure. The accessory olfactory bulb thus has both cortical and subcortical efferent projections. Subcortical projections from the main olfactory bulb have been reported in mammals but remain controversial (cf. 14,42,74,89,90,92,236).

In addition to the peripheral afferents, the olfactory bulb receives centrifugal afferents from more central regions of the nervous system. The existence of centrifugal inputs to the main olfactory bulb has been known since the classic Golgi studies of Ramon y Cajal (197–199). However, only recently has the massiveness of these inputs come to be appreciated (15,17,34,38,42,44–46,49,88,90, 134,135,146,184,187,208,219,232). The main olfactory bulb receives projections from neurons lying throughout the following structures: the anterior olfactory nucleus, the ventral hippocampal rudiment, the dorsal peduncular cortex, the piriform cortex (see Fig. 14), the nucleus of the lateral olfactory tract, the medial septum/diagonal band complex (i.e., the anterior pole of the medial septal area, vertical limb of the diagonal band, and nucleus of the horizontal limb of the diagonal band) (Fig. 5 and also see Fig. 15), the lateral, dorsal, and posterior hypothalamic areas, the dorsal and median raphe nuclei, and the locus ceruleus. The extensiveness of projections to the main olfactory bulb from the central nervous system rivals or indeed exceeds that from the periphery.

The accessory olfactory bulb also receives prominent centrifugal inputs (17,44,46,135,213). The accessory olfactory bulb is reciprocally connected with all of its central projection targets. The main olfactory bulb is similarly reciprocally connected with most of its central projection targets (see above). The findings that the centrifugal afferents of the main and accessory olfactory bulbs from the piriform lobe are distinct and that they parallel the organization of efferent projections have been interpreted as additional morphological support for the concept of a dual olfactory system (cf. 44,213). However, it is likely that both the main and accessory olfactory bulbs receive subcortical centrifugal afferents from the medial septum/diagonal band complex, hypothalamus, raphe nuclei, and locus ceruleus (cf. 134) and from a unique group of LHRH-immunoreactive neurons positioned along the medial surface of the cerebral hemisphere (see below). Because many of the subcortical centrifugal fibers destined for the main olfactory bulb pass through the accessory olfactory bulb, it has proven difficult to assess whether these fibers also have terminal fields within the accessory olfactory bulb.

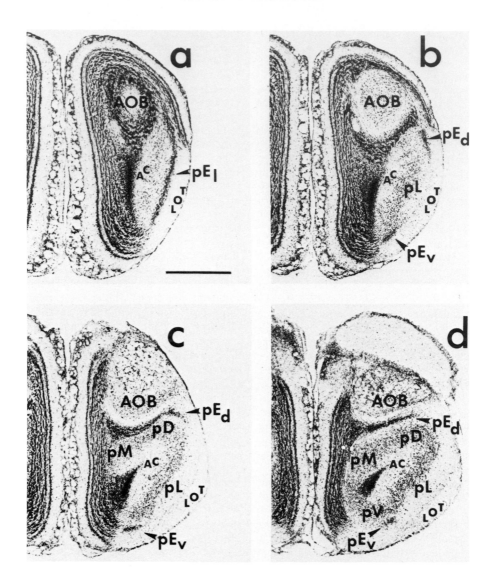

FIG. 3. Coronal sections through progressively more caudal levels of the retrobulbar area in the hamster. The accessory olfactory bulb is positioned dorsally, the caudal part of the main olfactory bulb extends medially, and the rostral part of the anterior olfactory nucleus lies laterally in the retrobulbar area. Part of the retrobulbar area (**d**) lies ventral to the frontal pole. *Bar,* 1 mm. (For abbreviations, see Fig. 1, legend.) (Adapted from Davis and Macrides, ref. 42.)

The morphological findings of extensive projections to the olfactory bulb from limbic cortical regions and from subcortical regions that are also associated with the limbic system may help to explain reports that the responses of olfactory bulb neurons can vary in relation to nutritional, hormonal, or motivational states and that these responses often appear to be related to functional attributes of chemosensory stimuli (25,130,131, 133,169,170,172). Furthermore, the recent findings of reciprocal interconnections between the ol-

factory bulb and limbic structures have fostered reconsideration of its functional relationship to the limbic system. Historical and critical reviews of the notion that the olfactory bulb is an integral component of the limbic system appear elsewhere (24,130,213).

Intrinsic Neurons and Synaptic Organization

The main olfactory bulb is organized into six distinct layers (i.e., the olfactory nerve layer, glomer-

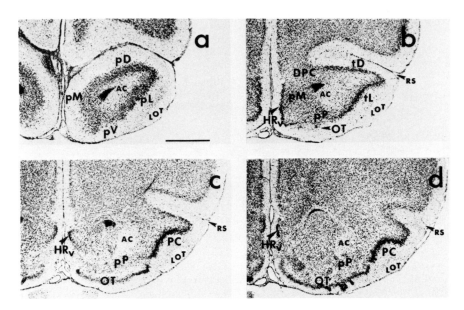

FIG. 4. Coronal sections through the olfactory peduncle (**a**), the transitional zones of the anterior olfactory nucleus (**b**), and the anterior levels of the piriform cortex (**c, d**) in the hamster. In their transitional zones, pars dorsalis and pars lateralis of the anterior olfactory nucleus exhibit cytoarchitectonic features similar to those of the piriform cortex. These transitional zones project bilaterally to the main olfactory bulb, whereas the centrifugal projections from the piriform cortex are strictly ipsilateral. At its caudal levels, pars medialis of the anterior olfactory nucleus is positioned deep to the ventral hippocampal rudiment and dorsal peduncular cortex (**b**). Pars posterior of the anterior olfactory nucleus lies deep to the rostral one-third of the olfactory tubercle (**b,c,d**). *Bar,* 1 mm. (For abbreviations, see Fig. 1, legend.) (From David and Macrides, ref. 42, with permission.)

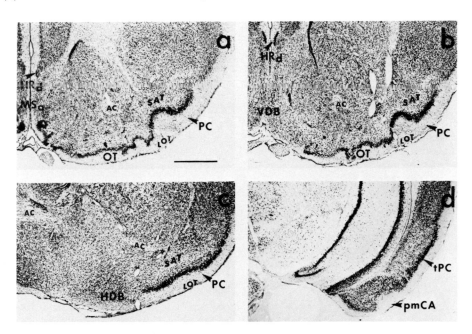

FIG. 5. Coronal sections through the piriform cortex at middle levels of the olfactory tubercle (**a,b**), at the level of the crossing of the anterior commissure (**c**), and at the level of the posteromedial division of the cortical amygdaloid nucleus (**d**) in the hamster. At its caudal levels, the piriform cortex exhibits cytoarchitectonic features similar to those of the entorhinal cortex. This transitional zone of the piriform cortex is reciprocally connected with the main olfactory bulb, whereas the entorhinal cortex receives projections from the main olfactory bulb but does not return centrifugal afferents. The posteromedial division of the cortical amygdaloid nucleus is reciprocally connected with the accessory olfactory bulb. *Bar,* 1 mm. (For abbreviations, see Fig. 1, legend.) (From Davis and Macrides, ref. 42, with permission.)

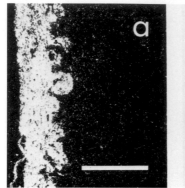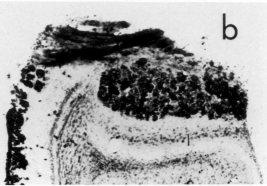

FIG. 6. Laminar organization of peripheral afferent projections to the main (**a,b**) and accessory (**b**) olfactory bulbs. **Panel a** illustrates autoradiographic labeling of the olfactory nerve layer and the glomeruli of the main olfactory bulb following nasal irrigation with tritiated β-alanine. (Adapted from Burd et al., ref. 23; see text.) **Panel b** illustrates labeling of the olfactory and vomeronasal nerve layers and of the glomeruli in the main and accessory olfactory bulbs following nasal irrigation with horseradish peroxidase. Epinephrine was injected intraperitoneally prior to nasal irrigation with solutions of tracers so as to facilitate the vomeronasal pumping mechanism that draws fluids into the vomeronasal organ (see text). *Bar,* 400 μm for **a**; 250 μm for **b.**

ular layer, external plexiform layer, mitral body layer, internal plexiform layer, and granule cell layer) which surround the ependymal zone rostrally (Fig. 1c) and are positioned medially in the retrobulbar area (Fig. 3). The accessory olfactory bulb exhibits a similar laminar organization, but its external plexiform layer is reduced and indistinct (Fig. 2b). In macrosomatic mammals, the accessory olfactory bulb is considerably smaller than the main olfactory bulb and is embedded within it dorsally in the retrobulbar area (Fig. 3).

Although Golgi studies of both the main and accessory olfactory bulbs have been conducted by classical neuroanatomists (9,26,71,110,197–199,240), contemporary studies of their intrinsic neurons and synaptic organization have focused primarily on the main olfactory bulb (cf. 63,176–180,183,186,188–190,195,196,214, 215,239,245,247). In both structures, the second-order neurons receive axodendritic synapses from peripheral afferents within specialized regions of neuropil called glomeruli (Fig. 6). These second-order neurons are the mitral cells, whose somata form the mitral body layer, the tufted cells, and the periglomerular cells.

Tufted cells have their somata in the external plexiform layer and in the periglomerular region of the glomerular layer. They are a major class of neurons in the main olfactory bulb but appear to be rare or absent in the accessory olfactory bulb. Although the nature of tufted cell axonal projections was controversial for many years (123, 124,162,199,217,238), recent studies (see below)

have demonstrated that a large proportion of tufted cells are true output neurons, as are the mitral cells.

The periglomerular cells (Fig. 9) are a major class of interneurons whose somata are located in the periglomerular region. Granule cells (Fig. 8) are the most numerous class of interneurons. Their somata form the granule cell layer but are also present in the internal plexiform and mitral body layers. Six additional morphologically distinct classes of interneurons are present in the main olfactory bulb (Figs. 7–9). These latter classes have not been reported and might not be present in the accessory olfactory bulb.

Contemporary studies on the cell types and synaptology of the main olfactory bulb support the concept that mechanisms of neuronal integration in the olfactory bulb are organized into two morphological and functional tiers of lateral and recurrent interactions controlling mitral and tufted cell excitability (cf. 42,176,215,222). Specifically, periglomerular cells control output neuron excitability in the glomerular layer through serial and reciprocal dendrodendritic synaptic contacts with the primary (i.e., intraglomerular) dendrites of mitral and tufted cells and via axodendritic synapses onto the mitral and tufted cell primary dendritic shafts (178,179). Deeper, in the external plexiform layer, granule cells mediate lateral and recurrent interactions through serial and reciprocal dendrodendritic synaptic contacts with the secondary (i.e., nonglomerular) dendrites of mitral and tufted cells (195). The granule cells are amacrine interneu-

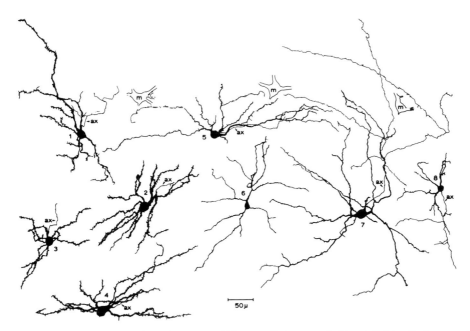

FIG. 7. Camera lucida drawings of Golgi-impregnated Blanes cells (neurons 1–4) and Golgi cells (neurons 5–8) in the main olfactory bulb of the hamster. Blanes cells have a greater density of dendritic spines than do the other classes of deep short-axon cells. In this and the next two figures, outlines of mitral cell somata (m) are drawn to illustrate the predominant locations of the various classes of interneurons relative to the mitral body layer. *Bar*, 50 μm. (From Schneider and Macrides, ref. 215, with permission.)

rons. They bear short proximal dendrites which arborize near the soma and support a lengthy, radially oriented distal dendrite which arborizes in the external plexiform layer.

Considerable electrophysiological evidence ex-

ists for the view that the granule cells and output neurons interact primarily via their dendrodendritic synapses in the external plexiform layer, that the output neurons are excitatory to granule cells, and that the granule cells are inhibitory to output

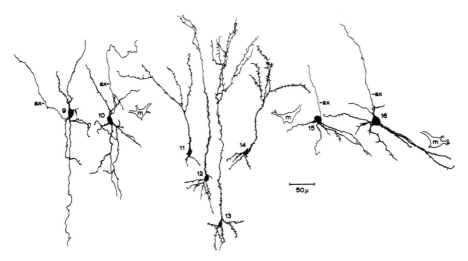

FIG. 8. Camera lucida drawings of Golgi-impregnated Cajal cells (neurons 9 and 10), granule cells (neurons 11–14), and horizontal cells (neurons 15 and 16) in the main olfactory bulb of the hamster. *Bar*, 50 μm (From Schneider and Macrides, ref. 215, with permission.)

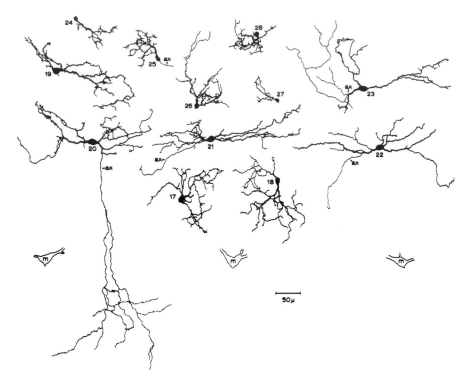

FIG. 9. Camera lucida drawings of Golgi-impregnated Van Gehuchten cells (neurons 17 and 18), superficial short-axon cells (neurons 19–23), and periglomerular cells (neurons 24–28) in the main olfactory bulb of the hamster. *Bar,* 50 μm. (From Schneider and Macrides, ref. 215, with permission.)

neurons (68,103,152,153,161,173,195,252). Although it is likely that the periglomerular cells also are excited by mitral and tufted cells and mediate lateral and recurrent inhibition in the glomerular layer (67,223,254), the electrophysiological evidence for this view suffers from methodological difficulties (see below). The peripheral inputs to the olfactory bulb appear to be excitatory, on the basis of studies employing electrical stimulation of the olfactory (e.g., 164) or vomeronasal (e.g., 150) nerves.

The other six classes of interneurons exhibit a great diversity in their form and laminar organization. Consistent with the concept of a two-tiered organization of intrinsic circuits, they can be categorized into deep and superficial groups based on their predominant interconnections with granule cells or periglomerular cells, respectively (cf. 196,215). The Blanes cells and Golgi cells are multipolar short-axon cells located most commonly in the granule cell layer but also in the internal plexiform and mitral body layers and are distinguished by their markedly different spine densities (Fig. 7). They are thought to form axosomatic and axoden-dritic synapses onto granule cells and onto short axon cells in the deep layers (188). Two classes of oriented short-axon cells, the vertical cells of Cajal and the horizontal cells, are located most commonly in the internal plexiform and mitral body layers (Fig. 8). These interneurons are thought to form axodendritic synapses onto the distal dendrites of granule cells (188,190). The Van Gehuchten cells are diffusely arborizing neurons located in the internal plexiform and mitral body layers and most commonly in the external plexiform layer (Fig. 9). No information is available on their synaptic connections, although they are in a position to interact with the distal dendrites of granule cells (cf. 215). The deep short-axon cells as a group are thought to be inhibitory to granule cells, to receive excitatory inputs from mitral and tufted cell axon collaterals and/or centrifugal fibers, and thereby to provide pathways for disinhibition of mitral and tufted cells (27,186,188,215,252).

The superficial short-axon cells (Fig. 9) have only recently been discovered (63,177,215). They are located in the periglomerular region and in the superficial region of the external plexiform layer.

Their dendritic arbors are restricted to these regions and form clasp-like branchings around the glomeruli. Their axons ramify predominantly in the periglomerular region and at the border between the glomerular and external plexiform layers, but they occasionally extend as deep as the granule cell layer. Electron microscopic studies indicate that the superficial short-axon cells receive symmetrical axodendritic and axosomatic synapses from periglomerular cells and to a lesser degree from other short-axon cells, that they receive asymmetrical axodendritic and axosomatic synapses from tufted cell collaterals and/or centrifugal fibers, and that they in turn form symmetrical axodendritic and axosomatic synapses onto periglomerular cells (177–179). On the basis of their synaptic ultrastructure and by analogy to the deeper layers, the superficial short-axon cells thus might mediate disinhibitory mechanisms in the glomerular layer.

Electron microscopic studies indicate that the centrifugal afferents terminate predominantly on interneurons (180,183,186,190). The more central regions of the nervous system thus modulate the synaptic integrations of mitral and tufted cells through influences on granule cells, periglomerular cells, and the superficial and deep short-axon cells. The centrifugal projections from the various cortical and subcortical structures exhibit marked differences in their laminar patterns of terminations within the olfactory bulb (16,38,42,146). These differences not only determine the intrabulbar circuits and classes of interneurons through which the central structures can influence the integrations of mitral and tufted cells but can also provide experimental advantages in attempts to characterize the neurotransmitters or neuromodulators associated with these pathways and intrinsic circuits (see below).

Heterogeneity of Mitral and Tufted Cells

In his descriptions of the main olfactory bulb, Ramon y Cajal (199) subdivided tufted cells into three broad classes based on the laminar distributions of their somata. External tufted cells have their somata in the periglomerular region or at the border between the glomerular and external plexiform layers. The somata of middle tufted cells are located deep to these regions in the superficial two-thirds of the external plexiform layer. Internal tufted cells have their somata in the deep one-third of the external plexiform layer just superficial to the mitral body layer. These classes of tufted cells

and the mitral cells exhibit marked differences in the spatial organization of their dendritic fields and in their likely patterns of lateral and recurrent interactions with granule cells and/or periglomerular cells (cf. 137). For example, the mitral and internal tufted cells have relatively numerous secondary dendrites which are sparsely branched but extremely lengthy and which extend tangentially along the deep portion of the external plexiform layer in relatively symmetric radial patterns from their parent somata (110,137,214). The secondary dendritic fields of individual mitral and internal tufted cells thus envelop substantial proportions of the external plexiform layer. Through their dendrodendritic interactions with granule cells, individual mitral and internal tufted cells integrate synaptic activity over wide regions of the olfactory bulb. At the other extreme, many of the external tufted cells, and particularly those located in the superficial two-thirds of the glomerular layer, have no secondary dendrites; all of their dendrites arborize within a single or within adjacent glomeruli (137,177). Because most of these neurons are not in positions where they could receive synaptic contacts from granule cells, they are likely to receive interneuronal input predominantly from periglomerular cells.

In a recent quantitative Golgi study of the hamster main olfactory bulb (137), we also observed systematic differences in the secondary dendritic fields of middle tufted cells and of external tufted cells located at the border between the glomerular and external plexiform layers. Most of these neurons have sparsely branched secondary dendrites which extend tangentially in the external plexiform layer. The lengths, number per neuron, and laminar distributions of the secondary dendrites within the external plexiform layer are correlated with the depths of their somata. There are progressive decreases in the overall size of the secondary dendritic fields and a striking increase in their degree of spatial asymmetry with increasing distance from the mitral body layer. Many of the tufted cells in the superficial one-third of the external plexiform layer have asymmetric secondary dendritic fields. The trunks and branches of their secondary dendrites all extend tangentially in the same direction from the parent soma. Furthermore, we found clear differences in the sizes of glomerular arbors among mitral and tufted cells. The mitral and internal tufted cells and the external tufted cells that lack secondary dendrites have the largest glomerular arbors. Those of the middle tufted cells and the external tufted cells with secondary dendrites tend to be much smaller. We also observed a category of external tufted cells and a few very superficially situated middle tufted cells distinctive for their short, densely branched secondary dendrites. Their compact secondary dendritic fields stand in marked contrast to the much more elongated and often asymmetric fields of tufted cells with sparsely branched secondary dendrites. The substantial differences in the sizes and symmetries of mitral and tufted cell dendritic fields are likely to impart different functional characteristics to these neurons.

Recent retrograde tracing studies employing injections of horseradish peroxidase into the projection targets of the main olfactory bulb have demonstrated that the mitral and tufted cells differ in their central projection patterns (75,137,228). The mitral and internal tufted cells have the most extensive projections. As a group, they project to all of the central targets discussed above. The central projections of middle tufted cells and some of the external tufted cells located at the border between the glomerular and external plexiform layers are restricted to the anterior olfactory nucleus, the ventral hippocampal rudiment, the dorsal peduncular cortex, the olfactory tubercle, and the anterior sector of the piriform cortex adjacent to the olfactory tubercle. Progressively more of the middle and external tufted cells are labeled with more anterior injections of tracer. Most of the external tufted cells do not appear to project caudal to the retrobulbar area. This differential but overlapping spatial organization of bulbofugal projections from mitral and tufted cells in the main olfactory system is reminiscent of the differential but overlapping organization of retinofugal projections from morphologically and functionally distinguishable retinal ganglion cells in the visual system (cf. 231). Together with the morphological differences discussed above, these findings suggest that the mitral and tufted cells may be organized into functionally defined parallel pathways (cf. 137,228).

These findings also make it necessary to reconsider the results of many electrophysiological studies on the synaptic organization of the olfactory bulb. Such studies have employed antidromic stimulation of the lateral olfactory tract to distinguish recordings from output neurons or from interneurons. The antidromic electrode placements used in these studies (i.e., typically at the level of the olfactory tubercle or at caudal levels in the olfactory peduncle) permit the antidromic activation of mitral and internal tufted cells and many middle tufted cells. However, not all of the middle tufted cells and few if any external tufted cells are activated. In such studies, single units that were recorded in the glomerular layer and could not be driven antidromically but exhibited short-latency excitation to orthodromic stimulation of the olfactory nerve have been categorized as periglomerular cells (e.g., 65,67,222,253). We now know that many of these recordings in fact could have been from external tufted cells.

This might help to explain a recent claim that periglomerular cells mediate lateral excitation rather than lateral inhibition (64,65). Although mitral and tufted cells are now thought to receive extraglomerular synaptic contacts predominantly from granule cells and periglomerular cells, there is some evidence that the axon collaterals of external tufted cells might terminate on the primary dendritic shafts of mitral and tufted cells (179). External tufted cells thus might mediate the posited lateral excitation in the glomerular layer. Of course, now that the spatial organization of efferent projections from the main olfactory bulb is better known, appropriate placements of antidromic stimulation electrodes can be employed to distinguish mitral cells and classes of tufted cells on the basis of their central projection patterns and to evaluate the hypothesis that they differ in their functional characteristics (cf. 217).

Pathways and Laminar Organization of Efferents and Centrifugal Afferents

In rodents, the efferents of the main olfactory bulb proceed caudally in the superficial regions of the granule cell layer, then pass through the internal plexiform layer of the accessory olfactory bulb or exit directly from the granule cell layer of the main olfactory bulb, and collect laterally in the retrobulbar area and olfactory peduncle to form the main body of the lateral olfactory tract (cf. 44,48). The efferents of the accessory olfactory bulb collect into a compact bundle embedded within the main body of the lateral olfactory tract. This bundle has been termed the accessory olfactory tract (14). Most of the centrifugal afferents enter directly into the granule cell layer of the main olfactory bulb or enter via the internal plexiform layer of the accessory olfactory bulb regardless of the pathways by which they reach the retrobulbar area (Figs. 10 and 11); therefore, these two sites of entry and exit have been termed the final common bulbar pathway (42).

The efferents and centrifugal afferents of the main olfactory bulb are almost totally segregated caudal to the final common bulbar pathway (cf.

42). This separation of efferents and afferents makes it practical to manipulate one or the other in anatomical, neurochemical, electrophysiological, or behavioral experiments (e.g.,47,69,70,134, 136,144,158,254). The efferents travel in the main body of the lateral olfactory tract and on the surface of the olfactory peduncle and basal forebrain. They terminate in the superficial half of the superficial plexiform layer (i.e., layer IA) (Fig. 11b) of their various cortical targets (14,44,185). The associational projections among these cortical targets terminate in the deep half of the superficial plexiform layer (i.e., layer IB) (Fig. 11d) and in the cellular layers (185). The centrifugal projections from the piriform cortex initially travel in the sagittal association tract (see Fig. 5) and enter the anterior limb of the anterior commissure at the level of the olfactory peduncle. The axons of the laterally, dorsally, and ventrally situated subdivisions of the anterior olfactory nucleus also travel in the anterior commissure. In contrast, the centrifugal fibers from the medially situated cortices travel rostrally in the cellular layer of the olfactory peduncle (Fig. 11c). The subcortical centrifugal afferents also travel predominantly in the cellular layer and enter the olfactory peduncle from the anterior continuation of the medial forebrain bundle. The pathway taken by the centrifugal projections from the nucleus of the lateral olfactory tract has not been described. Based on our studies in the hamster, these fibers probably travel initially in the stria terminalis and then proceed rostrally in the region of the precommissural fornix. Some of the centrifugal afferents from subcortical regions and from the anterior sector of the piriform cortex travel along the deep border of the lateral olfactory tract in the olfactory peduncle. However, contrary to earlier thought (187,197), the lateral olfactory tract does not appear to be a principal pathway for axons coming from any of the major sources of centrifugal afferents to the main olfactory bulb (cf. 42,135). The pathways taken by the centrifugal projections to the accessory olfactory bulb have not been studied as extensively. Those from the amygdala probably travel initially in the stria terminalis, then join those from the bed nucleus of the stria terminalis, and continue rostrally in the region of the precommissural fornix (cf. 34,89). As discussed below, the LHRH-immunoreactive system of neurons associated with the olfactory bulb is a noteworthy exception to the generalization that its efferents and afferents are segregated.

Although the spatial organization of centrifugal afferent terminations in the olfactory bulb is complex, some generalizations can be made (cf. 42). The laminar termination patterns of cortical afferents to the ipsilateral main olfactory bulb are correlated with the mediolateral axis of the olfactory peduncle and the rostrocaudal axis of the piriform cortex. The projections from the laterally situated subdivisions of the anterior olfactory nucleus (i.e., pars lateralis, dorsalis, ventralis, and posterior) have heavy terminations in the deep layers but also exhibit a prominent terminal field in the glomerular layer (Fig. 10). In contrast, the medially situated cortical regions (i.e., the ventral hippocampal rudiment and pars medialis of the anterior olfactory nucleus) have terminal fields exclusively in the granule cell layer. The projections from the anterior sector of the piriform cortex terminate predominantly in the superficial half of the granule cell layer but do extend into the external plexiform layer to its border with the glomerular layer. The centrifugal projections from progressively more posterior regions of the piriform cortex terminate progressively deeper (Fig. 12a,b), and those from the posterior sector terminate exclusively in the granule cell layer. This laminar organization of terminations is, in turn, correlated with the spatial organization of associational connections among the olfactory cortices. The anterior regions of the piriform cortex are extensively interconnected with the laterally situated subdivisions of the anterior olfactory nucleus, whereas the posterior regions of the piriform cortex are extensively interconnected with the medially situated cortical regions (76,77). Thus, the olfactory cortical regions that are most heavily interconnected by associational projections have similar laminar patterns of centrifugal projections to the main olfactory bulb.

The laminar organization of centrifugal terminations also is correlated with the spatial organization of efferent projections from the main olfactory bulb to the laterally situated olfactory cortices. The output neurons that project to posterior regions of the piriform cortex are exclusively mitral and internal tufted cells (see above). The posterior piriform cortex, in turn, can influence the integrations of mitral and internal tufted cells through its centrifugal projections onto granule cells and/or deep short-axon cells. The posterior piriform cortex does not receive projections from external tufted cells, and, because its centrifugal projections do not reach the glomerular layer, it is unlikely to exert much influence on the integrations of external tufted cells (cf. 42). In contrast, the laterally situated subdivisions of the anterior olfactory nucleus do appear to receive projections from external tufted cells as well as from the deeper lying output neurons, and, through their projections to the glomerular layer as well as to the deeper layers, these subdivisions appear to be capable of influencing all classes of mitral and tufted cells. The centrifugal projections of these cortical regions thus may serve to regulate the lateral and recurrent interactions among those classes of olfactory bulb output neurons from which they receive efferent projections.

Similar reasoning can be applied to the pathways by which the main olfactory bulb interacts with the hippocampal formation. The entorhinal cortex receives direct olfactory bulb projections exclusively from the mitral and internal tufted cells. The posterior piriform cortex and the posterolateral division of the cortical amygdaloid nucleus also send heavy projections to the entorhinal cortex (113) and themselves receive direct projections exclusively from the mitral and internal tufted cells. The regions of entorhinal cortex that receive olfactory bulb efferents have been demonstrated to support projections to the dentate gyrus, hippocampus, and subiculum (229,230). The ventral subiculum and adjoining transitional area with the hippocampal field CA_1 project to the medial cortical regions of the olfactory peduncle (46,76,77,233), whose centrifugal projections terminate exclusively in the granule cell layer (see above). Thus, the most direct pathways to the hippocampal formation from the main olfactory bulb originate from the deep output neurons, and the most direct pathways from the hippocampal formation to the main olfactory bulb terminate on those interneurons that mediate the lateral and recurrent interactions among the deep output neurons. These various connectional relationships provide additional morphological support for the notion that the mitral and tufted cells, and their central circuits, are organized into functionally defined parallel pathways.

Although the centrifugal projections exhibit prominent laminar patterns of terminations, most of these projections do not appear to be topographically organized in the conventional sense of being restricted to particular sectors, as opposed to laminae, of the olfactory bulb (42). The projections from pars externa of the anterior olfactory nucleus are a noteworthy exception. In contrast to the other subdivisions of the anterior olfactory nucleus, whose centrifugal projections are predominantly ipsilateral, pars externa projections almost exclusively to the contralateral main olfactory bulb (42,44,46,77,219). These contralateral projections have a narrow terminal field just deep to the internal plexiform layer and appear to be topographically organized (Fig. 13). Pars externa is a narrow band of cells circumferentially distributed in the retrobulbar area. The efferents of the main olfactory bulb are topographically organized as they exit in the final common bulbar pathway and pass through the superficial plexiform layer of pars externa (191,225). Pars externa thus is in an ideal position to receive topographically organized projections and might mediate topographically organized interactions between the olfactory bulbs (cf. 42).

→

FIG. 10. The final common bulbar pathway. Panels **a** and **b** are dark-field photomontages of coronal sections approximately at the levels illustrated in Figs. 3a,b, respectively. Tritiated amino acids were injected ipsilaterally into pars lateralis of the anterior olfactory nucleus, and the centrifugal projections to the main olfactory bulb from this subdivision have been visualized autoradiographically. Labeled fibers exiting from the anterior commissure either enter directly into the granule cell layer of the main olfactory bulb or proceed rostrally through the internal plexiform layer of the accessory olfactory bulb. These same two routes are taken by centrifugal afferents regardless of how they reach the retrobulbar area (i.e., whether or not they travel in the anterior commissure) and by the efferents of the main olfactory bulb as they exit into the retrobulbar area (see text). The superficial and deep borders of the external plexiform layer in the main olfactory bulb are indicated *(arrowheads)*. The ipsilateral centrifugal afferents from pars lateralis extend into the deep regions of the glomerular layer. *Bar,* 1 mm. (Adapted from Davis and Macrides, ref. 42.)

FIG. 11. Segregation of efferents and centrifugal afferents caudal to the final common bulbar pathway. The bright-field photomicrograph (**a**) and autoradiographs (**b,c,d**) are from coronal sections approximately at the level illustrated in Fig. 3d. **Panel b** illustrates efferent projections in a hamster that received an injection of tritiated amino acids into the main olfactory bulb. The labeled axons are concentrated in the main body of the lateral olfactory tract and have terminal fields exclusively in layer IA. In contrast, the centrifugal and associational projections from the piriform cortex (**d**) travel in the anterior commissure, and the associational projections terminate predominantly in layer IB. **Panel c** is from a hamster that received an injection centered in pars medialis of the anterior olfactory nucleus with modest involvement of the ventral hippocampal rudiment. The centrifugal projections from these medially situated olfactory cortical regions travel in the cellular layer rather than in the anterior commissure. Their associational projections are predominantly to the posterior olfactory cortical regions, and no labeling is evident in layer IB of the rostrolateral region illustrated in this figure. *Bar,* 500 μm. (Adapted from David et al., ref.44, and Davis and Macrides, ref. 42.)

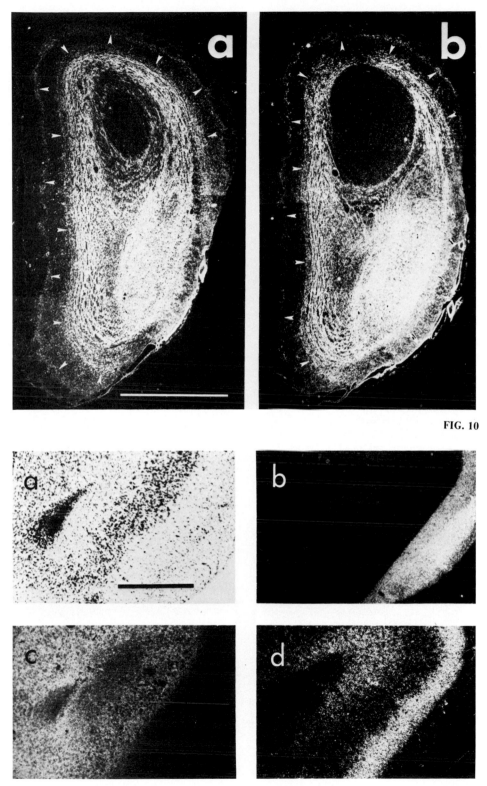

FIG. 10

FIG. 11

FIG. 12

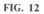

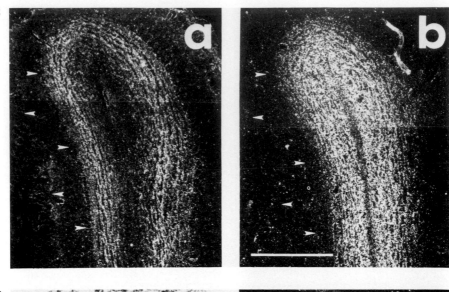

FIG. 13

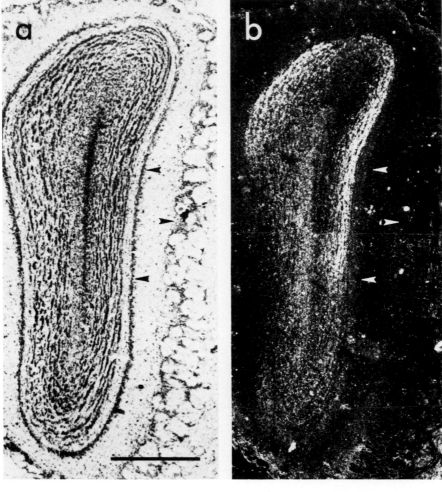

NEUROCHEMICAL ORGANIZATION

Cholinergic Systems

On the basis of electrophysiological studies (5,10,11,209), it has been known for some time that acetylcholine and its antagonists can affect the activity of neurons in the main olfactory bulb. Iontophoresis of acetylcholine generally suppress output neuron activity, but excitatory effects suggestive of disinhibitory influences also have been observed. Ligand-binding studies indicate that both muscarinic (157) and nicotinic (99) receptors are present in the main olfactory bulb. Choline acetyltransferase (ChAT) and acetylcholinesterase (AChE) also are present, predominantly in the glomerular layer and in the internal plexiform layer (70,100,102,134,159,221,242). Electron microscopic studies of the accessory olfactory bulb have visualized AChE-positive terminals in its deep layers, but, in contrast to the main olfactory bulb, AChE activity does not appear to be present in the glomerular layer of the accessory olfactory bulb (28). The possibility that mitral and tufted cells are cholinergic has been entertained (cf. 99). However, the ChAT and AChE contents of the olfactory bulb are drastically reduced or eliminated following destruction of its centrifugal inputs (70,134,243,244). The cholinergic activity in the olfactory bulb thus appears to be of extrinsic origin.

In their classical studies using AChE histochemistry, Shute and Lewis (227) described a prominent presumably cholinergic system of projections to the olfactory peduncle and olfactory bulb which they termed the olfactory radiation. Because the labeled fibers could be observed to enter the olfactory peduncle from the region deep to the olfactory tubercle, which itself is densely labeled in AChE histochemical material, they described the olfac-

tory radiation as originating in the olfactory tubercle. However, subsequent neuroanatomical tracing studies indicated that the olfactory tubercle does not support centrifugal projections to the olfactory bulb (Figs. 14a,15b) or associational projections to other olfactory cortical regions (42,44,75,76,134). The origin of the olfactory radiation had to be sought elsewhere.

Correlations among neuroanatomical, histochemical, immunocytochemical, and biochemical findings now indicate that the olfactory radiation originates in the medial septum/diagonal band complex and that this subcortical region is the major source of cholinergic inputs to the olfactory bulb (16,70,101,109,120,134,243,244). The anterior septal component, vertical limb (Fig. 15a), and predominantly the horizontal limb (Fig. 15b) of this complex are sources of ipsilateral centrifugal projections to the olfactory bulb. The laminar termination pattern of the projections (Fig. 16a) corresponds well to the laminar distribution pattern of AChE (Fig. 16b) and ChAT in the olfactory bulb. The somata of neurons in this complex contain AChE histochemical activity and ChAT immunoreactivity. Finally, lesions in the vertical limb of the diagonal band and particularly in the nucleus of the horizontal limb markedly reduce the levels of AChE and ChAT in the ipsilateral olfactory bulb, whereas control lesions positioned caudal to the horizontal limb in the lateral and dorsal hypothalamus have no significant effect on the content of ChAT in olfactory bulb and do not alter the histochemically visualized distribution of AChE in the rostral forebrain (cf. 134).

The septal component and vertical limb of the medial septum/diagonal band complex are thought to be the subcortical sources of cholinergic projections to the hippocampal formation (I. Walaas, *this volume*). The vertical and horizontal limbs are now known to be sources of projections to cortical

---

FIG. 12. Laminar termination patterns of the centrifugal projections from the piriform cortex. **Panel a** shows the pattern of labeling within the main olfactory bulb for a hamster that received an injection of tritiated amino acids into the piriform cortex approximately at the level illustrated in Fig. 5b. **Panel b** is from a case with a more caudal injection, approximately at the level illustrated in Fig. 5c. The *arrowheads* indicate the superficial and deep borders of the external plexiform layer. The terminal fields of the centrifugal projections from progressively more caudal regions of the piriform cortex are restricted to progressively deeper regions of the main olfactory bulb. *Bar,* 500 μm. (Adapted from Davis and Macrides, ref. 42.)

FIG. 13. Topographically organized contralateral projections to the main olfactory bulb from pars externa of the anterior olfactory nucleus. Panels **a** and **b** are a bright-field photomicrograph and matching dark-field photomontage, respectively, of the contralateral main olfactory bulb in a hamster that received an injection of tritiated amino acids into the dorsal sector of pars externa. The *arrowheads* indicate the superficial and deep borders of the external plexiform layer. A dense, narrow, discontinuous band of labeling is present immediately deep to the internal plexiform layer in the dorsal sector of the granule cell layer. The additional, more diffuse labeling in the granule cell layer may be attributed to involvement of pars dorsalis in the injection. *Bar,* 500 μm. (From Davis and Macrides, ref. 42, with permission.)

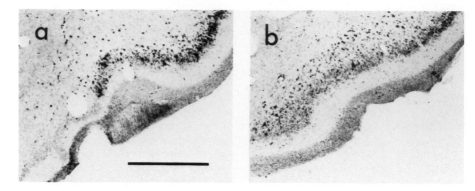

FIG. 14. Anterograde and retrograde labeling in the piriform cortex following an injection of horseradish peroxidase into the main olfactory bulb. Panels **a** and **b** are photomicrographs of coronal sections approximately at the levels illustrated in Figs. 5b and 5c, respectively. The efferents of the main olfactory bulb exhibit anterograde labeling in the main body of the lateral olfactory tract and in layer IA of the olfactory tubercle (*lower left* in **a**) and piriform cortex. Numerous retrogradely labeled neurons are present in layers II and III of the piriform cortex. In contrast, the neurons of the olfactory tubercle are not labeled. *Bar,* 500 μm.

regions that receive olfactory bulb efferents (6,17,49,53,127). Lesions in the vertical and horizontal limbs markedly reduce or eliminate AChE histochemical activity not only in the olfactory bulb but also in all of the olfactory cortical and amygdaloid regions (134,243,244). The medial septum/diagonal band complex thus appears to be a source of cholinergic inputs to most of the olfactory system and thereby could modulate the inter-

actions among the olfactory bulb, the olfactory cortices, and the related structures of the limbic system (cf., 135).

Monoaminergic Systems

Like acetylcholine, norepinephrine and serotonin generally suppress but occasionally elevate output neuron activity when they are iontophoretically in-

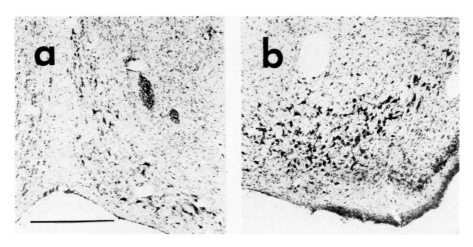

FIG. 15. Retrograde neuronal labeling in the vertical limb (**a**) and nucleus of the horizontal limb (**b**) of the diagonal band following an injection of horseradish peroxidase into the main olfactory bulb. **Panel a** corresponds to the level illustrated in Fig. 5b. Neurons scattered throughout the septal and basal portions of the vertical limb exhibit retrograde labeling. **Panel b** is from a section slightly rostral to the level illustrated in Fig. 5c. The caudal part of the olfactory tubercle is still present *(lower right),* and anterograde labeling is evident in layer IA. Most of the neurons in the horizontal limb are densely labeled, but the neurons of the olfactory tubercle do not contain reaction product. *Bar,* 400 μm. (Adapted from Macrides et al., ref. 135.)

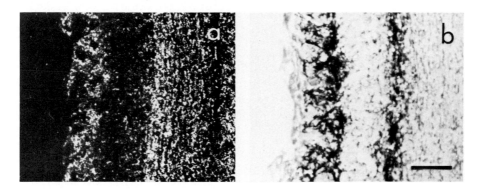

FIG. 16. Comparison of the projections from the nucleus of the horizontal limb of the diagonal band to the main olfactory bulb (**a**) and the distribution of AChE histochemical activity (**b**). Following an injection of tritiated amino acids into the horizontal limb, autoradiographic labeling within the main olfactory bulb is concentrated throughout the periglomerular region and in the internal plexiform layer. This distribution of label corresponds well to the distribution of AChE reaction product. *Bar,* 150μm. (Adapted from Macrides et al., ref. 135.)

jected into the olfactory bulb (5,11). Both norepinephrine and serotonin are normally present (58,86,102,134,171) and have been reported to be released within the olfactory bulb during peripheral stimulation with odorants (30). Also, like acetylcholine, norepinephrine and serotonin are associated with centrifugal afferents (39,58,80,82). Based on correlations between morphological and

lesion studies (134), most of the noradrenergic input to the olfactory bulb can be attributed to the centrifugal projections from the locus ceruleus (Fig. 17b). The other known noradrenergic cell groups (O. Lindvall and A. Björklund, *this volume*) have not been revealed as sources of centrifugal afferents to the olfactory bulb in retrograde tracing studies. The noradrenergic fibers are con-

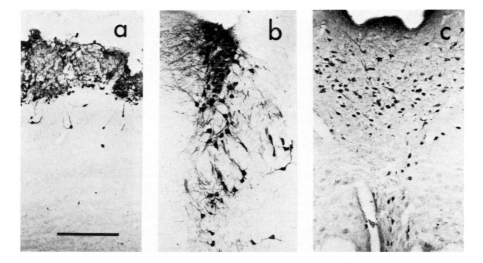

FIG. 17. Tyrosine hydroxylase-immunoreactive neurons in the main olfactory bulb (**a**) and in the locus ceruleus (**b**) and serotonin-immunoreactive neurons in the dorsal raphe nucleus (**c**) of the hamster. In the main olfactory bulb, the majority of external tufted cells, many middle tufted cells, and some periglomerular cells contain tyrosine hydroxylase immunoreactivity. These neurons are thought to synthesize dopamine (see text). Tyrosine hydroxylase immunoreactivity also is present within some small neurons in the deeper layers, but the mitral and internal tufted cells are not labeled. The locus ceruleus is the principal source of noradrenergic centrifugal afferents to the olfactory bulb, and the dorsal raphe nucleus is a source of serotonergic centrifugal afferents (see text). *Bar,* 250 μm.

centrated in the granule cell and internal plexiform layers of the main and accessory olfactory bulbs but also are present in the external plexiform layer and occasionally extend into the glomerular layer of the main olfactory bulb. On the basis of retrograde tracing studies employing injections of horseradish peroxidase (16,17,44,134) and tritiated serotonin (1,2) into the olfactory bulb, the serotonergic input appears to originate in the dorsal (Fig. 17c) and median raphe nuclei, with only a minor contribution, if any, from the other raphe cell groups (cf. 134). The serotonergic fibers are found throughout the deep layers and are prevalent in the glomerular layer.

The monoaminergic systems also have widespread projections to the piriform lobe (39,57–59,151,171) and, like the cholinergic system, could modulate the interactions among many of the olfactory and related limbic structures of the forebrain. Dopaminergic projections from the substantia nigra and ventral tegmental area to the piriform lobe have been reported to extend as far rostrally as the olfactory bulb (58). However, horseradish peroxidase injections that are restricted to the olfactory bulb have failed to demonstrate retrograde neuronal labeling in this subcortical region, and lesions that would be expected to interrupt these projections do not reduce the dopamine content of the olfactory bulb (cf. 134). The dopaminergic projections from this subcortical region to the olfactory system thus appear to become extremely sparse or be absent rostral to the retrobulbar area. Immunocytochemical findings suggest that catecholaminergic neurons are present in several other structures that support projections to the olfactory bulb, including the dorsal and median raphe nuclei, lateral and dorsal hypothalamus, medial septum/diagonal band complex, medial amygdaloid nucleus, dorsal peduncular cortex, ventral hippocampal rudiment, and anterior olfactory nucleus (cf. 43).

Recent studies in the rat using the immunofluorescence technique have provided evidence that intrinsic neurons of the main olfactory bulb synthesize dopamine (78–80,82,97,122). These neurons have been termed the A15 catecholamine cell group (cf. 122). Earlier studies indicated that small cells in the glomerular layer contain a catecholamine (39) and can accumulate exogenous norepinephrine (121). The immunofluorescence studies demonstrated that neurons in the glomerular layer and in the superficial regions of the external plexiform layer contain tyrosine hydroxylase and DOPA decarboxylase immunoreactivities but do not contain dopamine-β-hydroxylase immunoreactivity. These findings indicate that the neurons

can synthesize DOPA and convert it to dopamine but cannot convert the dopamine to norepinephrine. Electron microscopic analyses of serial sections have demonstrated that the tyrosine hydroxylase immunoreactivity is present in periglomerular cells and in superficially situated tufted cells (79). Thus, it appears that at least two distinct classes of intrinsic neurons synthesize dopamine. Autoradiographic studies similarly have shown that both periglomerular cells and superficially situated tufted cells accumulate catecholamines and precursors (80,192).

The reported incidences of dopamine-synthesizing periglomerular and tufted cells in the rat were rather low and appeared to favor the periglomerular cells. In a recent study in the hamster using the unlabeled antibody enzyme method, we similarly found that the incidence of tyrosine hydroxylase immunoreactive periglomerular cells is rather low (43). However, we found that the great majority of external tufted cells and many of the middle tufted cells contain tyrosine hydroxylase immunoreactivity (Fig. 17a). We also observed tyrosine hydroxylase immunoreactivity in some deep interneurons which appear to be primarily Van Gehuchten cells and small Golgi cells and in some tiny fusiform cells similar to the LHRH-immunoreactive plexus of neurons that extends into the olfactory bulb (see below). A recent study in the rat and mouse also has demonstrated a high incidence of tyrosine hydroxylase-positive neurons in the superficial layers, and a low incidence of labeling in small neurons of the deep layers (3a). Neither our studies in the hamster nor those in the rat and mouse have provided any evidence that mitral and internal tufted cells synthesize catecholamines. Thus, these deep output neurons appear to be functionally distinguishable from the superficially situated tufted cells on neurochemical grounds as well as on the morphological and connectional grounds discussed above. We rarely observe tyrosine hydroxylase immunoreactive neurons in the glomerular layer or external plexiform–mitral body layer of the accessory olfactory bulb. The latter observation is consistent with the low incidence of tyrosine hydroxylase immunoreactivity in periglomerular cells and the rarity or absence of tufted cells in the accessory olfactory bulb.

Luteinizing Hormone-Releasing Hormone

We recently reported a system of LHRH-immunoreactive neurons in the hamster that appear to be associated with the olfactory bulb (42,96). These observations have been confirmed and extended in several species of rodents (104,105, 174,216). The somata and processes of these neurons form plexes along the surface of the retrobulbar area and olfactory peduncle, i.e., in the vomeronasal and olfactory nerve layers and in layer IA of the anterior olfactory nucleus and ventral hippocampal rudiment. Although they are present in layer IA of the olfactory tubercle and anterior piriform cortex, the plexes are concentrated medially and extend caudally along the medial walls of the hemispheres in proximity to the main trunk and branches of the anterior cerebral artery. At the level at which the hemispheres join, the LHRH-immunoreactive somata and fibers are distributed within the medial septum/diagonal band complex.

In the hamster, but less so in the mouse and rat, a plexus of somata and fibers also extends rostrally from the septal region into the deep regions of the olfactory peduncle and retrobulbar area in proximity to the ependymal zone. The LHRH-immunoreactive neurons and fibers of this deep plexus extend medially into the granule cell layer of the main olfactory bulb and dorsally toward the accessory olfactory bulb but become extremely rare rostral to the retrobulbar area. Fibers from the superficial plexes enter the periglomerular regions of the main and accessory olfactory bulbs in the retrobulbar area and can be traced into the external plexiform layers but do not appear to reach the anterior regions of the main olfactory bulb. Radioimmunochemical findings similarly indicate that there is a much greater concentration of LHRH in the caudal half as compared to the rostral half of the olfactory bulb (50). Components of the superficial plexes remain associated with the vomeronasal and olfactory nerves and appear to pass through the cribriform plate. A recent study in the fetal guinea pig has demonstrated that the latter components do cross the cribriform plate and extend into the nasal epithelium and has provided compelling evidence that they are part of the nervus terminalis (216).

The LHRH-immunoreactive processes also are prevalent in olfactory cortical and related limbic structures of the piriform lobe, particularly in the amygdaloid regions that are associated with the accessory olfactory bulb (cf. 105,174). Dluzen et al. (51) have reported that female prairie voles exposed to a single drop of male urine on the snout show significant changes in the concentration of LHRH in the caudal olfactory bulb and that these changes are correlated with rapid elevations of serum luteinizing hormone in these induced ovulators. These various morphological and endocrinological findings have aroused considerable speculation that in addition to its direct role in mediating pituitary gonadotropin release, LHRH may play a neurotransmitter or neuromodulatory role in nasal chemoreception, in the effects of sex-related chemosensory stimuli on gonadotropin secretion, and/or in the effects of circulating hormones on the activity and evoked responses of neurons in the olfactory system.

Substance P

Moderate concentrations of substance P have been reported in the rat olfactory bulb (20,175). In the hamster, we have localized substance P immunoreactivity within intrinsic neurons of the main olfactory bulb and within centrifugal afferents (40,41,43). We have recently determined that the substance P immunoreactivity corresponds to the genuine undecapeptide (R. M. Kream, B. J. Davis, T. Kuwano, F. L. Margolis, and F. Macrides, *unpublished*), but to our knowledge the physiological actions of substance P in the olfactory bulb have not been studied.

The somata of the substance P-immunoreactive neurons are located exclusively in the periglomerular region and at the border between the glomerular and external plexiform layers (Fig. 18a). Their dendrites arborize within the glomeruli (Fig. 18b,c). Based on light microscopic comparisons between our immunocytochemical and Golgi material, the substance P-immunoreactive neurons appeared to be external tufted cells. Their somata were too large to be those of periglomerular cells, and the dendrites of superficial short-axon cells do not enter glomeruli (Fig. 9). Of course, we could not confirm that every substance P-immunoreactive neuron in the glomerular layer bears a dendrite with an intraglomerular arborization, and therefore, we could not exclude the possibility that superficial short-axon cells also might contain substance P immunoreactivity. However, our subsequent electron microscopic studies have confirmed that substance P immunoreactivity is present in external tufted cells, and we have found no ultrastructural evidence that it is present in periglomerular cells or in superficial short-axon cells (21,22). We find no substance P-immunoreactive neurons in the accessory olfactory bulb. The latter finding, together with the rarity of tyrosine hydroxylase-immunoreactive neurons (see above), provides neurochemical evidence that the accessory olfactory bulb contains few if any neurons that are functionally equivalent to the superficially situated tufted cells of the main olfactory bulb.

The incidence of substance P-immunoreactive

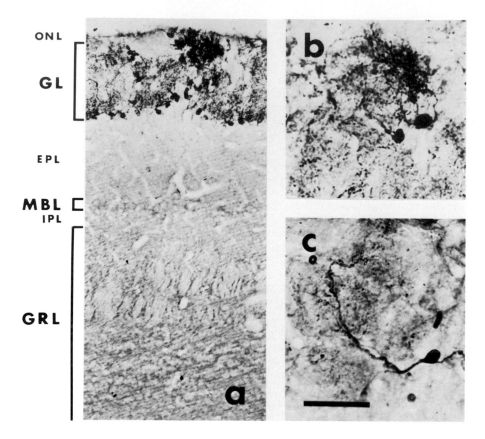

FIG. 18. Substance P-immunoreactive neurons in the main olfactory bulb of the hamster. Substance P immunoreactivity is localized within external tufted cells. It is also present in centrifugal afferents but has not been detected within any other class of intrinsic neurons (see text). *Bar,* 190 μm for **a**; 50 μm for **b** and **c**. (For abbreviations, see Fig. 1, legend.) (From Davis et al., ref. 41, with permission.)

external tufted cells in our material is less than the incidence of tyrosine hydroxylase-immunoreactive external tufted cells, but they are both sufficiently high to suggest that some of the external tufted cells may be catecholaminergic and may also contain substance P or a related compound. The middle tufted cells that contain tyrosine hydroxylase immunoreactivity do not appear to contain substance P. Using two independent antibodies raised against substance P (one purchased from Immuno-Nuclear Corporation and the other donated by Dr. Susan Leeman), we have failed to label middle tufted cells. Furthermore, pretreatment with colchicine (intended to block transport in neuronal processes) modestly increased the incidence of labeled tufted cells and resulted in more dense labeling of their somata but did not alter the laminar distributions of substance P or tyrosine hydroxylase immunoreactive neurons in the main olfactory

bulb. The superficially situated tufted cells thus appear to be heterogeneous populations on neurochemical grounds as well as on the morphological and connectional grounds discussed above.

The substance P-immunoreactive centrifugal fibers travel deep in the olfactory peduncle and enter the main and accessory olfactory bulbs. We also observe substance P-immunoreactive fibers in structures of the piriform lobe and in subcortical regions that are associated with the olfactory bulb. The most dense labeling is in the amygdaloid regions and in the locus ceruleus (Fig. 19a). Among the structures known to support centrifugal projections to the olfactory bulb, we observe unambiguous labeling of somata only in the dorsal (Fig. 19b) and median raphe nuclei. Recent studies have demonstrated that some raphe neurons contain both serotonin and substance P immunoreactivity (29,106). The possibility that this might also be true for some of the neurons in the dorsal or median raphe nuclei that project to the olfactory bulb merits investigation.

Glutamic and Aspartic Acid

Several lines of evidence suggest that glutamate and/or aspartate function as excitatory transmitters in the efferents of the olfactory bulb to the piriform cortex. Glutamate and aspartate exist in high concentrations in the piriform cortex (69,85,107). Their concentrations are reduced following olfactory bulbectomy or transection of the lateral olfactory tract, and these reductions occur preferentially in layer IA (13,69,85). Stimulation of the lateral olfactory tract produces calcium-dependent release of glutamate and aspartate (13,31,32,147,250,251). Both amino acids are excitatory on olfactory cortical neurons (33, 98,117,203). In contrast, the concentration of glycine in the piriform cortex is relatively low and does not appear to be affected by transections of the lateral olfactory tract (69). Although the differential distributions of efferent projections from mitral and tufted cells were not known or were not directly addressed in these studies, it is likely that their results deal predominantly with the efferents of mitral cells and the deeply situated tufted cells (see above). Glutamate and aspartate also are released from olfactory bulb synaptosomal fractions on electrical stimulation (168), as would be expected if these amino acids were transmitters in the intrinsic circuits of mitral and internal tufted cells. Furthermore, in isolated olfactory bulb preparations, application of glutamate results in pronounced hyperpolarization of mitral cells, and the hyperpolarization is prevented when synaptic transmission is blocked by cobalt (165). This finding is consistent with the hypothesis that glutamate is a transmitter in the dendrodendritic synapses of mitral cells onto inhibitory interneurons in the olfactory bulb.

Hori et al. (98) recently questioned the evidence that glutamate or aspartate serves as a transmitter in efferents of the olfactory bulb. They found that 2-amino-4-phosphonobutyric acid (APB), a presumed specific glutamate antagonist, blocked the field potentials and single-unit activity that are normally elicited in the piriform cortex by stimulation of the lateral olfactory tract. However, APB did not block the single-unit responses elicited by direct iontophoretic applications of glutamate or aspatate. Hori et al. suggested that these amino acids may be released at the same time as the endogenous transmitter but serve some role other than classical neurotransmission. Alternatively, they suggested that either of the amino acids might be the endogenous transmitter and that the postsynaptic neurons might have extrajunctional glutamate and aspartate receptors that are not sensitive to APB.

GABA

Extensive electrophysiological, morphological, and biochemical evidence supports the conclusion that GABA is an inhibitory transmitter in the dendrodendritic synapses of granule cells onto mitral and tufted cells (e.g., 3,149,163,167,168,194). This evidence has been well reviewed, most recently by Quinn and Cagan (194). In this section we briefly describe the immunocytochemical evidence for the synthesis of GABA by intrinsic neurons of the ol-

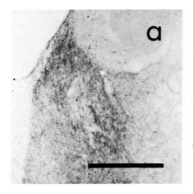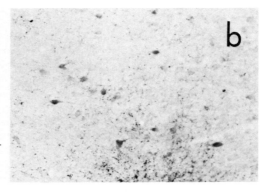

FIG. 19. Substance P immunoreactivity in sources of centrifugal afferents to the olfactory bulb. Numerous immunoreactive fibers but no labeled somata are present in the locus ceruleus (**a**). In contrast, many immunoreactive somata are present in the dorsal raphe nucleus (**b**). Some of the latter neurons may be the sources of substance P-immunoreactive centrifugal afferents in the olfactory bulb (see text). *Bar,* 150 μm.

factory bulb, and in the next section, we compare the distribution of GABA-synthesizing intrinsic neurons with the distribution of enkephalin-immunoreactive neurons.

Glutamate decarboxylase (GAD) synthesizes GABA and is the rate-limiting enzyme (204). Ribak and his colleagues (201,202) have localized GAD immunoreactivity within large proportions of both the granule cells and the periglomerular cells in the main olfactory bulb. Their ultrastructural studies have demonstrated that GAD immunoreactivity is present in the somata, dendritic shafts, and predominantly in the gemmules and spines of granule cells. The GAD immunoreactivity of periglomerular cells is distributed similarly throughout their cytoplasm and is concentrated in their dendritic spines. The dendrites and somata of mitral and tufted cells are devoid of GAD immunoreactivity. The distribution of GAD immunoreactivity in the accessory olfactory bulb was not examined. The somata of deep and superficial short-axon cells in the main olfactory bulb were not observed to contain GAD immunoreactivity. However, in contrast to the other types of neurons in the olfactory bulb, the short-axon cells do not have presynaptic dendrites, and in such neurons GAD tends to be concentrated in the axon terminals (248). Halász et al. (81,83) recently demonstrated selective neuronal uptake of tritiated GABA into granule cells and periglomerular cells, into some short-axon cells (particularly into their terminals), and into the terminals of some centrifugal afferents. As would be expected (cf. 73), most of the uptake was into glial cells and pericytes. It thus appears that most of the granule cells and periglomerular cells are GABAergic; some of the short-axon cells and centrifugal afferents might also be GABAergic, but the mitral and tufted cells are not.

Opioid Peptides

The presence of methionine-enkephalin in the olfactory bulb was first reported on the basis of radioimmunochemical measurements (253). Its presence recently has been confirmed in the mouse by a high-performance liquid chromatographic procedure (141). Enkephalin immunoreactivity has been localized within neuronal perikarya of the rat olfactory bulb using antibodies that react with both methionine- and leucine-enkephalin (12,62). Our studies in the hamster indicate that this immunoreactivity is relatively specific to methionine-enkephalin (40,41).

Both in the rat and in the hamster (Fig. 20a), enkephalin-immunoreactive neurons are widely distributed in the main olfactory bulb. Our electron microscopic studies in the hamster (21) have demonstrated that the enkephalin immunoreactivity in the glomerular layer is localized within the somata, dendritic shafts, and intraglomerular arbors of periglomerular cells. We have not found any evidence that it is present in external tufted cells, in the primary dendritic arbors of the deeper tufted cells and mitral cells, or in the peripheral afferents. Thus, whereas most of the external tufted cells and some of the periglomerular cells appear to be catecholaminergic, substance P and enkephalin immunoreactivities are distributed differently in these two broad classes of intrinsic neurons (see above). Furthermore, the incidence of enkephalin-immunoreactive periglomerular cells is extremely high (Fig. 20b), and it is therefore likely that methionine-enkephalin coexists with GABA or dopamine in some periglomerular cells.

In the deeper layers, enkephalin immunoreactivity similarly is associated with interneurons. Most of these neurons appear to be granule cells (Fig. 20c). Although the absolute number of labeled granule cells in our material is large, they represent a small percentage of the total number of granule cells in the main olfactory bulb. The enkephalin-immunoreactive granule cells could thus be an entirely different population from the GABAergic granule cells. We also observe enkephalin immunoreactivity within deep interneurons that clearly are not granule cells. They have dendritic morphologies similar to those of Van Gehuchten cells, Cajal cells, horizontal cells, and some small Golgi cells (e.g., neurons 6 and 8 in Fig. 7). The somata of the latter immunoreactive interneurons are smaller than those of Blanes cells and most Golgi cells. Thus, enkephalin appears to be present in many but not all categories of deep short-axon cells. Deep short-axon cells also have been reported to contain enkephalin immunoreactivity in the rat (12).

We rarely observe enkephalin-immunoreactive neurons in the glomerular layer of the accessory olfactory bulb. The few that have been observed are in tissue sections processed with anti-methionine-enkephalin and appear to be periglomerular cells. The granule cells of the accessory olfactory bulb are labeled routinely in sections processed with anti-methionine-enkephalin, and the percentage of labeled granule cells is similar to that in the main olfactory bulb. In addition, we routinely observe faint labeling of the mitral cells in the accessory olfactory bulb. The latter labeling is eliminated by prior adsorption of the antibody with synthetic methionine-enkephalin and is not present in sections processed with anti-leucine-enkephalin. In an autoradiographic study of opiate receptors, Herkenham

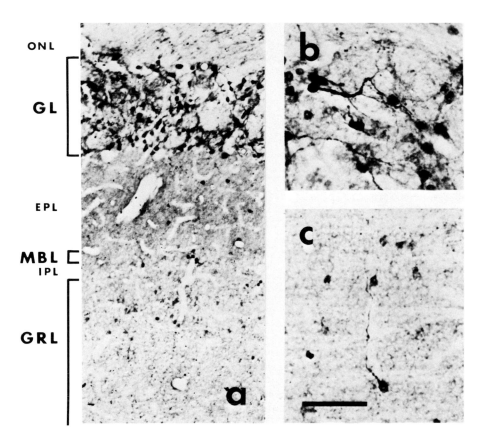

FIG. 20. Methionine-enkephalin-immunoreactive neurons in the main olfactory bulb of the hamster. The majority of periglomerular cells contain methionine-enkephalin immunoreactivity. This immunoreactivity also is present in a large number, but a relatively small percentage, of granule cells and in several classes of deep short-axon cells (see text). Methionine-enkephalin immunoreactivity has not been detected in the mitral or tufted cells of the main olfactory bulb. *Bar,* 190 μm for **a;** 50 μm for **b** and **c.** (For abbreviations, see Fig. 1, legend.) (From Davis et al., ref. 41, with permission.)

and Pert (91) observed particularly heavy ligand binding in the amygdaloid regions where the efferents of the accessory olfactory bulb have their terminal fields. They suggested that the mitral cells of the accessory olfactory bulb contain an opioid peptide. Although our observations might be interpreted as evidence that these output neurons contain methionine-enkephalin, the faintness of the reaction product under conditions that produce dense labeling of other neurons in the olfactory bulb makes us concerned that we are observing some form of cross reactivity. For example, we might be visualizing an endorphin-like compound. The reported concentrations of β-endorphin and β-lipotropin in the olfactory bulb are extremely low (193) but are based on the tissue weight of the entire olfactory bulb and probably a portion of the olfactory peduncle. Their concentrations would be

considerably higher if they were assumed to be located in the accessory olfactory bulb and the calculations were based on the tissue weight of the accessory olfactory bulb alone.

We also observe enkephalin immunoreactivity in centrifugal afferents and neuronal labeling in olfactory structures that support centrifugal projections to the main olfactory bulb (41). The most consistent labeling of somata occurs in pars externa and pars medialis of the anterior olfactory nucleus and in the ventral hippocampal rudiment (Fig. 21). We occasionally observe neuronal labeling in the medial amygdaloid nucleus, a source of centrifugal afferents to the accessory olfactory bulb. Enkephalin-immunoreactive neurons also have been reported in the medial amygdaloid nucleus of the rat (62). In our hamster material and in the rat (241), enkephalin-immunoreactive fibers

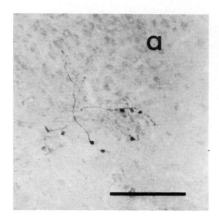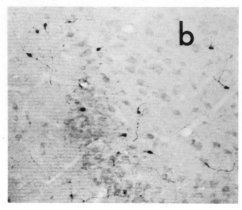

FIG. 21. Methionine-enkephalin immunoreactivity in sources of centrifugal afferents to the olfactory bulb. Many of the neurons in pars externa of the anterior olfactory nucleus contain methionine-enkephalin immunoreactivity. **Panel a** illustrates such neurons in the ventral sector of pars externa. Methionine-enkephalin-immunoreactive neurons also are common in pars medialis of the anterior olfactory nucleus and in the ventral hoppocampal rudiment. **Panel b** illustrates such neurons at a level corresponding to Fig. 4b. *Bar,* 150 μm

are present in the piriform cortex. Their distribution corresponds to the associational projections from pars medialis and the ventral hippocampal rudiment. These observations may help to explain the recent finding that bilateral olfactory bulbectomy results in a reduction of opiate ligand binding in the piriform cortex and that unilateral olfactory bulbectomy significantly reduces opiate ligand binding in the contralateral olfactory bulb (93). The lesions are likely to have involved the whole of the retrobulbar area and a portion of the olfactory peduncle, thereby interrupting the associational projections of pars medialis and the contralateral centrifugal projections of pars externa.

In summary, enkephalin immunoreactivity is present in many classes of intrinsic neurons that are known or suspected to utilize GABA as a transmitter. Enkephalin immunoreactivity also is associated with centrifugal afferents, and some centrifugal afferents have been shown to take up GABA. Enkephalin immunoreactivity and GABA are likely to coexist in periglomerular cells but could be distributed differentially in subclasses of granule cells and short-axon cells.

Somatostatin

Somatostatin is widely distributed in the olfactory system (8,18,19,41,61,206,226). Numerous neurons in the cellular regions of the olfactory peduncle and piriform cortex contain somatostatin immunoreactivity (Fig. 22). Many of these neurons are sources of centrifugal afferents. Their labeled axons can be traced into the anterior commissure and, in parasagittal sections, can be traced rostrally into the granule cell layer of the main olfactory bulb (41). Somatostatin-immunoreactive neurons are scattered throughout the vertical and horizontal limbs of the diagonal band (61,226). In our hamster material, these are not as plentiful as those in the olfactory cortical regions. The somatostatin-immunoreactive neurons in the diagonal band may be sources of centrifugal afferents (see above), but experimental procedures will be required to evaluate this possibility.

Somatostatin immunoreactivity also is present in intrinsic neurons of the main olfactory bulb (Fig. 23). These neurons are located exclusively in the granule cell layer. Based on comparisons with our

FIG. 22. Somatostatin-immunoreactive neurons in the olfactory cortical regions. Low-power (**a, c**) and companion high-power (**b, d**) photomicrographs illustrate somatostatin-immunoreactive neurons in the deep cellular regions. Many of these neurons are sources of somatostatin-immunoreactive centrifugal afferents in the olfactory bulb (see text). *Bar,* 500 μm for **a** and **c**; 150 μm for **b** and **d**.

FIG. 23. Somatostatin-immunoreactive neurons in the main olfactory bulb of the hamster. These neurons are located exclusively in the granule cell layer and appear to be large, deep short-axon cells (see text). *Bar,* 160 μm for **a**; 50 μm for **b** and **c**. (For abbreviations, see Fig. 1, legend.) (From Davis et al., ref. 41, with permission.)

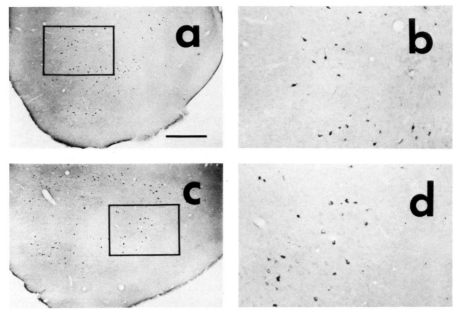

FIG. 22

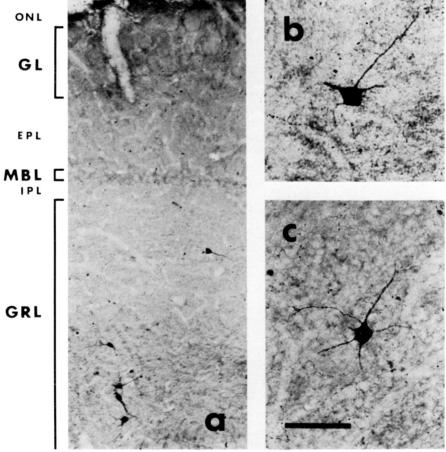

ONL
GL
EPL
MBL
IPL
GRL

FIG. 23

Golgi material (Fig. 7), they appear to be Blanes cells and/or large Golgi cells. Both in the olfactory bulb and in the olfactory cortical regions, the somatostatin-immunoreactive neurons have considerably larger somata than the enkephalin-immunoreactive neurons. In the olfactory cortices, the somata of enkephalin-immunoreactive neurons often lie in layer II and layer IB, whereas the somata of somatostatin-immunoreactive neurons are almost entirely restricted to layer III. The somatostatin- and enkephalin-immunoreactive neurons in the olfactory system thus appear to be morphologically distinct populations.

Somatostatin has been associated with the pancreas and may participate in the regulation of insulin secretion (154). It is interesting to note, therefore, that insulin has been reported to be present in the olfactory bulb of the rat at more than 30 times its concentration in plasma, and insulin immunoreactivity has been localized within intrinsic neurons (87). Although these neurons were not identified, in the published photomicrograph they appear to be granule cells. Electrophysiological studies in the rat have shown that during food deprivation the responses of single units in the olfactory bulb to food-related odors are selectively facilitated (170), and the facilitation can be simulated in sated rats by injections of insulin (25,181). Lesions of the anterior commissure and adjacent regions of the olfactory peduncle reduce the facilitation in the ipsilateral but not the contralateral olfactory bulb, indicating that the facilitation is mediated by centrifugal afferents (169). Based on the published illustrations of these lesions, they would be expected to have interrupted many of the somatostatin-immunoreactive projections to the olfactory bulb. Somatostatin thus might interact with insulin in regulating neuronal responses in the olfactory bulb. However, the presence of insulin in the central nervous system is controversial, and marked species differences have been reported (cf. 54).

Carnosine

In addition to neuropeptides that are widely distributed in the central nervous system, the olfactory system contains a relatively uncommon dipeptide. The concentrations of carnosine (β-alanyl-L-histidine) in the olfactory epithelium and olfactory bulb are 10 to 50 times greater than those in any other region of the forebrain (60,138). Biochemical and lesion studies in the mouse indicate that carnosine is synthesized by the peripheral olfactory receptor neurons. The levels of carnosine

and carnosine synthetase in the olfactory bulb decline rapidly following destruction of the olfactory receptor neurons and subsequent degeneration of their axons and terminals, whereas the level of carnosinase, the degradative enzyme for carnosine, is relatively unaffected (84,140). In a recent autoradiographic and biochemical study in the hamster (23), we found that following nasal irrigation with tritiated β-alanine, both the olfactory and vomeronasal receptor neurons took up the labeled precursor and transported the label in their axons to their terminals in the main (see Fig. 6a) and accessory olfactory bulbs, respectively. At 6 and 24 hr after the nasal irrigation, greater than 86% of the radioactivity in the olfactory bulb was present in carnosine, and less than 3% was present in macromolecules. Carnosine thus appears to be associated with the peripheral afferents of both the main and accessory olfactory systems. However, separate determinations of carnosine levels in the main and accessory olfactory bulbs have not been performed.

An extensive series of biochemical studies conducted by Margolis and his colleagues (cf. 138–140,142,143) suggests that carnosine is released in the olfactory bulb and may function as a transmitter or neuromodulator in the peripheral inputs. Depolarizing potassium concentrations cause release of carnosine from olfactory bulb synaptosomes, and this release is calcium dependent (205). Binding of carnosine to olfactory bulb membrane preparations is saturable, reversible, stereospecific, and occurs with high affinity at physiologically significant concentrations (94,95). The carnosine binding is localized to the glomerular layer (157). In our autoradiographic study with labeled precursor (23), we found that at the time of maximum labeling in the olfactory nerve and glomeruli, a moderate amount of labeling also was present in glial cells, pericytes, and in the ependymal zone, but no labeling was evident in the second-order neurons. This observation also suggests that carnosine is released from the nerve terminals and that its metabolites are cleared by nonneuronal elements as is thought to be the case for other neuropeptides (cf. 73).

The existing electrophysiological studies on the actions of carnosine in the olfactory bulb are difficult to interpret and illustrate some of the problems that are likely to be encountered in attempts to characterize the functions of putatively neuroactive compounds in this structure. In an extracellular single-unit study in the rat olfactory bulb (128), iontophoretic application of carnosine was reported to have either no obvious effect or variable and predominantly suppressive effects on the activity of antidromically identified output neurons. The injections were made at the recording sites, and, therefore, many of the injections were in the mitral body and external plexiform layers rather than in the glomerular layer where the peripheral afferents have their terminal fields. However, similar results were obtained using glomerular applications of carnosine in the gecko olfactory bulb (235). Based on analyses of averaged evoked and spontaneous slow potentials during injections of carnosine into the glomerular layer of the rabbit olfactory bulb, Gonzáles-Estrada and Freeman (72) concluded that carnosine has an excitatory action on the mitral and tufted cells and that this action is accompanied by a secondary increase in granule cell inhibitory activity. An increase in recurrent and lateral inhibition might explain the results of the extracellular single-unit studies.

However, using intracellular recording from mitral cells in isolated turtle and frog olfactory bulbs, Nicoll et al. (165) failed to observe any hyperpolarization or any initial depolarization following surface applications of carnosine. Under similar conditions, they found that glutamate does produce hyperpolarization (which is prevented when synaptic transmission is blocked by cobalt; see above), indicating that the recurrent and lateral inhibitory circuits onto mitral cells remain intact in these preparations. Also, orthodromic or antidromic stimulation excites mitral cells in these preparations, and the excitation is followed by inhibitory postsynaptic potentials. In the turtle preparations, they found that (D-Ala)^2-Met^5-enkephalinamide (DALA), a stable enkephalin analog, had little effect on the resting membrane properties of mitral cells but attenuated the inhibitory postsynaptic potentials elicited by orthodromic, antidromic, or direct depolarizing stimulation. This attenuation could be reversed by naloxone and was interpreted as a disinhibitory effect resulting from an inhibitory action of DALA on interneurons. Excitatory, inhibitory, and disinhibitory mechanisms that influence the activity of mitral cells thus appear to remain intact in these preparations, and the failure to observe an effect of carnosine is strong evidence that carnosine does not mediate classical neurotransmission in mitral cells.

On the other hand, Nowycky et al. (166) have recently shown in the isolated turtle olfactory bulb that when recurrent and lateral inhibition is blocked with bicuculline, orthodromic stimulation elicits a slow, long-lasting (i.e., up to 1,600 msec) depolarization in mitral cells that does not occur in response to antidromic stimulation. This might re-

flect a slow modulatory effect of carnosine release. Also, an appreciable number of single units did respond reliably to carnosine in the *in vivo* studies (see above). In the rat, carnosine was described as a "particularly effective inhibitor of periglomerular cells" (128, p. 187). Of 33 units categorized as periglomerular cells (i.e., units recorded in the glomerular layer that could not be driven antidromically), 24 (73%) were suppressed by carnosine, and none were excited. Of 52 units categorized as output neurons, 18 (35%) were suppressed, and 11 (21%) showed reliable increases in their activity. For reasons discussed above, it is likely that the units categorized as periglomerular cells were a mixed population of periglomerular and external tufted cells and that those categorized as output neurons predominantly were mitral cells and deeply situated tufted cells. Although this apparent trend toward a higher incidence of responses by the superficially situated neurons may have been caused by injections of carnosine closer to their synaptic junctions with the peripheral afferents, these findings, together with those in the *in vitro* studies, suggest that carnosine might not exert pronounced electrochemical effects on all classes of second-order neurons in the olfactory bulb or might have different effects on the various classes. Our studies in the hamster (cf. 41) indicate that the peripheral afferents, the periglomerular cells, and the external tufted cells form a triad of synaptically interacting neuronal elements each associated with a specific neuropeptide: carnosine, methionine-enkephalin, and substance P, respectively. It is intriguing to speculate that these neuropeptides might regulate the actions of classical neurotransmitters (e.g., GABA and dopamine) in the glomerular layer.

Other Putative Transmitters or Neuromodulators

High concentrations of CCK have been reported in the olfactory bulb and piriform lobe (7,116,200). A neuroactive molecular form of CCK is thus likely to be of major importance in the olfactory system. Similarly, TRH is likely to play a major role. The amount of TRH in the olfactory bulbs of the rat is 56% of that in the hypothalamus (112). Another neuropeptide that is abundant in the olfactory system is VIP. It is present in the olfactory bulb (56), and VIP-immunoreactive neurons have been localized throughout structures of the piriform lobe including the anterior olfactory nucleus, piriform cortex, amygdaloid regions, and entorhinal cortex (125). The immunoreactive neurons in the piriform and entorhinal cortices are concentrated in layer II and thus are likely to receive synaptic contacts from efferents of the olfactory bulb. Numerous neurons in layers II and III of the piriform cortex send centrifugal projections to the olfactory bulb (Fig. 14), as do many of the neurons in the anterior olfactory nucleus and in some amygdaloid regions (see above). Thus, like other neuropeptides (i.e., LHRH, substance P, methionine-enkephalin, and somatostatin) and several of the classical transmitter substances discussed above, VIP may be present in centrifugal afferents of the olfactory bulb. The parasympathetic innervation of the nasal epithelium also has been shown to contain VIP immunoreactivity, and VIP appears to coexist with acetylcholine in neurons of the sphenopalatine ganglion (126). Thus, VIP may interact with acetylcholine to regulate vascular and secretory processes in the nasal cavity and thereby may influence the access and egress of chemosensory stimuli (see above). Vasopressin also has been reported in the olfactory bulb, but in low concentrations (52).

This chapter has not exhausted the list of compounds that have been suggested as possible transmitters or neuromodulators in the olfactory bulb, and this list is still growing steadily. Indeed, based on the morphological and neurochemical organizations that we have discussed, virtually every transmitter substance and neuropeptide that is thought to play an important role in sensory, behavioral, neuroendocrine, or affective functions merits investigation in the olfactory bulb.

ACKNOWLEDGMENTS

Personal work reported here was supported by grant number NS12344 from the National Institutes of Health and by grants numbers BNS78-06248 and BNS81-18767 from the National Science Foundation.

REFERENCES

1. Araneda, S., Bobillier, P., Buda, M., and Pujol J. (1980): Retrograde axonal transport following injection of [³H]serotonin in the olfactory bulb. I. Biochemical study. *Brain Res.,* 196:405–415.
2. Araneda, S., Gamrani, H., Font, C., Calas, A., Pujol, J., and Bobillier, P. (1980): Retrograde axonal transport following injections of [³H] serotonin into the olfactory bulb. II. Radioautographic study. *Brain Res.,* 196:417–427.
3. Austin, L., Recasens, M., and Mandel, P. (1979): GABA in the olfactory bulb and olfactory nucleus of the rat: The distribution of γ-aminobutyric acid,

glutamic acid decarboxylase, GABA transaminase and succinate semialdehyde dehydrogenase. *J. Neurochem.,* 32:1473–1477.
3a. Baker, H., Kawano, T., Margolis, F. L., and Joh, T. H. (1983): Transneuronal regulation of tyrosine hydroxylase expression in olfactory bulb of mouse and rat. *J. Neurosci.,* 3:69–78.
4. Barber, P. C., and Field, P. M. (1975): Autoradiographic demonstration of afferent connections of the accessory olfactory bulb in the mouse. *Brain Res.,* 85:201–203.
5. Baumgarten, R. von, Bloom, F. E., Oliver, A. P., and Salmoiraghi, G. C. (1963): Response of individual olfactory nerve cells to microelectrophoretically administered chemical substances. *Pfluegers Arch.,* 227:125–140.
6. Beckstead, R. M. (1978): Afferent connections of the entorhinal area in the rat as demonstrated by retrograde cell-labeling with horseradish peroxidase. *Brain Res.,* 152:249–264.
7. Beinfeld, M. C., Meyer, D. K., Eskay, R. L., Jensen, R. T., and Brownstein. M. J. (1981): The distribution of cholecystokinin immunoreactivity in the central nervous system of the rat as determined by radioimmunoassay. *Brain Res.,* 212:51–57.
8. Bennett-Clarke, C., Romagnano, M. A., and Joseph, S. A. (1980): Distribution of somatostatin in the rat brain: Telencephalon and diencephalon. *Brain Res.,* 188:473–486.
9. Blanes, T. (1980): Sobre algunos puntos dudosos de la estructura del bulbo olfatorio. *Revta. Trimest. Microgr.,* 3:99–127.
10. Bloom, F. E., Baumgarten, R. von, Oliver, A. P., Costa, E., and Salmoiraghi, G. C. (1964): Studies of adrenergic mechanisms of rabbit olfactory neurons. *Life Sci.,* 3:131–136.
11. Bloom, F. E., Costa, E., and Salmoiraghi, G. C. (1964): Analysis of individual rabbit olfactory bulb neuron responses to the microelectrophoresis of acetylcholine, norepinephrine and serotonin synergists and antagonists. *J. Pharmacol. Exp. Ther.,* 146:16–23.
12. Bogan, N., Brecha, N., Gall, C., and Karten, H. J. (1982): Distribution of enkephalin-like immunoreactivity in the rat main olfactory bulb. *Neuroscience,* 7:895–906.
13. Bradford, H. F., and Richards, C. D. (1976): Specific release of endogenous glutamate from piriform cortex stimulated *in vitro. Brain Res.,* 105:168–172.
14. Broadwell, R. D. (1975): Olfactory relationships of the telencephalon and diencephalon in the rabbit. I. An autoradiographic study of the efferent connections of the main and accessory olfactory bulbs. *J. Comp. Neurol.,* 163:329–346.
15. Broadwell, R. D. (1975): Olfactory relationships of the telencephalon and diencephalon in the rabbit. II. An autoradiographic and horseradish peroxidase study of the efferent connections of the anterior olfactory nucleus. *J. Comp. Neurol.,* 164:389–410.
16. Broadwell, R. D. (1977): Neurotransmitter pathways in the olfactory system. In: *Society for Neuroscience Symposia. III. Aspects of Behavioral*

Neurobiology, edited by J. A. Ferrendelli and G. Gurvitch, pp. 131–166. Society for Neuroscience, Bethesda.

17. Broadwell, R. D., and Jacobowitz, D. M. (1976): Olfactory relationships of the telencephalon and diencephalon in the rabbit. III. The ipsilateral centrifugal fibers to the olfactory bulbar and retrobulbar formations. *J. Comp. Neurol.,* 170:321–346.

18. Brownstein, M. J. (1977): Biologically active peptides in the mammalian central nervous system. In: *Peptides in Neurobiology,* edited by H. Gainer, pp. 145–170. Plenum Press, New York.

19. Brownstein, M., Arimura, A., Sato, H., Schally, A. V., and Kizer, J. S. (1975): The regional distribution of somatostatin in the rat brain. *Endocrinology,* 96:1456–1461.

20. Brownstein, J., Mroz, A., Kizer, J., Palkovits, M., and Leeman, S. E. (1976): Regional distribution of substance P in the brain of the rat. *Brain Res.,* 116:299–305.

21. Burd, G. D., Davis, B. J., and Macrides, F. (1981): Ultrastructure of substance P and methionine–enkephalin immunoreactive neurons in the glomerular layer of the hamster olfactory bulb. *Soc. Neurosci. Abstr.,* 7:100.

22. Burd, G. D., Davis, B. J., and Macrides, F. (1982): Ultrastructural identification of substance P immunoreactive neurons in the main olfactory bulb of the hamster. *Neuroscience,* 7:2697–2704.

23. Burd, G. D., Davis, B. J., Macrides, F., Grillo, M., and Margolis, F. L. (1982): Carnosine in primary afferents of the olfactory system: An autoradiographic and biochemical study. *J. Neurosci.,* 2:244–255.

24. Cain, D. P. (1972): The role of the olfactory bulb in limbic mechanisms. *Psychol. Bull.,* 81:654–671.

25. Cain, D. P. (1975): Effects of insulin injection on responses of olfactory bulb and amygdala single units to odors. *Brain Res.,* 99:69–83.

26. Calleja, C. (1893): *La Región Olfactoria del Cerebro.* N. Moya, Madrid.

27. Callens, M. (1967): *Peripheral and Central Regulatory Mechanisms of the Excitability in the Olfactory System.* Editions Arscia S.A., Brussels.

28. Carson, K. A., and Burd, G. D. (1980): The localization of acetylcholinesterase in the main and accessory olfactory bulbs of the mouse by light and electronmicroscopic histochemistry. *J. Comp. Neurol.,* 191:358–371.

29. Chan-Palay, V. (1979): Combined immunocytochemistry and autoradiography after *in vivo* injections of monoclonal antibody to substance P and ³H-serotonin: Coexistence of two putative transmitters in single raphe cells and fiber plexuses. *Anat. Embryol.,* 156:241–254.

30. Chase, T. N., and Kopin, I. J. (1968): Stimulus-induced release of substances from olfactory bulb using the push–pull cannula. *Nature,* 217:466–467.

31. Collins. G. G. S. (1979): Evidence of a neurotransmitter role for aspartate and gamma-aminobutyric acid in the rat olfactory cortex. *J. Physiol. (Lond.),* 291:51–60.

32. Collins, G. G. S., Anson, J., and Probett, G. A. (1981): Patterns of endogenous amino acid release from slices of rat and guinea pig olfactory cortex. *Brain Res.,* 204:103–120.

33. Collins, G. G. S., and Probett, G. A. (1981): Aspartate and not glutamate is the likely transmitter of the rat lateral olfactory tract fibres. *Brain Res.,* 209:231–234.

34. Conrad, L. C. A., and Pfaff, D. W. (1976): Efferents from medial basal forebrain and hypothalamus in the rat. I. An autoradiographic study of the medial preoptic area. *J. Comp. Neurol.,* 189:185–220.

35. Costanzo, R. M., and Mozell, M. M. (1976): Electrophysiological evidence for a topographical projection of the nasal mucosa onto the olfactory bulb of the frog. *J. Gen. Physiol.,* 68:297–312.

36. Costanzo, R. M. and O'Connell, R. J. (1978): Spatially organized projections of hamster olfactory nerves. *Brain Res.,* 139:327–332.

37. Costanzo, R. M., and O'Connell, R. J. (1980): Receptive fields of second-order neurons in the olfactory bulb of the hamster. *J. Gen. Physiol.,* 76:53–68.

38. Cragg, B. G. (1962): Centrifugal fibres to the retina and olfactory bulb and composition of the supraoptic commissures in the rabbit. *Exp. Neurol.,* 5:406–427.

39. Dahlström, A., Fuxe, K., Olson, L., and Ungerstedt, U. (1965): On the distribution and possible function of monoamine nerve terminals in the olfactory bulb of the rabbit. *Life Sci.,* 4:2071–2074.

40. Davis, B. J., Burd, G. D., and Macrides, F. (1980): Distribution of met-enkephalin, substance P and somatostatin immunoreactive neurons in the main olfactory bulb in the hamster. *Soc. Neurosci. Abstr.,* 6:244.

41. Davis, B. J., Burd, G. D., and Macrides, F. (1982): Localization of methionine-enkephalin, substance P and somatostatin immunoreactivities in the main olfactory bulb of the hamster. *J. Comp. Neurol.,* 204:377–383.

42. Davis, B. J., and Macrides, F. (1981): The organization of centrifugal projections from the anterior olfactory nucleus, ventral hippocampal rudiment, and piriform cortex to the main olfactory bulb in the hamster: An autoradiographic study. *J. Comp. Neurol.,* 203:475–493.

43. Davis, B. J., and Macrides, F. (1983): Tyrosine hydroxylase immunoreactive neurons and fibers in the olfactory system of the hamster. *J. Comp. Neurol.,* 214:427–440.

44. Davis, B. J., Macrides, F., Youngs, W. M., Schneider, S. P., and Rosene, D. L. (1978): Efferents and centrifugal afferents of the main and accessory olfactory bulbs in the hamster. *Brain Res. Bull.,* 3:59–72.

45. Dennis, B. J., and Kerr, D. I. B. (1976): Origins of olfactory bulb centrifugal fibres in the cat. *Brain Res.,* 110:593–600.

46. DeOlmos, J., Hardy, H., and Heimer, L. (1978): The afferent connections of the main and the accessory olfactory bulb formations in the rat: An experimental HRP study. *J. Comp. Neurol.,* 181:213–244.

47. Devor, M. (1973): Components of mating dissociated by lateral olfactory tract transection in male
hamsters. *Brain Res.*, 64:437–441.

48. Devor, M. (1976): Fiber trajectories of olfactory
bulb efferents in the hamster. *J. Comp. Neurol.*,
166:31–48.

49. Divac, I. (1975): Magnocellular nuclei of the basal
forebrain project to neocortex, brain stem, and olfactory bulb. Review of some functional correlates.
Brain Res., 93:385–398.

50. Dluzen, D. E., and Ramirez, V. D. (1981): Presence
and localization of immunoreactive luteinizing hormone-releasing hormone (LHRH) within the olfactory bulbs of adult male and female rats. *Peptides*,
2:493–496.

51. Dluzen, D. E., Ramirez, V. D., Carter, C. S., and
Getz, L. L. (1981): Male vole urine changes luteinizing hormone-releasing hormone and norepinephrine in female olfactory bulb. *Science*, 212:573–
575.

52. Dogsterom, J., and Buijs, R. M. (1980): Vasopres-
sin and oxytocin distribution in rat brains: Radioim-
munoassay and immunocytochemical studies. In:
Neuropeptides and Neural Transmission, edited by
C. Ajmone and W. Z. Traczyk, pp. 307–314. Raven
Press, New York.

53. Domesick, V. B. (1978): Projections of the nucleus
of the diagonal band of Broca in the rat. *Anat. Rec.*,
184:391–392.

54. Dorn, A., Bernstein, H.-G., Hahn, H.-J., Ziegler,
M., and Rummelfänger, H. (1981): Insulin immunohistochemistry of rodent CNS: Apparent species
differences but good correlation with radioimmunological data. *Histochemistry*, 71:609–616.

55. Estes, R. D. (1972): The role of the vomeronasal
organ in mammalian reproduction. *Mammalia*,
36:315–341.

56. Fahrenkrug, J. (1980): Vasoactive intestinal polypeptide. *Trends Neurosci.*, 3:1–4.

57. Fallon, J. H., Koziell, D. A., and Moore, R. Y.
(1978): Catecholamine innervation of the basal
forebrain. II. Amygdala, suprarhinal cortex and entorhinal cortex. *J. Comp. Neurol.*, 180:509–532.

58. Fallon, J. H., and Moore, R. Y. (1978): Catecholamine innervation of basal forebrain. III. Olfactory
bulb, anterior olfactory nuclei, olfactory tubercle
and piriform cortex. *J. Comp. Neurol.*, 180:533–
544.

59. Fallon, J. H., and Moore, R. Y. (1978): Catecholamine innervation of the basal forebrain. IV. Topography of the dopamine projection to the basal
forebrain and neostriatum. *J. Comp. Neurol.*,
180:545–580.

60. Ferriero, D., and Margolis, F. L. (1975): Denerva-
tion in the primary olfactory pathway of mice. II.
Effects on carnosine and other amine compounds.
Brain Res., 94:75–86.

61. Finley, J. C. W., Grossman, G. H., Dimeo, P., and
Petrusz, P. (1978): Somatostatin-containing neurons in the rat brain: Widespread distribution revealed by immunocytochemistry after pretreatment
with pronase. *Am. J. Anat.*, 153:483–488.

62. Finley, J. C. W., Maderut, J. L., and Petrusz, P.
(1981): The immunocytochemical localization of

enkephalin in the central nervous system of the rat.
J. Comp. Neurol., 198:541–565.

63. Freeman, W. J. (1972): Depth recording of averaged evoked potentials of olfactory bulb. *J. Neurophysiol.*, 35:780–796.

64. Freeman, W. J. (1974): A model for mutual excitation in a neuron population in olfactory bulb.
IEEE Trans. Biomed. Eng., 21:358–364.

65. Freeman, W. J. (1974): Relation of glomerular
neuronal activity to glomerular transmission attenuation. *Brain Res.*, 65:91–107.

66. Freeman, W. J. (1974): Topographic organization
of primary olfactory nerve in cat and rabbit as
shown by evoked potentials. *Electroencephalogr.
Clin. Neurophysiol.*, 36:33–45.

67. Getchell, T. V., and Shepherd, G. M. (1975): Short
axon cells in the olfactory bulb: Dendrodendritic
synaptic interactions. *J. Physiol. (Lond.)*, 251:523–
548.

68. Getchell, T. V., and Shepherd, G. M. (1975): Synaptic actions on mitral and tufted cells elicited by
olfactory nerve volleys in the rabbit. *J. Physiol.
(Lond.)*, 251:497–522.

69. Godfrey, D. A., Ross, C. D., Carter, J. A., Lowry,
O. H., and Matschinsky, F. M. (1980): Effect of in-
tervening lesions on amino acid distributions in rat
olfactory cortex and olfactory bulb. *J. Histochem.
Cytochem.*, 28:1157–1169.

70. Godfrey, D. A., Ross, C. D., Herrmann, A. D., and
Matschinsky, F. M. (1980): Distribution and derivation of cholinergic elements in the rat olfactory
bulb. *Neuroscience*, 5:273–292.

71. Golgi, C. (1975): *Sulla Fina Struttura dei Bulbi
Olfacttori*. Reggio-Emilia, Rome.

72. González-Estrada, M. T., and Freeman, W. J.
(1980): Effects of carnosine on olfactory bulb EEG,
evoked potentials and DC potentials. *Brain Res.*,
202:373–386.

73. Grafstein, B.. and Forman, D. S. (1980): Intracellular transport in neurons. *Physiol. Rev.*, 60:1168–
1283.

74. Gurdjian, E. S. (1925): Olfactory connections in the
albino rat, with special reference to the stria medullaris and the anterior commissure. *J. Comp. Neurol.*, 38:127–163.

75. Haberly, L. B., and Price, J. L. (1977): The axonal
projection patterns of the mitral and tufted cells of
the olfactory bulb in the rat. *Brain Res.*, 129:152–
157.

76. Haberly, L. B., and Price, J. L. (1978): Association
and commissural fiber systems of the olfactory cortex of the rat. I. Systems originating in the piriform-
cortex and adjacent areas. *J. Comp. Neurol.*,
178:711–740.

77. Haberly, L. B., and Price, J. L. (1978): Association
and commissural fiber systems of the olfactory cortex of the rat. II. Systems originating in the olfactory peduncle. *J. Comp. Neurol.*, 181:781–808.

78. Halász, N., Hökfelt, T., Ljungdahl, Å., Johannson,
O., and Goldstein, M. (1977): Dopamine neurons in
the olfactory bulb. In: *Advances in Biochemical
Psychopharmacology*, Vol. 16, edited by E. Costa
and G. L. Gessa, pp. 169–177. Raven Press, New
York.

79. Halász, N., Johansson, O., Hökfelt, T., Ljungdahl, Å., and Goldstein, M. (1981): Immunohistochemical identification of two types of dopamine neurons in the rat olfactory bulb as seen by serial sectioning. *J. Neurocytol.,* 10:251–259.

80. Halász, N., Ljungdahl, Å., and Hökfelt, T. (1978): Transmitter histochemistry of the rat olfactory bulb. II. Fluorescence, histochemical, autoradiographic and electron microscopic localization of monoamines. *Brain Res.,* 154:253–271.

81. Halász, N., Ljungdahl, Å., and Hökfelt, T. (1979): Transmitter histochemistry of the rat olfactory bulb. III. Autoradiographic localization of ³H-GABA. *Brain Res.,* 167:221–240.

82. Halász, N., Ljungdahl, Å., Hökfelt, T., Johansson, O., Goldstein, M., Park, D., and Biberfeld, P. (1977): Transmitter histochemistry of the rat olfactory bulb. I. Immunohistochemical localization of monoamine synthesizing enzymes. Support for intrabulbar, periglomerular dopamine neurons. *Brain Res.,* 126:455–474.

83. Halász, N., Parry, D. M., Blackett, N. M., Ljungdahl, Å., and Hökfelt, T. (1981): [³H]γ-Aminobutyrate autoradiography of the rat olfactory bulb: Hypothetical grain analysis of the distribution of silver grains. *Neuroscience,* 6:473–479.

84. Harding, J., and Margolis, F. L. (1976): Denervation in the primary olfactory pathway of mice. III. Effect on enzymes of carnosine metabolism. *Brain Res.,* 110:351–360.

85. Harvey, J. A., Scholfield, L. T., Graham, L. T., and Aprison, M. H. (1975): Putative transmitter in denervated olfactory cortex. *J. Neurochem.,* 24:445–449.

86. Haubrich, D. R., and Denzer, J. S. (1973): Simultaneous extraction and fluoremetric measurement of brain serotonin, catecholamines, 5-hydroxyindoleacetic acid and homovanillic acid. *Anal. Biochem.,* 55:306–312.

87. Havrankova, J., Schemechel, D., Roth, J., and Brownstein, M. (1978): Identification of insulin in rat brain. *Proc. Natl. Acad. Sci. U.S.A.,* 75:5737–5741.

88. Heimer, L. (1968): Synaptic distribution of centripetal and centrifugal nerve fibers in the olfactory system of the rat. An experimental anatomical study. *J. Anat.,* 103:413–432.

89. Heimer, L. (1976): The olfactory cortex and the ventral striatum. In: *Limbic Mechanisms: The Continuing Evolution of the Limbic System Concept,* edited by K. E. Livingston and O. Hornykiewicz, pp. 95–189. Plenum Press, New York.

90. Heimer, L., Van Hoesen, G. W., and Rosene, D. L. (1977): The olfactory pathways and the anterior perforated substance in the primate brain. *Int. J. Neurol.,* 12:42–52.

91. Herkenham, M., and Pert, C. B. (1980): *In vitro* autoradiography of opiate receptors in rat brain suggests loci of "opiatergic" pathways. *Proc. Natl. Acad. Sci. U.S.A.,* 77:5532–5536.

92. Herrick, C. J. (1924): The nucleus olfactorius anterior of the opposum. *J. Comp. Neurol.,* 37:317–359.

93. Hirsch, J. D. (1980): Opiate and muscarinic ligand binding in five limbic areas after bilateral olfactory bulbectomy. *Brain Res.,* 198:271–283.

94. Hirsch, J. D., Grillo, M., and Margolis, F. L. (1978): Ligand binding studies in the mouse olfactory bulb: Identification and characterization of a L-[³H]carnosine binding site. *Brain Res.,* 158:407–422.

95. Hirsch, J. D., and Margolis, F. L. (1979): L-[³H]Carnosine binding in the olfactory bulb. II. Biochemical and biological studies. *Brain Res.,* 174:81–94.

96. Hoffman, G. E., Davis, B. J., and Macrides, F. (1979): LHRH perikarya send axons to the olfactory bulb in the hamster. *Soc. Neurosci. Abstr.,* 5:1779.

97. Hökfelt, T., Halász, N., Ljungdahl, Å., Johansson, O., Goldstein, M., and Park, D. (1975): Histochemical support for a dopaminergic mechanism in the dendrites of certain periglomerular cells in the rat olfactory bulb. *Neurosci. Lett.,* 1:85–90.

98. Hori, N., Auker, C. R., Braitman, D. J., and Carpenter, D. O. (1981): Lateral olfactory tract transmitter: Glutamate, aspartate or neither? *Cell. Mol. Neurobiol.,* 1:115–120.

99. Hunt, S., and Schmidt, J. (1977): Are mitral cells cholinergic? In: *Society for Neuroscience Symposia. III. Aspects of Behavioral Neurobiology,* edited by J. A. Ferrendelli and G. Gurvitch, pp. 204–218. Society for Neuroscience, Bethesda.

100. Ishii, Y. (1957): The histochemical studies of cholinesterase in the central nervous system of the rat. I. Normal distribution in rodents. *Arch. Histol. Jpn.,* 12:587–612.

101. Jacobowitz, D. M., and Palkovits, M. (1974): Topographic atlas of catecholamine and acetylcholinesterase-containing neurons in the rat brain. I. Forebrain (telencephalon, diencephalon). *J. Comp. Neurol.,* 157:13–28.

102. Jaffé, E. H., and Cuello, A. C. (1980): The distribution of catecholamines, glutamate decarboxylase and choline acetyltransferase in layers of the rat olfactory bulb. *Brain Res.,* 186:232–237.

103. Jahr, C. E., and Nicoll, R. A. (1980): Dendrodendritic inhibition: Demonstration with intracellular recording. *Science,* 207:1473–1475.

104. Jennes, L., and Stumpf, W. E. (1980): LHRH-neuronal projections to the inner and outer surface of the brain. *Neuroendocrinol. Lett.,* 4:241–245.

105. Jennes, L., and Stumpf, W. E. (1980): LHRH-systems in the brain of the golden hamster. *Cell Tissue Res.,* 209:239–256.

106. Johansson, O., Hökfelt, T., Pernow, B., Jeffcoate, S. L., White, N., Steinbusch, H. W. M., Verhofstad, A. A. J., Emson, P. C., and Spindel, E. (1981): Immunohistochemical support for three putative transmitters in one neuron: Coexistence of 5-hydroxytryptamine, substance P- and thyrotropin releasing hormone-like immunoreactivity in medullary neurons projecting to the spinal cord. *Neuroscience,* 6:1857–1881.

107. Johnson, J. L., and Aprison, M. H. (1971): The distribution of glutamate and total free amino acids in thirteen specific regions of the cat central nervous system. *Brain Res.,* 26:141–148.

108. Kauer, J. S. (1981): Olfactory receptor cell staining using horseradish peroxidase. *Anat. Rec.*, 200:331–336.

109. Kimura, H., McGeer, P. L., Peng, F., and McGeer, E. G. (1980): Choline acetyltransferase-containing neurons in rodent brain demonstrated by immunohistochemistry. *Science,* 208:1057–1059.

110. Koelliker, A. (1896): *Handbuch der Gewebelehre des Menschen,* Vol. 2. Verlag Wilhelm Englemann, Leipzig.

111. Kosel, K. C., Van Hoesen, G. W., and West, J. R. (1981): Olfactory bulb projections to the parahippocampal area of the rat. *J. Comp. Neurol.,* 198:467–482.

112. Krieder, M. S., Winokur, A., and Kreiger, N. R. (1981): The olfactory bulb in rich in TRH immunoreactivity. *Brain Res.,* 217:69–77.

113. Krettek, J. E., and Price, J. L. (1977): Projections from the amygdaloid complex and adjacent olfactory structures to the entorhinal cortex and to the subiculum in the rat and cat. *J. Comp. Neurol.,* 172:723–752.

114. Land, L. J. (1973): Localized projection of olfactory nerves to rabbit olfactory bulb. *Brain Res.,* 63:153–166.

115. Land, L. J., and Shepherd, G. M. (1974): Autoradiographic analysis of olfactory receptor projections in the rabbit. *Brain Res.,* 70:506–510.

116. Larsson, L.-I., and Rehfeld, J. F. (1979): Localization and molecular heterogeneity of cholecystokinin in the central and peripheral nervous system. *Brain Res.,* 165:201–218.

117. Legge, K. F., Randic, M., and Straughan, D. W. (1966): The pharmacology of neurons in the pyriform cortex. *Br. J. Pharmacol.,* 26:87–107.

118. LeGros Clark, W. E., and Meyer, M. (1947): The terminal connections of the olfactory tract in the rabbit. *Brain,* 70:304–328.

119. LeGros Clark, W. E. (1951): The projection of the olfactory epithelium on the olfactory bulb in the rabbit. *J. Neurol. Neurosurg. Psychiatry,* 14:1–10.

120. Lehmann. J., Nagy, J. I., Atmadja, S., and Fibiger, H. C. (1980): The nucleus basalis magnocellularis: The origin of a cholinergic projection to the neocortex of the rat. *Neuroscience,* 5:1161–1174.

121. Lichtensteiger, W. (1966): Uptake of norepinephrine in periglomerular cells of the olfactory bulb of the mouse. *Nature,* 210:955–956.

122. Ljungdahl, Å., Hökfelt, T., Halász, N., Johansson, O., and Goldstein, M. (1977): Olfactory bulb dopamine neurons—the A15 catecholamine cell group. *Acta. Physiol. Scand. [Suppl],* 452:31–35.

123. Lohman, A. H. M. (1963): The anterior olfactory lobe of the guinea pig. A descriptive and experimental anatomical study. *Acta Anat. (Basel), [Suppl.],* 49:1–109.

124. Lohman, A. H. M., and Mentink, G. M. (1969): The lateral olfactory tract, the anterior commissure and the cells of the olfactory bulb. *Brain Res.,* 12:396–413.

125. Lorén, I., Emson, P. C., Fahrenkrug, J., Björklund, A., Alumets, J., Hakannson, R., and Sundler, F. (1979): Distribution of vasoactive intestinal polypeptide in the rat and mouse brain. *Neuroscience,* 4:1953–1976.

126. Lundberg, J. M., Änggård, A., Emson, P., Fahrenkrug, J., and Hökfelt, T. (1981): Vasoactive intestinal polypeptide and cholinergic mechanisms in cat nasal mucosa: Studies on choline acetyltransferase and release of vasoactive intestinal polypeptide. *Proc. Natl. Acad. Sci. U.S.A.,* 78:5255–5259.

127. Luskin, M. B., and Price, J. L. (1982): The distribution of axon collaterals from the olfactory bulb and the nucleus of the horizontal limb of the diagonal band to the olfactory cortex, demonstrated by double retrograde labeling techniques. *J. Comp. Neurol.,* 209:249–263.

128. MacLeod, N. K., and Straughan, D. W. (1979): Responses of olfactory bulb neurons to the dipeptide carnosine. *Exp. Brain Res.,* 34:183–188.

129. Macrides, F. (1975): Temporal relationships between hippocampal slow waves and exploratory sniffing in hamsters. *Behav. Biol.,* 14:295–308.

130. Macrides, F. (1976): Olfactory influences on neuroendocrine functions in mammals. In: *Mammalian Olfaction, Reproductive Processes, and Behavior,* edited by R. L. Doty, pp. 29–65. Academic Press, New York.

131. Macrides, F. (1977): Dynamic aspects of central olfactory processing. In: *Chemical Signals in Vertebrates,* edited by D. Müller-Schwarze and M. M. Mozell, pp. 499–514. Plenum Press, New York.

132. Macrides, F., Bartke, A., Fernandez, F., and D'Angelo, W.(1974): Effects of exposure to vaginal odor and receptive females on plasma testosterone in the male hamster. *Neuroendocrinology,* 15:355–364.

133. Macrides, F., and Chorover, S. L. (1972): Olfactory bulb units: Activity correlated with inhalation cycles and odor quality. *Science,* 175:84–87.

134. Macrides, F., Davis, B. J., Youngs, W. M., Nadi, N. S., and Margolis, F. L. (1981): Cholinergic and catecholaminergic afferents to the olfactory bulb in the hamster: A neuroanatomical, biochemical and histochemical investigation. *J. Comp. Neurol.,* 203:497–516.

135. Macrides, F., Eichenbaum, H. B., and Forbes, W. B. (1982): Temporal relationship between sniffing and the limbic θ rhythm during odor discrimination reversal learning. *J. Neurosci.,* 2:1705–1717.

136. Macrides. F., Firl, A. C., Schneider, S. P., Bartke, A., and Stein, D. G. (1976): Effects of one-stage or serial transections of the lateral olfactory tracts on behavior and plasma testosterone levels in male hamsters. *Brain Res.,* 109:97–109.

137. Macrides, F., and Schneider, S. P. (1982): Laminar organization of mitral and tufted cells in the main olfactory bulb of the adult hamster. *J. Comp. Neurol.,* 208:419–430.

138. Margolis, F. L. (1975): Biochemical markers of the primary olfactory pathway: A model neural system. In: *Advances in Neurochemistry,* Vol. 1, edited by B. Agranoff and M. Aprison, pp. 193–246. Plenum Press, New York.

139. Margolis, F. L. (1977): Biochemical studies of the primary olfactory pathway. In: *Society for Neuroscience Symposia. III. Aspects of Behavioral Neurobiology,* edited by J. A. Ferrendelli and G. Gurvitch, pp. 167–188. Society for Neuroscience, Bethesda.

140. Margolis, F. L. (1980): Carnosine: An olfactory

neuropeptide. In: *Role of Peptides in Neuronal Function,* edited by J. L. Barker and T. Smith, pp. 545–572. Marcel Dekker, New York.

141. Margolis, F. L. (1981): Neurotransmitter biochemistry of the mammalian olfactory bulb. In: *Biochemistry of Taste and Olfaction,* edited by R. Cagan, pp. 369–394. Academic Press, New York.

142. Margolis, F. L., and Grillo, M. (1977): Axoplasmic transport of carnosine (β-alanyl-L-histidine) in the mouse olfactory pathway. *Neurochem. Res.,* 2:507–519.

143. Margolis, F. L., Keller, A., and Ferriero, D. (1975): The olfactory pathway as a model cerebral system. In: *Metabolic Compartmentation and Neurotransmission,* edited by S. Berl, D. D. Clarke, and D. Schneider, pp. 137–143. Plenum Press, New York.

144. Marques, D. M., O'Connell, R. J., Benimoff, N., and Macrides, F. (1982): Delayed deficits in behavior after transections of the olfactory tracts in hamsters. *Physiol. Behav.,* 28:353–365.

145. Mascitti, T. A., and Ortega, S. N. (1966): Efferent connection of the olfactory bulb in the cat. An experimental study with silver impregnation methods. *J. Comp. Neurol.,* 127:121–136.

146. Mascitti, T. A., Vaccarezza, R. R., Caruso, R. C., and Pavia, M. A. (1971): Centrifugal olfactory fibers in the cat. I. Site of termination. An experimental study with silver impregnation methods. *Acta Physiol. Lat. Am.,* 21:216–228.

147. Matsui, S., and Yamamoto, C. (1975): Release of radioactive glutamic acid from thin sections of guinea-pig olfactory cortex *in vitro. J. Neurochem.,* 24:245–250.

148. McCotter, R. E. (1912): The connection of the vomeronasal nerves with the accessory olfactory bulb in the opposum and other mammals. *Anat. Rec.,* 6:299–318.

149. McLennan, H. (1971): The pharmacology of inhibition of mitral cells in the olfactory bulb. *Brain Res.,* 29:177–184.

150. Meredith, M., and O'Connell, R. J. (1979): Efferent control of stimulus access to the hamster vomeronasal organ. *J. Physiol. (Lond.),* 286:301–316.

151. Moore, R. Y. (1978): Catecholamine innervation of the basal forebrain. I. The septal area. *J. Comp. Neurol.,* 177(4):655–681.

152. Mori, K., and Takagi, S. F. (1978): An intracellular study of dendrodendritic inhibitory synapses on mitral cells in the rabbit olfactory bulb. *J. Physiol. (Lond.),* 279:569–588.

153. Mori, K., Nowycky, M. C., and Shepherd, G. M. (1981): Electrophysiological analysis of mitral cells in the isolated turtle olfactory bulb. *J. Physiol. (Lond.),* 314:281–294.

154. Mortimer, C. H. (1977): Growth-hormone release-inhibiting hormone (GH-RIH, somatostatin). In: *Clinical Neuroendocrinology,* edited by L. Martini and G. M. Besser, pp. 279–294. Academic Press, New York.

155. Mozell, M. M., and Jagodowicz, M. (1973): Chromatographic separation of odorants by the nose: Retention times measured across *in vivo* olfactory mucosa. *Science,* 191:1247–1249.

156. Nachbar, R. B., and T. H. Morton (1981): A gas chromatographic (GLPC) model for the sense of smell. Variation of olfactory sensitivity with conditions of stimulation. *J. Theor. Biol.,* 89:387–407.

157. Nadi, N. S., Hirsch, J. D., and Margolis, F. L. (1980): Laminar distribution of putative neurotransmitter amino acids and ligand sites in the dog olfactory bulb. *J. Neurochem.,* 34:138–146.

158. Nakashima, M., Mori, K., and Takagi, S. (1978): Centrifugal influence on olfactory bulb activity in the rabbit. *Brain Res.,* 154:301–316.

159. Nandy, K. (1965): Histochemical study of the olfactory bulb in the rodent. *Ann. Histochem.,* 10:245–256.

160. Negus, V. (1958): *The Comparative Anatomy and Physiology of the Nose and Paranasal Sinuses.* Churchill Livingston, Edinburgh.

161. Nicoll, R. A. (1969): Inhibitory mechanisms in the rabbit olfactory bulb: Dendrodendritic mechanisms. *Brain Res.,* 14:157–172.

162. Nicoll, R. A. (1970): Identification of tufted cells in the olfactory bulb. *Nature,* 227:623–625.

163. Nicoll, R. A. (1971): Pharmacological evidence for GABA as the transmitter in granule cell inhibition in the olfactory bulb. *Brain Res..* 35:137–149.

164. Nicoll, R. A. (1972): Olfactory nerves and their excitatory action in the olfactory bulb. *Exp. Brain Res.,* 14:185–197.

165. Nicoll, R. A., Alger, B. E., and Jahr, C. E. (1980): Peptides as putative excitatory neurotransmitters: Carnosine, enkephalin, substance P and TRH. *Proc. R. Soc. Lond. [Biol.],* 210:133–149.

166. Nowycky, M. C., Mori, K., and Shepherd, G. M. (1981): Blockade of synaptic inhibition reveals long-lasting synaptic excitation in isolated turtle olfactory bulb. *J. Neurophysiol.,* 46:649–658.

167. Nowycky, M. C., Mori, K., and Shepherd, G. M. (1981): GABAergic mechanisms of dendrodendritic synapses in isolated turtle olfactory bulb. *J. Neurophysiol.,* 46:639–648.

168. Osborne, R. H., Duce, I. R., and Keer, P. (1976): Amino acids in "light" and "heavy" synaptosome fractions from rat olfactory lobes and their release by electrical stimulation. *J. Neurochem.,* 27:1483–1488.

169. Pager, J. (1974): A selective modulation of olfactory input suppressed by lesions of the anterior limb of the anterior commissure. *Physiol. Behav.,* 13:523–526.

170. Pager, J., Giachetti, I., Holley, A., and LeMagnen, J. (1972): A selective control of olfactory bulb electrical activity in relation to food deprivation and satiety in rats. *Physiol. Behav.,* 9:573–579.

171. Palkovits, M., Záborszky, L., Brownstein, M. J., Fekete, M. I. K., Herman, J. P., and Kanyicska, B. (1979): Distribution of norepinephrine and dopamine in cerebral cortical areas of the rat. *Brain Res. Bull.,* 4:593–601.

172. Pfaff, D. W., and Gregory, E. (1971): Olfactory coding in olfactory bulb and medial forebrain bundle of normal and castrated male rats. *J. Neurophysiol.,* 34:208–216.

173. Phillips, C. G., Powell, T. P. S., and Shepherd, G. M. (1963): Responses of mitral cells to stimulation of the lateral olfactory tract in the rabbit. *J. Physiol. (Lond.),* 168:65–88.

174. Phillips, H. S., Hostetter, G., Kerdelhue, B., and Kozlowski, G. P. (1980): Immunocytochemical localization of LHRH in central olfactory pathways of hamster. *Brain Res.,* 193:574–579.

175. Phillis, J. W. (1980): Substance P in the central nervous system. In: *The Role of Peptides in Neuronal Function,* edited by J. L. Barker and T. G. Smith, Jr., pp. 615–652. Marcel Dekker, New York.

176. Pinching, A. J. (1972): Spatial aspects of the neuronal connections in the rat olfactory bulb. In: *Olfaction and Taste IV. Proceedings of the Fourth International Symposium,* edited by D. Schneider, pp. 40–48. Wissenschaftliche, Stuttgart.

177. Pinching, A. J., and Powell, T. P. S. (1971): The neuron types of the glomerular layer of the olfactory bulb. *J. Cell. Sci.,* 9:305–345.

178. Pinching, A. J., and Powell, T. P. S. (1971): The neuropil of the glomeruli of the olfactory bulb. *J. Cell. Sci.,* 9:347–377.

179. Pinching, A. J., and Powell, T. P. S. (1971): The neuropil of the periglomerular region of the olfactory bulb. *J. Cell. Sci.,* 9:379–409.

180. Pinching, A. J., and Powell, T. P. S. (1972): The terminations of the centrifugal fibres in the glomerular layer of the olfactory bulb. *J. Cell. Sci.,* 10:621–625.

181. Potter, H. (1977): The role of nucleus basalis in olfactory bulb responses to odors in rabbits. *Soc. Neurosci. Abstr.,* 3:82.

182. Powers, J. B., Fields, R. B., and Winans, S. S. (1979): Olfactory and vomeronasal system participation in male hamster's attraction to female vaginal secretions. *Physiol. Behav.,* 22:77–84.

183. Price, J. L. (1968): The termination of centrifugal fibers in the olfactory bulb. *Brain Res.,* 7:483–486.

184. Price, J. L. (1969): The origin of the centrifugal fibers to the olfactory bulb. *Brain Res.,* 14:542–545.

185. Price, J. L. (1973): An autoradiographic study of complementary laminar patterns of termination of afferent fibers to the olfactory cortex. *J. Comp. Neurol.,* 150:87–108.

186. Price, J. L., and Powell, T. P. S. (1970): An electron microscopic study of the termination of the afferent fibres to the olfactory bulb from the cerebral hemisphere. *J. Cell Sci.,* 7:157–187.

187. Price, J. L., and Powell, T. P. S. (1970): An experimental study of the origin and the course of the centrifugal fibres to the olfactory bulb in the rat. *J. Anat.,* 107:215–237.

188. Price, J. L., and Powell, T. P. S. (1970): The mitral and short axon cells of the olfactory bulb. *J. Cell Sci.,* 7:631–651.

189. Price, J. L., and Powell, T. P. S. (1970): The morphology of the granule cells of the olfactory bulb. *J. Cell Sci.,* 7:91–123.

190. Price, J. L., and Powell, T. P. S. (1970): The synaptology of the granule cells of the olfactory bulb. *J. Cell Sci.,* 7:125–155.

191. Price, J. L., and Sprich, W. W. (1975): Observations on the lateral olfactory tract of the rat. *J. Comp. Neurol.,* 162:321–336.

192. Priestly, J. V., Kelly, J. S., and Cuello, A. C.

(1979): Uptake of (^{3}H)dopamine in periglomerular cells of the rat olfactory bulb: An autoradiographic study. *Brain Res.,* 165:149–155.

193. Przewlocki, R., Gramsch, C., Höllt, V., Millon, M. J., Osborne, H., and Herz, A. (1980): The distribution and release of β-endorphin in relation to certain possible functions. In: *Neuropeptides and Neurotransmission,* edited by C. Ajmone and W. Z. Traczk, pp. 245–256. Raven Press, New York.

194. Quinn, M. R., and Cagan, R. H. (1981): Neurochemical studies of the γ-aminobutyric acid system in the olfactory bulb. In: *Biochemistry of Taste and Olfaction,* edited by R. H. Cagan and M. R. Kare, pp. 395–415. Academic Press, New York.

195. Rall, W., Shepherd, G. M., Reese, T. S., and Brightman, M. W. (1966): Dendrodendritic synaptic pathway for inhibition in the olfactory bulb. *Exp. Neurol.,* 14:44–56.

196. Ramon-Moliner, E. (1977): The reciprocal synapses of the olfactory bulb: Questioning the evidence. *Brain Res.,* 128:1–20.

197. Ramon y Cajal, S. (1890): Origen y terminación de las fibres nerviosas olfactorias. *Gac. Sanit. Barcelona,* pp. 133–212.

198. Ramon y Cajal, S. (1911): *Histologie du Systeme Nerveux de l'Homme et des Vertebres.* Maloine, Paris.

199. Ramon y Cajal, S. (1955): *Studies on the Cerebral Cortex (Limbic Structures),* translated by L. M. Kraft. Year Book Publishers, Chicago.

200. Rehfeld, J. F. (1978): Immunochemical studies on cholecystokinin. II. Distribution and molecular heterogeneity in the central nervous system and small intestine of man and hog. *J. Biol. Chem.,* 253:4022–4030.

201. Ribak, C. E. (1977): The GABAergic neurons of the olfactory bulb in the rat. In: *Society for Neuroscience Symposia. III. Aspects of Behavioral Neurobiology,* edited by J. A. Ferrendelli and G. Gurvitch, pp. 189–203. Society for Neuroscience, Bethesda.

202. Ribak, C. E., Vaughn, J. E., Saito, K., Barber, R., and Roberts, E. (1977): Glutamate decarboxylase localization in neurons of the olfactory bulb. *Brain Res.,* 126:1–18.

203. Richards, C. D., Russell, W. J., and Smaje, J. C. (1975): The action of ether and methoxyflorane on synaptic transmission in isolated preparations of the mammalian cortex (guinea-pig). *J. Physiol. (Lond.),* 248:121–142.

204. Roberts, E., and Kuriyama, K. (1968): Biochemical-physiological correlations in studies of the γ-aminobutyric acid system. *Brain Res.,* 8:1–35.

205. Rochel, S., and Margolis, F. L. (1982): Carnosine release from olfactory bulb synaptosomes is calcium dependent and depolarization stimulated. *J. Neurochem.,* 38:1505–1514.

206. Rorstad, O. P., Martin, J. C., and Terry, L. C. (1980): Somatostatin and the nervous system. In: *The Role of Peptides in Neuronal Function,* edited by J. L. Barker and T. G. Smith, Jr., pp. 573–614. Marcel Dekker, New York.

207. Rosene, D. L., and Heimer, L. (1977): Olfactory

bulb efferents in the rhesus monkey. *Anat. Rec.*, 187–698.

208. Rosene, D. L., Heimer, L., and Van Hoesen, G. W. (1978): Centrifugal efferents to the olfactory bulb in the rhesus monkey. *Proc. Soc. Neurosci.*, 4:91.

209. Salmoiraghi, G. C., Bloom, F. E., and Costa, E. (1964): Adrenergic mechanisms in rabbit olfactory bulb. *Am J. Physiol.*, 207:1417–1424.

210. Scalia, F. (1968): A review of recent experimental studies on the distribution of the olfactory tracts in mammals. *Brain Behav. Evol.*, 1:101–123.

211. Scalia, F. (1966): Some olfactory pathways in the rabbit brain. *J. Comp. Neurol.*, 126:285–310.

212. Scalia, F., and Winans, S. S. (1975): The differential projections of the olfactory bulb and accessory olfactory bulb in mammals. *J. Comp. Neurol.*, 161:31–56.

213. Scalia, F., and Winans, S. S. (1976): New Perspectives on the morphology of the olfactory system: Olfactory and vomeronasal pathways in mammals. In: *Mammalian Olfaction, Reproductive Processes, and Behavior*, edited by R. L. Doty, pp. 8–28. Academic Press, New York.

214. Scheibel, M. E., and Scheibel, A. B. (1975): Dendritic bundles, central programs and the olfactory bulb. *Brain Res.*, 95:407–421.

215. Schneider, S. P., and Macrides, F. (1978): Laminar distributions of interneurons in the main olfactory bulb of the adult hamster. *Brain Res. Bull.*, 3(1):73–82.

216. Schwanzel-Fukuda, M., and Silverman, A. J. (1980): The nervus terminalis of the guinea pig: A new luteinizing hormone-releasing hormone (LHRH) neuronal system. *J. Comp. Neurol.*, 191:213–225.

217. Scott, J. W. (1981): Electrophysiological identification of mitral and tufted cells and distributions of their axons in olfactory system of the rat. *J. Neurophysiol.*, 46:918–931.

218. Scott, J. W., McBride, R. L., and Schneider, S. P. (1980): The organization of projections to the piriform cortex and olfactory tubercle in the rat. *J. Comp. Neurol.*, 194:519–534.

219. Shafa, F., and Meisami, E. (1977): A horseradish peroxidase study of the origin of central projections to the rat olfaction *(sic)* bulb. *Brain Res.*, 136:355–359.

220. Shammah-Lagnado, S. J., and Negrão, N. (1981): Efferent connections of the olfactory bulb in the opossum *(Didelphis marsupialis aurita)*: A. Fink-Heimer study. *J. Comp. Neurol.*, 201:51–63.

221. Sharma, N. N. (1968): Studies on the histochemical distribution of simple esterase and cholinesterases in the olfactory bulb of the rat. *Acta Anat.*, 69:168–175.

222. Shepherd, G. M. (1970): The olfactory bulb as a simple cortical system: Experimental analysis and functional implications. In: *The Neurosciences: Second Study Program*, edited by F. O. Schmitt, pp. 539–552. Rockefeller University Press, New York.

223. Shepherd, G. M. (1971): Physiologic evidence for dendrodendritic synaptic interactions in the rabbit's olfactory glomerulus. *Brain Res.*, 32:212–217.

224. Shepherd, G. M. (1972): Synaptic organization of the mammalian olfactory bulb. *Physiol Rev.*, 52:864–917.

225. Shepherd, G. M., and Haberly, L. B. (1970): Partial activation of olfactory bulb: Analysis of field potentials and topographical relation between bulb and lateral olfactory tract. *J. Neurophysiol.*, 33:643–653.

226. Shiosaka, S., Takatsuki, K., Sakanaka, M., Inagaki, S., Takagi, H., Senba, E., Kawai, Y., Iida, H., Minagawa, H., Hara, Y., Matsuzaki, T., and Tohyama, M. (1982): Ontogeny of somatostatin-containing neuron systems of the rat: Immunohistochemical analysis. II. Forebrain and diencephalon. *J. Comp. Neurol.*, 204:211–224.

227. Shute, C. C. D., and Lewis, P. R. (1967): The ascending cholinergic reticular system: Neocortical, olfactory and subcortical projections. *Brain*, 90:497–520.

228. Skeen, L. C., and Hall, W. C. (1977): Efferent projections of the main and accessory olfactory bulb in the tree shrew *(Tupaia glis)*. *J. Comp. Neurol.*, 172:1–36.

229. Steward, O. (1976): Topographical organization of the projections from the entorhinal area to the hippocampal formation of the rat. *J. Comp. Neurol.*, 167:285–314.

230. Steward, O., and Scoville, S. A. (1976): Cells of origin of entorhinal cortical afferents to the hippocampus and fascia dendata of the rat. *J. Comp. Neurol.*, 169:347–370.

231. Stone, J., Dreher, B., and Leventhal, A. (1979): Hierarchical and parallel mechanisms in the organization of visual cortex. *Brain Res. Rev.*, 1:345–394.

232. Swanson, L. W. (1976): An autoradiographic study of the efferent connections of the preoptic region in the rat. *J. Comp. Neurol.*, 167:227–256.

233. Swanson, L. W., and Cowan, W. M. (1977): An autoradiographic study of the organization of the efferent connections of the hippocampal formation in the rat. *J. Comp. Neurol.*, 172:49–84.

234. Tucker, D. (1963): Physical variables in the olfactory stimulation process. *J. Gen. Physiol.*, 46:453–489.

235. Tonosaki, K., and Shibuya, T. (1979): Action of some drugs on gecko olfactory bulb mitral cell responses to odor stimulation. *Brain Res.*, 167:180–184.

236. Turner, B. H., Gupta, K. C., and Mishkin, M. (1978): The locus and cytoarchitecture of the projection areas of the olfactory bulb in *Macaca mulatta*. *J. Comp. Neurol.*, 177:381–396.

237. Turner, B. H., Gupta, K., Mishkin, M., and Kapp, M. (1977): The projections of the olfactory bulb in the monkey *(Macaca mulatta)*. *Anat. Rec.*, 187:733.

238. Valverde, F. (1964): The commissura anterior, pars bulbaris. *Anat. Rec.*, 148:406–407.

239. Valverde, F. (1965): *Studies on the Piriform Lobe*. Harvard University Press, Cambridge.

240. Van Gehuchten, A., and Martin, I. (1891): Le bulbe olfactif chez quelques mammiferes. *La Cellule*, 5:205–237.

241. Wamsley, J. K., Young, W. S., III, and Kuhar, M.

J. (1980): Immunohistochemical localization of enkephalin in rat forebrain. *Brain Res.,* 190:153–174.

242. Wenk, H., Meyer, U., and Bigl, V. (1976): Zur Histochemie cholinerger Systeme im ZNS. II. Topo-
chemische und quantitative Veränderungen cholinerger Transmitter-enzyme (AChE, ChAc) im
olfactorischen System bei Ratten nach Zwischen-
hirnläsion. *Z. Mikrosk. Anat. Forsch.,* 90:940–
958.

243. Wenk, H., Meyer, U., and Bigl, V. (1977): Centrifugal cholinergic connections in the olfactory system
of rats. *Neuroscience,* 2:797–800.

244. Wenk, H., Ritter, J., and Meyer, V. (1975): Histochemistry of cholinergic systems in the CNS. I.
Topochemical and quantitative changes in acetylcholinesterase activity in the limbic cortex after
septal lesions in the rat. *Acta Histochem.,* 53:77–
92.

245. White, E. L. (1973): Synaptic organization of the
mammalian olfactory glomerulus: New findings including an intraspecific variation. *Brain Res.,*
60:299–313.

246. White, L. E., Jr. (1965): Olfactory bulb projections
of the rat. *Anat. Rec.,* 152:465–480.

247. Willey, T. J. (1973): The ultrastructure of the cat
olfactory bulb. *J. Comp. Neurol.,* 152:211–232.

248. Wood, J. G., McLaughlin, B. J., and Vaughn, J. E.
(1975): Immunocytochemical localization of GAD
in electron microscopic preparations of rodent
CNS. In: *GABA in Nervous System Function,* edited by E. Roberts, T. N. Chase, and D. B. Tower,
pp. 133–148. Raven Press, New York.

249. Wysocki, C. J., Wellington, J. L., and Beauchamp,
G. K. (1980): Access of urinary nonvolatiles to the
mammalian vomeronasal organ. *Science,* 207:781–
783.

250. Yamamoto, C., and Matsui, S. (1974): Facilitated
release of glutamic acid from olfactory cortex slices
by stimulation of excitatory input. *Proc. Jpn.
Acad.,* 50:653–657.

251. Yamamoto, C., and Matsui, S. (1976): Effect of
stimulation of excitatory nerve tract on release of
glutamic acid from olfactory cortex slices *in vitro.
J. Neurochem.,* 26:487–491.

252. Yamamoto, C., Yamamoto, Y., and Iwana, K.
(1963): The inhibitory systems in the olfactory bulb
studied by intracellular recording. *J. Neurophysiol.,* 26:403–415.

253. Yang, H. Y., Hong, J. S., Fratin, W., and Costa, E.
(1978): Rat brain enkephalins: Distribution and
biosynthesis. *Adv. Biochem. Psychopharmacol.,*
18:149–159.

254. Youngs, W. M., Macrides, F., Schneider, S., and
Davis, B. (1977): Some response properties of single
units in the outer layers of the hamster olfactory
bulb. *Soc. Neurosci. Abstr.,* 3:85.

Chemical Neuroanatomy, edited by P.C. Emson,
Raven Press, New York © 1983.

Biochemical Anatomy of the Striatum

Ann M. Graybiel and Clifton W. Ragsdale, Jr.

*Department of Psychology and Brain Science, Massachusetts Institute of Technology,
Cambridge, Massachusetts 02139*

The chemoarchitecture of the striatum became a focus for work on neurotransmitter distributions in the forebrain in the 1950s and 1960s when the caudate–putamen complex was found to have the highest content of acetylcholine and dopamine in the forebrain (104,311,412). At that time, methods for studying the anatomical distributions of neurotransmitter-related compounds were limited to classic histochemical techniques (226,576), assays of small dissected samples (396), and, beginning in 1962, the Falck–Hillarp method for the detection of catecholamines and indoleamines in histological preparations (195). By now, immunohistochemistry, a variety of autoradiographic tagging methods including ligand binding to receptors, and combinations of these techniques with axon transport, fiber degeneration, and Golgi and classic histochemical methods have dramatically expanded possibilities for studying the anatomical distributions of compounds related to neural transmission (266,279,696,841). In addition, neurochemical microassay methods have been perfected and allow a far greater range of compounds to be analyzed than before.

It is remarkable that even with the increased perspective these new methods have brought, the striatum, and more generally the basal ganglia, continue to stand out as having an extremely rich content of known neurotransmitter-related compounds compared with many other parts of the brain. Efforts to learn more about these compounds have been enhanced because of the suspected linkage between abnormal amounts of certain neurotransmitters and disease states including psychiatric disorders and disorders of movement (55,59,132,341). Consequently, knowledge derived from neuropharmacological studies has come to have an important influence on the directions taken by morphological studies of the striatum. By the same token, neuroanatomical studies of pathways in the basal ganglia have become recognized as crucial to the neurotransmitter work.

Clearly, the disposition of the cells of origin and termination of these pathways, together with local connections intrinsic to the striatum, must account for the morphological patterning in the distributions of neurotransmitters in the striatum. Information is only now becoming available about the precise localization of these neurotransmitters, however, partly because the organization of the pathways has been difficult to study and is not yet fully understood, partly because the architecture of the striatum is turning out to be more complex than previously suspected, and partly because combinations of individually demanding techniques must be applied to obtain definitive identifications of the neurotransmitter-related compounds within striatal cells and fibers. To make as sharp a distinction as possible between direct and indirect evidence for such identifications, we have focused on recent findings bringing together the pathway anatomy and cytology of the striatum with histochemical demonstrations of its chemoarchitecture. We have also, where possible, correlated these observations with findings based on regional microassays, which are especially important as a prime source of information about neurotransmitter systems in the basal ganglia of the human brain in health and disease.

TISSUE ARRANGEMENTS IN THE STRIATUM

The tissue of the striatum is noncortical in type and is divided into dorsal and ventral districts which have distinguishable input–output connections and, to a degree, different histochemistries. The dorsal striatum includes the caudate nucleus and putamen (the "caudoputamen" of the rat and other small mammals); it receives dense afferent connections from the neocortex, the substantia nigra, pars compacta, and elsewhere (275) and projects mainly to the pallidum. The designation ventral striatum is given to the nucleus accumbens septi, olfactory tubercle, and associated parts of the basal forebrain (315,316). These regions are in direct physical continuity with the caudate–putamen, have close affiliations with the hippocampal formation and elements of the limbic system, and receive dopaminergic inputs mainly from the ventral tegmental area. As shown in Fig. 1, the boundaries between these two different components of the striatum are not everywhere clear, and until attention was drawn to the distinction between them, most biochemical measurements of striatal neurotransmitters and enzymes were made without reference to the subdivision. This is still reflected in a lack of precise information about the differential neurotransmitter content of these two districts. There are also uncertain borders between the striatum and at least two adjoining regions: the bed nucleus of the stria terminalis (see Fig. 1D) and parts of the amygdaloid complex (not illustrated). To a striking degree, however, there are characteristics of striatal cytology and histochemistry that serve as defining characteristics of the striatum and that set it apart both from the neocortex and from other parts of the hemisphere (275,316). These are noted below.

NEURONS IN THE STRIATUM

On the basis mainly of indirect evidence from lesion studies combined with biochemical assays, striatal neurons are thought to contain (a) acetylcholine (ACh), (b) γ-aminobutyric acid (GABA), (c) taurine and, especially in the ventral striatum–nucleus accumbens, some aspartate or glutamate, (d) a variety of neuropeptides, and (e) certain enzymes related to these compounds and perhaps to other substrates as well. Major efforts are being made to visualize these compounds by histochemistry and to relate such cytochemical findings to anatomical classifications of striatal neurons.

The anatomical categories have developed mainly from light microscopic studies carried out with Golgi impregnation methods, which reveal fine details of the morphology of single cells (for example, dendritic branching patterns, presence or absence of spines), and from ultrastructural studies, which reveal intracellular detail (e.g., patterns of disposition of the endoplasmic reticulum, presence or absence of indentations in the nuclear membrane). More recently, it has been possible with intracellular markers, applied locally or trans-

ported to the cell bodies by retrograde axonal flow, to ask whether given cell types are projection neurons or interneurons. What has evolved from this work is a system of classification of neurons in the striatum based on a combination of morphological characteristics. Inferences about the neurotransmitter content of different cell types depend critically on recognition of these characteristics in histochemical, immunohistochemical, and ligand-binding studies. The morphological cell types are accordingly introduced in some detail as a basis for reviewing findings regarding their cytochemistry.

Morphological Cell Types

The neurons in the striatum are mostly of medium size. More than 95% have diameters of 10 to 20 μm. Large neurons (20–60 μm diameter) occur in low density (2–3%) scattered among the medium cells (391,574). Some Golgi studies (142,391,392,476,500,574) include as a third group small neurons ($\leq$10 μm diameter), but others consider these as a subtype of glial cell (108,161,162,219,222). As these small cells lack axons and are apparently only rarely seen in Golgi preparations, the confusion in the literature is understandable. Markers specific for glia [e.g., glial fibrillary acidic protein (67)] or for neurons [e.g., ran-1(613)] should help in establishing their proper classification.

The large neurons were for many years considered to be the main output cells of the striatum, and most medium-sized cells were classified as short-axon neurons. In particular, the influential Golgi studies by Kemp and Powell (391) and Fox and his colleagues (220) identified as an interneuron the main cell of medium size, the so-called medium spiny cell, which constitutes, according to Kemp and Powell, some 96% of all striatal neurons. Beginning with Grofová's report in 1975 (285) however, experimental retrograde transport studies have established unequivocally that many if not most of the medium spiny neurons are projection neurons (28,93,203,276,410,608,697,739). For example, in a quantitative retrograde tracer study, Bolam et al. (72) estimated that nearly 70% of the neurons in striatum project to the substantia nigra, nearly all of them medium-sized spiny cells (see below). Thus, the Golgi classification of the medium-sized striatal cells as being mainly interneurons turned out to be an error, probably attributable to incomplete Golgi impregnation of the axons of the medium cells beyond their local collateral arbors [see Pasik et al. (574) for a review].

This misinterpretation is emphasized here be-

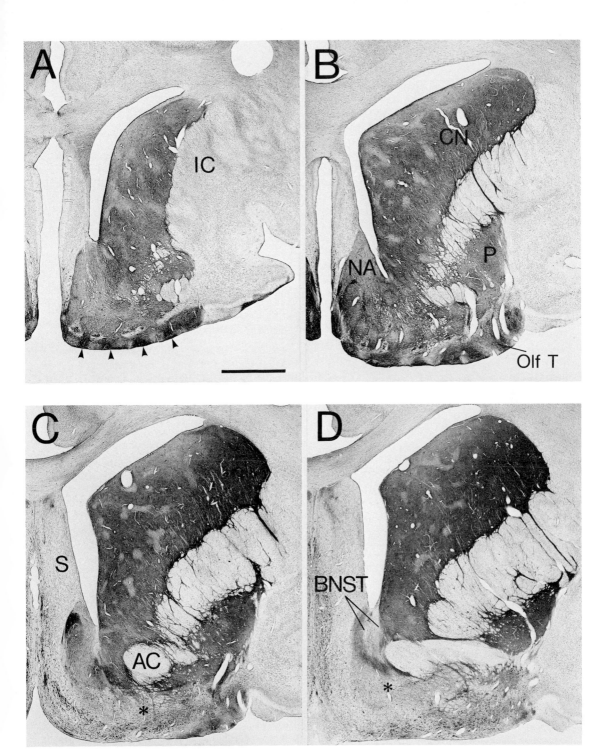

FIG. 1. The distribution of acetylcholinesterase (AChE, *dark stain*) in the dorsal and ventral striatum of the cat is shown in sections taken at four transverse levels through the caudate nucleus (CN) and putamen (P). The cat was treated with diisopropylfluorophosphate (DFP) 6 hr before perfusion. At rostral levels (**A,B**), the nucleus accumbens septi (NA) and olfactory tubercle (Olf T) are prominent. At more caudal levels (**C,D**), these are displaced by the bed nucleus of the stria terminalis (BNST), ventral pallidum *(asterisks)*, and cell groups of the basal forebrain including the diagonal band of Broca (e.g., see AChE-positive neurons in **C**). Striosomes (variably shaped 300–600-μm-wide zones of low acetylcholinesterase activity) are visible in the caudate nucleus. Note prominent periodicity of AChE-positive zones in the olfactory tubercle (see *arrowheads* in **A**). AC, anterior commissure; IC, internal capsule; S, septum. See Graybiel and Ragsdale (277). *Scale marker,* 2 mm.

cause it was important in shaping concepts about neurochemical interactions in the striatum. For example, most cells were thought to be cholinergic interneurons because most cells were thought to be interneurons and there were known to be high levels of ACh in the striatum (493). It should be stressed, however, that the Golgi-based descriptions of the cell bodies, dendritic trees, and local axonal arbors of striatal neurons, including those of the medium-sized spiny neurons, have proved crucial in attempts to classify cell types in the striatum, and several such descriptions have now been confirmed by intracellular tracer filling of the neuronal types in question (60,819). The Golgi method as modified by Fairén et al. (194) (so-called Golgi gold toning) now also serves as a direct way for extending light microscopic identification of different cell types to the electron microscopic level.

Medium-Sized Neurons

Most authors recognize on the basis of Golgi studies at least four types of medium-sized neuron (Table 1). A number of terminologies have been proposed for these cell types (108,391,574), and the Golgi observations have been made in different species including the monkey (161,220,221), cat (391), dog (743), and rat (108,142,162,476,500). Many, but not all, observations can be fit to the schemes of Kemp and Powell (391) and DiFiglia et al. (161). Both classifications include two types of spiny neuron and two types of aspiny neuron and are based on correlated observations by light and electron microscopy.

TABLE 1. *Morphological cell types in the striatum*

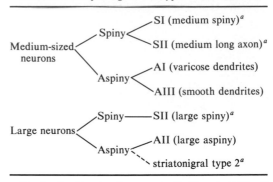

[a]In the classification drawn up by Pasik et al. (574), all striatal projection neurons are spiny neurons. Bolam et al. (71) have, in addition, identified a presumably rare aspiny ("striatonigral type 2") projection neuron.

The spiny I neuron (161) [medium spiny neuron of Kemp and Powell (391)] has a dense population of spines on its distal but not on its proximal dendrites and a rich local axonal arbor (Fig. 2). This cell type corresponds to the medium-sized type I of Dimova et al. (162), type I of Chang et al. (108), and MS1 of Bishop et al. (60). The spiny I neuron can be recognized at the electron microscopic level as the only medium cell type with an unindented nucleus (60,160,162,220,391,697,819) and with a nucleus lacking nuclear inclusions (162). Figure 4G shows one such neuron in a Golgi–Cox preparation of the cat's caudate nucleus.

The spiny II neuron (161) [medium long axon neuron (391)] has sparsely distributed spines on

---

FIG. 2. Photomicrographs illustrating medium spiny striatal projection neurons and their processes (**A–E**) and a second type of striatonigral projection neuron (**F,G**) in the caudoputamen of the rat. **A:** Partial photomontage of Golgi-stained and gold-toned, medium-sized densely spiny neuron that has been identified as a striatonigral projection neuron by retrograde transport of labeled horseradish peroxidase (HRP) from the substantia nigra. Three granules of HRP reaction product are indicated by *small arrows* and are also visible in **B**, which shows a 1-μm plastic section cut through the same neuron. Two other structures common to both micrographs are the capillary (c) and an HRP-labeled perikaryon (n). **C:** Electron micrograph of part of the dendrite that is indicated in **A** *(large arrow)*. The dendrite (d), identified by the electron-dense gold deposit, emits a spine (S). **D:** High-power electron micrograph of the same spine (s). An electron-dense degenerating bouton (db) originating from the cortex is in asymmetrical synaptic contact with the spine of the striatonigral neuron. **E:** Electron micrograph of a gold-toned bouton (b) that arose from a local axon collateral of the medium-sized densely spiny striatonigral neuron. The neuron was in synaptic contact with a degenerating bouton whose axon originated in the cortex. The bouton (b) contains large, clear, round and pleomorphic vesicles and is in symmetrical synaptic contact with a dendritic shaft (d). **F,G:** Light (**F**) and electron (**G**) micrographs illustrating a second type of striatonigral neuron labeled with HRP following injection of the substantia nigra. The HRP reaction product is amorphous and dark when viewed at the light-microscopic level. This neuron type differs from the medium-sized densely spiny striatonigral neuron in that it is larger, has an indented nucleus *(arrows)*, and has a heavy axosomatic synaptic input. The neuron (n) and the capillary (c) are common to both micrographs. **H:** Partial photomontage of a Golgi-impregnated neuron that was indirectly correlated with the second type of striatonigral neuron. The neuron had a size, ultrastructure, and synaptic input similar to those of the identified second type of striatonigral neuron. The major dendrites *(arrows)* extended more than 500 μm from the perikaryon. Note difference in magnification between **A** and **H**. See refs. 71 and 695. *Scale markers,* **A,** 10 μm; **B,** 10 μm; **C,** 1 μm; **D,** 0.2 μm; **E,** 0.5 μm; **F,** 12.5 μm; **G,** 4 μm; **H,** 50 μm. (Photomicrographs kindly supplied by Dr. J. P. Bolam and colleagues.)

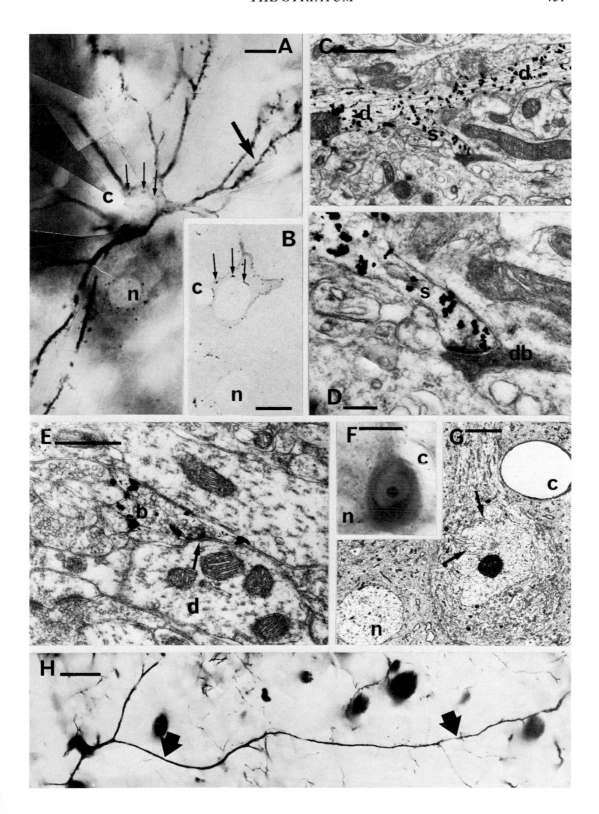

mary as well as higher-order dendrites, primary dendrites branching closer to the cell body than those of the spiny I neuron, and a less dense local axonal arbor than that of the spiny I cells. This cell type corresponds to the medium-sized II of Dimova et al. (162), MS2 of Bishop et al. (60), and probably type II of Chang et al. (108).

The aspiny I neuron (161) [cell with varicose dendrites (391)] has varicose and often curved dendrites which branch close to the the cell body and a beaded axon which forms a rich local plexus. According to Kemp and Powell (391) and DiFiglia et al. (161), this cell has a deeply indented nuclear envelope. It probably corresponds to type V of Chang and Kitai (108) (see Fig. 3).

The aspiny III neuron (161) [medium-sized smooth cell (391)] has long, slender, nearly spineless dendrites and an axon that branches locally to form a beaded local collateral arbor.

According to DiFiglia and the Pasiks (161,574), both spiny types have long axons, and both aspiny types have short axons. This conclusion is in close agreement with the earlier Golgi observations of Lentovich (438), who is to be credited with first clearly recognizing that most medium spiny neurons have long axons. The generalization has been further supported by several experimental studies: retrograde or iontophoretic marking of cells projecting to the substantia nigra and globus pallidus regularly labels medium spiny I neurons but not neurons clearly belonging to the medium aspiny groups (110,608,695–697). Bak et al. (28; cf.60) have suggested that spiny II neurons project to the substantia nigra, but this claim has not yet been confirmed experimentally. It should be noted that the cells of medium size have been shown in retrograde transport studies to project to all three of the major targets of striatal efferent projections, viz., the substantia nigra and the two segments of the globus pallidus, but have not been shown to participate in either the sparse projection from the striatum to the neocortex (357) (see below) or the recently described interhemispheric connection from one caudoputamen to the other (27).

Large Neurons

Most workers distinguish either one or two types of large neuron in the striatum. There is less agreement about these types than about the medium-cell categories. DiFiglia and the Pasiks (161) have suggested the existence of two classes of large cells (cf. 108,513,614,743).

Spiny II neurons are considered to be the large-cell counterpart of the medium spiny II neurons

and are distinguished from them because of their larger size. The large spiny II neurons have an elongated cell body and sparse spines on the primary and higher-order dendrites. They may correspond to the single class of large cells recognized by Kemp and Powell (391) (their "giant cell," characterized as being similar to the medium long-axon cell).

Aspiny II neurons, the largest neurons of the striatum, have an oval cell body and many smooth varicose dendrites. The Pasiks and DiFiglia have suggested that this cell type is a large version of the aspiny I neuron (161).

In a recent study of the striatum in the rat, Dimova et al. (162) concluded that the large cells form a single class. It is a testimony to the difficulties of classification that they could not clearly identify them with either of the two types described by DiFiglia and the Pasiks [or by Mori (513)]. However, Chang and Kitai, in another recent study in the rat, were able to distinguish two large cell types on the basis of Golgi and electron microscopic observations (109).

Pasik et al. (574) suggest that the large spiny cells but not the large aspiny cells are striatal projection neurons. This would mean that the spiny neurons, whether large or small, are the long-axon cells of the striatum and that the aspiny neurons, again regardless of size, are the short-axon cells. It is extremely difficult to sample large numbers of neurons identified with respect both to their axonal trajectories and to their somatic and dendritic morphologies, and so it is too early to make a definitive generalization. However, at least one exception to the Pasiks' view has apparently been demonstrated by Bolam et al. (71) who have identified a large (20–30 μm) aspiny neuron in the rat striatum by retrograde transport of horseradish peroxidase (HRP) from the substantia nigra and have compared the type so identified with neuron types identified by Golgi gold toning (see Fig. 2F–H). These aspiny "striatonigral type 2" neurons—evidently lacking varicosities—may constitute a third category of large neuron, but Bolam et al. found them only rarely and only in the ventral part of the rat caudoputamen (cf. 28,284,739). Large neurons in the ventral part of the caudate nucleus of the cat and in the cat's putamen have also been singled out in HRP studies as projecting to the cortex (see below) (357,619,627), but nothing is yet known of their Golgi morphology or ultrastructure. Nor are there cytological descriptions available for the large neurons that have been found labeled on occasion after injections of retrograde tracer into the medial pallidum (see Fig. 11) (276,495).

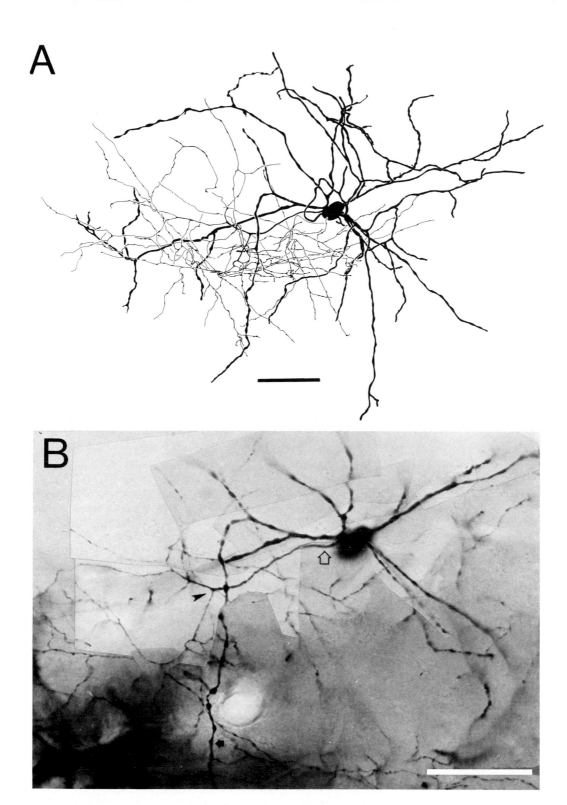

FIG. 3. Camera lucida drawing (**A**) and photomicrograph (**B**) illustrate rich local axonal plexus of a medium-size neuron in the striatum of the rat [type V in the classification of Chang et al. (108)]. The neuron has varicose dendrites (*solid arrow*). The *open arrow* and *arrowhead* point, respectively, to the main axon and its first bifurcation. See Chang et al. (108). *Scale markers,* 50 μm. (Drawing and micrograph kindly supplied by Dr. H. T. Chang and colleagues.)

In addition to this sparse projection to the neocortex and a projection of uncertain magnitude to the substantia nigra (28,71,284,739), a third striatal efferent system has been reported to originate from large neurons, namely, an interhemispheric projection from one caudate–putamen to the other. According to Bak et al. (27), the cells in question are large spiny neurons with lobulated nuclei and perikaryal diameters of 30 to 50 μm.

Neurotransmitter-Related Compounds Associated with Individual Cell Types

With few exceptions, identification of neurotransmitter-related compounds in striatal neurons depended until recently on evidence obtained by comparing measurements of the compound's concentration or activity in the normal striatum with measurements made after destruction of striatal afferents by distant lesions or destruction of striatal parenchyma by the local introduction of neurotoxins. In such experiments, preservation of normal levels of the compound after damage to afferents, or decreases in these levels after intrastriatal lesions, are interpreted as evidence that the compound is synthesized within neurons (or, in certain instances, glia) of the striatum.

There are acknowledged difficulties in interpreting findings obtained in such lesion studies, among the problems being transneuronal effects and compensatory metabolic changes in the striatum and unintended sparing of tissue. Gradually, it has become possible (though it is not yet routine) to identify neurotransmitter-related compounds within striatal tissue by immunohistochemistry and other methods that provide direct anatomical evidence of the compounds' intraperikaryal location. In addition, certain classic histochemical methods are valuable in identifying enzymes associated with these candidate neurotransmitters. There are pitfalls associated with these morphological techniques also (for example, cross reactivity in the immunohistochemical studies), but when applied with care, these methods greatly increase the likelihood of accuracy in identifying neurotransmitters (or at least members of particular families of neurotransmitters, as may be the case with neuropeptide localizations).

The sections that follow emphasize such direct morphological evidence concerning neurotransmitter-related compounds thought to be associated with particular morphological cell types in the striatum, with striatal projection cells in particular, and with striatal afferent fiber populations. Table 2 provides a more comprehensive summary of neurotransmitter-related compounds present in the striatum and leans heavily on studies of the regional distributions of these compounds carried out with biochemical assay methods.

Acetylcholine and Related Enzymes

Because of the high concentrations of ACh in the striatum (116), and because of clinical evidence that cholinergic neurotransmission is essential for normal striatal function (58,490,709), great efforts have been made to determine which neurons and fibers in the striatum contain ACh. Biochemical assays combined with lesions of striatal afferent and efferent pathways suggest that most of the ACh in the striatum is in intrinsic neurons, not in projection neurons or afferent fibers (see below; 99,493). There is no fully satisfactory histochemical method for localizing ACh itself, however, so that indirect methods involving the histochemical localization of the synthetic and degradative enzymes of the cholinergic mechanism have been used as substitutes. The potentially valuable anatomical method of examining the distribution of [^{3}H]choline uptake (26) has not yet been applied to the striatum.

Choline Acetyltransferase.

Acetylcholine is synthesized from choline and acetyl coenzyme A by the action of choline acetyltransferase (CAT). Because CAT has a high degree of substrate specificity, identification of this enzyme within the soma of a neuron should establish that neuron as cholinergic. Early attempts to visualize CAT by histochemistry proved unsuccessful, but more recently developed immunohistochemical methods in which tissue slices are reacted with an antibody raised against CAT should clearly be reliable for light and electron microscopic studies given proof of the antibody's specificity [see Sternberger (724)]. Several laboratories have claimed success in raising monoclonal or polyclonal antibodies against CAT (114,176, 402,439,491,570). For most of these antibodies, however, immunospecificity has been questioned or is yet to be fully tested (636,638). This problem may account for the lack of consistency in the findings of the McGeers and associates who, in their early studies with a polyclonal antibody (305), suggested that the cholinergic neurons were medium-sized cells with unindented nuclei, some at least with spines, but with another polyclonal antibody have more recently identified as CAT-positive large neurons with long dendrites having few spines (401,402).

TABLE 2. *Neuroactive compounds and related substances in the striatum: Their nature, levels, distribution, and disposition in disease states[a]*

Compound or macromolecule	Nature	Levels[a]	Histochemical localization	Disease states[a]
1. Dopamine (DA)	Monoamine (catecholamine)	Highest* in brain	Dense; patchy after drug pretreatment and in neonate	HD: unchanged or increased* PD: decreased*
2. Tyrosine hydroxylase (TOH)	Synthetic enzyme for catecholamines	Very high	Dense; patchy in ventral striatum	HD: unchanged PD: decreased
3. Aromatic amino acid decarboxylase (AAD)	Synthetic enzyme for many monoamines	Moderate* to high		PD: decreased
4. Dopamine binding sites	DA receptors	Highest* in brain	Very dense; patchy	HD: decreased PD: D_3-decreased; D_2-increased; decreased or unchanged* in patients treated with L-DOPA therapy
5. DA-sensitive adenylate cyclase	Synthetic enzyme for cyclic AMP, acts in presence of DA	Very high*		
6. DA uptake	Presumed reuptake system for DA	High*		
7. Norepinephrine (NE)	Monoamine (catecholamine)	Very low*; low to moderate in ventral striatum	A few fibers*	HD: unchanged or increased PD: decreased
8. Dopamine-β-hydroxylase (DBH)	Synthetic enzyme for NE	Low	Fibers in ventral striatum	HD: unchanged
9. α-Adrenergic binding sites	Probably NE receptors	Substantial	Low to moderate density	
10. β-Adrenergic binding sites	Probably NE receptors	Intermediate (primate); β_1: extremely high (rat)	Highest density (rat)	HD: unchanged or decreased
11 Epinephrine	Monoamine (catecholamine)	Not detectable (rat); very low (c-p) to low (n. acc.) (human)		
12. Phenylethanolamine-N-methyltransferase (PNMT)	Synthetic enzyme for epinephrine	Not detectable (rat); intermediate (primate)		
13. Catechol-O-methyltransferase (COMT)	Degradative enzyme for catecholamines	Moderate	Nonneuronal	HD: unchanged PD: unchanged
14. β-Phenylethylamine	Trace monoamine (arylalkylamine)	Moderate to very high		
15. Phenylethanolamine	Trace monoamine	Moderate to high		
16. p-, m-Tyramine	Trace monoamine	Very high		
17. Octopamine	Trace monoamine	Low		
18. Serotonin (5-HT)	Monoamine (indoleamine)	Moderate*	Low* to moderate density	HD: unchanged or increased PD: decreased
19. Tryptophan hydroxylase	Synthetic enzyme for 5-HT	Moderate to high		
20. 5-HT binding sites	5-HT receptors	High	Moderate* density	HD: decreased PD: unchanged or decreased*
21. 5-HT uptake	Presumed reuptake system for 5-HT	Moderate*		
22. Tryptamine	Trace monoamine (arylalkylamine)	High		

[a]Asterisk indicates that compound exhibits clear regional variation.

Abbreviations: c-p, caudate–putamen; n. acc., nucleus accumbens; HD, Huntington's disease; PD, Parkinson's disease; AD, Alzheimer's disease; WD, Wilson's disease.

Compound or macromolecule	Nature	Levels	Histochemical localization	Disease states
23. Histamine	Monoamine (imidazole amine)	Moderate		
24. Histidine decarboxylase	Synthetic enzyme for histamine	Moderate		
25. Histamine binding sites	Histamine receptors	H_1: low* to moderate H_2: highest in brain	H_1: low density	
26. Histamine methyltransferase	Degradative enzyme for histamine	Moderate to high		
27. Monoamine oxidase (MAO)	Degradative enzyme for monoamines	Moderate to high	Low to moderate density	HD: unchanged or increased (MAO type B) PD: unchanged
28. γ-Aminobutyric acid (GABA)	γ-Amino acid	Moderate; high in n. acc.		HD: decreased
29. Glutamic acid decarboxylase (GAD)	Synthetic enzyme for GABA	Moderate* to high; very high in n. acc.	Moderate* density; patchy neurons	HD: decreased PD: decreased *Note:* affected by agonal state (decreased) and L-DOPA therapy (increased)
30. GABA binding sites	GABA receptors	Moderate* to high	Low to moderate density (high-affinity sites)	HD: decreased or unchanged PD: unchanged
31. Benzodiazepine binding sites	Valium® may act here; related to GABA receptors	Low (type 1) to intermediate (type 2)	Low to moderate density; mostly type 2 sites	HD: decreased (peripheral-type binding sites unchanged or increased)
32. GABA uptake	Presumed reuptake system for GABA	Intermediate	Neurons	
33. GABA transaminase (GABA-T)	Degradative enzyme for GABA	Moderate to high	Moderate density; occasional neurons	HD: unchanged
34. Succinic semialdehyde dehydrogenase (SSADH)	Degradative enzyme for GABA	High		
35. γ-Hydroxybutyric acid (GHB)	Carboxylic acid	High		HD: increased
36. Succinic semialdehyde reductase	Synthetic enzyme for GHB	Moderate		
37. GHB uptake	Presumed reuptake system for GHB	Highest in brain		
38. Taurine	β-Amino acid (contains sulfonic acid)	High		HD: unchanged or increased PD: unchanged
39. Cysteine sulfinic acid decarboxylase (CSAD)	Synthetic enzyme for taurine	Very high		HD: decreased
40. Taurine uptake	Presumed reuptake system for taurine	Moderate		
41. Glutamate (Glu)	Amino acid	High		HD: decreased
42. Aspartate (Asp)	Amino acid	Low		
43. L-Glutamate binding sites	Relation to kainate, quisqualate, NMDA and Asp/Glu receptors unclear	High		
44. Kainic acid binding sites	Glu may act here	Highest in brain		HD: decreased
45. D-Aspartate and glutamate uptake	Presumed reuptake system for Glu and Asp	High*, lower in ventral striatum	High density	
46. Glycine	Amino acid	Low		

Compound or macromolecule	Nature	Levels	Histochemical localization	Disease states
47. Glycine binding sites	Glycine receptors	Very low	Very low density	
48. Triiodothyronine (T_3) binding sites	T_3, an amino acid, accumulates here	Low to moderate	Present*	
49. Homocarnosine	GABA-histidine (dipeptide)	Low to intermediate		HD: decreased
50. Homocarnosine synthetase	Synthetic enzyme for homocarnosine	Low to moderate		
51. Homocarnosinase	Degradative enzyme for homocarnosine	Moderate to high		
52. β-Endorphin/ ACTH/β-lipotropin	Pro-opiocortin peptides	Not detected or very low	Possibly fibers in n. acc.	
53. α-Melanocyte-stimulating hormone (α-MSH)	Pro-opiocortin peptide	Low	Possibly fibers	
54. Met-Enkephalin-Arg^6-Phe^7	Peptide	Moderate	Neurons	
55. Enkephalin convertase	Cleaves ENK precursors to produce ENK (carboxypeptidase)	High		
56. Met-Enkephalin (m-ENK)	Peptide	High; much more m-ENK than either l-ENK or m-ENK-arg-phe	Moderate* density; somewhat heavier in n. acc.; patchy neurons	HD: unchanged (decreased in striatal efferent sites)
57. Leu-Enkephalin (l-ENK)	Peptide	High	Neurons*	
58. Dynorphin-8,-13,-17/α-neoendorphin	Peptides	Dyn-8,-13 moderate; Dyn-17 and α-n-end high	A few fibers	
59. FRMF-amide	Peptide	Low	Possibly fibers in n. acc.	
60. μ-Opiate binding sites	Morphine binds here; possibly ENK receptors	Moderate to high	Low* density; patchy (patches very dense)	
61. δ-Opiate binding sites	DADL-ENK binds here; ENK receptors	Moderate to high	Moderate density; high density in ventral striatum; patchy	
62. κ-Opiate binding sites	Ketocyclazocine binds here; possibly dynorphin receptors	Moderate	Low density; possibly patchy	
63. σ-Opiate binding sites	N-Allynorcyclazocine binds here	Moderate		
64. Phencyclidine (PCP) binding sites	Ketamine and "angel dust" may act here; probably same as σ-opiate receptors	Moderate to high	Moderate density	
65. Enkephalinase	Degradative enzyme for enkephalin	Very high		
66. Angiotensin II (AII)	Peptide	High	Occasional* fibers; dense in n. acc.	
67. Renin	Synthetic enzyme for Angiotensin I (endopeptidase)	Low to intermediate	Possibly neurons	

Compound or macromolecule	Nature	Levels	Histochemical localization	Disease states
68. Angiotensin-converting enzyme (ACE)	Cleaves AI to produce AII	Highest* in brain	Apparently nonneuronal	HD: decreased
69. Angiotensin II binding sites	AII receptors	Low; higher in n. acc.		
70. (Avian) Pancreatic polypeptide (APP)	Peptide		Neurons; fibers, heavy in ventral striatum	
71. Bombesin binding sites	Bombesin receptors	Intermediate		
72. Bradykinin	Peptide		Occasional* fibers	
73. Colecystokinin (CCK)-8 and other forms	Peptide	High	Moderate* density; patchy	HD: unchanged (decreased in striatal efferent sites) PD: unchanged
74. CCK-33 binding sites	CCK receptors	High		HD: decreased
75. Insulin binding sites	Insulin receptors	Moderate		
76. Neurotensin	Peptide	Low to moderate; higher in ventral striatum	Low density; dense in n. acc.; patchy	
77. Neurotensin binding sites	Neurotensin receptors	Intermediate	Moderate* density; heavier in n. acc.	
78. Secretin	Peptide	Low		
79. Somatostatin (SOM)	Peptide	Low* to moderate; higher in n. acc.	Fibers*, especially in ventral striatum; patchy neurons	HD: increased
80. Somatostatin binding sites	SOM receptors	Intermediate		
81. Substance P (SP)	Peptide	Moderate*	Moderate* density; heavier in n. acc.; patchy neurons	HD: decreased
82. Substance P binding sites	SP receptors	Moderate		
83. Thyrotropin-releasing hormone (TRH)	Peptide	Moderate*, high in n. acc.	Very dense in n. acc.	HD: increased
84. TRH binding sites	TRH receptors	Low; moderate in n. acc.		
85. Cyclo(His–Pro)	Cyclic dipeptide— possible metabolite of TRH	Moderate		
86. Vasoactive intestinal polypeptide (VIP)	Peptide	Low to moderate	Low density; heavy in n. acc.; patchy; occasional neurons	HD: unchanged
87. VIP binding sites	VIP receptors	Highest in brain		
88. Vasopressin	Peptide	Very low (rat); not detected (c-p) to low (n. acc.) (human)		
89. Cathepsin D	Degradative enzyme for peptides (endopeptidase)		Neurons	
90. Acetylcholine	Monoamine (choline ester)	Very high*		

Compound or macromolecule	Nature	Levels	Histochemical localization	Disease states
91. Choline acetyltrans-ferase (CAT)	Synthetic enzyme for ACh	Very high*	Neurons	HD: decreased or unchanged* PD: unchanged, increased, or decreased* AD: decreased in CN
92. Pyruvate dehydrogenase	Synthetic enzyme for acetyl-CoA in Krebs cycle; may be associated with cholinergic systems			HD: decreased
93. Muscarinic ACh binding sites	Quinuclidinyl benzi-late (QNB) binds here; muscarinic ACh receptors	Highest* in brain	Dense; patchy in neonate; mostly low affinity sites in c-p; both low and high affinity sites in n. acc.	HD: decreased PD: unchanged or increased*
94. Non-muscarinic ACh binding sites	Presumably nicotinic ACh receptors	Intermediate		
95. α-Bungarotoxin binding sites	Related to nicotinic ACh receptors	Low to moderate	Moderate* (mouse) to very low (rat) density	
96. High-affinity choline uptake	Uptake system asso-ciated with cholin-ergic systems	Very high*		
97. Acetylcholinesterase (AChE)	Degradative enzyme for ACh	Highest in brain	Very dense*; patchy neurons	HD: unchanged PD: unchanged
98. Butyrylcholinesterase (BuChE)	Degradative enzyme	High	Moderate* den-sity; patchy	
99. Adenosine binding sites	Adenosine (or P_1) receptors	A_1: highest in brain	A_1: moderate* density	
100. Adenosine-sensitive adenylate cyclase	Synthetic enzyme for cyclic AMP; acts in presence of adenosine	Very high*		
101. Cyclic adenosine monophosphate (cAMP)	Cyclic nucleotide; possible "second messenger"	Very high	Neurons	
102. Cyclic guanosine monophosphate (cGMP)	Cyclic nucleotide; possible "second messenger"	Moderate	Fibers associ-ated with small neurons or glia	
103. Steroid binding sites	17-β-Estradiol accu-mulates here		Lightly labeled neurons in ventral striatum	
104. Succinate dehydrogenase	Enzyme in Krebs cycle	High	Dense; patchy in neonate; lightly labeled large neurons	HD: decreased
105. NADH-diaphorase (NADH-d)	Enzymatic activity responsible for oxi-dizing NADH in NADH-linked dehydrogenase systems	High	Dense; patchy in neonate; occasional large neurons	
106. NADPH-diaphor-ase (NADPH-d)	Enzymatic activity responsible for oxi-dizing NADPH in NADPH-linked		"Solitary active cells"	

TABLE 2. *(continued) Neuroactive compounds and related substances in the striatum: Their nature, levels, distribution, and disposition in disease states*[a]

Compound or macromolecule	Nature	Levels	Histochemical localization	Disease states
107. Glucose-6-phosphate dehydrogenase	dehydrogenase systems Enzyme in pentose phosphate pathway involved in NADPH generation	High	"Solitary active cells"	HD: unchanged
108. Copper (Cu)	Trace element	Moderate		HD: decreased WD: accumulates
109. Iron (Fe)	Trace element	Very high	Fibers and glial elements; possibly some neurons	HD: decreased
110. Zinc (Zn)	Trace element	Moderate		HD: decreased

[a]References consulted in compiling this table are listed according to item number and grouped according to column of entry. The species used in the studies cited here are noted by the letters following the reference number. The abbreviations are: B, rabbit; Ba, baboon; C, cow; D, dog; F, cat; G, guinea pig; Ha, hamster; H, human; M, monkey; Ms, mouse; P, pig; R, rat; S, sheep. Species is not designated when the data concern human disease states or when the study was done solely on rats. The instruction *cf. text* cites unpublished material discussed in the text.

(1) 88, 104, 131M, 179H, 296, 709H, 729, 732H, 744, 780; 271F, 355, 539H, 553H, 554, 749B; 51, 58, 191, 179, 497, 709. (2) 130M, 248H, 286H, 490H, 655, 661, 667; 236, 271F; 58, 248, 490, 492. (3) 69D, 131M, 214–216, 421F, 463H, 490H, 654; 458, 462, 464. (4) 385; 68, 96C, 208HR, 347, 610; 333, 406, 556; 186, 429, 430, 621–623. (5) 68, 347, 610. (6) 254, 694, 744. (7) 88, 191H, 201H, 421F, 709H, 729, 780; 449; 191, 201, 460, 709. (8) 286H, 655; 288, 733; 54. (9) 765C; 840. (10) 2, 100MR, 186H; 559, 187, 188.

(11) 494H, 767. (12) 441HM, 652. (13) 24M, 81, 286H, 381, 656; 381; 389, 458, 462. (14) 595; 140, 175, 382, 595, 596H, 816. (15) 658, 816. (16) 140, 382, 596H, 742. (17) 22H, 92. (18) 69DF, 191H, 296, 421F, 657, 751FR; 718; 50, 191, 460. (19) 69DF, 87, 150, 593F. (20) 186H, 580BGR; 53, 496, 556; 187, 188, 622.

(21) 751RF, 821. (22) 596H, 597, 693. (23) 450H, 746. (24) 32H, 670, 746. (25) 31, 112CGHR, 324G, 560, 745F; 558. (26) 23M, 31, 656, 746. (27) 69D, 131M, 178, 230, 286H, 529H, 656; cf. 226BGMsR; 458, 462, 482, 712, 252. (28) 29, 149M, 193M, 440, 549BaBGR, 588F, 589H, 640H, 769MsR; 58, 587, 708, 710, 766. (29) 131M, 186H, 189M, 214–216, 248H, 459H, 475BM, 490H, 517H, 667, 700P, 709H, 729; 579, 629, cf. text; 58, 188, 248, 459, 461, 490, 492, 581, 583, 708, 709, 712, 766, 825. (30) 38, 186H, 189MR, 291, 454H, 692, 814, 847; 107, 557; 187, 188, 454, 455, 457, 552, 622.

(31) 76H, 77, 465C, 508, 624H, 705H; 763, 838, 839; 620, 624, 668. (32) 73, 189M, 214, 331, 440; 70, 331, 727. (33) 662M, 675H; 783, 785; 766, 825. (34) 505H. (35) 165GHM; 10. (36) 651. (37) 42. (38) 123, 290, 380, 468, 588F, 589H; 584, 585. (39) 700P; 825. (40) 33F, 123, 380, 467.

(41) 149M, 361F, 440, 588F, 589H; 586. (42) 149M, 588F, 589H. (43) 363; 62. (44) 470, 683; 37, 469. (45) 33F, 214, 440, 789; 213. (46) 149M, 588F, 589H, 674. (47) 836; 844. (48) 170; 169. (49) 374H, 403H, 588F, 589H; 587, 766. (50) 403H, 534.

(51) 403H. (52) 265H, 415, 779; 397, 577, 798, 801. (53) 190, 545; 173, 293, 354, 397, 545. (54) 637; 64; 815. (55) 46, 338; 224. (56) 184H, 265H, 317, 335, 336, 344, 448C, 506, 637, 679C, 680M, 723, 779, 829; 210, 272F, 297M, 329, 428G, 601, 665, 681, 792, 802, cf. text; 184. (57) 317, 344, 416H, 448C, 506, 829; 159M, 181, 210, 428G, 601, 665, 681. (58) 332, 507, 803; 804. (59) 163, 164BR; 163, 164, 805. (60) 74H, 111, 186H, 420HM, 503B, 537C, 820; 21, 263, 320, 510DHMMsR, 592, 791M, 841.

(61) 74H, 111, 537C, 820; 263. (62) 115, 127; 342, 351H, 503B, 820; 261, 611. (63) 351H, 820, 845. (64) 612, 845; 781, 846; 612. (65) 264, 453H, 480, 735. (66) 687; 83, 113, 238, 245. (67) 144H, 243, 244, 442; 245, 690. (68) 19BHR, 442, 605H, 653, 830; 83, 633; 18, 20. (69) 43CR, 688. (70) 473, 782, cf. text.

(71) 509, 591. (72) 129. (73) 40, 427; 327, 349, 427, 472, 634, 768; 183, 730. (74) 348, 660; 310. (75) 308. (76) 125H, 182, 383M, 409, 481H, 758C, 759CR, 761C; 634, 756, 760. (77) 758C, 759; 837. (78) 543. (79) 86, 125H, 147H, 409, 711; 44, 180, 204G, 211, 272F, 360, 634, 782; 126. (80) 711.

(81) 85, 125H, 184H, 379, 667; 137, 272F, 451, 634, 667, cf. text; 91. (82) 302, 522B. (83) 89, 511, 512M; 330, 360; 707. (84) 95, 747S. (85) 511, 512M. (86) 52, 251; 231DFGMsR, 237, 471MsR, 634, 684MsR; 185. (87) 748. (88) 309, 642H. (89) 809. (90) 116, 296, 340.

(91) 11H, 116, 186H, 192M, 214–216, 248H, 296, 311DHS, 340, 459H, 490H, 618, 640H, 663BMsR, 667, 709H, 729, 741, 787, 795H, 796H, 826; 401, 402, cf. text; 11, 57, 58, 148, 188, 248, 459, 490, 492, 622, 623, 640, 650, 698, 709, 712, 795, 796. (92) 431, 582; 698. (93) 186H, 407Ms, 408, 618, 663BCMsR, 795H, 796H, 826, 827, 828M; 78F, 418, 419, 644, 645, 793, cf. text; 187, 188, 323, 622, 650, 795, 796. (94) 671. (95) 103, 664; 373, 514, 515, 663BCMsR, 706; 16Ms, 346, 672. (96) 618, 699, 741. (97) 94D, 131M, 212H, 340; 98, 277FHM, 321, 350H, 355, 412, 478, 565F, 567F, 603M, 826; 492, 712. (98) 94D, 212H, 555; 225FHMR, 412, cf. text. (99) 813; 262, 444. (100) 607.

(101) 721Ms; 12. (102) 721Ms; 12. (103) 386M, 594. (104) 94D; 227, 229G; 712. (105) 228H; 98, 228H, 350H. (106) 576HaH, 752BHaHMMsR. (107) 56H; 576HaH; 56. (108) 753; 133, 485. (109) 326; 223, 736; 133. (110) 326, 343H; 133.

The confusion should soon be resolved. Eckenstein and colleagues have now fully purified CAT (176) and have developed a rigorously tested antibody against this enzyme that should allow definitive identification of the cholinergic cell types in the striatum and elsewhere. Work with this antiserum in our own laboratory (A. M. Graybiel, M.-F. Chesselet, and F. Eckenstein, *in preparation*) suggests that the CAT-containing neurons of the striatum include both medium and large cell types.

Acetylcholinesterase.

In the absence of antisera to CAT, most attempts to identify the cholinergic neurons of the striatum have been based on localizing acetylcholinesterase (AChE), the degradative enzyme of the cholinergic mechanism responsible for hydrolysis of ACh. There are reliable histochemical methods for visualizing this enzyme in tissue sections from both fixed and fresh specimens (249,412) and for studying its distribution at the electron microscopic level (301,411,445). The appearance of AChE within a neuron, however, does not mean that the neuron is cholinergic. Acetylcholinesterase apparently is synthesized by cholinoceptive as well as cholinergic neurons, and the enzyme may have functions other than those related to the cholinergic mechanism (412,678). Acetylcholinesterase has recently been shown to hydrolyze certain neuropeptides [substance P and met and leu-enkephalin, but not somatostatin, β-endorphin, neurotensin, angiotensin II, oxytocin, or vasopressin (121,122)]. Even before these studies on alternate substrates, it was clear that the distributions of AChE and CAT do not match everywhere (678). For example, the substantia nigra has high concentrations of AChE but low levels of CAT (see 116,561). The localization of AChE-positive neurons can thus be taken, at most, as helpful in suggesting which neuronal types may be cholinergic.

It is well documented that part of the AChE in the striatum is contained in afferent fibers (including, as discussed below, dopaminergic nigrostriatal fibers), but as much as 50% of the AChE is thought to be synthesized within striatal neurons (435). To observe these neurons, it is usually necessary in adults (but not neonates) to treat the animals with an irreversible AChE inhibitor, e.g., diisopropylfluorophosphate (DFP) some hours before perfusion (478). This pretreatment blocks the enzymatic activity of AChE present at the time of injection so that newly synthesized (hence perikaryal) AChE can be visualized (See Fig. 1). All studies by this method indicate that AChE-positive neurons are scattered through the caudate–putamen and make up a small percentage (ca. 3%) of the total population (97,271,318,478,565,567,603,822; and A. M. Graybiel, M.-F. Chesselet, and F. Eckenstein, *in preparation*). It seems remarkable that so small a group of neurons could account for half the AChE in the striatum, and further study of this point is in order.

Most investigators agree that there are both large and medium-sized AChE-positive neurons in the striatum (see Fig. 4A,B). With the DFP method, Butcher and Hodge (98) and Woolf and Butcher (822) have identified in the rat's striatum medium-sized and large neurons that synthesize large amounts of AChE. In a careful ultrastructural study also carried out in the rat's caudoputamen, Henderson (318) identified "large" (21 ± 4 μm diameter) and "small" (12 ± 2 μm diameter) AChE-positive neurons and showed that both types have indented nuclei (see also 369). Like Butcher and his colleagues, Henderson found no AChE-positive medium spiny I neurons (i.e., neurons with unindented nuclei). Butcher and colleagues (97,435,603,822) and Parent et al. (565,567) suggest that both the large and medium-sized AChE-positive neurons are aspiny neurons.

Three studies combining AChE histochemistry with retrograde transport—Henderson's electron microscopic HRP–AChE study (318), the light microscopic AChE/DPF–fluorescence retrograde labeling study of Woolf and Butcher (28,822), and the light microscopic AChE/DFP–HRP study by Parent et al. (566)—indicate that the AChE-positive neurons may be interneurons, because no such cells were labeled following injections of tracer into the substantia nigra or pallidum (globus pallidus and entopeduncular nucleus of rat, cat). In a single discrepant study, Kaiya and colleagues (370) report finding retrograde labeling of medium-sized AChE-positive neurons in the rat's caudoputamen after injecting HRP into the substantia nigra. Though at odds with the results of other tracer work, their findings are in accord with the earlier claim by Olivier et al. (551) that striatonigral and striatopallidal fibers contain AChE.

Interest in the issue of whether AChE-positive neurons are projection neurons or interneurons has been further spurred by Parent et al. (566) who recently have shown with combined HRP and AChE/DFP staining that at least some of the large AChE-positive neurons in the cat's putamen project to the neocortex. As the cortical injections in their experiments were confined to the auditory cortex [after the original description of this striatocortical projection by Jayaraman (357; see Cajal (101)], it is an open question whether the restriction of retrograde labeling mainly to the putamen

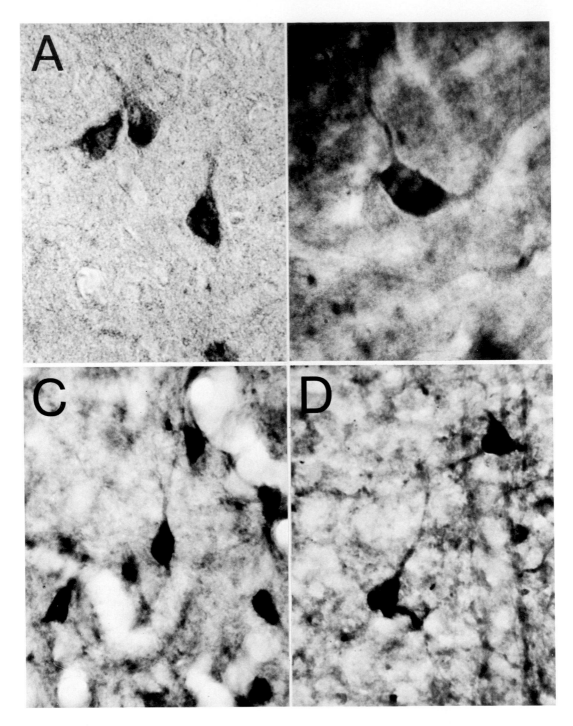

FIG. 4. Examples of medium-sized (**A,C–G**) and large (**B**) neurons of the cat's caudate nucleus stained for acetylcholinesterase (**A,B**) and neuropeptide immunoreactivity (**C–F**) and shown at the same magnification as the Golgi-impregnated medium spiny neuron in **G. A,B:** Acetylcholinesterase-positive neurons from DFP-pretreated cat. **C:** Neurons showing met-enkephalin-like immunoreactivity. **D:** Neurons expressing substance P-like immunoreactivity from a cholchicine-pretreated cat.

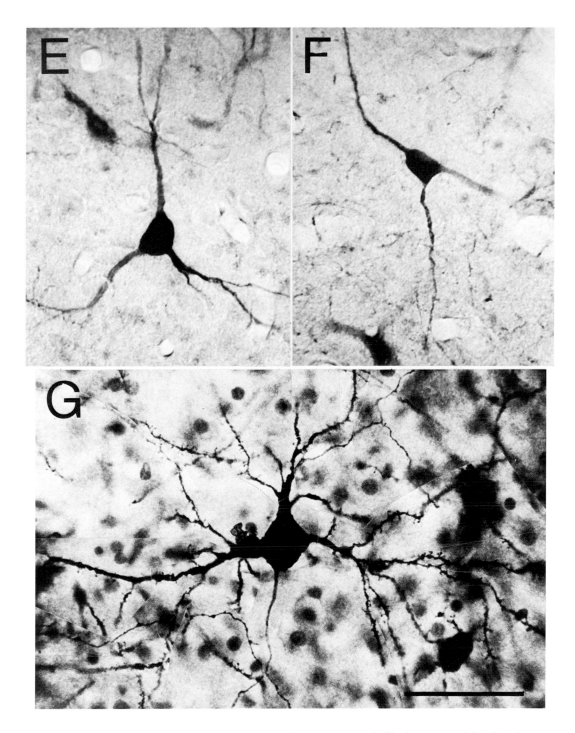

FIG. 4. *(continued)* **E:** Neurons with varicose dendrites showing somatostatin-like immunoreactivity. **F:** Avian pancreatic polypeptide-like immunoreactivity in medium-sized neuron with varicose dendrites. **G:** Photomontage illustrating a spiny I (medium spiny) neuron stained by the Golgi–Cox method. Immunoreactive neurons visualized by the peroxidase–antiperoxidase method (272). *Scale marker,* 50 μm. (From M.-F. Chesselet and A. M. Graybiel, *in preparation.*)

reflects the topography of the striatocortical projection or a difference in the connections of large
neurons in the putamen and caudate nucleus. Even
with large injections of HRP in a number of other
cortical regions, however, Reinoso-Suarez and colleagues (619) have found HRP labeling in a similarly restricted zone of the cat's striatum including
the putamen and cell bridges joining it with the
caudate nucleus. This zone adjoins the pallidum, in
which labeled neurons were also found. As Reinoso-Suarez and colleagues point out, the striatocortical fiber projection may therefore be associated with the massive corticopetal projection
originating in the basal forebrain continuum
formed by neurons of the diagonal band, substantia
innominata, nucleus basalis, and pallidum
(177,353,364,390,436,502,676,677,807; cf. 75,148,
569,583,640,641,810).

It should be noted that there have so far been no
reports in rats or monkeys of striatal neurons projecting to the neocortex. The large AChE-positive
striatal neurons found to do so in the cat may
therefore not be representative of the striatal
AChE-positive cell population in general but instead of neurons in another basal forebrain group.
Even in the cat, the large-celled projection from
the putamen and associated cell bridges to the neocortex does not account for the majority of AChE-
positive neurons in the striatum, which lie in the
caudate nucleus (565,567). We thus are still left
with the question of whether these neurons are interneurons or projection neurons.

Summary and comments on clinical findings.

The view is emerging that (a) a population of
large, probably aspiny, neurons of the striatum
contains AChE; that (b) a small population of medium-sized, probably aspiny, neurons also contains
AChE; that (c) these neurons may not project in
large numbers (if at all) to the substantia nigra or
globus pallidus; and that (d) at least some of the
large AChE-positive neurons may project to the
neocortex. Findings from work now in progress (A.
M. Graybiel, M.-F. Chesselet, and F. Eckenstein)
suggest that (e) most if not all of these AChE-positive neurons contain CAT and that (f) CAT-containing AChE-positive neurons in the cat's putamen, putamino–caudate cell bridges, and, rarely,
the caudate nucleus, project to the neocortex.

These findings have a high priority from the
standpoint of clinical work on extrapyramidal disorders. The level of CAT activity (but, evidently,
not AChE activity) is markedly reduced in the
brains of most but not all patients dying with a diagnosis of Huntington's chorea, and this loss is
thought to result from a specific but perhaps non-

uniform loss of cholinergic neurons in the striatum
(11,54,58,490,710,712). As discussed further
below, an animal "model" for choreic striatum has
been proposed by Coyle and Schwarcz (134) and
by McGeer and McGeer (489), who showed that
intrastriatal injections of the glutamate analog
kainic acid destroy neurons but not afferent or
transit fibers in the striatum and result in large
losses of CAT and AChE. It is curious that in Huntington's disease, large neurons are reported to be
spared relative to medium-sized neurons (90), yet
at least some of the large cells are presumably cholinergic, judging from findings in experimental animals (A. M. Graybiel, M.-F. Chesselet, and F.
Eckenstein, *in preparation*). No such differential
survival of large cells is claimed for kainic acid
effects.

Choline acetyltransferase activity has also been
reported to decrease in the striatum in a familial
subtype of Alzheimer's disease (57,640). In Parkinsonian brains, CAT activity is reported to be elevated in the nucleus accumbens, normal in the
caudate nucleus, and possibly decreased in the putamen (248,459,490,622,650).

Drug treatments considered to affect the striatum also are thought to modify CAT activity in
cholinergic neurons in the striatum, both directly
and indirectly. An indirect effect is indicated in the
etiology of tardive dyskinesia following prolonged
treatment with neuroleptics. Bird and Iversen's
measurements on brains of patients with Huntington's disease (58) are pertinent: higher levels of
CAT activity were found in the putamen of Huntingtonian patients who had been treated with a
phenothiazine such as thoridazine (Melleril®) than
in the putamen of patients not so treated; conversely, lower levels of CAT were found in the putamen of patients who had taken anticholinergic
drugs.

γ-Aminobutyric Acid and Related Enzymes and Substrates

There is direct morphological evidence that the
inhibitory neurotransmitter GABA and its synthetic enzyme, glutamic acid decarboxylase
(GAD), are localized in medium-sized neurons of
the striatum (70,629). Indirect evidence from lesion studies suggests that many of these cells are
projection neurons giving rise to the striatonigral
and striatopallidal (including striatoentopeduncu-
lar) pathways (84, 215, 216, 218, 241, 306, 358,
384, 400, 520, 547, 628, 713, 788). Three methods
have been applied to identify the cell type of the
GABAergic neurons, with different results.

Ribak and colleagues (629) carried out a light

and electron microscopic immunohistochemical study of the rat's striatum with the well-characterized GAD antiserum of the Roberts group. This method allows identification of neurons that contain GAD and that therefore synthesize GABA. To visualize immunoreactive neurons in the striatum, it was necessary to inject into the ventricular system the drug colchicine, which blocks axonal transport and thus increases the concentration of transportable compounds in the perikaryon. Ribak et al. (629) identified many GAD-positive perikarya as well as GAD-positive spines, axons, and axon terminals and characterized the neurons as the medium-sized neurons of Kemp and Powell (391) [i.e., the spiny I or, possibly, spiny II neurons of DiFiglia et al. (161)].

Somogyi et al. (695) have taken issue with this identification because Ribak et al. (629) illustrated an electron micrograph of a GAD-positive neuron with abundant cytoplasm, a ruffled and indented nuclear membrane, and a prominent nuclear inclusion. As Somogyi et al. point out, the cardinal ultrastructural characteristics of the medium spiny neurons are lack of abundant cytoplasm, lack of nuclear inclusions, and a smooth nuclear envelope (see above). Somogyi and colleagues suggest that the GAD-positive neurons of Ribak et al. must be of a class other than medium spiny projection cells, perhaps a class of interneurons.

Bolam, Somogyi, and their colleagues (70) have presented evidence for just such a GABAergic cell type. They injected [³H]GABA directly into the striatum and identified the neurons heavily labeled by this procedure as medium-sized aspiny neurons with prominent nuclear invaginations. Pertinent here is Panula's report that in cell cultures of striatal tissue from the rat, putative GABAergic (GAD-positive) neurons also have nuclear invaginations (563).

Given the strong evidence from lesion studies that all three of the main striatal output pathways are at least in part GABAergic, it is remarkable that no medium spiny neurons were labeled in the [³H]GABA uptake experiments of Bolam et al. (70). The result is all the more surprising because Streit and his colleagues (728) have succeeded in labeling "numerous" medium-sized striatal neurons following injections of [³H]GABA into the substantia nigra. These neurons were not analyzed by electron microscopy but are clearly at least candidates for the medium spiny class. Further, Ribak et al. (629) reported and illustrated GAD-containing dendritic spines in their study, so that some spiny neurons (spiny I or II) were immunoreactive. With the uncertainty about which cell types were represented by the majority of immunoreactive

perikarya observed by these authors, however, we still lack direct proof that medium densely spiny (spiny I) neurons are GABAergic.

The absence of a straightforward demonstration of medium spiny GABAergic neurons in the local [³H]GABA uptake experiments could reflect a problem related to technique; for example, the GABA uptake mechanism in neurons of this particular cell type could make them especially difficult to demonstrate. The alternative, that there are few GABAergic medium spiny projection neurons, can almost certainly be discounted. It is important to clarify the situation not only because GABA inhibition is considered to have a major influence on transmission of information through the striatum but also because the GABA-containing neurons appear to be highly vulnerable in extrapyramidal disorders in man. In Huntington's disease, GAD activity in the striatum is decreased by as much as 75% (58,490,492,708–710,766,825), and striatal GAD activity is also decreased in parkinsonism (248,459,490). Levels of GABA itself and of metabolically related compounds, e.g., homocarnosine (GABA-histidine) and glutamate (see below), are also abnormal in the striatum of Huntington brains (586,587,766).

In addition to GAD, there are other enzymes related to the metabolism of GABA that are found in high concentrations in the striatum. These include GABA transaminase (GABA-T), which acts on GABA to produce a succinic semialdehyde; succinic semialdehyde dehydrogenase (SSADH), which acts on the semialdehyde and is part of the "GABA shunt" leading into the Krebs cycle; and succinic semialdehyde reductase, which acts on the semialdehyde to produce γ-hydroxybutyrate (GHB) (see below).

GABA transaminase and succinic semialdehyde dehydrogenase.

GABA transaminase is the major degradative enzyme of GABA and can be localized histochemically (776). Vincent and collaborators have applied the van Gelder histochemical method to demonstrate dense GABA-T activity in the neuropil and in occasional neurons of the dorsal and ventral striatum of the rat (783,785). They have further shown that this staining virtually disappears following intrastriatal injection of kainic acid and that under these conditions GABA-T activity is also reduced in the ipsilateral globus pallidus, entopeduncular nucleus, and substantia nigra (targets of striatal efferents) and in the lateral hypothalamus (a target of fibers from the nucleus accumbens) (525,783–785). On the basis of these results, Vincent et al. (783) suggest that GABA-T histochemistry may serve as a marker for GABA-ergic pathways. Caution is clearly necessary, however, as GABA-T may appear also in glia (cf. 30). Assays of GABA-T in postmortem specimens suggest that there are normal levels of this enzyme in Huntington's disease (766,825).

The distribution of SSADH has not yet been mapped out in the striatum, although a histochemical method has been developed by Sims et al. for demonstrating this enzyme in frozen sections (685).

Succinic semialdehyde reductase and γ-hydroxybutyrate.

Succinic semialdehyde reductase acts on succinic semialdehyde to form γ-hydroxybutyrate. The lactone derivative of GHB is γ-butyrolactone (GBL), which is measured for quantitative assessments of GHB levels (165). These compounds are of particular interest not only because GHB levels in the striatum, pallidum, and substantia nigra are high relative to other parts of the brain (165) but also because GHB has been shown to have an inhibitory effect on dopaminergic neurons including those of the substantia nigra. Walters, Roth, and their colleagues have shown that systemic injection of GHB causes a dose-dependent (and, in high concentration, total) inhibition of firing of neurons in the pars compacta of the substantia nigra (643). Along with this suppression of activity, they found decreases in striatal levels of dopamine and a dopamine metabolite, dihydroxyphenyl acetic acid (DOPAC) (790). Generalized behavior depression (an anesthetic or sleep-like state) also results from systemic injection of high concentrations of GHB or GBL (790).

These studies suggest, though they clearly do not prove, that GHB is a neuroactive compound. Accordingly, the control of its synthesis from GABA via succinic semialdehyde (651), exerted by specific succinic semialdehyde reductase, could be important in modulation of the nigrostriatal dopamine pathway.

γ-Hydroxybutyrate has been measured in the striatum of persons dying with a diagnosis of Huntington's disease and has been found to be increased relative to normal control values (10; cf. 9). This may be an important clue to the location and function of GHB, as few other compounds are found in increased concentration in the striatum in this disease.

Homocarnosine and other GABA derivatives.

Much remains to be learned about the remarkably large number of compounds derived from the metabolism of GABA. One that should be mentioned here because of its potential importance in striatal mechanisms is homocarnosine (GABA-histidine). This compound is a dipeptide thought to be derived from GABA that is synthesized from putrescine (itself suspected of being a neuroactive compound) rather than from GABA synthesized from glutamate through the action of GAD (cf. 403). Homocarnosine has been reported to occur in the striatum in low levels (374,403,589), but concentrations of its synthetic enzyme (homocarnosine–carnosine synthetase) and especially of its degradative enzyme (homocarnosinase) are considerably higher (403,534). In the substantia nigra and globus pallidus, high levels of homocarnosine have been reported (589,403).

Striatal homocarnosine is stressed here because subnormal levels of this dipeptide have been found in the striatum (and substantia nigra) of patients with a diagnosis of Huntington's disease who died (587,766). The physiological role of homocarnosine is unknown, but the related dipeptide, carnosine, is considered a neurotransmitter candidate in the olfactory bulb (483). Further work on location and function of homocarnosine in the striatum is clearly warranted.

Brief mention should also be made of other compounds related to GABA such as γ-aminobutyryl-lysine (GABA-lysine) and γ-aminobutyrylcholine (GABA-choline), which may have functions independent of GABA itself (35,426,589). For the most part, assays have not been carried out to establish the regional concentrations of these substances, and the enzymes related to their synthesis and degradation have not yet been identified. GABA-choline, however, is known to be hydrolyzed at low rates by butyrylcholinesterase (pseudocholinesterase) (334), and this enzyme is of interest because it is present in very high levels in the striatum (94,225,226,555) and is now known to occur in a highly patterned distribution within the caudate nucleus (C. W. Ragsdale, Jr. and A. M. Graybiel, *in preparation;* see below). A link between this butyrylcholinesterase activity and GABA metabolites in the striatum is by no means certain; for example, butyrylcholinesterase also has been reported to have peptidase activity (466).

Glutamic Acid, Aspartic Acid, and Taurine

In addition to GABA, other presumed amino acid transmitters have been identified in the striatum, including glutamic acid and aspartic acid, both excitatory amino acids, and taurine, an inhibitory amino acid. As reviewed below, there is strong evidence that at least glutamate is a neurotransmitter in the corticostriatal projection to the caudate–putamen (217,488) and in the fiber projection from the hippocampal formation (probably from the subiculum) to the nucleus accumbens septi (789). This evidence is based on the finding of (a) large decreases in the high-affinity uptake of glutamate in the rat's striatum following lesions disrupting these afferent pathways and (b) decreases in the concentration of glutamate but not aspartate in the caudoputamen and nucleus accumbens after such lesions. It is the latter set of measurements that Fonnum and collaborators (213) have used to identify glutamate, in particular, as the neurotransmitter in these afferent-fiber systems: the high-affinity uptake channels for glutamate and aspartate are considered to be indistinguishable (and an apparent technical consequence of this is that the metabolically inert [^{3}H]-D-aspartate can be used to mark the uptake).

At least in the nucleus accumbens, there are probably also glutaminergic or aspartergic neurons. Walaas and Fonnum (789) found that after intrastriatal injections of kainic acid (which, it is claimed, destroys neurons but not afferent fibers, passing fibers, or glia), about 50% of the high-affinity uptake of glutamate in the nucleus accumbens was abolished. By adding lesions of the fornix, they obtained large further decreases in uptake so that the kainic acid effect could not be attributed to unexpected afferent-fiber damage. Walaas and Fonnum did not extend this study to the dorsal striatum (caudoputamen proper), but large decreases in glutamate (40–50%) and aspartate (35–40%) levels were observed there by Nicklas et al. (535) following comparable kainate lesions. These investigators suggested that the glutamate and aspartate may be in GABAergic neurons of the caudoputamen (there was a concomitant 60% to 70% drop in striatal GABA levels), but the alternate interpretation, that the caudoputamen contains glutamatergic or aspartergic neurons, should receive serious consideration in the light of Walaas and Fonnum's findings on the nucleus accumbens.

Antibodies have now been raised against aspartate aminotransferase and have been used to demonstrate putative aspartergic/glutamatergic neurons and terminals in the auditory and visual systems (3,4). Although glial and GABAergic neural labeling could be a complication, this immunohistochemical method should help in settling the question of whether there are intrinsic glutamatergic/aspartergic neurons in the striatum. The claim for transmitter-specific retrograde labeling

by [^{3}H]-D-aspartate or [^{3}H]-glutamate (cf. 34) suggests that injection of efferent targets of the caudate–putamen might also help in identifying such neurons. Streit and his colleagues, however, failed to see labeled cells after injecting ^{3}H-glutamic acid into the substantia nigra (727). It should be noted that in Huntingtonian brains, Perry et al. (587) have found abnormally low levels of glutamate in the striatum but not in the substantia nigra.

Taurine has been suggested as an amino acid transmitter candidate in the striatum by Nicklas et al. (535), who found a consistent 20% to 30% decrease in taurine levels in the rat caudoputamen following intrastriatal injections of kainic acid. In similar lesion studies with kainic acid, decreases of up to 64% in striatal taurine levels have been reported (715). Subnormal levels of the synthetic enzyme for taurine, cysteine sulfinate decarboxylase, have been reported in the striatum of choreic brains, whereas taurine itself has been found in greater than normal amounts (584,585,825). Immunohistochemical and radiolabel-uptake methods are now available for labeling putative taurinergic neurons (105,106,824) but have not yet been applied to the striatum.

Other Enzymes and Related Compounds Localized Within Striatal Neurons

Enzymes related to the metabolism of many of the known or putative neurotransmitters in the striatum have, not surprisingly, been detected in biochemical and histochemical assays of striatal tissue. Some of these have already been mentioned, and others not localized specifically to cell bodies in the striatum are indicated in Table 2. Two additional enzymes, cathepsin D and nicotinamide adenine dinucleotide phosphate diaphorase (NADPH-d), are of great interest because they have been unequivocally localized to the cell bodies of striatal neurons but have not been definitely associated with neurotransmitter substrates. Though direct morphological proof is still lacking, a third enzyme, angiotensin-converting enzyme (ACE), also is thought to occur in striatal neurons and to be related to neuropeptide metabolism.

Nicotinamide adenine dinucleotide phosphate-diaphorase.

This enzyme, formerly known as TPN-diaphorase, is one of a group of oxidative enzymes that can be observed by tetrazolium salt histochemistry (226,519). Thomas and Pearse (576,752) have described NADPH-d-positive "solitary active cells" in the striatum (and cerebral cortex) and have suggested that they have a "neurosecretory function" by virtue of their high content of NADPH-d and glucose-6-phosphate dehydrogenase. Pearse and his colleagues have further demonstrated that these cells are highly resistant to toxic effects such as anoxia and have suggested that they may be the so-called residual cells observed in some pathological states.

Given these findings, NADPH-d histochemistry should be applied to Huntington brains. Bird and colleagues (56) have already noted that striatal glucose-6-phosphate dehydrogenase levels are normal in Huntington's disease. Study of the possible coexistence of NADPH with known neurotransmitter candidates clearly also has high priority. It is interesting in this regard to note that somatostatin-containing neurons (or processes) might be residual elements in the striatum of Huntingtonian brains (see below). A second candidate that should be considered is GHB, because the synthetic enzyme for GHB, specific succinic semialdehyde reductase, requires NADPH for its activity (651), and, as noted earlier, striatal levels of GHB are high in Huntington's disease.

Cathepsin D.

Cathepsin D is a lysosomal enzyme with peptidase activity. Whitaker and his colleagues have produced an antiserum to this enzyme and have demonstrated that "large" neurons of the rat's caudoputamen express strong cathepsin D-like immunoreactivity (809). The distribution of these neurons has not yet been plotted in detail, and it is also not yet known whether cathepsin D is co-localized with neurotransmitters or related compounds (for large neurons, AChE and ACh come to mind as candidates, but there are also fairly large neurons containing somatostatin-like immunoreactivity; see below). Cathepsin D is broadly but selectively distributed elsewhere in the brain and in the spinal cord (809).

Cathepsin D is no longer thought to be the "isorenin of brain tissue" (see 325,754) and appears to have a broad spectrum of peptidase activity. This enzyme has been reported to act not only on angiotensinogen but also on angiotensin I, β-lipotropin and β-endorphin, substance P, and somatostatin (47,809). Given the strikingly specific cellular localization of cathepsin-D-like immunoreactivity within the striatum, further work on this enzyme should be given high priority, including study of whether it coexists with one or more of the known neuropeptides or other neurotransmitter candidates.

Angiotensin-converting enzyme.

This enzyme is a component of the renin–angiotensin mechanism in the kidney but is also found in the brain, where it appears to function in relation to the control of drinking and electrolyte balance. Angiotensin-converting enzyme is concentrated in the choroid plexus and circumventricular tissues but, aside from these sites, its activity in the brain tissue is highest in the striatum, with the pallidum and substantia nigra having the second highest levels (19,605,653,830). Arregui and his colleagues (17,18,20) have demonstrated remarkably large reductions of ACE activity in the basal ganglia of Huntington brains: 70% to 90% in the globus pallidus and 60% to 70% in the caudate nucleus and putamen.

Arregui and Iversen and their co-workers (17) have suggested that ACE is contained within neural perikarya in the striatum, in particular, within neurons projecting to the substantia nigra. Their evidence is indirect. First, they have demonstrated that lesions of the striatum induced with kainic acid lead to a marked (60%) reduction of ACE activity in the substantia nigra (18). Second, they have made systematic measurements of ACE activity in the brains of persons who had suffered Huntington's disease and compared these with values in matched controls and have found reductions in the Huntington brains that were specific to the striatum and its two main target structures (the substantia nigra, pars reticulata and the pallidum) (18,20). There is still doubt about the cellular localization of striatal ACE. The levels of ACE activity in the caudoputamen itself were reported by Arregui and colleagues to be insensitive to kainic acid injected directly into the striatum (17,18), but in a later study, the McGeer group succeeded in producing reductions in ACE activity with large injections of this neurotoxin (232,686). Antisera directed against ACE have so far failed to elicit immunohistochemical labeling of striatal neurons (or pallidal or nigral neurons), even in animals pretreated with colchicine (83).

The substrate for striatal ACE has not been identified with certainty; ACE is a generally active peptidase that cleaves dipeptides from the carboxy-terminal end of its substrates. There is evidence that ACE is effective in acting on enkephalin and bradykinin (168,264,735) as well as on angiotensin I (the known substrate for ACE in the renal renin–angiotensin system). Angiotensin-converting enzyme is reported to be different from enkephalinase (735). Its most likely substrate in the central nervous system, as in the periphery, is angiotensin I, which it converts to angiotensin II. Various components of the renin–angiotensin system have been detected in the striatum, but cross reactivities are apparently a serious problem (83,113,442,687), and findings are contradictory. For example, angiotensin II-like immunoreactivity is present in the striatum as measured by radioimmunoassay (687), but no more than a few scattered immunoreactive fibers, if that, have been seen in the striatum, even in colchicine-pretreated rats (83,113,238,245). There are moderate levels of angiotensinogen (the prohormone for angiotensin I) in striatal tissue, and angiotensinogenase activity (which may include ACE activity) is reported to be higher in the striatum than anywhere else in the brain (442). Finally, there are some reports of an intrastriatal localization of renin (the specific protease which converts angiotensinogen to angiotensin I) (144,243,244). Interestingly, single neuroblastoma cells from stable lines have been shown to coexpress renin and the angiotensins (550).

Neuropeptides

As many as 18 neuropeptides or neuropeptide families have been identified in homogenates of striatal tissue (see Table 2), but only four of these have yet been shown by immunohistochemistry to occur within cell bodies of the caudate–putamen and nucleus accumbens. These include peptides that display immunoreactivity to antisera (usually polyclonal) raised against opiate peptides, substance P, somatostatin, and avian pancreatic polypeptide (APP). It seems likely that other neuropeptides will be demonstrated to have an intraperikaryal location within the striatum. For example, indirect evidence both from kainic acid lesion studies and from postmortem assays of Huntington brains suggests that the striatum may contain neurons synthesizing cholecystokinin (183) and angiotensin (see above). Homocarnosine is another peptide that should be considered because of its low concentrations in the striatum in Huntington's disease (see above). With none of these peptides, however, is there direct immunohistochemical evidence for perikaryal localization.

Opiate-like Immunoreactivity

Three groups of opiate peptides have been identified in the central and peripheral nervous system: the enkephalins (met- and leu-enkephalin and met-enkephalin-arg[6]-phe[7]); pro-opiocortin compounds including β-endorphin and α-MSH; and the neoendorphins and dynorphin. There is excellent evidence that these peptides occur in separate fiber systems (for immunohistochemical evidence, see 63,800; for radioimmunoassay and biochemical studies, see 446,639; for evidence from cloning, see 124,289,371,521,540). Until very recently, it was thought that opiates in the striatum were principally enkephalins, but Barchas and colleagues (803) have now shown that dynorphin[1–8] occurs in very high concentration in the striatum of the rat. As yet, no dynorphin- or α-neoendorphin-containing cell bodies have been detected in the striatum by immunohistochemistry (804). The report of a dense network of dynorphin-positive fibers in the substantia nigra (804), however, has raised the possibility of a major dynorphin-containing nigral afferent system, and the striatum is an obvious candidate for its origin. There are also low levels of α-MSH (293,545) and β-endorphin (779,801) reported in the striatum and these may derive from hypothalamic afferents (see below).

Enkephalin-like immunoreactivity has been unequivocally identified at the light and electron microscopic levels in medium-sized spiny neurons of the rat's striatum (159,601). Medium-sized neurons with enkephalin-like immunoreactivity have been observed in a number of other light microscopic studies (181,210,329,428,665,792; see Fig. 4C). With an antiserum to leu-enkephalin, DiFiglia et al. (159) classified the immunoreactive neurons as spiny I cells (see Fig. 5). The immunoreactive neurons observed earlier by Pickel et al. (601) with an antiserum to met-enkephalin also appear to be spiny I neurons because they lack indentations of the nuclear membrane. There is a puzzling point of disagreement between these two studies, however, for Pickel et al. found that the immunoreactive neurons make asymmetric synapses with other neurons in the striatum, whereas DiFiglia et al. state that the neurons make symmetric synapses (see Fig. 5). The fact that the two groups had different antisera at their disposal could explain this discrepancy; and though it is by no means clear that the crucial differences would be between met- and leu-enkephalin substrates, it should be noted that Larsson et al. (428) claim to have identified separate leu- and met-enkephalin-containing neurons in the caudoputamen of the guinea pig.

A third enkephalin, met-enkephalin-arg[6]-phe[7], also has been found in high concentration in the striatum (723), and according to Udenfriend and his co-workers (637), levels of this variant of met-enkephalin in the human striatum are five times higher than those of leu-enkephalin. On the basis of immunohistochemical findings in the rat, Williams and Dockray (815) have suggested that met-

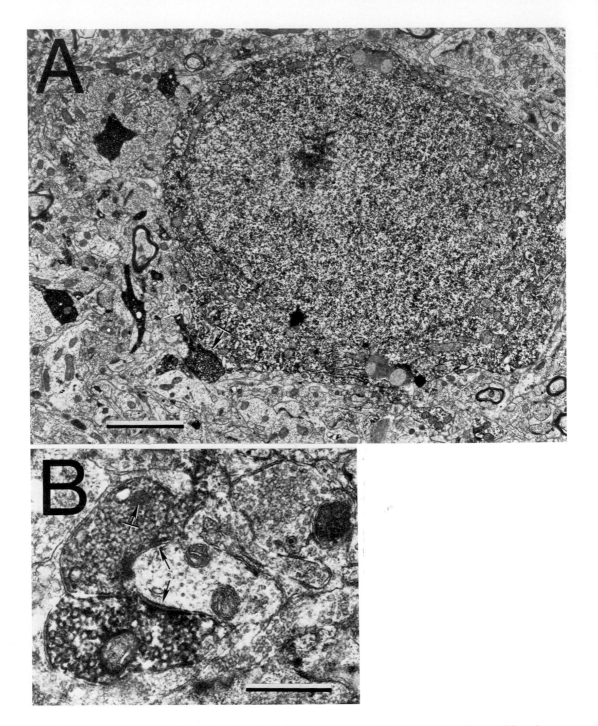

FIG. 5. Electron micrographs illustrating leu-enkephalin-like immunoreactivity in neural perikaryon (**A**) and axon terminals (**A,B**) visualized by the peroxidase–antiperoxidase method in the striatum of the macaque monkey. **A** shows reaction product present in the nucleus and cytoplasm. The cytologic features of the immunoreactive neuron are similar to those of medium-sized spiny neurons. An enkephalin-positive axon synapses with the immunoreactive neuron at *crossed arrow*. Note that the surrounding neuropil contains labeled axons and dendritic spines. *Scale marker,* 2 μm. See DiFiglia et al. (159). In **B,** both immunoreactive axon terminals shown contain numerous clear round and ovoid vesicles which are rimmed by a dense peroxidase precipitate. A large granular vesicle also appears in one of the boutons *(crossed arrow).* The axon terminals form synaptic contact *(arrows)* with the same dendrite. An unlabeled profile with clear vesicles appears at upper right. *Scale marker,* 0.5 μm. (Micrographs kindly supplied by Dr. M. DiFiglia.)

enkephalin-arg[6]-phe[7] may be a transient precursor of met-enkephalin. They find immunoreactive cell bodies in the caudoputamen when they react the striatal tissue sections with antiserum to met-enkephalin-arg[6]-phe[7], yet, when they react comparable sections with antiserum to met-enkephalin, they do not observe immunoreactive cell bodies but, instead, immunoreactive efferent fibers entering the globus pallidus (cf. 805). The substantia nigra, the second major target of striatal efferent fibers (see below), was not analyzed.

Substance P-like immunoreactivity.

There is strong evidence from lesion studies that substance P (SP) is a neurotransmitter in the striatonigral and striatoentopenduncular pathways. Large lesions of the caudoputamen in the rat result in at least a 70% to 75% loss of SP in the ipsilateral substantia nigra and a 50% to 60% decrease in the entopeduncular nucleus (41,84,241,337,358, 375,378,516,562,575,713). Comparable losses of SP in the internal segment of the globus pallidus and in the substantia nigra occur in Huntington's disease (91,184,240,377) and are attributed to the vulnerability of SP-containing neurons in the choreic striatum.

Although this evidence makes it virtually certain that SP is contained in a population of medium spiny striatal projection neurons, no classification of the SP neurons can yet be made because these neurons have not yet been identified at the electron microscopic level. In light microscopic studies, SP immunoreactivity has been reported in "small" and "medium"-sized striatal neurons in the rat (137,451), and Ljungdahl et al. (451) also report some "large" SP-immunoreactive neurons. In the cat (see Fig. 4D), SP-positive neurons are round or triangular, have little cytoplasm around the nucleus, and fall in the medium-size (10–20 μm diameter) range of Kemp and Powell (M.-F. Chesselet and A. M. Graybiel, *in progress*).

Somatostatin-like immunoreactivity.

Somatostatin-like immunoreactivity has been identified in medium-sized neurons in the striatum of the rat (44,211,360), cat (272), and guinea pig (204) and is of great interest because of the recent report that striatal somatostatin levels are increased in Huntington's disease (126). Electron microscopic evidence (M. DiFiglia and N. Aronin, *in preparation*; G. D. Burd, P. E. Marshall, and D. M. D. Landis, *in preparation;* see Fig. 6) suggests that the somatostatin neurons are of the aspiny I type because they have nuclear indentations and varicose dendrites. Even at the light microscopic

level, the dendritic varicosities are clearly visible (Fig. 4E), and an additional identifying feature is the presence of a stout and sometimes bulbous dendritic extension which bifurcates into much thinner processes (117). Evidence from experiments combining retrograde labeling with immunohistochemical identification suggests that the somatostatin-containing neurons do not project to the substantia nigra, pallidum, or neocortex (M.-F. Chesselet and A. M. Graybiel, *in preparation*). This fits well with their classification as aspiny I cells.

Both in the rat (782) and cat (M.-F. Chesselet and A. M. Graybiel, *in preparation*) some somatostatin-containing neurons in the caudate–putamen complex have been shown to express immunoreactivity to a second neuropeptide, avian pancreatic polypeptide (APP). It is not clear whether these represent a special subclass of somatostatin neurons or whether every neuron in the caudate–putamen that possesses immunoreactivity to one of these peptides also possesses immunoreactivity to the other. A further interesting question that remains to be answered is whether any of the somatostatin-containing neurons contain GAD immunoreactivity. A subtype of somatostatin-immunoreactive GAD-positive neurons has been identified in the thalamic reticular nucleus (546), and somatostatin and GABA have been reported to affect dopamine release in similar ways (117,253).

Avian pancreatic polypeptide-like immunoreactivity.

The cooccurrence of APP and somatostatin-like immunoreactivity just mentioned implies that at least some APP neurons (473,782) may correspond to the aspiny I cells of Golgi classification. A photomicrograph of APP-positive neurons in the caudate nucleus of the cat is shown in Fig. 4F. The APP neurons also appear to be interneurons since they are not retrogradely labeled following injections of tracer into the neocortex, substantia nigra, or pallidum (M.-F. Chesselet and A. M. Graybiel, *in preparation*).

Striatal Projection Neurons: Neurotransmitters and Transmitter Candidates Associated with the Efferent Connections of the Striatum

There are three massive efferent conduction routes leading away from the striatum: the striatopallidal pathways to the external and to the internal segments of the globus pallidus ("globus pallidus" and "entopeduncular nucleus," respectively, in nonprimates) and the striatonigral path-

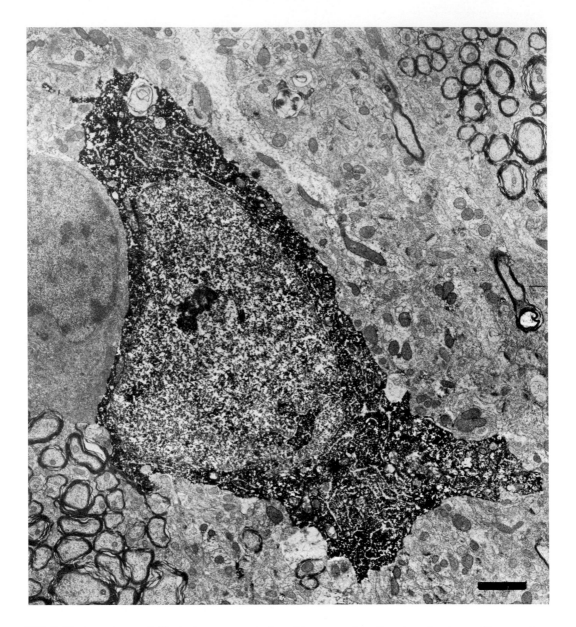

FIG. 6. Electron micrograph illustrating a somatostatin-positive neuron from the rat caudoputamen. Note prominent indentation in the nuclear envelope, a characteristic feature of these neurons (G. D. Burd, P. E. Marshall, and D. M. D. Landis, *unpublished data*). Compare with Fig. 4E. *Scale marker,* 2 μm. (Micrograph kindly supplied by Dr. G. D. Burd and colleagues.)

pathway to the pars reticulata of the substantia nigra (275). GABA is thought to be a neurotransmitter in all three pathways. Each also is associated with a neuropeptide, mainly enkephalin for the fiber projection from the striatum to the external segment of the globus pallidus, and mainly substance P for the fiber projections to the internal pallidum and substantia nigra, pars reticulata (Table 3). Whether GABA and one or more neuropeptides coexist in the fibers making up these efferent pathways is still unknown. The enkephalin-containing striatopallidal connection is the only one of these pathways so far demonstrated unequivocally by the combination of retrograde tracer labeling with immunohistochemistry (80,128,135,151; cf.352,713). Lesion studies combined with immunohistochemistry, biochemical assays, or binding studies provide evidence for occurrence of GABA and SP in striatal efferents, and for GABA there is additional corroborative evidence from the transmitter-specific retrograde labeling studies of Streit and colleagues (see above).

The known peptidergic content of these pathways strongly suggests that the internal pallidum and substantia nigra form a unit by virtue of being regulated by a major SP-containing connection originating in the striatum and that this unit may be functionally distinguishable from the external pallidum which receives a major enkephalin-containing input. This distinction may well be a crucial one, because it parallels natural divisions drawn on the basis of the efferent connections of these nuclei: the external pallidum projects almost entirely into the pallido–subthalamo–pallidal loop system and is thereby distinct from the internal pallidum and pars reticulata of the substantia nigra, which together give rise to the long efferent pathways of the pallidonigral mechanism leading to the thalamus, superior colliculus, and tegmentum (275).

Although this parallel suggests that the SP-containing neurons in the striatum may have some special importance in affecting the long efferents of the corpus striatum and that the enkephalin-containing neurons may play a role in controlling the pallido–subthalamic loop, the generalization remains to be tested. The fact that there is enkephalin as well as SP-like immunoreactivity in the sub-

TABLE 3. *Neurotransmitter-related compounds associated with striatal input–output connections*

Neurotransmitter-related compounds associated with efferent connections		Neurotransmitter-related compounds associated with afferent connections	
Compound	Pathway	Compound	Pathway
Certain		*Certain*	
GABA	Striatonigral and striopallidal	Dopamine	Nigrostriatal and tegmentostriatal pathways from cell groups A8,9,10; raphe–striatal from B7; possibly subthalamostriatal
Enkephalin	Striatopallidal to GP$_e$		
Substance P	Striatopallidal to GP$_i$ and strionigral		
Acetylcholine	In the cat, putaminocortical	Serotonin	Fibers from raphe nuclei, principally cell group B7
		Norepinephrine	Afferents from cell groups A1/A2,A5, and A6 (locus cerulus)
Uncertain			
Angiotensin I/II	Strionigral and striopallidal	Glutamate; Aspartate	Corticostriatal (from neocortex and hippocampal formation); possibly thalamostriatal
Angiotensin converting enzyme			
Homocarnosine	Strionigral	Cholecystokinin	Fibers from the SN and VTA; fibers from the amygdala; fibers from the claustrum or the piriform cortex or both
Cholecystokinin	Strionigral and striopallidal		
Acetylcholinesterase	Strionigral	Acetylcholinesterase	Nigrostriatal
		Histamine	Via medial forebrain bundle
		Vasoactive intestinal polypeptide	Via medial forebrain bundle
		α-MSH; β-Lipotropin/ACTH	Hypothalamostriatal
		Uncertain	
		Acetylcholine	Thalamostriatal
		Monoamine (e.g., phenylethylamine)	Subthalamostriatal
		GABA	Pallidostriatal or nigrostriatal
		Somatostatin	?

stantia nigra's pars reticulata (210,297,362,757), for example, raises the possibility that there may be an opiatergic strionigral pathway. In this regard, it is noteworthy that in Huntington's disease enkephalin levels are abnormal in the substantia nigra as well as in the pallidum (184). A similar argument holds also for the two segments of the globus pallidus: the internal segment of the globus pallidus, though predominantly expressing SP-like immunoreactivity, has a band of enkephalin-like immunoreactivity in its inner half (136,297). Because the inputs to the pallidum are limited (275), an enkephalergic striatopallidal pathway to this part of the internal segment seems likely. There is, conversely, some SP-immunoreactivity in the external pallidal segment, mainly along its margins (297). This may also be accounted for by a restricted striatopallidal connection, though in the rat (but not yet in the cat or monkey) SP-like immunoreactivity has been reported in pallidal neurons (137). An interesting possibility to consider is that the restricted districts of the striatopallidal system with overlapping SP and enkephalin immunoreactivities may be related in terms of their fiber connections. The fact that the ventral pallidum is just such a district (298,736) may indicate a limbic association.

There are further histochemical subdivisions to be drawn both in the pars reticulata and in the two segments of the pallidum, and it is probable that there will be parallels in the differentiated anatomical connections of these districts. The discovery of different immunoreactivities in the inner and outer parts of the internal pallidal segment is a case in point: Carpenter and his colleagues had already found that the two parts have distinguishable efferent projections (399), and a marked division of the internal pallidum in the human had also been noted (275).

In trying to assess the possible functional significance of these immunohistochemically distinct output pathways of the striatum, it becomes essential to know how the peptidergic pathways are related to those containing GABA. This problem has been studied mainly with respect to the strionigral pathway because the physical separation of the striatum and pars reticulata makes it possible to evaluate the effects of lesions and other treatments of the striatum without directly affecting the substantia nigra by the intervention itself. Such studies strongly suggest that the GABAergic and SP-containing pathways from striatum to substantia nigra are distinct (84,241,358), but direct proof is not yet available and would require double immunofluorescence combined with retrograde tracer marking. In the rat, the SP pathway is thought to

arise in the rostral part of the caudoputamen (241,358,451, but see 667), whereas the GABA-ergic pathway is reported to originate from the caudal half or to exhibit no marked gradient in its origin (215,241,358,520,667).

In electrophysiological studies, Kanazawa and Yoshida (376,606,833) succeeded in differentiating excitatory and inhibitory strionigral effects in the substantia nigra and have attributed these, respectively, to the SP- and GABA-containing pathways. After recording inhibition evoked in the cat's substantia nigra by stimulation of the caudoputamen, they blocked GABA-mediated inhibition by injecting picrotoxin into the systemic circulation and thereby uncovered an excitatory strionigral influence that itself was sensitive to systemic injection of baclofen, a putative antagonist of SP-induced excitation (see also 146). Given that GABA-mediated inhibition also dominates striopallidal transmission (832), it would be of interest to learn whether the effects of enkephalin and SP in the pallidum could be monitored with this infusion technique as well.

Another important consideration in assessing the function of these fiber pathways is the degree to which they are formed by collaterals branching from single neurons in the striatum. Apparently, medium-sized projection cells can be subdivided according to whether they project both to the pallidum and to the substantia nigra or to one of these districts alone (737; A. M. Graybiel and M.-F. Chesselet, *in progress*). Even among medium spiny neurons projecting to the external pallidum, there are neurons exhibiting different patterns of intrapallidal arborization (110; cf. 312,817): one type has a diffuse arbor; the second has two distinct fields of terminal ramification. It remains to be seen whether these subgroups are also distinguishable by immunohistochemistry.

In addition to these three major efferent pathways of the striatum, two other apparently sparse fiber projections have been noted: a projection from neurons scattered mainly in the putamen to the neocortex and a commissural pathway. Nothing is known about the neurotransmitter-related histochemistry of these pathways other than that, as discussed above, the corticopetal projection contains AChE and CAT.

Neurotransmitters and Transmitter Candidates Associated with the Afferent Connections of the Striatum

The evidence just reviewed suggests that of the neurotransmitter-related compounds in the striatum, the neuropeptides somatostatin and avian pancreatic polypeptide are probably contained in interneurons, whereas enkephalin and substance P are probably in projection neurons; that ACh and GABA are probably contained in both projection neurons and interneurons; and that at least some of the glutamate and aspartate in the nucleus accumbens (and possibly taurine in the striatum) are in intrinsic neurons (whether these are interneurons or projection neurons is unknown). There are many other neuroactive compounds in the striatum (see Table 2). Some of these may yet be found in neural cell bodies, but a number are already known to be associated with afferent pathways leading into the striatum. These include biogenic amines (dopamine, serotonin, probably histamine, and, in low concentrations, norepinephrine), amino acids (glutamate, aspartate, and possibly GABA), AChE and possibly ACh, and neuropeptides (cholecystokinin and vasoactive intestinal polypeptide). The neuropeptides neurotensin, α-MSH, and somatostatin may also be associated with afferent-fiber projections to the caudoputamen, and β-lipotropin and ACTH with projections to the nucleus accumbens (Table 3).

Afferents from the Midbrain and Hindbrain: Substantia Nigra, Ventral Tegmental Area, and Related Cell Groups

The fiber projections from the mesencephalic dopamine-containing cell groups to the striatum are probably the most studied pathways in the brain. The cells of origin in and around the substantia nigra were identified in 1964 by Dahlström and Fuxe (139), who established for them the well-known classification scheme distinguishing three main groups: A8, retrorubral nucleus; A9, substantia nigra, pars compacta; A10, ventral tegmental area of Tsai. This scheme has been confirmed and extended in subsequent studies (5–7,239,449,762). Retrograde labeling of neurons in each of these cell groups has been demonstrated by modern anatomical tracing methods after injections of tracer compounds into the striatum (198,202,525,527, 648,727,738,774,778). The median and near-midline dopamine-containing cell groups include the classic ventral tegmental area of Tsai (equivalent to the dorsolateral nucleus parabrachialis pigmentosis and ventromedial nucleus paranigralis) and also the nucleus interfascicularis just dorsal to the interpeduncular nucleus, the central and rostral linear raphe nuclei, and part of the dorsal raphe nucleus (7,449,542,561,599). Phillipson (599) has presented an excellent argument for considering

the interfascicular nucleus and the nucleus linearis as part of A10 or "the ventral tegmental area," although these terms are often used to denote a more restricted district.

The intrastriatal distribution of dopaminergic fibers originating in these cell groups has been studied by cathecholamine fluorescence and at both light and electron microscopic levels by immunohistochemistry with antisera raised against tyrosine hydroxylase (see Fig. 7) (236,239,449,600, 602). The appearance of the innervation as seen with fluorescence methods is fairly uniform but can be modified so as to appear patchy by pretreatment of the animal with a tyrosine hydroxylase inhibitor, α-methylparatyrosine (554). According to Fuxe and colleagues (234,554), the "dopamine islands" represent an early developing system of fluorescing processes having dotted fluorescence, whereas the more evenly distributed dopamine innervation develops later and shows diffuse fluorescence. The dotted (patchy) system is said to exhibit lower rates of tyrosine hydroxylase turnover (235,554) and may account for the patchiness of the nigrostriatal system seen by autoradiography following injections of tritiated amino acids into the substantia nigra (823). The dopamine islands are probably also related to other inhomogeneities in striatal chemoarchitecture (see below) (267) including the patchy distribution of [^{3}H]spiriperidol binding observed by Höllt and Schubert (333).

The intensity of catecholamine fluorescence is greater in the ventral striatum (nucleus accumbens and olfactory tubercle) than in the caudate nucleus and putamen. In the rat, levels of dopamine are also reported to be higher in the ventral striatum than in the caudoputamen proper (780). In the human, however, Bird and co-workers have found similar levels of dopamine in the nucleus accumbens and dorsal striatum (caudate nucleus and putamen) but have reported that the ratio of homovanillic acid to dopamine (i.e., of dopamine metabolite to dopamine) is higher in the nucleus accumbens than in the caudate nucleus or putamen (*personal communication*).

Early in the study of the dopaminergic projection to the striatum, a distinction was made between a mesolimbic system originating in cell group A10 and a nigrostriatal system originating in cell group A9 (7,762). The disposition of the connections now seems more complicated (39,275,437,525,526). Fallon et al. (199,200) and Fallon and Moore (197,198) have argued that the pars compacta of the substantia nigra should be divided into (a) a dorsal sheet of cells that are fusiform in shape, have horizontally directed dendrites, and project to the ventral striatum and to

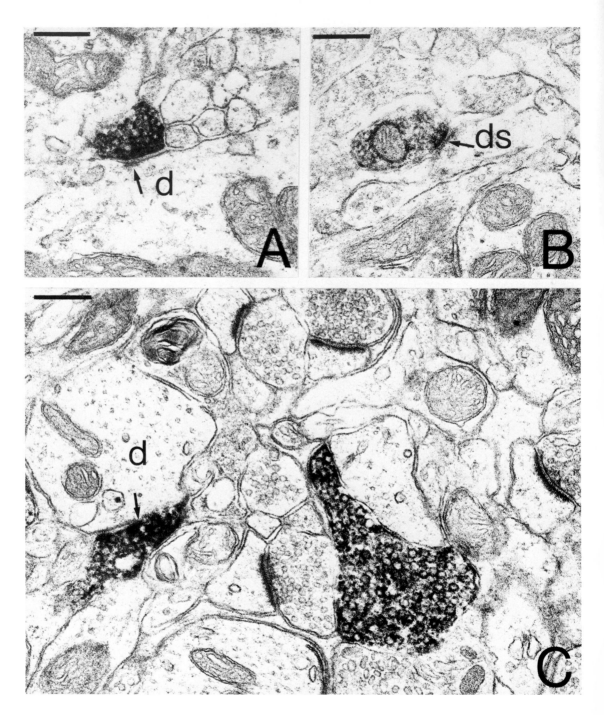

FIG. 7. Electron micrographs illustrating tyrosine hydroxylase-like immunoreactivity in axon terminals in the rat's caudoputamen. **A,B:** Type I terminals of Pickel et al. (600) making symmetric synaptic junctions with dendrite (d) and dendritic spine (ds). **C:** Type I (left) and type II (right) tyrosine hydroxylase-positive terminals. The type II terminal is rare compared to the type I; its junction lacks the membrane-density specializations typical of the type I. *Scale markers,* 1 μm. See Pickel et al. (600). (Micrographs kindly supplied by Dr. V. M. Pickel.)

the amygdala and piriform cortex and (b) a ventral sheet of cells that are pyramidal in shape, have dendrites extending into the pars reticulata, and project to more dorsal parts of the striatum and to the septum (see 368). The ventral tegmental area can similarly be separated into a dorsal nucleus parabrachialis pigmentosus and a ventral nucleus paranigralis on connectional criteria (198,599). Based on a study of Golgi-impregnated material, Phillipson (598) considers the ventral tegmental area to be continuous only with the dorsal sheet of pars compacta neurons.

Fallon (196) has suggested that a crucial difference between the neurons of the ventral tegmental area and those of the adjoining medial part of the pars compacta may be the degree of collateralization of their efferent projections: labeling patterns evoked by placement of distinguishable retrograde tracers in several locations (caudoputamen, septum, neocortex) demonstrate that cells of the medial part of the pars compacta have widely branched axons, whereas those in the ventral tegmented area do not. The electrophysiological studies of Deniau et al. offer support for this distinction (152). It is interesting, however, that in a study of these connections in the rabbit, retrograde tracers placed in the nucleus accumbens and caudate nuclei did not double label neurons in either the pars compacta or the ventral tegmental area (119).

Several lines of evidence suggest that a component of the nigrostriatal system—possibly as little as 5%—is nondopaminergic (49,207,294,295, 452,771,794). These neurons have been found in the ventral tegmental area, the pars reticulata of the substantia nigra, and in the medial part of the pars compacta. Hedreen (314) has described a trajectory for a nondopaminergic nigrostriatal connection in the rat that is different from the route followed by the dopaminergic fibers. The fibers initially travel with the nigrothalamic tract, although most probably do not give off collaterals to the thalamus or tectum (45,202; see below). The identity of the neurotransmitter in the nondopaminergic system is unknown, but neurotransmitter-related substances other than dopamine and associated compounds have been localized within neurons of the pars compacta and ventral tegmental area.

First, there is clear immunohistochemical evidence for the presence of cholecystokinin (CCK) in many of the mesencephalic dopaminergic neurons of cell groups A8, A9, and A10 both in the rat and in the human. There evidently are also some CCK neurons that do not contain dopamine (327, 328,768). The neurons containing both CCK and dopamine are most numerous in the classic ventral tegmental area but also occur elsewhere along the midline (e.g., nucleus interfascicularis) and in the pars lateralis of the substantia nigra (327). Skirboll et al. (689) have reported that CCK can affect the physiological activity of at least some of these mesencephalic dopaminergic neurons. Retrograde transport studies and lesion studies with the neurotoxin 6-hydroxydopamine (6-OHDA), which selectively destroys dopaminergic neurons, indicate that in the rat the CCK-containing neurons of A10 project to the ventral striatum (dorsomedial part of the caudal nucleus accumbens and medial part of the olfactory tubercle) and the periventricular part of the caudoputamen and also to the bed nucleus of the stria terminalis and central amygdaloid nucleus (327). Though only low levels of CCK have been detected in the substantia nigra (40), and no changes in these levels have been found in the caudoputamen following lesions (504), Studler et al. (730) have reported a "slight but significant decrease" in CCK in the substantia nigra of parkinsonian brains. Nondopaminergic neurons containing CCK and neurons with neurotensin-like immunoreactivity have been found in the ventral tegmental area and central linear nucleus of the raphe. The efferent projections of these cells have not yet been specified but could include the nucleus accumbens, which has high levels of neurotensin and CCK (327,760).

Neurons containing serotonin (5-HT) have been localized within the ventral tegmental area by immunohistochemistry (716,718), and retrograde labeling of neurons in the substantia nigra has also been reported to occur after injection of [3H]-5-HT into the caudoputamen (727). Priestly et al. (609) did not find double labeling of cells in the substantia nigra when they combined 5-HT immunohistochemistry with retrograde tracing following HRP injections into the caudoputamen, but a combination of fluorescent dye tracer and immunofluorescence histochemistry might prove more sensitive to the presence of serotonergic projection neurons.

Glutamate decarboxylase-positive and therefore presumably GABAergic neurons have been observed in the substantia nigra by Ribak and Oertel and their colleagues (547,628), and the possibility of a GABAergic pathway from substantia nigra to striatum has been raised by Streit's finding (727) that injections of [3H]GABA into the rat's caudoputamen elicit some weak perikaryal labeling in the pars compacta. The presence of such a GABAergic projection would be in accord with evidence that a small population of nigrostriatal fibers is composed of collaterals of nigrothalamic fibers, themselves thought to be inhibitory (153,295,720; 154,158,479,834). Also pertinent here are reports (459,461,490) that in Parkinson's disease, where the primary deficit affects catecholaminergic neurons, there is a decline in striatal GAD. This reduction need not be a direct effect, for it could reflect a transsynaptic regulation of the enzyme, a diminution of GAD after protracted illness, or other factors (581,786). It is interesting that Hornykiewicz and co-workers have found the decrease in GAD levels to be partly reversible by treatment with L-DOPA (461; cf. 456,458).

Acetylcholinesterase is contained in dopaminergic neurons of the pars compacta (97,318, 435,436,561) and almost certainly is a prominent marker of the early developing dopamine-island system (see Fig. 8) (98,271). According to Lehmann and Fibiger (436; cf. 677), about 10% of the AChE in the caudate–putamen complex derives from the substantia nigra. The function of this AChE is unknown. Greenfield and her colleagues (281) have reported that AChE is released in the ipsilateral substantia nigra and is decreased in the ipsilateral caudoputamen on stimulation of the substantia nigra. Opposite effects were recorded contralaterally. This asymmetric release of AChE does not parallel the pattern of release of dopamine induced by the same stimulation, for the release of dopamine is increased bilaterally both in the substantia nigra and in the caudoputamen. Pseudocholinesterase levels are not changed (253,281). Greenfield and co-workers have further demonstrated that iontophoretically applied AChE can have a direct physiological effect on nigral neurons (280).

Dorsal raphe nucleus.

Next to the nigrostriatal projection, the second largest fiber projection from the brainstem to the caudate nucleus and putamen is from the dorsal raphe nucleus [including the so-called B7 group (139)]. This afferent projection predictably includes a large serotonergic component, and, in fact, nearly all of the serotonin in the caudate nucleus and putamen arises from the B7 complex (7, 25, 65, 66, 356, 387, 432, 474, 648, 727, 738, 762, 778). A sparse projection to the striatum has also

been reported to arise from the adjoining serotonergic B8 group, including the central superior nucleus and caudal part of the central linear nucleus (604,738,811). As much as a quarter of the projection from the dorsal raphe nucleus to the striatum may be nonserotonergic, to judge from retrograde transport studies in the rat (1,356,571,609,719).

Steinbusch (717,718) divides the (rostral) B7 group into dorsomedian, ventromedial, and lateral sectors, all of which project to the striatum (as does the caudal part of B7), and has suggested that it is mainly from the ventromedial sector that the nonserotonergic projection derives (719). Ochi and Shimizu (542) report the presence of dopaminergic neurons in this ventromedial part of the nucleus. Steinbusch and co-workers were unable to confirm this by catecholamine immunohistochemistry (717), but Descarries and colleagues (155) have recently confirmed Streit's observation (727) of cell labeling in the dorsal raphe nucleus following injection of [^{3}H]dopamine into the rat's caudoputamen and have demonstrated that the raphe neurons so labeled lie in a ventromedial zone that is resistant to pretreatment with 5-HT. There are also neurons expressing CCK, substance P, enkephalin, and norepinephrine immunoreactivity in the dorsal raphe nucleus, but Steinbusch, van der Kooy, and colleagues have argued that these do not occur in the regions projecting to the caudoputamen (717,770). GABA (242) could be a neurotransmitter in the projection neurons of the nucleus.

The fiber projection from the dorsal raphe nucleus to the striatum is bilateral and apparently includes sizeable collateral offsets to the substantia nigra (772) and other regions of the forebrain (773). Within the caudoputamen of the rat, fibers expressing serotonin-like immunoreactivity are mainly found laterally and ventrally, especially near the pallidum (718).

Locus ceruleus.

There is a puzzling discrepancy between measures of noradrenergic receptors and noradrenergic fibers in the striatum. On the basis of ligand-binding studies, levels of β-adrenergic receptors in the striatum of the rat are reported to be the highest in the brain (2,100,559), and levels of α-adrenergic

$\longrightarrow$

FIG. 8. A: Patches ("dopamine islands") formed by catecholamine-induced glyoxylic acid fluorescence in the caudate nucleus (CN) of a kitten at embryonic day E50. **B:** The identical field is photographed a second time after the fluorescence section had been stained for acetylcholinesterase (AChE), thus showing that the dopamine islands are AChE-positive. Note detailed match between the AChE and fluorescence patch patterns. IC, internal capsule. See Graybiel et al. (271). *Scale marker, 500 μm.*

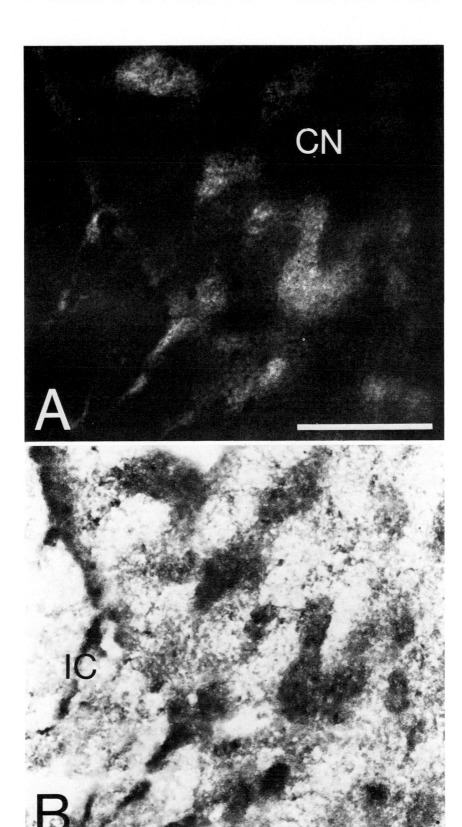

receptors to be at least "low to moderate" (as visualized by autoradiography) or "substantial" (as measured by scintillation counting) (765,840). By contrast, histofluorescence methods give negative results with respect to a noradrenergic innervation of the striatum or demonstrate only a weak and restricted innervation (239,449); immunohistochemical marking with antisera to dopamine-β-hydroxylase (DBH) also gives negative results in the caudoputamen and suggests the presence of at most a few fibers in the ventral striatum (288,733). There is only one report (486) of more than sporadic cell labeling in the locus ceruleus after injections of retrograde tracer into the striatum (283,727).

Jacobowitz and colleagues have studied this problem systematically in the rat and have found that the levels of norepinephrine in the striatum, though low, can be altered by lesions of the hindbrain. They conclude, first, that the dorsal noradrenergic bundle, which originates in the locus ceruleus (A6), is the source of part of the noradrenergic innervation of the caudoputamen and nucleus accumbens (544). Similar evidence has been obtained by others (365), but this result is not in accord with the findings of Ross and Reis (635) who found no decrease in striatal DBH following lesions of the locus ceruleus. The second conclusion of the Jacobowitz group is that neurons of norepinephrine-containing cell groups caudal to the locus ceruleus also project (via the ventral bundle) to the caudoputamen: cell group A5 to the dorsal striatum, and cell groups A1 and A2 to the nucleus accumbens but not to the caudoputamen (544,702). These pathways are reported to be bilateral. The autoradiographic findings of Ricardo and Koh (631) probably bear directly on this last point: they observed anterograde labeling of the nucleus accumbens after injections of tracer into the nucleus of the solitary tract, where neurons of the A2 group lie.

In the human, levels of norepinephrine are reported to be low in the caudate nucleus but moderate in the nucleus accumbens (191,201). They are reported to decrease in Parkinson's disease (179,191).

Epinephrine and the enzyme controlling its synthesis from norepinephrine (phenylethanolamine-*N*-methyltransferase, PNMT) are hardly detectable in the striatum of the rat (652,767), but in the monkey and human brain, PNMT, but not epinephrine, is apparently more widely distributed and is found in moderate concentrations in the striatum (and also in the globus pallidus and substantia nigra) (441,494). The presence of PNMT is presumably a selective indicator of epinephrine synthesis, so the difference in levels between PNMT and epinephrine is puzzling. Additional work in the monkey seems to be required.

Medial forebrain bundle.

Most if not all of the ascending fiber systems already discussed (notably those containing the biogenic amines) join the medial forebrain bundle on their way to the striatum. In addition, two striatal afferent systems containing histamine and vasoactive intestinal polypeptide (VIP) are also thought to follow the medial forebrain bundle, though the cells of origin of these two pathways have not yet been identified.

The evidence for the histaminergic afferents is of two sorts. First, the levels of histamine in the striatum decrease following lesions of the medial forebrain bundle (246,247). Second, following kainic acid lesions of the striatum, histamine binding decreases, and levels of the synthetic enzyme, histidine decarboxylase, are transiently reduced, but histamine levels increase (704). This increase in histamine levels is dependent on the integrity of the medial forebrain bundle (704). Clarifying information on the origin of the histaminergic innervation should come with use of new antisera raised against histamine (812) and histidine decarboxylase (755).

The evidence for a VIP-containing afferent fiber system is also indirect: VIP is present in low to moderate amounts to the striatum (52,471) and can be found in striatal synaptosomes (251). Taylor and Pert (748) report that VIP binding in the striatum is the highest in the brain. Immunohistochemical studies suggest that VIP-positive fibers are distributed in a patchy manner in the striatum (237,634) and are most heavily concentrated in the nucleus accumbens (237,471,684). According to Sims et al. (684), striatal cell bodies expressing VIP immunoreactivity are present only in the olfactory tubercle. In a recent abstract, however, Fukui and colleagues (231) report that VIP-positive neurons appear "occasionally" in the "striatum," presumably the dorsal striatum.

Marley et al. (484) report that levels of VIP in the nucleus accumbens and elsewhere, but not in the dorsal striatum, decrease following lesions of the medial forebrain bundle. They suggest as a possible source of ascending VIP-containing axons the group of VIP-positive neurons that lie in the ventral part of the central gray substance in the vicinity of the dorsal raphe nucleus (471,484,684). Neurons in this region have been reported to project to the nucleus accumbens (532).

Afferent Connections Originating in the Forebrain

Cerebral cortex.

The entire cerebral cortex projects onto the striatum in a highly ordered arrangement, with the neocortex sending fibers to the caudoputamen, and the olfactory and hippocampal formations sending fibers to the ventral striatum (275,282,394, 532,647,806). In the neocortex, two classes of cells are involved: large fast-conducting cells in layer V that project to the brainstem and give off collaterals to the striatum (167,313,359,367,404,778) and slowly conducting cells that project only to the striatum and are located both in layer V and in layer VI and supragranular layers (359,404,548, 647,669).

There has been intensive study of potential neurotransmitters for the corticostriatal pathway, and there is now near consensus that both the neocortical and hippocampal (probably subicular) projections use the excitatory amino acid glutamate and possibly aspartate. In 1976, Spencer (703) showed that excitation of striatal cells evoked by cortical stimulation could be antagonized by glutamic acid diethylester (GDEE), a drug that acts at L-glutamate/aspartate receptors. There followed a series of studies in which it was shown that high-affinity uptake for glutamate and aspartate in the striatum is sensitive to cortical lesions (214, 217,488,787,789,835), that potassium-evoked release of newly synthesized glutamate (from labeled glutamine) and aspartate (from labeled asparagine) decreases following cortical lesions (172, 625,626,646; see 255), and that the levels of glutamate (but not aspartate) in the dorsal and ventral striatum decrease after corresponding lesions of the neocortex or subiculum (172,214, 398,538,789). Streit has further reported that injections of [^{3}H]-D-aspartate into the striatum produce labeling of medium-sized pyramidal cells in layer V of the neocortex, presumably by transmitter-specific retrograde labeling (727). Some neurons in layer VI were labeled by intrastriatal injections of [^{3}H]-DL-glutamate, but this could have reflected labeling from uptake by fibers of passage [cf. Hedreen (313)].

Much of the interest in the apparently massive glutamatergic (aspartergic) input from the neocortex stems from the findings that neurotoxins such as kainic acid, which kill striatal neurons, are thought to do so by an excitotoxic action in which they bring to final metabolic exhaustion neurons that receive a glutamatergic/aspartergic input, i.e., neurons that have glutamate/aspartate receptors. The mechanism of kainate toxicity is still not understood but is under intensive study because of the possibility that this toxicity may provide a model for destruction of striatal neurons in Huntington's disease (134,489). Originally, it was thought that the kainic acid binding sites were the receptors for endogenous glutamate/aspartate, but this has been questioned because the neurotoxicity of kainic acid in the striatum seems to depend on the presence of an intact corticostriatal innervation (61,487). This effect is not understood.

Henke and Cuénod (319) point out that cortical ablation results in a 20% decrease in kainic acid binding and suggest that the effect is postsynaptic [cf. Hattori and Fibiger (304)]. The presence of such indirect effects is a serious concern in all such studies (see below). The most recent evidence suggests that kainate toxicity may involve both a presynaptic effect (induced release of glutamate and/or aspartate) and a postsynaptic effect (direct stimulation of receptors) (206). The preservation of striatal tissue imparted by deafferentation has been thought to indicate a specific mechanism involving corticostriatal afferents. Thus, Campochiaro and Coyle (102) have reported, and Lehmann and Fibiger (434) have confirmed, that the development of kainate toxicity in the rat parallels that of presumed glutamatergic corticostriatal innervation. It now seems unlikely that the cortical afferents are unique in this respect, however, because Hornykiewicz and collaborators have demonstrated a sparing effect on kainate toxicity of treatments removing the serotonergic innervation of the striatum (48).

Multiple mechanisms for the excitatory actions of glutamate, aspartate, and their analogs are to be expected, because evidence has accumulated for as many as four subclasses of receptors related to glutamate: (a) a kainate receptor, which may prefer an extended conformation of glutamate; (b) a quisqualate receptor, where glutamate diethyl ester may act as an antagonist; (c) an N-methyl-D-aspartate (NMDA) receptor, at which 2-amino-5-phosphonovalerate (APV) is a blocking agent; and (d) an L-aspartate/L-glutamate receptor, which may be the major binding site for L-glutamate (363,477,797). There is physiological evidence for the presence of all of these sites in the rat striatum (256,477,703,725,740). The striatum exhibits very high levels of the kainic acid binding site (62,470,683), which is thought to account for as much as 10% of the L-glutamate binding. No such measures have yet been made with NMDA and quisqualate as ligands (see 691). Whether or not glutamate itself acts on kainate receptors is unclear, but the antagonistic action of GDEE and the excitatory action of L-aspartate apparently do not depend on kainate receptors (300,470,797). Luini et al. (477) have reported that an unidentified excitatory compound is released from striatal slices under high-potassium conditions and that this compound may act preferentially on the *N*-methyl-D-aspartate site.

Amygdala.

The basolateral nucleus of the amygdala projects to the caudatoputamen (388,648,778) and to the nucleus accumbens (283,414,532). The termination of this fiber system is patchy and bilateral (388). Additional components of the amygdalostriatal projection arise from the basomedial and lateral nuclei (388). The neurotransmitters associated with these pathways are unknown, but Roberts et al. (634) have reported that many of the fibers running between the amygdala and caudatoputamen contain immunoreactivity to somatostatin, somewhat fewer fibers with CCK- and neurotensin-like immunoreactivity, and still fewer with VIP-like immunoreactivity. The CCK immunoreactivity, in particular, is present in some cells in the basolateral and basomedial nuclei of the amygdala, and lesions of the amygdala are reported to lead to a 30% reduction in striatal CCK (504). No comparable measurements have yet been reported for somatostatin, neurotensin, or VIP in the striatum after destruction of the amygdala, but there are cell bodies expressing immunoreactivity for each of these neuropeptides in the amygdaloid complex.

Globus pallidus.

Nauta (524) has reported autoradiographic evidence for a projection from the globus pallidus to the caudate nucleus and putamen of the cat. In addition, Staines et al. (714) have reported that neuronal labeling is elicited in the pallidum by intrastriatal injections of a horseradish peroxidase–wheatgerm agglutinin conjugate. The injection sites in these HRP experiments may have implicated pallidal or peripallidal fibers en route to the cortex (353,433,524,566), but Staines et al. report that the labeled pallidal neurons are those that do not stain intensely for AChE (as do the neurons projecting to the cortex, see above).

The neurotransmitter for the pallidostriatal pathway is not known, but the findings just cited make it unlikely that AChE is contained in the pallidostrial fibers, and this is in accord with the observations of McGeer et al. (493) who described only a small decline in AChE and no decline in CAT in the striatum following pallidal lesions. The

loss of striatal AChE observed by Shute and Lewis (676) after pallidal destruction may have reflected damage to fibers ascending from the brainstem. Based on immunohistochemical studies of neurons in the pallidum (137,378,628,629), a more likely candidate for the neurotransmitter in this pallidostriatal pathway would be GABA (or substance P).

Claustrum and piriform cortex.

Meyer et al. (504) have suggested that a major source of CCK in the caudoputamen is the claustrum or adjoining piriform cortex, because knife cuts separating these basolateral forebrain structures from the striatum result in a 70% decrease in CCK levels in the striatum. The precise origin of the suggested CCK pathway has not been specified, but there are known to be CCK-positive neurons in the piriform cortex and claustrum (40,349,504). Krettek and Price (414) have reported autoradiographic evidence in the rat for a pathway to the ventral caudoputamen from the endopiriform nucleus (the presumed equivalent of the claustrum), but they could not exclude involvement of the deepest layers of the adjoining cortex.

Thalamus.

The main thalamic projection to the striatum originates in the intralaminar nuclei (275,366, 527,648,778). Other small thalamostriatal fiber projections have also been reported to arise from the mediodorsal nucleus (666,808), from parts of the ventral tier including the ventromedial nucleus (322,669,727,778), from midline, lateral, and anterior nuclei (648,666,778), and from the posterior nuclear group (157,275,778). The intralaminar projection is massive and terminates in an ordered patchy pattern (see below), and at least some of the cells of origin send axon collaterals to the neocortex (578,722). The neurotransmitter of the intralaminar projection has not yet been identified. The parafascicular nucleus is reported to contain moderately high levels of ACh, AChE, and CAT (340,568,677), and Saelens et al. (659,682) have observed decreases in CAT and ACh in the striatum following lesions of the parafascicular nucleus. However, the McGeers and colleagues have not found such a lowering of CAT levels (or lowering of AChE levels) in the striatum even after large thalamic lesions (488,493), and from the early studies of Shute and Lewis (676), it appears that at least part of the AChE in the parafascicular nucleus [and the CAT—(339)] is of extrinsic origin because there are sharp declines in the levels of these enzymes following lesions of the dorsal tegmental pathway at the level of the nucleus cuneiformis. Kimura et al. (401) found no immunoreactive cell bodies in the intralaminar nucleus in their study with the putative anti-CAT antiserum discussed above.

Another possibility raised by Streit is that the thalamostriatal fibers from the intralaminar nuclei use glutamate or aspartate as their neurotransmitter. After [³H]-D-aspartate injection into the caudoputamen, Streit (727) found retrograde labeling of neurons in the intralaminar complex and parts of the ventrolateral nucleus but not elsewhere. Other evidence is needed, however, because the McGeers and co-workers (488) have claimed that glutamate uptake levels in the striatum are not affected by thalamic lesions, and the specificity of the retrograde transport is still at issue (see 138). The nature of the neurotransmitters used by thalamic neurons is a general problem; there is little if any labeling of cell bodies in the thalamus with any of the known neurotransmitter-specific markers.

Subthalamic region.

In a study of striatal afferents by the ¹²⁵I-tetanus toxin retrograde transport method, Schwab and co-workers (669) reported "pronounced labeling" of neurons in the subthalamic region in the rat, specifically in the zona incerta and Forel's field H₂. Newman and Winans (532,533) have also reported cell labeling in this region after placing deposits of HRP into the nucleus accumbens and olfactory tubercle of the hamster. The only report of anterograde labeling of the striatum after tracer injections in the subthalamic region is that of Ricardo (630), who attributed the striatal labeling he saw to incidental involvement of the cortex in his experiments. No information is available about the neurotransmitter substances associated with this pathway, but Schwab and his colleagues (669) observed that the subthalamic cell labeling was sensitive to 6-OHDA pretreatment. This raises the possibility that some striatal dopamine may arise from the A13 cell system (449).

An alternative, however, is that these subthalamic neurons may be among the noncatecholaminergic, nonserotonergic neurons that contain aromatic amino acid decarboxylase and accumulate L-DOPA (which could account for the 6-OHDA toxicity)(447). The neurotransmitter of these neurons is unknown, but it could be one of the trace monoamines, for example, phenylethylamine, which are in their highest concentrations in the striatum and hypothalamus, or possibly histamine (see above). This same subthalamic district also appears to correspond to the region containing many of the extraarcuate α-MSH-positive neurons (397) (see below).

Hypothalamus.

There is at most a weak innervation of the striatum by endorphin-containing fiber systems originating in the hypothalamus. A β-lipotropin/β-endorphin/ACTH system and one of two known α-MSH systems arise from neurons in and around the arcuate nucleus of the hypothalamus (545,799,800). The two subclasses of pro-opiocortin peptides are thought to coexist in the same neurons (521,799), and these neurons are thought to be distinct from those containing LHRH (63; cf. 673). Watson et al. (798,801) have reported immunohistochemical evidence for β-lipotropin and ACTH in the nucleus accumbens, and it has been suggested very recently that a second sparse α-MSH fiber system reaches the caudoputamen from dorsolateral hypothalamic neurons which may be characterized by a different processing of pro-opiocortin (293,397; cf. 843). Both fiber projections are apparently very weak; in fact, Jacobowitz and O'Donohue (354,545) reported on the basis of immunohistochemical and radioimmunoassay evidence that α-MSH fibers are not present in either the caudoputamen or the nucleus accumbens but skirt the medial edge of the nucleus accumbens on their way to the medial septal nucleus.

RECEPTORS FOR STRIATAL NEUROTRANSMITTERS AND THEIR ANALOGS

The locations of sites capable of binding known and putative neurotransmitter substances and their analogs have been studied intensively in the striatum by autoradiographic procedures involving exposure of frozen tissue sections to radiolabeled ligands. Such anatomical studies have a great advantage over assays of dissected samples because they allow the distribution of receptor binding sites to be identified in detail. This is important not only for accuracy in charting regional distributions (for example, the span from caudate nucleus to nucleus accumbens to olfactory tubercle can be surveyed without artificial borders set by microdissection) but also because local patterning in the distributions of receptors can be detected (for example, within the caudate nucleus, the patchy distribution of opiate receptors mentioned below and illustrated in Fig. 9).

As shown in Table 2, the striatum contains the highest levels of binding for a number of neurotransmitters and neurotransmitter-related compounds, including ACh (muscarinic cholinergic), norepinephrine (β₁-adrenergic), dopamine, histamine (H₂), kainic acid, and vasoactive intestinal polypeptide. At least moderate binding levels have

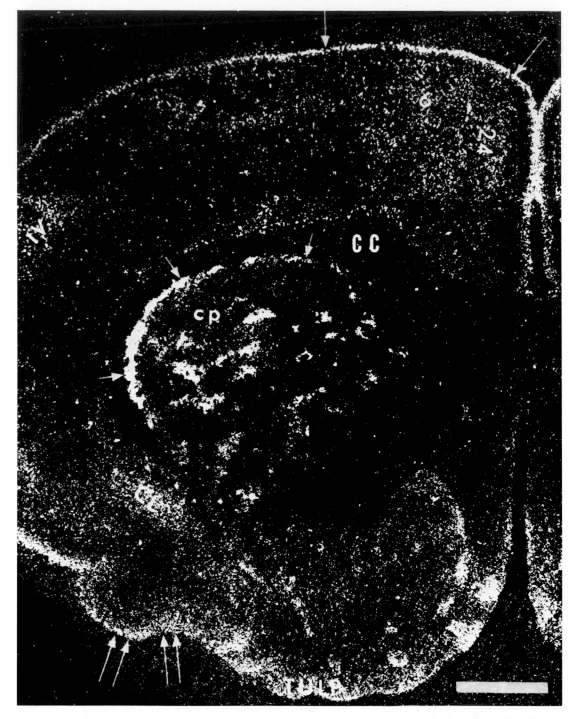

FIG. 9. Dark-field photomicrograph illustrating the clustering of opiate receptors in the rat's caudoputamen visible when tissue sections are exposed to the radiolabeled ligand [^{3}H]dihydromorphine and prepared for autoradiography. cp, caudoputamen; CC, corpus callosum; TUL, olfactory tubercle; 24,6, cortical areas 24 and 6; IV, cortical layer IV; CL, claustrum. *Scale marker,* 100 μm. (This photomicrograph was modified from Young and Kuhar, ref. 841, and was kindly supplied by Dr. M. J. Kuhar.)

been reported for a number of other substances listed in Table 2. In interpreting such receptor-binding studies, several points should be kept in mind. First, there may be binding sites with high and low affinities for a particular ligand, and these may be functionally distinct. Second, the concentration or distributions of receptor sites and of apparently corresponding neurotransmitter molecules do not always match. The contrast between the levels of β-adrenergic binding in the striatum (highest in the brain) and the levels of norepinephrine and epinephrine themselves (very low) has already been mentioned. Third, definitive identification of receptor subtypes can be difficult or controversial (e.g., in the case of opiate receptor subtypes), and these problems reflect back on attempts to match localizations of neurotransmitters and receptors. A fourth and particularly serious problem is that receptors are themselves transported by axonal flow (842) and may apparently occur anywhere in or on the neuron, including locations devoid of synaptic junctions (cf. 36,145,345). A striking example is the report of opiate and histamine-H_1 receptors associated with neurons of the dorsal root ganglia (536). In addition to the distinction between junctional and nonjunctional receptors, differences in the location of junctional receptors (presynaptic, postsynaptic) must clearly be crucial from the functional point of view yet are virtually impossible to demonstrate by current methods (see Fig. 10) (304).

Careful studies need to be made of the precise distribution of receptor binding sites in relation to distributions of neurotransmitters. For at least some ligands, the newly reported method for combined immunohistochemistry and ligand binding (443) should help in this effort. Kuhar, Stumpf, and their colleagues, however, have documented reasons for caution in applying other than exacting dry-section processing, which is difficult to combine with immunohistochemistry (417,731).

HISTOCHEMICAL COMPARTMENTALIZATION OF THE STRIATUM

There is now compelling evidence that the neuropil of the striatum is organized into chemoarchitecturally distinct tissue compartments related to the organization of striatal afferent and efferent connections and to the disposition of a number of the neurotransmitter-related compounds discussed above. Every major striatal afferent pathway studied by autoradiography has been shown to terminate in a patchy manner. This patterning in striatal

afferents was discovered by Künzle in his study of corticostriatal fiber projections in the monkey (422–425; see Fig. 11; 259,615,777,831) and has since been described for the thalamostriatal (266,321,372,649), amygdalostriatal (388), and nigrostriatal (250,823) pathways. No clear evidence is available about the distribution of the less massive inputs to the striatum from pallidum, subthalamus, and the raphe, though according to Steinbusch, serotonergic fibers in the striatum may be unevenly distributed (718).

Cell bodies in the striatum labeled in retrograde transport experiments after injections in the pallidum and substantia nigra also show marked clustering, with distinct pockets of sparse retrograde labeling interrupting larger fields and bands of dense labeling (276; see Fig. 12). Clustering of striatal neurons can even be seen in Nissl preparations (257,269,564), though it is only during development that the cell clustering is as obvious as the patterning visible in the input–output connections and the chemoarchitecture of the mature striatum [120,258,498; and C. W. Ragsdale, Jr., and A. M. Graybiel, *in preparation*—see Graybiel (266)].

The histochemical compartmentalization of striatal tissue has been demonstrated for a variety of neuropeptides and neurotransmitter-related enzymes in the neuropil of the striatum. As shown in Figs. 1 and 13 (cat) and Fig. 11 (monkey), cross sections stained lightly for AChE are marked by 300- to 600-μm-wide zones of low AChE activity which stand out against an otherwise AChE-rich background. These zones of low AChE activity are called "striosomes" and have been observed in many mammalian species including the human (277,278). Serial-section reconstructions demonstrate that the striosomes form highly connected labyrinths running through the striatum (277). These labyrinths are in turn related to the distribution of opiate peptides in the striatum. In the cat, the AChE-poor striosomes correspond spatially to patches of high opiate-like immunoreactivity (272,274). In the monkey (Fig. 11), the striosomes also correspond to opiate patches, but these often have a ring-and-hollow form (A. M. Graybiel and C. W. Ragsdale, Jr., *unpublished data*). In the rat, the striosomes have further been shown to correspond to regions of high opiate-receptor density (321; see refs. 21,320,592,841).

These correspondences appear to express a general tissue organization in the striatum. Matches between the AChE-poor striosomes and patches of high or low SP immunoreactivity have been made (272), and GAD-like immunoreactivity also has

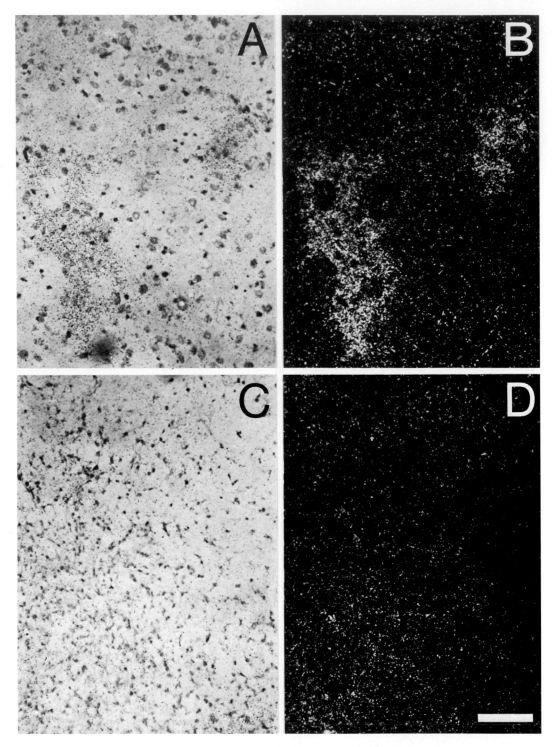

FIG. 10. Photomicrographs illustrating (**A,B**) clusters of [³H]diprenorphine-labeled opiate receptors in the caudoputamen of an adult rat and (**C,D**) virtual absence of clusters in the contralateral caudoputamen in which kainic acid had been injected 2 weeks previously. *Scale marker,* 100 μm. (Kindly provided by Dr. M. J. Kuhar and colleagues; see Murin et al., ref. 518.)

been found to express a striosomal organization (A. M. Graybiel, M.-F. Chesselet, and J.-Y. Wu, *in preparation*). In kittens, the AChE-poor striosomes have been shown to correspond to patches of high tyrosine hydroxylase immunoreactivity and high catecholamine fluorescence (the dopamine "islands") (A. M. Graybiel and T. H. Joh, *in preparation*). In certain species (e.g., the squirrel), the striosomes correspond to regions of high pseudocholinesterase activity (C. W. Ragsdale, Jr., and A. M. Graybiel, *in preparation*). Patchy distributions of VIP, CCK, and neurotensin have been reported, but these have not yet related to the striosomes (see Table 2).

Direct serial-section comparisons of these histochemical compartments with the patchy ordering of striatal connections have been made in the rat, cat, and monkey. Cortiocostriatal fibers (from the frontal cortex) have been shown to fill in or just avoid the striosomes (Fig. 11); both patterns have been seen in individual cases, suggesting a heterogeneity in the functional affiliations of different parts of the striosomal system (615,616). Thalamic fibers mainly avoid the striosomes (266,321), whereas the early incoming dopaminergic fibers mainly fill them in (A. M. Graybiel and T. H. Joh, *in preparation*). In retrograde labeling experiments (276), zones of low retrograde labeling have been correlated with the striosomes, as though the striosomes represented regions with a high density of interneurons (see Fig. 12). Double- and triple-label experiments are needed to decide whether certain projection cells might lie in the striosomes and other projection cells outside of them.

There are strong indications that the striosomal architecture visible in the histochemistry and connections of the striatum is related to patterns established early in development. Dopamine and AChE (which appear to coexist in at least a subset of the nigrostriatal fibers; see refs. 97,271,436; Fig. 8) are distributed in small patches in the fetal and neonatal striatum (98,271,273,539,553,554,617, 749), and there are also patches of high muscarinic and opiate receptor binding (395,645,764; and M. Nastuk and A. M. Graybiel, *in preparation*) and high enkephalin and substance P immunoreactivity (270,272). Moreover, there is evidence from [^{3}H]thymidine studies that medium-sized neurons with similar birthdates (possibly together with labeled daughter cells) come to lie in clusters (see Fig. 13) (8,79,166,205,269). The dopamine islands, patches of muscarinic receptor binding and neuropeptide immunoreactivity, and the clusters of thymidine-labeled cells are probably all related to the AChE patch-patterns seen in the immature striatum (cf. 98,269–271).

A remarkable transition in the chemoarchitecture of the striatum occurs in the perinatal period. The patches of high AChE activity, high muscarinic receptor binding, and high tyrosine hydroxylase immunoreactivity and catecholamine fluorescence become obliterated or obscured in the adult, leaving the striosomal (enzyme-poor) patch-pattern in the AChE stain and only faint inhomogeneity in the muscarinic receptor binding, tyrosine hydroxylase immunohistochemistry, and catecholamine fluorescence (78,98,554,617,644,645). The fact that some patches visible in the fetal brain are maintained in the adult [e.g., patches of high enkephalin-like immunoreactivity (270) and matching thymidine-labeled clusters (269; A. M. Graybiel and T. H. Joh, *in preparation*)] strongly suggests that despite the maturational changes, a basic three-dimensional matrix is maintained throughout development.

In addition to these distinctly bounded tissue compartments which tend to be periodic in their arrangement (272), there are gradients in the distribution of neurotransmitters and neurotransmitter-related compounds that are visible in the striatal neuropil in histochemical and immunohistochemical preparations and measurable in samples dissected for biochemical assays. For example, in the rat, assays suggest that 5-HT and GAD levels are highest in the caudal part of the caudoputamen (214,667,718,751), whereas substance P, acetylcholine and dopamine and their related compounds and D-aspartate uptake are most concentrated rostrally (68, 84, 214, 241, 296, 358, 413, 451, 618, 667, 729, 741, 744, 787). The cholinergic markers tend to be denser in the lateral part of the caudoputamen than in the medial part (296,618,729), and in both rat (210,601,681,792) and cat (272), enkephalin-like immunoreactivity is strongest ventrally. Even the striosomal patterns show marked gradients. For example, in the cat the AChE-poor striosomes are least distinct in the dorsolateral and caudal part of the caudate nucleus (272,277); in the human, the striosomes are less clearly defined in the putamen than in the caudate nucleus (277). These histochemical gradients appear to be related to developmental gradients in the time at which AChE activity, tyrosine-hydroxylase immunoreactivity, and catecholamine fluorescence appear in striatal neuropil and also to the birth dates of striatal neurons (8, 98, 143, 166, 205, 269, 273, 539, 553, 554, 617, 701, 734, 749). They are of special interest from the clinical standpoint because of comparable gradients in the appearance of histological abnormalities in the striatum in Huntington's disease (J.-P. von Sattel and E. P. Richardson, *in preparation*).

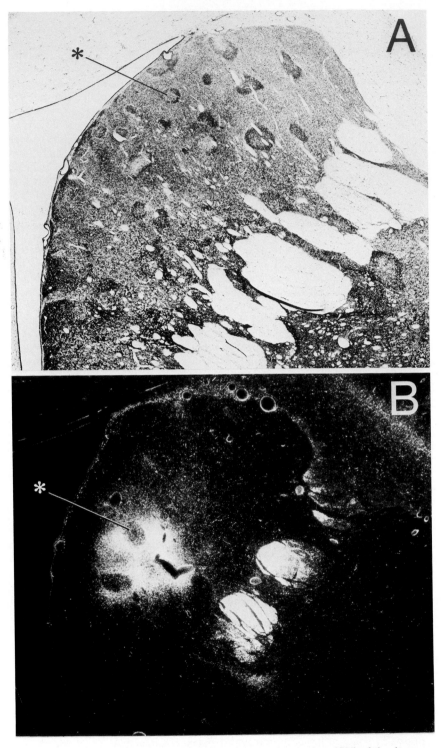

FIG. 11. Pairs of serially adjacent transverse sections through the caudate nucleus (CN) of the rhesus macaque illustrating the striosomal architecture of the striatum. **A,A′**: Correspondence of acetylcholinesterase (AChE)-poor striosomes (**A′**) with met-enkephalin-immunoreactive patches and ring-and-hollow formations (**A**). One such correspondence is marked *(asterisks)* (A. M. Graybiel and C. W. Ragsdale, Jr., *unpublished data*). **B,B′**: Correspondence

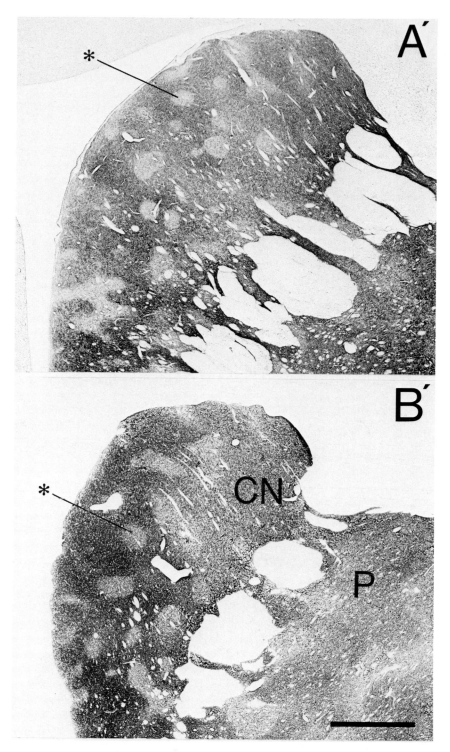

between the AChE-poor striosomes (**B′**) and pockets avoided by prefrontostriatal fibers made visible in anterograde autoradiographic experiments (**B**). One matching pair of patches is marked *(asterisks)*. Labeled fibers appear white in dark-field photograph of **B**. P, putamen. See Ragsdale and Graybiel (615). *Scale marker,* 2 mm.

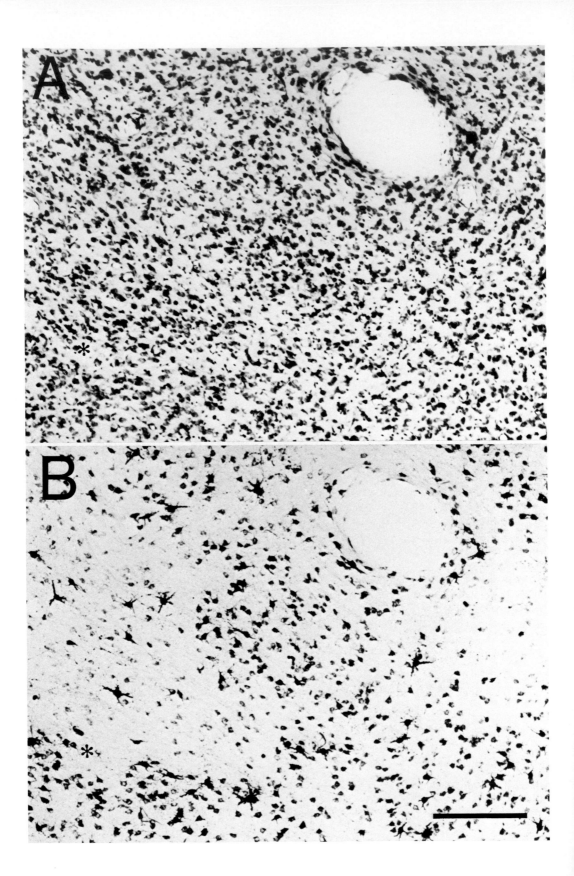

Though local patterning in the chemoarchitecture of the striatum has been studied mainly with respect to the caudate nucleus, there is also marked inhomogeneity in the distribution of neurotransmitter-related compounds in the ventral striatum, both in the nucleus accumbens septi and in the olfactory tubercle (272,277,327,837). Figure 14 gives an idea of this by illustrating the lobulated appearance of enkephalin- and substance P-like immunoreactivity and AChE staining in the olfactory tubercle (see also Fig. 1) and the striking subdivisions found in the nucleus accumbens by these substances, e.g., a dorsal zone that is rich in substance P but poor in enkephalin and that shows a pronounced mediolateral gradient in AChE activity. Equally marked subdistricts within the ventral striatum are visible in sections prepared for tyrosine hydroxylase immunohistochemistry and catecholamine fluorescence (236,271,554; and *unpublished observations*).

A related subject that needs study is the degree to which the caudate nucleus and putamen should be considered as distinct from one another in terms of their neurotransmitter-related anatomy. Most biochemical studies have been performed on the rat, in which a differentiation between caudate nucleus and putamen is problematic, and there is accordingly only limited information on this important point. There are hints from biochemical assays of the human striatum that there may be differences in the chemical composition of these two subdivisions, however, and in cat and monkey, striking differences have been observed in the histochemistry and immunohistochemistry of the caudate nucleus and putamen (272,277). Given the different afferent affiliations of the caudate nucleus and putamen in the monkey (see refs. 425,777), distinctions between these two subdivisions in terms of their content of neurotransmitter-related compounds might have important functional consequences. It may also be possible now to relate such neurochemical variations to the somatotopic maps in the striatum observed directly by electrophysiological recording (632) and indirectly by analysis of topographic corticostriatal connections (394, 423,425,806).

INTERACTIONS AMONG NEUROTRANSMITTERS IN THE STRIATUM

Appreciation of the diversity of neurotransmitter-related substances in the brain is still so fresh that studies of striatal transmitter systems have as a first goal the establishment of accurate inventories of the transmitter-related compounds present. Table 2, summarizing current information on this matter, was prepared to emphasize the breadth of representation within the striatum of different neurotransmitter classes. The striatum stands out as extreme in this respect. Only a few known neurotransmitters or neurotransmitter candidates are poorly represented, striking examples being norepinephrine, glycine, octopamine, and the neuropeptides vasopressin and β-endorphin.

Given the complexity of the anatomical organization of the striatum, it should not be surprising that its neurotransmitter systems interact extensively with one another. What has been unexpected, however, is the type and breadth of the interactions. For example, the release of newly synthesized dopamine from nigrostriatal terminals in the striatum can be influenced by applying one or another of a growing list of neurotransmitter-related compounds to striatal tissue *in vivo* or *in vitro* (118), and such alterations in neurotransmitter release can be shown to have distant effects (253). These observations suggest the existence of either presynaptic inputs to control the dopamine fiber terminals or extensive circuits designed to have a similar effect. Other findings implicate multiple neurotransmitter systems in disease states that affect the striatum directly or indirectly. These are far more extensive than initially thought, involving constellations of neurotransmitters, neurotransmitter-related compounds, and their receptors rather than simple balances (for example, between dopamine and acetylcholine). Finally, in

---

←

FIG. 12. Photomicrographs illustrating neurons in the cat's caudate nucleus stained for Nissl substance (**A**) and for horseradish peroxidase (HRP) (**B**) following retrograde transport of the enzyme from an injection site centered in the entopeduncular nucleus. The same field of neurons is shown in **A** and **B**: the tissue was first processed for retrograde HRP cell labeling and photographed (**B**), was then treated to remove the HRP reaction product, and was finally restained with cresylecht violet and rephotographed (**A**). The pockets of low retrograde labeling in **B** coincide with acetylcholinesterase-poor striosomes [not shown; see Graybiel et al. (276)]. Note that there is a parvocellular septum visible in the Nissl stain that surrounds the weakly labeled striosome appearing at the lower left in **B**. (See matching asterisks.) *Scale marker,* 200 μm.

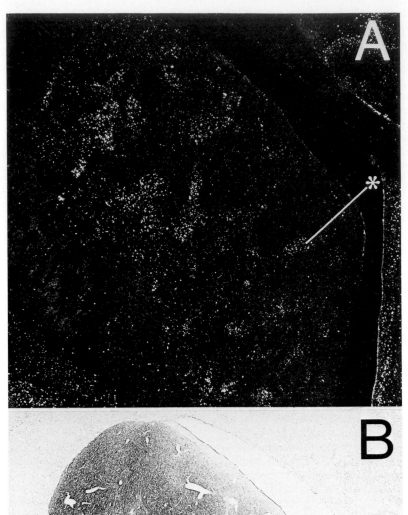

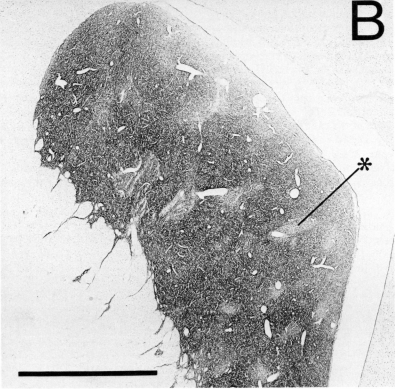

behavioral studies, the effects of serial and parallel pharmacological manipulations suggest that functional representations in the basal ganglia depend on a complex of chemically specified effector channels, most involving links with the striatum (174,530,531,541).

All of these new findings emphasize the need for bringing together information about the functional organization of striatal tissue with information about its neurochemistry. We have reviewed here two groups of findings that bear directly on this point. First, attempts to distinguish which neurotransmitter-related compounds are housed in cell bodies of the striatum, which within its afferent fibers, and which within both suggest that the complex pathways associated with the striatum may be divided into subgroups according to their neurotransmitter content. This means that fiber connections once thought to be single can now be considered as multiple lines marked by different neuroactive substances. Second is the finding that the striatum is itself divided up into small compartments having distinguishable histochemistries and connections. This has led to the realization that the diversity of neurotransmitter-related compounds in the striatum should not be considered as acting *en masse* but as acting within architectural constraints that segregate certain groups of neurotransmitters from others.

Crucial information is still lacking about the distribution of neurotransmitter-related compounds at the ultrastructural level. This is reflected by present uncertainties about the types of synapses made by different classes of afferent fiber (13–15,156,287,307,393,572,600,602,696,750; see Fig. 7), about the interconnections among striatal neurons with known neurotransmitter content (159,601), and about the presence or absence of nonconventional forms of neural interaction (159,287,600,601,750). It is not even yet known whether the detailed organization of the neuropil within particular striosomal compartments is similar to the organization of striatal neuropil elsewhere. What sets this period apart from those before, however, is that the methods are now available for working on nearly all of these problems. It is such work, relating the chemoarchitecture of the striatum to the communication lines established within it, that should help to clarify the functions of its diverse neurotransmitter systems.

ACKNOWLEDGMENTS

It is a pleasure to thank our colleagues Drs. Suzanne Roffler-Tarlov and Marie-Françoise Chesselet and Ms. Mary Nastuk for their comments on the manuscript; Ms. Lana Gilbert for her efforts in its typing; and Mr. Henry F. Hall for his skilled photographic work. We also wish to express our gratitude to colleagues who kindly made available illustration of their work: Dr. J. P. Bolam and his colleagues (Fig. 2), Dr. H. T. Chang and his colleagues (Fig. 3), Dr. M. DiFiglia and her colleagues (Fig. 5), Dr. G. D. Burd and her colleagues (Fig. 6), Dr. V. M. Pickel and her colleagues (Fig. 7), and Dr. M. J. Kuhar and his colleagues (Figs. 9 and 10). Preparation of this review and experiments cited that were carried out in our laboratory were funded by grants from the Scottish Rite Foundation, the National Science Foundation (# BNS 81-12125), and the National Aeronautics and Space Administration (#NAG2-124).

ADDENDUM

Since submission of the manuscript, observations on several neurotransmitter systems have been extended.

1. *CAT*: Correspondence of CAT-positive and AChE-positive neurons in striatum has been confirmed (Levey et al., *Neurosci. Abstr.*, 8:134).

2. *Dynorphin (DYN) and Enkephalin (ENK)*: Small DYN-positive striatal neurons have now been observed in the rat and there are DYN-positive fibers in the pallidum (especially the entopeduncular n. and ventral pallidum). Striosomes appear in ENK but not in DYN preparations in the cat. (Vincent et al., *Neurosci. Lett.*, 33:185; M. F. Chesselet and A. M. Graybiel, *in press*). Bovine adrenal medullary enkephalin-precursor (BAM-22P)-immunoreactive neurons have been observed

---

FIG. 13. A: Dark-field photomicrograph of [³H]thymidine-labeled neurons forming clusters in the caudate nucleus of an adult cat that had been exposed as a 29-day-old fetus to a pulse injection of [³H]thymidine. The labeled neurons are visible as white dots in the autoradiogram. **B:** Serially adjacent section stained for acetylcholinesterase (AChE) to show the AChE-poor striosomes. By comparing the patterns in **A** and **B**, one can see that the [³H]-thymidine clusters correspond to the AChE-poor striosomes (see *asterisks*). *Scale marker,* 2 mm. (Modified from Graybiel and Hickey, ref. 269.)

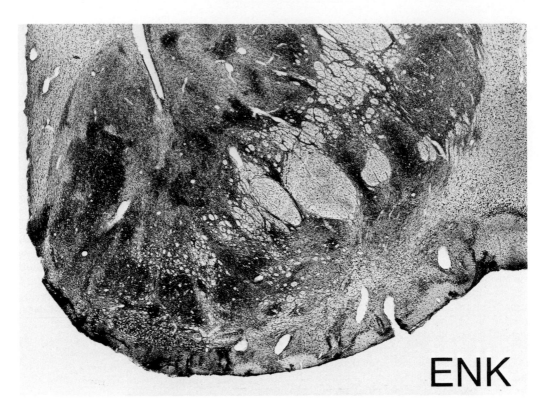

ENK

FIG. 14. (*above and facing page*) Transverse sections through the ventral striatum of the cat illustrating the complex chemoarchitecture of this region visible in sections stained for immunoreactivity to met-enkephalin (ENK) and substance P (SP) and for acetylcholinesterase activity (AChE). See Graybiel et al. (272). *Scale marker,* 1 mm.

in the caudoputamen in the rat (Khachaturian et al., *Life Sci.,* 31:1879). Leu-ENK-immunoreactive processes have been shown to contact neurons identified as medium spiny neurons and the striatonigral type-2 neurons, and to ensheath the perikaryon and dendrites of the latter type (Somogyi et al., *J. Neuroctyol.,* 11:779).

3. *Somatostatin (SOM):* SOM-positive striatal neurons have been identified as medium aspiny neurons (DiFiglia and Aronin, *Neurosci. Abstr.,* 8:507; *J. of Neurosci.,* 2:1267; Burd et al., *Neurosci. Abstr.,* 8:507). Immunostaining has been seen with SOM-28(1-14) as well as with SOM-14 antiserum in striatal neurons in the cat (A. M. Graybiel and R. P. Elde, *in press*). An increase in striatal SOM in Huntington's disease has been confirmed (Nemeroff et al., *Neurosci. Abstr.,* 8:153). and attributed to SOM-positive fibers (Marshall et al., *Neurosci. Abstr.,* 8:507). The hypothalamus was suggested as a source of SOM-containing fibers in the rat's caudoputamen and nucleus accumbens in a paper by Palkovits et al.

(*Brain Res.,* 195:499) which we missed in our initial review.

4. *Cyclic GMP and cyclic AMP:* cGMP, guanylate cyclase, and cGMP-dependent protein kinase have been demonstrated in medium spiny striatal neurons by immunohistochemistry (Ariano, *Neurosci. Abstr.,* 8:344) and such neurons as well as cyclic AMP-positive neurons have been shown by double-labeling to project to the substantia nigra (Ufres and Ariano, *Neurosci. Abstr.,* 8:961). The cyclic GMP-immunoreactive neurons were distinguished from the cyclic AMP-immunoreactive neurons as being similar in appearance to substance P (SP) and GAD-containing neurons.

5. *Substance P (SP) and enkephalin (ENK):* Immunohistochemically identified SP and ENK neurons have been retrogradely labeled by injections of tracer into the substantia nigra (Bradley and Kitai, *Neurosci. Abstr.,* 8:172; also M.-F. Chesselet and A. M. Graybiel, *in preparation*).

6. *Neurotensin (NT):* NT-immunoreactive cell bodies (as well as NT-immunoreactive fibers) have

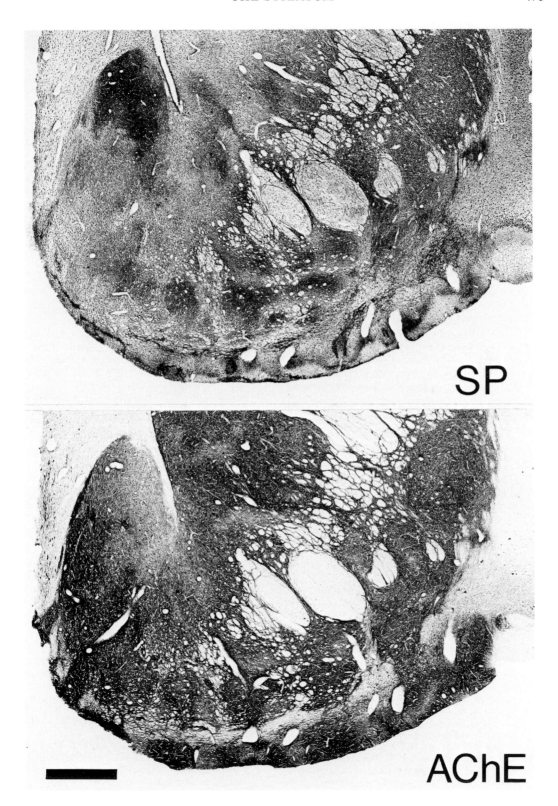

SP

AChE

been reported to occur in the ventral caudoputamen of the rat (Jennes et al., *J. comp. Neurol.*, 210:211). Neurotensin levels in the caudate nucleus were found to be elevated in brains from patients with Huntington's disease (Nemeroff et al., *Neurosci. Abstr.*, 8:153)

7. *Delta sleep-inducing peptide (DSIP), corticotropin-releasing factor (CRF)*: Immuno-reactivity to DSIP has been noted in neurons of the rat's caudoputamen (Feldman and Kastin, *Neurosci. Abstr.*, 8:809) and CRF-positive cell bodies have been observed in the n. accumbens of the rat (Merchenthaler et al., *Am. J. Anat.*, 165:385).

8. *Bombesin (BOM), ranatensin (RT)*: With antibodies to RT not crossreacting appreciably with BOM, RT has not been reported in the striatum (O'Donohue et al., *Neurosci. Abstr.*, 8:587) but in an article overlooked in our initial review, low levels of BOM have been reported (Moody and Pert, *Biochem. Biophys. Res. Comm.*, 90:7).

9. *γ-Hydroxybutyric acid (GHB)*: Binding sites for [^{3}H]-GHB have been found in intermediate levels in homogenates of rat striatum (Benavides et al., *Life Sci.*, 30:953). A possible source of striatal succinic semialdehyde reductase (SSAR) is the dorsal raphe nucleus where SSAR-positive neurons have been found (Weissmann-Nanopoulos et al., *Neurochem. Int.*, 4:523).

REFERENCES

1. Aghajanian. G. K., Wang, R. Y., and Baraban, J. (1978): Serotonergic and non-serotonergic neurons of the dorsal raphe: Reciprocal changes in firing induced by peripheral nerve stimulation. *Brain Res.*, 153:169–175.
2. Alexander, R. W., Davis, J. N., and Lefkowitz, R. J. (1975): Direct identification and characterization of β-adrenergic receptors in rat brain. *Nature*, 258:437–440.
3. Altschuler, R. A., Mosinger, J. L., Harmison, G. G., Parakkal, M. H., and Wenthold, R. J. (1982): Aspartate aminotransferase-like immunoreactivity as a marker for aspartate/glutamate in guinea pig photoreceptors. *Nature*, 298:657–659.
4. Altschuler, R. A., Neises, G. R., Harmison, G. C., Wenthold, R. J., and Fex, J. (1981): Immunocytochemical localization of aspartate aminotransferase immunoreactivity in cochlear nucleus of the guinea pig. *Proc. Natl. Acad. Sci. U.S.A.*, 78:6553–6557.
5. Andén, N. E., Carlsson, A., Dahlström, A., Fuxe, K., Hillarp, N. A., and Larsson, K. (1964): Demonstration and mapping out of nigro-neostriatal dopamine neurons. *Life Sci.*, 3:523–530.
6. Andén, N. E., Dahlström, A., Fuxe, K., and Larsson, K. (1965): Further evidence for the presence of nigro-neostriatal dopamine neurons in the rat. *Am. J. Anat.*, 116:329–333.
7. Andén, N. E., Dahlström, A.. Fuxe, K., Larsson, K., Olson, L., and Ungerstedt, U. (1966): Ascending monoamine neurons to the telencephalon and diencephalon. *Acta. Physiol. Scand.*, 67:313–326.
8. Angevine, J. B., Jr., and McConnell, J. A. (1974): Time of origin of striatal neurons in the mouse: An autoradiographic study. *Anat. Rec.*, 178:300.
9. Ando, N., Simon, J. R., and Roth, R. H. (1979): Inverse relationship between GABA and γ-hydroxybutyrate levels in striatum of rat injected with kainic acid. *J. Neurochem.*, 32:621–625.
10. Ando, N., Gould, B. I., Bird, E. D., and Roth, R. H. (1979): Regional brain levels of γ-hydroxybutyrate in Huntington's disease. *J. Neurochem.*, 32:617–622.
11. Aquilonius, S. M., Eckernas, S. A., and Sundwall, A. (1975): Regional distribution of choline acetyltransferase in the human brain: Changes in Huntington's chorea. *J. Neurol. Neurosurg. Psychiatry*, 38:669–677.
12. Ariano, M. A., Butcher, L. L., and Appleman, M. M. (1980): Cyclic nucleotides in the rat caudate–putamen complex: Histochemical characterization and effects of deafferentation and kainic acid infusion. *Neuroscience*, 5:1269–1276.
13. Arluison, M., and De La Manche, I. S. (1980): High-resolution radioautographic study of the serotonin innervation of the rat corpus striatum after intraventricular administration of (^{3}H) 5-hydroxytryptamine. *Neuroscience*, 5:229–240.
14. Arluison, M., Agid, Y., and Javoy, F. (1978): Dopaminergic nerve endings in the neostriatum of the rat. I. Identification by intracerebral injections of 5-hydroxydopamine. *Neuroscience*, 3:657–673.
15. Arluison, M., Agid, Y., and Javoy, F. (1978): Dopaminergic nerve endings in the neostriatum of the rat. 2. Radioautographic study following local microinjections of tritiated dopamine. *Neuroscience*, 3:675–683.
16. Armatsu, Y., Seto, A., and Amano, T. (1981): An atlas of α-bungarotoxin binding sites and structures containing acetylcholinesterase in the mouse central nervous system. *J. Comp. Neurol.*, 198:603–631.
17. Arregui, A., Iversen, L. L., Spokes, E. G. S., and Emson, P. C. (1979): Alterations in postmortem brain angiotensin-converting enzyme activity and some neuropeptides in Huntington's disease. In: *Advances in Neurology*, vol. 23, edited by T. N. Chase, N. S. Wexler, and A. Barbeau, pp. 517–525. Raven Press, New York.
18. Arregui, A., Emson, P. C., and Spokes, E. G. (1978): Angiotensin-converting enzyme in substantia nigra: Reduction of activity in Huntington's disease and after intrastriatal kainic acid in rats. *Eur. J. Pharmacol.*, 52:121–124.
19. Arregui, A., and Iversen, L. L. (1978): Angiotensin-converting enzyme: Presence of high activity in choroid plexus of mammalian brain. *Eur. J. Pharmacol.*, 52:147–150.
20. Arregui, A., Bennett, J. P., Jr., Bird, E. D., Yamamura, H. I., Iversen, L. L., and Snyder, S. H. (1977): Huntington's chorea: Selective depletion of activity of angiotensin converting enzyme in the corpus striatum. *Ann. Neurol.*, 2:294–298.

21. Atweh, S. F., and Kuhar, M. (1977): Autoradiographic localization of opiate receptors in rat brain. III. The telencephalon. *Brain Res.*, 134:393–405.

22. Axelrod, J., and Saavedra, J. (1976): Trace amines in the brain. In: *Trace Amines and the Brain*, edited by E. Usdin and M. Sandler, pp. 1–20. Marcel Dekker, New York.

23. Axelrod, J., MacLean, P. D., Albers, R. W., and Weissbach, H. (1961): Regional distribution of methyl transferase enzymes in the nervous system and glandular tissues. In: *Regional Neurochemistry*, edited by S. S. Kety and J. Elkes, pp. 307–311. Pergamon Press, New York.

24. Axelrod, J., Albers, W., and Clemente, C. D. (1959): Distribution of catechol-*O*-methyl transferase in the nervous system and other tissues. *J. Neurochem.*, 5:68–72.

25. Azmitia, E. C., and Segal, M. (1978): An autoradiographic analysis of the differential ascending projections of the dorsal and median raphe nuclei in the rat. *J. Comp. Neurol.*, 179:641–668.

26. Bagnoli, P., Beaudet, A., Stella, M., and Cuénod, M. (1981): Selective retrograde labeling of cholinergic neurons with (^{3}H)choline. *J. Neurosci.*, 1:691–695.

27. Bak, I. J., Markham, C. H., and Morgan, E. S. (1981): A striato–striatal connection in rats. *Neurosci. Abstr.*, 7:193.

28. Bak, I. J., Markham, C. H., Cook, M. L., and Stevens, J. G. (1978): Ultrastructural and immunoperoxidase study of striatonigral neurons by means of retrograde axonal transport of herpes simplex virus. *Brain Res.*, 143:361–368.

29. Balcom, G. J., Lenox, R. H., and Meyerhoff, J. L.(1974): Regional γ-aminobutyric acid levels in rat brain determined after microwave fixation. *J. Neurochem.*, 24:609–613.

30. Barber, R., and Saito, K. (1976): Light microscopic visualization of GAD and GABA-T in immunocytochemical preparations of rodent CNS. In: *GABA in Nervous System Function*, edited by E.Roberts, T. N. Chase, and D. B. Tower, pp. 113–132. Raven Press, New York.

31. Barbin, C. J., Palacios, J. M., Rodergas, E., Schwartz, J. C., and Garbarg, M. (1980): Characterization of the high-affinity binding sites of (^{3}H)histamine in rat brain. *Mol. Pharmacol.*, 18:1–10.

32. Barbin, G., Palacios, J. M., Garbarg, J., Schwartz, J. C., Gaspar, P., Javoy- Agid, F., and Agid, Y. (1980): L-Histidine decarboxylase in the human brain: Properties and localization. *J. Neurochem.*, 35:400–406.

33. Battistin, L., Grynbaum, A., and Lajtha, A. (1969): Distribution and uptake of amino acids in various regions of the cat brain *in vitro. J. Neurochem.*, 16:1439–1468.

34. Baughman, R. W., and Gilbert, C. D. (1981): Aspartate and glutamate as possible neurotransmitters in the visual cortex. *J. Neurosci.*, 1:427–439.

35. Baxter, C. F. (1970): The nature of γ-aminobutyric acid. In: *The Handbook of Neurochemistry*, Volume 3, edited by A. Lajtha, pp. 289–354. Plenum Press, New York.

36. Beaudet, A., and Descarries, L. (1978): The monoamine innervation of rat cerebral cortex: Synaptic and nonsynaptic axon terminals. *Neuroscience*, 3:851–860.

37. Beaumont, K., Maurin, Yl, Reisine. T. D., Fields, J. Z., Spokes, E., Bird, E. D., and Yamamura, H. I. (1979): Huntington's disease and its animal model: Alterations in kainic acid binding. *Life Sci.*, 24:809–816.

38. Beaumont, K., Chilton, W. S., Yamamura, H. I., and Enna, S. J. (1978): Muscimol binding in rat brain: Association with synaptic GABA receptors. *Brain Res.*, 148:153–162.

39. Beckstead, R. M., Domesick, V. B., and Nauta, W. J. H. (1979): Efferent connections of the substantia nigra and ventral tegmental area in the rat. *Brain Res.*, 175:191–217.

40. Beinfeld, M. C., Meyer, D. K., Eskay, R. L., Jensen, R. T., and Brownstein, M. J. (1981): The distribution of cholecystokinin immunoreactivity in the central nervous system of the rat as determined by radioimmunoassay. *Brain Res.*, 212:51–57.

41. Ben-Ari, Y., Pradelles, P., Oros, C., and Dray, F. (1979): Identification of authentic substance P in striatonigral and amygdaloid nuclei using combined high performance liquid chromatography and radioimmunoassay. *Brain Res.*, 173:360–363.

42. Benavides, J., Rumigny, J. F., Bourgingnon, J. J., Wermuth, C. G., Mandel, P., and Maitre, M. (1982): A high-affinity, NA$^+$-dependent uptake system for γ-hydroxybutyrate in membrane vesicles prepared from rat brain. *J. Neurochem.*, 38:1570–1575.

43. Bennett, J. P., Jr., and Snyder, S. H. (1976): Angiotensin II binding to mammalian brain membranes. *J. of Biol. Chem.*, 251:7423–7430.

44. Bennet-Clarke, C., Romagnano, M. A., and Joseph, S. A. (1980): Distribution of somatostatin in the rat brain: Telencephalon and diencephalon. *Brain Res.*, 188:473–486.

45. Bentivoglio, M., van der Kooy, D., and Kuypers, H. G. J. M. (1979): The organization of the efferent projections of the substantia nigra in the rat. A retrograde fluorescent double labeling study. *Brain Res.*, 174:1–17.

46. Benuck, M., Berg, M. J., and Marks, N. (1981): Met-enkephalin-Arg^6-Phe^7 metabolism: Conversion to met-enkephalin by brain and kidney dipeptidyl carboxypeptidases. *Biochem. Biophys. Res. Commun.*, 99:630–636.

47. Benuck, M., Grynbaum, A., and Marks, N. (1977): Breakdown of somatostatin and substance P by cathepsin D purified from cell brain by affinity chromotography. *Brain Res.*, 143:181–185.

48. Berger, M., Sperk, G., and Hornykiewicz, O. (1982): Serotonergic denervation partially protects rat striatum from kainic acid toxicity. *Nature*, 299:284–286.

49. Berger, B., Nguyen-Legros, J., and Thierry, A. M. (1978): Demonstration of horseradish peroxidase and fluorescent catecholamines in the same neuron. *Neurosci. Lett.*, 9:297–302.

50. Bernheimer, H., Birkmayer, W., and Hornykiewicz, O. (1961): Verteilung des 5-Hydroxytryptam-

ins (Serotonin) im Gehirn des Menschen und sein Verhalten bei Patientem mit Parkinson-Syndrom. *Wien. Klin. Wochenschr.,* 39:1056–1059.

51. Bernheimer, H., Birkmayer, W., Hornykiewicz, O., Jellinger, K., and Settelberger, F. (1973): Brain dopamine and the syndromes of Parkinson and Huntington: Clinical, morphological and neurochemical correlations. *J. Neurol. Sci.,* 20:415–425.

52. Besson, J., Rotszien, W., LaBurthe, M., Epelbaum, J., Beaudet, A., Kordon, C., and Rosselin, G. (1979): Vasoactive intestinal peptide (VIP): Brain distribution subcellular localization and effect of deafferentation of the hypothalamus in male rats. *Brain Res.,* 165:79–85.

53. Biegon, A., Rainbow, T. C., and McEwen, B. S. (1982): Quantitative autoradiography of serotonin receptors in the rat brain. *Brain Res.,* 242:197–204.

54. Bird, E. D., and Kaus, L. J. (1981): Transmitter biochemistry of Huntington's disease. In: *Transmitter Biochemistry of Human Brain Tissue,* edited by P. Rieder and E. Usdin, pp. 201–220. MacMillan Press, New York.

55. Bird, E. D., Spokes, E. G. S., and Iversen, L. L. (1979): Increased dopamine concentration in limbic areas of brain from patients dying with schizophrenia. *Brain,* 102:347–360.

56. Bird, E. D., Gale, J. S., and Spokes, E. G. (1977): Huntington's chorea: Post mortem activity of enzymes involved in cerebral glucose metabolism. *J. Neurochem.,* 29:539–545.

57. Bird, E. D. (1978): The clinical significance of disturbances in the central GABA system. In: *Neurotransmission and Disturbed Behavior,* edited by H. M. van Prang and J. Bruinvels, pp. 140–149. Spectrum Publications, New York.

58. Bird, E. D., and Iversen, L. L. (1974): Huntington's chorea. Post-mortem measurement of glutamic acid decarboxylase, choline acetyltransferase and dopamine in basal ganglia. *Brain,* 97:457–472.

59. Birkmayer, V. W., and Hornykiewicz, O. (1961): Der L-3,4-Dioxyphenylalanin (= DOPA)-Effekt bei der Parkinson-Akinese. *Wiener Klin. Wochenschr.,* 73:787–788.

60. Bishop, G. A., Chang, H. T., and Kitai, S. T. (1982): Morphological and physiological properties of neostriatal neurons: An intracellular horseradish peroxidase study in the rat. *Neuroscience,* 7:179–191.

61. Biziere, K., and Coyle, J. T. (1978): Influence of cortico-striatal afferents on striatal kainic acid neurotoxicity. *Neurosci. Lett.,* 8:303–310.

62. Biziere, K., Thompson, H., and Coyle, J. T. (1980): Characterization of specific high-affinity binding sites for L-(^{3}H)glutamic acid in rat brain membranes. *Brain Res.,* 183:421–433.

63. Bloom, F., Battenberg, E., Rossier, J., Ling, N., and Guillemin, R. (1978): Neurons containing β-endorphin in rat brain exist separately from those containing enkephalin: Immunocytochemical studies. *Proc. Natl. Acad. Sci. U.S.A.,* 75:1591–1595.

64. Boarder, M. R., Lockfeld, A. J., and Barchas, J. D. (1982): Measurement of methionine-enkephalin [Arg[6],Phe[7]] in rat brain by specific radioimmunoas-

say directed at methionine sulphoxide enkephalin [Arg[6],Phe[7]]. *J. Neurochem.,* 38:299–304.

65. Bobillier, P., Seguin, S., Petitjean, F., Salvert, D., Touret, M., and Jouvet, M. (1976): The raphe nuclei of the cat brain stem: A topographical atlas of their efferent projections as revealed by autoradiography. *Brain Res.,* 113:449–486.

66. Bobillier, P., Petitjean, F., Salvert, D., Ligier, M., and Seguin, S. (1975): Differential projections of the nucleus raphe dorsalis and nucleus raphe centralis as revealed by autoradiography. *Brain Res.,* 85:205–210.

67. Bock, E. (1978): Nervous system specific proteins. *J. Neurochem.,* 30:7–14.

68. Bockaert, J., Premont, J., Glowinski, J., Thierry, A. M., and Tassin, J. P. (1979): Topographical distribution of dopaminergic innervation and of dopaminergic receptors in the rat striatum. II. Distribution and characteristics of dopamine adenylate cyclase interaction of D-LSD with dopaminergic receptors. *Brain Res.,* 107:303–315.

69. Bogdanski, D. F., Weissbach, H., and Undenfriend, S. (1957): The distribution of serotonin, 5-hydroxytryptophan decarboxylase, and monoamine oxidase in brain. *J. Neurochem.,* 1:272–278.

70. Bolam, J. P., Freund, T. P., Hammond, D. J., Smith, A. D., and Somogyi, P. (1982): Morphological characterization of (^{3}H)GABA accumulating neurons in the rat neostriatum by golgi-staining and electron microscopy. *Br. J. Pharmacol.,* 75:46P.

71. Bolam, J. P., Somogyi, P., Totterdell, S., and Smith, A. D. (1981): A second type of striatonigral neuron: A comparison between retrogradely labeled and Golgi-stained neurons at the light and electron microscopic levels. *Neuroscience,* 6:2141–2157.

72. Bolam, J. P., Powell, J. F., Totterdell, S., and Smith, A. D. (1981): The proportion of neurons in the rat neostriatum that project to the substantia nigra demonstrated using horseradish peroxidase conjugated with wheat-germ agglutinin. *Brain Res.,* 220:339–343.

73. Bond, P. A. (1973): The uptake of [^{3}H]γ-aminobutyric acid by slices from various regions of rat brain and the effect of lithium. *J. Neurochem.,* 20:511–517.

74. Bonnet, K. A., Groth, J., Gioannini, T., Cortes, M., and Simon, E. J. (1981): Opiate receptor heterogeniety in human brain regions. *Brain Res.,* 221:437–440.

75. Bowen, D. M., Smith, C. B., White, P., and Davison, A. N. (1976): Neurotransmitter-related enzymes and indices of hypoxia in senile dementia and other abiotrophies. *Brain,* 99:459–496.

76. Braestrup, C., Albrechtsen, R., and Squires, R. F. (1977): High densities of benzodiazepine receptors in human cortical areas. *Nature,* 269:702–704.

77. Braestrup, C., and Squires, R. F. (1977): Specific benzodiazepine receptors in rat brain characterized by high-affinity [^{3}H]diazepam binding. *Proc. Natl. Acad. Sci. U.S.A.,* 74:3805–3809.

78. Brand, S. (1980): A comparison of the distribution of acetylcholinesterase and muscarinic cholinergic receptors in the feline neostriatum. *Neurosci. Lett.,* 17:113–117.

79. Brand, S., and Rakic, P. (1979): Genesis of the primate neostriatum: [³H]thymidine autoradiographic analysis of the time of neuron origin in the rhesus monkey. *Neuroscience,* 4:767–778.

80. Brann, M. R., and Emson, P. C. (1980): Microionophoretic injection of fluorescent tracer combined with simultaneous immunofluorescent histochemistry for the demonstration of efferents from the caudate–putamen projecting to the globus pallidus. *Neurosci. Lett.,* 16:61–65.

81. Broch, O. J., and Fonnum, F. (1972): The regional and subcellular distribution of catechol-*O*-methyl transferase in the rat brain. *J. Neurochem.,* 19:2049–2055.

82. Brockhaus, H. (1942): Zur feineren Anatomie des Septum und des Striatum. *J. Psychol. Neurol.,* 51:1–56.

83. Brownfield, M. S., Reid, I. A., Ganten, D., and Ganong, W.F. (1982): Differential distribution of immunoreactive angiotensin and angiotensin-converting enzyme in rat brain. *Neuroscience,* 7:1759–1769.

84. Brownstein, M. J., Mroz, E. A., Tappaz, M. L., and Leeman, S. E. (1977): On the origin of substance P and glutamatic acid decarboxylase (GAD) in the substantia nigra. *Brain Res.,* 135:315–323.

85. Brownstein, M. J., Mroz, E. A., Kizer, J. S., Palkovits, M., and Leeman, S. (1976): Regional distribution of substance P in the brain of the rat. *Brain Res.,* 116:299–303.

86. Brownstein, M., Arimura, A., Sato, H., Schally, A. V., and Kizer, J. S. (1975): The regional distribution of somatostatin in the rat brain. *Endocrinology,* 96:1456–1461.

87. Brownstein, M. J., Palkovits, M., Saavedra, J. M., and Kizer, J. S. (1975): Tryptophan hydroxylase in the rat brain. *Brain Res.,* 97:161–166.

88. Brownstein, M., Saavedra, J. M., and Palkovits, M. (1974): Norepinephrine and dopamine in the limbic system of the rat. *Brain Res.,* 79:431–436.

89. Brownstein, M. J., Palkovits, M., and Saavedra, J. M. (1974): Thyrotropin-releasing hormone in specific nuclei of rat brain. *Science,* 185:267–269.

90. Bruyn, G. W., Bots, G. T. A. M., and Dom, R. (1979): Huntington's chorea: Current neuropathological status. In: *Advances in Neurology,* Vol. 23, edited by T. N. Chase, N. S. Wexler, and A. Barbeau, pp. 83–93. Raven Press, New York.

91. Buck, S. H., Burke, T. F., Yamamura, H. I., Bird, E. D., Rossor, M., and Brown, M. R. (1980): Decreased striatal and nigral substance P levels in Huntington's disease. *Neurosci. Abstr.,* 6:600.

92. Buck, S. H., Murphy, R. C., and Molinoff, P. B. (1977): The normal occurrence of octopamine in the central nervous system of the rat. *Brain Res.,* 122:281–297.

93. Bunney, B. S., and Aghajanian, G. K. (1976): The precise localization of nigral afferents in the rat as determined by a retrograde tracing technique. *Brain Res.,* 117:423–436.

94. Burgen, A. S. V., and Chipman, L. M. (1951): Cholinesterase and succinic dehydrogenase in the central nervous system of the dog. *J. Physiol. (Lond.),* 114:296–305.

95. Burt, D. R., and Snyder, S. H. (1975): Thyrotropin releasing hormone (TRH): Apparent receptor binding in rat brain membranes. *Brain Res.,* 93:309–328.

96. Burt, D. R., Creese, I., and Snyder, S. H. (1976): Properties of [³H]haloperidol and [³H]dopamine binding associated with dopamine receptors in calf brain membranes. *Mol. Pharmacol.,* 12:800–812.

97. Butcher, L. L., and Marchand, R. (1978): Dopamine neurons in pars compacta of the substantia nigra contain acetylcholinesterase: Histochemical correlations on the same brain section. *Eur. J. Pharmacol.,* 52:415–417.

98. Butcher, L. L., and Hodge, G. K. (1976): Postnatal development of acetylcholinesterase in the caudate–putamen and substantia nigra of rats. *Brain Res.,* 106:223–240.

99. Butcher, S. G., and Butcher, L. L. (1974): Origin and modulation of acetylcholine activity in the neostriatum. *Brain Res.,* 71:167–171.

100. Bylund, D. B., and Snyder, S. H. (1976): Beta adrenergic receptor binding in membrane preparations from mammalian brain. *Mol. Pharmacol.,* 12:568–580.

101. Cajal, S. Ramon y (1911): *Histologie du Système Nerveux de l'Homme et des Vertébrés.* J. Maloine, Paris.

102. Campochiaro, P., and Coyle, J. T. (1978): Ontogenetic development of kainate neurotoxicity: Correlates with glutamatergic innervation. *Proc. Natl. Acad. Sci. U.S.A.,* 75:2025–2029.

103. Carbonetto, S. T., Fambrough, D. M., and Muller, K. J. (1978): Nonequivalence of α-bungarotoxin receptors and acetylcholine receptors in chick sympathetic neurons. *Proc. Natl. Acad. Sci. U.S.A.,* 75.1016–1020.

104. Carlsson, A. (1959): The occurrence, distribution and physiological role of catecholamines in the nervous system. *Pharmacol. Rev.,* 11:490–493.

105. Chan-Palay, V., Lin, C.-T., Palay, S., Yamamoto, M., and Wu, J.-Y. (1982): Taurine in the mammalian cerebellum: Demonstration by autoradiography with [³H]taurine and immunocytochemistry with antibodies against the taurine-synthesizing enzyme, cysteine-sulfinic acid decarboxylase. *Proc. Natl. Acad. Sci. U.S.A.,* 78:2695–2699.

106. Chan-Palay, V., Palay, S. L., and Wu, J.-Y. (1982): Sagittal cerebellar microbands of taurine neurons: Immunocytochemical demonstration by using antibodies against the taurine-synthesizing enzyme cysteine sulfinic acid decarboxylase. *Proc. Natl. Acad. Sci. U.S.A.,* 79:4221–4225.

107. Chan-Palay, V. (1978): Autoradiographic localization of γ-aminobutyric acid receptors in the rat central nervous system by using [³H]muscimol. *Proc. Natl. Acad. Sci. U.S.A.,* 75:1024–1028.

108. Chang, H. T., Wilson, C. J., and Kitai, S. T. (1982): A Golgi study of rat neostriatal neurons: Light microscopic analysis. *J. Comp. Neurol.,* 208:107–126.

109. Chang, H. T., and Kitai, S. T. (1982): Large neostriatal neurons in the rat: An electron microscopic study of gold-toned Golgi-stained cells. *Brain Res. Bull.,* 8:631–643.

110. Chang, H. T., Wilson, C. J., and Kitai, S. T. (1981): Single neostriatal efferent axons in the globus pallidus: A light and electron microscopic study. *Science*, 213:915–918.

111. Chang, K. J., Cooper, B. R., Hazum, E., and Cuatrecasas, P. (1979): Multiple opiate receptors: Different regional distribution in the brain and differential binding of opiates and opioid peptides. *Mol. Pharmacol.*, 16:91–104.

112. Chang, R. S. L., Tran, V. T., and Snyder, S. H. (1979): Heterogeneity of histamine H_1-receptors: species variations in [^{3}H]mepyramine binding of brain membranes. *J. Neurochem.*, 32:1653–1663.

113. Changaris, D. G., Severs, W. B., and Kehl, L. C. (1978): Localization of angiotensin in rat brain. *J. Histochem. Cytochem.*, 26:593–607.

114. Chao, L., Kan, K. S. K., and Hung, F. (1982): Immunohistochemical localization of choline acetyltransferase in rabbit forebrain. *Brain Res.*, 235:65–82.

115. Chavkin, C., James, I. F., and Goldstein, A. (1982): Dynorphin is a specific endogenous ligand of the κ opioid receptor. *Science*, 215:413–415.

116. Cheney, D. L., LeFevre, H. F., and Racagni, G. (1975): Choline acetyltransferase activity and mass fragmentographic measurement of acetylcholine in specific nuclei and tracts of rat brain. *Neuropharmacology*, 14:801–809.

117. Chesselet, M.-F., Reisine, T. D., Glowinski, J., and Graybiel, A. M. (1982): Striatal somatostatin: Immunohistochemistry and effects on dopaminergic transmission. *Neurosci. Abstr.*, 8:287.

118. Chesselet, M.-F., Cheramy, A., Reisine, T., Lubetzki, C., and Glowinski, J. (1982): Presynaptic regulation of striatal dopamine release, *in vivo* and *in vitro* studies. *J. Physiol. (Paris) (in press)*.

119. Chronister, R. B. (1981): A double label analysis of tegmental efferents to caudate and accumbens. *Anat. Rec.*, 199:51A–52A.

120. Chronister, R. B., Farnell, K. E., Marco, L. A., and White, L. E. (1976): The rodent neostriatum: A Golgi analysis. *Brain Res.*, 108:37–46.

121. Chubb, I. W., Hodgson, A. J., and White, G. H. (1980): Acetylcholinesterase hydrolyzes substance P. *Neuroscience*, 5:2065–2072.

122. Chubb, I. W., Ranieri, E., Hodgson, A. J., and White, G. H. (1982): The hydrolysis of leu- and met-enkephalin by acetylcholinesterase. *Neurosci. Lett. [Suppl.]*, 8:S39.

123. Collins, G. G. S. (1974): The rates of synthesis uptake and disappearance of [^{14}C]-taurine in eight areas of the rat central nervous system. *Brain Res.*, 76:447–459.

124. Comb, M., Seeburg, P. H., Adelman, J., Eiden, L., and Herbert, E. (1982): Primary structure of the human met- and leu-enkephalin precursor and its mRNA. *Nature*, 295:663–666.

125. Cooper, P. E., Fernstrom, M. H., Rorstad, O. P., Leeman, S. E., and Martin, J. B. (1981): The regional distribution of somatostatin, substance P and neurotensin in human brain. *Brain Res.*, 218:219–232.

126. Cooper, P. E., Aronin, N., Bird, E. D., Leeman, S. E., and Martin, J. B. (1981): Increased somatostatin in basal ganglia of Huntington's disease. *Neurology (N.Y.)*, 31:64.

127. Corbett, A. D., Paterson, S. J., McKnight, A. T., Magnan, J., and Kosterlitz, H. W. (1982): Dynorphin$_{1-8}$ and dynorphin$_{1-9}$ are ligands for the κ-subtype of opiate receptor. *Nature*, 299:79–81.

128. Corrêa, F. M. A., Innis, R. B., Hester, L. D., and Snyder, S. H. (1981): Diffuse enkephalin innervation from caudate to globus pallidus. *Neurosci. Lett.*, 25:63–68.

129. Corrêa, F. M. A., Innis, R. B., Uhl, G. R., and Snyder, S. H. (1979): Bradykinin-like immunoreactive neuronal systems localized histochemically in rat brain. *Proc. Natl. Acad. Sci. U.S.A.*, 76:1489–1493.

130. Côté, L. J., and Fahn, S. (1968): Properties of tyrosine hydroxylase in brain and its distribution in rhesus monkey brain. *Fed. Proc.*, 27:752.

131. Côté, L. J., and Fahn, S. (1967): Some aspects of the biochemistry of the substantia nigra of the rhesus monkey. *Prog. Neurogenet.*, 1:311–317.

132. Cotzias, G. C., Papavasiliou, P. S., and Gellene, R. (1969): Modification of parkinsonism—chronic treatment with L-dopa. *N. Engl. J. Med.*, 280:337–345.

133. Courville, C. B.,Nusbaum, R. E., and Buti, E. M. (1963): Changes in trace metals in brain in Huntington's chorea. *Arch. Neurol.*, 8:481–489.

134. Coyle, J. T., and Schwarcz, R. (1976): Lesion of striatal neurones with kainic acid provides a model for Huntington's chorea. *Nature*, 263:244–245.

135. Cuello, A. C., and Paxinos, G. (1978): Evidence for a long leu-enkephalin striopallidal pathway in rat brain. *Nature*, 271:178–180.

136. Cuello, A. C. (1978): Endogenous opioid peptides in neurons of the human brain. *Lancet*, 2:291–293.

137. Cuello, A. C., and Kanazawa, I. (1978): The distribution of substance P immunoreactive fibers in the rat central nervous system. *J. Comp. Neurol.*, 178:129–156.

138. Cuénod, M., Bagnoli, P., Beaudet, A., Rustioni, A., Wiklund, L., and Streit, P. (1982): Transmitter-specific retrograde labeling of neurons. In: *Cytochemical Methods in Neuroanatomy*, edited by V. Chan-Palay and S. Palay, pp. 17–44. Alan R. Liss, New York.

139. Dahlström, A., and Fuxe, K. (1964): Evidence for the existence of monoamine containing neurons in the central nervous system. I. Demonstration of monoamines in the cell bodies of brain stem neurons. *Acta Physiol. Scand.*, 62[Suppl. 232]:1–55.

140. Danielson, T. J., Wishart, T. B., and Boulton, A.A. (1976): Effect of acute and chronic injections of amphetamine on intracranial self-stimulation (ICS) and some aryl aklyl amines in the rat brain. *Life Sci.*, 18:1237–1244.

141. Danner, H., and Pfister, C. (1982): Wietere Untersuchungen zur Zytoarchitekionik des Nucleus accumbens septi der Ratte. *J. Hirnofrsch.*, 23:87–99.

142. Danner, H., and Pfister, C. (1979): Untersuchungen zur Struktur des Neostriatum der Ratte. *J. Hirnforsch.*, 20:285–301.

143. Das, G. D. and Altman, J. (1970): Postnatal neu-

rogenesis in the caudate nucleus and nucleus accumbens septi in the rat. *Brain Res.*, 21:122–127.

144. Daul, C. B., Heath, R. G., and Garey, R. E. (1975): Angiotensin-forming enzyme in human brain. *Neuropharmacology*, 14:75–80.

145. Davies, J., Evans, R. H., Francis, A. A., and Watkins, J. C. (1979): Excitatory amino acid receptors and synaptic excitation in the mammalian central nervous system. *J. Physiol. (Paris)*, 75:641–654.

146. Davies, J., and Dray, A. (1976): Substance P in the substantia nigra. *Brain Res.*, 107:623–627.

147. Davies, P., Josef, J., and Thompson, A. (1981): Anterior to posterior variations in the concentration of somatostatin-like immunoreactivity in human basal ganglia. *Brain Res. Bull.*, 7:365–368.

148. Davies, P., and Maloney, A. J. F. (1976): Selective loss of central cholinergic neurons in Alzheimer's disease. *Lancet*, 2:1403.

149. DeFeudis, F. V., Delgado, J. M. R., and Roth, R. H. (1970): Content, synthesis and collectability of amino acids in various structures of the brains of rhesus monkeys. *Brain Res.*, 18:15–23.

150. Deguchi, T., and Barchas, J. (1972): Regional distribution and developmental change of tryptophan hydroxylase activity in rat brain. *J. Neurochem.*, 19:927–929.

151. DelFiacco, M., Paxinos, G., and Cuello, A. C. (1982): Neostriatal enkephalin-immunoreactive neurones project to the globus pallidus. *Brain Res.*, 231:1–17.

152. Deniau, J. M., Thierry, A. M., and Feger, J. (1980): Electrophysiological identification of mesencephalic ventromedial tegmental (VMT) neurons projecting to the frontal cortex, septum and nucleus accumbens. *Brain Res.*, 189:315–326.

153. Deniau, J. M., Hammond, C., Riszk, A., and Feger, J. (1978): Electrophysiological properties of identified output neurons of the rat substantia nigra (pars compacta and pars reticulata): Evidences for the existence of branched neurons. *Exp. Brain Res.*, 32:409–422.

154. Deniau, J. M., Lackner, D., and Feger, J. (1978): Effect of substantia nigra stimulation on identified neurons in the VL–VA thalamic complex: Comparison between intact and chronically decorticated cats. *Brain Res.*, 145:27–35.

155. Descarries, L., Berthelet, F., and Garcia, S. (1981): Axophoresis of (³H)DA and (³H)NA by central catecholaminergic neurons in rat brain: Radioautographic demonstration. *Neurosci. Abstr.*, 7:802.

156. Descarries, L., Bosler, O., Berthelet, F., and Des Rosiers, M. H. (1980): Dopaminergic nerve endings visualized by high-resolution autoradiography in adult rat neostriatum. *Nature*, 284:620–622.

157. DeVito, J. L., Anderson, M. E., and Walsh, K. E. (1980): A horseradish peroxidase study of afferent connections of the globus pallidus in *Macaca mulatta*. *Exp. Brain Res.*, 38:65–73.

158. DiChiara, G., Proceddu, M. L., Morelli, M., Mulas, M. L., and Gessa, G. L. (1979): Evidence for a GABAergic projection from the substantia nigra to the ventromedial thalamus and to the superior colliculus of the rat. *Brain Res.*, 176:273–284.

159. DiFiglia, M., Aronin, N., and Martin, J. B. (1982):

Light and electron microscopic localization of immunoreactive leu-enkephalin in the monkey basal ganglia. *J. Neurosci.*, 2:303–320.

160. DiFiglia, M., Pasik, T., and Pasik, P. (1980): Ultrastructure of Golgi-impregnated and gold-toned spiny and aspiny neurons in the monkey neostriatum. *J. Neurocytol.*, 9:471–492.

161. DiFiglia, M., Pasik, P., and Pasik, T. (1976): A Golgi study of neuronal types in the neostriatum of monkeys. *Brain Res.*, 114:245–256.

162. Dimova, R., Vuillet, J., and Seite, R. (1980): Study of the rat neostriatum using a combined Golgi-electron microscope technique and serial sections. *Neuroscience*, 5:1581–1596.

163. Dockray, G. J., and Williams, R. G. (1981): FMRFamide immunoreactivity in rat brain: A new mammalian neuropeptide. *Neurosci. Lett.* [Suppl.], 7:S452.

164. Dockray, G. J., Vaillant, C., and Williams, R. G. (1981): New vertebrate brain–gut peptide related to a molluscan neuropeptide and an opioid peptide. *Nature*, 293:656–657.

165. Doherty, J. D., Hattox, S. E., Snead, O. C., and Roth, R. H. (1978): Identification of endogenous γ-hydroxybutyrate in human and bovine brain and its regional distribution in human, guinea pig and rhesus monkey brain. *J. Pharmacol Exp. Ther.*, 207:130–139.

166. Donkelaar, H. J., and Dederen, P. J. W. (1979): Neurogenesis in the basal forebrain of the Chinese hamster. *Anat. Embryol.*, 156:331–348.

167. Donoghue, J. P., and Kitai, S. T. (1981): A collateral pathway to the neostriatum from corticocofugal neurons of the rat sensory–motor cortex: An intracellular HRP study. *J. Comp. Neurol.*, 201:1–13.

168. Dorer, F. E., Kahn, J. R., Lentz, K. E., Levine, M., and Skeggs, L. T. (1974): Hydrolysis of bradykinin by angiotensin-converting enzyme. *Circ. Res.*, 34:824–827.

169. Dratman, M. B., Futaesaku, Y., Crutchfield, F. L., Berman, N., Payne, B., Sar, M., and Stumpf, W. E. (1982): Iodine-125-labeled triiodothyronine in rat brain: Evidence for localization in discrete neural systems. *Science*, 215:309–312.

170. Dratman, M. B., and Crutchfield, F. L. (1978): Synaptosomal [¹²⁵I]triiodothyronine after intravenous [¹²⁵I]thyroxine. *Am. J. Physiol.*, 235:E638–E647.

171. Dray, A. (1979): The striatum and substantia nigra: A commentary on their relationships. *Neuroscience*, 4:1407–1439.

172. Druce, D., Peterson, D., DeBelleroche, J., and Bradford, H. F. (1982): Differential amino acid neurotransmitter release in rat neostriatum following lesioning of the cortico–striatal pathway. *Brain Res.*, 247:303–307.

173. Dube, D., Lissitzky, J. C., LeClerc, R., and Pelletier, G. (1978): Localization of α-melanocyte-stimulating hormone in rat brain and pituitary. *Endocrinology*, 102:1283–1291.

174. Dunnett, S. B., and Iversen, S. D. (1980): Regulatory impairments following selective kainic acid lesions of the neostriatum. *Behav. Brain Res.*, 1:497–506.

175. Durden, D. A., Philips, S. R., and Boulton, A. A. (1973): Identification and distribution of β-phenylethylamine in the rat. *Can. J. Biochem.,* 51:995–1002.

176. Eckenstein, F., Barde, Y.-A., and Thoenen, H. (1981): Production of specific antibodies to choline acetyltransferase purified from pig brain. *Neuroscience,* 6:993–1000.

177. Edstrom, J. P., and Phillis, J.W. (1980): A cholinergic projection from the globus pallidus to cerebral cortex. *Brain Res.,* 189:524–529.

178. Edwards, D. J. (1976): Monoamine oxidases in brain and platelets: Implications for the role of trace amines and drug action. In: *Trace Amines and the Brain,* edited by E. Usdin and M. Sandler, pp. 59–81. Marcel Dekker, New York.

179. Ehringer, H., and Hornykiewicz, O. (1960): Verteilung von Noradrenalin und Dopamin (3-Hydroxytyramin) im Gehirn des Menschen und ihr Verhalten bei Erkrankungen des extrapyramidalen Systems. *Wien. Klin. Wochenschr.,* 38:1236–1239.

180. Elde, R., Hökfelt, T., and Johansson, O. (1978): Cellular localization of somatostatin. *Metabolism,* 27:1151–1159.

181. Elde, R., Hökfelt, T., Johansson, O., and Terenius, L. (1976): Immunohistochemical studies using antibodies to leucine-enkephalin: Initial observations on the nervous system of the rat. *Neuroscience,* 1:349–351.

182. Emson, P. C., Goedert, M., Horsfield, P., Rioux, F., and St. Pierre, S. (1982): The regional distribution and chromatographic characterization of neurotensin-like immunoreactivity in the rat central nervous system. *J. Neurochem.,* 38:992–999.

183. Emson, P. C., Rehfeld, J. F., Langevin, H., and Rossor, M. (1980): Reduction in cholecystokinin-like immunoreactivity in the basal ganglia in Huntington's disease. *Brain Res.,* 198:497–500.

184. Emson, P. C., Arregui, A., Clement-Jones, V., Sandberg, B. E. B., and Rossor, M. (1980): Regional distribution of methionine-enkephalin and substance P-like immunoreactivity in normal human brain and in Huntington's disease. *Brain Res.,* 199:147–160.

185. Emson, P. C., Fahrenkrug, J., and Spokes, E. G. (1979): Vasoactive intestinal polypeptide (VIP): Distribution in normal human brain and in Huntington's disease. *Brain Res.,* 173:174–178.

186. Enna, S. J., Bennett, J. P., Bylund, D. B., Creese, I., Burt, D. R., Charness, M. E., Yamamura, H. I., Simantov, R., and Snyder, S. H. (1977): Neurotransmitter receptor binding: Regional distribution in human brain. *J. Neurochem.,* 28:233–236.

187. Enna, S. J., Bennett, J. P., Bylund, D. B., Snyder, S. H., Bird, E. D., and Iversen, L. L. (1976): Alterations of brain neurotransmitter receptor binding in Huntington's chorea. *Brain Res.,* 116:531–537.

188. Enna, S. J., Bird, E. D., Bennett, J. P., Bylund, D. B., Yamamura, H. I., Iversen, L. L., and Snyder, S. H. (1976): Huntington's chorea. Changes in neurotransmitter receptors in the brain. *N. Engl. J. Med.,* 294:1305–1309.

189. Enna, S. J. (1978): Regional variation and characteristics of GABA-receptors in the mammalian CNS. In: *GABA—Biochemistry and CNS Func-* tions, edited by P. Mandel and F. V. DeFeudis, pp. 323–337. Plenum Press, New York.

190. Eskay, R. L., Giraud, P., Oliver, C., and Brownstein, M. J. (1979): Distribution of α-melanocyte-stimulating hormone in the rat brain: Evidence that α-MSH-containing cells in the arcuate region send projections to extrahypothalamic areas. *Brain Res.,* 178:55–67.

191. Fahn, S., Libsch, L. R., and Cutler, R. W. (1971): Monoamines in the human neostriatum: Topographic distribution in normals and in Parkinson's disease and their role in akinesia, rigidity, chorea and tremor. *J. Neurol. Sci.,* 14:427–455.

192. Fahn, S., and Côté, L. J. (1968): Regional distribution of choline acetylase in the brain of the rhesus monkey. *Brain Res.,* 7:323–325.

193. Fahn, S., and Côté, L. J. (1968): Regional distribution of γ-aminobutyric acid (GABA) in brain of rhesus moneky. *J. Neurochem.,* 15:209–213.

194. Fairén, A., Peters, A.,and Saldanha, J. (1977): A new procedure for examining Golgi impregnated neurons by light and electron microscopy. *J. Neurocytol.,* 6:311–337.

195. Falck, B., Hillarp, N. A., Thieme, G., and Torp, A. (1962): Fluorescence of catechol amines and related compounds condensed with formaldehyde. *J. Histochem. Cytochem.,* 10:348–354.

196. Fallon, J. H. (1981): Collateralization of monoamine neurons: Mesotelencephalic dopamine projections to caudate, septum, and frontal cortex. *J. Neurosci.,* 1:1361–1368.

197. Fallon, J. H., and Moore. R. Y. (1978): Catecholamine innervation of the basal forebrain. III. Olfactory bulb, anterior olfactory nuclei, olfactory tubercle and piriform cortex. *J. Comp. Neurol.,* 180:533–544.

198. Fallon, J. H., and Moore, R. Y. (1978): Catecholamine innervation of the basal forebrain. IV. Topography of the dopamine projection to the basal forebrain and neostriatum. *J. Comp. Neurol.,* 180:545–580.

199. Fallon, J. H., Koziell, D. A., and Moore, R. Y. (1978): Catecholamine innervation of the basal forebrain. II. Amygdala, suprarhinal cortex and entorhinal cortex. *J. Comp. Neurol.,* 180:509–532.

200. Fallon, J. H., Riley, J. N., and Moore, R. Y. (1978): Substantia nigra dopamine neurons: Separate populations project to neostriatum and allocortex. *Neurosci. Lett.,* 7:157–162.

201. Farley, I. J., and Hornykiewicz, O. (1977): Noradrenaline distribution in subcortical areas of the human brain. *Brain Res.,* 126:53–62.

202. Faull, R. L. M., and Mehler, W. R. (1978): The cells of origin of nigrotectal, nigrothalamic and nigrostriatal projections in the rat. *Neuroscience,* 3:989–1002.

203. Faull, R. L. M., and Mehler, W. R. (1976): Studies of the fiber connections of the substantia nigra in the rat using the method of retrograde transport of horseradish peroxidase. *Neurosci. Abstr.,* 2:62.

204. Feldman, S. C., Silverman, A. J., and Lichtenstein, E. (1979): Distribution of somatostatin-containing neurons in the guinea pig forebrain. *Neurosci. Abstr.,* 5:526.

205. Fentress, J. C., Stanfield, B. B., and Cowan, W. M.

(1981): Observations on the development of the striatum in mice and rats. *Anat. Embryol.,* 163:275–298.

206. Ferkany, J. W., Zaczek, R., and Coyle, J. T. (1982): Kainic acid stimulates excitatory amino acid neurotransmitter release at presynaptic receptors. *Nature,* 298:757–759.

207. Fibiger, H. C., Pudritz, R. E., McGeer, P. L., and McGeer, E. G. (1972): Axonal transport in nigrostriatal and nigro–thalamic neurons: Effects of medial forebrain bundle lesions and 6-hydroxydopamine. *J. Neurochem.,* 19:1697–1708.

208. Fields, J. Z., Reisine, T. D., and Yamamura, H. I. (1977): Biochemical demonstration of dopaminergic receptors in rat and human brain using [^{3}H]spiroperidol. *Brain Res.,* 136:578–584.

209. Filion, M., and Harnois, C. (1978): A comparison of projections of entopeduncular neurons to the thalamus, the midbrain and the habenula in the cat. *J. Comp. Neurol.,* 181:763–780.

210. Finley, J. C. W., Manderdrut, J. L., and Petrusz, P. (1981): The immunocytochemical localization of enkephalin in the central nervous system of the rat. *J. Comp. Neurol.,* 198:541–565.

211. Finley, J. C. W., Maderdrut, J. L., Roger, L. J., and Petrusz, P. (1981): The immunocytochemical localization of somatostatin-containing neurons in the rat central nervous system. *Neuroscience,* 6:2173–2192.

212. Foldes, F. F., Zsigmond, E. K., Foldes, V. M., and Erdos, E. G. (1962): The distribution of acetylcholinesterase and butyrylcholinesterase in the human brain. *J. Neurochem.,* 9:559–572.

213. Fonnum, F., Soeride, A., Kvale, I., Walker, J., and Walaas, I. (1981): Glutamate in cortical fibers. In: *Glutamate as a Neurotransmitter,* edited by G. DiChiara and G. L. Gessa, pp. 29–41. Raven Press, New York.

214. Fonnum, F., Storm-Mathisen, J., and Divac, I. (1981): Biochemical evidence for glutamate as neurotransmitter in corticostriatal and corticothalamic fibers in rat brain. *Neuroscience,* 6:863–873.

215. Fonnum, F., Gottesfeld, Z, and Grofová, I. (1978): Distribution of glutamate decarboxylase, choline acetyl-transferase and aromatic amino acid decarboxylase in the basal ganglia of normal and operated rats. Evidence for striatopallidal, striatoentopenduncular and striatonigral gabaergic fibers. *Brain Res.,* 143:125–138.

216. Fonnum, F., Walaas, I., and Iversen, L. (1977): Localization of gabaergic, cholinergic and aminergic structures in the mesolimbic system. *J. Neurochem.,* 29:221–230.

217. Fonnum, F., and Storm-Mathisen, J. (1977): High affinity uptake of glutamate in terminals of corticostriatal axons. *Nature,* 266:377–378.

218. Fonnum, F., Grofová, I., Rinvik, E., Storm-Mathisen, J., and Walberg, F. (1974): Origin and distribution of glutamate decarboxylase in substantia nigra of the cat. *Brain Res.,* 71:77–92.

219. Fox, C. A., Lu Qui, I. J., and Rafols, J. A. (1974): Further observations on Ramon y Cajal's "dwarf" or "neurogliaform" neurons and the oligodendroglia in the primate striatum. *J. Hirnforsch.,* 15:517–527.

220. Fox, C. A., Andrade, A., Hillman, D. E., and Schwyn, R. C. (1971/72): The spiny neurons in the primate striatum: A Golgi and electron microscopic study. *J. Hirnforsch.,* 13:181–201.

221. Fox, C. A., Andrade, A. N., Schwyn, R. C., and Rafols, J. A. (1971/72): The aspiny neurons and the glia in the primate striatum: A Golgi and electron microscopic study. *J. Hirnforsch.,* 13:341–362.

222. Fox, C. A., and Rafols, J. A. (1971/72): Observations on the oligodendroglia in the primate striatum. Are they Ramon y Cajal's "dwarf" or "neurogliaform" neurons? *J. Hirnforsch.,* 13:331–340.

223. Francois, C., Nguyen-Legros, J., and Percheron, G. (1981): Topographical and cytological localization of iron in rat and monkey brains. *Brain Res.,* 215:317–322.

224. Fricker, L. D., and Snyder, S. H. (1982): Enkephalin convertase: Purification and characterization of a specific enkephalin-synthesizing carboxypeptidase localized to adrenal chromaffin granules. *Proc. Natl. Acad. Sci. U.S.A.,* 79:3886–3890.

225. Friede, R. L. (1967): A comparative histochemical mapping of the distribution of butyryl cholinesterase in the brains of four species of mammals, including man. *Acta Anat.,* 66:161–177.

226. Friede, R. L. (1966): *Topographic Brain Chemistry.* Academic Press, New York.

227. Friede, R. L. (1959): Histochemical investigations on succinic dehydrogenase in the central nervous system. I. The postnatal development of rat brain. *J. Neurochem.,* 4:101–110.

228. Friede, R. L., and Fleming, L. M. (1962): A mapping of oxidative enzymes in the human brain. *J. Neurochem.,* 9:179–198.

229. Friede, R. L. (1961): Histochemical investigations on succinic dehydrogenase in the central nervous system-V. The diencephalon and basal telecephalic centres of the guinea pig. *J. Neurochem.,* 6:190–199.

230. Fuentes, J. A. (1978): Inhibition of 2-phenylethylamine metabolism in brain by type B monoamine oxidase blockers. In: *Noncatecholic Phenylethylamines,* edited by A. D. Moshaim and M. E. Wolf, pp. 47–61. Marcel Dekker, New York.

231. Fukui, K., Kato, N., Kimura, H., Tange, A., Okamura, H., Obata, H. L., Ibata, Y., and Yanaihara, N. (1982): The distribution of vasoactive intestinal polypeptide (VIP) in central nervous system, studied by immunohistochemistry. *Neurosci. Lett.* [Suppl.], 9:S96.

232. Fuxe, K., Ganten, D., Köhler, C., Schüll, B., and Speck, G. (1980): Evidence for differential localization of angiotensin-I converting enzyme and renin in the corpus striatum of rat. *Acta Physiol. Scand.,* 110:321–323.

233. Fuxe, K., Ganten, D., Hökfelt, T., Locatelli, V., Poulsen, K., Stock, G., Rix, E., and Taugner, R. (1980): Renin-like immunocytochemical activity in the rat and mouse brain. *Neurosci. Lett.,* 18:245–250.

234. Fuxe, K., Anderson, K., Schwarcz, R., Agnati, L. F., Perez de la Mora, M., Hökfelt, T., Goldstein, M., Ferland, L., Possani, L., and Tapia, R. (1979): Studies on different types of dopamine nerve terminals in the forebrain and their possible interac-

tions with hormones and with neurons containing GABA, glutamate, and opioid peptides. In: *Advances in Neurology*, Vol. 24, edited by L. J. Poirier, T. L. Sourkes, and P. J. Richard, pp. 199–215. Raven Press, New York.

235. Fuxe, K., Fredholm, B. B., Agnati, L. F., and Corrodi, H. (1978): Dopamine receptors and ergot drugs. Evidence that an ergolene derivative is a differential agonist at subcortical limbic dopamine receptors. *Brain Res., 146*:295–311.

236. Fuxe, K., Hökfelt, T., Agnati, L. F., Johannson, O., Goldstein, M., Pérez de la Mora, M., Possani, L., Tapia, R., Teran, L., and Palacios, R. (1978): Mapping out central catecholamine neurons: Immunohistochemical studies on catecholamine-synthesizing enzymes. In: *Psychopharmacology: A Generation of Progress*, edited by M. A. Lipton, A. DiMascio, and K. F. Killam, pp. 67–94. Raven Press, New York.

237. Fuxe, K., Hökfelt, T., Said, S. I., and Mutt, V. (1977): Vasoactive intestinal polypeptide and the nervous system: Immunohistochemical evidence for localization in central and peripheral neurons, particularly intracortical neurons of the cerebral cortex. *Neurosci. Lett., 5*:241–246.

238. Fuxe, K., Ganten, D., Hökfelt, T., and Bolme, P. (1976): Immunohistochemical evidence for the existence of angiotensin II-containing nerve terminals in the brain and spinal cord in the rat. *Neurosci. Lett., 2*:229–234.

239. Fuxe, K. (1965): Evidence for the existence of monoamine neurons in the central nervous system. IV. Distribution of monoamine nerve terminals in the central nervous system. *Acta Physiol. Scand., 64*:39–85.

240. Gale, J. S., Bird, E. D., Spokes, E. G., Iversen, L. L., and Jessell, T. (1978): Human brain substance P: Distribution in controls and Huntington's chorea. *J. Neurochem., 30*:633–634.

241. Gale, K., Hong, J. S., and Guidotti, A. (1977): Presence of substance P and GABA in separate striatonigral neurons. *Brain Res., 136*:371–375.

242. Gamrani, H., Calas, A., Belin, M. F., Aguera, M., and Pujol, J. F. (1979): High resolution radioautographic identification of [³H]GABA labeled neurons in the rat nucleus raphe dorsalis. *Neurosci. Lett., 15*:43–48.

243. Ganten, D., Boucher, R., and Genest, J. (1971): Renin activity in brain tissue of puppies and adult dogs. *Brain Res., 33*:557–559.

244. Ganten, D., Minnich, J. L., Granger, P., Hayduk, K., Brecht, H. M., Barbeau, A., Boucher, R., and Genest, J. (1971): Angiotensin-forming enzyme in brain tissue. *Science, 173*:64–65.

245. Ganten, D., Fuxe, K., Phillips, M. I., Mann, J. F. E., and Ganten, U. (1978): The brain isorenin-angiotensin system: Biochemistry, localization, and possible role in drinking and blood pressure regulation. In: *Frontiers in Neuroendocrinology*, edited by W. F. Ganong and L. Martini, pp. 61–100. Raven Press, New York.

246. Garbarg, M., Barbin, G., Bischoff, S., Pollard, H., and Schwartz, J. C. (1976): Dual localization of histamine in an ascending neuronal pathway and in

non-neuronal cells evidenced by lesions in the lateral hypothalamic area. *Brain Res., 106*:333–348.

247. Garbarg, M., Barbin, G., Feger, J., and Schwartz, J.-C. (1974): Histaminergic pathway in rat brain evidenced by lesions of the medial forebrain bundle. *Science, 186*:833–835.

248. Gaspar, P., Javoy-Agid, F., Ploska, A., and Agid, Y. (1980): Regional distribution of neurotransmitter synthesizing enzymes in the basal ganglia of human brain. *J. Neurochem., 34*:278–283.

249. Geneser-Jensen, F. A., and Blackstad, J. W. (1971): Distribution of acetylcholinesterase in the hippocampal region of the guinea pig. I. Entorhinal area, para subiculum, and presubiculum. *Z. Zellforsch. Mikrosk. Anat., 114*:460–481.

250. Gerfen, C. R., Staines, W. A., Arbuthinott, G. W., and Fibiger, H. C. (1982): Crossed connections of the substantia nigra in the rat. *J. Comp. Neurol., 207*:283–303.

251. Giachetti, A., Said, S. I., Reynolds, R. C., and Koniges, F. C. (1977): Vasoactive intestinal polypeptide in brain: Localization in and release from isolated nerve terminals. *Proc. Natl. Acad. Sci. U.S.A., 74*:3424–3428.

252. Glover, V.. Sandler, M., Owen, F., and Riley, G. J. (1977): Dopamine is a monoamine oxidase B substrate in man. *Nature, 265*:80–81.

253. Glowinski, J. (1981): *In vivo* release of transmitters in the cat basal ganglia. *Fed. Proc., 40*:135–141.

254. Glowinski, J., and Iversen, L. L. (1966): Regional studies of catecholamines in the rat brain. I. The disposition of [³H]norepinephrine, [³H]dopamine and [³H]DOPA in various regions of the brain. *J. Neurochem., 13*:655–669.

255. Godukhin, O. V., Zharikova, A. D., and Novoselov, V. I. (1980): The release of labeled L-glutamic acid from rat neostriatum *in vivo* following stimulation of frontal cortex. *Neuroscience, 5*:2151–2154.

256. Goldberg, O., Luini, A., and Teichberg, V. I. (1981): Lactones derived from kainic acid: Novel selective antagonists of amino acid-induced Na⁺ fluxes in rat striatum slices. *Neurosci. Lett., 23*:187–191.

257. Goldman-Rakic, P. S. (1982): Cytoarchitectonic heterogeneity of the primate neostriatum: Subdivision into island and matrix cellular compartments. *J. Comp. Neurol., 205*:398–413.

258. Goldman-Rakic, P. S. (1981): Prenatal formation of cortical input and development of cytoarchitectonic compartments in the neostriatum of the rhesus monkey. *J. Neurosci., 1*:721–735.

259. Goldman, P. S., and Nauta, W. J. H. (1977): An intricately patterned prefronto-caudate projection in the rhesus monkey. *J. Comp. Neurol., 171*:369–386.

260. Goldschmidt, R. B., and Heimer, L. (1980): The rat olfactory tubercle: Its connections and relation to the strio–pallidal system. *Neurosci. Abstr., 6*:271.

261. Goodman, R. R., and Snyder, S. H. (1982): Autoradiographic localization of kappa opiate receptors to deep layers of the cerebral cortex may explain unique sedative and analgesic effects. *Life Sci., 31*:1291–1294.

262. Goodman, R. R., and Snyder, S. H. (1981): The

light microscopic *in vitro* autoradiographic localization of adenosine (A1) receptors. *Neurosci. Abstr.,* 7:613.

263. Goodman, R. R., Snyder, S. H., Kuhar, M. J., and Young, W. S. III (1980): Differentiation of delta and mu opiate receptor localizations by light microscopic autoradiography. *Proc. Natl. Acad. Sci. U.S.A.,* 77:6239–6243.

264. Gorenstein, C., and Snyder, S. H. (1980): Enkephalinases. *Proc. R. Soc. Lond. [Biol.],* 210:123–132.

265. Gramsch, C., Höllt, V., Mehraein, P., Pasi, A., and Herz, A. (1979): Regional distribution of methionine–enkephalin- and beta-endorphin-like immunoreactivity in human brain and pituitary. *Brain Res.,* 171:216–270.

266. Graybiel, A. M. (1982): Correlative studies of histochemistry and fiber connections in the central nervous system. In: *Cytochemical Methods in Neuroanatomy,* edited by V. Chan-Palay and S. Palay, pp. 46–67. Alan R. Liss, New York.

267. Graybiel, A. M. (1982): Compartmental organization of the mammalian striatum. In: *Molecular and Cellular Interactions Underlying Higher Brain Function,* edited by J.-P. Changeux. Elsevier, New York (*in press*).

268. Graybiel, A. M., and Ragsdale, C. W. (1982): Pseudocholinesterase staining in the primary visual pathway of the macaque monkey. *Nature,* 299:439–442.

269. Graybiel, A. M., and Hickey, T. L. (1982): Chemospecificity of ontogenic units in the striatum: Demonstration by combining [^{3}H]thymidine neuronography and histochemical staining. *Proc. Natl. Acad. Sci. U.S.A.,* 79:198–202.

270. Graybiel, A. M., Pickel, V. M., Joh, T. H., Reis, D. J., and Elde, R. P. (1981): Discontinuous distribution of tyrosine hydroxylase immunoreactivity in the striatum of the fetal and neonatal cat and its relation to compartments of acetylcholinesterase staining and met-enkephalin immunoreactivity. *Neurosci. Lett. [Suppl.],* 7:S476.

271. Graybiel, A. M., Pickel, V. M., Joh, T. H., Reis, D. J., and Ragsdale, C. W. (1981): Direct demonstration of a correspondence between the dopamine islands and acetylcholinesterase patches in the developing striatum. *Proc. Natl. Acad. Sci. U.S.A.,* 78:5871–5875.

272. Graybiel, A. M., Ragsdale, C. W., Yoneoka, E. S., and Elde, R. P. (1981): An immunohistochemical study of enkephalins and other neuropeptides in the striatum of the cat with evidence that the opiate peptides are arranged to form mosaic patterns in register with the striosomal compartments visible by acetylcholinesterase staining. *Neuroscience,* 6:377–397.

273. Graybiel, A. M., and Ragsdale, C. W. (1980): Clumping of acetylcholinesterase activity in the developing striatum of the human fetus and young infant. *Proc. Natl. Acad. Sci. U.S.A.,* 77:1214–1218.

274. Graybiel, A. M., Ragsdale, C. W., Yoneoka, E. S., and Elde, R. P. (1980): Opioid peptides, substance P and somatostatin in the striatum. An immunohis-

tochemical study in the cat and kitten. *Neurosci. Abstr.* 6:342.

275. Graybiel, A. M., and Ragsdale, C. W. (1979): Fiber connections of the basal ganglia. In: *Development and Chemical Specifity of Neurons,* edited by M. Cuénod, G. W. Kreutzberg, and F. E. Bloom, pp. 239–283. Elsevier, Amsterdam.

276. Graybiel, A. M., Ragsdale, C. W., and Moon Edley, S.(1979): Compartments in the striatum of the cat observed by retrograde cell-labeling. *Exp. Brain Res.,* 34:189–195.

277. Graybiel, A. M., and Ragsdale, C. W. (1978): Histochemically distinct compartments in the striatum of human, monkey and cat demonstrated by acetylcholinesterase staining. *Proc. Natl. Acad. Sci. U.S.A.,* 75:5723–5726.

278. Graybiel, A. M., and Ragsdale, C. W. (1978): Striosomal organization of the caudate nucleus. I. Acetylcholinesterase histochemistry of the striatum in the cat, rhesus monkey and human being. *Neurosci. Abstr.,* 4:44.

279. Graybiel, A. M. (1975): Wallerian degeneration and anterograde tracer methods. In: *The Use of Axonal Transport for Studies of Neuronal Connectivity,* edited by W. M. Cowan and M. Cuenod, pp. 174–216. Elsevier, Amsterdam.

280. Greenfield, S. A., Stein, J. F., Hodgson, A. J., and Chubb, I. W. (1981): Depression of nigral pars compacta cell discharge by exogenous acetylcholinesterase. *Neuroscience,* 6:2287–2295.

281. Greenfield, S., Cheramy, A., Leviel, V., and Glowinski, J. (1980): *In vivo* release of acetycholinesterase in cat substantia nigra and caudate nucleus. *Nature,* 284:355–357.

282. Groenewegen, H. J., Room, P., Witter, M. P., and Lohman, A. H. M. (1982). Cortical afferents of the nucleus accumbens in the cat, studied with anterograde and retrograde transport techniques. *Neuroscience,* 7:977–995.

283. Groenewegen, H. J., Becker, N. E. H. M., and Lohman, A. H. M. (1980): Subcortical afferents of the nucleus accumbens septi in the cat, studied with retrograde axonal transport of horseradish peroxidase and bisbenzimid. *Neuroscience,* 5:1903–1916.

284. Grofová, I. (1979): Types of striatonigral neurons labeled by retrograde transport of horseradish peroxidase. *Appl. Neurophysiol.,* 42:25–28.

285. Grofová, I. (1975): The identification of striatal and pallidal neurons projecting to substantia nigra. An experimental study by means of retrograde axonal transport of horseradish peroxidase. *Brain Res.,* 91:286–291.

286. Grote, S. S., Moses, S. G., Robins, E., Hudgens, R. W., and Croninger, A. B. (1974): A study of selected catecholamine metabolizing enzymes: A comparison of depressive suicides and alcoholic suicides with controls. *J. Neurochem.,* 23:791–802.

287. Groves, P. M. (1980): Synaptic endings and their postsynaptic targets in neostriatum: Synaptic specializations revealed from analysis of serial sections. *Proc. Natl. Acad. Sci. U.S.A.,* 77:6926–6929.

288. Grzanna, R., Morrison, J. H., Coyle, J. T., and Molliver, M. E. (1977): The immunohistochemical demonstration of noradrenergic neurons in the rat

brain: The use of homologous anti-serum to dopamine-β-hydroxylase. *Neurosci. Lett.,* 4:127–134.

289. Gubler, U., Seeburg, P., Hoffman, B. J., Gage, L. P., and Udenfriend, S. (1982): Molecular cloning establishes proenkephalin as precursor of enkephalin-containing peptides. *Nature,* 295:206–208.

290. Guidotti, A., Badiani, G., and Pepeu, G. (1972): Taurine distribution in cat brain. *J. Neurochem.,* 19:431–435.

291. Guidotti, A., Gale, K., Suria, A., and Toffano, G. (1979): Biochemical evidence for two classes of GABA receptors in rat brain. *Brain Res.,* 172:566–571.

292. Gurewitsch, M. (1930): Cytoarchitektonische Gliederung des Neostriatum der Saeugetiere. *Z. Anat.,* 93:723–742.

293. Guy, J., Vaudry, H., and Pelletier, G. (1981): Differential projections of two immunoreactive α-melanocyte stimulating hormone (α-MSH) neuronal systems in the rat brain. *Brain Res.,* 230:199–202.

294. Guyenet, P. G., and Crane, J. K. (1981): Non-dopaminergic nigrostriatal pathway. *Brain Res.,* 213:291–305.

295. Guyenet, P. G., and Aghajanian, G. K. (1978): Antidromic identification of dopaminergic and other output neurons of the rat substantia nigra. *Brain Res.,* 150:69–84.

296. Guyenet, P., Euvrard, C., Javoy, F., Herbet, A., and Glowinski, J. (1977): Regional differences in the sensitivity of cholinergic neurons to dopaminergic drugs and quipazine in the rat striatum. *Brain Res.,* 136:487–500.

297. Haber, S., and Elde, R. (1982): The distribution of enkephalin immunoreactive fibers and terminals in the monkey central nervous system: An immunohistochemical study. *Neuroscience,* 7:1049–1095.

298. Haber, S., and Nauta, W. J. H. (1981): Substance P, but not enkephalin immunoreactivity distinguishes ventral from dorsal pallidum. *Neurosci. Abstr.,* 7:916.

299. Haber, S., and Elde R. (1981): Correlation between met-enkephalin and substance P immunoreactivity in the primate globus pallidus. *Neuroscience,* 6:1291–1297.

300. Hall, J. G., Hicks, T. P., and McLennan, H. (1978): Kainic acid and the glutamate receptor. *Neurosci. Lett.,* 8:171–175.

301. Hanker, J. S., Thornburg, L. P., Yates, P. E., and Moore, H. G. III (1973): The demonstration of cholinesterases by the formation of osimium blacks at the sites of Hatchett's brown. *Histochemie,* 37:223–242.

302. Hanley, M. R., Sandberg, B. E. B., Lee, C. M., Iversen, L. L., Bruncish, D. E., and Wade, R. (1980): Specific binding of ^{3}H-substance P to rat brain membranes. *Nature,* 286:810–813.

303. Hassler, R. (1979): Electronmicroscopic differentiation of the extrinsic and intrinsic types of nerve cells and synapses in the striatum and their putative transmitters. In: *Advances in Neurology,* Vol. 24, edited by L. J. Poirier, T. L. Sourkes, and P. J. Bédard, pp. 93–108. Raven Press, New York.

304. Hattori, T., and Fibiger, H. C. (1982): On the use of lesions of afferents to localize neurotransmitter

receptor sites in the striatum. *Brain Res.,* 238:245–250.

305. Hattori, T., Singh, V. K., McGeer, E. G., and McGeer, P. L. (1976): Immunohistochemical localization of choline acetyltransferase containing neostriatal neurons and their relationship with dopaminergic synapses. *Brain Res.,* 102:164–173.

306. Hattori, T., McGeer, P. L., Fibiger, H. C., and McGeer, E. G. (1973): On the source of GABA containing terminals in the substantia nigra. Electron microscopic, autoradiographic and biochemical studies. *Brain Res.,* 54:103–114.

307. Hattori, T., Fibiger, H. C., McGeer, P. L., and Maler, L. (1973): Analysis of the fine structure of the dopaminergic nigrostriatal projection by electron microscopic autoradiography. *Exp. Neurol.,* 41:599–611.

308. Havrankova, J., and Roth, J. (1978): Insulin receptors are widely distributed in the central nervous system of the rat. *Nature,* 272:827–829.

309. Hawthorn, J., Vincent, T. Y., and Jenkins, J. S. (1980): Localization of vasopressin in the rat brain. *Brain Res.,* 197:75–81.

310. Hays, S. E., Goodwin, F. K., and Paul, S. M. (1981): Cholecystokinin receptors are decreased in basal ganglia and cerebral cortex of Huntington's disease. *Brain Res.,* 225:452–456.

311. Hebb, C. O., and Silver, A. (1956): Choline acetylase in the central nervous system of man and some other mammals. *J. Physiol. (Lond.),* 134:718–728.

312. Hedreen, J., Holm, G., Delong, M., Crutcher, M., and Branch, M. (1980): Projection of neostriatum to globus pallidus and substantia nigra in macaques. *Anat. Rec.,* 196:79A.

313. Hedreen, J. C. (1977): Corticostriatal cells identified by the peroxidase method. *Neurosci. Lett.,* 4:1–7.

314. Hedreen, J. C. (1971): Separate demonstration of dopaminergic and non-dopaminergic projections of substantia nigra in the rat. *Anat. Rec.,* 169:338.

315. Heimer, L. (1976): The olfactory cortex and the ventral striatum. In: *Limbic Mechanisms: The Continuing Evolution of the Limbic System Concept,* edited by K. E. Livingston and O. Hornykiewicz, pp. 95–187. Plenum Press, New York.

316. Heimer, L., and Wilson, R. D. (1975): The subcortical projections of the allocortex: Similarities in the neural associations of the hippocampus, the piriform cortex, and the neocortex. In: *Golgi Centennial Symposium,* edited by M. Santini, pp. 177–193. Raven Press, New York.

317. Henderson, G., Hughes, J., and Kosterlitz, H. W. (1978): *In vitro* release of leu- and met-enkephalin from the corpus striatum. *Nature,* 271:677–679.

318. Henderson, Z. (1981): Ultrastructure and acetylcholinesterase content of neurones forming connections between the striatum and substantia nigra of rat. *J. Comp. Neurol.,* 197:185–196.

319. Henke, H., and Cuénod, M. (1979): L-Glutamate specific [^{3}H]kainic acid binding in the rat neostriatum after degeneration of the cortico–striatal pathway. *Neurosci. Lett.,* 11:341–345.

320. Herkenham, M., and Pert, C. B. (1982): Light microscopic localization of brain opiate receptors: A

general autoradiographic method which preserves tissue quality. *J. Neurosci.,* 2:1129–1149.

321. Herkenham, M., and Pert, C. B. (1981): Mosaic distribution of opiate receptors, parafascicular projections and acetylcholinesterase in rat striatum. *Nature,* 291:415–418.

322. Herkenham, M. (1979): The afferent and efferent connections of the ventromedial thalamic nucleus in the rat. *J. Comp. Neurol.,* 183:487–518.

323. Hiley, C. R., and Bird, E. D. (1974): Decreased muscarinic receptor concentration in post-mortem brain in Huntington's chorea. *Brain Res.,* 80:355–358.

324. Hill, S. J., Emson, P. C., and Young, J. M. (1978): The binding of [^{3}H]mepyramine to histamine H_1 receptors in guinea-pig brain. *J. Neurochem.,* 31:997–1004.

325. Hirose, S., Yokosawa, H., and Inagami, T. (1978): Immunochemical identification of renin in rat brain and distinction from acid proteases. *Nature,* 274:392–393.

326. Höck, A., Demmel, U., Schicha, H., Kasperek, K., and Feinendegen, L. E. (1975): Trace element concentration in human brain. Activation analysis of cobalt, iron, rubidium, selenium, zinc, chromium, silver, cesium, antimony and scandium. *Brain,* 98:49–64.

327. Hökfelt, T., Skirboll, L., Rehfeld, M. F., Goldstein, M., Markey, K., and Dann, O. (1980): A subpopulation of mesencephalic dopamine neurons projecting to limbic areas contains a cholecystokinin-like peptide: Evidence from immunohistochemistry combined with retrograde tracing. *Neuroscience,* 5:2093–2124.

328. Hökfelt, T., Rehfeld, J. F., Skirboll, L., Ivemark, B., Goldstein, M., and Markey, K. (1980): Evidence for coexistence of dopamine and CCK in meso-limbic neurons. *Nature,* 285:476–478.

329. Hökfelt, T., Elde, R., Johansson, O., Terenius, L., and Stein, L. (1977): The distribution of enkephalin-immunoreactive cell bodies in the rat central nervous system. *Neurosci. Lett.,* 5:25–31.

330. Hökfelt, T., Fuxe, K., Johansson, O., Jeffocate, S., and White, N. (1975): Distribution of thyrotropin-releasing hormone (TRH) in the central nervous system as revealed with immunohistochemistry. *Eur. J. Pharmacol.,* 34:389–392.

331. Hökfelt, T., Johnson, C., and Ljungdahl, Å. (1970): Regional uptake and subcellular localization of [^{3}H]-gamma-aminobutyric acid (GABA) in rat brain slices. *Life Sci.,* 9:202–212.

332. Höllt, V., Haarmann, I., Bovermann, K., Jerlicz, M., and Herz, A. (1980): Dynorphin-related immunoreactive peptides in rat brain and pituitary. *Neurosci. Lett.,* 18:149–153.

333. Höllt, V., and Schubert, P. (1978): Demonstration of neuroleptic receptor sites in mouse brain by autoradiography. *Brain Res.,* 151:149–153.

334. Holmstedt, B., and Sjöqvist, F. (1960): Pharmacological properties of γ-aminobutyrylcholine, a supposed inhibitory neutrotransmitter. *Biochem. Pharmacol.,* 3:297–304.

335. Hong, J. S., Yang, H.-Y. T., Fratta, W., and Costa, E. (1977): Determination of methionine enkephalin in discrete regions of rat brain. *Brain Res.,* 134:383–386.

336. Hong, J. S., Yang, H.-Y., and Costa, E. (1977): On the location of methionine enkephalin neurons in rat striatum. *Neuropharmacology,* 16:451–453.

337. Hong, J. S., Yang, H.-Y. T., Racagni, G., and Costa, E. (1977): Projections of substance P containing neurons from neostriatum to substantia nigra. *Brain Res.,* 122:541–544.

338. Hook, V. Y. H., Elden, L. E., and Brownstein, M. J. (1982): A carboxypeptidase processing enzyme for enkephalin precursors. *Nature,* 295:341–342.

339. Hoover, D. B., and Jacobowitz, D. M. (1979): Neurochemical and histochemical studies of the effect of a lesion of the nucleus cuneiformis on the cholinergic innervation of discrete areas of the rat brain. *Brain Res.,* 170:113–122.

340. Hoover, D. B., Muth, E. A., and Jacobowitz, D. M. (1978): A mapping of the distribution of acetylcholine, choline acetyltransferase and acetylcholinesterase in discrete areas of rat brain. *Brain Res.,* 153:295–306.

341. Hornykiewicz, O. (1963): Die topische lokalisation und das Verhalten von Noradrenalin und Dopamin (3-Hydroxytyramin) in der Substantia nigra des normalen und Parkinson-kranken Menschen. *Wiener Klin. Wochenschr.,* 75:309–312.

342. Howlett, W., Akii, H., Carlini, W., and Barchas J. D. (1982): Tritiated ethylketocylazocine binding in rat brain: Differential distribution of binding sites across brain regions. *Life Sci.,* 31:1351–1354.

343. Hu, K. H., and Friede, R. L. (1968): Topographic determination of zinc in human brain by atomic absorption spectrophotometry. *J. Neurochem.,* 15:677–685.

344. Hughes, J., Kosterlitz, H. W., and Smith, T. W. (1977): The distribution of methionine-enkephalin and leucine-enkephalin in the brain and peripheral tissues. *Br. J. Pharmacol.,* 61:639–647.

345. Hunt, S. P., Kelly, J. S., and Emson, P. C. (1980): The electron microscopic localization of methionine-enkephalin within the superficial layers (I and II) of the spinal cord. *Neuroscience,* 5:1871–1890.

346. Hunt, S., and Schmidt, J. (1978): Some observations on the binding patterns of α-bungarotoxin in the central nervous system of the rat. *Brain Res.,* 157:213–232.

347. Hyttel, J. (1978): Effects of neuroleptics on [^{3}H]-haloperidol and ^{3}H-CIS (2)-flupenthixol binding and on adenylate cyclase activity *in vitro. Life Sci.,* 23:351–356.

348. Innis, R. B., and Snyder, S. H. (1980): Distinct cholecystokinin receptors in brain and pancreas. *Proc. Natl. Acad. Sci. U.S.A.,* 77:6917–6921.

349. Innis, R. B., Corrêa, F. M. A., Uhl, G. R., Schneider, B., and Snyder, S. H. (1979): Cholecystokinin octapeptide-like immunoreactivity: Histochemical localization in rat brain. *Proc. Natl. Acad. Sci. U.S.A.,* 76:521–525.

350. Ishii, T., and Friede, R. L. (1967): A comparative histochemical mapping of the distribution of acetylcholinesterase and nicotinamide adenine dinucleotide-diaphorase activities in the human brain. In: *International Review of Neurobiology,* Volume 10,

edited by C. C. Pfeiffer and J. R. Smythies, pp. 231–275. Academic Press, New York.

351. Itzhak, Y., Bonnet, K. A., Groth, J., Miller, J. M., and Simon, E. J. (1982): Multiple opiate binding sites in human brain regions: Evidence for κ and σ sites. *Life Sci.*, 31:1363–1366.

352. Iversen, L. L., Iversen, S. D., Bloom, F. E., Vargo, T., and Guillemin, R. (1978): Release of enkephalin from rat globus pallidus *in vitro*. *Nature*, 271:679–681.

353. Jackson, A., and Crossman, A. R. (1981): Subthalamic nucleus efferent projection to the cerebral cortex. *Neuroscience*, 6:2367–2377.

354. Jacobowitz, D. M., and O'Donohue, T. L. (1978): α-Melanocyte stimulating hormone: Immunohistochemical identification and mapping in neurons of rat brain. *Proc. Natl. Acad. Sci. U.S.A.*, 78:6300–6304.

355. Jacobowitz, D. M., and Palkovits, M. (1974): Topographic atlas of catecholamine and acetylcholinesterase-containing neurons in the rat brain. I. Forebrain (telecephalon, diencephalon). *J. Comp. Neurol.*, 157:13–28.

356. Jacobs, B. L., Foote, S. L., and Bloom, F. E. (1978): Differential projections of neurons within the dorsal raphe nucleus of the rat: A horseradish peroxidase (HRP) study. *Brain Res.*, 147:149–153.

357. Jayaraman, A. (1980): Anatomical evidence for cortical projections from the striatum in the cat. *Brain Res.*, 195:29–36.

358. Jessell, T. M., Emson, P. C., Paxinos, G., and Cuello, A. C. (1978): Topographic projections of substance P and GABA pathways in the striato- and pallido-nigral system: A biochemical and immunohistochemical study. *Brain Res.*, 152:487–498.

359. Jinnai, K., and Matsuda, Y. (1979): Neurons of the motor cortex projecting commonly on the caudate nucleus and the lower brain stem in the cat. *Neurosci. Lett.*, 13:121–126.

360. Johannson, O., and Hökfelt, T. (1980): Thyrotropin-releasing hormone, somatostatin, and enkephalin: Distribution studies using immunohistochemical techniques. *J. Histochem. Cytochem.*, 28:364–366.

361. Johnson, J. L., and Aprison, M. H. (1970): The distribution of glutamate and total free amino acids in thirteen specific regions of the cat central nervous system. *Brain Res.*, 26:141–148.

362. Johnson, R. P., Sar, M., and Stumpf, W. E. (1980): A topographic localization of enkephalin on the dopamine neurons of the rat substantia nigra and ventral tegmental area demonstrated by combined histofluorescence-immunocytochemistry. *Brain Res.*, 194:566–571.

363. Johnston, G. A. R. (1979): Central nervous system receptors for glutamic acid. In: *Glutamic Acid: Advances in Biochemistry and Physiology*, edited by L. J. Filer, Jr., S. Garattini, M. R. Karc, W. A. Reynolds, and R. J. Wurtman, pp. 177–185. Raven Press, New York.

364. Johnston, M. V., McKinney, M., and Coyle, J. T. (1979): Evidence for a cholinergic projection to neocortex from neurons in basal forebrain. *Proc. Natl. Acad. Sci. U.S.A.*, 76:5392–5396.

365. Jones, B. E., Halaris, A. E., McIlhany, M., and Moore, R. Y. (1977): Ascending projections of the locus coeruleus in the rat. I. Axonal transport in central noradrenaline neurons. *Brain Res.*, 127:1–21.

366. Jones, E. G., and Leavitt, R. Y. (1974): Retrograde axonal transport and the demonstration of non-specific projections to the cerebral cortex and striatum from the thalamic intralaminar nuclei in the rat, cat and monkey. *J. Comp. Neurol.*, 154:349–378.

367. Jones, E. G., Coulter, J. D., Burton, H., and Porter, R. (1977): Cells of origin and terminal distribution of corticostriatal fibers arising in the sensory–motor cortex of monkeys. *J. Comp. Neurol.*, 173:53–80.

368. Juraska, J. M., Wilson, C. J., and Groves, P. M. (1977): The substantia nigra in the rat: A Golgi study. *J. Comp. Neurol.*, 172:585–600.

369. Kaiya, H., Kreutzberg, G. W., and Namba, M. (1980): Ultrastructure of acetylcholinesterase synthesizing neurons in the neostriatum. *Brain Res.*, 187:369–382.

370. Kaiya, H., Okinaga, M., Namba, M., Shoumura, K., and Watanabe, S. (1979): Ultrastructure of acetylcholinesterase containing striato–nigral neurons transporting HRP retrogradely. *Neurosci. Lett.*, 14:7–11.

371. Kakidani, H., Furutani, Y., Takahashi, H., Noda, M., Morimoto, Y., Hirose, T., Asai, M., Inayama, S., Nakanishi, S., and Numa, S. (1982): Cloning and sequence analysis of cDNA for procine β-neoendorphin/dynorphin precursor. *Nature*, 298:245–249.

372. Kalil, K. (1978): Patch-like termination of thalamic fibers in the putamen of the rhesus monkey: An autoradiographic study. *Brain Res.*, 140:333–339.

373. Kamiya, H., Takano, Y., Kusunoki, T., Uchimura, K., Kohjimoto, Y., Honda, K., and Sakurai, Y. (1982): Studies on ^{125}I-α-bungarotoxin binding sites in rat brain. *Brain Res. Bull.*, 8:431–433.

374. Kanazawa, A., and Sano, I. (1967): A method of determination of homocarnosine and its distribution in mammalian tissues. *J. Neurochem.*, 14:211–214.

375. Kanazawa, I., Mogaki, S., Muramoto, O., and Kuzuhara, S. (1980): On the origin of substance P-containing fibers in the entopeduncular nucleus and the substantia nigra of the rat. *Brain Res.*, 184:481–485.

376. Kanazawa, I., and Yoshida, M. (1980): Electrophysiological evidence for the excitatory fibers in the caudato–nigral pathway in the cat. *Neurosci. Lett.*, 20:301–306.

377. Kanazawa, I., Bird, E., O'Connell, R., and Powell, D. (1977): Evidence for a decrease in substance P content of substantia nigra in Huntington's chorea. *Brain Res.*, 120:387–392.

378. Kanazawa, I., Emson, P. C., and Cuello, A. C. (1977): Evidence for the existence of substance P-containing fibres in striato–nigral and pallido-nigral pathways in rat brain. *Brain Res.*, 119:447–453.

379. Kanazawa, I., and Jessell, T. (1976): Post mortem changes and regional distribution of substance P in the rat and mouse nervous system. *Brain Res.*, 117:362–367.

380. Kandera, J., Levi, G., and Lajtha, A. (1968): Con-

trol of cerebral metabolite levels. II. Amino acid uptake and levels in various areas of the rat brain. *Arch. Biochem. Biophys.,* 126:219–260.

381. Kaplan, G. P., Hartman, B. K., and Creveling, C. R. (1979): Immunohistochemical demonstration of catechol-*O*-methyltransferase in mammalian brain. *Brain Res.,* 167:241–250.

382. Karoum, F., Nasballah, H., Potkin, S., Chuang, L., Moyer-Schwing, J., Phillips, I., and Wyatt, R. J. (1979): Mass fragmentography of phenylethylamine, *m*- and *p*-tyramine and related amines in plasma, cerebrospinal fluid, urine, and brain. *J. Neurochem.,* 33:201–212.

383. Kataoka, K., Mizuno, N., and Frohman, L. A. (1979): Regional distribution of immunoreactive neurotensin in monkey brain. *Brain Res. Bull.,* 4:57–60.

384. Kataoka, K., Bak, I. J., Hassler, R., Kim, J. S., and Wagner, A. (1974): L-Glutamate decarboxylase and choline acetyltransferase activity in the substantia nigra and striatum after surgical interruption of strio–nigral fibers of the baboon. *Exp. Brain Res.,* 19:217–227.

385. Kebebian, J. W., and Calne, D. B. (1979): Multiple receptors for dopamine. *Nature,* 277:93–96.

386. Keefer, D. A., and Stumpf, W. E. (1975): Atlas of estrogen-concentrating cells in the central nervous system of the squirrel monkey. *J. Comp. Neurol.,* 160:419–442.

387. Kellar, K. J., Brown, P. A., Madrid, J., Bernstein, M., Vernikos-Danellis, J., and Mehler, W. R. (1977): Origins of serotonin innervation of forebrain structures. *Exp. Neurol.,* 56:52–62.

388. Kelley, A. E., Domesick, V. B., and Nauta, W. J. H. (1982): The amygdalostriatal projection in the rat—an anatomical study by anterograde and retrograde tracing methods. *Neuroscience,* 7:615–630.

389. Kelly, P. H., Moore, K. E., Spokes, E. G., and Bird, E. D. (1979): Catechol-*O*-methyltransferase in the kainic-acid-treated rat striatum and in the basal ganglia in Huntington's disease. In: *Advances in Neurology,* Vol. 23, edited by T. N. Chase, N. S. Wexler, and A. Barbeau, pp. 625–632. Raven Press, New York.

390. Kelly, P. H., and Moore, K. E. (1978): Decrease of neocortical choline acetyltransferase after lesion of the globus pallidus in the rat. *Exp. Neurol.,* 61:479–484.

391. Kemp, J. M., and Powell, T. P. S. (1971): The structure of the caudate nucleus of the cat: Light and electron microscopy. *Phil. Trans. R. Soc. Lond.* [*Biol.*], 262:383–401.

392. Kemp, J. M., and Powell, T. P. S. (1971): The synaptic organization of the caudate nucleus. *Phil. Trans. R. Soc. Lond.* [*Biol.*], 262:403–412.

393. Kemp, J. M., and Powell, T. P. S. (1971): The site of termination of afferent fibers in the caudate nucleus. *Phil. Trans. R. Soc. Lond.* [*Biol.*], 262:413–427.

394. Kemp, J. M., and Powell, T. P. S. (1970): The cortico–striate projection in the monkey. *Brain,* 93:525–546.

395. Kent, J. L., Pert, C. B., and Herkenham, M. (1982): Ontogeny of opiate receptors in rat forebrain: Visualization by *in vitro* autoradiography. *Dev. Brain Res.,* 2:487–504.

396. Kety, S. S., and Elkes, J. (1981): *Regional Neurochemistry.* Pergamon Press, New York.

397. Khachaturian, H., Tsou, K., and Watson, S. (1981): β-Endorphin and α-MSH in the rat brain: A comparative immunocytochemical analysis. *Neurosci. Abstr.,* 7:93.

398. Kim, J., Hassler, R., Haug, P., and Paik, K. (1977): Effect of frontal cortex ablation on striatal glutamic acid level in rat. *Brain Res.,* 132:370–374.

399. Kim, R., Nakano, K., Jayaraman, A., and Carpenter, M. B. (1976): Projections of the globus pallidus and adjacent structures: An autoradiographic study in the monkey. *J. Comp. Neurol.,* 169:263–290.

400. Kim, J. S., Bak, I. J., Hassler, R., and Okada, Y. (1971): Role of γ-aminobutyric acid (GABA) in the extrapyramidal motor system. 2. Some evidence for the existence of a type of GABA-rich strionigral neuron. *Exp. Brain Res.,* 14:95–104.

401. Kimura, H., McGeer, P. L., Peng, J. H., and McGeer, E. G. (1981): The central cholinergic system studied by choline acetyltransferase immunohistochemistry in the cat. *J. Comp. Neurol.,* 200:151–201.

402. Kimura, H., McGeer, P. L., Peng, J. H., and McGeer, E. G. (1980): Choline acetyltransferase-containing neurons in rodent brain demonstrated by immunohistochemistry. *Science,* 208:1057–1059.

403. Kish, S. J., Perry, T. L., and Hansen, S. (1979): Regional distribution of homocarnosine, homocarnosine–carnosine synthetase and homocarnosinase in human brain. *J. Neurochem.,* 32:1629–1636.

404. Kitai, S. T., Kocsis, J. D., and Wood, J. (1976): Origin and characteristics of the cortico–caudate afferents: An anatomical and electrophysiological study. *Brain Res.,* 118:137–141.

405. Kitai, S. T., Kocsis, J. D., Preston, R. J., and Sugimori, M. (1976): Monosynaptic inputs to caudate neurons identified by intracellular injection of horseradish peroxidase. *Brain Res.,* 109:601–606.

406. Klemm, N., Murrin, L. C., and Kuhar, M. J. (1979): Neuroleptic and dopamine receptors: Autoradiographic localization of [^{3}H]spiperone in rat brain. *Brain Res.,* 169:1–9.

407. Kloog, Y., Egozi, Y., and Sokolovsky, M. (1978): Regional heterogeneity of muscarinic receptors of mouse brain. *FEBS Lett.,* 97:265–268.

408. Kobayashi, R. M., Palkovits, M., Hruska, R. E., Rothschild, R., and Yamamura, H. I. (1978): Regional distribution of muscarinic cholinergic receptors in rat brain. *Brain Res.,* 154:13–23.

409. Kobayashi, R. M., Brown, M., and Vale, W. (1977): Regional distribution of neurotensin and somatostatin in rat brain. *Brain Res.,* 126:584–588.

410. Kocsis, J. D., Sugimori, M., and Kitai, S. T. (1977): Convergence of excitatory synaptic inputs to caudate spiny neurons. *Brain Res.,* 124:403–413.

411. Koelle, G. B., Davis, R., Smyri, E. G., and Fine, A. V. (1974): Refinement of the bis-(thioacetoxy)aurate (1) method for the electron microscopic localization of acetylcholinesterase and nonspecific cholinesterase. *J. Histochem. Cytochem.,* 22:252–259.

412. Koelle, G. B. (1954): The histochemical localiza-

tion of cholinesterase in the central nervous system of the rat. *J. Comp. Neurol.,* 100:211–236.

413. Koslow, S. H., Racagni, G., and Costa, E. (1974): Mass fragmentographic measurement of norepinephrine, dopamine, serotonin and acetylcholine in seven discrete nuclei of the rat tel–diencephalon. *Neuropharmacology,* 13:1123–1130.

414. Krettek, J. E., and Price, J. L. (1978): Amygdaloid projections to subcortical structures within the basal forebrain and brainstem in the rat and cat. *J. Comp. Neurol.,* 178:225–254.

415. Krieger, D. T., Liotta, A., and Brownstein, M. J. (1972): Presence of corticotropin in limbic system of normal and hypophysectomized rats. *Brain Res.,* 128:575–579.

416. Kubek, M. J., and Wilber, J. F. (1980): Regional distribution of leucine-enkephalin in hypothalamic and extrahypothalamic loci of the human nervous system. *Neurosci. Lett.,* 18:153–161.

417. Kuhar, M. J., and Unnerstall, J. R. (1982): *In vitro* labeling receptor autoradiography: Loss of label during ethanol dehydration and preparative procedures. *Brain Res.,* 244:178–181.

418. Kuhar, M. J., and Yamamura, H. I. (1976): Localization of cholinergic muscarinic receptors in rat brain by light microscopic radioautography. *Brain Res.,* 110:229–243.

419. Kuhar, M. J., and Yamamura, H. I. (1975): Light autoradiographic localization of cholinergic muscarinic receptors in rat brain by specific binding of a potent antagonist. *Nature,* 253:560–561.

420. Kuhar, M. J., Pert, C. B., and Snyder, S. H. (1973): Regional distribution of opiate receptor binding in monkey and human brain. *Nature,* 245:447–450.

421. Kuntzman, R., Shore, P. A., Bogdanski, D., and Brodie, B. B. (1961): Microanalytical procedures for fluorometric assay of brain DOPA–5HTP decarboxylase, norepinepherine and serotonin, and a detailed mapping of decarboxylase activity in brain. *J. Neurochem.,* 6:226–232.

422. Künzle, H. (1978): An autoradiographic analysis of the efferent connections from premotor and adjacent prefrontal regions (areas 6 and 9) in *Macaca fascicularis. Brain Behav. Evol.,* 15:185–234.

423. Künzle, H. (1977): Projections from the primary somatosensory cortex to basal ganglia and thalamus in the monkey. *Exp. Brain Res.,* 30:481–492.

424. Künzle, H., and Akert, K. (1977): Efferent connections of cortical area 8 (frontal eye field) in *Macaca fascicularis.* A reinvestigation using the autoradiographic method. *J. Comp. Neurol.,* 173:147–164.

425. Künzle, H. (1975): Bilateral projections from precentral motor cortex to the putamen and other parts of the basal ganglia. *Brain Res.,* 88:195–210.

426. Kuriaki, K., Yakushiji, T., Noro, T., Shimizu, T., and Saji, S. (1958): Gamma-aminobutyrylcholine. *Nature,* 181:1336–1337.

427. Larsson, L.-I., and Rehfeld, J. F. (1979): Localization and molecular heterogeneity of cholecystokinin in the central and peripheral nervous system. *Brain Res.,* 165:201–218.

428. Larsson, L.-I., Childers, S., and Snyder, S. H. (1979): Met- and leu-enkephalin immunoreactivity in separate neurones. *Nature,* 282:407–410.

429. Lee, T., Seeman, P., Hornykiewicz, O., Bilbao, J., Deck, J., and Tourtellotte, W. W. (1981): Parkinson's disease: Low density and presynaptic location of D_3 dopamine receptors. *Brain Res.,* 212:494–498.

430. Lee, T., Seeman, P., Rajput, A., Farley, I. J.. and Hornykiewicz, O. (1978): Receptor basis for dopaminergic supersensitivity in Parkinson's disease. *Nature,* 273:59–61.

431. Lefresne, P., Beacjouan, J. C., and Glowinski, J. (1978): Origin of the acetyl moiety of acetylcholine in rat striatal synaptosomes: A specific pyruvate dehydrogenase involved in ACh synthesis? *Biochemie,* 60:479–487.

432. Leger, L., Pujol, J.-F., Bobillier, P., and Jouvet, M. (1977): Transport axoplasmique de la serotonine par voie retrograde dans les neurones mono-aminergiques centraux. *C. R. Acad. Sci. [D] (Paris),* 285:1179–1182.

433. Lehmann, J., Nagy, J. I., Atmada, S., and Fibiger, H. C. (1980): The nucleus basalis magnocellularis: The origin of a cholinergic projection to the neocortex of the rat. *Neuroscience,* 5:1161–1174.

434. Lehmann, J., and Fibiger, H. C. (1979): Acetylcholinesterase and the cholinergic neuron. *Life Sci.,* 25:1939–1947.

435. Lehmann, J., Fibiger, H. C., and Butcher, L. L. (1979): The localization of acetylcholinesterase in the corpus striatum and substantia nigra of the rat following kainic acid lesion of the corpus striatum: A biochemical and histochemical study. *Neuroscience,* 4:217–225.

436. Lehmann, J., and Fibiger, H. C. (1978): Acetylcholinesterase in the substantia nigra and caudate-putamen of the rat: Properties and localization in dopaminergic neurons. *J. Neurochem.,* 30:615–624.

437. Lénárd, L., and Nauta, W. J. H. (1979): Neostriatal and limbic projection of cell group A8. *Neurosci. Lett. [Suppl.],* 3:S70.

438. Lentovich, T. A. (1954): [Fine structure of subcortical ganglia.] *Z. Neuropatol. Psikh.,* 54:168–178.

439. Levey, A. I., and Wainer, B. H. (1981): Monoclonal antibodies against choline acetyltransferase (ChAT): Intraspecies and interspecies reactivities. *Neurosci. Abstr.,* 7:121.

440. Levi, G., Bertollini, A., Chen, J., and Ratteri, M. (1974): Regional differences in the synaptosomal uptake of ^3H-γ-aminobutyric acid and ^{14}C-glutamate and possible role of exchange processes. *J. Pharmacol. Exp. Ther.,* 188:429–438.

441. Lew, J. Y., Matsumoto, Y., Pearson, J., Goldstein, M., Hökfelt, T., and Fuxe, K. (1977): Localization and characterization of phenylethanolamine N-methyl transferase in the brain of various mammalian species. *Brain Res.,* 119:199–210.

442. Lewicki, J. A., Fallon, J. H., and Printz, M. P. (1978): Regional distribution of angiotensinogen in rat brain. *Brain Res.,* 138:339–371.

443. Lewis, M. E., Khachaturian, H., and Watson, S. J. (1982): Visualization of opiate receptors and opioid peptides in sequential brain sections. *Life Sci.,* 31:1347–1350.

444. Lewis, M. E., Patel, J., Moon Edley, S., and Marangos, P. J. (1981): Autoradiographic visualization

of rat brain adenosine receptors using N[6]-cyclohexyl[³H]adenosine. *Eur. J. Pharmacol.,* 73:109–110.

445. Lewis, P. R., and Shute, C. C. D. (1969): An electron microscopic study of cholinesterase distribution in the rat adrenal medulla. *J. Microsci.,* 89:191–193.

446. Lewis, R. V., Stein, S., Gerber, L. D., Rubinstein, M., and Udenfriend, S. (1978): High molecular weight opioid-containing proteins in striatum. *Proc. Natl. Acad. Sci. U.S.A.,* 75:4021–4023.

447. Lidbrink, P., Jonsson, C., and Fuxe, K. (1974): Selective reserpine-resistant accumulation of catecholamines in central dopamine neurones after DOPA administration. *Brain Res.,* 67:439–456.

448. Lindberg, I., Smythe, S. J., and Dahl, J. L. (1979): Regional distribution of enkephalin in bovine brain. *Brain Res.,* 168:200–204.

449. Lindvall, O., and Björklund, A. (1978): Organization of catecholamine neurons in the rat central nervous system. In: *Handbook of Psychopharmacology,* edited by L. L. Iversen, S. D. Iversen, and S. H. Snyder, pp. 139–231. Plenum Press, New York.

450. Lipinski, J. F., Schaumburg, H. M., and Baldessarini, R. J. (1973): Regional distribution of histamine in human brain. *Brain Res.,* 52:403–408.

451. Ljungdahl, Å., Hökfelt, T., and Nilsson, G. (1978): Distribution of substance P-like immunoreactivity in the central nervous system of the rat. I. Cell bodies and nerve terminals. *Neuroscience,* 3:861–944.

452. Ljungdahl, Å., Hökfelt, T., Goldstein, M., and Park, D. (1975): Retrograde peroxidase tracing of neurons combined with transmitter histochemistry. *Brain Res.,* 84:313–319.

453. Llorens, C., Malfroy, B., Schwartz, J.-C., Gacel, G., Roques, B. P., Roy, J., Morgat, J. L., Javoy-Agid, F., and Agid, Y. (1982): Enkephalin dipeptidyl carboxypeptidase (enkephalinase) activity: Selective radioassay, properties, and regional distribution in human brain. *J. Neurochem.,* 39:1081–1089.

454. Lloyd, K. G., and Dreksler, S. (1979): An analysis of [³H]gamma-aminobutyric acid (GABA) binding in the human brain. *Brain Res.,* 163:77–87.

455. Lloyd, K. G., Shiemen, L., and Hornykiewicz, O. (1977): Distribution of high affinity sodium-independent [³H]gamma-aminobutyric acid ([³H]GABA) binding in the human brain: Alterations in Parkinson's disease. *Brain Res.,* 127:269–278.

456. Lloyd, K. G., and Hornykiewicz, O. (1977): Effect of chronic neuroleptic or L-DOPA administration on GABA levels in the rat substantia nigra. *Life Sci.,* 21:1489–1496.

457. Lloyd, K. G., Drekeler, S., and Bird, E. D. (1977): Alterations in ³H-GABA binding in Huntington's chorea. *Life Sci.,* 21:747–754.

458. Lloyd, K. G., Davidson, L., and Hornykiewicz, O. (1975): The neurochemistry of Parkinson's disease: Effect of L-DOPA therapy. *J. Pharmacol. Exp. Ther.,* 195:453–464.

459. Lloyd, K. G., Mohler, H., Heitz, P., and Bartholini, G. (1975): Distribution of choline acetyltransferase and glutamate decarboxylase within the substantia nigra and in other brain regions from control and Parkinsonian patients. *J. Neurochem.,* 25:789–795.

460. Lloyd, K. G., and Hornykiewicz, O. (1974): Dopamine and other monoamines in the basal ganglia: Relation to brain dysfunctions. In: *Frontiers in Neurology and Neuroscience Research,* edited by P. Seeman and G. M. Brown, pp. 26–35. University of Toronto Press, Toronto.

461. Lloyd, K. G., and Hornykiewicz, O. (1973): L-Glutamic acid decarboxylase in Parkinson's disease: Effect of L-DOPA therapy. *Nature,* 243:521–523.

462. Lloyd, K. G., Davidson, L., and Hornykiewicz, O. (1973): Metabolism of levodopa in the human brain. *Adv. Neurol.,* 3:173–188.

463. Lloyd, K. G., and Hornykiewicz, O. (1972): Occurrence and distribution of aromatic L-amino acid (L-DOPA) decarboxylase in the human brain. *J. Neurochem.,* 19:1549–1559.

464. Lloyd, K. G., and Hornykiewicz, O. (1970): Parkinson's disease: Activity of L-DOPA decarboxylase in discrete brain regions. *Science,* 170:1212–1213.

465. Lo, M. M. S., Strittmatter, S. M., and Snyder, S. H. (1982): Physical separation and characterization of two types of benzodiazepine receptors. *Proc. Natl. Acad. Sci. U.S.A.,* 79:680–684.

466. Lockridge, O. (1982): Substance P hydrolysis by human serum cholinesterase. *J. Neurochem.,* 39:106–110.

467. Lombardini, J. B. (1978): High-affinity transport of taurine in the mammalian central nervous system. In: *Taurine and Neurological Disorders,* edited by A. Barbeau and R. J. Huxtable, pp. 119–135. Raven Press, New York.

468. Lombardini, J. B. (1976): Regional and subcellular studies on taurine in the rat central nervous system. In: *Taurine,* edited by R. Huxtable and A. Barbeau, pp. 311–326. Raven Press, New York.

469. London, E. D., Yamamura, H. I., Bird, E. D., and Coyle, J. T. (1981): Decreased receptor-binding sites for kainic acid in brains of patients with Huntington's disease. *Biol. Psychiatry,* 16:155–162.

470. London, E. D., and Coyle, J. T. (1979): Specific binding of [³H]kainic acid to receptor sites in rat brain. *Mol. Pharmacol.,* 15:492–506.

471. Lorén, I., Emson, P. C., Fahrenkrug, J., Björklund, A., Alumets, J., Håkanson, R., and Sundler, F. (1979): Distribution of vasoactive intestinal polypeptide in the rat and mouse brain. *Neuroscience,* 4:1953–1976.

472. Lorén, I., Alumets, J., Håkanson, R., and Sundler, F. (1979): Distribution of gastrin and CCK-like peptides in rat brain. *Histochemistry,* 59:249–257.

473. Lorén, I., Alumets, J., Håkanson, R., and Sundler, F. (1979): Immunoreactive pancreatic polypeptide (PP) occurs in the central and peripheral nervous system: Preliminary immunocytochemical observations. *Cell Tissue Res.,* 200:179–186.

474. Lorens, S. A., and Guldberg, H. C. (1974): Regional 5-hydroxytryptamine following selective midbrain raphe lesions in the rat. *Brain Res.,* 78:45–56.

475. Lowe, I. P., Robins, E., and Everman, G. S. (1958): The fluormetric measurement of glutamic decar-

boxylase and its distribution in brain. *J. Neurochem.*, 3:8–18.

476. Lu, E. J., and Brown, W. J. (1977): The developing caudate nucleus in the euthyroid and hypothyroid rat. *J. Comp. Neurol.*, 171:261–284.

477. Luini, A., Goldberg, O., and Teichberg, V. I. (1981): Distinct pharmacological properties of excitatory amino acid receptors in the rat striatum: Study of Na$^+$ efflux assay. *Proc. Natl. Acad. Sci. U.S.A.*, 78:3250–3254.

478. Lynch, G. S., Lucas, P. A., and Deadwyler, S. A. (1972): The demonstration of acetylcholinesterase containing neurons within the caudate nucleus of the rat. *Brain Res.*, 45:617–621.

479. MacLeod, N. K., James, T. A., Kilpatrick, I. C., and Starr, M. S. (1980): Evidence for a GABAergic nigrothalamic pathway in the rat. *Exp. Brain Res.*, 40:55–61.

480. Malfroy, B., Swerts, J. P., Guyon, A., Roques, B. P., and Schwartz, J. C. (1978): High affinity enkephalin-degrading peptidase in brain is increased after morphine. *Nature*, 276:523–526.

481. Manberg, P. J., Younghood, W. W., Nemeroff, C. B., Rossor, M. N., Iversen, L. L., Prange, A. J., Jr., and Kizer, J. S. (1982): Regional distribution of neurotensin in human brain. *J. Neurochem.*, 38:1777–1780.

482. Mann, J. J., Stanley, M., Gershon, S., and Rossor, M. (1980): Mental symptoms in Huntington's disease and a possible primary aminergic neuron lesion. *Science*, 210:1369–1371.

483. Margolis, F. L. (1974): Carnosine in the primary olfactory pathway. *Science*, 184:909–911.

484. Marley, P. D., Emson, P. C., Hunt, S. P., and Fahrenkrug, J. (1981): A long ascending projection in the rat brain containing vasoactive intestinal polypeptide. *Neurosci. Lett.*, 27:261–266.

485. Martin, J. P. (1968): Wilson's disease. In: *Handbook of Clinical Neurology*, Vol. 6, edited by P. J. Vinken and G. W. Bruyn, pp. 279–297. North Holland, Amsterdam.

486. Mason, S. T., and Fibiger, H. C. (1979): Regional topography within the noradrenergic locus coeruleus as revealed by retrograde transport of horseradish peroxidase. *J. Comp. Neurol.*, 187:703–724.

487. McGeer, E. G., McGeer, P. L., and Singh, K. (1978): Kainate-induced degeneration of neostriatal neurons: Dependency upon corticostriatal tract. *Brain Res.*, 139:381–383.

488. McGeer, P. L., McGeer, E. G., Scherer, U., and Singh, K. (1977): A glutamatergic corticostrital path? *Brain Res.*, 128:369–373.

489. McGeer, E. G., and McGeer, P. L. (1976): Duplication of biochemical changes of Huntington's chorea by intrastriatal injections of glutamic and kainic acids. *Nature*, 263:517–518.

490. McGeer, P. L., and McGeer, E. G. (1975): Enzymes associated with the metabolism of catecholamines, acetylcholine and GABA in human controls and patients with Parkinson's disease and Huntington's chorea. *J. Neurochem.*, 26:65–76.

491. McGeer, P. L., McGeer, E. G., Singh, V. K., and Chase, W. H. (1974): Choline acetyltransferase localization in the central nervous system by immunohistochemistry. *Brain Res.*, 81:373–379.

492. McGeer, P. L., McGeer, E. G., and Fibiger, H. C. (1973): Choline acetylase and glutamic acid decarboxylase in Huntington's chorea. *Neurology (Minneap.)*, 23:912–917.

493. McGeer, P. L., McGeer, E. G., Fibiger, H. C., and Wickson, V. (1971): Neostriatal choline acetylase and cholinesterase following selective brain lesions. *Brain Res.*, 35:308–314.

494. Mefford, I., Oke, A., Keller, R., Adams, R. N., and Jonsson, G. (1978): Epinephrine distribution in human brain. *Neurosci. Lett.*, 9:227–231.

495. Mehler, W. R. (1981): The basal ganglia—circa 1982. A review and commentary. *Appl. Neurophysiol.*, 44:261–290.

496. Meibach, R. C., Maayani, S., and Green, J. P. (1980): Characterization and radioautography of [^{3}H]LSD binding by rat brain slices *in vitro:* The effect of 5-hydroxytryptamine. *Eur. J. Pharmacol.*, 67:571–582.

497. Melamed, E., Hefti, F., and Bird, E. D. (1982): Huntington chorea is not associated with hyperactivity of nigrostriatal dopaminergic neurons: Studies in postmortem tissues and in rats with kainic acid lesions. *Neurology, N.Y.*, 32:645–650.

498. Mensah, P. L. (1977): Cell clustering in early and late postnatal mouse striatum. *Neurosci. Abstr.*, 3:42.

499. Mensah, P. L. (1977): The internal organization of the mouse caudate nucleus: Evidence for cell clustering and regional variation. *Brain Res.*, 137:53–66.

500. Mensah, P. L., and Deadwyler, S. (1974): The caudate nucleus of the rat: Cell types and the demonstration of a commissural system. *J. Anat.*, 177:281–293.

501. Mesulam, M.-M. (1978): Tetramethyl benzidine for horseradish peroxidase neurohistochemistry: A non-carcinogenic blue reaction product with superior sensitivity for visualizing neural afferents and efferents. *J. Histochem. Cytochem.*, 26:106–117.

502. Mesulam, M.-M., and Van Hoesen, G. W. (1976): Acetylcholinesterase-rich projections from the basal forebrain of the rhesus monkey to neocortex. *Brain Res.*, 109:152–157.

503. Meunier, J. C. (1982): Mu and kappa opiate binding sites in the rabbit CNS. *Life Sci.*, 31:1327–1330.

504. Meyer, D. K., Beinfeld, M. C., Oertel, W. H., and Brownstein, M. J. (1982): Origin of the cholecystokinin-containing fibers in the rat caudatoputamen. *Science*, 215:187–188.

505. Miller, A. L., and Pitts, F. N., Jr. (1967): Brain succinate semialdehyde dehydrogenase. III. Activities in twenty-four regions of human brain. *J. of Neurochem.*, 14:579–584.

506. Miller, R. J., Chang, K. J., Cooper, B., and Cuatrecasas. P. (1978): Radioimmunoassay and characterization of enkephalins in rat tissues. *J. Biol. Chem.*, 253:531–538.

507. Minamino, N., Kitamura, K., Hayashi, Y., Kangawa, K., and Matsuo, H. (1981): Regional distribution of α-neo-endorphin in rat brain and pituitary. *Biochem. Biophys. Res. Commun.*, 102:226–234.

508. Möhler, H., and Okada, T. (1977): Benzodiazepine

receptor: Demonstration in the central nervous system. *Science*, 198:849–851.

509. Moody, T. W., Pert, C. B., Rivier, J., and Brown, M. R. (1978): Bombesin: Specific binding to rat brain membranes. *Proc. Natl. Acad. Sci. U.S.A.*, 75:5372–5376.

510. Moon Edley, S., Herkenham, M., and Pert, C. B. (1981): Variations in opiate receptor distribution in the mammalian striatum. *Neurosci. Abstr.*, 7:502.

511. Mori, M., Prasad, C., and Wilber, J. F. (1982): Regional dissociation of histidyl-proline diketopiperazine [cyclo-(His–Pro)] and thyrotropin-releasing hormone (TRH) in the rat brain. *Brain Res.*, 231:451–453.

512. Mori, M., Jayaraman, A., Prasad, C., Pegues, J., and Wilber, J. F. (1982): Distribution of histidyl-proline diketopiperazine [cyclo (His–Pro)] and thyrotropin-releasing hormone (TRH) in the primate central nervous system. *Brain Res.*, 245:183–186.

513. Mori, S. (1966): Some observations on the fine structure of the corpus striatum of the rat brain. *Z. Zellforsch. Mikrosk. Anat.*, 70:461–488.

514. Morley, B. J., and Kemp, G. E. (1981): Characterization of a putative nicotinic acetylcholine receptor in mammalian brain. *Brain Res. Rev.*, 3:81–104.

515. Morley, B. J., Lorden, J. F., Brown, G. B., Kemp, G. E., and Bradley, R. J. (1977): Regional distribution of nicotinic acetylcholine receptor in rat brain. *Brain Res.*, 134:161–166.

516. Mroz, E. A., Brownstein, M. J., and Leeman, S. E. (1977): Evidence for substance P in the striato-nigral tract. *Brain Res.*, 125:305–311.

517. Müller, P. B., and Langemann, H. (1982): Distribution of glutamic acid decarboxylase activity in human brain. *J. Neurochem.*, 9:399–401.

518. Murrin, L. C., Coyle, J. T., and Kuhar, M. J. (1980): Striatal opiate receptors: Pre- and postsynaptic localization. *Life Sci.*, 27:1175–1183.

519. Nachlas, M. M., Tsou, K. C., DeSouza, E., Cheng, C. S., and Seligman, A. M. (1957): Cytochemical demonstration of succinic dehydrogenase by the use of a new *P*-nitrophenyl substituted ditetrazole. *J. Histochem. Cytochem.*, 5:420–436.

520. Nagy, J. I., Carter, D. A., and Fibiger, H. C. (1978): Anterior striatal projections to the globus pallidus, entopeduncular nucleus and substantia nigra in the rat: The GABA connection. *Brain Res.*, 158:15–29.

521. Nakanishi, S., Inoue, A., Kita, T., Nakamura, M., Chang, A. C. Y., Cohen, S. N., and Numa, S. (1979): Nucleotide sequence of cloned cDNA for bovine corticotropin-β-lipotropin precursor. *Nature*, 278:423–427.

522. Nakata, Y., Kusaka, Y., Segawa, T., Yajima, H., and Kitagawa, K. (1977): Substance P: Regional distribution and specific binding to synaptic membranes in rabbit central nervous system. *Life Sci.*, 22:259–268.

523. Namba, M. (1957): Cytoarchitektonische Untersuchungen am Striatum. *J. Hirnforsch.*, 3:24–48.

524. Nauta, H. J. W. (1979): Projections of the pallidal complex: An autoradiographic study in the cat. *Neuroscience*, 4:1853–1873.

525. Nauta, W. J. H., and Domesick, V. B. (1978): Crossroads of limbic and striatal circuitry: Hypo-

thalamonigral connections. In: *Limbic Mechanisms*, edited by K. E. Livingston and O. Hornykiewicz, pp. 75–93. Plenum Press, London.

526. Nauta, W. J. H., Smith, G. P., Faull, R. L. M., and Domesick, V. B. (1978): Efferent connections and nigral afferents of the nucleus accumbens septi in the rat. *Neuroscience*, 3:385–401.

527. Nauta, H. J. W., Pritz, M. B., and Lasek, R. J. (1974): Afferents to the rat caudoputamen studied with horseradish peroxidase. An evaluation of a retrograde neuroanatomical research method. *Brain Res.*, 67:219–238.

528. Nauta, W. J. H., and Haymaker, W. (1969): Hypothalamic nuclei and fiber connections. In: *The Hypothalamus*, edited by W. Haymaker, E. Anderson, and W. J. H. Nauta, pp. 136–209. Charles C. Thomas, Springfield, Illinois.

529. Neff, N. H., Garrison, C. K., and Fuentes, J. (1976): Trace amines and the monoamine oxidases. In: *Trace Amines and the Brain*, edited by E. Usdin and M. Sandler, pp. 41–57. Marcel Dekker, New York.

530. Neill, D. B., Peay, L. A., and Gold, M. S. (1978): Identification of a subregion within rat neostriatum for the dopaminergic modulation of lateral hypothalamic self-stimulation. *Brain Res.*, 153:515–528.

531. Neill, D. B., and Herndon, J. G., Jr. (1978): Anatomical specificity within rat striatum for the dopaminergic modulation of DRL responding and activity. *Brain Res.*, 153:529–538.

532. Newman, R., and Winans, S. S. (1980): An experimental study of the ventral striatum of the golden hamster. I. Neuronal connections of the nucleus accumbens. *J. Comp. Neurol.*, 191:167–192.

533. Newman, R., and Winans, S. S. (1980): An experimental study of the ventral striatum of the golden hamster. II. Neuronal connections of the olfactory tubercle. *J. Comp. Neurol.*, 191:193–212.

534. Ng, R. H., and Marshall, F. D. (1978): Regional and subcellular distribution of homocarnosine–carnosine synthetase in the central nervous system of rats. *J. Neurochem.*, 30:187–190.

535. Nicklas, W. J., Duvoisin, R. C., and Berl, S. (1979): Amino acids in rat neostriatum: Alteration by kainic acid lesion. *Brain Res.*, 167:107–117.

536. Ninkovic, M., Hunt, S. P., and Cleave, R. W. (1982): Localization of opiate and histamine H_1-receptors in the primate sensory ganglia and spinal cord. *Brain Res.*, 241:197–206.

537. Ninkovic, M., Hunt, S. P., Emson, P. C., and Iversen, L. L. (1981): The distribution of multiple opiate receptors in bovine brain. *Brain Res.*, 214:163–167.

538. Nitsch, C., Hassler, R., Kim, J.-K., and Paik, K.-S. (1979): Glutamic acid as a possible neurotransmitter of neo- and allocortical projections to the fundus striati. In: *Advances in Neurology*, Vol. 29, edited by L. J. Poirier, T. L. Sourkes, and P. J. Bedard, pp. 37–43. Raven Press, New York.

539. Nobin, A., and Björklund, A. (1973): Topography of the monoamine neuron system in the human brain as revealed in fetuses. *Acta. Physiol. Scand.* [*Suppl.*], 388:1–40.

540. Noda, M., Furutani, Y., Takahashi, H., Toyosato,

M., Hirose, T., Inayama, S., Nakanishi, S., and Numa, S. (1982): Cloning and sequence analysis of cDNA for bovine adrenal preproenkephalin. *Nature*, 295:202–206.

541. Oberg, R. G. E., and Divac, I. (1975): Dissociative effects of selective lesions in the caudate nucleus of cats and rats. *Acta Neurobiol. Exp.*, 35:647–659.

542. Ochi, J., and Shimizu, K. (1978): Occurrence of dopamine-containing neurons in the midbrain raphe nuclei of the rat. *Neurosci. Lett.*, 8:317–320.

543. O'Donohue, T. L., Charlton, C. G., Miller, R. L., Boden, G., and Jacobowitz, D. M. (1981): Identification, characterization, and distribution of secretin immunoreactivity in rat and pig brain. *Proc. Natl. Acad. Sci. U.S.A.*, 78:5221–5224.

544. O'Donohue, T. L., Crowley, W. R., and Jacobowitz, D. M. (1979): Biochemical mapping of the noradrenergic ventral bundle projection sites: Evidence for a noradrenergic–dopaminergic interaction. *Brain Res.*, 172:87–100.

545. O'Donohue, T. L., Miller, R. L., and Jacobowitz, D. M. (1979): Identification, characterization and stereotaxic mapping of intraneuronal α-melanocyte stimulating hormone-like immunoreactive peptides in discrete regions of the rat brain. *Brain Res.*, 176:101–123.

546. Oertel, W., Graybiel, A. M., Mugnaini, E., Elde, R., Schmechel, D., and Kopin, I. (1981): Coexistence of glutamate decarboxylase immunoreactivity and somatostatin-like immunoreactivity in neurons of nucleus reticularis thalami of the cat. *Neurosci. Abstr.*, 7:223.

547. Oertel, W. H., Schmechel, D. E., Brownstein, M. J., Tappaz, M. L., Ransom, D. H., and Kopin, I. J. (1981): Decrease of glutamate decarboxylase (GAD)-immunoreactive nerve terminals in the substantia nigra after kainic acid lesion of the striatum. *J. Histochem. Cytochem.*, 29:977–980.

548. Oka, H. (1980): Organization of the cortico–caudate projections. A horseradish peroxidase study in the cat. *Exp. Brain Res.*, 40:203–208.

549. Okada, Y., Nitsch-Hassler, C., Kim, J. S., Bak, I. J., and Hassler, R. (1971): Role of γ-aminobutyric acid (GABA) in the extrapyramidal motor system. I. Regional distribution of GABA in rabbit, rat, guinea pig and baboon CNS. *Exp. Brain Res.*, 13:514–518.

550. Okamura, T., Clemens, D. L., and Inagami, T. (1981): Renin, angiotensins, and angiotensin-converting enzyme in neuroblastoma cells: Evidence for intracellular formation of angiotensins. *Proc. Natl. Acad. Sci. U.S.A.*, 78:6940–6943.

551. Olivier, A., Parent, A., Simard, H., and Poirier, L. J. (1970): Cholinesterasic striatopallidal and striatonigral efferents in the cat and monkey. *Brain Res.*, 18:273–282.

552. Olsen, R. W., Van Ness, P. C., and Tourtellotte, W. W. (1979): Gamma-aminobutyric acid receptor binding curves for human brain regions: Comparison of Huntington's disease and normal. In: *Advances in Neurology*, Vol. 23, edited by T. N. Chase, N. S. Wexler, and A. Barbeau, pp. 697–704. Raven Press, New York.

553. Olson, L., Boréus, L. O., and Seiger, Å. (1973): Histochemical demonstration and mapping of 5-hydroxytryptamine- and catecholamine-containing neuron systems in the human fetal brain. *Z. Anat. Entwickl. Gesch.*, 139:259–282.

554. Olson, L., Seiger, Å., and Fuxe, K. (1972): Heterogeneity of striatal and limbic dopamine innervation: Highly fluorescent islands in developing and adult rats. *Brain Res.*, 44:283–288.

555. Ord, M. G., and Thompson, R. H. S. (1951): Pseudocholinesterase activity in the central nervous system. *Biochem. J.*, 51:245–251.

556. Palacios, J. M., Niehoff, D. L., and Kuhar, M. (1981): [^{3}H]Spiperone binding sites in brain: Autoradiographic localization of multiple receptors. *Brain Res.*, 213:277–289.

557. Palacios, J. M., Wamsley, J. K., and Kuhar, M. J. (1981): High affinity GABA receptors—autoradiographic localization. *Brain Res.*, 222:285–307.

558. Palacios, J. M., Wamsley, J. K., and Kuhar, M. J. (1981): The distribution of histamine H_1-receptors in the rat brain: An autoradiographic study. *Neuroscience*, 6:15–37.

559. Palacios, J. M., and Kuhar, M. J. (1980): Beta-adrenergic-receptor localization by light microscopic autoradiography. *Science*, 208:1378–1380.

560. Palacios, J. M., Schwartz, J.-C., and Garbarg, M. (1978): High affinity binding of ^{3}H-histamine in rat brain. *Eur. J. Pharmacol.*, 50:443–444.

561. Palkovits, M., and Jacobowitz, D. M. (1974): Topographic atlas of catecholamine and acetylcholinesterase-containing neurons in the rat brain. II. Hindbrain (mesencephalon, rhombencephalon). *J. Comp. Neurol.*, 157:29–42.

562. Palkovits, M., Mroz, E. A., Brownstein, M. J., and Leeman, S. E. (1978): Descending substance P-containing pathway: A component of the ansa lenticularis. *Brain Res.*, 156:124–128.

563. Panula, P., Wu, J. Y., and Emson, P. (1981): Ultrastructure of GABA-neurons in cultures of rat neostriatum. *Brain Res.*, 219:202–207.

564. Papez, J. W. (1929): *Comparative Neurology*. Thomas Y. Crowell, New York.

565. Parent, A., and O'Reilly-Fromentin, J. (1982): Distribution and morphological characteristics of acetylcholinesterase-containing neurons in the basal forebrain of the cat. *Brain Res. Bull.*, 8:183–196.

566. Parent, A., Boucher, R., and O'Reilly-Fromentin, J. (1981): Acetylcholinesterase-containing neurons in cat pallidal complex: Morphological characteristics and projection towards the neocortex. *Brain Res.*, 230:356–361.

567. Parent, A., O'Reilly-Fromentin, J., and Boucher, R. (1980): Acetylcholinesterase-containing neurons in cat neostriatum: A morphological and quantitative analysis. *Neurosci. Lett.*, 20:271–276.

568. Parent, A., Poirier, L. J., Boucher, R., and Butcher, L. L. (1977): Morphological characteristics of acetylcholinesterase-containing neurons in the CNS of DFP-treated monkeys. 2. Diencephalic and medial telencephalic structures. *J. Neurol. Sci.*, 32:9–28.

569. Parhad, I. M., Clark, A. W., Folstein, S., Whitehouse, P. J., Hedreen, J. C., Price, D. L., and Chase, G. A. (1982): The nucleus basalis in Huntington disease. *Neurology (N.Y.)*, 32:A168.

570. Park, D. H., Ross, M. E., Baker, H., Reis, D. J., and Joh, T. H. (1981): Production and characterization of antibodies to choline acetyltransferase of rat striata for immunochemistry and immunocytochemistry. *Neurosci. Abstr.,* 7:493.

571. Park, M. R., Gonzales-Vegas, J. A., and Kitai, S. T. (1982): Serontonergic excitation from dorsal raphe stimulation recorded intracellularly from rat caudate–putamen. *Brain Res.,* 243:49–58.

572. Pasik, P., Pasik, T., and Saavedra, J. (1982): Immunocytochemical localization of serotonin at the ultrastructural level. *J. Histochem. Cytochem.,* 30:760–764.

573. Pasik, P., Pasik, T., Saavedra, P. J., and Holstein, G. R. (1981): Light and electron microscopic immunocytochemical localization of serotonin in the basal ganglia of cats and monkeys. *Anat. Rec.,* 199:194A.

574. Pasik, P., Pasik, T., and DiFiglia, M. (1979): The internal organization of the neostriatum in mammals. In: *The Neostriatum,* edited by I. Divac and R. G. E. Oberg, pp. 5–36. Pergammon Press, New York.

575. Paxinos, G., Emson, P. C., and Cuello, A. C. (1978): Substance P projections to the entopeduncular nuclcus, the medial preoptic area and the lateral septum. *Neurosci. Lett.,* 7:133–136.

576. Pearse, A. G. E. (1967): Fundamentals of functional neurochemistry. *Brain Res.,* 4:125–134.

577. Pelletier, G., and LeClerc, R. (1979): Immunohistochemical localization of adrenocorticotropin in the rat brain. *Endocrinology,* 104:1426–1433.

578. Penny, G.R., and Itoh, K. (1981): Overlap between the distribution of thalamostriatal neurons and reticulothalamic projections in the intralaminar nuclei of the cat. *Anat. Rec.,* 199:199A.

579. Perez de la Mora, M., Possani, L. D., Tapia, R., Teran, L., Palacios, R., Fuxe, K., Hökfelt, T., and Ljungdahl, Å. (1981): Demonstration of central γ-aminobutyrate-containing nerve terminals by means of antibodies against glutamate decarboxylase. *Neuroscience,* 6:875–895.

580. Peroutka, S. J. and Snyder, S. H. (1981): Two distinct serotonin receptors: Regional variations in receptor binding in mammalian brain. *Brain Res.,* 208:339–347.

581. Perry, E. K., Perry, R. H., and Tomlinson, B. E. (1982): The influence of agonal status on some neurochemical activities of postmortem human brain tissue. *Neurosci. Lett.,* 29:303–307.

582. Perry, E. K., Perry, R. H., Tomlinson, B. E., Blessed, G., and Gibson, P. H. (1980): Coenzyme A-acetylating enzymes in Alzheimer's disease: Possible cholinergic "compartment" of pyruvate dehydrogenase. *Neurosci. Lett.,* 18:105–110.

583. Perry, E. K., Gibson, P. H., Blessed, G., Perry, R. H., and Tomlinson, B. (1977): Neurotransmitter enzyme abnormalities in senile dementia. *J. Neurol. Sci.,* 34:247–265.

584. Perry, T. L. (1978): Taurine in dominantly inherited cerebellar atrophies and other human neurological disorders. In: *Taurine and Neurological Disorders,* edited by A. Barbeau and R.J. Huxtable, pp. 441–451. Raven Press, New York.

585. Perry, T. L. (1976): Hereditary mental depression with taurine deficiency: Further studies, including a therapeutic trial of taurine administration. In: *Taurine,* edited by R. Huxtable and A. Barbeau, pp. 365–374. Raven Press, New York.

586. Perry, T. L. (1982): Normal cerebrospinal fluid and brain glutamate levels in schizophrenia do not support the hypothesis of glutamatergic neuronal dysfunction. *Neurosci. Lett.,* 28:81–85.

587. Perry, T. L., Hansen, S., and Kloster, M. (1973): Huntington's chorea: Deficiency of γ-aminobutyric acid in brain. *N. Engl. J. Med.,* 288:337–342.

588. Perry, T. L., Sanders, H. D., Hansen, S., Lesk, D., Kloster, M., and Gravlin, L. (1972): Free amino acids and related compounds in five regions of biopsied cat brain. *J. Neurochem.,* 19:2651–2656.

589. Perry, T. L., Berry, K., Hansen, S., Diamond, S., and Mok, C. (1971): Regional distribution of amino acids in human brain obtained at autopsy. *J. Neurochem.,* 18:513–519.

590. Perry, T. L., Kish, S. J., Sjaastad, O., Gjessing, L. R., Nesbakken, R., Schrader, H., and Loken, A. C. (1979): Homocarnosinosis: Increased content of homocarnosine and deficiency of homocarnosinase in brain. *J. Neurochem.,* 32:1637–1640.

591. Pert, A., Moody, T. W., Pert, C. B., DeWald, L. A., and Rivier, J. (1980): Bombesin: Receptor distribution in brain and effects on nociception and locomotor activity. *Brain Res.,* 193:209–220.

592. Pert, C. B., Kuhar, M. J., and Snyder, S. H. (1976): Opiate receptors: Autoradiographic localization in rat brain. *Proc. Natl. Acad. Sci. U.S.A.,* 73:3729–3733.

593. Peters, D. A. V., McGeer, P. L., and McGeer, F. G. (1968): The distribution of tryptophan hydroxylase in cat brain. *J. Neurochem.,* 15:1431–1435.

594. Pfaff, D., and Keiner, M. (1973): Atlas of estradiol-concentrating cells in the central nervous system of the female rat. *J. Comp. Neurol.,* 151:121–158.

595. Philips, S. R. (1978): β-Phenylethylamine: A metabolically and pharmacologically active amine. In: *Noncatecholic Phenylethylamines,* edited by A. D. Mosnaim and M. E. Wolf, pp. 113–138. Marcel Dekker, New York.

596. Philips, S. R., Rozdilsky, B., and Boulton, A. A. (1978): Evidence for the presence of *m*-tyramine, *p*-tyramine, tryptamine, and phenylethylamine in the rat brain and several areas of the human brain. *Biol. Psychiatry,* 13:51–57.

597. Philips, S. R., Durden, D. A., and Boulton, A. A. (1974): Identification and distribution of tryptamine in the rat. *Can. J. Biochem.,* 52:447–451.

598. Phillipson, O. T. (1979): A Golgi study of the ventral tegmental area of Tsai and interfasicular nucleus in the rat. *J. Comp. Neurol.,* 187:99–116.

599. Phillipson, O. T. (1979): The cytoarchitecture of the interfascicular nucleus and ventral tegmental area of Tsai in the rat. *J. Comp. Neurol.,* 187:85–98.

600. Pickel, V. M., Beckley, S. C., Joh, T. H., and Reis, D. J. (1981): Ultrastructural immunocytochemical localization of tyrosine hydroxylase in the neostriatum. *Brain Res.,* 225:373–385.

601. Pickel, V. M., Sumal, K. K., Beckley, S. C., Miller,

R. J., and Reis, D. J. (1980): Immunocytochemical localization of enkephalin in the neostriatum of rat brain: A light and electron microscopic study. *J. Comp. Neurol.*, 189:721–740.

602. Pickel, V. M., Joh, T. H., and Reis, D. J. (1977): Regional and ultrastructural localization of tyrosine hydroxylase by immunocytochemistry in dopaminergic neurons of the mesolimbic and nigroneostriatal systems. In: *Advances in Biochemical Psychopharmacology*, Vol. 16, edited by E. Costa and G. L. Gessa, pp. 321–325. Raven Press, New York.

603. Poirier, L. J., Parent, A., Marchand, R., and Butcher, L. L. (1977): Morphological characteristics of the acetylcholinesterase-containing neurons in the CNS of DFP-treated monkeys. 2. Extrapyramidal and related structures. *J. Neurol. Sci.*, 31:181–198.

604. Poitras, D., and Parent, A. (1978): Atlas of the distribution of monoamine-containing nerve cell bodies in the brain stem of the cat. *J. Comp. Neurol.*, 179:699–718.

605. Poth, M. M., Heath, R. G., and Ward, M. (1975): Angiotensin-covering enzyme in human brain. *J. Neurochem.*, 25:83–85.

606. Precht, W., and Yoshida, M. (1971): Blockage of caudate-evoked inhibition of neurons in the substantia nigra by picrotoxin. *Brain Res.*, 32:229–233.

607. Prémont, J., Perez, M., Blanc, G., Tassin, J.-P., Thierry, A. M., Hervé, D., and Bockaert, J. (1979): Adenosine-sensitive adenylate cyclase in rat brain homogenates. Kinetic characteristics, specificity, topographical, subcellular and cellular distribution. *Mol. Pharmacol.*, 16:790–804.

608. Preston, R. J., Bishop, G. A., and Kitai, S. T. (1980): Medium spiny neuron projection from the rat striatum: An intracellular horseradish peroxidase study. *Brain Res.*, 183:253–263.

609. Priestly, J. V., Somogyi, P., and Cuello, A. C. (1981): Neurotransmitter-specific projection neurons revealed by combining PAP immunohistochemistry with retrograde transport of HRP. *Brain Res.*, 239:231–240.

610. Quik, M., and Iversen, L. L. (1979): Regional study of ^{3}H-spiperone binding and the dopamine-sensitive adenylate cyclase in rat brain. *Eur. J. Pharmacol.*, 56:323–330.

611. Quirion, R., Herkenham, M., and Pert, C. B. (1981): Characterization and visualization of the "κ" opiate receptor in rat brain. *Neurosci. Abstr.*, 7:434.

612. Quirion, R., Hammer, R. P., Jr., Herkenham, M., and Pert, C. B. (1981): Phencyclidine (angel dust)/σ "opiate" receptor: Visualization by tritium-sensitive film. *Proc. Natl. Acad. Sci. U.S.A.*, 78:5881–5885.

613. Raff, M. C., Fields, K. L., Hakomori, S., Mirsky, R., Pruss, R. M., and Winter, J. (1979): Cell-type-specific markers for distinguishing and studying neurons and the major classes of glial cells in culture. *Brain Res.*, 174:283–308.

614. Rafols, J. A., and Fox, C. A. (1979): Fine structure of the primate striatum. *Appl. Neurophysiol.*, 42:13–16.

615. Ragsdale, C. W., and Graybiel, A. M. (1981): The fronto-striatal projection in the cat and monkey and its relationship to inhomogeneities established by acetylcholinesterase histochemistry. *Brain Res.*, 208:259–266.

616. Ragsdale, C. W., and Graybiel, A. M. (1979): Striosomal organization of the caudate nucleus. III. Distribution of afferents from the frontal cortex of the cat. *Neurosci. Abstr.*, 4:78.

617. Ragsdale, C. W., and Graybiel, A. M. (1979): Acetylcholinesterase staining in the striatum of the fetal and neonatal cat. *Neurosci. Lett. [Suppl.]*, 3:S26.

618. Rea, M. S., and Simon, J. R. (1981): Regional distribution of cholinergic parameters within the rat striatum. *Brain Res.*, 219:317–326.

619. Reinoso-Suarez, F., Llamas, A., and Avendaño, C. (1982): Pallido–cortical projections in the cat studied by means of the horseradish peroxidase retrograde transport technique. *Neurosci. Lett.*, 29:255–229.

620. Reisine, T. D., Wastek, G. J., Speth, R. C., Bird, E. D., and Yamamura, H. I. (1979): Alterations in the benzodiazepine receptor of Huntington's diseased human brain. *Brain Res.*, 165:183–187.

621. Reisine, T. D., Fields, J. Z., Bird, E. D., Spokes, E., and Yamamura, H. I. (1978): Characterization of brain dopaminergic receptors in Huntington's disease. *Commun. Psychopharmacol.*, 2:79–84.

622. Reisine, T. D., Fields, J. Z., Yamamura, H. I., Bird, E. D., Spokes, E., Schreiner, P. S., and Enna, S. J. (1977): Neurotransmitter receptor alterations in Parkinson's disease. *Life Sci.*, 21:335–344.

623. Reisine, T. D., Fields, J. Z., Stern, L. Z., Johnson, P. C., Bird, E. D., and Yamamura, H. I. (1977): Alterations in dopaminergic receptors in Huntington's disease. *Life Sci.*, 21:1123–1128.

624. Reisine, T. D., Overstreet, D., Gale, K., Rossor, M., Iversen, L., and Yamamura, H. (1980): Benzodiazepine receptors: The effect of GABA on their characteristics in human brain and their alteration in Huntington's disease. *Brain Res.*, 199:79–88.

625. Reubi, J. C., Toggenburger, G., and Cuénod, M. (1980): Asparagine as precursor for transmitter aspartate in corticostriatal fibers. *J. Neurochem.*, 35:1015–1017.

626. Reubi, J. C., and Cuénod, M. (1979): Glutamate release *in vitro* from corticostriatal terminals. *Brain Res.*, 176:185–188.

627. Ribak, C. E., and Kramer, W. G. III (1982): Cholinergic neurons in the basal forebrain of the cat have direct projections to the sensorimotor cortex. *Exp. Neurol.*, 75:453–465.

628. Ribak, C. E., Vaughn, J. E., and Roberts, E. (1980): GABAergic nerve terminals decrease in the substantia nigra following hemitransections of the striatonigral and pallidonigral pathways. *Brain Res.*, 192:413–420.

629. Ribak, C. E., Vaughn, J. E., and Roberts, E. (1979): The GABA neurons and their axon terminals in rat corpus striatum as demonstrated by GAD immunocytochemistry. *J. Comp. Neurol.*, 187:281–284.

630. Ricardo, J. A. (1981): Efferent connections of the subthalamic region in the rat. II. The zona incerta. *Brain Res.*, 214:43–60.

631. Ricardo, J. A., and Koh, E. T. (1978): Anatomical evidence of direct projections from the nucleus of the solitary tract to the hypothalamus, amygdala, and other forebrain structures in the rat. *Brain Res.,* 153:1–26.

632. Richards, C. D., and Taylor, D. C. M. (1982): Electrophysiological evidence for a somatotopic sensory projection to the striatum of the rat. *Neurosci. Lett.,* 30:235–240.

633. Rix, E., Ganten, D., Schull, R., Unger, T., and Taugner, R. (1981): Converting-enzyme in the choroid plexus, brain, and kidney: Immunocytochemical and biochemical studies in rats. *Neurosci. Lett.,* 22:125–130.

634. Roberts, G. W., Woodhams, P. L., Polak, J. M., and Crow, T. J. (1982): Distribution of neuropeptides in the limbic system of the rat: The amygdaloid complex. *Neuroscience,* 7:99–131.

635. Ross, R. A., and Reis, D. J. (1974): Effects of lesions of locus coeruleus on regional distribution of dopamine-β-hydroxylase activity in rat brain. *Brain Res.,* 73:161–166.

636. Rossier, J. (1981): Serum monospecificity: A prerequisite for reliable immunohistochemical localization of neuronal markers including choline acetyltransferase. *Neuroscience,* 6:989–991.

637. Rossier, J., Audigier, Y., Ling, N., Cros, J., and Udenfriend, S. (1980): Met-enkephalin-Arg[6]-Phe[7], present in high amounts in brain of rat, cattle and man, is an opioid agonist. *Nature,* 288:88–90.

638. Rossier, J. (1975): Immunohistochemical localization of choline acetyltransferase: Real or artefact? *Brain Res.,* 98:619–622.

639. Rossier, J., Vargo, T. M., Minick, S., Ling, N., Bloom, F. E., and Guillemin, R. (1977): Regional dissociation of β-endorphin and enkephalin contents in rat brain and pituitary. *Proc. Natl. Acad. Sci. U.S.A.,* 74:5162–5165.

640. Rossor, M. N., Garrett, N. J., Johnson, A. L., Mountjoy, C. Q., Roth, M., and Iversen, L. L. (1982): A post-mortem study of the cholinergic and GABA systems in senile dementia. *Brain,* 105:313–350.

641. Rossor, M. N., Svendsen, C., Hunt, S. P., Mountjoy, C. Q., Roth, M., and Iversen, L. L. (1982): The substantia innominata in Alzheimer's disease: An histochemical and biochemical study of cholinergic marker enzymes. *Neurosci. Lett.,* 28:217–222.

642. Rossor, M. N., Iversen, L. L., Hawthorn, J., Ang, V. T. Y., and Jenkins, S. (1981): Extrahypothalamic vasopressin in human brain. *Brain Res.,* 214:349–355.

643. Roth, R. H., Doherty, J. D., and Walters, J. R. (1980): Gamma-hydroxybutyrate: A role in the regulation of central dopaminergic neurons? *Brain Res.,* 189:556–560.

644. Rotter, A., Birdsall, N. J. M., Burgen, A. S. V., Field, P.M., Hulme, E. C., and Raisman, G. (1979): Muscarinic receptors in the central nervous system of the rat. I. Technique for autoradiographic localization of the binding of [3H]propylbenzilylcholine mustard and its distribution in the forebrain. *Brain Res., Rev.,* 1:141–165.

645. Rotter, A., Field, P. M., and Raisman, G. (1979): Muscarinic receptors in the central nervous system

of the rat. III. Postnatal development of binding of [3H]propylbenzilylcholine mustard. *Brain Res. Rev.,* 1:185–205.

646. Rowlands, G. J., and Roberts, P. J. (1980): Specific calcium-dependent release of endogenous glutamate from rat striatum is reduced by destruction of the cortico–striatal tract. *Exp. Brain Res.,* 39:239–240.

647. Royce, G. J. (1982): Laminar origin of cortical neurons which project upon the caudate nucleus: A horseradish peroxidase investigation in the cat. *J. Comp. Neurol.,* 205:8–29.

648. Royce, G. J. (1978): Cells of origin of subcortical afferents to the caudate nucleus: A horseradish peroxidase study in the cat. *Brain Res.,* 153:465–475.

649. Royce, G. J. (1978): Autoradiographic evidence for a discontinuous projection to the caudate nucleus from the centromedian nucleus in the cat. *Brain Res.,* 146:145–150.

650. Ruberg, M., Ploska, A., Javoy-Agid, F., and Agid, V. (1982): Muscarinic binding and choline acetyltransferase activity in Parkinsonian subjects with reference to dementia. *Brain Res.,* 232:129–139.

651. Rumigny, J. F., Maitre, M., Cash, C., and Mandel, P. (1981): Regional and subcellular localization in rat brain of the enzymes that can synthesize γ-hydroxybutyric acid. *J. Neurochem.,* 36:1433–1438.

652. Saavedra, J. M., Palkovits, M., Brownstein, M. J., and Axelrod, J. (1974): Localization of phenylethanolamine N-methyl transferase in the rat brain nuclei. *Nature,* 248:695–696.

653. Saavedra, J. M., Fernandez-Pardal, J., and Chevillard, C. (1982): Angiotensin-converting enzyme in discrete areas of the rat forebrain and pituitary gland. *Brain Res.,* 245:317–325.

654. Saavedra, J. M. (1976): 5-Hydroxy-*l*-tryptophan decarboxylase activity: Microassay and distribution in discrete rat brain nuclei. *J. Neurochem.,* 26.585–589.

655. Saavedra, J. M., and Zivin, J. (1976): Tyrosine hydroxylase and dopamine-β-hydroxylase: Distribution in discrete areas of the rat limbic system. *Brain Res.,* 105:517–524.

656. Saavedra, J. M., Brownstein, M. J., and Palkovits, M. (1976): Distribution of catechol-O-methyltransferase, histamine N-methyltransferase and monoamine oxidase in specific areas of the rat brain. *Brain Res.,* 118:152–156.

657. Saavedra, J. M., Brownstein, M., and Axelrod, J. (1973): A specific and sensitive enzymatic–isotopic microassay for serotonin in tissues. *J. Pharmacol. Exp. Ther.,* 186:508–515.

658. Saavedra, J. M., and Axelrod, J. (1973): Demonstration and distribution of phenylethanolamine in brain and other tissues. *Proc. Natl. Acad. Sci. U.S.A.,* 70:769–772.

659. Saelens, J. K., Edwards-Neale, S., and Simke, J. P. (1979): Further evidence for cholinergic thalamo-striatal neurons. *J. Neurochem.,* 32:1093–1094.

660. Saito, A., Sankaran, H., Goldfine, I. D., and Williams, J. A. (1980): Cholecystokinin receptors in the brain: Characterization and distribution. *Science,* 208:1155–1156.

661. Saito, M., Hirano, M., Uchimura, H., Nakahara, T., and Ito, M. (1977): Tyrosine hydroxylase activ-

ity in the catecholamine nerve terminals and cell bodies of the rat brain. *J. Neurochem.*, 29:161–165.

662. Salvador, R. A., and Albers, R. W. (1958): The distribution of glutamic-γ-aminobutyric transaminase in the nervous system of the rhesus monkey. *J. Biol. Chem.*, 234:922–925.

663. Salvaterra, P. M., and Foders, R. M. (1979): [125I]α-Bungarotoxin and [3H]quinuclidinylbenzilate binding in central nervous systems of different species. *J. Neurochem.*, 32:1509–1517.

664. Salvaterra, P. M., and Mahlers, H. R. (1976): Nicotinic acetylcholine receptor from rat brain. *J. Biol. Chem.*, 251:6327–6334.

665. Sar, M., Stumpf, W. E., Miller, R. J., Chang, K. J., and Cuatrecasas, P. (1978): Immunohistochemical localization of enkephalin in rat brain and spinal cord. *J. Comp. Neurol.*, 182:17–38.

666. Sato, M., Itoh, K., and Mizuno, N. (1979): Distribution of thalamocaudate neurons in the cat as demonstrated by horseradish peroxidase. *Exp. Brain Res.*, 34:143–153.

667. Scally, M. C., Ulus, I. H., Wurtman, R. J., and Pettibone, D. J. (1978): Regional distribution of neurotransmitter-synthesizing enzymes and substance P within the rat corpus striatum. *Brain Res.*, 143:556–560.

668. Schoemaker, H., Morelli, M., Deshmukh, P., and Yamamura, H. I. (1982): [3H]Ro5-4864 benzodiazepine binding in the kainate lesioned striatum and Huntington's diseased basal ganglia. *Brain Res.*, 248:396–401.

669. Schwab, M., Agid, Y., Glowinski, J., and Thoenen, H. (1977): Retrograde axonal transport of 125I-tetanus toxin as a tool for tracing fiber connections in the central nervous system: Connections of the rostral part of the rat neostriatum. *Brain Res.*, 126:211–224.

670. Schwartz, J.-C., Lampart, C., and Rose, C. (1970): Properties and regional distribution of histidine decarboxylase in rat brain. *J. Neurochem.*, 17:1527–1534.

671. Schwartz, R. D., McGee, R., Jr., and Kellar, K. J. (1982): Nicotinic cholinergic receptors labeled by [3H]acetylcholine in rat brain. *Mol. Pharmacol.*, 22:56–62.

672. Segal, M., Dudai, Y., and Amsterdam, A. (1978): Distribution of an α-bungarotoxin-binding cholinergic nicotinic receptor in rat brain. *Brain Res.*, 148:105–119.

673. Selmanoff, M. K., Wise, P. M., and Barraclough, C. A. (1980): Regional distribution of luteinizing hormone-releasing hormone (LH-RH) in rat brain determined by microdissection and radioimmunoassay. *Brain Res.*, 192:421–432.

674. Shank, R. P., and Aprison, M. H. (1970): The metabolism *in vivo* of glycine and serine in eight areas of the rat central nervous system. *J. Neurochem.*, 17:1461–1475.

675. Sheridan, J. J., Sims, K. L., and Pitts, F. N., Jr. (1967): Brain γ-aminobutyrate-α-oxoglutarate transaminase. II. Activities in twenty-four regions of human brain. *J. Neurochem.*, 14:571–578.

676. Shute, C. C. D., and Lewis, P. R. (1967): The as-

cending cholinergic reticular system: Neocortical, olfactory and subcortical projections. *Brain*, 90:497–521.

677. Shute, C. C. D., and Lewis, P. R. (1963): Cholinesterase-containing systems of the brain of the rat. *Nature*, 199:1160–1164.

678. Silver, A. (1974): *The Biology of Cholinesterases.* Elsevier, Amsterdam.

679. Simantov, R., and Snyder, S. H. (1976): Morphine-like peptides in mammalian brain: Isolation, structure elucidation, and interactions with the opiate receptor. *Proc. Natl. Acad. Sci. U.S.A.*, 73:2515–2519.

680. Simantov, R., Kuhar, M. J., Pasternak, G. W., and Snyder, S. H. (1976): The regional distribution of a morphine-like factor enkephalin in monkey brain. *Brain Res.*, 106:189–197.

681. Simantov, R., Kuhar, M. J., Uhl, G. R., and Snyder, S. H. (1977): Opioid peptide enkephalin: Immunohistochemical mapping in rat central nervous system. *Proc. Natl. Acad. Sci. U.S.A.*, 74:2167–2171.

682. Simke, J. P., and Saelens, J. K. (1977): Evidence for a cholinergic fiber tract connecting the thalamus with the head of the striatum of the rat. *Brain Res.*, 126:487–495.

683. Simon, J. R., Contrera, J. F., and Kuhar, M. J. (1976): Binding of [3H]kainic acid, an analogue of L-glutamate, to brain membranes. *J. Neurochem.*, 26:141–147.

684. Sims, K. B., Hoffman, D. L., Said, S., and Zimmerman, E. A. (1980): Vasoactive intestinal polypeptide (VIP) in mouse and rat brain: An immunocytochemical study. *Brain Res.*, 186:165–183.

685. Sims, K. L., Weitsen, H. A., and Bloom, F. E. (1971): Histochemical localization of brain succinic semialdehyde dehydrogenase—a γ-aminobutyric acid degradative enzyme. *J. Histochem. Cytochem.*, 19:408–415.

686. Singh, E. A., and McGeer, E. G. (1978): Angiotensin converting enzyme in kainic acid-injected striata. *Ann. Neurol.*, 4:85–86.

687. Sirett, N. E., Bray, J. J., and Hubbard, J. I. (1981): Localization of immunoreactive angiotensin in the hippocampus and striatum of the brain. *Brain Res.*, 217:405–411.

688. Sirett, N. E., McLean, A. S., Bray, J. J., and Hubbard, J. I. (1977): Distribution of angiotensin II receptors in rat brain. *Brain Res.*, 122:299–312.

689. Skirboll, L. R., Grace, A. A., Hommer, D. W., Rehfeld, J., Goldstein, M., Hökfelt, T., and Bunney, B. S. (1981): Peptide–monoamine coexistence: Studies of the actions of cholecystokinin-like peptide on the electrical activity of midbrain dopamine neurons. *Neuroscience*, 6:2111–2124.

690. Slater, E. E., Defendini, R., and Zimmerman, E. A. (1980): Wide distribution of immunoreactive renin in nerve cells of human brain. *Proc. Natl. Acad. Sci. U.S.A.*, 77:5458–5460.

691. Snodgrass, S. R. (1979): *In vitro* binding studies with 3H-N-methyl aspartate. *Neurosci. Abstr.*, 5:572.

692. Snodgrass, S. R. (1978): Use of 3H-muscimol for GABA receptor studies. *Nature*, 273:392–394.

693. Snodgrass, S. R., and Horn, A. S. (1973): An assay procedure for tryptamine in brain and spinal cord using its [³H]dansyl derivative. *J. Neurochem.*, 21:687–696.

694. Snyder, S. H., and Coyle, J. T. (1969): Regional differences in ³H-norepinephrine and ³H-dopamine uptake into rat brain homogenates. *J. Pharmacol. Exp. Ther.*, 165:78–86.

695. Somogyi, P., Bolam, J. P., and Smith, A. D. (1981): Monosynaptic cortical input and local axon collaterals of identified striatonigral neurons. A light and electron microscopic study using the Golgi–peroxidase transport–degeneration procedure. *J. Comp. Neurol.*, 195:567–584.

696. Somogyi, P., Hodgson, A. J., and Smith, A. D. (1979): An approach to tracing neuron networks in the cerebral cortex and basal ganglia. Combination of Golgi staining, retrograde transport of horseradish peroxidase and anterograde degeneration of synaptic boutons in the same material. *Neuroscience*, 4:1805–1852.

697. Somogyi, P., and Smith, A. D. (1979): Projection of neostriatal spiny neurons to the substantia nigra. Application of a combined Golgi-staining and horseradish peroxidase transport procedure at both light and electron microscopic levels. *Brain Res.*, 178:3–15.

698. Sorbi, S., Bird, E. D., and Blass, J. P. (1981): Low activity of the pyruvate dehydrogenase complex as well as of choline acetyltransferase in Huntington caudate and putamen. *Neurosci. Abstr.*, 7:494.

699. Sorimachi, M., and Kataoka, K. (1974): Choline uptake by nerve terminals: A sensitive and a specific marker of cholinergic innervation. *Brain Res.*, 72:350–353.

700. Spears, R. M., and Martin, D. L. (1982): Resolution and brain regional distribution of cysteine sulfinate decarboxylase isoenzymes from hog brain. *J. Neurochem.*, 38:985–991.

701. Specht, L. A., Pickel, V. M., Joh, T. H., and Reis, D. J. (1981): Light-microscopic immunocytochemical localization of tyrosine hydroxylase in prenatal rat brain. II. Late ontogeny. *J. Comp. Neurol.*, 199:255–276.

702. Speciale, S. G., Crowley, W. R., O'Donohue, T. L., and Jacobowitz, D. M. (1978): Forebrain catecholamine projections of the A5 cell group. *Brain Res.*, 154:128–133.

703. Spencer, H. J. (1976): Antagonism of cortical excitation of striatal neurons by glutamic acid diethyl ester: Evidence for glutamic acid as an excitatory transmitter in the rat striatum. *Brain Res.*, 102:91–101.

704. Sperk, G., Hörtnagl, H., Reuther, H., and Hornykiewicz, O. (1981): Changes in histamine in the rat striatum following local injection of kainic acid. *Neuroscience*, 7:2669–2675.

705. Speth, R. C., Wastek, G. J., Johnson, P. C., and Yamamura, H. I. (1978): Benzodiazepine binding in human brain: Characterization using [³H]flunitrazepam. *Life Sci.*, 22:859–866.

706. Speth, R. C., Chen, F. M., Lindstrom, J. M., Kobayashi, M., and Yamamura, H. I. (1977): Nicotinic cholinergic receptors in rat brain identified by

[¹²⁵I] *Naja naja siamensis* α-toxin binding. *Brain Res.*, 131:350–355.

707. Spindel, E. R., Wurtman, R. J., and Bird, E. D. (1980): Increased TRH content of the basal ganglia in Huntington's disease. *N. Engl. J. Med.*, 303:1235–1236.

708. Spokes, E. G. S., Garrett, N. J., Rossor, M. N., and Iversen, L. L. (1980): Distribution of GABA in post-mortem brain tissue from control, psychotic and Huntington's chorea subjects. *J. Neurol. Sci.*, 48:303–313.

709. Spokes, E. G. S. (1980): Neurochemical alterations in Huntington's chorea. A study of post-mortem brain tissue. *Brain*, 103:179–210.

710. Spokes, E. G. S., Garrett, N. J., and Iversen, L. L. (1979): Differential effects of agonal status on measurements of GABA and glutamate decarboxylase in human post-mortem brain tissue from control and Huntington's chorea subjects. *J. Neurochem.*, 33:773–778.

711. Srikant, C. B., and Patel, Y. C. (1981): Somatostatin receptors: Identification and characterization in rat brain membranes. *Proc. Natl. Acad. Sci. U.S.A.*, 78:3930–3934.

712. Stahl, W. L., and Swanson, P. D. (1974): Biochemical abnormalities in Huntington's chorea brains. *Neurology (Minneap.)*, 24:813–819.

713. Staines, W. A., Nagy, J. I., Vincent, S. R., and Fibiger, H. C. (1980): Neurotransmitters contained in the efferents of the striatum. *Brain Res.*, 194:391–402.

714. Staines, W. A., Atmadja, S., and Fibiger, H. C. (1980): Demonstration of a pallidostriatal pathway by retrograde transport of HRP-labeled lectin. *Brain Res.*, 206:446–450.

715. Staines, W. A., Benjamin, A. M., and McGeer, E. G. (1978): Striatal cysteinesulfinic acid decarboxylase. *Neurosci. Abstr.*, 4:50.

716. Steinbusch, H. W. M., Verhofstad, A. A. J., Joosten, H. W. J., and Goldstein, M. (1982): Serotonin-immunoreactive cell bodies in the nucleus dorsomedialis hypothalami, in the substantia nigra and area ventralis tegmentalis of Tsai: Observations after pharmacological manipulations in the rat. In: *Cytochemical Methods in Neuroanatomy*, edited by V. Chan-Palay and S. Palay, pp. 407–421. Alan R. Liss, New York.

717. Steinbusch, H. W. M., Nieuwenhuys, R., Verhofstad, A. A. J., and van der Kooy, D. (1981): The nucleus raphe dorsalis of the rat and its projection upon the caudatoputamen: A combined cytoarchitectonic, immunohistochemical and retrograde transport study. *J. Physiol. (Paris)*, 77:157–174.

718. Steinbusch, H. W. M. (1981): Distribution of serotonin-immunoreactivity in the central nervous system of the rat cell bodies and terminals. *Neuroscience*, 6:557–618.

719. Steinbusch, H. W. M., van der Kooy, D., Verhofstad, A. A. J., and Pellegrino, A. (1980): Serotonergic and non-serotonergic projections from the nucleus raphe dorsalis to the caudate-putamen complex in the rat, studied by a combined immunofluorescence and fluorescent retrograde axonal labeling technique. *Neurosci. Lett.*, 19:137–142.

720. Steindler, D. A., and Deniau, J. M. (1980): Anatomical evidence for collateral branching of substantia nigra neurons: A combined horseradish peroxidase and [³H]wheat germ agglutinin axonal transport study in the rat. *Brain Res.*, 196:228–236.

721. Steiner, A. L., Ferrendelli, A., and Kipnis, D. M. (1972): Radioimmunoassay for cyclic nucleotides: Effect of ischemia, changes during development and regional distribution of adenosine 3′,5′ monophosphate and guanosine 3′,5′ monophosphate in mouse brain. *J. Biol. Chem.*, 247:1121–1124.

722. Steriade, M., and Glenn, L. L. (1982): Neocortical and caudate projections of intralaminar thalamic neurons and their synaptic excitation from midbrain reticular core. *J. Neurophysiol.*, 48:352–371.

723. Stern, A. S., Lewis, R. V., Kimura, S., Rossier, J., Gerber, L. D., Brink, L., Stein, S., and Udenfriend, S. (1979): Isolation of the opioid heptapeptide met-enkephalin (Arg⁶, Phe⁷) from bovine adrenal medullary granules and striatum. *Proc. Natl. Acad. Sci. U.S.A.*, 76:6680–6683.

724. Sternberger, L. A. (1979): *Immunocytochemistry.* John Wiley & Sons, New York.

725. Stone, T. W. (1979): Amino acids as neurotransmitters of corticofugal neurones in the rat: A comparison of glutamate and aspartate. *Br. J. Pharmacol.*, 67:545–551.

726. Strassman, G. (1945): Hemosiderin and tissue iron in the brain, its relationship, occurrence and importance. *J. Neurol. Pathol. Exp. Neurol.*, 4:393–400.

727. Streit, P. (1980): Selective retrograde labeling indicating the transmitter of neuronal pathways. *J. Comp. Neurol.*, 191:429–463.

728. Streit, P., Knecht, E., and Cuénod, M. (1979): Transmitter specific retrograde labeling in the striato-nigral and raphe-nigral pathways. *Science,* 205:306–308.

729. Strong, R., Samorajski, T., and Gottesfeld, Z. (1982): Regional mapping of neostriatal neurotransmitter systems as a function of aging. *J. Neurochem.*, 39:831–836.

730. Studler, J. M., Javoy-Agid, F., Cesselin, F., Legrand, J. C., and Agid, Y. (1982): CCK-8-immunoreactivity distribution in human brain: Selective decrease in the substantia nigra from Parkinsonian patients. *Brain Res.*, 243:176–179.

731. Stumpf, W. E., and Roth, L. G. (1966): High resolution autoradiography with dry mounted, freeze-dried frozen sections. Comparative study of six methods using two diffusible compounds [³H]estradiol and [³H]mesobilirubinogen. *J. Histochem. Cytochem.*, 14:274–287.

732. Suzuki, Y., Shibuya, M., Okada, T., Mutsuga, N., Kageyama, N., and Ogura, K. (1981): Regional distribution of monoamines and their metabolites in the human basal ganglia and thalamus. *Applied Neurophysiol.*, 44:379.

733. Swanson, L. W., and Hartman, B. K. (1975): The central adrenergic system. An immunofluoroescence study of the location of cell bodies and their efferent connections in the rat utilizing dopamine-β-hydroxylase as a marker. *J. Comp. Neurol.*, 163:467–506.

734. Swanson, L. W., and Cowan, W. M. (1975): A note on the connections and development of the nucleus accumbens. *Brain Res.*, 92:324–330.

735. Swerts, J. P., Perdrisot, R., Patey, G., de la Baume, S., and Schwartz, J.-C. (1979): "Enkephalinase" is distinct from brain "angiotensin-converting enzyme." *Eur. J. Pharmacol.*, 57:279–281.

736. Switzer, R. C. III, Hill, J., and Heimer, L. (1982): The globus pallidus and its rostroventral extension into the olfactory tubercle of the rat: A cyto- and chemoarchitectural study. *Neuroscience,* 7:1891–1904.

737. Szabo, J. (1981): Retrograde double labeling experiments on the striatal efferents in cat and monkey. *Anat. Rec.,* 199:251A.

738. Szabo, J. (1980): Distribution of striatal afferents from the mesencephalon in the cat. *Brain Res.,* 188:3–21.

739. Szabo, J. (1979): Strionigral and nigrostriatal connections. *Appl. Neurophysiol.,* 42:9–12.

740. Tai, N., Goldberg, O., Luini, A., and Teichberg, V. I. (1982): An evaluation of γ-glutamyl dipeptide derivatives as antagonists of amino acid-induced Na⁺ fluxes in rat striatum slices. *J. Neurochem.,* 39:574–576.

741. Takano, Y., Kohjimoto, Y., Uchmura, K., and Kamiya, H. (1980): Mapping of the distribution of high affinity choline uptake and choline acetyltransferase in the striatum. *Brain Res.,* 194:583–587.

742. Tallman, J. F., Saavedra, J. M., and Axelrod, J. (1976): A sensitive enzymatic-isotopic method for the analysis of tyramine in brain and other tissues. *J. Neurochem.,* 27:463–469.

743. Tanaka, D. (1980): Development of spiny and aspiny neurons in the caudate nucleus of the dog during the first postnatal month. *J. Comp. Neurol.,* 192:247–263.

744. Tassin, J. P., Cheramy, A., Blanc, G., Thierry, A. M., and Glowinski, J. (1976): Topographical distribution of dopaminergic innervation and of dopaminergic receptors in the rat striatum. I. Microestimate of [³H]dopamine uptake and dopamine content in microdiscs. *Brain Res.,* 194:291–301.

745. Taylor, J. E., Vakshi, T. L., and Richelson, E. (1982): Histamine H₁ receptors in the brain and spinal cord of the cat. *Brain Res.,* 243:391–394.

746. Taylor, K. M., and Snyder, S. H. (1972): Isotopic microassay of histamine, histidine, histidine decarboxylase and histamine methyltransferase in brain tissue. *J. Neurochem.* 19:1343–1358.

747. Taylor, R. L., and Burt, D. R. (1981): Properties of [³H] (3-Me-His²)TRH binding to apparent TRH receptors in the sheep central nervous system. *Brain Res.,* 218:207–217.

748. Taylor, D. P., and Pert, C. B. (1979): Vasoactive intestinal polypeptide: Specific binding to rat brain membranes. *Proc. Natl. Acad. Sci. U.S.A.,* 76:660–664.

749. Tennyson, V. M., Barrett, R. E., Cohen, G., Côté, L., Heikkila, R., and Mytilneou, C. (1972): The developing neostriatum of the rabbit: Correlation of fluorescence histochemistry, electron microscopy, endogenous dopamine levels, and [³H] dopamine uptake. *Brain Res.,* 46:251–285.

750. Tennyson, V. M., Heikkila, R., Mytilineou, C., Côté, L., and Cohen, G. (1974): 5-Hydroxydopamine "tagged" neuronal boutons in rabbit neostriatum: Interrelationship between vesicles and axonal membrane. *Brain Res., 82*:341–348.

751. Ternaux, J. P., Héry, F., Bourgoin, S., Adrien, J., Glowinski, J., and Hamon, M. (1977): The topographical distribution of sertoninergic terminals in the neostriatum of the rat and the caudate nucleus of the cat. *Brain Res., 121*:311–326.

752. Thomas, E., and Pearse, A. G. E. (1964): The solitary active cells. Histochemical demonstration of damage-resistant nerve cells with a TPN-diaphorase reaction. *Acta Neuropathol., 3*:238–249.

753. Thompson, R. H. S. (1960): The regional distribution of copper in human brain. In: *Regional Neurochemistry*, edited by S. S. Kety and J. Elkes, pp. 103–106. Pergamon Press, New York.

754. Tonnaer, J. A. D. M., Wiegant, V. M., and deJong, W. (1982): Subcellular localization in rat brain of angiotensin I-generating endopeptidase activity distinct from cathepsin D. *J. Neurochem., 38*:1356–1364.

755. Tran, V. T., and Snyder, S. H. (1981): Histidine decarboxylase. Purification from fetal rat liver, immunologic properties, and histochemical localization in brain and stomach. *J. Biol. Chem., 256*:680–686.

756. Uhl, G. R., Goodman, R. R., and Snyder, S. H. (1979): Neurotensin-containing cell bodies, fibers and nerve terminals in the brain stem of the rat: Immunohistochemical mapping. *Brain Res., 167*:77–91.

757. Uhl, G. R., Goodman, R. R., Kuhar, M. J., Childers, S. R., and Snyder, S. H. (1979): Immunohistochemical mapping of enkephalin containing cell bodies, fibers and nerve terminals in the brain stem of the rat. *Brain Res., 166*:75–94.

758. Uhl, G. R., and Snyder, S. H. (1977): Neurotensin receptor binding, regional and subcellular distributions favor transmitter role. *Eur. J. Pharmacol., 41*:89–91.

759. Uhl, G. R., Bennett, J. P., Jr., and Snyder, S. H. (1977): Neurotensin, a central nervous system peptide: Apparent receptor binding in brain membranes. *Brain Res., 130*:299–313.

760. Uhl, G. R., Kuhar, M. J., and Snyder, S. H. (1977): Neurotensin: Immunohistochemical localization in rat central nervous system. *Proc. Natl. Acad. Sci. U.S.A., 74*:4059–4063.

761. Uhl, G. R., and Snyder, S. H. (1976): Regional and subcellular distributions of brain neurotensin. *Life Sci., 19*:1827–1832.

762. Ungerstedt, U. (1971): Stereotaxic mapping of the monamine pathways in the rat brain. *Acta Physiol. Scand., 197*:1–48.

763. Unnerstall, J. R., Niehoff, D. L., Kuhar, M. J., and Palacios, J. M. (1982): Quantitative receptor autoradiography using [^{3}H]Ultrofilm: Application to multiple benzodiazepine receptors. *J. Neurosci. Methods, 6*:59–73.

764. Unnerstall, J. R., Molliver, M. E., Kuhar, M. J., and Palacios, J. M. (1982): Ontogeny of opiate binding sites in the hippocampus, olfactory bulb and other regions of the rat forebrain by autoradiographic methods. *Brain Res. (in press).*

765. U'Prichard, D. C., Greenbers, D. A., Sheehan, P., and Snyder, S. H. (1977): Regional distribution of α-noradrenergic receptor binding in calf brain. *Brain Res., 138*:151–158.

766. Urquhart, N., Perry, T. L., Hansen, S., and Kennedy, J. (1975): GABA content and glutamic acid decarboxylase activity in brain of Huntington's chorea patients and control subjects. *J. Neurochem., 24*:1071–1075.

767. van der Gugten, J., Palkovits, M., Wunen, H. L. J. M., and Versteeg, H. G. (1976): Regional distribution of adrenaline in rat brain. *Brain Res., 107*:171–175.

768. Vanderhaeghen, J. J., Lotstra, F., De Mey, J., and Gilles, C. (1980): Immunohistochemical localization of cholecystokinin- and gastrin-like peptides in the brain and hypophysis of the rat. *Proc. Natl. Acad. Sci. U.S.A., 77*:1190–1194.

769. van der Heyden, J. A. M., and Korf, J. (1978): Regional levels of GABA in the brain: Rapid semiautomated assay and prevention of postmortem increases by 3-mercapto-propionic acid. *J. Neurochem., 31*:197–203.

770. van der Kooy, D., Hunt, S. P., Steinbusch, H. W. M., and Verhofstad, A. A. M. (1981): Separate populations of cholecystokinin and 5-hydroxytryptamine-containing neuronal cells in the rat dorsal raphe, and their contribution to the ascending raphe projections. *Neurosci. Lett., 26*:25–30.

771. van der Kooy, D., Coscina, D. V., and Hattori, T. (1981): Is there a non-dopaminergic nigrostriatal pathway? *Neuroscience, 6*:345–357.

772. van der Kooy, D., and Hattori, T. (1980): Dorsal raphe cells with collateral projections to the caudate–putamen and substantia nigra: A fluorescent retrograde double labeling study in the rat. *Brain Res., 186*:1–7.

773. van der Kooy, D., and Kuypers, H. G. J. M. (1979): Fluorescent retrograde double labeling: Axonal branching in the ascending raphe and nigral projections. *Science, 204*:873–875.

774. Vandermaelen, C. P., Kocsis, J. D., and Kitai, S. T. (1978): Caudate afferents from the retrorubral nucleus and other midbrain areas in the cat. *Brain Res. Bull., 3*:639–644.

775. Vandesande, F. (1979): A critical review of immunocytochemical methods for light microscopy. *J. Neurosci. Methods, 1*:3–24.

776. van Gelder, N. M. (1965): The histochemical demonstration of γ-aminobutyric acid metabolism by reduction of a tetrazolium salt. *J. Neurochem., 12*:231–237.

777. Van Hoesen, G. W., Yeterian, E. H., and Lavizzo-Mourey, R. (1981): Widespread corticostriate projections from temporal cortex of the rhesus monkey. *J. Comp. Neurol., 199*:205–219.

778. Veening, J. G., Cornelissen, F. M., and Lieven, P. A. J. M. (1980): The topical organization of the afferents to the caudatoputamen of the rat. A horseradish peroxidase study. *Neuroscience, 5*:1233–1268.

779. Verhoef, J., Wiegant, V. M., and DeWied, D.

(1982): Regional distribution of α- and γ-type endorphins in rat brain. *Brain Res.*, 231:454–460.

780. Versteeg, D. H. G., van der Gugten, de Jong, W., and Palkovits, M. (1976): Regional concentrations of noradrenaline and dopamine in rat brain. *Brain Res.*, 113:563–574.

781. Vincent, J. P., Kartalowski, H., Geneste, P., Kamenka, J. M., and Lazdunski, M. (1979): Interaction of phencyclidine ("angel dust") with a specific receptor in rat brain membranes. *Proc. Natl. Acad. Sci. U.S.A.*, 76:4678–4682.

782. Vincent, S. R., Skirboll, L., Hökfelt, T., Johansson, O., Lundberg, J. M., Elde, R. P., Terenius, L., and Kimmel, J. (1982): Coexistence of somatostatin- and avian pancreatic polypeptide (APP)-like immunoreactivity in some forebrain neurons. *Neuroscience*, 7:439–446.

783. Vincent, S. R., Kimura, H., and McGeer, E. G. (1981): The histochemical localization of GABA-transaminase in the efferents of the striatum. *Brain Res.*, 222:198–203.

784. Vincent, S. R., Lehmann, J., and McGeer, E. G. (1980): The localization of GABA-transaminase in the striato–nigral system. *Life Sci.*, 27:593–601.

785. Vincent, S. R., Kimura, H., and McGeer, E. G. (1979): Pharmacohistochemical procedure for GABA-transaminase: Implications for basal ganglia anatomy. *Neurosci. Abstr.*, 5:80.

786. Vincent, S. R., Nagy, J. I., and Fibiger, H. C. (1978): Increased striatal glutamate decarboxylase after lesions of the nigrostriatal pathway. *Brain Res.*, 143:168–173.

787. Walaas, I. (1981): Biochemical evidence for overlapping neocortical and allocortical glutamate projections to the nucleus accumbens and rostral caudatoputamen in the rat brain. *Neuroscience*, 6:399–405.

788. Walaas, I., and Fonnum, F. (1980): Biochemical evidence for γ-aminobutyrate containing fibers from the nucleus accumbens to the substantia nigra and ventral tegmental area in the rat. *Neuroscience*, 5:63–72.

789. Walaas, I., and Fonnum, F. (1979): The effects of surgical and chemical lesions on neurotransmitter candidates in the nucleus accumbens of the rat. *Neuroscience*, 4:209–216.

790. Walters, J. R., and Roth, R. H. (1972): Effect of gamma-hydroxybutyrate on dopamine and dopamine metabolites in the rat striatum. *Biochem. Pharmacol.*, 21:2111–2121.

791. Wamsley, J. K., Zarbin, M. A., Young, W. S. III, and Kuhar, M. J. (1982): Distribution of opiate receptors in the monkey brain: An autoradiographic study. *Neuroscience*, 7:595–613.

792. Wamsley, J. K., Young, W. S. III, and Kuhar, M. (1980): Immunohistochemical localization of enkephalin in rat forebrain. *Brain Res.*, 190:153–174.

793. Wamsley, J. K., Zarbin, M. A., Birdsall, N. J. M., and Kuhar, M. J. (1980): Muscarinic cholinergic receptors: Autoradiographic localization of high and low affinity agonist binding sites. *Brain Res.*, 200:1–12.

794. Wang, R. Y. (1981): Dopaminergic neurons in the

rat ventral tegmental area. I. Identification and characterization. *Brain Res. Rev.*, 3:123–140.

795. Wastek, G. J., and Yamamura, H. I. (1978): Biochemical characterization of the muscarinic cholinergic receptor in human brain. Alterations in Huntington's disease. *Mol. Pharmacol.*, 14:768–780.

796. Wastek, G. J., Stern, L. Z., Johnson, P. C., and Yamamura, H. I. (1976): Huntington's disease: Regional alteration in muscarinic cholinergic receptor binding in human brain. *Life Sci.*, 19:1033–1040.

797. Watkins, J. C., Davies, J., Evans, R. H., Francis, A. A., and Jones, A. W. (1981): Pharmacology of receptors for excitatory amino acids. In: *Glutamate as a Neurotransmitter*, edited by G. DiChiara and G. L. Gessa, pp. 263–273. Raven Press, New York.

798. Watson, S. J., Richard, C. W. III, and Barchas, J. D. (1978): Adrenocorticotropin in rat brain: Immunocytochemical localization in cells and axons. *Science*, 200:1180–1181.

799. Watson, S. J., and Akil, H. (1980): α-MSH in rat brain: Occurrence within and outside of β-endorphin neurons. *Brain Res.*, 182:217–223.

800. Watson, S. J., Akil, H., Richard, C. W. III, and Barchas, J.D. (1978): Evidence for two separate opiate peptide neuronal systems. *Nature*, 275:226–228.

801. Watson, S. J., Barchas, J. D., and Li, C. H. (1977): β-Lipotropin: Localization of cells and axons in rat brain immunohistochemistry. *Proc. Natl. Acad. Sci. U.S.A.*, 74:5155–5158.

802. Watson, S. J., Akil, H., Sullivan, S., and Barchas, J. D. (1977): Immunocytochemical localization of methionine enkephalin: Preliminary observations. *Life Sci.*, 21:733–738.

803. Weber, E., Evans, C. J., and Barchas, J. D. (1982): Predominance of the amino-terminal octapeptide fragment of dynorphin in rat brain regions. *Nature*, 299:77–79.

804. Weber, E., Roth, D. A., and Barchas, J. D. (1982): Immunohistochemical distribution of α-neo-endorphin/dynorphin neuronal systems in rat brain: Evidence for colocalization. *Proc. Natl. Acad. Sci. U.S.A.*, 79:3062–3066.

805. Weber, E., Evans, C. J., Samuelsson, S. J., and Barchas, J. D. (1981): Novel peptide neuronal system in rat brain and pituitary. *Science*, 214:1248–1251.

806. Webster, K. E. (1965): The cortico–striatal projection in the cat. *J. Anat.*, 99:329–337.

807. Wenk, H., Bigl, V., and Meyer, U. (1980): Cholinergic projections from magnocellular nuclei of the basal forebrain to cortical areas in rats. *Brain Res. Rev.*, 2:295–316.

808. West, C. H. K., Jackson, J. C., and Benjamin, R. M. (1979): An autoradiographic study of subcortical forebrain projections from mediodorsal and adjacent midline thalamic nuclei in the rabbit. *Neuroscience*, 4:1977–1988.

809. Whitaker, J. N., Terry, L. C., and Whetsell, W. O., Jr., (1981): Immunocytochemical localization of cathepsin D in rat neural tissue. *Brain Res.*, 216:109–124.

810. Whitehouse, P. J., Price, D. L., Clark, A. W., Coyle, J. T., and DeLong, M. R. (1980): Alzheimer

disease: Evidence for selective loss of cholinergic neurons in the nucleus basalis. *Ann. Neurol.,* 10:122–126.

811. Wiklund, L., Léger, L., and Persson, M. (1981): Monoamine cell distribution in the cat brainstem. A fluorescence histochemical study with quantification of indolaminergic and locus coeruleus cell groups. *J. Comp. Neurol.,* 203:613–648.

812. Wilcox, B. J., and Seybold, V. S. (1982): Localization of neuronal histamine in rat brain. *Neurosci. Lett.,* 29:105–110.

813. Williams, M., and Risley, E. A. (1980): Biochemical characterization of putative central purinergic receptors by using 2-choro[^{3}H]adenosine, a stable analog of adenosine. *Proc. Natl. Acad. Sci. U.S.A.,* 77:6892–6896.

814. Williams, M., and Risley, E. A. (1978): Characterization of the binding of [^{3}H]muscimol, a potent γ-aminobutyric acid agonist, to rat brain synaptosomal membranes using a filtration assay. *J. Neurochem.,* 32:713–718.

815. Williams, R. G., and Dockray, G. J. (1982): Differential distribution in rat basal ganglia of met-enkephalin- and met-enkephalin Arg^6 Phe^7-like peptides revealed by immunohistochemistry. *Brain Res.,* 240:167–170.

816. Willner, J., LeFevre, H., and Costa, E. (1974): Assay by multiple ion detection of phenylethylamine and phenylethanolamine in rat brain. *J. Neurochem.,* 23:857–859.

817. Wilson, C. J., and Phelan, K. D. (1982): Dual topographic representation of neostriatum in the globus pallidus of rats. *Brain Res.,* 243:354–359.

818. Wilson, C. J., Chang, H. T., and Kitai, S. T. (1982): Origins of postsynaptic potentials evoked in identified rat neostriatal neurons by stimulation in substantia nigra. *Exp. Brain Res.,* 45:157–167.

819. Wilson, C. J., and Groves, P. M. (1980): Fine structure and synaptic connections of the common spiny neuron of the rat neostriatum: A study employing intracellular injection of horseradish peroxidase. *J. Comp. Neurol.,* 194:599–615.

820. Wolozin, B. L., Nishimura, S., and Pasternak, G. W. (1982): The binding of κ- and σ-opiates in rat brain. *J. Neurosci.,* 2:708–713.

821. Wong, D. T., Bymaster, F. P., Horng, J. S., and Molloy, B. B. (1975): A new selective inhibitor for uptake of serotonin into synaptosomes of rat brain: 3-(*p*-trifluoromethylphenoxy)-*N*-methyl-3-phenylpropylamine. *J. Pharmacol. Exp. Ther.,* 193:804–811.

822. Woolf, N. J., and Butcher, L. L. (1981): Cholinergic neurons in the caudate–putamen complex proper are intrinsically organized: A combined Evans blue and acetylcholinesterase analysis. *Brain Res. Bull.,* 7:487–507.

823. Wright, A. K., and Arbuthnott, G. W. (1981): The pattern of innervation of the corpus striatum by the substantia nigra. *Neuroscience,* 6:2063–2067.

824. Wu, J.-Y. (1982): Purification and characterization of cysteic acid and cysteine sulfinic acid decarboxylase from bovine brain. *Proc. Natl. Acad. Sci. U.S.A.,* 70:4270–4274.

825. Wu, J.-Y., Bird, E. D., Chen, M. S., and Huang,

W. M. (1979): Abnormalities of neurotransmitter enzymes in Huntington's chorea. *Neurochem. Res.,* 4:575–586.

826. Yamamura, H. I. and Snyder, S. H. (1974): Muscarinic cholinergic binding in rat brain. *Proc. Natl. Acad. Sci. U.S.A.,* 71:1725–1729.

827. Yamamura, H. I., Kuhar, M. J., and Snyder, S. H. (1974): *In vivo* identification of muscarinic cholinergic receptor binding in rat brain. *Brain Res.,* 80:170–176.

828. Yamamura, H. I., Kuhar, M. J., Greenberg, D., and Snyder, S. H. (1974): Muscarinic cholinergic receptor binding: Regional distribution in monkey brain. *Brain Res.,* 66:541–546.

829. Yang, H.-Y., Hong, J. S., and Costa, E. (1977): Regional distribution of leu and met enkephalin in rat brain. *Neuropharmacology,* 16:303–307.

830. Yang, H.-Y. T., and Neff, N. H. (1972): Distribution and properties of angiotensin converting enzyme of rat brain. *J. Neurochem.,* 19:2443–2450.

831. Yeterian, E. H. and Van Hoesen, G. W. (1978): Cortico–striate projections in the rhesus monkey: The organization of certain cortico–caudate connections. *Brain Res.,* 139:43–63.

832. Yoshida, M., Rabin, A., and Anderson, M. (1974): Monosynaptic inhibition of pallidal neurons by axon collaterals of caudato–nigral fibers. *Exp. Brain Res.,* 15:333–347.

833. Yoshida, M., and Precht, W. (1971): Monosynaptic inhibition of neurons of the substantia nigra by caudato–nigral fibers. *Brain Res.,* 32:225–228.

834. Yoshida, M., and Omata, S. (1979): Blocking by picrotoxin of nigra-evoked inhibition of neurons of ventromedial nucleus of the thalamus. *Experientia,* 35:794.

835. Young, A. B., Bromberg, M. B., and Penney, J. B., Jr., (1981): Decreased glutamate uptake in subcortical areas deafferented by sensorimotor cortical ablation in the cat. *J. Neurosci.,* 1:241–249.

836. Young, A. B., and Snyder, S. H. (1973): Strychnine binding associated with glycine receptors of the central nervous system. *Proc. Natl. Acad. Sci. U.S.A.,* 70:2832–2836.

837. Young, W. S. III, and Kuhar, M. J. (1981): Neurotensin receptor localization by light microscopic autoradiography in rat brain. *Brain Res.,* 206:273–285.

838. Young, W. S. III, and Kuhar, M. J. (1981): Radiohistochemical localization of benzodiazepine receptors in rat brain. *J. Pharmacol. Exp. Ther.,* 212:337–346.

839. Young, W. S. III, Niehoff, D., Kuhar, M. J., Beer, B., and Lipps, A. S. (1980): Multiple benzodiazepine receptor localization by light microscopic radiohistochemistry. *J. Pharmacol. Exp. Ther.,* 216:425–430.

840. Young, W. S. III, and Kuhar, M. J. (1980): Noradrenergic α_1 and α_2 receptors: Light microscopic autoradiographic localization. *Proc. Natl. Acad. Sci. U.S.A.,* 77:1696–1700.

841. Young, W. S. III, and Kuhar, M. J. (1979): A new method for receptor autoradiography: [^{3}H]Opioid receptors in rat brain. *Brain Res.,* 179:255–270.

842. Young, W. S. III, Wamsley, J. K., Zarbin, M. A.,

and Kuhar, M. J. (1980): Opiate receptors undergo axonal flow. *Science,* 210:76–77.

843. Zakarian, S., and Smyth, D. G. (1982): β-Endorphin is processed differently in specific regions of rat pituitary and brain. *Nature,* 296:280–282.

844. Zarbin, M. A., Wamsley, J. K., and Kuhar, M. J. (1981): Glycine receptor: Light microscopic autoradiographic localization with [³H]strychnine. *J. Neurosci.,* 1:532–547.

845. Zukin, R. S., and Zukin, S. R. (1981): Demonstra-

tion of [³H]cyclazocine binding to multiple opiate receptor sites. *Mol. Pharmacol.,* 20:246–254.

846. Zukin, S. R., and Zukin, R. S. (1979): Specific [³H]phencyclidine binding in rat central nervous system. *Proc. Natl. Acad. Sci. U.S.A.,* 76:5372–5376.

847. Zukin, S. R., Young, A. B., and Snyder, S. H. (1974): Gamma-aminobutyric acid binding to receptor sites in the rat central nervous system. *Proc. Natl. Acad. Sci. U.S.A.,* 71:4802–4807.

Chemical Neuroanatomy, edited by P.C. Emson,
Raven Press, New York © 1983.

The Cerebral Cortex

*John G. Parnavelas and **John K. McDonald

*Departments of *Cell Biology and **Physiology, The University of Texas Health Science Center,
Dallas, Texas 75235*

Investigations of the cerebral cortex began in the eighteenth century, but the earliest microscopical studies, performed by Baillarger, occurred during the early part of the following century and were published in 1840 [see Polyak (359) for historical overview]. Early efforts were hampered by the lack of adequate staining techniques. However, the invention of the Golgi method provided investigators with a powerful tool that permitted visualization of the morphology of individual neurons and the relations that may exist between nerve fibers and cells. Santiago Ramón y Cajal and his pupil, Lorente de Nó, seized upon this new technique, and, by the latter part of the nineteenth and early twentieth century, they had provided detailed morphological descriptions of cortical organization. Systematic analyses of Golgi-stained cortical cell types continued over the years and particularly during the past decade. These studies together with ultrastructural observations of synaptic connections have shed new light on the neuronal architecture of the cerebral cortex.

Although studies of cortical function began long ago, it was not until the introduction of microelectrode recording that electrophysiologists were able to characterize the properties of individual neurons and elucidate the functional organization of the neocortex. One area of research that has consistently lagged behind neuroanatomy and neurophysiology is the field of neurochemistry. Recently, the development of sensitive and reliable microassays for enzymes, putative neurotransmitters, and receptors, and the generation of specific antisera for use in radioimmunoassay and immunocytochemistry have caused an explosion in our knowledge of cortical neurochemistry.

To date, most reviews have focused on either the structural (259,412,436), functional (27,172), or neurochemical (93) organization of the neocortex. The aim of this review is to present an account of the morphological organization of a cortical region and describe what is known about the chemical properties of its constituent neurons and connections.

It would be a monumental task to attempt an adequate morphological and chemical description of the entire cerebral cortex. We have, therefore, concentrated on the visual cortex of the rat, an area that has been the focal point of extensive anatomical, physiological, and, more recently, chemical investigations. We shall briefly mention observations on the structure and chemistry of other cortical regions in the rat and other mammals.

NEURONAL ORGANIZATION

Cytology

The primary visual cortex (area 17; striate cortex) of the rat occupies a relatively large portion of the occipital region of the cerebral hemisphere (220,469). It is bordered medially by area 18 and laterally and caudally by area 18a (54,220,401). Areas 18 and 18a together make up the peristriate cortex. Nissl-stained coronal sections through area 17 of the rat reveal six horizontal layers, a feature common to the neocortex of other mammals (259). Neurons in each layer, aside from showing considerable morphological diversity, have distinct perikaryal form, size, and packing density (221). In the rat visual cortex, individual layers are clearly delineated, with the exception of layers II and III which are not separated by a discrete border (331,469) (Fig. 1). A feature that distinguishes area 17 from the peristriate areas is the increased thickness of layer IV which primarily contains closely packed neurons of small size (221,469) (Fig. 1). It is interesting to note that area 17 as defined by cytoarchitectonic criteria corresponds to

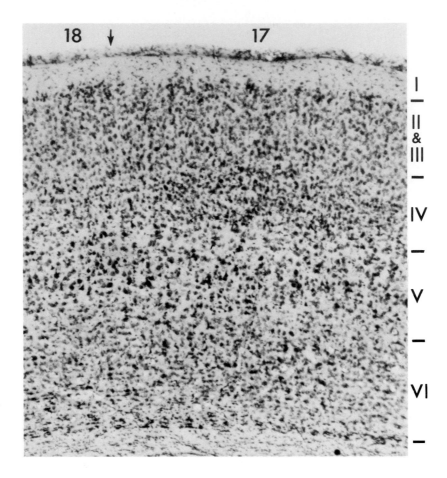

FIG. 1. Nissl-stained coronal section of rat visual cortex. *Arrow* demarcates areas 17 and 18. The approximate boundaries of layers are indicated. ×70.

the primary visual cortex determined electrophysiologically (291).

Types of Neurons

The morphology and organization of neurons in the mammalian cerebral cortex have been investigated with the Golgi methods for almost a century (46,259). Although much was known in this field by the early 1900s, the last decade has witnessed a notable revival of interest in the use of the Golgi methods to further analyze cortical organization (108,194,261,331,349,411,435,450,451). The strength of the Golgi methods lies in their ability to allow visualization of the neuronal cell body and its processes, some of which may be traced for a few millimeters in favorable preparations. However, these techniques demand, as was so brilliantly achieved by Cajal and Lorente de Nó, that the in-

vestigator be able to synthesize a complete picture from a small number of individually stained neurons.

A variety of morphological criteria have been used over the years to classify cortical neurons on the basis of Golgi preparations, and these have resulted in diverse classification schemes (46, 194,258,261,319,435). Despite the efforts of so many investigators, there is still no agreement concerning the morphological features that should be used in cell classification. However, there is general agreement that two main types of neurons exist in the mammalian neocortex: the pyramidal and the nonpyramidal neurons.

Pyramidal Neurons

Pyramidal cells comprise approximately two-thirds of the neuronal population in the rat visual cortex (331,468) and are present in all cortical layers except layer I. Their perikarya are typically pyramidal in shape, and their dendrites, which are richly endowed with spines, display a fairly consistent morphology (Fig. 2). These morphological characteristics include (a) a prominent apical dendrite, which emanates from the apex of the soma and extends towards the pial surface, giving off several oblique and horizontal branches, and (b) two or more primary dendrites, which arise from the base of the cell body and, together with their branches, comprise the basal dendritic field. The apical dendrites frequently branch near the border of layers I and II to form an apical tuft. The axons of pyramidal neurons arise either from the base of the cell body or from the proximal portion of one of the basal dendrites and emit a number of collaterals as they course towards the white matter.

Included in the pyramidal cell category are pyramid-like cells and inverted pyramidal cells, both concentrated in layers V and VI, which lack some of the stereotypical features of classical pyramidal neurons. Pyramid-like cells display round or spindle-shaped perikarya and an apical dendrite directed sideways or towards the pial surface at an angle (Fig. 3a). Inverted pyramidal cells resemble

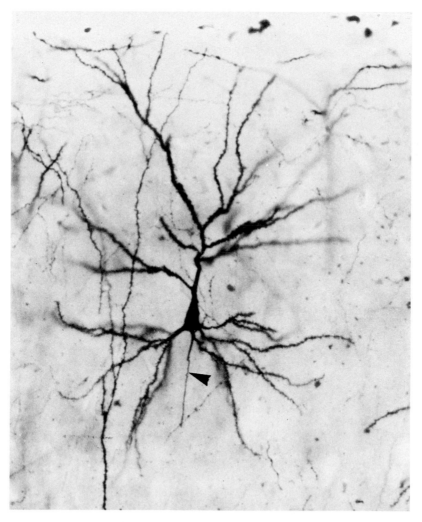

FIG. 2. Pyramidal neuron in layer II stained with the rapid Golgi method. Its short apical dendrite forms an extensive terminal tuft in layers I and II. *Arrowhead* points to the axon which arises from the proximal portion of a basal dendrite and is directed towards the subcortical white matter. ×320. (From Parnavelas et al., ref. 331, with permission.)

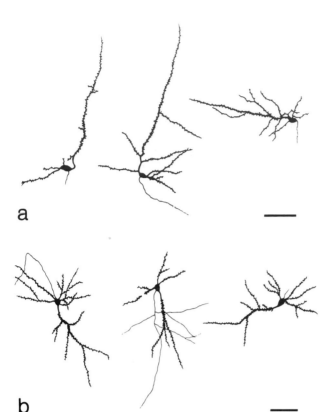

a

b

FIG. 3. Camera lucida drawings of typical pyramid-like cells (**a**) and inverted pyramidal cells (**b**) commonly encountered in layers V and VI. *Bars,* 100 μm. (From Parnavelas et al., ref. 331, with permission.)

typical pyramids except, as their name suggests, they appear upside down, so that their "apical" dendrite is directed towards the subcortical white matter (Fig. 3b).

Pyramidal cells have been identified with the electron microscope in the visual cortex of the rat (332,468). Their ultrastructural features closely resemble previous descriptions of pyramidal cells in the cerebral cortex of other mammals (58,127,197,420,442). Their perikarya vary considerably in size, with the Meynert cells of layer V being the largest (331,468). Pyramidal neurons possess a large pale nucleus containing evenly distributed heterochromatin and, with the exception of Meynert cells, have relatively small amounts of perinuclear cytoplasm which includes a variety of loosely packed organelles (332,468).

Electron microscopic examination of Golgi-impregnated pyramidal cells shows that they receive exclusively Gray's (144) type II synaptic contacts on their perikarya, type I contacts on their dendritic spines, and both synaptic types (type II predominating) on their dendritic shafts (332). Pyramidal cell axons may be either myelinated or unmyelinated (341), and their collaterals in the cortex have been observed to form type I synapses with dendritic spines and occasionally with dendritic shafts of unknown origin (332,424) (Fig. 4a,b).

Nonpyramidal Neurons

Neurons that do not possess the features outlined for pyramidal neurons are referred to as nonpyramidal cells. In Golgi preparations of rat visual cortex, nonpyramidal cells comprise a heteromorphic population displaying a wide range of variation in dendritic geometry and in perikaryal size, form, and orientation (108,331,470). A common morphological feature of these cells is that their axons are distributed entirely within the cortex (331), although the axons of a few nonpyramidal neurons have been seen to enter the white matter (108,274).

Feldman and Peters (108) have used dendritic geometry and the presence or absence of dendritic spines to classify nonpyramidal neurons in the visual cortex of the rat. On the basis of dendritic form, cells were classified as multipolar, bitufted, and bipolar, and based on the frequency of spines, they were subdivided into spinous, sparsely spinous, and spine-free. Spinous dendrites appear to be associated only with multipolar neurons, whereas sparsely spinous and spine-free dendrites are associated with each of the three dendritic forms.

Approximately 60% of the nonpyramidal neurons encountered in the visual cortex are multipo-

lar. Found in all cortical layers, their perikarya may be spherical, ovoid, or irregular in shape. Their dendrites, three or more in number, may originate from any point on the soma and extend in any direction (Figs. 5–7). Multipolar cells with spinous dendrites are predominantly present in layer IV, and the sparsely spinous and spine-free

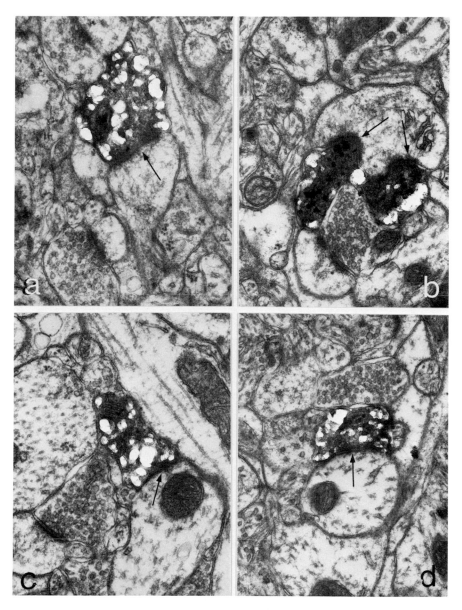

FIG. 4. a,b: Golgi-impregnated terminals of axon collaterals of two layer III pyramidal cells forming Gray's type I synapses *(arrows)* with dendritic spines. ×32,000; **c,d:** Golgi-impregnated axon terminals of a spine-free nonpyramidal neuron of layer III. These terminals establish type II synaptic contacts *(arrows)* with dendritic shafts. **c,** ×30,000; **d,** ×30,500. (From Parnavelas et al., ref. 332, with permission.)

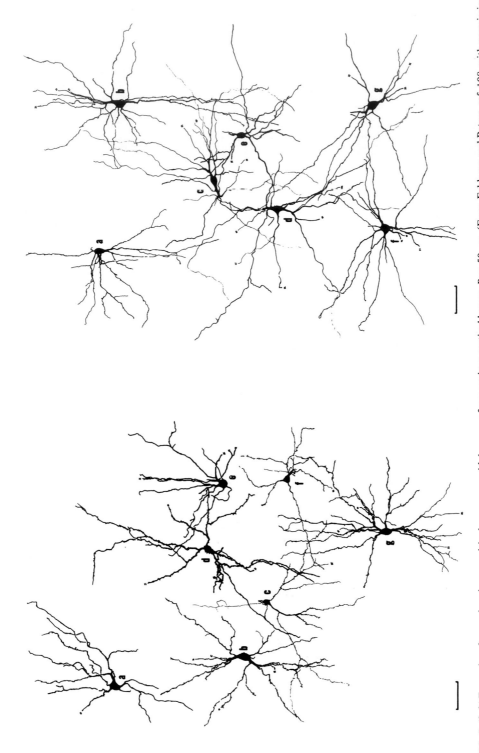

FIG. 5. (*left*) Examples of sparsely spinous nonpyramidal neurons from various cortical layers. *Bar*, 50 μm. (From Feldman and Peters, ref. 108, with permission.)

FIG. 6. (*right*) Examples of spine-free multipolar nonpyramidal neurons from various cortical layers. *Bar*, 50 μm. (From Feldman and Peters, ref. 108, with permission.)

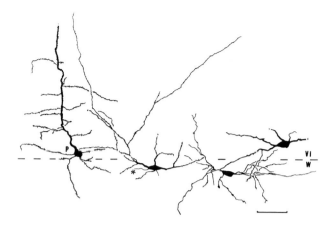

FIG. 7. Three sparsely spinous multipolar nonpyramidal neurons located in deep layer VI or in the uppermost portion of the white matter (W). These cells display horizontally oriented perikarya and dendrites. Cell P is a pyramidal neuron. *Asterisk* identifies the initial portion of the axon of one of the nonpyramidal cells. *Bar*, 50 μm. (From Feldman and Peters, ref. 108, with permission.)

forms are fairly evenly distributed throughout the cortex. Multipolar cells exhibit variable dendritic patterns. The majority are stellate, with dendrites radiating in all orientations from the cell body. However, an appreciable number of cells display a degree of dendritic polarization (cells c, e, and g, Fig. 5). Common among this group are nonpyramidal neurons, concentrated in layer VI, with horizontally oriented dendrites (Fig. 7).

Multipolar cell axons may emerge from the superficial or deep surface of the cell body or from one of the proximal dendrites. Their distribution is highly diverse, although the majority form an elaborate local plexus. Axons of spinous multipolar cells arise from the deep surface of the perikarya or from one of the descending dendrites and consistently course towards the lower layers (108). In no case has an axon been traced into the subcortical white matter as has been reported for other species (46,435).

Bitufted cells comprise approximately 20% of the impregnated nonpyramidal neurons in the visual cortex of the rat and are most frequently observed in layers IV and V (108). They typically exhibit elongated perikarya, with their long axes directed vertically. One or more dendrites arise from each pole of the soma and tend to branch repeatedly near the soma, forming a superficial and a deep dendritic tuft of almost equal length (Fig. 8). Their dendrites may be sparsely spinous or spine-free, and the overall dendritic field exhibits a vertical orientation. The axons of bitufted cells arise from the cell body or from one of the primary dendrites and may ascend or descend. One group of nonpyramidal neurons, composed of multipolar and bitufted cells, are known as chandelier cells. They have received special attention because of the characteristic appearance of their terminal axonal

arbors—they look like candles in a chandelier—and the abundance of axoaxonal contacts they form with the axon initial segments of pyramidal neurons (341,423).

Bipolar cell perikarya are predominantly present in layers II, III, and IV. Most perikarya are vertically elongated, although a few round forms are also recognized. One and occasionally two dendrites emerge from each pole and extend vertically for a considerable distance. The elongated dendritic envelopes of many bipolar cells span most of the cortex from layer I to deep layer V (Fig. 9). The ascending dendrites of bipolar cells are frequently observed to give rise to several branches near the border of layers I and II, forming a subpial tuft. The descending dendrites, similar to the ascending dendrites, arborize at some distance from the soma, with the daughter branches displaying oblique or horizontal orientations. Axons usually arise from a major dendrite and exhibit a predominantly vertical orientation.

In addition to the nonpyramidal cell types described so far, which are present in all cortical layers, there exist other cell forms that are unique to cortical layer I (Fig. 10). These unique neurons of layer I of the rat visual cortex include the Retzius–Cajal cells, persisting horizontal cells, vertical cells, and cells without axons (34). Retzius–Cajal cells (also known as fetal horizontal cells) (Fig. 10a) are only present in the perinatal period. Early observations of Golgi material (46,271) and a more recent examination with the electron microscope (89) suggest that these cells undergo morphological transformation later in life and become indistinguishable from typical nonpyramidal neurons of layer I. Persisting horizontal cells possess horizontally elongated perikarya which usually give rise to two primary dendrites from opposite poles. These

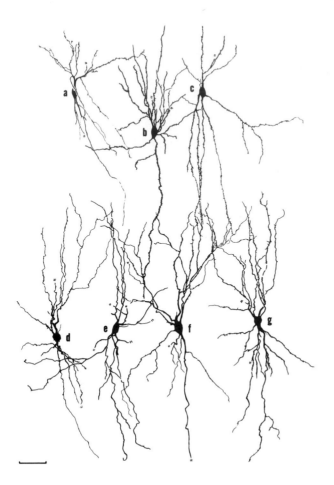

FIG. 8. Examples of bitufted nonpyramidal neurons from various cortical layers. *Bar,* 50 μm. (From Feldman and Peters, ref. 108, with permission.)

dendrites, which may be spinous or sparsely spinous, ramify into oblique branches (Fig. 10c). Vertical cells have their perikarya located in the superficial aspect of layer I. Emerging from their cell bodies are usually one or two short, horizontally oriented dendrites and a thick primary dendrite which is directed perpendicularly towards layer II. This primary dendrite frequently ramifies into several obliquely oriented branches (Fig. 10d). Finally, a small number of cells without recognizable axons have been consistently observed in layer I (34).

Examination of Golgi-impregnated neurons in different cortical areas and species reveals no notable differences in the morphology of pyramidal cells (46,137,259,261,319,331,435), but the overall morphology of nonpyramidal neurons appears to be "simpler" in lower mammals than in carnivores and primates. For example, the visual and other cortical areas of rodents lack nonpyramidal neurons with the more elaborate axonal and dendritic patterns typically observed in higher mammals.

Among these neurons are spinous stellate cells whose axons project to the white matter (435), "basket" cells (46,319,435), "midget" cells (127,435), and "double bouquet" cells which appear frequently in Golgi preparations of cat and monkey cerebral cortex (46,194,319,435).

Electron microscopic investigations in the visual cortex have provided detailed accounts of the ultrastructural features of nonpyramidal neurons and their synaptic organization (332,345,348,468). Nonpyramidal cell nuclei appear more electron dense than those of most pyramidal cells, and their outline displays a number of invaginations. The amount of perinuclear cytoplasm varies among neurons, being relatively sparse in small nonpyramidal cells and abundant in larger neurons. Their ultrastructural features resemble the descriptions of nonpyramidal cells in the cerebral cortex of other mammals (127,197,420,442).

Ultrastructural analyses of Golgi-impregnated nonpyramidal cells reveal that they receive both Gray's type I and type II synapses on their somata

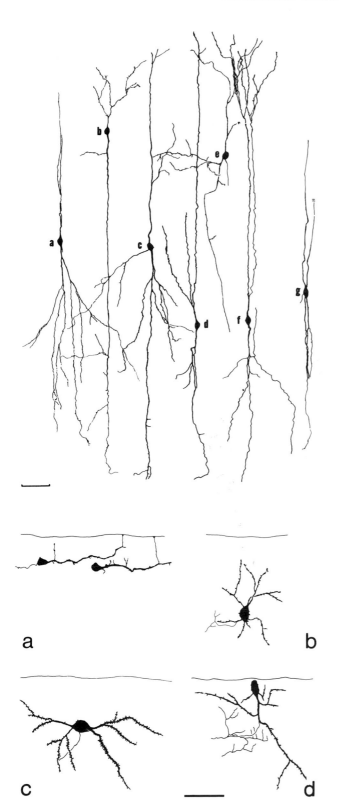

FIG. 9. Examples of bipolar nonpyramidal neurons from various cortical layers. *Bar,* 50 μm. (From Feldman and Peters, ref. 108, with permission.)

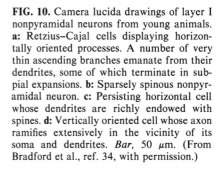

FIG. 10. Camera lucida drawings of layer I nonpyramidal neurons from young animals. **a:** Retzius–Cajal cells displaying horizontally oriented processes. A number of very thin ascending branches emanate from their dendrites, some of which terminate in sub-pial expansions. **b:** Sparsely spinous nonpyramidal neuron. **c:** Persisting horizontal cell whose dendrites are richly endowed with spines. **d:** Vertically oriented cell whose axon ramifies extensively in the vicinity of its soma and dendrites. *Bar,* 50 μm. (From Bradford et al., ref. 34, with permission.)

and dendrites (332,345). The axons of nonpyramidal neurons may be myelinated or unmyelinated (341,347). Axons of sparsely spinous and spine-free multipolar neurons and of bitufted cells have been observed to form type II synaptic contacts with pyramidal and nonpyramidal neurons in the visual cortex (332,341,345) (Fig. 4c,d). Unlike most nonpyramidal neurons, the axons of some bipolar cells have been recently reported to form type I synapses with dendrites of pyramidal cells and with perikarya and dendrites of other nonpyramidal neurons in the visual cortex (348).

CONNECTIONS

Subcortical Afferents

Thalamic Input

Thalamocortical relationships have been the subject of intensive investigations since the end of the last century (45). But only in recent years have new techniques enabled investigators to precisely localize the termination sites of thalamic afferents and identify the cortical neurons that are involved in thalamocortical synapses.

In his classical Golgi studies of rodent neocortex, Lorente de Nó (259) distinguished two types of thalamic fibers. One type, conveying specific information, originates in one of the sensory relay nuclei of the thalamus and forms dense terminal arbors in layer IV and the adjacent portion of layer III. The other type contains nonspecific afferents which are generally thinner axons that give rise to a diffuse pattern of collaterals throughout the cortex and eventually ascend to layer I (213). The intralaminar nuclei of the thalamus have been traditionally considered the source of nonspecific afferents (196,213). However, evidence suggests that these fibers arise not only from the intralaminar nuclei but also from a number of other sources including specific thalamic nuclei (47,156,196,307,335).

Investigations of the thalamic afferents to the visual cortex have emphasized the specific projection that originates in the dorsal lateral geniculate nucleus. The early studies of Lashley (240,241), performed in the rat, have demonstrated that this nucleus projects solely to the striate cortex (area 17), but recent autoradiographic studies have shown that this projection also extends into portion of area 18a (66,173,374). The distribution of the geniculocortical afferents in the visual cortex of the rat has been carefully examined with degeneration and autoradiographic techniques (173,342,374,

402,403). These studies have shown that the major site of termination within area 17 is in layer IV and the adjacent portion of layer III, with secondary sites located in layer VI and the uppermost portion of layer I. A comparable pattern of termination has been reported for the geniculocortical projection in the visual cortex of other mammals (20, 86,121,128,142,171,203,383) and for the projections of other relay nuclei to corresponding primary sensory cortical areas (85,121,195,199,213). It should be mentioned, however, that the termination sites are different in cortical areas other than the primary sensory areas (121,156,196,199).

The neuronal elements in the visual cortex of the rat that synapse with geniculocortical fibers have been thoroughly investigated by Peters and colleagues (343,344,346). These authors concluded that all cell perikarya and dendrites contained in layer IV and deep layer III that are capable of forming Gray's type I synapses can receive some portion of their input from the thalamus. This apparent lack of specificity of geniculocortical connections is not consistent with the reported precise representation of the retina in area 17 (291) and with the presence of neurons in the visual cortex that possess well-defined receptive field properties (334). The observations of Peters and colleagues concerning the fine organization of geniculocortical projections in the rat are consonant with descriptions of thalamocortical terminations in the visual cortex and other sensory cortical areas in several species (35,167,198,421,435,466,467).

Other afferents to the rat visual cortex originate from the following thalamic nuclei: lateral posterior, posterior, ventromedial, ventral anterolateral, and central medial. The lateral posterior nucleus provides a dense projection to layers I and IV of areas 18 and 18a and a more sparse projection to layer I and the superficial portion of layer V of area 17 (56,173,317,335,399,403). Projections from the posterior complex of the thalamus and the ventromedial nucleus appear to terminate chiefly in layer I (155,156,335), whereas afferents from the ventral anterolateral nucleus terminate in layers I and VI of area 17 (156). Finally, afferents from the central medial nucleus project primarily to layer VI of cortical area 17 (156). Nothing is known about the synaptic organization of these thalamic afferents in the visual cortex.

Other Subcortical Inputs

It is now well documented that the visual cortex and, in fact, the entire cortex of the rat and other species receives afferents (predominantly ipsilateral) from the magnocellular nuclei in the basal forebrain. The nuclei concerned include the nucleus of the diagonal band, the preoptic nucleus, and the nucleus basalis (2,78,153,191,192, 201,243,414,464). These afferents provide the cholinergic innervation of the mammalian neocortex (see the section Acetylcholine below).

The visual cortex is also innervated by two widely distributed axonal systems in the brain. These systems, which provide the noradrenergic and serotonergic innervation to the central nervous system (CNS), arise in the locus ceruleus in the pons and in the midbrain medial and dorsal raphe nuclei (69). The locus ceruleus provides the noradrenergic input, and its projections to the cortex (predominantly ipsilateral) have received a great deal of attention (119,123,129,193,250,355,380, 447). The raphe nuclei give rise to the serotonergic innervation (also predominantly ipsilateral), which has been traced to the mammalian cerebral cortex with various methods (6,31,122,246,295,330). Finally, there is some indirect evidence to suggest a weak projection from the ventral tegmental area of the midbrain to the visual cortex (391,443). A major projection from the ventral tegmentum to other cortical areas is well documented (14,48,125,251,252).

Corticocortical Afferents

Callosal Input

Detailed studies of the organization of callosal connections in the rat visual cortex have recently appeared in the literature (54,66). These authors utilized the Fink–Heimer degeneration technique after sectioning the corpus callosum and described complex forms of callosal connections that resemble somewhat the patterns described in other animals. Their findings show only a sparse termination of callosal afferents in area 17 but major terminations near the borders of area 17 and adjacent areas 18 and 18a. These observations are consistent with previous degeneration and autoradiographic studies in the visual and other areas of rodent neocortex (1,115,152,186,262,372,471, 476). It is interesting to note that anatomical (187,188,372) and electrophysiological (143) data suggest that there are reciprocal callosal projections in the cortex such that cells in the superficial layers project to the upper layers of the contralateral hemisphere, whereas neurons in the deeper layers project to the contralateral deeper layers.

The electron microscopic study of Lund and Lund (262) in the rat occipital cortex has established that callosal fibers form type I synapses with somata and dendrites of nonpyramidal neurons as well as with shafts and spines of dendrites that could not be traced to the parent cells. Similar findings have been reported for the termination of callosal fibers in the visual cortex and in other functional areas in cat and monkey (115,198,421,435). Experiments that utilized the retrograde transport of horseradish peroxidase have shown that the cells that give rise to callosal connections in the rat and other species are present in layers II through VI but tend to be concentrated in layers III and V (136,168,188,403,413,471).

Ipsilateral Input

The degeneration studies of Nauta and Bucher (306) were the first to describe the connections between the striate (area 17) and peristriate areas (areas 18 and 18a) of the rat visual cortex. More recently, studies utilizing degeneration, autoradiography, and horseradish peroxidase histochemistry have shown that the extrastriate areas are reciprocally connected to the striate cortex (290, 292,318). An autoradiographic study by Ribak (372) has also demonstrated an ipsilateral corticocortical projection from area 18a to area 18.

Cortical Efferents

The corticofugal fibers arising in the rat visual cortex (striate and peristriate) have a wide distribution. Their target areas, which have been examined with various techniques, include the following structures: dorsal and ventral lateral geniculate nucleus, lateral posterior nucleus, thalamic reticular nucleus, zona inserta, superior colliculus, pretectal area, nucleus of the optic tract, pontine nuclei, and striatum (141,247,260,284, 306,316,372,399,408,463). The retrograde, horseradish peroxidase technique has been used to demonstrate the cells of origin of the descending fibers from the visual cortex. Fibers that descend to the dorsal lateral geniculate nucleus and the thalamic reticular nucleus arise from pyramidal neurons of layer VI (408), whereas fibers projecting to the superior colliculus, pons, and ventral lateral geniculate nucleus originate from pyramidal cells of layer V (284,400,408). It is not yet known whether an individual neuron projects to more than one subcortical area. Comparable patterns of termination have been reported for descending fibers in other sensory cortical areas of the rat (284,472) and in various sensory systems of other species (3,36, 135,165,166,200,211,263,400).

PUTATIVE NEUROTRANSMITTERS

Acetylcholine

Acetylcholine (ACh) has been studied extensively for many years. Consequently, there is a vast volume of literature on the distribution, function, and chemistry of the cholinergic system, which has been summarized in several reviews (60,93,116, 224,279,464).

The synthesis of ACh involves the transfer of an acetyl group from acetyl-CoA to choline; the reaction is catalyzed by choline acetyltransferase (ChAT). Acetylcholine is hydrolyzed by cholinesterase to form acetate and choline which is taken up and reused in the cholinergic terminal. Acetylcholinesterase (AChE) is found in all cholinergic and in some noncholinergic neurons. Contrary to the distribution of AChE, ChAT is restricted to cholinergic cells and their axons (386). Thus, the localization of ChAT is preferred as a marker for cholinergic neurons, not only because of the greater specificity but also because biochemical analysis reveals that the activity of this enzyme is considered to reflect changes in cholinergic activity. Recent studies have described the distribution of ChAT in the mammalian brain using immunocytochemical techniques (216,217). Based on these investigations and other anatomical and biochemical studies, it has been established that the magnocellular nuclei of the basal forebrain contain the cell bodies that provide the cholinergic innervation to the cerebral cortex (see above).

In 1963, Hebb and colleagues (151) reported that undercutting the cortex reduced ChAT activity by 90%. Furthermore, immunocytochemical studies performed in rat and cat (216,217) revealed a significant terminal innervation and several cholinoceptive neurons (cells with labeled ChAT terminals on the perikarya and proximal dendrites) but no labeled cell bodies in the cerebral cortex. We have recently measured ChAT activity in individual layers of the rat visual cortex (J. K. McDonald, S. G. Speciale, and J. G. Parnavelas, *unpublished observations*). The results show that layer V exhibits a slightly higher level of ChAT activity than the other cortical layers (Table 1). However, examination of the distribution of ChAT in the rat sensorimotor cortex has revealed greater activity in the more superficial layers (15). To date, nothing is known about the ultrastructural features of the cholinergic terminals.

It is likely that the ChAT-immunoreactive terminals observed by Kimura et al. (217) form synaptic contacts in the cerebral cortex. Several re-

TABLE 1. *Localization of GAD and ChAT activity in rat cortex*[a]

Layer	GAD	ChAT
I	945 ± 364	270 ± 43
II, III	1242 ± 199	249 ± 22
IV	1531 ± 132	244 ± 19
V	1166 ± 102	288 ± 17
VI	1058 ± 203	233 ± 42

[a]Glutamate decarboxylase (GAD) activity (dpm/µg protein/60 min) and choline acetyltransferase (ChAT) activity (dpm/µg protein/30 min) in laminae of the rat visual cortex. Each value represents the mean ± standard deviation of duplicate determinations of laminae from each of five rats.

ports describe the properties of cortical cholinergic synaptosomes (116,202). Briefly, evidence indicates that there is a low- and a high-affinity, sodium-dependent uptake mechanism for choline into synaptosomes (231). The high-affinity system is involved in providing choline for rapid synthesis of new ACh in the terminal (475). In addition, ACh can be released from cortical slices in the presence of calcium by electrical stimulation or potassium depolarization (70,116,230).

Investigators have attempted to examine the distribution of muscarinic receptors in the cortex using autoradiographic techniques (456,457) (Fig. 11). Results suggest that muscarinic sites are concentrated in layer IV of the rat parietal cortex. Recently, Westlind et al. (465) have reported that septal lesions or chronic atropine treatment increases the number of muscarinic receptors in the hippocampus. It would be interesting to determine if this type of muscarinic supersensitivity also occurs in the cerebral cortex and what effect this may have on cortical function. The cortex also contains a relatively low concentration of nicotinic receptors which vary in density among cortical regions (297) [see Morley and Kemp (296) for a review].

The neurophysiological effects of ACh on cortical neurons have been examined in detail (224,226,227,427,433). Iontophoretic studies indicate that cholinergic excitation of cortical cells is primarily muscarinic in character, is most clearly observed in cells located below layer III, and is especially exhibited by pyramidal cells (228). In contrast, some cells in the superficial layers of the cortex are depressed by ACh (64,227).

There is some evidence that supports an interaction between the cholinergic and noradrenergic systems in the brain. Neonatal 6-hydroxydopamine treatment has been reported to increase ChAT ac-

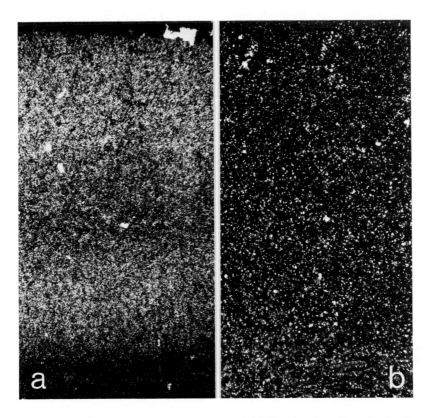

FIG. 11. Autoradiographic localization of muscarinic cholinergic binding sites throughout the visual cortex. **a:** Total binding in a section incubated with 1 nM tritiated *N*-methylscopolomine; layer V appears to have the lowest density of total binding sites. **b:** Section incubated with 1 nM tritiated *N*-methylscopolomine and 1 μM atropine to displace the specific binding of the label. ×60. (Courtesy of J. K. Wamsley.)

tivity in the brainstem and cortex of the rat (28,189). However, our observations indicate that neonatal 6-hydroxydopamine treatment does not affect the normal development of ChAT activity in the visual cortex or dorsal lateral geniculate nucleus of the rat (J. K. McDonald, S. G. Speciale, and J. G. Parnavelas, *unpublished observations*). Some studies suggest that norepinephrine may affect the synthesis (159) and release (11,455) of ACh in the cerebral cortex. Norepinephrine, dopamine, and serotonin have been reported to decrease the excitatory response of cortical neurons to ACh (366), although other studies suggest that norepinephrine facilitates cholinergic transmission in the cortex (461). Recently, Palmer et al. (329) have observed that cholinergic stimulation of cortical slices increases cyclic guanosine monophosphate (cyclic GMP) production and inhibits the norepinephrine-induced accumulation of cyclic adenosine monophosphate (cyclic AMP). Further research is needed to clarify this hypothesized as-

sociation between adrenergic and cholinergic systems in the cortex.

Acetylcholine has been found to stimulate the release of somatostatin from cerebral cortical neurons in culture (379). The cerebral cortex contains several types of peptide-containing neurons (see below). The regulation of peptide release by ACh and other putative neurotransmitters promises to be an interesting area of investigation which may provide clues concerning the functional relationships of these substances in the cortex.

Amino Acids

Gamma-aminobutyric Acid

The evidence that suggests that γ-aminobutyric acid (GABA) is a major inhibitory neurotransmitter in the cerebral cortex has been summarized in a number of excellent books and review articles (65,181,224,310,376).

The pathway for the synthesis of GABA in the nervous system involves the decarboxylation of glutamic acid by the enzyme glutamate decarboxylase (GAD). Glutamate decarboxylase exhibits a high degree of substrate specificity and requires pyridoxal phosphate as a cofactor. Catabolism of GABA is accomplished primarily through transamination with α-ketoglutarate by the enzyme GABA α-ketoglutarate aminotransferase, which is known as GABA-transaminase (GABA-T). This enzyme is found in mitochondria of neurons and glial cells, in contrast to GAD which has been localized in cell bodies and axons of neurons that synthesize GABA (181).

Glutamate decarboxylase activity and GABA have been measured in the cortex of several species (68,158,273). In an early study, Hirsch and Robins (158) reported relatively equal concentrations of GABA throughout the superficial layers and significantly reduced amounts in the lower layers of the monkey visual cortex. Recent measurements of GAD activity in individual layers of the rat visual cortex (J. K. McDonald, S. G. Speciale, and J. G. Parnavelas, *unpublished observations*) indicate a fairly even distribution throughout the cortex, with somewhat higher levels in layer IV (Table 1). Ribak (373), using immunocytochemical methods, has localized GAD in somata, dendrites, and axon terminals of nonpyramidal neurons in the visual cortex of the rat (Figs. 12,13). Labeled cells are fairly evenly distributed throughout all cortical layers in rats injected with colchicine, but very few immunoreactive somata are seen in rats without prior colchicine treatment. In contrast, clear laminar differences in the distribution of GAD-positive cell bodies and terminals have been observed in the visual cortex of the monkey (154). Ribak's findings show that labeled cells possess round or fusiform cell bodies of various orientations. Round somata are associated with dendrites that radiate in all directions, whereas fusiform perikarya often exhibit a bipolar dendritic appearance (Fig. 12). Accurate correlations between the appearance of GAD-positive cells and Golgi descriptions of nonpyramidal neurons can not be accomplished because staining is limited to perikarya and proximal dendrites. The GAD-positive terminals commonly form type II synaptic contacts with dendritic shafts and perikarya of pyramidal and nonpyramidal neurons and occasionally with dendritic spines and axon initial segments of pyramidal neurons (Fig. 13a). In view of recent reports that describe the coexistence of GAD-like and motilin-like immunoreactivities in cerebellar Purkinje neurons (49), it would be interesting to examine the possible coexistence of GAD and various peptides observed in cortical nonpyramidal cells (274–277).

Another approach used to examine GABA-containing neurons utilizes cortical superfusion or injection of tritiated GABA followed by autoradiography (51–53,161,425,426). This technique, when combined with the Golgi method, allows for visualization of the morphology of labeled neurons (425). Overall, these uptake studies support the immunocytochemical observations of Ribak (373).

A variety of techniques have been applied to examine the release of GABA from the cerebral cortex (55,67,70,130,204,288). In 1971, Iversen and associates (183) demonstrated the release of GABA from the cat visual cortex during electrical stimulation. This finding was later supported by studies in the rat visual cortex (55,57) that showed a calcium-dependent release of GABA during spreading depression, potassium stimulation, electrical stimulation of the contralateral cortex, and stimulation with calcium ionophores. Veratridine and potassium stimulation of tissue slices of rat visual cortex evoke a pronounced release of GABA which can be blocked by low calcium/high magnesium or tetrodotoxin (10).

The uptake of GABA at the synapse appears to be the major mode of inactivation (22,182,235, 384). This net uptake of GABA by a high-affinity mechanism is sodium and energy dependent as well as temperature sensitive. The binding of GABA to postsynaptic receptors isolated from the cortex has been examined in several reports (71,103,146,244) [see also Nistri and Constanti (310) for an excellent review]. Recently, Wamsley et al. (457) have attempted to visualize high-affinity GABA receptor sites in the cerebral cortex of the rat using tissue slices exposed to tritiated muscimol and subsequently processed for autoradiography. They reported a high concentration of tritiated muscimol binding sites in layers I through IV, with fewer sites distributed over layers V and VI.

The neurophysiological effects of GABA in the cerebral cortex have been examined by several investigators. These findings support a role for GABA as a major cortical inhibitory transmitter (224,225). Much of this work has been performed in the visual cortex of the cat (157,382,415, 416,444), where GABA appears to exert inhibitory influences on the response properties of cells. Iontophoretic application of the GABA antagonist bicuculline decreases orientation and direction specificity of simple and complex cells and affects the inhibitory end zones of hypercomplex neurons

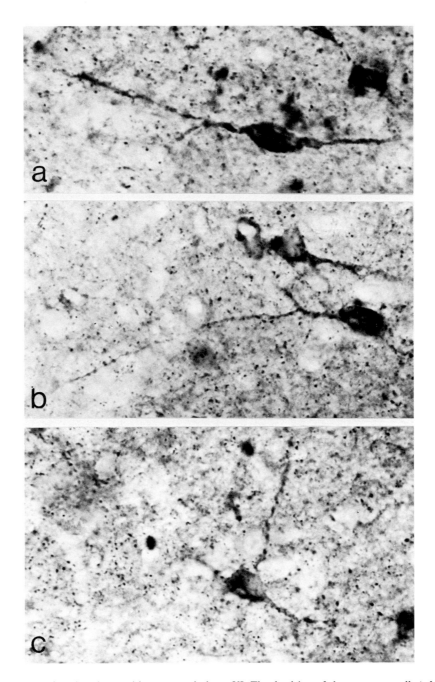

FIG. 12. Glutamate decarboxylase-positive neurons in layer VI. The dendrites of the upper two cells (**a,b**) are horizontally oriented, whereas the dendrites of the lower cell (**c**) are directed radially. ×750. (From Ribak, ref. 373, with permission.)

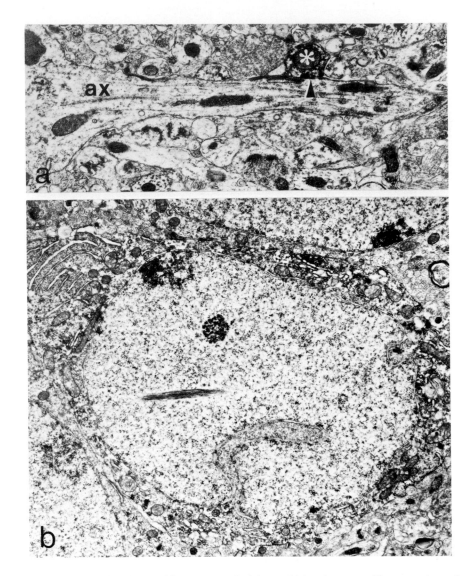

FIG. 13. a: Glutamate decarboxylase-positive axon terminal *(asterisk)* forming a type II synapse *(arrowhead)* with an initial axon segment (ax) of a layer II pyramidal cell. ×13,500. **b:** A GAD-positive soma containing reaction product in the perinuclear cytoplasm. ×8,200. (From Ribak, ref. 373, with permission.)

(350,382,415–417,444). Additional reports indicate that GABA may also be involved in the ocular dominance shift that occurs in the cat visual cortex following mononular eyelid suture (87,336).

Glutamate

The research that supports a role for glutamate as an excitatory neurotransmitter in the nervous system is quite extensive and has been reviewed by several authors (65,93,105,224).

Glutamate is rapidly produced from glucose via the Krebs cycle (279), and recent evidence, obtained in the hippocampus, indicates that glutamine uptake and the activity of glutaminase may be important in the rate of glutamate synthesis in the readily releasable pool (147,148). Glutamate is metabolized via several routes which include decarboxylation by GAD to GABA and transamination by glutamine synthetase to glutamine (65,224). Cortical synaptosomes possess a high-affinity, sodium-dependent uptake mechanism for glutamate and aspartate (22,254,384). Glutamate can be released by electrical or potassium stimulation of cortical slices (67) or by potassium stimulation of the exposed cerebral cortex in the intact rat (298). Jasper and Koyama (190) observed an increase in measured cortical glutamate release in response to stimulation of the reticular formation but not following stimulation of the medial thalamus in the spinal cat. A few descriptions of glutamate receptors have appeared in the literature (377,395,409), but there are several problems associated with measurements of these receptors (310,409). The location and distribution of glutamate receptors in the cerebral cortex has not been investigated.

Iontophoretic application of small amounts of glutamate to cortical neurons has been shown repeatedly to produce a rapid and strong excitation (223,225,226). The excitatory effects of glutamate have been verified in cat visual cortex (157). The reported effects include an increase in the diameter of the cells' excitatory receptive fields and an enhancement of the response amplitudes within the excitatory receptive fields. Using the cortical cup technique, Clark and Collins (55) observed a calcium-dependent, potassium-stimulated release of glutamate in the rat visual cortex. These investigators also reported that electrical stimulation of the visual cortex ipsilateral to the cortical cup results in a significant increase in the release of glutamate, whereas stimulation of the contralateral side produces a decline. Stimulation of glutamate release from the rat visual cortex by calcium ionophores has also been observed (57). The subcellular distribution of glutamate in homogenates of monkey occipital cortex provides additional support for glutamate as a putative neurotransmitter in this region (361).

A few studies have examined glutamate and aspartate as possible neurotransmitters contained in corticofugal fibers (9,10,37,117,264). Lund-Karlsen and Fonnum (264) found that unilateral ablation of the visual cortex in the rat results in a decline in the high-affinity uptake of D-aspartate and L-glutamate in the ipsilateral lateral geniculate nucleus and superior colliculus, although uptake in the contralateral visual cortex was unaffected. These authors also reported that the levels of L-glutamate were reduced significantly in the ipsilateral superior colliculus and lateral geniculate nucleus following unilateral ablation of the visual cortex, although the level of L-aspartate remained unchanged. These findings suggest that L-glutamate is the transmitter in these corticofugal fibers. In contrast, the work of Baughman and Gilbert (9,10)

in the cat and rat suggests that corticofugal fibers to the superior colliculus do not utilize glutamate or aspartate as a neurotransmitter. However, injection of these substances (labeled D-aspartate and D-glutamate) into the lateral geniculate nucleus results in labeling of layer VI pyramidal neurons. In addition, potassium or veratridine stimulation of rat visual cortical slices stimulates the release of glutamate and aspartate which can be blocked by low calcium/high magnesium or tetrodotoxin. The results of these studies suggest that layer VI pyramids that project to the lateral geniculate nucleus may use glutamate or aspartate as their transmitter.

Aspartate

Much of the research concerning the localization of aspartate in the brain has been performed in conjunction with studies on glutamate, and often there are striking similarities in the distribution, uptake, release, and neurophysiological effects of these two substances (65,93,105,224). Iontophoretic application of aspartate excites cortical neurons (226), and, like glutamate, it is released from the cerebral cortex of the spinal cat following stimulation of the reticular formation (190). Aspartate is released from the intact rat visual cortex by a calcium-dependent potassium depolarization, by calcium ionophores, and by electrical stimulation (55,57). Stimulation of the contralateral cortex significantly decreases the release of aspartate (55). Aspartate release has also been demonstrated in cortical synaptosomes (70). These synaptosomes possess a high-affinity sodium- and energy-dependent mechanism for aspartate uptake which may be involved in its rapid inactivation (22,105,254, 385). Stimulation of rat visual cortical slices with veratridine or potassium produces a marked release of aspartate into the medium (10). Although the evidence listed above suggests that aspartate may be a cortical neurotransmitter, unequivocal evidence demonstrating responsiveness in physiological situations remains to be established.

Taurine

Although some evidence indicates that taurine may possess features exhibited by other putative neurotransmitters, its role in the nervous system remains unknown. Taurine is found in high concentrations in the cortex and can be released by electrical stimulation and potassium depolarization of the visual cortex (10,190,205). However, results concerning taurine release are somewhat controversial (9,10,55,57). A possible explanation for the contradictory findings may be due to difficulties encountered in the measurement of taurine. Tachiki and Baxter (437) have recently claimed that glycerophosphoryl ethanolamine is a major contaminant of the taurine peak measured by ion-exchange chromatography.

Autoradiographic studies indicate that taurine is taken up by neurons and glia in the central nervous system (32,169). Recent research suggests that this amino acid may play an important role in development. Studies in monkey occipital cortex (361) show that taurine is present in large amounts in early life and declines gradually later in development (131,434).

Monoamines

Norepinephrine

The basic biochemistry and physiology of norepinephrine (NE) have been reviewed extensively by Van Dongen (452), Dahlström (68), and Cooper et al. (60). The biosynthesis of NE from tyrosine occurs in several stages. First, tyrosine is converted to L-DOPA by the action of tyrosine hydroxylase which is the rate-limiting step in the biosynthetic pathway. DOPA decarboxylase synthesizes dopamine from L-DOPA, after which dopamine is rapidly converted to NE by dopamine-β-hydroxylase which is found in noradrenergic cell bodies, axons, and axon terminals. Norepinephrine is stored in vesicles which provide protection against degradation by monoamine oxidase. Once released, NE can either combine with a pre- or postsynaptic α or β receptor, be metabolized by catechol-O-methyltransferase, or be rapidly inactivated by uptake into the presynaptic terminal for subsequent utilization.

The noradrenergic fibers originate in the locus ceruleus in the pons and follow various pathways to enter the neocortex where they undergo extensive arborization [see Emson and Lindvall (93), and Moore and Bloom (294) for reviews of pathways]. The distribution and orientation of the noradrenergic axons in the rat neocortex have been examined by the use of the Falck–Hillarp formaldehyde method (122,123), the glyoxylic acid method (245,252), and, recently, by immunofluorescence (300,302). These studies show that the orientation of fibers displays fairly consistent features throughout the cortex. Specifically, layer VI is characterized by predominantly horizontal fibers, layers IV and V exhibit primarily obliquely oriented fibers, and layers II and III contain radially oriented axons. Many of these axons appear to

continue into layer I where they arborize into horizontal branches that form a dense plexus (Fig. 14).

Attempts have been made by many investigators to precisely describe the density of the noradrenergic innervation in various layers of the mammalian neocortex. Existing studies show that the noradrenergic innervation varies in density and laminar distribution from area to area. For example, Morrison and colleagues (300) have observed that the outer half of the rat visual cortex is more densely innervated than the infragranular layers, which is opposite to the pattern observed in somatosensory and motor cortices. Careful analysis of immunocytochemical preparations of rat visual cortex by Molliver and Grzanna (M. E. Molliver, personal communication) has shown that within this cortical area, layer V consistently has the lowest density of noradrenergic axons (Fig. 14). In cat visual cortex, measurement of endogenous norepinephrine by a radiometric assay (365) as well as glyoxylic acid histofluorescence (179) have both shown the highest levels to be in the superficial layers. The primate cerebral cortex appears to exhibit far greater laminar and regional differences in the pattern of innervation than the rat cortex (39,138,301,304,364). In a recent immunocytochemical study using an antiserum directed against dopamine-β-hydroxylase, Morrison et al. (304) has shown that the overall noradrenergic innervation is low in area 17 compared to other primary sensory areas of the monkey neocortex. Their results show that layers III, V, and VI receive the heaviest NE innervation, whereas layer IV contains extremely few noradrenergic fibers. The innervation of layer I is relatively sparse.

Despite extensive efforts by several laboratories, descriptions of the ultrastructural features of noradrenergic axon terminals in the cerebral cortex remain controversial. Four techniques have been used to visualize these terminals in the cortex and in other areas of the central nervous system: (a) potassium permanganate fixation (160,219), (b) pretreatment with a histochemical marker, 5-hydroxydopamine (29,375), (c) superfusion or intraventricular injection of tritiated norepinephrine followed by electron microscopic autoradiography (73), and (d) dopamine-β-hydroxylase immunocytochemistry (322). Descarries and colleagues (74,76,238) have reported that superfusion of the rat cortex (frontoparietal) with tritiated norepinephrine selectively labels cortical axons and terminals. Of the labeled terminals, only 5% form synapses with specialized membrane appositions. In cat visual cortex, Itakura et al. (179), using tissue fixed with glyoxylic acid perfusion followed by

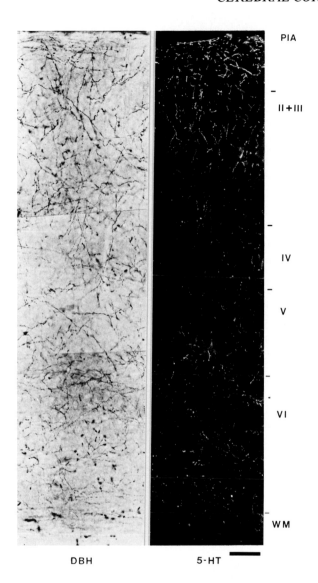

PIA

II + III

IV

V

VI

WM

DBH   5-HT

FIG. 14. Monoaminergic innervation of visual cortex in the albino rat. Serotonin (5-HT) immunofluorescence (**right**) shows a medium density of labeled axons in layer I and somewhat less in II and III. The infragranular layers have a lower density than elsewhere in the cortex, and, in area 17, layer IV has the lowest density. The noradrenergic innervation is shown by dopamine-β-hydroxylase (DBH) immunocytochemistry (**left**) using the peroxidase–antiperoxidase technique. There is a moderate density of varicose positive axons ramifying in all cortical layers, and there are considerably more noradrenergic than serotonergic axons in layer IV. Analysis of many sections indicates that within the visual cortex, layer V consistently has the lowest density of noradrenergic axons. *Bar*, 100 μm. (Courtesy of M. E. Molliver and R. Grzanna.)

immersion in potassium permanganate, reported that a similarly low percentage (10%) of noradrenergic terminals form conventional synapses.

However, studies that utilized administration of exogenous catecholaminergic markers or immunocytochemistry have produced significantly different findings. In the cerebral cortex of the immature rat, systemic administration of 5-hydroxydopamine reveals presumptive noradrenergic terminals as identified by the presence of small granular vesicles. In these young animals (less than 1 week of age), the majority of terminals form Gray's type I synapses with dendritic elements (63,289,480).

More recently, Olschowka et al. (322,324) employed dopamine-β-hydroxylase immunocyto-chemistry to examine the ultrastructural features of noradrenergic terminals in various areas of the adult rat brain including the cerebral cortex. Their findings show that the majority of all labeled terminals form axodendritic synapses characterized by synaptic vesicles and specialized membrane appositions. These authors concluded, contrary to the reports of others, that formation of synaptic contacts is a general feature of the noradrenergic innervation in the brain.

We have recently undertaken the task of repeating the experiments of Descarries and co-workers in the visual cortex of the rat. We have used both topical and intraventricular administration of tritiated norepinephrine to examine labeled terminals with the electron microscope. Our findings, in accordance with the immunocytochemical observations of Olschowka et al. (322,324), show that these axon terminals are scattered throughout the cortex, with the majority forming type I synapses with spines and dendritic shafts of unknown origin

(Fig. 15a,b) (J. G. Parnavelas and H. C. Moises, *unpublished data*).

Neurochemists, neuropharmacologists, and neurophysiologists have compiled an enormous body of data concerning noradrenergic receptors in the brain, and many of these studies have focused spe-

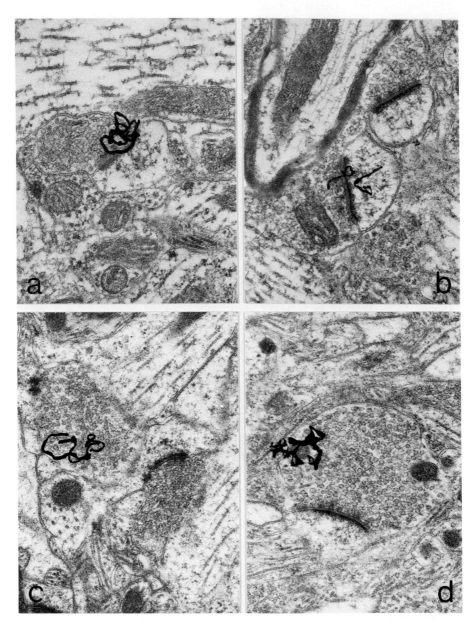

FIG. 15. a,b: Labeled terminals in the visual cortex after superfusion of the cortex with tritiated norepinephrine. Both terminals establish type I synapses with dendritic spines. **c,d:** Labeled terminals after superfusion of the cortex with tritiated serotonin. One of the terminals (**d**) forms a type I synapse with a dendritic spine. ×32,000. (From J. G. Parnavelas and H. C. Moises, *unpublished data*.)

cifically on the cerebral cortex (237,369,405). Both α- and β-adrenergic receptors have been described in the cortex (369), and these classes have been further subdivided into α_1, α_2, β_1, and β_2 receptors (44,237,285,286,299,369,444). Existing reports suggest that cortical β receptors are predominantly postsynaptic in location and that the β_1 subclass is responsive to changes in noradrenergic input, whereas the β_2 subclass is often called "nonneuronal" and may be responsive to other signals (287). The β_1 receptors predominate in the cortex (44) and comprise about 85% of the total β-receptor population (285–287). The α_1 receptors have been thought to be postsynaptic, and the α_2 receptor presynaptic in location (237), although recent findings (369) indicate that α_2 receptors may also be postsynaptic.

The few anatomical studies that have attempted to localize adrenergic receptors in specific layers of the cortex have used autoradiography to visualize binding sites for tritiated ligands (325,457) or β antagonists labeled with fluorescent markers (282). Recent reports have described a fairly uniform distribution of binding sites with a slightly higher concentration in layers I and III (325,457). In contrast, Melamed and colleagues (282) observed labeling extending from the deep aspect of layer II to layer VI, whereas the superficial part of layer II and layer I exhibited negligible fluorescence. These contradictory findings may be caused by nonspecific binding of ligands to other receptors. In an autoradiographic examination of noradrenergic α_1 and α_2 receptors, Young and Kuhar (477) observed moderate to low levels of cortical binding for each ligand, with slightly higher labeling for tritiated aminoclonidine (α_2 ligand) in the superficial layers.

Although regional differences in NE concentrations have been reported in the cerebral cortex (39,138,364), little is known about variations in receptor density that may exist among cortical areas. A recent comparison of β-adrenergic receptors in samples of rat visual cortex and whole cortex using the high-affinity ligand [^{125}I]cyanopindolol (100) revealed no significant differences in the affinity or density of these receptors (278).

Beta-adrenergic receptors respond to a variety of substances and particularly to NE. Noradrenergic denervation causes an increase in the density of cortical β receptors and a supersensitivity of adenylate cyclase to β-receptor stimulation (180, 328,428,429). Recently, Schliebs et al. (398) observed no changes in the affinity or density of β receptors in the visual cortex of rats following monocular deprivation; however, striking changes were

measured in the lateral geniculate nucleus. The effects of various manipulations of normal visual input on cortical α receptors have not been reported. The response of cortical α receptors to adrenergic denervation is somewhat controversial (170,419,448) and awaits final clarification.

The action of norepinephrine on cortical neurons has been investigated repeatedly during the last two decades. Most cells in the mammalian cerebral cortex either increase or decrease their spontaneous discharges following iontophoretic application of norepinephrine [see Krnjević (224) and Van Dongen (452) for reviews; also see refs. 118,266,267,362,366,473]. Interest in the role of norepinephrine in cortical information processing has never been greater than at present. This spurt of interest has come about partly by the fascinating suggestion of Kasamatsu and colleagues (206, 208,209) that neuronal plasticity in young kittens is controlled, at least to some extent, by the noradrenergic system. Furthermore, norepinephrine has been found to exert an influence in the process of synapse formation in early life (30,333). The cellular mechanisms responsible for these effects during development remain unknown.

Efforts to elucidate the mechanisms responsible for the observed cortical plasticity have concentrated on understanding the way norepinephrine influences the functional properties of single cells in the visual cortex. In the cat, these cells either increase, decrease, or do not change their visual responsiveness following iontophoretic application of norepinephrine (207). Simple cells tend to be more sensitive to norepinephrine than complex cells, a finding similar to that reported briefly for cells in rat visual cortex following stimulation of the locus ceruleus (266). Most cells that alter their visual responsiveness display a relative enhancement of signal-to-noise ratio, a result consistent with the suggestion that norepinephrine modulates neuronal firing by suppressing background spontaneous activity more than evoked activity (118,120,366, 460,473). Recent experiments suggest that NE may facilitate excitatory ACh transmission within the cortex through postsynaptic α receptors (461) and that NE may enhance inhibitory (GABA) synaptic mechanisms by stimulating β receptors (462).

Serotonin

Little is known about the organization and function of the serotonergic system in the cerebral cortex compared to the catecholamine projection systems. The following is a brief account of the biosynthetic pathway of serotonin. Tryptophan is taken up by neurons and converted to 5-hydroxytryptophan by the enzyme tryptophan hydroxylase, the rate-limiting enzyme in the synthesis of serotonin [see Mandell (270) for review]. 5-Hydroxytryptophan decarboxylase rapidly converts 5-hydroxytryptophan to serotonin which is then metabolized primarily by monoamine oxidase A to 5-hydroxyindoleacetaldehyde; this substance is converted to 5-hydroxyindoleacetic acid or 5-hydroxytryptophol.

It is well established that serotonergic terminals contain tryptophan hydroxylase and an efficient uptake system for serotonin. Furthermore, lesions produce a marked decrease in tryptophan hydroxylase and high-affinity uptake (41,232–234,422). Serotonin can be released from synaptosomes by a calcium-dependent potassium stimulation (339) or by electrical stimulation of cortical slices (90,91). Serotonin release and synthesis may be closely linked to the ionic nature of depolarization (90,91) and may not be as dependent on tryptophan availability as previously thought.

Serotonergic fibers originate in the medial and dorsal raphe nuclei and ascend to the neocortex via the medial forebrain bundle (4,6,59,246,295,330). The serotonergic innervation of the rat cerebral cortex has been examined with immunocytochemistry (246). This study shows that serotonin-containing axons are finer and more dense and tortuous than noradrenergic fibers. Although regional differences have been reported in the rat (363,364), the innervation of most cortical areas including the visual cortex appears to be uniform except for a slight preponderance of axons in layer I (246). This differs from earlier reports that indicate that this projection is primarily concentrated in layer I (124). A recent examination that concentrated on the visual cortex has shown that layer IV contains the lowest density of serotonergic fibers (Fig. 14) (M. E. Molliver, *personal communication*). The pattern of serotonin innervation in the rat differs considerably from that in the primate. A recent immunocytochemical study in the monkey visual cortex by Morrison et al. (304) has shown the projection to be sparse in layers V and VI but very dense in layer IV, a pattern complementary to that exhibited by the noradrenergic innervation.

Descarries and colleagues (12,13,75) have reported that prolonged topical application of tritiated serotonin on the rat cortex (frontoparietal) labels axonal processes in layers I through V, which exhibit regularly spaced varicosities. Only a small proportion (5%) of these varicosities have been reported to display features of typical synaptic terminals. We have recently sought to investigate the ultrastructural features of serotonin-containing terminals in the visual cortex of rats after topical or intraventricular injections of tritiated serotonin. Our findings clearly show, contrary to the reports of Descarries and colleagues, that serotonin is present in large vesicle-containing terminals which form type I synapses with spines and dendritic shafts throughout the cortex (Fig. 15c,d) (J. G. Parnavelas and H.C. Moises, *unpublished data*).

Serotonin receptors are present in high concentrations in the cortex (23,24). They appear to be enriched in synaptosome fractions (111) and are associated with a serotonin-sensitive adenylate cyclase (101,102,453). Several studies indicate that serotonin denervation resulting from administration of the neurotoxin 5,7-dihydroxytryptamine or lesions of the midbrain raphe nuclei produces a supersensitivity response with an increase in the number of high-affinity binding sites or in the sensitivity of neurons to the application of serotonin (110,149,308,321,407,459). However, De Montigny et al. (72) have suggested that these effects may not apply to all regions of the brain, as they were not observed in hippocampal pyramidal cells. Additional research has shown that repeated treatment with D-fenfluramine (392), which releases serotonin, or with monoamine oxidase inhibitors (396) decreases the number of binding sites in the cortex. However, inhibition of serotonin uptake with fluoxitine appears inadequate to cause subsensitivity (268).

There are few reports concerning the laminar or cellular distribution of serotonin receptors in the cortex. A recent autoradiographic study indicates a higher density of sites in layers III and IV at which labeling could be blocked by serotonin (281). Additional biochemical and anatomical research is needed to elucidate the laminar distribution of serotonin receptors.

Neurophysiological studies suggest that iontophoresis of serotonin decreases the spontaneous activity of cortical neurons (110,362). This response is enhanced by prior treatment with 5,7-dihydroxytryptamine or *para*-chlorophenylalanine. There is some evidence to suggest that alterations in serotonin availability affect the responsiveness of cortical neurons to other neurotransmitters (110,474), although opposite effects have been observed in the amygdala (459).

Dopamine

In contrast to the widespread innervation to all cortical regions by noradrenergic and serotonergic fibers, the dopaminergic innervation appears to be primarily restricted to frontal and limbic areas [see Moore and Bloom (293) and Emson and Lindvall (93) for reviews]. Recent biochemical studies have measured only small amounts of dopamine within the visual cortex (327,364). The reader is referred to the reviews of Emson and Lindvall (93) and Moore and Bloom (293) for details concerning this projection system.

Histamine

It appears that histamine may be another transmitter candidate in the cerebral cortex (8,93,404,406). Convincing immunocytochemical descriptions of histamine in the cerebral cortex have not appeared in the literature. One study (326) has attempted to visualize H_1 receptors using autoradiography to examine the distribution of tritiated mepyramine binding in rat brain slices. Results suggest a prominent band of labeling located in layer IV that is higher in rostral and temporal cortical areas and lower in more caudal areas. The exact contribution of nonneuronal elements to the overall binding of tritiated mepyramine in the cortex is not clear.

Peptides

Somatostatin

Somatostatin (SRIF) activity was first observed in hypothalamic extracts from rat and sheep (229,272), and its chemical nature was subsequently determined (35,43,449). It is composed of 14 amino acids and may be derived from a larger precursor molecule composed of 28 amino acids, SRIF-28 (242,337,338,381,397). Somatostatin has been localized in a variety of sites throughout the gut and central nervous system by radioimmunoassay and immunocytochemistry (5,25,40, 61,104,112,113,162,218,438). Several investigators have demonstrated the presence of SRIF in the neocortex. These immunocytochemical studies have provided divergent views regarding the cellular localization and distribution of SRIF-like immunoreactivity (25,109,113,222,236,303,438). Our observations in the visual cortex of the rat indicate that SRIF-immunoreactive neurons are present in layers II through VI and are concentrated in layers II and III (274). These cells exhibit morphologies typical of multipolar and bitufted forms of nonpyramidal neurons (Fig. 16).

Multipolar neurons comprise the majority of SRIF-immunoreactive neurons and display considerable variation in perikaryal form, size, and dendritic morphology. Based on dendritic morphology, three subgroups of multipolar neurons may be distinguished. The first subgroup includes cells whose dendrites radiate in all directions from the cell body (Fig. 16a; also see Figs. 5 and 6). Notable within this subgroup of SRIF-immunoreactive neurons are large cells scattered throughout layer V. The second subgroup exhibits a conspicuous absence of descending dendrites (Fig. 16c; also cell e in Fig. 5). The third subgroup includes multipolar cells, found predominantly in the deeper layers, which display an overall horizontal orientation (see Fig. 7). The axons of some of these horizontal cells appear to enter the subcortical white matter.

Other investigators (25,236) have reported that SRIF immunoreactivity is not only localized in nonpyramidal neurons but also in cortical pyramidal cells. Controversy also exists regarding the laminar distribution of SRIF-immunoreactive neurons in various layers of the cortex. Some investigators (25,274,303) have observed labeled neurons in layers II through VI with the highest concentration in layers II and III, whereas others have indicated no laminar differences (109) or high concentrations mainly in layers V and VI (113,438). These variations may be attributed to differences in antisera employed, fixation procedures, or cortical areas examined.

Although the precise role of SRIF in the cerebral cortex is unknown, evidence suggests that SRIF may affect synaptic transmission. Relevant data include the presence of SRIF in synaptosomes, the effect of potassium on stimulating SRIF release, and the influence of somatostatin on calcium uptake (21,104,184,439). Furthermore, Peterfreund and Vale (340) have reported that SRIF-28 is a major secretory product of dispersed cortical cells. Biogenic amines have been demonstrated to affect the release of SRIF, and some studies indicate that SRIF itself may release biogenic amines (440). It has been observed recently (77,379) that dispersed cortical cells increase the secretion of SRIF following cholinergic stimulation and decrease SRIF secretion in response to GABA. Cortical receptors have been demonstrated for SRIF and the larger precursor form, SRIF-28 (371,430,431).

Neurophysiological experiments utilizing iontophoresis have provided contradictory results. Whereas some studies have reported excitatory effects of SRIF on cortical pyramidal cells (178,320), others have observed inhibitory effects on parietal cortical neurons (370). Both effects have been observed in the hippocampus (81,358).

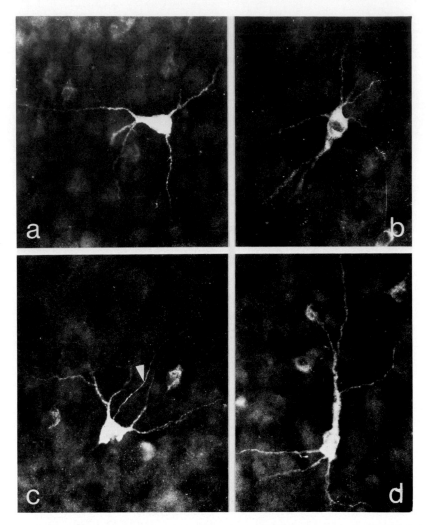

FIG. 16. Examples of somatostatin-immunoreactive neurons in the visual cortex of young rats. Labeled with the immunofluorescence technique. *Arrowhead* points to an axon. ×450. (From McDonald et al., ref. 274, with permission.)

The role of SRIF in the cerebral cortex awaits final clarification.

Vasoactive Intestinal Polypeptide

Vasoactive intestinal polypeptide (VIP) was originally isolated from the porcine duodenum by Said and Mutt (387,388). It contains 28 amino acids (305) and resembles secretin, glucagon, and gastric inhibitory peptide in composition/size (79).

Several investigators have measured high concentrations of VIP in the neocortex (26, 94,107,164,255,280,393,394), and some have examined the cells that exhibit VIP immunoreactivity (94,126,164,255,269,275,303,418). Immuno-

cytochemical studies in our laboratory have recently shown that neurons that display VIP immunoreactivity comprise approximately 3% of the neuronal population in the visual cortex (275). Their cell bodies are located in layers II through VI but are concentrated in layers II and III. These are all nonpyramidal neurons and are predominantly of the bipolar variety (Fig. 17a). Bipolar neurons, which resemble some bipolar forms described in Golgi preparations (108) (see Fig. 9), display a vertical orientation. These cells possess an ascending dendrite that commonly forms a subpial tuft in layers I and II (Fig. 17b) and a descending dendrite that gives rise to branches oriented obliquely or at right angles as it courses through layers IV and V (Fig. 17c). These results are in general agreement with the findings of Lorén et al. (255).

The other group of VIP-labeled cells are small multipolar neurons distributed in layers II through VI but predominantly located in layers II and VI. These cells, which have not been described in the studies of Morrison et al. (303), tend to have small perikarya and short dendrites which radiate from the cell body in several directions. Comparable

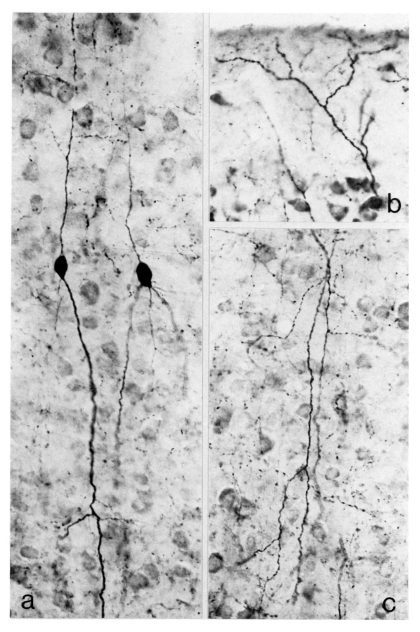

FIG. 17. a: Typical VIP-immunoreactive bipolar neuron in layer IV of an adult animal. **b:** Portion of a subpial tuft formed by the ascending process of a bipolar cell. **c:** Typical descending processes of bipolar cells displaying the characteristic branching pattern in layers IV and V. Peroxidase–antiperoxidase technique. ×450. (From McDonald et al., ref. 275, with permission.)

cells have been observed by Lorén et al. (255) in their preparations of rodent brain.

The results of several studies support a role for VIP as a potential neuromodulator or neurotransmitter (95,106,389). Cortical VIP has been found in synaptosomes and can be released by a calcium-dependent potassium depolarization (133,134). Furthermore, VIP receptors and a VIP-sensitive adenylate cyclase have been described (33, 360,378,441), and a few studies indicate that VIP exerts excitatory effects when iontophoretically applied to cortical and hippocampal neurons (83,352,354). Although these neurochemical and electrophysiological investigations suggest that VIP may influence synaptic transmission, its precise role in the cortex remains unknown.

Cholecystokinin

Cholecystokinin (CCK) is yet another "gut peptide" that has been found in abundance throughout the brain (7,16–19,92,98,132,145,276,367). In fact, the cerebral cortical concentration of CCK is the highest in the body (80,367). Biochemical studies indicate that CCK undergoes considerable enzymatic processing in the cortex from the CCK-variant form of 39 amino acids (which contains a hexapeptide extension on the amino terminal of CCK-33) though the CCK form containing 33 residues to the subsequent carboxyl terminal fragments 12, 8, and 4 amino acids in length (80, 139,140,367,368). The predominant form of CCK (depending on the method of cortical extraction) appears to be the octapeptide CCK-8.

Our studies in the rat visual cortex indicate that CCK-immunoreactive cells comprise approximately 1% of the neuronal population in this region (276). They are nonpyramidal cells whose perikarya are distributed in all cortical layers, with the majority identified in layers II and III. Most CCK-labeled cells are of the bitufted variety of nonpyramidal neurons (Fig. 18a,b), although a substantial number of multipolar cells are also present (Fig. 18c,d). Bitufted cells may be found in all layers but are more frequently seen in layers II and III. One or two dendrites extend from each pole of the vertically oriented perikaryon and usually divide close to the soma into branches that form superficial and deep dendritic tufts of almost equal length (Fig. 18a,b). The axons of these bitufted neurons and their collaterals form a fine network throughout the cortex which is particularly dense in layers II and III. Cholecystokinin-immunoreactive neurons are observed routinely in layer I which is sparsely populated by nerve cells. The bitufted

and multipolar varieties of labeled cells are present in this layer. In addition, other forms unique to layer I are identified. They include the persisting horizontal cells (Fig. 18d; see also Fig. 10c) and the vertically oriented neurons (see Fig. 10d). A few studies have briefly described CCK-labeled neurons in the cerebral cortex of the rat and guinea pig, and these descriptions agree in some respects with the observations presented here (95,97,175, 239,256).

The precise function of CCK in the cortex is unknown at the present time. Newly synthesized CCK-8 and CCK-4 have been localized in cortical synaptosomes (139,140) and can be released by calcium-dependent potassium depolarization (84, 96,356,357). The CCK-8 appears to be the major form that is released from rat and cat cortex *in vitro* and *in vivo* (283,458). Several studies indicate a high concentration of CCK receptors in the cerebral cortex (150,176,390,432,479), and recently, Innis et al. (177), using autoradiographic techniques, have demonstrated a high density of CCK receptors in layers IV and VI of the cerebral cortex. Finally, a preliminary investigation suggests that iontophoretic application of CCK excites cerebral cortical neurons (354). Similar effects have been observed in the hippocampus (82,212).

Avian Pancreatic Polypeptide

Avian pancreatic polypeptide (APP) was originally isolated from the chicken pancreas by Kimmel and associates, and its sequence was determined soon thereafter (214,215). Porcine, bovine, and human pancreatic polypeptides (PPB, BPP, HPP) have been examined by Lin and Chance (248,249). All of the pancreatic polypeptides thus far studied are composed of 36 amino acids, and the mammalian forms differ in only one or two amino acids at specific locations in the molecule. In contrast, APP and BPP are similar at 15 of 36 positions. Antisera have been generated against APP and BPP, and, given the variation in composition noted above, it is not surprising that APP antiserum does not cross react with BPP (277). In fact, some investigators have been unable to demonstrate neuronal immunoreactivity with the BPP antiserum, although a recent report has described BPP-like immunoreactivity throughout the rat brain (323).

Several studies have reported APP-like immunoreactivity in various regions of the nervous system (163,174,257,265), including the cerebral cortex (257,277,454). We have recently examined the morphology and distribution of APP-like immu-

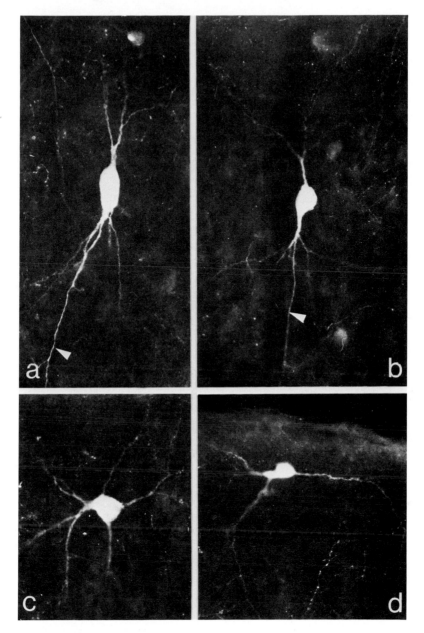

FIG. 18. Examples of CCK-immunoreactive neurons in the visual cortex of rats 14 days of age. Labeled with the immunofluorescence technique. *Arrowheads* point to axons. ×450. (From McDonald et al., ref. 276, with permission.)

noreactivity in identified neurons of the adult and developing visual cortex of the rat (277). Labeled cells comprise roughly 1% to 2% of the neurons in the visual cortex of the rat and are distributed in layers II to VI. They are predominantly nonpyramidal neurons (multipolar, bitufted, and bipolar forms) (Fig. 19), although a very small number of pyramidal cells are also present. A prominent group of multipolar neurons consists of cells in layer VI whose dendritic envelope displays a horizontal orientation (Fig. 19b; see also Fig. 7). It is interesting to mention that the morphology of a

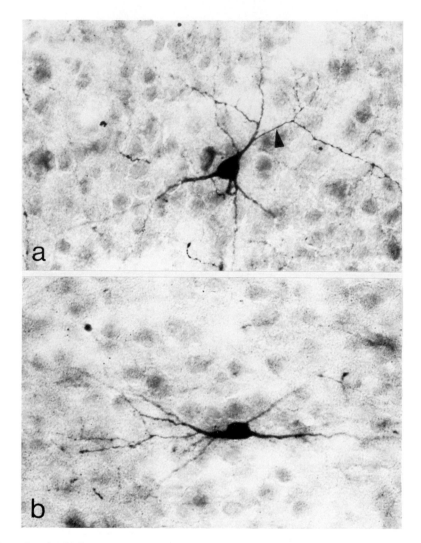

FIG. 19. Examples of APP-immunoreactive neurons in the visual cortex of rats 14 days of age. Labeled with the peroxidase–antiperoxidase technique. *Arrowhead* points to axon. ×450. (From McDonald et al., ref. 277, with permission.)

number of APP-immunoreactive neurons resembles the perikaryal and dendritic appearance of some somatostatin-labeled cells (274). In this regard, coexistence of APP and somatostatin in some cortical and hippocampal neurons has recently been documented (454). A recent study of Olschowka et al. (323) has reported BPP-like immunoreactivity in cortical neurons, and it is likely that both APP- and BPP-directed antisera visualize a recently isolated neuropeptide, neuropeptide Y (440a), which is similar in structure to both APP and BPP.

Other Peptides

Several other peptides have been measured in the cortex by radioimmunoassay and immunocytochemistry, although their low concentrations often impede accurate measurements and descriptions.

Neurotensin-like immunoreactivity has been measured in low amounts in the cortex of the rat, monkey, and cat (99,210,218,445) and appears to be somewhat unevenly distributed among different areas of the cortex (99,210,445). Immunocytochemistry reveals a thin band of sparse fluorescence near the pial surface and a thicker band of labeling in deeper cortical layers (446). Finally, autoradiography shows a moderate density of tritiated neurotensin binding sites in layer VI of the cortex (478). The function of neurotensin in the cerebral cortex remains obscure.

Very low amounts of substance P in the rat cerebral cortex have been reported (42,309). Immunocytochemistry has revealed the presence of a few labeled fibers throughout the medial aspects of the frontal cortex (253), and excitatory effects of substance P on cortical Betz cells have been described (351).

O'Donahue and associates (315) have observed that the cerebral cortex of the rat contains the second highest concentration of motilin in the brain, surpassed only by the cerebellum. To date, only a single abstract (50) has mentioned the existence of motilin-positive cells in the cortex, but this observation has not been confirmed in a subsequent study in the rat (185). The discrepancies between radioimmunoassay and immunocytochemical studies of motilin-like reactivity in the cortex are intriguing and await further examination. One physiological report has described excitatory effects of motilin applied iontophoretically to cortical neurons (353).

Low levels of met-enkephalin have been reported in the rat and bovine frontal cortex (88), and recently, Finley et al. (114) have reported enkephalin-like immunoreactivity in the cortex. Small labeled cells have been observed throughout layers II to VI, but further research is needed to precisely determine the morphology, distribution, and function of these enkephalin-immunoreactive neurons.

Finally, very low but detectable amounts of immunoreactive secretin (314), bombesin (38), α-melanocyte-stimulating hormone (α-MSH) (311,313), and γ₃-melanocyte-stimulating hormone (410) have been measured in the rat and bovine cerebral cortex. Lesions of the arcuate nucleus of the hypothalamus, which contains α-MSH cell bodies, eliminates α-MSH immunoreactivity in the cortex (312). The localization and functions of these peptides in the cortex remain unknown.

ACKNOWLEDGMENTS

We wish to thank Mrs. Alicia B. Benitez for typing several drafts of this chapter. We are grateful to Drs. M. E. Molliver, R. Grzanna, M. L. Feldman, C. E. Ribak, and J. K. Wamsley for providing illustrations of their material and to Drs. N. Brecha, J. I. Koenig, J. Walsh, G. Rosenquist, and J. R. Kimmel for making available the antisera used in our immunocytochemical studies. Support by the United States Public Health Service (Grants EY02964 and EY03783) is gratefully acknowledged.

REFERENCES

1. Akers, R. M., and Killackey, H. P. (1978): Organization of corticocortical connections in the parietal cortex of the rat. *J. Comp. Neurol.*, 181:513–538.
2. Albus, K. (1981): Hypothalamic and basal forebrain afferents to the cat's visual cortex: A study with horseradish peroxidase. *Neurosci. Lett.*, 24:117–121.
3. Albus, K., Donate-Oliver, F., Sanides, D., and Fries, W. (1981): The distribution of pontine projection cells in visual and association cortex of the cat: An experimental study with horseradish peroxidase. *J. Comp. Neurol.*, 201:175–189.
4. Andén, N.-E., Dahlström, A., Fuxe, K., Larsson, K., Olson, L., and Ungerstedt, U. (1966): Ascending monoamine neurons to the telencephalon and diencephalon. *Acta Physiol. Scand.*, 67:313–326.
5. Aubert, M. L., Grumbach, M. M., and Kaplan, S. L. (1977): The ontogenesis of human fetal hormones. IV. Somatostatin, luteinizing hormone releasing factor, and thyrotropin releasing factor in hypothalamus and cerebral cortex of human fetuses 10–22 weeks of age. *J. Clin. Endocrinol. Metab.*, 44:1130–1141.
6. Azmitia, E. C., and Segal, M. (1978): An autoradiographic analysis of the differential ascending projections of the dorsal and medial raphe nuclei in the rat. *J. Comp. Neurol.*, 179:641–668.
7. Barden, N., Mérand, Y., Rouleau, D., Moore, S., Dockray, G. J., and Dupont, A. (1981): Regional distributions of somatostatin and cholecystokinin-like immunoreactivities in rat and bovine brain. *Peptides*, 2:229–302.
8. Baudry, M., Martres, M. P., and Schwartz, J. C. (1973): The subcellular localization of histidine decarboxylase in various regions of rat brain. *J. Neurochem.*, 21:1301–1309.
9. Baughman, R. W., and Gilbert, C. D. (1980): Aspartate and glutamate as possible neurotransmitters of cells in layer 6 of the visual cortex. *Nature*, 287:848–850.
10. Baughman, R. W., and Gilbert, C. D. (1981): Aspartate and glutamate as possible neurotransmitters in the visual cortex. *J. Neurosci.*, 1:427–439.
11. Beani, L., Bianchi, C., Giacomelli, A., and Tamberi, F. (1978): Noradrenaline inhibition of acetylcholine release from guinea-pig brain. *Eur. J. Pharmacol.*, 48:179–193.
12. Beaudet, A., and Descarries, L. (1976): Quantitative data on serotonin nerve terminals in adult rat neocortex. *Brain Res.*, 111:301–309.

13. Beaudet, A., and Descarries, L. (1978): The mono-amine innervation of rat cerebral cortex: Synaptic and nonsynaptic axon terminals. *Neuroscience,* 3:851–860.

14. Beckstead, R. M. (1976): Convergent thalamic and mesencephalic projections to the anterior medial cortex in the rat. *J. Comp. Neurol.,* 166:403–416.

15. Beesley, P. W., and Emson, P. C. (1975): Distribution of transmitter related enzymes in rat sensorimotor cortex. *Biochem. Soc. Trans.,* 3:936–939.

16. Beinfeld, M. C., and Palkovits, M. (1981): Distribution of cholecystokinin in the hypothalamus and limbic system of the rat. *Neuropeptides,* 2:123–129.

17. Beinfeld, M. C., and Palkovits, M. (1982): Distribution of cholecystokinin (CCK) in the rat lower brain stem nuclei. *Brain Res.,* 238:260–265.

18. Beinfeld, M. C., Meyer, D. K., and Brownstein, M. J. (1980): Cholecystokinin octapeptide in the rat hypothalamo–neurohypophysial system. *Nature,* 288:376–378.

19. Beinfeld, M. C., Meyer, D. K., Eskay, R. L., Jensen, R. T., and Brownstein, M. J. (1981): The distribution of cholecystokinin immunoreactivity in the central nervous system of the rat as determined by radioimmunoassay. *Brain Res.,* 212:51–57.

20. Benevento, L. A., and Ebner, F. F. (1971): The contribution of the dorsal lateral geniculate nucleus to the total pattern of thalamic terminations in striate cortex of the Virginia opossum. *J. Comp. Neurol.,* 143:243–260.

21. Bennett, G. W., Edwardson, J. A., Marcano de Cotte, D., Berelowitz, M., Pimstone, B. L., and Kronheim, S. (1979): Release of somatostatin from rat brain synaptosomes. *J. Neurochem.,* 32:1127–1130.

22. Bennett, J. P., Logan, W. J., and Snyder, S. H. (1973): Amino acids as central nervous transmitters: The influence of ions, amino acid analogues, and ontogeny on transport systems for L-glutamic and L-aspartic acid and glycine into central nervous synaptosomes of the rat. *J. Neurochem.,* 21:1533–1550.

23. Bennett, J. P., and Snyder, S. H. (1975): Stereospecific binding of D-lysergic acid diethylamide (LSD) to brain membranes: Relationship to serotonin receptors. *Brain Res.,* 94:523–544.

24. Bennett, J. P., and Snyder, S. H. (1976): Serotonin and lysergic acid diethylamide binding in rat brain membranes: Relationship to postsynaptic serotonin receptors. *Mol. Pharmacol.,* 12:373–389.

25. Bennett-Clarke, C., Romagnano, M. A., and Joseph, S. A. (1980): Distribution of somatostatin in the rat brain: Telencephalon. *Brain Res.,* 188:473–486.

26. Besson, J., Rotsztejn, W., Laburthe, M., Epelbaum, J., Beaudet, A., Kordon, C., and Rosselin, G. (1979): Vasoactive intestinal peptide (VIP): Brain distribution, subcellular localization and effect of deafferentation of the hypothalamus in male rats. *Brain Res.,* 165:79–85.

27. Bindman, L., and Lippold, O. (1981): *The Neurophysiology of the Cerebral Cortex.* University of Texas Press, Austin.

28. Black, I. B., Hendry, I. A., and Iversen, L. L. (1972): The role of post-synaptic neurones in the biochemical maturation of presynaptic cholinergic nerve terminals in a mouse sympathetic ganglion. *J. Physiol. (Lond.),* 221:149–159.

29. Bloom, F. (1973): Ultrastructural identification of catecholamine-containing central synaptic terminals. *J. Histochem. Cytochem.,* 21:333–348.

30. Blue, M. E., and Parnavelas, J. G. (1982): The effect of neonatal 6-hydroxydopamine treatment on synaptogenesis in the visual cortex of the rat. *J. Comp. Neurol.,* 205:199–205.

31. Bobilier, P., Seguin, S., Petitjean, F., Salvert, D., Touret, M., and Jouvet, M. (1976): The raphe nuclei of the cat brain stem: A topographical atlas of their efferent projections as revealed by autoradiography. *Brain Res.,* 113:449–486.

32. Borg, J., Ramaharobandro, N., Mark, J., and Mandel, P. (1980): Changes in the uptake of GABA and taurine during neuronal and glial maturation. *J. Neurochem.,* 34:1113–1122.

33. Borghi, C., Nicosia, S., Giachetti, A., and Said, S. I. (1979): Vasoactive intestinal polypeptide (VIP) stimulates adenylate cyclase in selected areas of rat brain. *Life Sci.,* 24:65–70.

34. Bradford, R., Parnavelas, J. G., and Lieberman, A. R. (1977): Neurons in layer I of the developing occipital cortex of the rat. *J. Comp. Neurol.,* 176:121–132.

35. Brazeau, P., Vale, W., Burgus, R., Ling, N., Butcher, M., Rivier, J., and Guillemin, R. (1973): Hypothalamic polypeptide that inhibits the secretion of immunoreactive pituitary growth hormone. *Science,* 179:77–79.

36. Brodal, P. (1979): The pontocerebellar projection in rhesus monkey: An experimental study with retrograde axonal transport of horseradish peroxidase. *Neuroscience,* 4:193–208.

37. Bromberg, M. B., Penney, J. B., Jr., Stephenson, B. S., and Young, A. B. (1981): Evidence for glutamate as the neurotransmitter of corticothalamic and corticorubral pathways. *Brain Res.,* 215:369–374.

38. Brown, M., Allen, R., Villareal, J., Rivier, J., and Vale, W. (1978): Bombesin-like activity: Radioimmunologic assessment in biological tissue. *Life Sci.,* 23:2721–2728.

39. Brown, R. M., Crane, A. M., and Goldman, P. S. (1979): Regional distribution of monoamines in the cerebral cortex and subcortical structures of the rhesus monkey: Concentration and *in vivo* synthesis rates. *Brain Res.,* 168:133–150.

40. Brownstein, M., Arimura, A., Sato, H., Schally, A. V., and Kizer, J. S. (1975): The regional distribution of somatostatin in the rat brain. *Endocrinology,* 96:1456–1461.

41. Brownstein, M. J., Palkovits, M., Saavedra, J. M., and Kizer, J. S. (1975): Tryptophan hydroxylase in the rat brain. *Brain Res.,* 97:163–166.

42. Brownstein, M. J., Mroz, E. A., Kizer, J. S., Palkovitz, M., and Leeman, S. E. (1976): Regional distribution of substance P in the brain of the rat. *Brain Res.,* 116:299–305.

43. Burgus, R., Ling, N., Butcher, M., and Guillemin,

R. (1973): Primary structure of somatostatin, a hypothalamic peptide that inhibits the secretion of pituitary growth hormone. *Proc. Natl. Acad. Sci. U.S.A.*, 70:684–688.

44. Bylund, D. B., and Snyder, S. H. (1976): Beta adrenergic receptor binding in membrane preparations from mammalian brain. *Mol. Pharmacol.*, 12:568–580.

45. Cajal, S. R. (1899): Comparative study of the sensory areas of the human cortex. In: *Clark University Decennial Celebration,* edited by W. E. Storey, pp. 311–359. Norwood Press, Norwood, Massachusetts.

46. Cajal, S. R. (1911): *Histologie due Systieme de l'Homme et des Vertébrés,* Vol. 2 (translated by S. Azoulay). Maloine, Paris.

47. Carey, R. G., Fitzpatrick, D., and Diamond, I. T. (1979): Layer I of striate cortex of *Tupaia glis* and *Galago senegalensis.* Projections from thalamus and claustrum revealed by retrograde transport of horseradish peroxidase. *J. Comp. Neurol.*, 186:393–438.

48. Carter, D. A., and Fibiger, H. C. (1977): Ascending projections of presumed dopamine-containing neurons in the ventral tegmentum of the rat as demonstrated by horseradish peroxidase. *Neuroscience,* 2:569–576.

49. Chan-Palay, V., Nilaver, G., Palay, S. L., Beinfeld, M. C., Zimmerman, E. A., Wu, J. Y., and O'Donohue, T. L. (1981): Chemical heterogeneity in cerebellar Purkinje cells: Existence and coexistence of glutamic acid decarboxylase-like and motilin-like immunoreactivities. *Proc. Natl. Acad. Sci. U.S.A.*, 78:7787–7791.

50. Chey, W. Y., Escoffery, R., Roth, F., Chang, T. M., and Yajima, H. (1980): Motilin-like immunoreactivity (MLI) in the gut and neurons of peripheral and central nervous system. *Regul. Peptides [Suppl.],* 1:519.

51. Chronwall, B. M., and Wolff, J. R. (1978): Classification and location of neurons taking up ^{3}H-GABA in the visual cortex of rats. In: *Amino Acids as Chemical Transmitters,* edited by F. Fonnum, pp. 297–303. Plenum Press, New York.

52. Chronwall, B., and Wolff, J. R. (1980): Prenatal and postnatal development of GABA-accumulating cells in the occipital neocortex of rat. *J. Comp. Neurol.*, 190:187–208.

53. Chronwall, B. M., and Wolff, J. R. (1981): Development of GABA-accumulating neurons and glial cells in the rat visual cortex. In: *Amino Acid Neurotransmitters,* edited by F. V. De Feudis and P. Mandel, pp. 453–458. Raven Press, New York.

54. Cipolloni, P. B., and Peters, A. (1979): The bilaminar and banded distribution of the callosal terminals in the posterior neocortex of the rat. *Brain Res.*, 176:33–47.

55. Clark, R. M., and Collins, G. G. S. (1976): The release of endogenous amino acids from the rat visual cortex. *J. Physiol. (Lond.),* 262:383–400.

56. Coleman, J., and Clerici, W. J. (1980): Extrastriate projections from thalamus to posterior occipital–temporal cortex in rat. *Brain Res.*, 194:205–209.

57. Collins, G. G. S. (1977): The release of endogenous amino acids from rat visual cortex by calcium ions in the presence of the calcium ionophores X537A and A23187. *J. Neurochem.*, 28:461–463.

58. Colonnier, M. (1968): Synaptic patterns on different cell types in the different laminae of the cat visual cortex. An electron microscope study. *Brain Res.*, 9:268–287.

59. Conrad, L. C. A., Leonard, C. M., and Pfaff, D. W. (1974): Connections of the median and dorsal raphe nuclei in the rat: An autoradiographic and degeneration study. *J. Comp. Neurol.*, 156:179–206.

60. Cooper, J. R., Bloom, F. E., and Roth, R. H. (1978): *The Biochemical Basis of Neuropharmacology.* Oxford Press, New York.

61. Cooper, P. E., Fernstrom, M. H., Rorstad, O. P., Leeman, S. E., and Martin, J. B. (1981): The regional distribution of somatostatin, substance P and neurotensin in human brain. *Brain Res.*, 218:219–232.

62. Coyle, J. T., and Enna, S. J. (1976): Neurochemical aspects of the ontogenesis of gabanergic neurons in the rat brain. *Brain Res.*, 111:119–133.

63. Coyle, J. T., and Molliver, M. E. (1977): Major innervation of newborn rat cortex by monoaminergic neurons. *Science,* 196:444–447.

64. Crawford, J. M. (1970): The sensitivity of cortical neurones to acidic amino acids and acetylcholine. *Brain Res.*, 17:287–296.

65. Curtis, D. R., and Johnston, G. A. R. (1974): Amino acid transmitters in the mammalian central nervous system. *Ergeb. Physiol.*, 69:98–188.

66. Cusick, C. G., and Lund, R. D. (1981): The distribution of the callosal projection to the occipital visual cortex in rats and mice. *Brain Res.*, 214:239–259.

67. Cutler, R. W. P., and Dudzinski, D. S. (1975): Release of [^{3}H]GABA and [^{14}C]glutamic acid from rat cortex slices, the relationship between the tissue pool size and rates of spontaneous and electrically induced release. *Brain Res.*, 88:415–423.

68. Dahlström, A. (1973): Aminergic transmission. Introduction and short review. *Brain Res.*, 62:441–460.

69. Dahlström, A., and Fuxe, K. (1964): Evidence for the existence of monoamine-containing neurons in the central nervous system. I. Demonstration of monoamines in the cell bodies of brain stem neurons. *Acta Physiol. Scand.*, 62(Suppl. 232):1–55.

70. DeBelleroche, J. S., and Bradford, H. F. (1972): Metabolism of beds of mammalian cortical synaptosomes: Response to depolarizing influences. *J. Neurochem.*, 19:585–602.

71. DeFeudis, F. V., Maitre, M., Ossola, L., Elkouby, A., and Mandel, P. (1979): Bicuculline-sensitive GABA binding to a synaptosome-enriched fraction of rat cerebral cortex in the presence of a physiological concentration of sodium. *Gen. Pharmacol.*, 10:193–194.

72. De Montigny, C., Wang, R. Y., Reader, T. A., and Aghajanian, G. K. (1980): Monoaminergic denervation of the rat hippocampus: Microiontophoretic studies on pre- and postsynaptic supersensitivity to norepinephrine and serotonin. *Brain Res.*, 200:363–376.

73. Descarries, L., and Droz, B. (1970): Intraneural distribution of exogenous norepinephrine in the central nervous system of the rat. *J. Cell Biol.*, 44:385–399.

74. Descarries, L., and Lapierre, Y. (1973): Noradrenergic axon terminals in the cerebral cortex of rat. I. Radioautographic visualization after topical application of DL-[³H]norepinephrine. *Brain Res.*, 51:141–160.

75. Descarries, L., Beaudet, A., and Watkins, K. C. (1975): Serotonin nerve terminals in adult rat neocortex. *Brain Res.*, 100:563–588.

76. Descarries, L., Watkins, K. C., and Lapierre, Y. (1977): Noradrenergic axon terminals in the cerebral cortex of rat. III. Topometric ultrastructural analysis. *Brain Res.*, 133:197–222.

77. Dichter, M. A., and Delfs, J. R. (1981): Somatostatin and cortical neurons in cell culture. In: *Neurosecretion and Brain Peptides,* edited by J. B. Martin, S. Reichlin, and K. L. Bick, pp. 145–157. Raven Press, New York.

78. Divac, I. (1975): Magnocellular nuclei of the basal forebrain project to neocortex, brain stem, and olfactory bulb. Review of some functional correlates. *Brain Res.*, 93:385–398.

79. Dockray, G. J. (1977): Molecular evolution of gut hormones: Application of comparative studies on the regulation of digestion. *Gastroenterology,* 72:344–358.

80. Dockray, G. H. (1980): Cholecystokinin in rat cerebral cortex: Identification, purification and characterization by immunochemical methods. *Brain Res.,* 188:155–165.

81. Dodd, J., and Kelly, J. S. (1978): Is somatostatin an excitatory transmitter in the hippocampus? *Nature,* 273:674–675.

82. Dodd, J., and Kelly, J. S. (1981): The actions of cholecystokinin and related peptides on pyramidal neurons of the mammalian hippocampus. *Brain Res.,* 205:337–350.

83. Dodd, J., Kelly, J. S., and Said, S. I. (1979): Excitation of CA1 neurons of the rat hippocampus by the octacosapeptide, vasoactive intestinal polypeptide (VIP). *Br. J. Pharmacol.,* 66:125P.

84. Dodd, P. R., Edwardson, J. A., and Dockray, G. J. (1980): The depolarization-induced release of cholecystokinin C-terminal octapeptide (CCK-8) from rat synaptosomes and brain slices. *Regul. Peptides,* 1:17–29.

85. Donohue, J. P., and Ebner, F. F. (1981): The laminar distribution and ultrastructure of fibers projecting from three thalamic nuclei to the somatic sensory–motor cortex of the opossum. *J. Comp. Neurol.,* 198:389–420.

86. Dräger, U. C. (1974): Autoradiography of tritiated proline and fucose transported transneuronally from the eye to the visual cortex in pigmented and albino mice. *Brain Res.,* 82:284–292.

87. Duffy, F. H., Snodgrass, S. R., Burchfiel, J. L., and Conway, J. (1976): Bicuculline reversal of deprivation amblyopia in the cat. *Nature,* 260:256–257.

88. Dupont, A., Lépine, J., Langelier, P., Mérand, Y., Rouleau, P., Vaudry, H., Gros, C., and Barden, N. (1980): Differential distribution of β-endorphin and enkephalins in rat and bovine brain. *Regu. Peptides,* 1:43–52.

89. Edmunds, S. M., and Parnavelas, J. G. (1982): Retzius–Cajal cells: An ultrastructural study in the developing visual cortex of the rat. *J. Neurocytol.,* 11:427–446.

90. Elks, M. L., Youngblood, W. W., and Kizer, J. S. (1979): Serotonin synthesis and release in brain slices: Independence of tryptophan. *Brain Res.,* 172:471–486.

91. Elks, M. L., Youngblood, W. W., and Kizer, J. S. (1979): Synthesis and release of serotonin by brain slices: Effect of ionic manipulations and cationic ionophores. *Brain Res.,* 172:461–469.

92. Emson, P. C. (1979): Peptides as neurotransmitter candidates in the mammalian CNS. *Prog. Neurobiol.,* 13:61–116.

93. Emson, P. C., and Lindvall, O. (1979): Distribution of putative neurotransmitters in the neocortex. *Neuroscience,* 4:1–30.

94. Emson, P. C., Gilbert, R. F. T., Lorén, I., Fahrenkrug, J., Sundler, F., and Schaffalitzky de Muckadell, O. B. (1979): Development of vasoactive intestinal polypeptide (VIP) containing neurons in the rat brain. *Brain Res.,* 177:437–444.

95. Emson, P. C., Hunt, S. P., Rehfeld, J. F., Golterman, N., and Fahrenkrug, J. (1980): Cholecystokinin and vasoactive intestinal polypeptide in the mammalian CNS: Distribution and possible physiological roles. In: *Neural Peptides and Neuronal Communication,* edited by E. Costa and M. Trabucchi, pp. 63–74. Raven Press, New York.

96. Emson, P. C., Lee, C. M., and Rehfeld, J. F. (1980): Cholecystokinin octapeptide: Vesicular localization and calcium dependent release from rat brain *in vitro. Life Sci.,* 26:2157–2163.

97. Emson, P. C., and Hunt, S. P. (1981): Anatomical chemistry of the cerebral cortex. In: *The Organization of the Cerebral Cortex,* edited by F. O. Schmitt, F. C. Worden, G. Adelman, and S. G. Dennis, pp. 325–345. MIT Press, Cambridge, Massachusetts.

98. Emson, P. C., Rehfeld, J. F., and Rossor, M. N. (1982): Distribution of cholecystokinin-like peptides in the human brain. *J. Neurochem.,* 38:1177–1179.

99. Emson, P. C., Goedert, M., Horsfield, P., Rioux, F., and St. Pierre, S. (1982): The regional distribution and chromatographic characterization of neurotensin-like immunoreactivity in the rat central nervous system. *J. Neurochem.,* 38:992–999.

100. Engel, G., Hoyer, D., Berthold, R., and Wagner, H. (1981): (±)[¹²⁵Iodo]Cyanopindolol, a new ligand for β-adrenoceptors in guinea pig. *Naunyn Schmiedebergs Arch. Pharmacol.,* 317:277–285.

101. Enjalbert, A., Bourgoin, S., Hamon, M., Adrien, J., and Bochaert, J. C. (1978): Postsynaptic serotonin-sensitive adenylate cyclase in the central nervous system. I. Development and distribution of serotonin and dopamine-sensitive adenylate cyclases in rat and guinea pig brain. *Mol. Pharmacol.,* 14:2–10.

102. Enjalbert, A., Hamon, M., Bourgoin, S., and Bochaert, J. (1978): Postsynaptic serotonin-sensitive

adenylate cyclase in the central nervous system. II. Comparison with dopamine- and isoproterenol-sensitive adenylate cyclases in rat brain. *Mol. Pharmacol.*, 14:11–23.

103. Enna, S. J., and Snyder, S. H. (1975): Properties of γ-aminobutyric acid (GABA) receptor binding in rat brain synaptic membrane fractions. *Brain Res.*, 100:81–97.

104. Epelbaum, J., Brazeau, P., Tsang, D., Brawer, J., and Martin, J. B. (1977): Subcellular distribution of radioimmunoassayable somatostatin in rat brain. *Brain Res.*, 126:309–323.

105. Fagg, G. E., and Lane, J. D. (1979): The uptake and release of putative amino acid neurotransmitters. *Neuroscience*, 4:1015–1036.

106. Fahrenkrug, J. (1979): Vasoactive intestinal polypeptide: Measurement, distribution and putative neurotransmitter function. *Digestion*, 19:149–169.

107. Fahrenkrug, J., and Schaffalitzky De Muckadell, O. B. (1978): Distribution of vasoactive intestinal polypeptide (VIP) in the porcine central nervous system. *J. Neurochem.*, 31:1445–1451.

108. Feldman, M. L., and Peters, A. (1978): The forms of non-pyramidal neurons in the visual cortex of the rat. *J. Comp. Neurol.*, 179:761–794.

109. Feldman, S. C., and Lichtenstein, E. (1980): Morphology and distribution of somatostatin-containing neurons in the guinea pig neocortex. *Anat. Rec.*, 196:55A.

110. Ferron, A., Descarries, L., and Reader, T. A. (1982): Altered neuronal responsiveness to biogenic amines in rat cerebral cortex after serotonin denervation or depletion. *Brain Res.*, 231:93–108.

111. Fillion, G. M. B., Rouselle, J. C., Fillion, M. P., Beaudoin, D. M., Goiny, M. R., Deniau, J. M., and Jacob, J. J. (1978): High-affinity binding of [³H]5-hydroxytryptamine to brain synaptosomal membranes: Comparison with [³H]lysergic acid diethylamide binding. *Mol. Pharmacol.*, 14:50–59.

112. Finley, J. C. W., Grossman, G. H., Dimeo, P., and Petrusz P. (1978): Somatostatin-containing neurons in the rat brain: Widespread distribution revealed by immunocytochemistry after pretreatment with pronase. *Am. J. Anat.*, 153:483–488.

113. Finley, J. C. W., Maderdrut, J. L., Roger, L. J., and Petrusz, P. (1981): The immunocytochemical localization of somatostatin-containing neurons in the rat central nervous system. *Neuroscience*, 6:2173–2192.

114. Finley, J. C., Maderdrut, J. L., and Petrusz, P. (1981): The immunocytochemical localization of enkephalin in the central nervous system of the rat. *J. Comp. Neurol.*, 198:541–565.

115. Fisken, R. A., Garey, L. J., and Powell, T. P. S. (1975): The intrinsic, association and commissural connections of area 17 of the visual cortex. *Phil. Trans. R. Soc. Lond. [Biol.]*, 272:487–536.

116. Fonnum, F. (1973): Recent developments in biochemical investigations of cholinergic transmission. *Brain Res.*, 62:497–507.

117. Fonnum, F., Storm-Mathisen, J., and Divac, I. (1981): Biochemical evidence for glutamate as neurotransmitter in corticostriatal and corticothalamic fibers in rat brain. *Neuroscience*, 6:863–873.

118. Foote, S. L., Freedman, R., and Oliver, A. P. (1975): Effects of putative neurotransmitters on neuronal activity in monkey auditory cortex. *Brain Res.*, 86:229–242.

119. Freedman, R., Foote, S. L., and Bloom, F. E. (1975): Histochemical characterization of a neocortical projection of the nucleus locus coeruleus in the squirrel monkey. *J. Comp. Neurol.*, 164:209–237.

120. Freedman, R., Hoffer, B. J., Woodward, D. J., and Puro, D. (1977): Interaction of norepinephrine with cerebellar activity evoked by mossy and climbing fibers. *Exp. Neurol.*, 55:269–288.

121. Frost, D. O., and Caviness, V. S., Jr. (1980): Radial organization of thalamic projections to the neocortex in the mouse. *J. Comp. Neurol.*, 194:369–393.

122. Fuxe, K. (1965): Evidence for the existence of monoamine neurons in the central nervous system. IV. Distribution of monoamine nerve terminals in the central nervous system. *Acta Physiol. Scand. [Suppl.]*, 247:36–85.

123. Fuxe, K., Hamberger, B., and Hökfelt, T. (1968): Distribution of noradrenaline nerve terminals in cortical areas of the rat. *Brain Res.*, 8:125–131.

124. Fuxe, K., Hökfelt, T., and Ungerstedt, U. (1968): Localization of indolealkylamines in CNS. In: *Advances in Pharmacology*, Vol. 6, Part A, edited by S. Garattini and P. A. Shore, pp. 235–251. Academic Press, New York.

125. Fuxe, K., Hökfelt, T., Johansson, O., Jonsson, G., Lidbrink, P., and Ljungdahl, Å. (1974): The origin of the dopamine nerve terminals in limbic and frontal cortex. Evidence for meso-cortical dopamine neurons. *Brain Res.*, 82:349–355.

126. Fuxe, K., Hökfelt, T., Said, S. I., and Mutt, V. (1977): Vasoactive intestinal polypeptide and the nervous system: Immunohistochemical evidence for localization in central and peripheral neurons, particularly intracortical neurons of the cerebral cortex. *Neurosci. Lett.*, 5:241–246.

127. Garey, L. J. (1971): A light and electron microscopic study of the visual cortex of the cat and monkey. *Proc. R. Soc. Lond. [Biol.]*, 179:21–40.

128. Garey, L. J., and Powell, T. P. S. (1971): An experimental study of the termination of the lateral geniculo–cortical pathway in the cat and monkey. *Proc. R. Soc. Lond. Biol.*, 179:41–63.

129. Gatter, K. C., and Powell, T. P. S. (1977): The projection of the locus coeruleus upon the neocortex in the macaque monkey. *Neuroscience*, 2:441–445.

130. Gauchy, C. M., Iversen, L. L., and Jessell, T. M. (1977): The spontaneous and evoked release of newly synthesized [¹⁴C]GABA from rat cerebral cortex, *in vitro*. *Brain Res.*, 138:374–379.

131. Gaull, C. E., and Rassin, D. K. (1979): Taurine and brain development: Human and animal correlates. In: *Neural Growth and Differentiation*, edited by E. Meisami and M. A. B. Brazier, pp. 461–477. Raven Press, New York.

132. Geola, F. L., Hershman, J. M., Warwick, R., Reeve, J. R., Walsh, J. H., and Tourtellotte, W. W. (1981): Regional distribution of cholecystokinin-like immunoreactivity in the human brain. *J. Clin. Endocrinol. Metab.*, 53:270–275.

133. Giachetti, A., Rosenberg, R. N., and Said, S. I. (1976): Vasoactive intestinal polypeptide in brain synaptosomes. *Lancet*, 2:741–742.

134. Giachetti, A., Said, S. I., Reynolds, R. C., and Koniges, F. C. (1977): Vasoactive intestinal polypeptide in brain: Localization in and release from isolated nerve terminals. *Proc. Natl. Acad. Sci. U.S.A.*, 74:3424–3428.

135. Gilbert, C. D., and Kelly, J. P. (1975): The projections of cells in different layers of the cat's visual cortex. *J. Comp. Neurol.*, 163:81–106.

136. Glickstein, M., and Whitteridge, D. (1976): Degeneration of layer III pyramidal cells in area 18 following destruction of callosal input. *Brain Res.*, 104:148–151.

137. Globus, A., and Scheibel, A. (1967): Pattern and field of cortical structure: The rabbit. *J. Comp. Neurol.*, 131:155–172.

138. Goldman-Rakic, P. S., and Brown, R. M. (1981): Regional changes of monoamines in cerebral cortex and subcortical structures of aging rhesus monkeys. *Neuroscience*, 6:177–187.

139. Golterman, N. R., Rehfeld, J. F., and Roigaard-Petersen, H. (1980): *In vivo* biosynthesis of cholecystokinin in rat cerebral cortex. *J. Biol. Chem.*, 255:6181–6185.

140. Golterman, N. R., Stengaard-Pedersen, K., Rehfeld, J. F., and Christensen, N. J. (1981): Newly synthesized cholecystokinin in subcellular fractions of the rat brain. *J. Neurochem.*, 36:959–965.

141. Gosavi, V. S., and Dubey, P. N. (1972): Projection of striate cortex to the dorsal lateral geniculate body in the rat. *J. Anat.*, 113:75–82.

142. Gould, H. J. III, Hall, W. C., and Ebner, F. F. (1978): Connections of the visual cortex in the hedgehog *(Paraechinus hypomelas)*. I. Thalamocortical projections. *J. Comp. Neurol.*, 177:445–472.

143. Grafstein, B. (1959): Organization of callosal connections in suprasylvian gyrus of cat. *J. Neurophysiol.*, 22:504–515.

144. Gray, E. G. (1959): Axo-somatic and axo-dendritic synapses of the cerebral cortex: An electron microscope study. *J. Anat.*, 93:420–433.

145. Greenwood, R. S., Godar, S. E., Reaves, T. A., and Hayward, J. N. (1981): Cholecystokinin in hippocampal pathways. *J. Comp. Neurol.*, 203:335–350.

146. Guidotti, A., Gale, K., Suria, A., and Toffaro, G. (1979): Biochemical evidence for two classes of GABA receptors in rat brain. *Brain Res.*, 172:566–571.

147. Hamberger, A. C., Chiang, G. H., Sandoval, E., Nylén, E. S., and Cotman, C. W. (1979): Glutamate as a CNS transmitter. I. Evaluation of glucose and glutamine as precursors for the synthesis of preferentially released glutamate. *Brain Res.*, 168:513–530.

148. Hamberger, A., Chiang, G. H., Sandoval, E., and Cotman, C. W. (1979): Glutamate as a CNS transmitter. II. Regulation of synthesis in the releasable pool. *Brain Res.*, 168:531–541.

149. Hamon, M., Mallat, M., Herbet, A., Nelson, D. L., Audinot, M., Pichat, L., and Glowinski, J. (1981): [³H]Metergoline: A new ligand of serotonin receptors in the rat brain. *J. Neurochem.*, 36:613–626.

150. Hays, S. E., Houston, S. H., Beinfeld, M. C., and Paul, S. M. (1981): Postnatal ontogeny of cholecystokinin receptors in rat brain. *Brain Res.*, 213:237–241.

151. Hebb, C. O., Krnjević, K., and Silver A. (1963): Effect of undercutting on the acetylcholinesterase and choline-acetyltransferase in the cat's cerebral cortex. *Nature*, 198:692.

152. Heimer, L., Ebner, F. F., and Norton, W. J. H. (1967): A note on the termination of commissural fibers in the neocortex. *Brain Res.*, 5:171–177.

153. Henderson, Z. (1981): A projection from acetylcholinesterase-containing neurones in the diagonal band to the occipital cortex of the rat. *Neuroscience*, 6:1081–1088.

154. Hendrickson, A. E., Hunt, S. P., and Wu, J.-Y. (1981): Immunocytochemical localization of glutamic acid decarboxylase in monkey striate cortex. *Nature*, 292:605–607.

155. Herkenham, M. (1979): The afferent and efferent connections of the ventromedial thalamic nucleus in the rat. *J. Comp. Neurol.*, 183:487–518.

156. Herkenham, M. (1980): Laminar organization of thalamic projections to the rat neocortex. *Science*, 207:532–535.

157. Hess, R., and Murata, K. (1974): Effects of glutamate and GABA on specific response properties of neurones in the visual cortex. *Exp. Brain Res.*, 21:285–297.

158. Hirsch, H. E., and Robins, E. (1962): Distribution of γ-aminobutyric acid in the layers of the cerebral and cerebellar cortex. Implications for its physiological role. *J. Neurochem.*, 9:63–70.

159. Ho, A. K., Singer, G., and Gershon, S. (1971): Biochemical evidence of adrenergic interaction with cholinergic function in the central nervous system of the rat. *Psychopharmacologia*, 21:238–246.

160. Hökfelt, T. (1967): On the ultrastructural localization of noradrenaline in the central nervous system of the rat. *Z. Zellforsch. Mikrosk. Anat.*, 79:110–117.

161. Hökfelt, T., and Ljungdahl, Å. (1972): Autoradiographic identification of cerebral and cerebellar cortical neurons accumulating labeled gamma-aminobutyric acid (³H-GABA). *Exp. Brain Res.*, 14:354–362.

162. Hökfelt, T., Efendic, S., Johansson, O., Luft, R., and Arimura, A. (1974): Immunohistochemical localization of somatostatin (growth hormone release-inhibiting factor) in the guinea pig brain. *Brain Res.*, 80:165–169.

163. Hökfelt, T., Lundberg, J. M., Terenius, L., Jancsó, G., and Kimmel, J. R. (1981): Avian pancreatic polypeptide (APP) immunoreactive neurons in the spinal cord and spinal trigeminal nucleus. *Peptides*, 2:81–87.

164. Hökfelt, T., Schultzberg, M., Lundberg, J. M., Fuxe, K., Mutt, V., Fahrenkrug, J., and Said, S. I. (1982): Distribution of vasoactive intestinal polypeptide in the central and peripheral nervous systems as revealed by immunocytochemistry. In: *Va-*

soactive Intestinal Peptide, edited by S. I. Said, pp. 65–90. Raven Press, New York.

165. Holländer, H. (1974): Projections from the striate cortex to the diencephalon in the squirrel monkey *(Saimiri sciureus)*. A light microscopic radioautographic study following intracortical injection of H³ leucine. *J. Comp. Neurol.,* 155:424–440.

166. Holländer, H. (1974): On the origin of corticotectal projections of the cat. *Exp. Brain Res.,* 21:433–440.

167. Hornung, J. P., and Garey, L. J. (1981): The thalamic projection to cat visual cortex: Ultrastructure of neurons identified by Golgi impregnation or retrograde horseradish peroxidase transport. *Neuroscience,* 6:1053–1068.

168. Hornung, J. P., and Garey, L. J. (1981): Ultrastructure of visual callosal neurons in cat identified by retrograde transport of horseradish peroxidase. *J. Neurocytol.,* 10:297–314.

169. Hösli, E., and Hösli, L. (1980): Cellular localization of the uptake of [³H]taurine and [³H]β-alanine in cultures of the rat central nervous system. *Neuroscience,* 5:145–152.

170. Huang, M., Ho, A. K. S., and Daly, J. W. (1973): Accumulation of adenosine cyclic 3′, 5′-monophosphate in rat cerebral cortical slices. *Mol. Pharmacol.,* 9:711–717.

171. Hubel, D. H., and Wiesel, T. N. (1972): Laminar and columnar distribution of geniculo–cortical fibers in the macaque monkey. *J. Comp. Neurol.,* 146:421–450.

172. Hubel, D. H., and Wiesel, T. N. (1977): Functional architecture of macaque monkey visual cortex. *Proc. R. Soc. Lond. [Biol.],* 198:1–59.

173. Hughes, H. C. (1977): Anatomical and neurobehavioral investigations concerning the thalamo–cortical organization of the rat's system. *J. Comp. Neurol.,* 175:311–336.

174. Hunt, S. P., Emson, P. C., Gilbert, R., Goldstein, M., and Kimmel, J. R. (1981): Presence of avian pancreatic polypeptide-like immunoreactivity in catecholamine and methionine-enkephalin-containing neurons within the central nervous system. *Neurosci. Lett.,* 21:125–130.

175. Innis, R. B., Correa, F. M. A., Uhl, G. R., Schneider, B., and Snyder, S. H. (1979): Cholecystokinin octapeptide-like immunoreactivity: Histochemical localization in rat brain. *Proc. Natl. Acad. Sci.,* 76:521–525.

176. Innis, R. B., and Snyder, S. H. (1980): Distinct cholecystokinin receptors in brain and pancreas. *Proc. Natl. Acad. Sci. U.S.A.,* 77:6917–6921.

177. Innis, R. B., Zarbin, M. A., Wamsley, J. K., Snyder, S. H., and Kuhar, M. J. (1981): Autoradiographic localization of cholecystokinin receptors in guinea pig brain. *Soc. Neurosci. Abstr.,* 7:430.

178. Ioffe, S., Havlicek, V., Friesen, H., and Chernick, V. (1978): Effect of somatostatin (SRIF) and L-glutamate on neurons of the sensorimotor cortex in awake habituated rabbits. *Brain Res.,* 153:414–418.

179. Itakura, T., Kasamatsu, T., and Pettigrew, J. D. (1981): Norepinephrine-containing terminals in kitten visual cortex: Laminar distribution and ultrastructure. *Neuroscience,* 6:159–175.

180. Iversen, L. L. (1977): Catecholamine-sensitive adenylate cyclases in nervous tissues. *J. Neurochem.,* 29:5–12.

181. Iversen, L. L. (1978): Biochemical psychopharmacology of GABA. In: *Psychopharmacology: A Generation of Progress,* edited by M. A. Lipton, A. Di Mascio, and K. F. William, pp. 25–28. Raven Press, New York.

182. Iversen, L. L., and Neal, M. J. (1968): The uptake of [³H]GABA by slices of rat cerebral cortex. *J. Neurochem.,* 15:1141–1149.

183. Iversen, L. L., Mitchell, J. F., and Srinivasan, V. (1971): The release of γ-aminobutyric acid during inhibition in the cat visual cortex. *J. Physiol. (Lond.),* 212:519–534.

184. Iversen, L. L., Iversen, S. D., Bloom, F., Douglas, C., Brown, M., and Vale, W. (1978): Calcium-dependent release of somatostatin and neurotensin from rat brain *in vitro. Nature,* 273:161–163.

185. Jacobowitz, D. M., O'Donohue, T. L., Chey, W. Y., and Chang, T. M. (1981): Mapping of motilin-immunoreactive neurons of the rat brain. *Peptides,* 2:479–487.

186. Jacobson, S. (1970): Distribution of commissural axon terminals in the rat neocortex. *Exp. Neurol.,* 28:193–205.

187. Jacobson, S. (1971): The laminar contributions to the callosal system in the albino rat. *Anat. Rec.,* 169:346.

188. Jacobson, S., and Trojanowski, J. W. (1974): The cells of origin of the corpus callosum in rat, cat and rhesus monkey. *Brain Res.,* 74:149–155.

189. Jaim-Etcheverry, G., Teitelman, G., and Zieher, L. M. (1975): Choline acetyltransferase activity increases in the brain stem of rats treated at birth with 6-hydroxydopa. *Brain Res.,* 100:699–704.

190. Jasper, H. H., and Koyama, I. (1969): Rate of release of amino acids from the cerebral cortex in the cat as affected by brainstem and thalamic stimulation. *Can. J. Physiol. Pharmacol.,* 47:889–905.

191. Johnston, M. V., McKinney, M., and Coyle, J. T. (1979): Evidence for a cholinergic projection to neocortex from neurons in basal forebrain. *Proc. Natl. Acad. Sci. U.S.A.,* 76:5392–5396.

192. Johnston, M. V., McKinney, M., and Coyle, J. T. (1981): Neocortical cholinergic innervation: A description of extrinsic and intrinsic components in the rat. *Exp. Brain Res.,* 43:159–172.

193. Jones, B. E., and Moore, R. Y. (1977): Ascending projections of the locus coeruleus in the rat. II. Autoradiographic study. *Brain Res.,* 127:23–53.

194. Jones, E. G. (1975): Varieties and distribution of non-pyramidal cells in the somatic sensory cortex of the squirrel monkey. *J. Comp. Neurol.,* 160:205–268.

195. Jones, E. G. (1975): Lamination and differential distribution of thalamic afferents within the sensory–motor cortex of the squirrel monkey. *J. Comp. Neurol.,* 160:167–204.

196. Jones, E. G. (1981): Functional subdivision and synaptic organization of the mammalian thalamus.

In: *International Review of Physiology, Vol. 25: Neurophysiology IV,* edited by R. Porter, pp. 173–245. University Park Press, Baltimore.

197. Jones, E. G., and Powell, T. P. S. (1970): Electron microscopy of the somatic sensory cortex of the cat. I. Cell types and synaptic organization. *Phil. Trans. R. Soc. Lond. [Biol.],* 257:1–11.

198. Jones, E. G., and Powell, T. P. S. (1970): An electron microscopic study of the laminar pattern and mode of termination of afferent fibre pathways in the somatic sensory cortex of the cat. *Phil. Trans. R. Soc. Lond. [Biol.],* 257:45–62.

199. Jones, E. G., and Burton, H. (1976): Areal differences in the laminar distribution of thalamic afferents in cortical fields of the insular, parietal and temporal regions of primates. *J. Comp. Neurol.,* 168:197–248.

200. Jones, E. G., and Wise, S. P. (1977): Size, laminar and columnar distribution of efferent cells in the sensory–motor cortex of monkeys. *J. Comp. Neurol.,* 175:391–438.

201. Jones, E. G., Burton, H., Saper, C. B., and Swanson, L.W. (1976): Midbrain, diencephalic and cortical relationships of the basal nucleus of Meynert and associated structures in primates. *J. Comp. Neurol.,* 167:385–420.

202. Jope, R. S. (1981): Acetylcholine turnover and compartmentation in rat brain synaptosomes. *J. Neurochem.,* 36:1712–1721.

203. Kaas, J. H., Hall, W. C., and Diamond, I. T. (1972): Visual cortex of the grey squirrel *(Sciurus carolinensis):* Architectonic subdivisions and connections from the visual thalamus. *J. Comp. Neurol.,* 145:273–306.

204. Kaczmarek, L. K., and Adey, W. R. (1973): The efflux of $^{45}Ca^{2+}$ and $[^{3}H]\gamma$-aminobutyric acid from cat cerebral cortex. *Brain Res.,* 63:331–342.

205. Kaczmarek, L. K., and Adey, W. R. (1974): Factors affecting the release of $[^{14}C]$taurine from cat brain: The electrical effects of taurine on normal and seizure prone cortex. *Brain Res.,* 76:83–94.

206. Kasamatsu, T., and Pettigrew, J. D. (1979): Preservation of binocularity after monocular deprivation in the striate cortex of kittens treated with 6-hydroxydopamine. *J. Comp. Neurol.,* 185:139–162.

207. Kasamatsu, T., and Heggelund, P. (1982): Single cell responses in cat visual cortex to visual stimulation during iontophoresis of noradrenaline. *Exp. Brain Res.,* 45:317–327.

208. Kasamatsu, T., Pettigrew, J. D., and Ary, M. (1979): Restoration of visual cortical plasticity by local microperfusion of norepinephrine. *J. Comp. Neurol.,* 185:163–182.

209. Kasamatsu, T., Pettigrew, J. D., and Ary, M. (1981): Cortical recovery from effects of monocular deprivation. Acceleration with norepinephrine and suppression with 6-hydroxydopamine. *J. Neurophysiol.,* 45:254–266.

210. Kataoka, K., Mizuro, N., and Frohman, L. A. (1979): Regional distribution of immunoreactive neurotensin in monkey brain. *Brain Res. Bull.,* 4:57–60.

211. Kawamura, S., Sprague, J. M., and Niimi, K. (1974): Corticofugal projections from visual cor-

tices to the thalamus, pretectum and superior colliculus in the cat. *J. Comp. Neurol.,* 158:339–362.

212. Kelly, J. S., and Dodd, J. (1981): Cholecystokinin and gastrin as transmitters in the mammalian central nervous system. In: *Neurosecretion and Brain Peptides,* edited by J. B. Martin, S. Reichlin, and K. L. Bick, pp. 133–144. Raven Press, New York.

213. Killackey, H. P., and Ebner, F. F. (1972): Two different types of thalamocortical projections to a single cortical area in mammals. *Brain Behav. Evol.,* 6:141–169.

214. Kimmel, J. R., Pollock, H. G., and Hazelwood, R. L. (1971): A new pancreatic polypeptide hormone. *Fed. Proc.,* 30:1318.

215. Kimmel, J. R., Hayden, L. J., and Pollock, H. G. (1975): Isolation and characterization of a new pancreatic polypeptide hormone. *J. Biol. Chem.,* 250:9369–9376.

216. Kimura, H., McGeer, P. L., Peng, F., and McGeer, E. G. (1980): Choline acetyltransferase-containing neurons in rodent brain demonstrated by immunohistochemistry. *Science,* 208:1057–1059.

217. Kimura, H., McGeer, P. L., Peng, J. H., and McGeer, E. G. (1981): The central cholinergic system studied by choline acetyltransferase immunohistochemistry in the cat. *J. Comp. Neurol.,* 200:151–201.

218. Kobayashi, R. M., Brown, M., and Vale, W. (1977): Regional distribution of neurotensin and somatostatin in rat brain. *Brain Res.,* 126:584–588.

219. Koda, L. Y., and Bloom, F. E. (1977): A light and electron microscopic study of noradrenergic terminals in the rat dentate gyrus. *Brain Res.,* 120:327–335.

220. Krieg, W. J. S. (1946): Connections of the cerebral cortex. I. The albino rat. A. Topography of the cortical areas. *J. Comp. Neurol.,* 84:221–276.

221. Krieg, W. J. S. (1946): Connections of the cerebral cortex. I. The albino rat. B. Structure of the cortical areas. *J. Comp. Neurol.,* 84:277–324.

222. Krisch, B. (1980): Differing immunoreactivities of somatostatin in the cortex and the hypothalamus of the rat. *Cell Tissue Res.,* 212:457–464.

223. Krnjević, K. (1964): Microiontophoretic studies on cortical neurons. *Int. Rev. Neurobiol.,* 7:41–98.

224. Krnjević, K. (1974): Chemical nature of synaptic transmission in vertebrates. *Physiol. Rev.,* 54:418–540.

225. Krnjević, K., and Schwartz, S. (1967): The action of γ-aminobutyric acid on cortical neurones. *Exp. Brain. Res.,* 3:320–336.

226. Krnjević, K., and Phillis, J. W. (1963): Iontophoretic studies of neurones in the mammalian cerebral cortex. *J. Physiol. (Lond.),* 165:274–304.

227. Krnjević, K., and Phillis, J. W. (1963): Acetylcholine-sensitive cells in the cerebral cortex. *J. Physiol. (Lond.),* 166:296–327.

228. Krnjević, K., and Phillis, J. W. (1963): Pharmacological properties of acetylcholine-sensitive cells in the cerebral cortex. *J. Physiol. (Lond.),* 166:328–350.

229. Krulich, L., Dhariwal, A. P. S., and McCann, S. M. (1968): Stimulatory and inhibitory effects of purified hypothalamic extracts on growth hormone re-

lease from rat pituitary in vitro. *Endocrinology*, 83:783–790.

230. Kuhar, M. J. (1976): The anatomy of cholinergic neurons. In: *Biology of Cholinergic Function*, edited by A. M. Goldberg and I. Hanin, pp. 3–27. Raven Press, New York.

231. Kuhar, M. J., and Murrin, L. C. (1978): Sodium-dependent, high affinity choline uptake. *J. Neurochem.*, 30:15–21.

232. Kuhar, M. J., Aghajanian, G. K., and Roth, R. H. (1972): Tryptophan hydroxylase activity and synaptosomal uptake of serotonin in discrete brain regions after midbrain raphe lesions: Correlations with serotonin levels and histochemical fluorescence. *Brain Res.*, 44:165–176.

233. Kuhar, M. J., Aghajanian, G. K., and Roth, R. H. (1974): Serotonin neurons: A synaptic mechanism for the reuptake of serotonin. *Adv. Biochem. Psychopharmacol.*, 10:287–295.

234. Kuhar, M. J., Shaskan, E. G., and Snyder, S. H. (1971): The subcellular distribution of endogenous and exogenous serotonin in brain tissue: Comparison of synaptosomes storing serotonin, norepinephrine, and γ-aminobutyric acid. *J. Neurochem.*, 18:333–343.

235. Kuriyama, K., Weinstein, H., and Roberts, E. (1969): Uptake of γ-aminobutyric acid by mitochondrial and synaptosomol fractions from mouse brain. *Brain Res.*, 16:479–492.

236. Laemle, L. K., Feldman, S. C., and Lichtenstein, E. (1981): Somatostatin-like immunoreactivity in the rodent visual system. *Soc. Neurosci. Abstr.*, 7:761.

237. Langer, S. Z. (1977): Presynaptic receptors and their role in the regulation of transmitter release. *Br. J. Pharmacol.*, 60:481–497.

238. Lapierre, Y., Baudet, A., Demianczuk, N., and Descarries, L. (1973): Noradrenergic axon terminals in the cerebral cortex of rat. II. Quantitative data revealed by light and electron microscope radioautography of the frontal cortex. *Brain Res.*, 63:175–182.

239. Larsson, L. I., and Rehfeld, J. F. (1979): Localization and molecular heterogeneity of cholecystokinin in the central and peripheral nervous system. *Brain Res.*, 165:201–218.

240. Lashley, K. S. (1934): The mechanism of vision. VIII. The projection of the retina upon the cerebral cortex of the rat. *J. Comp. Neurol.*, 60:57–80.

241. Lashley, K. S. (1941): Thalamo–cortical connections of the rat's brain. *J. Comp. Neurol.*, 75:67–121.

242. Lauber, M., Camier, M., and Cohen, P. (1979): Higher molecular weight forms of immunoreactive somatostatin in mouse hypothalamic extracts. *Proc Natl. Acad. Sci.*, 76:6004–6008.

243. Lehmann, J., Nagy, J. I., Atmadja, S., and Fibiger, H. C. (1980): The nucleus basalis magnocellularis: The origin of a cholinergic projection to the neocortex of the rat. *Neuroscience*, 5:1161–1174.

244. Lester, B. R., and Peck, E. J. (1979): Kinetic and pharmacologic characterization of gamma-aminobutyric acid receptive sites from mammalian brain. *Brain Res.*, 161:79–97.

245. Levitt, P., and Moore, R. Y. (1978): Noradrenaline

neuron innervation of the neocortex in the rat. *Brain Res.*, 139:219–231.

246. Lidov, H. G. W., Grzanna, R., and Molliver, M. E. (1980): The serotonin innervation of the cerebral cortex in the rat. An immunohistochemical analysis. *Neuroscience*, 5:207–227.

247. Lieberman, A. R., and Webster, K. E. (1974): Aspects of the synaptic organization of intrinsic neurons in the dorsal lateral geniculate nucleus. *J. Neurocytol.*, 3:677–710.

248. Lin, T. M. (1980): Pancreatic polypeptide: Isolation, chemistry, and biological function. In: *Gastrointestinal Hormones*, edited by B. J. Glass, pp. 275–306. Raven Press, New York.

249. Lin, T. M., and Chance, R. E. (1974): Bovine pancreatic polypeptide (BPP) and avian pancreatic polypeptide (APP). *Gastroenterology*, 67:737–738.

250. Lindvall, O., and Björklund, A. (1974): The organization of the ascending catecholamine neuron systems in the rat brain. *Acta Physiol. Scand.* [Suppl.], 412:1–48.

251. Lindvall, O., Björklund, A., Moore, R. Y., and Stenevi, U. (1974): Mesencephalic dopamine neurons projecting to neocortex. *Brain Res.*, 81:325–331.

252. Lindvall, O., Björklund, A., and Divac, I. (1978): Organization of catecholamine neurons projecting to the frontal cortex in the rat. *Brain Res.*, 142:1–24.

253. Ljungdahl, Å., Höfelt, T., and Nilsson, G. (1978): Distribution of substance P-like immunoreactivity in the central nervous system of the rat. I. Cell bodies and nerve terminals. *Neuroscience*, 3:861–943.

254. Logan, W. J., and Snyder, S. H. (1972): High affinity uptake systems for glycine, glutamic and aspartic acids in synaptosomes of rat central nervous tissues. *Brain Res.*, 42:413–431.

255. Lorén, I., Emson, P. C., Fahrenkrug, J., Björklund, A., Alumets, J., Håkanson, R., and Sundler, F. (1979): Distribution of vasoactive intestinal polypeptide in the rat and mouse brain. *Neuroscience*, 4:1953–1976.

256. Lorén, I., Alumets, J., Håkanson, R., and Sundler, F. (1979): Distribution of gastrin and CCK-like peptides in rat brain. *Histochemistry*, 59:249–257.

257. Lorén, I., Alumets, J., Håkanson, R., and Sundler, F. (1979): Immunoreactive pancreatic polypeptide (PP) occurs in the central and peripheral nervous system: Preliminary immunocytochemical observations. *Cell Tissue Res.*, 200:179–186.

258. Lorente de Nó, R. (1922): La corteza cerebral del raton. (Primera contribución. La corteza acústica). *Trab. Lab. Invest. Biol. (Madrid)*, 20:41–78.

259. Lorente de Nó, R. (1949): Cerebral cortex: Architecture, intracortical connections, motor projections. In: *Physiology of the Nervous System*, edited by J. F. Fulton, pp. 288–330. Oxford University Press, London.

260. Lund, R. D. (1966): The occipitotectal pathway of the rat. *J. Anat.*, 100:51–62.

261. Lund, J. S. (1973): Organization of neurons in the visual cortex, area 17, of the monkey *(Maccaca mulatta)*. *J. Comp. Neurol.*, 147:455–496.

262. Lund, J. S., and Lund, R. D. (1970): The termina-

tion of callosal fibers in the paravisual cortex of the rat. *Brain Res.,* 17:25–45.

263. Lund, J. S., Lund, R. D., Hendrickson, A. E., Bunt, A. H., and Fuchs, A. F. (1975): The origin of efferent pathways from the primary visual cortex, area 17, of the macaque monkey as shown by retrograde transport of horseradish peroxidase. *J. Comp. Neurol.,* 164:287–304.

264. Lund-Karlsen, R., and Fonnum, F. (1978): Evidence for glutamate as a neurotransmitter in the corticofugal fibers to the dorsal lateral geniculate body and the superior colliculus in rats. *Brain Res.,* 151:457–467.

265. Lundberg, J. M., Hökfelt, T., Änggåard, A., Kimmel, J., Goldstein, M., and Markey, K. (1980): Coexistence of an avian pancreatic polypeptide (APP) immunoreactive substance and catecholamines in some peripheral and central neurons. *Acta Physiol. Scand.,* 110:107–109.

266. Madar, Y., and Segal, M. (1980): The functional role of the noradrenergic system in the visual cortex. Activation of noradrenergic pathway. *Exp. Brain Res.,* 41:A14.

267. Madar, Y., Segal, M., and Kuhnt, U. (1980): The functional role of the noradrenergic system in the visual cortex. Microiontophoretic study. *Exp. Brain Res.,* 41:A14.

268. Maggi, A., U'Prichard, D. C., and Enna, S. J. (1980): Differential effects of antidepressant treatment on brain monoaminergic receptors. *Eur. J. Pharmacol.,* 61:91–98.

269. Magistretti, P. J., Morrison, J. H., Shoemaker, W. J., Sapin, V., and Bloom, F. E. (1981): Vasoactive intestinal polypeptide induces glycogenolysis in mouse cortical slices: A possible regulatory mechanism for the local control of energy metabolism. *Proc. Natl. Acad. Sci. U.S.A.,* 78:6535–6539.

270. Mandell, A. J. (1978): Redundant mechanisms regulating brain tyrosine and tryptophan hydroxylases. *Annu. Rev. Pharmacol. Toxicol.,* 18:461–493.

271. Marin-Padilla, M. (1972): Prenatal ontogenetic history of the principal neurons of the neocortex of the cat *(Felis domestica).* A Golgi study. II. Developmental differences and their significance. *Z. Anat. Entwickl. Gesch.,* 136:125–142.

272. McCann, S. M., Krulich, L., Negro-Vilar, A., Ojeda, S. R., and Vijayan, E. (1980): Regulation and function of panhibin (somatostatin). In: *Neural Peptides and Neuronal Communication,* edited by E. Costa and M. Trabucchi, pp. 131–143. Raven Press, New York.

273. McDonald, J. K., Speciale, S. G., and Parnavelas, J. G. (1981): The development of glutamic acid decarboxylase in the visual cortex and the dorsal lateral geniculate nucleus of the rat. *Brain Res.,* 217:364–367.

274. McDonald, J. K., Parnavelas, J. G., Karamanlidis, A., Brecha, N., and Koenig, J. I. (1982): The morphology and distribution of peptide-containing neurons in the adult and developing visual cortex of the rat. I. Somatostatin. *J. Neurocytol.,* 11:809–824.

275. McDonald, J. K., Parnavelas, J. G., Karamanlidis, A., and Brecha, N. (1982): The morphology and distribution of peptide-containing neurons in the adult and developing visual cortex of the rat. II. Vasoactive intestinal polypeptide. *J. Neurocytol.,* 11:825–837.

276. McDonald, J. K., Parnavelas, J. G., Karamanlidis, A., Brecha, N., and Rosenquist, G. (1982): The morphology and distribution of peptide-containing neurons in the adult and developing visual cortex of the rat. III. Cholecystokinin. *J. Neurocytol.,* 11:881–895.

277. McDonald, J. K., Parnavelas, J. G., Karamanlidis, A., and Brecha, N. (1982): The morphology and distribution of peptide-containing neurons in the adult and developing visual cortex of the rat. IV. Avian Pancreatic Polypeptide. *J. Neurocytol.,* 11:985–995.

278. McDonald, J. K., Petrovic, S. L., McCann, S. M., and Parnavelas, J. G. (1982): The development of beta-adrenergic receptors in the visual cortex of the rat. *Neuroscience,* 7:2649–2655.

279. McGeer, P. L., Eccles, J. C., and McGeer, E. G. (1978): *Molecular Neurobiology of the Mammalian Brain.* Plenum Press, New York.

280. McGregor, G. P., Woodhams, P. L., O'Shaughnessy, D. J., Ghatei, M. A., Polak, J. M., and Bloom, S. R. (1982): Developmental changes in bombesin, substance P, somatostatin and vasoactive intestinal polypeptide in the rat brain. *Neurosci. Lett.,* 28:21–27.

281. Meibach, R. C., Maayani, S., and Green, J. P. (1980): Characterization and radioautography of [^{3}H]LSD binding by rat brain slices *in vitro:* The effect of 5-hydroxytryptamine. *Eur. J. Pharmacol.,* 67:371–382.

282. Melamed, E., Lahev, M., and Atlas, D. (1977): β-Adrenergic receptors in rat cerebral cortex: Histochemical localization by a fluorescent β-blocker. *Brain Res.,* 128:379–384.

283. Micevych, P., Go, V. L. W., and Yaksh, T. (1981): Simultaneous measurement of VIP and CCK released from rat and cat cortical slices. *Soc. Neurosci. Abstr.,* 7:605.

284. Mihailoff, G. A., Watt, C. B., and Burne, R. A. (1981): Evidence suggesting that both the corticopontine and cerebellopontine systems are each composed of two separate neuronal populations: An electron microscopic and horseradish peroxidase study in the rat. *J. Comp. Neurol.,* 195:221–242.

285. Minneman, K. P., Hedberg, A., and Molinoff, P. B. (1979): Comparison of beta adrenergic receptor subtypes in mammalian tissues. *J. Pharmacol. Exp. Ther.,* 211:502–508.

286. Minneman, K. P., Dibner, M. D., Wolfe, B. B., and Molinoff, P. B. (1979): β_1- and β_2-adrenergic receptors in rat cerebral cortex are independently regulated. *Science,* 204:866–868.

287. Minneman, K. P., Hegstrand, L. R., and Molinoff, P. B. (1979): Simultaneous determination of beta-1 and beta-2-adrenergic receptors in tissue containing both receptor subtypes. *Mol. Pharmacol.,* 16:34–46.

288. Mitchell, J. F., and Srinivasan, V. (1969): Release of ^{3}Hγ-aminobutyric acid from the brain during synaptic inhibition. *Nature,* 224:663–666.

289. Molliver, M. E., and Kristt, D. A. (1975): The fine

structural demonstration of monoaminergic synapses in immature rat neocortex. *Neurosci. Lett.,* 1:305–310.

290. Montero, V. M. (1981): Comparative studies on the visual cortex. In: *Cortical Sensory Organization, Vol. 2: Multiple Visual Areas,* edited by C. N. Woolsey, pp. 33–81. Humana Press, Clifton, New Jersey.

291. Montero, V. M., Rojas, A., and Torrealba, F. (1973): Retinotopic organization of striate and peristriate visual cortex in the albino rat. *Brain Res.,* 53:197–201.

292. Montero, V. M., Bravo, H., and Fernandez, V. (1973): Striate–peristriate cortico–cortical connections in the albino and gray rat. *Brain Res.,* 53:202–207.

293. Moore, R. Y., and Bloom, F. E. (1978): Central catecholamine neuron systems: Anatomy and physiology of the dopamine systems. *Annu. Rev. Neurosci.,* 1:129–166.

294. Moore, R. Y., and Bloom, F. E. (1979): Central catecholamine neuron systems: Anatomy and physiology of the norepinephrine and epinephrine systems. *Annu. Rev. Neurosci.,* 2:113–168.

295. Moore, R. Y., Halaris, A. I., and Jones, B. C. (1978): Serotonin neurons of the midbrain raphe ascending projections. *J. Comp. Neurol.,* 180:417–438.

296. Morley, B. J., and Kemp, G. E. (1981): Characterization of a putative nicotinic acetylcholine receptor in mammalian brain. *Brain Res. Rev.,* 3:81–104.

297. Morley, B. J., Lorden, J. F., Brown, G. B., Kemp, G. E., and Bradley, R. J. (1977): Regional distribution of nicotinic acetylcholine receptors in rat brain. *Brain Res.,* 134:161–166.

298. Moroni, F., Corradetti, R., Casamenti, F., Moneti, G., and Pepeu, G. (1981): The release of endogenous GABA and glutamate from the cerebral cortex in the rat. *Naunyn Schmiedebergs Arch. Pharmacol.,* 316:235–239.

299. Morris, M. J., Dausse, J. P., Devynck, M. A., and Meyer P. (1980): Ontogeny of α_1 and α_2-adrenoceptors in rat brain. *Brain Res.,* 190:268–271.

300. Morrison, J. H., Grzanna, R., Molliver, M. E., and Coyle, J. T. (1978): The distribution and orientation of noradrenergic fibers in neocortex of the rat: An immunofluorescence study. *J. Comp. Neurol.,* 181:17–40.

301. Morrison, J. H., Molliver, M. E., Grzanna, R., and Coyle, J. T. (1979): Noradrenergic innervation patterns in three regions of medial cortex: An immunofluorescence characterization. *Brain Res. Bull.,* 4:849–857.

302. Morrison, J. H., Molliver, M. E., Grzanna, R., and Coyle, J. T. (1981): The intra-cortical trajectory of the coeruleo–cortical projection of the rat: A tangentially organized cortical afferent. *Neuroscience,* 6:139–158.

303. Morrison, J. H., Magistretti, P. J., Benoit, R., and Bloom, F. E. (1981): The immunohistochemical characterization of somatostatin (SS) and vasoactive intestinal polypeptide (VIP) neurons within the cerebral cortex. *Soc. Neurosci. Abstr.,* 7:99.

304. Morrison, J. H., Foote, S. L., Molliver, M. E.,

Bloom, F. E., and Lidov, H. G. W. (1982): Noradrenergic and serotonergic fibers innervate complementary layers in monkey primary visual cortex: An immunohistochemical study. *Proc. Natl. Acad. Sci. U.S.A.,* 79:2401–2405.

305. Mutt, V., and Said, S. I. (1974): Structure of the procine vasoactive intestinal octacosapeptide. The amino-acid sequence. Use of kallikrein in its determination. *Eur. J. Biochem.,* 42:581–589.

306. Nauta, W. J. H., and Bucher, V. M. (1954): Efferent connections of the striate cortex in the albino rat. *J. Comp. Neurol.,* 100:257–285.

307. Nauta, W. J. H., and Whitlock, D. G. (1954): An anatomical analysis of the nonspecific thalamic projection system. In: *Brain Mechanisms and Consciousness,* edited by J. F. Delafresnaye, pp. 81–116. Charles C. Thomas, Springfield, Illinois.

308. Nelson, D. L., Herbert, A., Bourgoin, S., Glowinski, J., and Hamon, M. (1978): Characteristics of central 5-HT receptors and their adaptive changes following intracerebral 5,7-dihydroxytryptaminc administration in the rat. *Mol. Pharmacol.,* 14:983–995.

309. Nicoll, R. A., Schenker, C., and Leeman, S. E. (1980): Substance P as a transmitter candidate. *Annu. Rev. Neurosci.,* 3:227–268.

310. Nistri, A., and Constanti, A. (1979): Pharmacological characterization of different types of GABA and glutamate receptors in vertebrates and invertebrates. *Prog. Neurobiol.,* 13:117–235.

311. O'Donohue, T. L., and Jacobowitz, D. M. (1980): Studies on α-melanotropin in the central nervous system. In: *Polypeptide Hormones,* edited by R. F. Beers, Jr. and E. G. Bassctt, pp. 203–222. Raven Press, New York.

312. O'Donohue, T. L., and Jacobowitz, D. M. (1980): Studies on α-MSH-containing nerves in the brain. In: *Progress in Biochemical Pharmacology,* edited by R. Paoletti, pp. 69–83. S. Karger, Basel.

313. O'Donohue, T. L., Miller, R. L., and Jacobowitz, D. M.(1979): Identification, characterization and stereotaxic mapping of intraneuronal α-melanocyte stimulating hormone-like immunoreactive peptides in discrete regions of the rat brain. *Brain Res.,* 176:101–123.

314. O'Donohue, T. L., Charlton, C. G., Miller, R. L., Boden, G., and Jacobowitz, D. M. (1981): Identification, characterization, and distribution of secretin immunoreactivity in rat and pig brain. *Proc. Natl. Acad. Sci. U.S.A.,* 78:5221–5224.

315. O'Donohue, T. L., Beinfeld, M. C., Chey, W. Y., Chang, T. M., Nilaver, G., Zimmerman, E. A., Yajima, H., Adachi, H., Poth, M., McDevitt, R. P., and Jacobowitz, D. M. (1981): Identification, characterization and distribution of motilin immunoreactivity in the rat central nervous system. *Peptides,* 2:467–477.

316. Ohara, P. T., and Lieberman, A. R. (1981): Thalamic reticular nucleus: Anatomical evidence that cortico–reticular axons establish monosynaptic contact with reticulo–geniculate projection cells. *Brain Res.,* 207:153–156.

317. Olavarria, J. (1979): A horseradish peroxidase study of the projections from the latero-posterior

nucleus to three lateral peristriate areas in the rat. *Brain Res.*, 173:137–141.

318. Olavarria, J., and Montero, V. M. (1981): Reciprocal connections between the striate cortex and extrastriate cortical visual areas in the rat. *Brain Res.*, 217:358–363.

319. O'Leary, J. L. (1941): Structure of the area striata of the cat. *J. Comp. Neurol.*, 75:131–164.

320. Olpe, H.-R., Balcar, V. J., Bittiger, H., Rink, H., and Sieber, P. (1980): Central actions of somatostatin. *Eur. J. Pharmacol.*, 63:127–133.

321. Olpe, H. R., Ortmann, R., Fehr, B., and Waldmeier, P. C. (1981): Experimentally induced supersensitivity of neocortical neurons to microiontophoretically administered serotonin. *Brain Res.*, 224:367–374.

322. Olschowka, J. A., Molliver, M. E., Grzanna, R., Rice, F. L., and Coyle, J. T. (1981): Ultrastructural demonstration of noradrenergic synapses in the rat central nervous system by dopamine-β-hydroxylase immunocytochemistry. *J. Histochem. Cytochem.*, 29:271–280.

323. Olschowka, J. A., O'Donohue, T. L., and Jacobowitz, D. M. (1981): The distribution of bovine pancreatic polypeptide-like immunoreactive neurons in rat brain. *Peptides*, 2:309–331.

324. Olschowka, J. A., Grzanna, R., and Molliver, M. E. (1980): The distribution and incidence of synaptic contacts of noradrenergic varicosities in the rat neocortex: An immunocytochemical study. *Soc. Neurosci. Abstr.*, 6:352.

325. Palacios J. M., and Kuhar, M. J. (1980): Beta-adrenergic-receptor localization by light microscopic autoradiography. *Science*, 208:1378–1380.

326. Palacios, J. M., Wamsley, J. K., and Kuhar, M. J. (1981): The distribution of histamine H_1-receptors in the rat brain. An autoradiographic study. *Neuroscience*, 6:15–37.

327. Palkovits, M., Zaborzky, L., Brownstein, M. J., Fekete, M. I. K., Herman, J. P., and Kanyicska, B. (1979): Distribution of norepinephrine and dopamine in cerebral cortical areas of the rat. *Brain Res. Bull.*, 4:593–601.

328. Palmer, G. C. (1972): Increased cyclic AMP response to norepinephrine in the rat brain following 6-hydroxydopamine. *Neuropharmacology*, 11:145–149.

329. Palmer, G. C., Chronister, R. B., and Palmer, S. J. (1980): Cholinergic agonists and dibutyryl cyclic guanosine monophosphate inhibit the norepinephrine-induced accumulation of cyclic adenosine monophosphate in the rat cerebral cortex. *Neuroscience*, 5:310–322.

330. Parent, A., Descarries, L., and Baudet, A. (1981): Organization of ascending serotonin systems in the adult rat brain. A radioautographic study after intraventricular administration [^{3}H]5-hydroxytryptamine. *Neuroscience*, 6:115–138.

331. Parnavelas, J. G., Lieberman, A. R., and Webster, K. E. (1977): Organization of neurons in the visual cortex, area 17, of the rat. *J. Anat.*, 124:305–322.

332. Parnavelas, J. G., Sullivan, K., Lieberman, A. R., and Webster, K. E. (1977): Neurons and their synaptic organization in the visual cortex of the rat. Electron microscopy of Golgi preparations. *Cell Tissue Res.*, 183:499–517.

333. Parnavelas, J. G., and Blue, M. G. (1982): The role of the noradrenergic system on the formation of synapses in the visual cortex of the rat. *Dev. Brain Res.*, 3:140–144.

334. Parnavelas, J. G., Burne, R. A., and Lin, C.-S. (1981): Receptive field properties of neurons in the visual cortex of the rat. *Neurosci. Lett.*, 27:291–296.

335. Parnavelas, J. G., Chatzissavidou, A., and Burne, R. A. (1981): Subcortical projections to layer I of the visual cortex, area 17, of the rat. *Exp. Brain Res.*, 41:184–187.

336. Patel, H. H., and Sillito, A. M. (1978): Inhibition and the normal ocular dominance distribution in cat visual cortex. *J. Physiol. (Lond.)*, 280:48–49P.

337. Patel, Y. C., and Reichlin, S. (1978): Somatostatin in hypothalamus, extrahypothalamic brain, and peripheral tissues of the rat. *Endocrinology*, 102:523–530.

338. Patel, Y. C., Wheatley, T., and Ning, C. (1981): Multiple forms of immunoreactive somatostatin: Comparison of distribution in neural and nonneural tissues and portal plasma of the rat. *Endocrinology*, 109:1943–1949.

339. Penn, P. E., and McBride, W. J. (1977): The effects of injections of *d,l*-5-hydroxytryptophan on the efflux of endogenous serotonin and 5-hydroxyindoleacetic acid from a synaptosomal fraction. *J. Neurochem.*, 28:765–769.

340. Peterfreund, R. A., and Vale, W. (1981): High molecular weight somatostatin secretion by cultured brain cells. *Soc. Neurosci. Abstr.*, 7:507.

341. Peters, A. (1981): Neuronal organization in rat visual cortex. In: *Progress in Anatomy*, Vol. 1, edited by R. J. Harrison, pp. 95–121. Cambridge University Press, Cambridge.

342. Peters, A., and Feldman, M. L. (1976): The projection of the lateral geniculate nucleus to area 17 of the rat cerebral cortex. I. General description. *J. Neurocytol.*, 5:63–84.

343. Peters, A., Feldman, M., and Saldanha, J. (1976): The projection of the lateral geniculate nucleus to area 17 of the rat cerebral cortex. II. Terminations upon neuronal perikarya and dendritic shafts. *J. Neurocytol.*, 5:85–107.

344. Peters, A., and Saldanha, J. (1976): The projection of the lateral geniculate nucleus to area 17 of the rat cerebral cortex. III. Layer VI. *Brain Res.*, 105:533–537.

345. Peters, A., and Fairén, A. (1978): Smooth and sparsely-spined stellate cells in the visual cortex of the rat: A study using a combined Golgi-electron microscope technique. *J. Comp. Neurol.*, 181:129–172.

346. Peters, A., Proskauer, C. C., Feldman, M. L., and Kimerer, L. (1979): The projection of the lateral geniculate nucleus to area 17 of the rat cerebral cortex. V. Degenerating axon terminals synapsing with Golgi impregnated neurons. *J. Neurocytol.*, 8:331–357.

347. Peters, A., and Proskauer, C. C. (1980): Smooth and sparsely-spined cells with myelinated axons in rat visual cortex. *Neuroscience*, 5:2079–2092.

348. Peters, A., and Kimerer, L. M. (1981): Bipolar neurons in rat visual cortex: A combined Golgi-electron microscope study. *J. Neurocytol.*, 10:921–946.

349. Peters, A., and Regidor, J. (1981): A reassessment of the forms of non-pyramidal neurons in area 17 of cat visual cortex. *J. Comp. Neurol.*, 203:685–716.

350. Pettigrew, J. D., and Daniels, J. D. (1973): Gamma-aminobutyric acid antagonism in visual cortex: Different effects on simple, complex and hypercomplex neurons. *Science*, 182:81–82.

351. Phillis, J. W., and Limacher, J. J. (1974): Substance P excitation of cortical Betz cells. *Brain Res.*, 69:158–163.

352. Phillis, J. W., Kirkpatrick, J. R., and Said, S. I. (1978): Vasoactive intestinal polypeptide excitation of central neurons. *Can. J. Physiol. Pharmacol.*, 56:337–340.

353. Phillis, J. W., and Kirkpatrick, J. R. (1979): Motilin excites neurons in the cerebral cortex and spinal cord. *Eur. J. Pharmacol.*, 58:469–472.

354. Phillis, J. W., and Kirkpatrick, J. R. (1980): The action of motilin, luteinizing hormone releasing hormone, cholecystokinin, somatostatin, vasoactive intestinal peptide, and other peptides on rat cerebral cortical neurons. *Can. J. Physiol. Pharmacol.*, 58:612–623.

355. Pickel, V., Segal, M., and Bloom, F. E. (1974): A radioautographic study of the efferent pathways of the nucleus locus coeruleus. *J. Comp. Neurol.*, 155:15–42.

356. Pinget, M., Straus, E., and Yalow, R. S. (1978): Localization of cholecystokinin-like immunoreactivity in isolated nerve terminals. *Proc. Natl. Acad. Sci. U.S.A.*, 75:6324–6326.

357. Pinget, M., Straus, E., and Yalow, R. S. (1979): Release of cholecystokinin peptides from a synaptosome-enriched fraction of rat cerebral cortex. *Life Sci.*, 25:339–342.

358. Pittman, Q. J., and Siggins, G. R. (1981): Somatostatin hyperpolarizes hippocampal pyramidal cells in vitro. *Brain Res.*, 221:402–408.

359. Polyak, S. (1957): *The Vertebrate Visual System*. The University of Chicago Press, Chicago.

360. Quik, M., Iversen, L. L., and Bloom, S. R. (1978): Effect of vasoactive intestinal peptide (VIP) and other peptides on cAMP accumulation in rat brain. *Biochem. Pharmacol.*, 27:2209–2213.

361. Rassin, D. K., Sturman, J. A., and Gaull, G. E. (1981): Sulfur amino acid metabolism in the developing rhesus monkey brain: subcellular studies of taurine, cysteinesulfinic acid decarboxylase, γ-aminobutyric acid, and glutamic acid decarboxylase. *J. Neurochem.*, 37:740–748.

362. Reader, T. A. (1978): The effects of dopamine, noradrenaline and serotonin in the visual cortex of the cat. *Experientia*, 34:1586–1588.

363. Reader, T. A. (1980): Serotonin distribution in rat cerebral cortex; radioenzymatic assays with thin-layer chromatography. *Brain Res. Bull.*, 5:609–613.

364. Reader, T. A. (1981): Distribution of catecholamines and serotonin in the rat cerebral cortex: Absolute levels and relative proportions. *J. Neural Transm.*, 50:13–27.

365. Reader, T. A., Masse, D., and de Champlain, J. (1979): The intracortical distribution of norepinephrine, dopamine and serotonin in the cerebral cortex of the cat. *Brain Res.*, 177:499–513.

366. Reader, T. A., Ferron, A., Descarries, L., and Jasper, H. H. (1979): Modulatory role for biogenic amines in the cerebral cortex. Microiontophoretic studies. *Brain Res.*, 160:217–229.

367. Rehfeld, J. F. (1978): Immunochemical studies on cholecystokinin II. Distribution and molecular heterogeneity in the central nervous system and small intestine of man and hog. *J. Biol. Chem.*, 253:4022–4030.

368. Rehfeld, J. F. (1981): Four basic characteristics of the gastrin–cholecystokinin system. *Am. J. Physiol.*, 240:G255–266.

369. Reisine, T. (1981): Adaptive changes in catecholamine receptors in the central nervous system. *Neuroscience*, 6:1471–1502.

370. Renaud, L. P., Martin, J. B., and Brazeau, P. (1975): Depressant action of TRH, LH-RH and somatostatin on activity of central neurons. *Nature*, 255:233–235.

371. Reubi, J.-C., Rivier, J., Perrin, M., Brown, M., and Vale, W. (1981): Somatostatin receptors in brain and pancreas: Different pharmacological properties. *Soc. Neurosci. Abstr.*, 7:431.

372. Ribak, C. E. (1977): A note on the laminar organization of rat visual cortical projections. *Exp. Brain Res.*, 27:413–418.

373. Ribak, C. E. (1978): Aspinous and sparsely-spinous stellate neurons in the visual cortex of rats contain glutamic acid decarboxylase. *J. Neurocytol.*, 7:461–478.

374. Ribak, C. E., and Peters, A. (1975): An autoradiographic study of the projections from the lateral geniculate body of the rat. *Brain Res.*, 92:341–368.

375. Richards, J. G., and Tranzer, J. P. (1970): The ultrastructural localization of amine storage sites in the central nervous system with the aid of a specific marker, 5-hydroxydopamine. *Brain Res.*, 17:463–469.

376. Roberts, E., Chase, T., and Tower, D. B. (1976): *GABA in Nervous System Function*. Raven Press, New York.

377. Roberts, P. J. (1974): Glutamate receptors in rat central nervous system. *Nature*, 252:399–401.

378. Robberecht, P., Deschodt-Lanckman, M., De Neef, P., and Christophe, J. (1979): Vasoactive intestinal peptide: levels and functional receptors in rat brain before and after weaning. *Life Sci.*, 25:1001–1008.

379. Robbins, R. J., Sutton, R. E., and Reichlin, S. (1982): Effects of neurotransmitters and cyclic AMP on somatostatin release from cultured cerebral cortical cells. *Brain Res.*, 234:377–386.

380. Room, P., Postema, F., and Korf, J. (1981): Divergent axon collaterals of rat locus coeruleus neurons: Demonstration by a fluorescent double labeling technique. *Brain Res.*, 221:219–230.

381. Rorstad, O. P., Epelbaum, J., Brazeau, P., and Martin, J. B. (1979): Chromatographic and biological properties of immunoreactive somatostatin in hypothalamic and extrahypothalamic brain regions of the rat. *Endocrinology,* 105:1083–1092.

382. Rose, D., and Blakemore, C. (1974): Effects of bicuculline on functions of inhibition in visual cortex. *Nature,* 249:375–377.

383. Rosenquist, A. C., Edwards, S. B., and Palmer, L. A. (1974): An autoradiographic study of the projections of the dorsal lateral geniculate nucleus and the posterior nucleus in the cat. *Brain Res.,* 80:71–93.

384. Roskoski, R. (1978): Net uptake of L-glutamate and GABA by high-affinity synaptosomal transport systems. *J. Neurochem.,* 31:493–498.

385. Roskoski, R. (1979): Net uptake of aspartate by a high-affinity rat cortical synaptosomal transport system. *Brain Res.,* 160:85–93.

386. Rossier, J. (1977): Choline acetyltransferases: A review with special reference to its celluar and subcellular localization. *Int. Rev. Neurobiol.,* 20:284–334.

387. Said, S. I., and Mutt, V. (1970): Polypeptide with broad biological activity: Isolation from small intestine. *Science,* 169:1217–1218.

388. Said, S. I., and Mutt, V. (1972): Isolation from porcine-intestinal wall of a vasoactive octacosapeptide related to secretin and to glucagon. *Eur. J. Biochem.,* 28:199–204.

389. Said, S. I., Giachetti, A., and Nicosia, S. (1980): VIP: Possible function as a neural peptide. In: *Neural Peptides and Neuronal Communication,* edited by E. Costa and M. Trabucchi, pp. 75–82. Raven Press, New York.

390. Saito, A., Sankaran, H., Goldfine, I. D., and Williams, J. A. (1980): Cholecystokinin receptors in the brain: Characterization and distribution. *Science,* 208:1155–1156.

391. Saldate, M. C., and Orrego, F. (1977): Electrically induced release of ³H-dopamine from slices obtained from different rat brain cortex regions. Evidence for a widespread dopaminergic innervation of the neocortex. *Brain Res.,* 130:483–494.

392. Samanin, R., Mennini, T., Ferraris, A., Bendotti, C., and Borsini, F. (1980): Hyper- and hyposensitivity of central serotonin receptors: [³H]Serotonin binding and functional studies in the rat. *Brain Res.,* 189:449–457.

393. Samson, W. K. (1982): Radioimmunological localization of VIP in the mammalian brain. In: *Vasoactive Intestinal Peptide,* edited by S. I. Said, pp. 91–105. Raven Press, New York.

394. Samson, W. K., Said, S. I., and McCann, S. M. (1979): Radioimmunologic localization of vasoactive intestinal polypeptide in hypothalamic and extrahypothalamic sites in the rat brain. *Neurosci. Lett.,* 12:265–269.

395. Sanderson, C., and Murphy, S. (1982): Glutamate binding in the rat cerebral cortex during ontogeny. *Dev. Brain Res.,* 2:329–339.

396. Savage, P. D., Mendels, J., and Frazer, A. (1980): Monoamine oxidase inhibitors and serotonin uptake inhibitors: Differential effects of [³H]serotonin binding sites in rat brain. *J. Pharmacol. Exp. Ther.,* 212:259–263.

397. Schally, A. V., Dupont, A., Arimura, A., Redding, T. W., Nishi, N., Linthicum, G. L., and Schlesinger, D. H. (1976): Isolation and structure of somatostatin from porcine hypothalami. *Biochemistry,* 15:509–514.

398. Schliebs, R., Burgoyne, R. D., and Bigl, V. (1982): The effect of visual deprivation on β-adrenergic receptors in the visual centers of the rat brain. *J. Neurochem.,* 38:1038–1043.

399. Schober, W. (1981): Efferente and afferente Verbindungen des Nucleus lateralis posterior thalami (Pulvinar) der Albinoratte. *Z. Mikrosk. Anat. Forsch.,* 95:827–844.

400. Schober, W. (1981): Zur Morphologie der funktionellen Spezialisation des visuellen Systems der Säugetiere. *Z. Mikrosk. Anat. Forsch.,* 95:395–400.

401. Schober, W., and Winkelmann, E. (1975): Der visuelle Kortex der Ratte Cytoarchitektonik and stereotaktische Parameter. *Z. Mikrosk. Anat. Forsch.,* 89:431–446.

402. Schober, W., and Winkelmann, E. (1977): Die geniculo–kortikale Projektion bei Albinoratten. *J. Hirnforsch.,* 18:1–20.

403. Schober, W., Lüth, H.-J, and Gruschka, H. (1976): Die Herkunft afferenter Axone im striären Kortex der Albinoratte. Eine Studie mit Meerrettich-Peroxidase. *Z. Mikrosk. Anat. Forsch.,* 90:399–415.

404. Schwartz, J. C., Lampart, C., and Rose, C. (1970): Properties and regional distribution of histidine decarboxylase in rat brain. *J. Neurochem.,* 17:1527–1534.

405. Schwartz, J. C., Costentin, J., Martres, M. P., Protais, P., and Baudry, M. (1978): Modulation of receptor mechanisms in the CNS: Hyper- and hyposensitivity to catecholamines. *Neuropharmacology,* 17:665–685.

406. Schwartz, J. C., Pollard, H., and Quach, T. T. (1980): Histamine as a neurotransmitter in mammalian brain: Neurochemical evidence. *J. Neurochem.,* 35:26–33.

407. Seeman, P., Westman, K., Coscina, P., and Warsh, J. J. (1980): Serotonin receptors in hippocampus and frontal cortex. *Eur. J. Pharmacol.,* 66:179–191.

408. Sefton, A. J., Mackay-Sim, A., Baur, L. A., and Cottee, L. J. (1981): Cortical projections to visual centres in the rat: An HRP study. *Brain Res.,* 215:1–13.

409. Sharif, N. A., and Roberts, P. J. (1980): Problems associated with the binding of L-glutamic acid to synaptic membranes: Methodological aspects. *J. Neurochem.,* 34:779–784.

410. Shibasaki, T., Ling, N., Guillemin, R., Silver, M., and Bloom, F. (1981): The regional distribution of γ₃-melanotropin-like peptides in bovine brain is correlated with adrenocorticotrophin immunoreactivity but not with β-endorphin. *Regul. Peptides,* 2:43–52.

411. Shkol'nik-Yarros, E. G. (1971): *Neurons and Interneuronal Connections of the Central Visual System.* Plenum Press, New York.

412. Sholl, D. A. (1967): *The Organization of the Cerebral Cortex.* Hafner Publishing, London.

413. Shoumura, K. (1974): An attempt to relate the origin and distribution of commissural fibers to the presence of large and medium pyramids in layer III in the cat's visual cortex. *Brain Res., 67:*13–25.

414. Shute, C. C. D., and Lewis, P. R. (1967): The ascending cholinergic reticular system: Neocortical, olfactory and subcortical projections. *Brain,* 90:497–520.

415. Sillito, A. M. (1975): The effectiveness of bicuculline as an antagonist of GABA and visually evoked inhibition in the cat's striate cortex. *J. Physiol. (Lond.),* 250:287–304.

416. Sillito, A. M. (1975): The contribution of inhibitory mechanisms to the receptive field properties of neurones in the striate cortex of the cat. *J. Physiol. (Lond.),* 250:305–329.

417. Sillito, A. M. (1977): Inhibitory processes underlying the directional specificity of simple, complex and hypercomplex cells in the cat's visual cortex. *J. Physiol. (Lond.),* 271:699–720.

418. Sims, K. B., Hoffman, D. L., Said, S. I., and Zimmerman, E. A. (1980): Vasoactive intestinal polypeptide (VIP) in mouse and rat brain: An immunocytochemical study. *Brain Res.,* 106:165–183.

419. Skolnick, P., Stalvey, L. P., Daly, J. W., Hoyler, E., and Davis, J. N. (1978): Binding of α- and β-adrenergic ligands to cerebral cortical membranes: Effect of 6-hydroxydopamine treatment and relationship to the responsiveness of cyclic-AMP generating systems in two rat brains. *Eur. J. Pharmacol.,* 47:201–210.

420. Sloper, J. J. (1973): An electron microscope study of the neurons of the primate motor and somatic sensory cortices. *J. Neurocytol.,* 2:351–359.

421. Sloper, J. J. (1973): An electron microscope study of the termination of afferent connections to the primary motor complex. *J. Neurocytol.,* 2:361–368.

422. Snyder, S. H., Hendley, E. D., and Gfeller, E. (1969): Regional differences in accumulation of tritium-labeled norepinephrine, 5-hydroxytryptamine and gamma-aminobutyric acid in brain slices and rhesus monkey. *Brain Res.,* 16:469–477.

423. Somogyi, P. (1977): A specific "axo-axonal" interneuron in the visual cortex of the rat. *Brain Res.,* 136:345–350.

424. Somogyi, P. (1978): The study of Golgi stained cells and of experimental degeneration under the electron microscope: A direct method for the identification in the visual cortex of three successive links in a neuron chain. *Neuroscience,* 3:167–180.

425. Somogyi, P., Cowey, A., Halász, N., and Freund, T. F. (1981): Vertical organization of neurones accumulating ^{3}H-GABA in visual cortex of rhesus monkey. *Nature,* 294:761–763.

426. Somogyi, P., Freund, T. F., Halász, and Kisvárday, Z. F. (1981): Selectivity of neuronal [^{3}H]GABA accumulation in the visual cortex as revealed by Golgi staining of the labeled neurons. *Brain Res.,* 225:431–436.

427. Spehlmann, R. (1963): Acetylcholine and prostigmine electrophoresis at visual cortical neurons. *J. Neurophysiol.,* 26:127–139.

428. Sporn, J. R., Harden, T. K., Wolfe, B. B., and Molinoff, P. B. (1976): β-Adrenergic receptor involvement in 6-hydroxydopamine-induced supersensitivity in rat cerebral cortex. *Science,* 194:624–626.

429. Sporn, J. R., Wolfe, B. B., Harden, T. K., and Molinoff, P. B. (1977): Supersensitivity in rat cerebral cortex: Pre- and postsynaptic effects of 6-hydroxydopamine at noradrenergic synapses. *Mol. Pharmacol.,* 13:1170–1180.

430. Srikant, C. B., and Patel, Y. C. (1981): Somatostatin analogs. Dissociation of brain receptor binding affinities and pituitary actions in the rat. *Endocrinology,* 108:341–343.

431. Srikant, C. B., and Patel, Y. C. (1981): Somatostatin receptors: Identification and characterization in rat brain membranes. *Proc. Natl. Acad. Sci. U.S.A.,* 78:3930–3934.

432. Steigerwalt, R. W., and Williams, J. A. (1981): Characterization of cholecystokinin receptors on rat pancreatic membranes. *Endocrinology,* 109:1746–1753.

433. Stone, T. W., Taylor, D. A., and Bloom, F. E. (1975): Cyclic AMP and cyclic GMP may mediate opposite neuronal responses in rat cerebral cortex. *Science,* 187:845–847.

434. Sturman, J. A., Rassin, D. K., and Gaull, G. E. (1978): Taurine in the development of the central nervous system. In: *Taurine and Neurological Disorders,* edited by A. Barbeau and R. J. Huxtable, pp. 49–71. Raven Press, New York.

435. Szentágothai, J. (1973): Synaptology of the visual cortex. In: *Handbook of Sensory Physiology,* Vol. VII/3, Part B, edited by R. Jung, pp. 269–324. Springer-Verlag, Berlin.

436. Szentágothai, J. (1978): The neuron network of the cerebral cortex: A functional interpretation. *Proc. R. Soc. Lond. [Biol.],* 201:219–248.

437. Tachiki, K. H., and Baxter, C. F. (1979): Taurine levels in brain tissue: A need for re-evaluation. *J. Neurochem.,* 33:1125–1129.

438. Takatsuki, K., Shiosaka, S., Sakanaka, M., Inagaki, S., Senba, E., Takagi, H., and Tohyama, M. (1981): Somatostatin in the auditory system of the rat. *Brain Res.,* 213:211–216.

439. Tan, A. T., Tsand, D., Renaud, L. P., and Martin, J. B. (1977): Effect of somatostatin on calcium transport in guinea pig cortex synaptosomes. *Brain Res.,* 123:193–196.

440. Tanaka, S., and Tsujimoto, A. (1981): Somatostatin facilitates the serotonin release from rat cerebral cortex, hippocampus and hypothalamus slices. *Brain Res.,* 208:219–222.

440a. Tatemoto, K., Carlquist, M., and Mutt, V. (1982): Neuropeptide Y—A novel brain peptide with structural similarities to peptide Y and pancreatic polypeptide. *Nature,* 286:659–660.

441. Taylor, D. P., and Pert, C. B. (1979): Vasoactive intestinal polypeptide: Specific binding to rat brain membranes. *Proc. Natl. Acad. Sci. U.S.A.,* 76:660–664.

442. Tömböl, T. (1974): An electron microscopic study of the neurons of the visual cortex. *J. Neurocytol.,* 3:525–531.

443. Török, I., and Turner, S. (1981): Histochemical ev-

idence for a catecholaminergic (presumably dopaminergic) projection from the ventral mesencephalic tegmentum to visual cortex in the cat. *Neurosci. Lett.*, 24:215–219.

444. Tsumoto, T., Eckart, W., and Creutzfeldt, O. D. (1979): Modification of orientation sensitivity of cat visual cortex neurons by removal of GABA-mediated inhibition. *Exp. Brain Res.*, 34:351–363.

445. Uhl, G. R., and Snyder, S. H. (1976): Regional and subcellular distribution of brain neurotensin. *Life Sci.*, 19:1827–1832.

446. Uhl, G. R., Kuhar, M. J., and Snyder, S. H. (1977): Neurotensin: Immunohistochemical localization in rat central nervous system. *Proc. Natl. Acad. Sci. U.S.A.*, 74:4059–4063.

447. Ungerstedt, U. (1971): Stereotaxic mapping of the monoamine pathways in the rat brain. *Acta Physiol. Scand. Suppl.*, 367:1–48.

448. U'Prichard, D. C., Bechtel, W. D., Rouot, B. M., and Snyder, S. H. (1979): Multiple apparent alpha-noradrenergic receptor binding sites in rat brain: Effect of 6-hydroxydopamine. *Mol. Pharmacol.*, 16:47–60.

449. Vale, W., Brazeau, P., Grant, G., Nussey, A., Burgus, R., Rivier, J., Ling, N., and Guillemin, R. (1972): Premières observations sur le mode d'action de la somatostatine, un facteur hypothalamique qui inhibe la sécrétion de l'hormone de croissance. *Acad. Sci. [D] (Paris)*, 275:2913–2916.

450. Valverde, F. (1976): Aspects of cortical organization related to the geometry of neurons with intra-cortical axons. *J. Neurocytol.*, 5:509–529.

451. Valverde, F. (1978): The organization of area 18 in the monkey. A Golgi study. *Anat. Embryol.*, 154:305–334.

452. Van Dongen, P. A. M. (1981): The central noradrenergic transmission and the locus coeruleus: A review of the data, and their implications for neuro-transmission and neuromodulation. *Prog. Neurobiol.*, 16:117–143.

453. Van Hungen, K., and Roberts, S. (1973): Adenylate-cyclase receptors for adrenergic neurotransmitters in rat cerebral cortex. *Eur. J. Biochem.*, 36:391–401.

454. Vincent, S. R., Skirboll, L., Hökfelt, T., Johansson, O., Lundberg, J. M., Elde, R. P., Terenius, L., and Kimmel, J. (1982): Coexistence of somatostatin- and avian pancreatic polypeptide (APP)-like immunoreactivity in some forebrain neurons. *Neuroscience*, 7:439–446.

455. Vizi, E. S. (1972): Modulation of cortical release of acetylcholine by noradrenaline released from nerves arising from the rat locus coeruleus. *Neuroscience*, 5:2139–2144.

456. Wamsley, J. K., Zarbin, M. A., Nigel, J. M., and Kuhar, M. J. (1980): Muscarinic cholinergic receptors: Autoradiographic localization of high and low affinity agonist binding sites. *Brain Res.*, 200:1–12.

457. Wamsley, J. K., Palacios, J. M., Young, W. S., and Kuhar, M. J. (1981): Autoradiographic determination of neurotransmitter receptor distribution in the cerebral and cerebellar cortices. *J. Histochem. Cytochem.*, 29:125–135.

458. Wang, J. Y., Jhamandas, K., Yaksh, T. L., and Go, V. L. W. (1981): *In vivo* studies of the resting and evoked release of cholecystokinin (CCK) and vaso-active intestinal peptide (VIP) from cat cerebral cortex and ventricles. *Soc. Neurosci. Abstr.*, 7:604.

459. Wang, R. Y., de Montigny, C., Gold, B. I., Roth, R. H., and Aghajanian, G. K. (1979): Denervation supersensitivity to serotonin in rat forebrain: Single cell studies. *Brain Res.*, 178:479–497.

460. Waterhouse, B. D., Moises, H. C., and Woodward, D. J. (1980): Noradrenergic modulation of somatosensory cortical neuronal responses to iontophoretically applied putative neurotransmitters. *Exp. Neurol.*, 69:30–49.

461. Waterhouse, B. C., Moises, H. C., and Woodward, D. J. (1981): Alpha-receptor-mediated facilitation of somatosensory cortical neuronal responses to excitatory synaptic inputs and iontophoretically applied acetylcholine. *Neuropharmacology*, 20:907–920.

462. Waterhouse, B. D., Moises, H. C., Yeh, H. H., and Woodward, D. J. (1982): Norepinephrine enhancement of inhibitory synaptic mechanisms in cerebellum and cerebral cortex: Mediation by beta adrenergic receptor. *J. Pharmacol. Exp. Ther.*, 221:495–506.

463. Webster, K. E. (1961): Cortico–striate interrelations in the albino rat. *J. Anat.*, 95:532–544.

464. Wenk, H., Bigl, V., and Meyer, U. (1980): Cholinergic projections from magnocellular nuclei of the basal forebrain to cortical areas in rats. *Brain Res. Rev.*, 2:295–316.

465. Westlind, A., Grynfarb, M., Hedlund, B., Bartfai, T., and Fuxe, K. (1981): Muscarinic supersensitivity induced by septal lesion or chronic atropine treatment. *Brain Res.*, 225:131–141.

466. White, E. L. (1978): Identified neurons in mouse SmI cortex which are postsynaptic to thalamocortical axon terminals: A combined Golgi–electron microscopic and degeneration study. *J. Comp. Neurol.*, 181:627–662.

467. Winfield, D. A., and Powell, T. P. S. (1976): The termination of the thalamocortical fibers in the visual cortex of the cat. *J. Neurocytol.*, 5:269–286.

468. Winfield, D. A., Gatter, K. C., and Powell, T. P. S. (1980): An electron microscopic study of the types and proportions of neurons in the cortex of the motor and visual areas of the cat and rat. *Brain*, 103:245–258.

469. Winkelmann, E., Kunz, G., and Winkelmann, A. (1972): Untersuchungen zur laminären Organisation des Cortex cerebri der Ratte unter besonderer Berücksichtigung der Sehrinde (area 17). *Z. Mikrosk. Anat. Forsch.*, 85:369–380.

470. Winkelmann, E., Hedlich, A., Lüth, H.-J., and Brauer, K. (1981): Zur neuronalen Organisation der Sehrinde. *Z. Mikrosk. Anat. Forsch.*, 95:369–380.

471. Wise, S. P., and Jones, E. G. (1976): The organization and postnatal development of the commissural projection of the rat somatic sensory cortex. *J. Comp. Neurol.*, 168:313–344.

472. Wise, S. P., and Jones, E. G. (1977): Cells of origin and terminal distribution of descending projections

of the rat somatic sensory cortex. *J. Comp. Neurol.*, 175:129–158.

473. Woodward, D. J., Moises, H. C., Waterhouse, B. D., Hoffer, B. J., and Freedman, R. (1979): Modulatory actions of norepinephrine in the mammalian central nervous system. *Fed. Proc.*, 38:59–66.

474. Woodward, D. J., Waterhouse, B. D., and Moises, H. C. (1980): Serotonergic suppression of somatosensory cortical neuronal responses to putative neurotransmitters and afferent synaptic inputs. *Soc. Neurosci. Abstr.*, 6:448.

475. Yamamura, H. I., and Snyder, S. H. (1973): High affinity transport of choline into synaptosomes of rat brain. *J. Neurochem.*, 21:1355–1364.

476. Yorke, C. H., Jr., and Caviness, V. S., Jr. (1975): Interhemispheric neocortical connections of the corpus callosum in the normal mouse: A study based on anterograde and retrograde methods. *J. Comp. Neurol.*, 164:233–246.

477. Young, W. S., and Kuhar, M. J. (1980): Noradrenergic α_1 and α_2 receptors: Light microscopic autoradiographic localization. *Proc. Natl. Acad. Sci. U.S.A.*, 77:1696–1700.

478. Young, W. S., and Kuhar, M. J. (1981): Neurotensin receptor localization by light microscopic autoradiography in rat brain. *Brain Res.*, 206:273–285.

479. Zarbin, M. A., Innis, R. B., Wamsley, J. K., Snyder, S. H., and Kuhar, M. J. (1981): Autoradiographic localization of CCK receptors in guinea pig brain. *Eur. J. Pharmacol.*, 71:349–350.

480. Zecevic, N. R., and Molliver, M. E. (1978): The origin of the monoaminergic innervation of immature rat neocortex: An ultrastructural analysis following lesions. *Brain Res.*, 150:387–397.

SUBJECT INDEX

Subject Index